Psychiatric Nursing

FOURTH EDITION

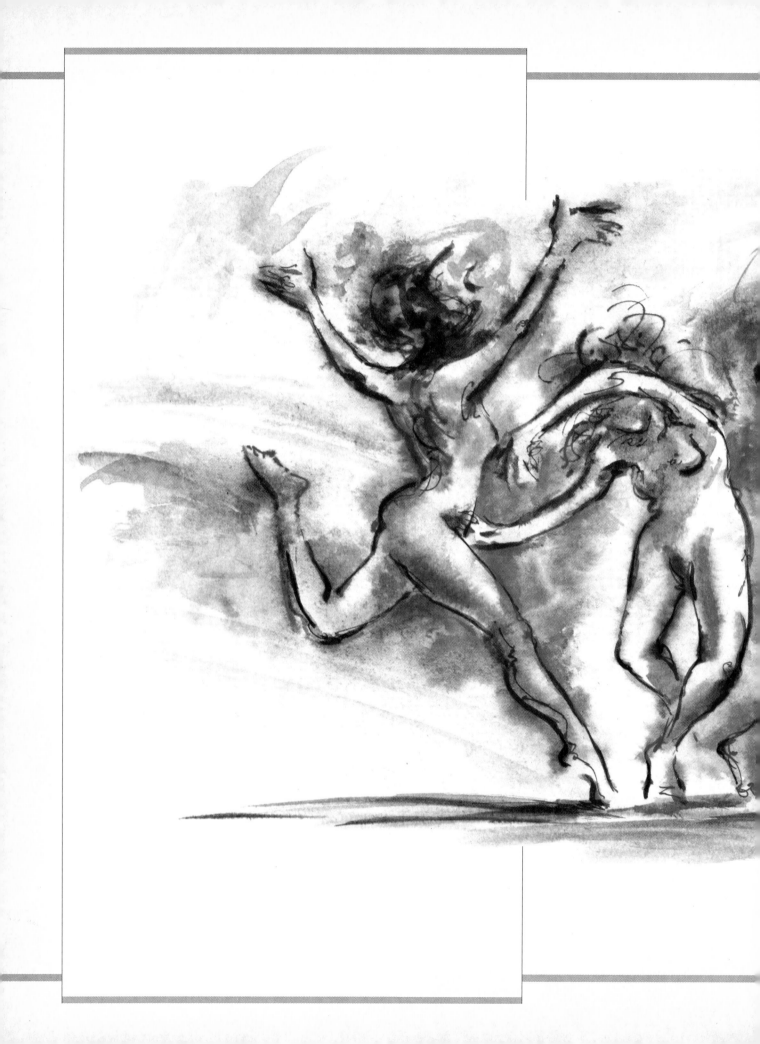

Psychiatric Nursing

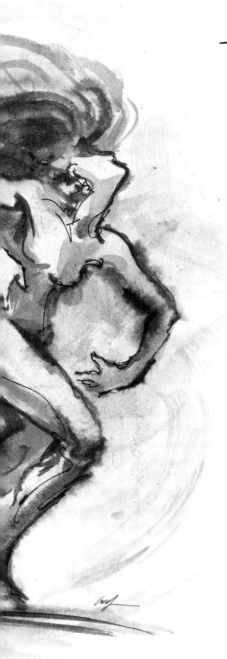

Holly Skodol Wilson
RN, PhD, FAAN

Carol Ren Kneisl
RN, CS, MS

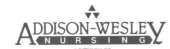

ADDISON-WESLEY
N U R S I N G
A DIVISION OF
THE BENJAMIN/CUMMINGS PUBLISHING COMPANY, INC.

Redwood City, California • Menlo Park, California
Reading, Massachusetts • New York • Don Mills, Ontario
Wokingham, UK • Amsterdam • Bonn • Sydney • Tokyo
Madrid • San Juan

Sponsoring editor: Mark McCormick
Production editor (freelance): Wendy Earl
Manuscript editor: Antonio Padial
Text designer: Paula Schlosser
Cover designer: Yvo Riezebos Design
Part opener illustrator: Alexander Laurant
Text illustrators: AYXA, Linda Harris, Shirley Bortoli
Editorial assistant: Wendy Gross
Production assistant: Frank Vaughn
Proofreader: John Hammett
Indexer: Ruthanne Lowe
Compositor: The Clarinda Company
Manufacturing supervisor: Casimira Kostecki
Text printer and binder: Courier/Westford

ISBN 0-8053-9400-1

Library of Congress Cataloging-in-Publication Data

Wilson, Holly Skodol.
    Psychiatric nursing / Holly Skodol Wilson, Carol Ren Kneisl.—
4th ed.
        p.   cm.
    Includes bibliographical references and index.
    ISBN 0-8053-9400-1
    1. Psychiatric nursing.   I.   Kneisl, Carol Ren.   II. Title.
    [DNLM: 1. Psychiatric Nursing.   WY 160 W748p]
RC440.W5   1992
610.73'68—dc20
DNLM/DLC   91-31707
for Library of Congress   CIP

5 6 7 8 9 10-MU-95 94

The cover illustration is from a quilt entitled "Challenges to the Blue Sky" by Setsuko Segawa of Brea, California.

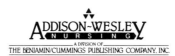

ADDISON-WESLEY
NURSING
A DIVISION OF
THE BENJAMIN/CUMMINGS PUBLISHING COMPANY, INC.

390 Bridge Parkway, Redwood City, California 94065

*We dedicate this book
to Holly's father, C. Harold Skodol,
and Carol's mother, Frances Ren.*

ABOUT THE AUTHORS

Holly Skodol Wilson, RN, PhD, FAAN, is a Professor in the Department of Mental Health, Community and Administrative Nursing, School of Nursing, University of California at San Francisco. She is also an affiliated Professor in the Women's Health and Healing Program, Department of Social and Behavior Sciences and Aging Health Policy Institute. Her clinical and research interests are in the fields of psychogerontology, particularly community care for the demented elderly. She has authored and coauthored 14 books, has contributed chapters to 3 others, and has published over 60 scientific articles in professional and scientific journals. Her Addison-Wesley text *Research in Nursing* (1989) won the *American Journal of Nursing* Book of the Year award. She is active as an international lecturer on topics ranging from research in nursing to the future of psychiatric nursing practice, education, and science.

Carol Ren Kneisl, RN, CS, MS, an internationally known nursing author, lecturer, and consultant, is President and Educational Director of Nursing Transitions, Inc., a nursing continuing education company in Williamsville, New York. During her twenty years as a nurse educator, she taught psychiatric nursing students at the diploma and baccalaureate levels and clinical specialists in psychiatric nursing at the master's level. Actively involved in clinical practice issues, she encourages psychiatric nurses through her writing, speaking, and consultation activities to provide expert, humanistic care in psychiatric-mental health nursing and to take active leadership roles in the AIDS era. She has authored and coauthored a total of 15 books in nursing, 10 of them in psychiatric nursing.

CONTRIBUTORS

CAROL BRADLEY-CORPUEL, RN, CS, MSN
Psychiatric Clinical Nurse Specialist
Nursing Education Department
Yale-New Haven Hospital
New Haven, Connecticut

JUDY BANKS CAMPBELL, RN, EdD, ARNP
Professor
Palm Beach Community College
Lake Worth, Florida

PAUL L. CERRATO, BS, MA
Director of Clinical Nutrition
Senior Editor, RN Magazine

LINDA CHAFETZ, RN, DNSc
Associate Professor
University of California at San
  Francisco
San Francisco, California

CATHERINE A. CHESLA, RN, DNSc
Adjunct Assistant Professor
University of California at San
  Francisco
San Francisco, California

KAY K. CHITTY, RN, CS, EdD
Associate Professor and Director,
  School of Nursing
The University of Tennessee at
  Chattanooga
Chattanooga, Tennessee

GAIL DeBOER, RN, MS
Samuel Merritt College
Oakland, California

JERRY D. DURHAM, RN, PhD, FAAN
Professor and
  Executive Associate Dean
  for Academic Programs
Indiana University School of Nursing
Indianapolis, Indiana

ANASTASIA FISHER, RN, MN, DNSc
Research and Case Manager
Kaiser-Permanente Medical Center
Oakland, California

KAREN FONTAINE, RN, MSN, AASECT
Associate Professor
Purdue University, Calumet Campus
Hammond, Indiana

CANDICE FURLONG, RN, CS, MSN
Faculty
School of Medicine
Department of Psychiatry
University of California at Davis
Davis, California

SUSAN HUNN GARRITSON, RN, DNSc
Director, Patient Care Services
Langley Porter Psychiatric Hospital
  and Clinics
San Francisco, California

SALLY HUTCHINSON, RN, PhD, FAAN
Professor
University of Florida
Jacksonville, Florida

JOANNE KEGLOVITS, RN, MSN
*Clinical Specialist and School Nurse
Practitioner
Pleasant Valley School District
Brodheadsville, Pennsylvania*

GLORIA KUHLMAN, RN, MSN
*Associate Professor
Ohlone College
Fremont, California
Doctoral Candidate
University of California at
San Francisco
San Francisco, California*

MAXINE LOOMIS, RN, CS, PhD, FAAN
*Professor and former Director
PhD Program in Nursing Science
University of South Carolina
Columbia, South Carolina*

COLLEEN CARNEY LOVE, RN, CS, MA
*Coordinator of Nursing Research
Atascadero State Hospital
Atascadero, California
Doctoral Candidate
University of California at
San Francisco
San Francisco, California*

GEOFFRY W. MCENANY, RN, MS
*Clinical Nurse Specialist
Turning Point Center
San Francisco, California
Predoctoral Fellow,
Neuroscience
University of California at
San Francisco
San Francisco, California*

MARYRUTH MORRIS, RN, CS, MS
*Supervisor, Geriatric Outreach
Treatment Team
Monsignor Carr Institute
Buffalo, New York*

BETH MOSCATO, RN, MS
*Doctoral Student in Epidemiology
Department of Social and
Preventive Medicine
State University of New York
at Buffalo
Buffalo, New York*

MARILYNN PETIT, RN, MS
*Consultant
Brockton Psychiatric Institute
Brockton, Massachusetts*

WILLIAM G. PHEIFER, RN, MS
*HIV Nursing Consultant and
Adjunct Clinical Assistant Professor
Old Dominion University
Norfolk, Virginia*

NOREEN KING POOLE, RN, CS, EdD, ARNP
*Professor
Palm Beach Community College
Lake Worth, Florida*

ELIZABETH A. RILEY, RN, CS, MS
*Program Director, Acute Adult Unit
Four Winds Hospital—Saratoga
Saratoga Springs, New York*

NAN RICH, RN, BA, MSN
*Clinical Nurse
Sequoia Hospital
Redwood City, California
Doctoral Student
University of California at
San Francisco
San Francisco, California*

BETH SIPPLE, RN, CS, MSN
*Child and Adolescent Clinical
Nurse Specialist
University of Maryland
Medical System
Baltimore, Maryland*

EILEEN TRIGOBOFF, RN, CS, MSN
*Clinical Specialist in Psychiatric
Nursing
Buffalo Psychiatric Center
Buffalo, New York*

PATRICIA UNDERWOOD, RN, MS DNSc, FAAN
*Professor of Clinical Nursing
University of California at
San Francisco
San Francisco, California*

REVIEWERS

Patricia Black, RN, BSN, MEd
Indiana University of Pennsylvania
Indiana, Pennsylvania

Robert Ertel, PhD
University of Pittsburgh
Pittsburgh, Pennsylvania

Anne Hopkins Fishel, RN, MSN, PhD
University of North Carolina
  at Chapel Hill
Chapel Hill, North Carolina

Mary Flickinger, BSN, MSN
University of Toledo
Toledo, Ohio

Karen Fontaine, RN, MSN
Purdue University, Calumet Campus
Hammond, Indiana

Jeanne Gelman, RN, BSN, MSN
Widener University
Chester, Pennsylvania

Valarie Hart-Smith, RN, BSN, MSN
University of Maine
Searsport, Maine

Barbara Holder, PhD
George Washington University
Washington, D.C.

Gloria Kuhlman, RN, BSN, MN
Ohlone College
Fremont, California

Delores Lesseig, RN, CS
Northeast Missouri State University
Kirksville, Missouri

Sheridan V. McCabe, RN, BSN, MSN
University of Virginia
Charlottesville, Virginia

Mary Ann Neihart, RN, BSN, MA
University of California at
  San Francisco
San Francisco, California

Shirley Noakes, RN, BSN, MEd
Oaks Treatment Center
Austin, Texas

Margaret Rafferty, RN, MA, MPH, CS
Long Island College Hospital
Brooklyn, New York

Mary Rode, RN, MSN
University of Evansville
Evansville, Indiana

Jerry Stamper, RNC, EdD
San Jose State University
San Jose, California

Ruth Staten, RN, MSN
University of Kentucky
Lexington, Kentucky

Norma Wilkerson, RN, PhD
University of Wyoming
Laramie, Wyoming

PREFACE

History and Philosophy

Psychiatric Nursing's first edition, published a dozen years ago in 1979, is recognized as a landmark in psychiatric nursing because it used cutting-edge knowledge from the humanities and social sciences to generate a unique humanistic–interactionist perspective for practice and research. Subsequent editions updated this trendsetting text, incorporating the American Nurses' Association Practice Standards, the American Psychiatric Association's most current nomenclature, the current thinking on psychiatric nursing diagnosis, application of the nursing process to psychiatric disorders, contemporary clinical problems such as the AIDS epidemic, a lifespan developmental focus, and a call to political awareness and activism. Acknowledgments of the value of this textbook throughout its prior editions are evident in its *American Journal of Nursing* "Book of the Year" awards, its translation into several languages, its many positive reviews, and its widespread international adoptions.

The Psychiatric Nursing Renaissance

With the publication of this fourth edition of *Psychiatric Nursing*, our nursing specialty embarks on a new decade. Declaration of the 1990s as the *Decade of the Brain* by the 101st United States Congress is intended to focus needed attention on research, treatment, care, and rehabilitation for the more than 50 million Americans affected each year by disorders and disabilities involving the brain. Integrating the knowledge innovation or paradigm shift reflected in the explosion of research findings from "biological psychiatry" challenges psychiatric nursing to expand our thinking beyond the familiarity of psychologic, behavioral, and psychodynamic frameworks. It challenges us to reframe our research and practice agenda toward a true biopsychosocial perspective that expands humanistic interactionism to include biologic vulnerabilities and interventions while continuing to consider interpersonal and environmental contexts. It challenges us to refine our knowledge base of the biological nature of mental disorders and thereby reduce the potential of dualistic approaches to clients.

Psychiatric nursing is poised for a renaissance—"a new leap forward." We have revised this text in its fourth edition to capture the spirit of that leap, that movement, and the ultimate balance required by psychiatric nurses:

• who must respond to the complex realities of growing populations of psychiatric clients such as the severely and persistently mentally ill, chemically addicted children and adults, the homeless mentally ill, elders suffering from the mind-wasting ravages of dementia, and the grief-torn families of AIDS patients;

• who must practice in health care systems characteristic of the aftermath of deinstitutionalization; and

• who must integrate rapidly expanding knowledge in the fields of neurobiology, genetics, endocrinology, immunology, brain imaging, and pharmacology with more familiar social and behavioral sciences and nursing's caring ethic.

Integrating Design and Content

Movement and balance are portrayed visually in the disciplined art of the dancers whose images serve as part opening art. Movement and balance capture our point of view as we attempt to integrate the knowledge explosion in psychobiology with psychological, social, and cultural influences on emotions and behavior to create a contemporary biopsychosocial synthesis. To do so is not to be equated with a retreat to a reductionist, disease-oriented biomedical model of psychiatric nursing care. Instead, we believe that the *Decade of the Brain* can offer a renaissance, an opportunity for socially responsible innovation for psychiatric nurses who are well-grounded in biologic, psychologic, interactional, and environmental sciences and who practice with the values and art of a humanist. The integration of research-based knowledge of the psychobiology of emotions, behaviors, and mental disorders can update and enrich our professional discipline, not displace it.

Retained in this Edition

Psychiatric Nursing in its fourth edition retains many of the strengths that have kept it on the cutting edge of the field for more than a decade.

• Content on mental disorders is organized in chapters using DSM-III-R nomenclature.

• The stages of the nursing process continue to provide the framework for discussing nursing care.

• Case studies, clinical examples, and nursing care plans illustrate the application of theory to real world practice with clients.

• Updated research notes briefly describe relevant published studies and relate them to clinical practice.

• Cross references at the beginning of each chapter refer students to related information elsewhere in the book.

• A comprehensive glossary of psychiatric nursing terms, a detailed table of contents, and a comprehensive index add to the book's utility for students.

New to this Edition

New features reflecting the theme of movement and balance in the fourth edition of *Psychiatric Nursing* include:

• Completely new chapters on codependence, suicide, and eating disorders.

- New features throughout the book:

   Nutrition boxes discuss the most up-to-date knowledge on how foods affect emotions, behavior, and mental disorders;

   Psychobiology boxes summarize current thinking on the mind-body connection and highlight interventions such as full-spectrum light treatments for mood disorders;

  Special boxes highlight information and tables on

   The Nursing Process (including Assessment, Nursing Diagnosis, and Intervention)

   Nursing Self-Awareness

   Client/Family Teaching

- A new, comprehensive psychotropic drug appendix. Drugs or therapeutic regimens are highlighted within the text with a marginal logo.

- A perforated, fold-out collection of pocket-sized drug cards for reference in the clinical setting summarize the information found in the appendix.

- A streamlined design using two colors enhances accessibility for students.

The Package

- A complete learning/teaching package includes a Test Bank/Resource Manual with over 500 multiple-choice questions in NCLEX format, an annotated bibliography on psychobiology, a Directory of Mental Health Resources, and an annotated listing of over 500 classroom resources that includes video and audio programs and computer software. A computerized test bank is also available.

- A video, free to adoptors, that explains the basic tenets of psychobiology. The video is designed to refresh the instructor while introducing the topic to the student. Your Addison-Wesley representative can provide more details on this exciting addition to the package.

Acknowledgments

Books are not the pure products of the imaginations of their authors. We welcome this opportunity to thank the many people who have been helpful in important ways.

We consider ourselves fortunate, indeed, that Wendy Earl was our production editor. She is scrupulously organized, ever graceful, and always eager. She has been encouraging and supportive. Her suggestions are woven with delicacy and tact. Wendy has been a calm guide through the many exciting and occasionally stormy moments associated with this fourth edition.

Our manuscript editor, Antonio Padial, has clarified our thoughts with a detective's eye and polished this text with his incisive writing craftsmanship while respecting our own and our contributors' needs.

The movement and grace of this beautiful book reflect the talent of Alexander Laurant, the artist whose dancers visually portray the exterior world of structure and the interior world of feelings. The inviting text design that eases the reader's way was created by Paula Schlosser. Their creativity enhances our work.

Mark McCormick, our sponsoring editor at Addison-Wesley, enthusiastically represented our project to his colleagues. He created an environment that removed all obstacles to working on this edition. Mark provided encouragement, good advice, and advocacy.

We also thank Wendy Gross, editorial assistant, and Frank Vaughn, production assistant, who were involved in the many day-to-day details that often go unobserved and unacknowledged. You are acknowledged and appreciated. We thank Wendy Gross for her contribution to the design and editing of the perforated drug cards.

Our deepest thanks go to this gifted set of publishing professionals.

We are indebted to our contributors for their rich diversity of clinical experience, their excitement about the potential of psychiatric nurses to blend the psychobiologic with the humanistic, and their commitment to this project.

Eileen Trigoboff and Nan Rich, besides contributing to the text, prepared the drug appendix. Eileen also wrote the Test Bank/Resource Manual, and was a constant source of support throughout the project.

Those with whom we share the most complex ties—our surviving parents, Harold Skodol and Frances Ren; and our children, Hillary, Emily, and Molly Wilson, and Kyle and Heidi Kneisl—nurtured us and have shared our frustrations and successes over the years. They remind us that intimacy can be a source of great joy and relationships a rich challenge.

And, how fortunate we are to have a relationship in which we energize and sustain one another throughout the best of times and the worst of times, despite the geographic distance that separates us.

We are sincerely grateful.

Holly Skodol Wilson
Carol Ren Kneisl

CONTENTS IN BRIEF

CONTENTS IN DETAIL

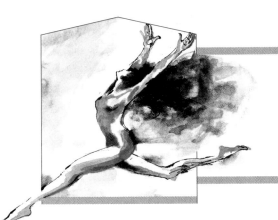

PART ONE

The Theoretic Basis for Psychiatric Nursing 1

CHAPTER
2

The Psychiatric Nurse and the Interdisciplinary Mental Health Team: Personal Integration and Professional Role 24

CHAPTER
3

Applying the Nursing Process 43

CHAPTER
4

Theories for Interdisciplinary Psychiatric Care 57

CHAPTER
5

Stress, Anxiety, and Coping 79

CHAPTER
6

Psychobiology 99

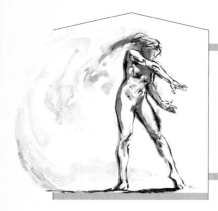

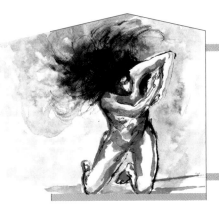

PART THREE

Human Responses to Distress and Disorder 182

CHAPTER

10

Applying the Nursing Process for Clients with Organic Mental Syndromes and Disorders 184

CHAPTER

11

Applying the Nursing Process for Clients with Psychoactive Substance Use Disorders 214

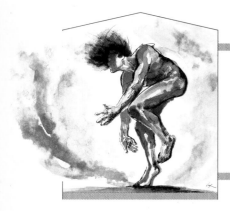

PART FOUR

Contemporary Clinical Concerns 418

CHAPTER

17

Psychosocial Rehabilitation with the Severely and Persistently Mentally Ill 420

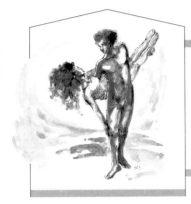

PART FIVE

Intervention Modes 612

CHAPTER
26
The One-to-One Relationship 614

CHAPTER
27
Stress Management 645

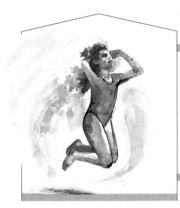

PART SIX

Applying the Nursing Process Across the Life Span 808

CHAPTER
33

Applying the Nursing Process with Children 810

CHAPTER
34

Applying the Nursing Process with Adolescents 839

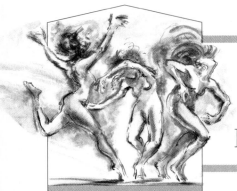

PART SEVEN

The Social, Political, Cultural, and Economic Environments for Care 900

SUMMARY OF SPECIAL FEATURES

ASSESSMENT BOXES

NURSING DIAGNOSIS BOXES

INTERVENTION BOXES

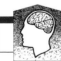

PSYCHOBIOLOGY BOXES

NUTRITION AND MENTAL HEALTH BOXES

CLIENT/FAMILY TEACHING BOXES

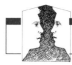

NURSING SELF-AWARENESS BOXES

THEORY BOXES

NURSING STANDARDS BOXES

ADVOCACY BOXES

CASE STUDIES

NURSING CARE PLANS

RESEARCH NOTES

 This logo appears in the margin next to key information about specific drugs or general information about drug interventions.

PART ONE

The Theoretic Basis for Psychiatric Nursing

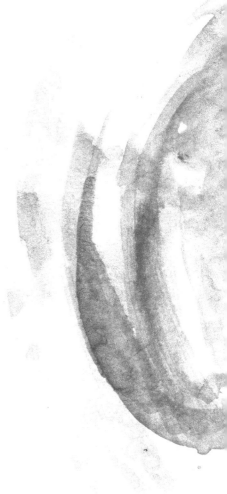

CONTENTS

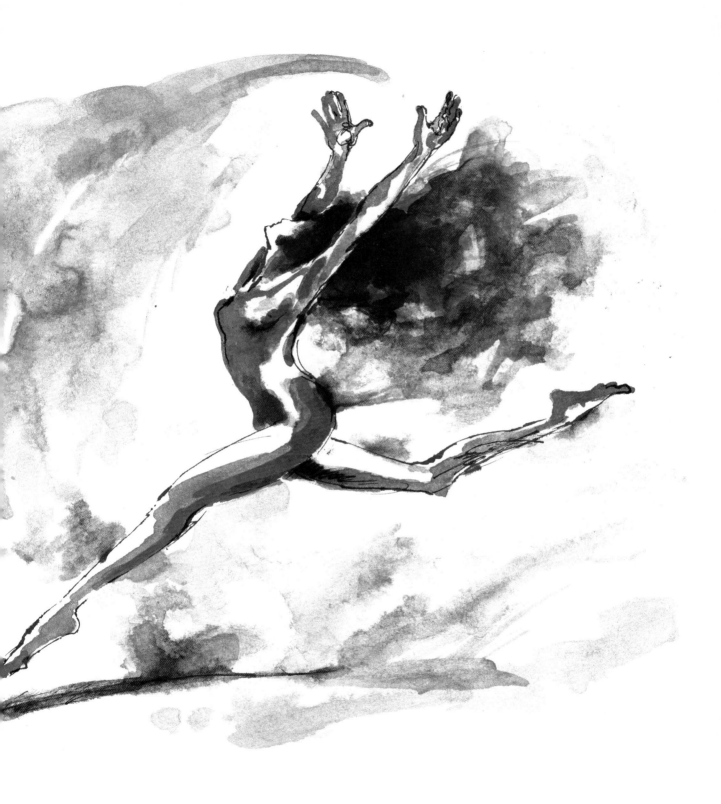

Dance—an affirmation of life through movement—has held an ageless magic for the world because it is a symbol of the performance of living.

Philosophic and Historical Perspectives

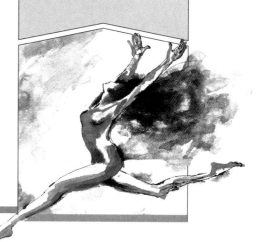

LEARNING OBJECTIVES

- Identify the major ideas of interactionism
- Identify the major principles of humanism
- Recognize the influence of the knowledge explosion in psychobiology
- Relate the premises of humanistic interactionism and psychobiology to the psychiatric nursing process
- Develop a personal philosophic framework for psychiatric nursing practice
- Describe the history of ideas about madness
- Correlate the history of psychiatric treatment with ideas about madness
- Describe the emergence of the discipline of psychiatric nursing
- Project directions for psychiatric nursing in the late 1990s

Holly Skodol Wilson
Carol Ren Kneisl

CROSS REFERENCES

Other topics relevant to this content are: Community mental health, Chapter 38; Conceptual frameworks for psychiatric treatment, Chapter 4; Contemporary roles of psychiatric nurses, Chapter 2; Cultural considerations in mental health care, Chapter 36; Ethics, Chapter 7; Legal aspects of confinement, Chapter 37; Psychobiology, Chapter 6.

THERE ARE MANY APPROACHES to understanding people. Each is like a searchlight that illuminates some of the facts while leaving others in shadow. Your approach to understanding is influenced by your philosophy of psychiatric nursing. This chapter introduces you to a philosophic perspective that encompasses humanism, interactionism, and the knowledge explosion in the field of psychobiology. This contemporary holistic philosophy is the basis for subsequent chapters in this text and, in the authors' opinions, offers psychiatric nursing new opportunities for practice and research in what is being called the "Decade of the Brain." The first part of Chapter 1 explains that philosophic perspective.

Madness has been recognized by many different faces throughout history. Clearly, the meaning assigned to madness has determined whether such persons are perceived as deranged and tragic heroes, to be valued and liberated, or as criminals, to be confined and modified. Through a comparative social history, we hope to offer perspectives on the odd courses human beings have run in the past. To understand the changing faces and future directions of psychiatric nursing, we must trace its historical development and understand how it evolved as a specialty. The second part of Chapter 1 summarizes this social history and concludes with directions for psychiatric nursing practice and clinical research in the 1990s.

Philosophic Perspectives

Psychiatric nurses and students might reasonably ask why issues of philosophy should even be considered. We believe that the guiding pattern in the lives of all psychiatric nurses is their philosophy, even though that philosophy may be demonstrated primarily in actions rather than systematically thought out. Philosophy teaches people to say what they mean and to mean what they say. It is an attempt to think through the fundamental issues of life and reach reasoned conclusions about society, human nature, action, and values. The practice of psychiatric nursing is grounded in certain philosophic assumptions about human nature, society, and values.

A psychiatric nurse's philosophic perspective influences every aspect of practice. This chapter introduces a perspective that combines *humanistic interactionism* with the rapidly growing field of *psychobiology*. We believe this perspective encompasses most of the variables that challenge today's psychiatric nurse, including the biologic explanations of feelings and behavior. We believe that a holistic philosophic perspective is crucial to psychiatric nursing. We hope that

readers will be moved to examine some basic philosophic questions and to formulate a philosophy of psychiatric nursing for their own personal and professional lives.

Introduction to Humanistic Interactionism and Psychobiology

Scope of Practice

All nurses are concerned with the quality of human life and its relationship to health. The psychiatric nurse is especially concerned with the relationship between the individual's optimal psychobiologic health and feelings of self-worth, personal integrity, self-fulfillment, and creative expression. Just as important are the satisfaction of basic living needs, comfortable relations with others, and the recognition of human rights. The psychiatric nurse's scope of practice is broad enough to include issues such as alienation, identity crises, sudden life changes, and troubled family interactions. It can encompass individual protests or mass confrontations. It deals with poverty and affluence, the experiences of birth and death, the loss of significant others, or the loss of body parts. It is concerned with sustaining and enhancing the individual and the group. Yet it also must address basic life issues of eating, sleeping, grooming, and hygiene.

This broad-ranging, humanistic, interactional, and psychobiologic view of the scope of psychiatric nursing is dramatically different from the exclusively medical or behavioral science orientation of the last forty years. The classic psychiatric and psychologic approaches have described and classified signs and symptoms of *illness*, then accounted for it by individual psychologic dynamics such as character disorder, weak ego, or failed defense mechanisms. The basis for this text is a new synthesis of the social-psychologic and the psychobiologic needed for practice in the 1990s.

Concepts of Mental Illness and Mental Health

We believe that concepts such as "mental illness" and "mental health" are interactional and derive their meaning not only from changes in brain biochemistry but also from the definitions given to certain acts by certain audiences. They do not arise exclusively from within the individual.

We advocate looking at the social conditions under which someone is labeled "mentally ill." Equally important are who applies the label and what the consequences are. Thus, we view mental illness and mental health as outgrowths of intra- and interpersonal processes.

Examined from this perspective, mental illness is not exclusively defined by particular character traits. Nor is it established purely by the nature of certain acts (*symptomatology*). Rather, it is a function of the individual's view of those acts, the reactions of others to them, and the overall cultural context in which they occur.

In short, the determination that someone is mentally ill is often a matter of judgment, even when brain chemicals are altered. The appropriateness of behavior depends on whether it is judged plausible or not according to a set of social, ethical, and legal rules that define the limits of appropriate behavior and reality. For example, if a man on a street corner says he is Napoleon, people will not believe him and will consider his statement symptomatic or disturbed. If a man at a masquerade party says he is Napoleon, people reach a different conclusion. Alterations in brain biochemistry may be present in both social contexts.

Mental Disorder and Psychiatric Nursing's Phenomena of Concern

With the publication of the third edition of the American Psychiatric Association's *Diagnostic and Statistical Manual of Mental Disorders* (DSM-III), psychiatric professionals accepted this definition of *mental disorder:* "A clinically significant behavioral or psychological syndrome or pattern that occurs in an individual that is typically associated with either a painful symptom (distress) or impairment in one or more important areas of functioning (disability)" (1980, p 6). This definition persists in the revised edition of DSM-III-R (1987) and in drafts of DSM-IV (1992–1993). Disturbances between an individual and society are acknowledged as conditions that may require therapy or treatment but are not themselves "mental disorders." Nor are mental disorders discrete, clearly delineated entities.

Psychiatric nurses are indeed concerned with care of clients with identified mental disorders. However, our phenomena of concern extend to the wide-ranging human responses to mental distress, disability, and disorder (ANA 1980, Loomis et al. 1987).

For example, an addicted parent may not only suffer from shame, unemployment, and abusive outbursts of anger but may also lose a sense of interconnectedness with life, lose a sense of purpose and meaning, and experience disturbed self-concept. These responses have detrimental effects for the health of children, partners, and other significant people. Individual, family, and community responses vary with individual interpretations of meaning and culture.

Faced with such a diverse array of human problems, the psychiatric nurse is challenged to synthesize a holistic philosophy for practice that can be the basis for care.

Basic Premises of Interactionism

One central idea in the approach we advocate above has come to be known as **symbolic interactionism,** a term introduced by Herbert Blumer (1969) to describe an approach to the study of human conduct. It is based on three philosophic premises:

1. Human beings act toward things (other people, events) on the basis of the meaning that the things have for them. Life experiences may have different meanings for different people.

2. The meaning of things in a person's life is derived from the social interactions that person has with others. We learn meanings during our experiences with others.

3. People handle and modify the meanings of the things they encounter through an interpretive process. They come to their own conclusions.

Implications of Premises for Psychiatric Nursing

The First Premise: Different Meanings for Different People The notion that people's actions in a situation are based on the unique meaning that situation has for them is all but ignored in many approaches to psychiatric nursing. Instead, human conduct is treated as the product of various factors that act on passive human beings—factors such as stimuli, unconscious motives, and character traits. This emphasis on factors thought to produce "symptoms" neglects the role of individual meaning in the formation of human behavior.

We believe that all behavior has meaning. The psychiatric nurse must be wary of interventions that ignore, discount, or discredit the meaning an experience has for the client in favor of the nurse's own definition of the situation. Thus, nurses need to develop skill in observing, interpreting, and responding to the client's lived experiences in the hope of arriving at a common ground of negotiated meanings and authentic communication.

The Second Premise: Meanings Arise in One's Social World In many conventional approaches to psychiatric nursing, meanings—such as the meaning of "normal," "mentally healthy," and "mentally ill"—are regarded as intrinsic to the nature of the behavior, the personality, or the disease. We believe meanings arise in the *process* of interaction with others. Meanings are social products formed in and through interpersonal communication and learning. It is essential, therefore, that psychiatric nurses take into account the social and cultural environment of each client. A holistic assessment of a client accounts for the interaction patterns in that person's social world.

A shaved head, black leather clothing, and tattoos may appear bizarre in a milieu of upper-middle-class bankers and businesspeople, yet they represent rather strict adherence to dress and demeanor codes of the "heavy metal" subculture. Individuals labeled "paranoid" or "neurotic" or "using alcohol or drugs as emotional crutches" cannot be understood outside their unique social context.

Similarly, it is within interpersonal interaction that clients can learn new definitions for life situations and new repertoires for action. This is the heart of the psychiatric nurse's therapeutic and caring role. The sensitive, intelligent, and humanistic use of self within interpersonal relationships is a key part of the psychiatric nurse's skill. Nurses have a particular potential for helping clients redefine their experiences in more satisfying ways, learn new patterns of coping with stress, and generally enhance the quality of their lives and social worlds.

The Third Premise: Meaning Is a Basis for Behavior We believe that people handle situations in terms of what they consider vitally important about the situation. To understand the actions of people, the psychiatric nurse must learn to identify the meanings those actions have for them.

Nurses need to keep this premise in mind when responding to an expression of human distress. A nurse may say, "I wouldn't worry about it," or "don't feel that way," "you are reacting inappropriately," or "it's not so bad." Such clichés are not usually helpful, not because they are inherently "untherapeutic" but because in voicing them the nurse neglects the basic premise that people interpret the world in their own way to act in a specific situation.

Interactionism offers psychiatric nursing a perspective of human beings as having purpose and control over their own lives even if they have altered brain chemistry and stressful environments. Interactionism as interpreted here provides the premises for a philosophy of caring with a strong humanistic cast. Interactionism acknowledges the interaction of psychology, biology, and sociocultural context.

Basic Premises of Humanism

One of the purposes of this chapter is to specify a philosophic basis for subsequent chapters. The three premises of interactionism provide us with a partial orientation. A theory of life centered on human beings, termed **humanism,** adds to the philosophic perspective.

The central proposition of humanism is that the chief end of human life is to work for well-being within the confines of life on this earth. Humanism is a philosophy of service to benefit humanity through reason, science, and democracy.

Humanism as a philosophic perspective can be clarified in eight central propositions:

1. The human being's mind is indivisibly connected with the body.

2. Human beings have the power or potential to solve their own problems.

3. Human beings, while influenced by the past, possess freedom of creative choice and action and are, within certain limits, masters of their own destinies.

4. Human values are grounded in life experiences and relationships, and our highest goal must be the happiness, freedom, and growth of all people.

5. Individuals attain well-being and a high quality of life by harmoniously combining personal satisfactions with activities that contribute to the welfare of the community.

6. We should develop art and awareness of beauty so that the aesthetic experience becomes a pervasive reality in people's lives.

7. We should apply reason, science, and democratic procedures in all areas of life.

8. We must continually examine our basic convictions—including those of humanism.

See Lamont (1967) for elaboration of these propositions.

The Meaning of Humanism for Psychiatric Nursing

As a philosophy underlying psychiatric nursing practice, humanism means devotion to the interests of human beings wherever they live and whatever their status. It reaffirms the spirit of compassion and caring toward others. It is a constructive philosophy that wholeheartedly affirms the joys, beauties, and values of human living.

The subsequent chapters in this text attempt to show how these basic premises can be put to use in psychiatric nursing practice. Some fundamental concepts are described briefly in the following sections.

Holistic View of Mind-Body Relations   There are two basic schools of thought about the relationship of the mind and the body. These two philosophic positions are called **monism** and **dualism.** The monistic view asserts that mind and body are one. The dualistic view asserts that mind and body are separate phenomena and may be (a) causally interrelated, (b) parallel but independent, or (c) unrelated.

Our humanistic interactionist view is neither monistic nor dualistic. We maintain that physical and mental factors are interrelated and that a change in one may result in a change in another. For example, anger may result in increased blood pressure. An invading organism, a decrease in a neurotransmitter, or a structural change in the body can alter thought processes. Low self-esteem can result in hunched shoulders and severe skeletal muscle contractures.

The implications for psychiatric nursing are clear. Healing and caring must be approached **holistically**. The psychiatric nurse deals with the biologic aspects of a primarily psychologic or emotional pattern and the psychologic or emotional aspects of biologic experiences. Psychiatric nursing care can be given not only in "mental hospitals" but also in general health care settings and may be directed toward clients whose immediate problems are primarily physical.

Expanded Role for Nurses The humanistic interactionist perspective on "mental illness" implies an expanded role for psychiatric nurse practitioners. Thus, the nurse can work in political or social arenas as well as with individual clients. When a person's behavior is viewed exclusively in terms of psychiatric symptoms, the emphasis is on intrapersonal variables, but we view behavior within an interpersonal field. For instance, in our opinion, no one can "have" schizophrenia all alone. Schizophrenia is experienced in a family context.

We believe that psychiatric nurses should be prepared to work for change within social and political systems. Psychiatric nursing can no longer be limited to client-oriented activities designed exclusively to control symptoms and increase the capability of individuals to adjust satisfactorily to the existing social condition. Instead, psychiatric nursing must be involved in social goals that advance health holistically. Because psychiatric nursing has political consequences, it is essential that nurses begin to develop a philosophic and ethical framework to guide and evaluate the political outcome of therapeutic intervention.

Decision Making A perspective that combines humanistic interactionism and psychobiologic knowledge suggests a different decision-making format from that of the traditional medical model. The medical model implies that the physician is the chief decision maker. In contrast, we do not advocate that any particular discipline provide leadership in psychiatric decision making. We prefer practical collaboration among interdisciplinary team participants to generate effective strategies.

Negotiation and Advocacy In this book's perspective, the model for intervention and change is one of negotiation and advocacy. The responsibility for change remains with the person who seeks psychiatric help or consultation. Clients are held accountable for their own behavior. They are not the passive recipients of care given by psychiatric professionals. Instead, they are supported in the process of developing new perspectives and encouraged to weigh alternatives and make self-directed choices. They and their families are educated about their disorder and their medications.

Basic Premises of the Psychobiologic Revolution

The last decade has seen major breakthroughs in knowledge about the brain, the mind, and behavior. This knowledge explosion has been termed *the biologic revolution* in psychiatry. Research has generated new understanding of how genetics, immunology, biorhythms, brain structure, and brain biochemistry influence mental disorders. New imaging techniques make it possible to see what has never been seen before. New drugs to correct biochemical imbalances in the brain are being studied. Researchers are exploring such psychobiologic interventions as exposure to bright light and white noise, and restriction of nutrients and non-nutrients believed to affect behavior.

Some authorities argue that psychiatric nurses should continue to focus on the human aspects of care as psychiatry moves toward "remedicalization." They fear that by embracing the biologic sciences we will diminish the art of psychiatric nursing. Others, including the authors of this text, contend that, to bring a contemporary holistic perspective to psychiatric nursing care, we need to integrate the rapidly accumulating knowledge in psychobiology. We do not give up our basic humanistic, psychosocial, and interactionist premises simply because we recognize the value of the breakthroughs being made in psychobiology. Instead, as we redefine the traditional art of psychiatric nursing care and caring in the "Decade of the Brain," our practice and research must integrate "high tech" and "high touch," nature and nurture, and the biologic sciences and the behavioral sciences.

Historical Perspectives

People who have been called "mentally ill" have been with us throughout history—to be feared, marveled at, ignored, banished, sheltered, laughed at, pitied, or tortured. A historical review on the place of the "mentally ill," however they have been defined in societies during different periods, brings up these central points:

• Dominant social attitudes and philosophic viewpoints have influenced the understanding and approach to "madness" throughout recorded history and probably before.

• Ideas that may be considered contemporary at one time often have roots in earlier centuries.

• The modern medical concept of "madness" as an illness is open to the same scrutiny as interpretations of the past, such as beliefs about witchcraft or mysticism.

Preliterate Times—Era of Magico-Religious Explanations

In preliterate cultures, mental and physical suffering were not differentiated. Both were attributed to forces acting outside the body. Consequently, no distinctions were made between medicine, magic, and religion. All were variously directed against some mortal or superhuman force that had cruelly inflicted suffering on another. Primitive healers quite logically dealt with the spirits of torment by appeal, reverence, prayer, bribery, intimidation, appeasement, confession, and punishment. These were expressed through exorcism, magical ritual, and incantation.

Most preliterate cultures held these beliefs:

• The liberation of supernatural (spiritual) forces by divine power or magical arts

• The principle of solidarity or contagion, which implies that human beings are continuous with, not separate from, their surroundings

• Sympathetic, imitative forms of magic occurring by telepathy and other interactions between similar elements

• The symbolism of certain substances, such as water, which played a purifying role

These beliefs about the nature of suffering gave rise to procedures based on the idea of *mimetic*, or imitative, magic. A medicine man would enact a person's illness and then slowly recover, thus prompting the person's own recovery. The principle of continuity was the belief in continued relationship between things that were once close but became separated. Thus, fingernail parings and afterbirths were seen as objects that could influence the lives of people from whom these things had been removed. Some approaches were based on substitution methods—i.e., transferring suffering to a scapegoat. Behavior considered to be "mental illness" by modern Western cultures was attributed in preliterate cultures to the violation of taboos, the neglect of ritual obligations, the loss of a vital substance from the body (such as the soul), the introduction of a foreign and harmful substance into the body (such as evil spirits), or witchcraft.

Early Civilization—Era of Organic Explanations

There are essentially three sources of the concept of madness in Greek and Roman cultures:

1. Earlier beliefs in the supernatural causation of mental suffering continued to be popularly held. This had no prescribed treatment.

2. A medical concept arose, centered on the interaction of four body "humors." It was explained in the writings of Hippocrates (fourth century B.C.).

3. The notion developed that violation of moral principles and subsequent punishment by the gods were part of human destiny. This notion is evident in the literary and philosophic works of the period.

What might be called the professional opinion on madness was summarized by Hippocrates, who lived from about 460 to 370 B.C. He rejected demonology and proposed that psychiatric illnesses were caused mainly by imbalances in body humors: blood, black bile, yellow bile, and phlegm. For example, an excess of black bile caused melancholy and could be corrected by purging or bloodletting. One important consequence of these beliefs was that psychiatric suffering came within the realm of medical practice.

Four ancient methods of psychotherapeutic intervention stand out because of their widespread use for many centuries in the cultures of the Near East and Mediterranean areas: the interpretation of dreams, ritual purifications, therapeutic use of the milieu, and catharsis. Both words and medicines were used in these methods. However, the need for supernatural explanations was so great that when cures were achieved, they were attributed to the interventions of the gods.

The Medieval Period—Era of Alienation

At the height of their civilization, the citizens of ancient Greece found their inner security in knowledge and reason. The Romans adopted the intellectual heritage of Greece but for their peace of mind relied more on their social institutions and the rational organization of society supported by law and military might. When these institutions disintegrated and the empire declined, fear tore apart the fabric of society.

The collapse of Rome signaled a general return to the magic, mysticism, and demonology from which people had retreated during Greek rationality. During the Middle Ages, the period between approximately 400 A.D. and the Renaissance (1300–1600), madness was seen as a dramatic encounter with secret powers. Troubled minds were thought to be influenced by the moon (*lunacy* literally means a disorder caused by the lunar body).

Mad people, left wandering on their own, were evidence of the greatness of God and the frailty of humans—a necessary, although sometimes annoying, part of the community. Many participated in religious wars, crusades, and long pilgrimages. Others embraced emotionally charged heretic movements, such as the dance epidemics of the fourteenth century.

In the Arab world, the insane were believed to be divinely inspired and not victims of demons. An asylum for the mentally ill was built in Fez, Morocco, early in the eighth century. Other asylums were soon established in Baghdad, Cairo, and Damascus. Hospital care in these asylums was usually benevolent and kindly.

By and large, through the thirteenth and fourteenth centuries, the human body and its organic afflictions were dealt with by lay physicians. During this period, the first European hospital devoted entirely to mental patients was built in 1409 in Valencia, Spain.

The problems of the mind, however, remained in the domain of clerical scholars. Two Dominican monks, Johann Sprenger and Heinrich Kraemer, summarized the ideas of the times in their book *Malleus Maleficarum* (*The Witches' Hammer*, 1487), a textbook of both pornography and supposed psychopathology. Witch-hunts became accepted as a system to maintain the status quo. The *Malleus* details the destruction of dissenters, heretics, and the "mentally ill," most of whom were women and all of whom were labeled *witches*. Theologic rationalizations and magical explanations were used to justify the burning at the stake of thousands of unfortunates.

The violent insane were shackled in prisons. Others were sent on a voyage of symbolic importance. The "ships of fools" were boatloads of mad people sent out to sea to search for their reason. In this phase of ritualized social exclusion, social abandonment was thought to provide the opportunity for spiritual reintegration.

The Renaissance—Era of Confinement

Whereas during the Middle Ages the insane were generally driven out of or excluded from community life, during the Renaissance they were confined. Tamed, retained, and maintained, madness was reduced to silence through a system of mutual obligation between the afflicted and society. Mad persons had the right to be fed but were morally constrained and physically confined.

Seventeenth-century society created enormous houses of confinement. In these asylums were gathered the mad, the poor, and various deviants. A landmark date is 1656, when by decree the Hôpital Générale in Paris was founded. It was not a medical establishment, but rather a threatening institution, complete with stakes, irons, prisons, and dungeons, established by the king to enforce the law. The "insane" were completely under the jurisdiction of the institution and had no recourse to appeal. The Hôpital Générale and others like it had little to do with any medical concept. They were institutions for the maintenance of social order. Michel Foucault (1973, p 71) describes the conditions in these terms:

The unfortunate whose entire furniture consisted of a straw pallet, lying with his head, feet and body pressed against the wall, could not enjoy sleep without being soaked by the water that trickled from that mass of stone. . . . In winter the waters of the Seine rose . . . and cells became a refuge for a swarm of huge rats. Madwomen have been found with feet, hands, and faces torn by bites.

In London, the hospital of Saint Mary of Bethlehem became famous as *Bedlam,* where, for the entertainment of visitors on Sunday excursions, mad persons were publicly beaten and tortured.

Madness thus was given the mask of the beast. Those chained to cell walls were no longer considered people who had lost their reason, but rather beasts seized by a frenzy. The animality in madness was seen as evidence that the mad person was not a sick person. Madness was less than ever linked to medicine in this period. It could be mastered only by discipline and brutality.

During the 1500s, 1600s, and 1700s, some physicians again began to consider psychiatric bases for mental disorders. Johann Weyer (1515–1588), a German physician, believed that "those illnesses whose origins are attributed to witches come from natural causes." He attributed a variety of so-called supernatural signs to natural factors. Weyer was a carefully observant clinician. He described a wide range of diagnostic categories with associated symptoms, including hysteria, paranoid reactions, toxic organic brain syndrome, epilepsy, folie à deux, depression, and delusions. His position on psychotherapy, however, is considered his most outstanding contribution. He insisted that the needs of individuals were more important than the rules of social institutions. He recognized the importance of the therapeutic relationship and stressed not only kindness but also a benevolent attitude based on careful observation and scientific principles. His approach was radical and completely alien to the thinking of his time. As a result, his work was met with hostility at first and then was simply ignored. In retrospect, his contributions are of such importance that he is called "the first psychiatrist."

Late Eighteenth and Early Nineteenth Centuries—Era of Moral Treatment

The continuous development of scientific ideas cannot be neatly divided into centuries. It has simply become a matter of convenience to label the eighteenth century the *Enlightenment*. Enlightenment there was, but the era was full of internal contradictions. Although the insane were unchained, the medical treatment they received consisted of torture by special paraphernalia. To grasp the incredible inhumanity with which the mentally disordered were treated in this era of enlightenment, consider the following:

• The nature of mental disorders could not be explained by any of the concepts—black humors could not be seen, demons or animal spirits could not be observed, and knowledge of anatomy could not be applied to the workings of the mind.

• Because mental disorders could not be satisfactorily explained, the deeply felt dread of the insane could not be removed.

• Mental disorders were believed to be incurable, and mad persons were thought to be dangerous.

Eventually, belief in reason replaced beliefs in faith and tradition. New medical and scientific data had become so overwhelming that synthesis and systematization became necessary. The Enlightenment witnessed the movement to classify mental disorders and unshackle the insane.

Eighteenth-century psychiatry typically emphasized the classification of symptoms of mental disorders. Even the most sensitive physicians did not try to understand the sources of mental suffering. Methods of psychiatric treatment were scarcely affected by these classifiers. Because they had no way to explain or understand these disorders, classification became overextended. There was a tendency to dismiss factual data that did not fit, and the system abounded with errors.

Among the classifiers was Hermann Boerhaave (1668–1738), a Dutch physician, for whom the practice of psychotherapy consisted of bloodletting, administering purgatives, dousing people in ice-cold water, or using other methods to put them in near shock. Boerhaave gave the medical profession one of its first shock instruments, a spinning chair that rendered its occupant unconscious. Another was William Cullen (1710–1790), who lectured at Edinburgh and was the first to use the term *neurosis* to denote diseases that are not accompanied by fever or localized symptoms. Cullen believed that neurosis was due to decay, either of the intellect or of the involuntary nervous system. By his time psychiatry had discarded the concept that a demon originating outside the person caused internal disharmony. Physicians now insisted that the cause was disordered physiology.

At the same time, doctors began subscribing to another movement characteristic of the Enlightenment—a zeal for social reform and moral enrichment. Rationalism, observation through experimentation, and classification were joined by a fourth approach—reform. In 1793, Philippe Pinel (1745–1826) became superintendent of the French institution Bicêtre for men and later of the Salpêtrière for women, where criminals, mentally retarded people, and the insane were housed. One of his first accomplishments was to release the inmates from their chains, abolish systematized brutality with chains and whips, open their windows, feed them nourishing food, and treat them with kindness. For this act, he himself was considered mad by his contemporaries. Many of the inmates were reported to improve dramatically.

Meanwhile in England, William Tuke (1732–1822), a Quaker tea merchant unhappy about the institutions available to treat mentally disordered Quakers, founded the York Retreat in England. The goal was to reconstruct around madness a milieu resembling the community of Quakers. Tuke's work focused on liberation of the insane, suppression of constraint, and establishment of a humane milieu. With the emergence of **moral treatment,** the asylum no longer punished the mad person's guilt. It did more; it organized that guilt. By becoming aware of their guilt, the mad became aware of themselves as responsible subjects and, consequently, were able to return to reason. At the York Retreat the suppression of physical freedom fostered "self-restraint" by inmates engaged in work under the observation of others.

The insane were among the clients of the first general hospital in the United States. Pennsylvania Hospital was opened through the efforts of the Quakers, Benjamin Franklin, and others in 1756. Treatment, rather than mere confinement of the mentally ill, was the stated goal, though the state of medical knowledge was such that treatment consisted of bleeding, blistering, and purging in the damp restraining cells of the hospital's cellar.

The treatment of psychiatric clients at the Pennsylvania Hospital in the United States was influenced by the ideas of Benjamin Rush (1746–1813), called "the father of American psychiatry," whose picture is reproduced on the seal of the American Psychiatric Association. Despite his association with humanitarianism and moral treatment, Rush was a major follower of Cullen's ideas in advocating bloodletting, the gyrating chair, and other inhumane devices.

The first American hospital devoted exclusively to the care and treatment of psychiatric clients opened in

Williamsburg, Virginia, in 1773. The only other colony to establish a hospital that accepted mentally disordered people in the eighteenth century was New York, which began building its first general hospital in 1774. The intention was to allot the cellar of the north wing to psychiatric clients. The Revolutionary War and a fire delayed the opening until 1792. As promised, the cellar of New York Hospital received these clients.

Moral treatment, by providing an alternative to mere confinement, played a major role in the development of institutional care and treatment of the mentally disordered in the United States. The growth of the mental hospital in the early nineteenth century was not a chance occurrence but the result of numerous social factors. It arose from the general spirit of reform and humanitarianism sweeping western Europe and the United States. Scientific and technologic advances, coupled with the successful struggle for political democracy in the United States and France, were proof to many people that humanity could tackle and conquer any problem.

Private philanthropy was largely responsible for the hospital movement in the early nineteenth century. In response to the needs brought on by increases in the population, hospitals were established in urban areas. These early corporate hospitals, such as McLean Asylum in Massachusetts (opened in 1818), Friends' Asylum in Frankfort, Pennsylvania (1817), Hartford Retreat in Connecticut (1824), and Bloomingdale Asylum in New York City (1818), were small and used "moral treatment" on a homogeneous population with an astounding degree of success.

It became clear in the mid-1820s that the corporate mental hospitals would be unable to meet the needs of all those requiring services. Responsibility for psychiatric clients, then, began gradually to shift away from the corporate hospitals (just as it had, to a certain extent, shifted away from the family and to the corporate hospital). It now moved to the new institution on the horizon—the public mental hospital.

Late Nineteenth and Early Twentieth Centuries

Era of Public Mental Hospitals   Strongly influenced by optimistic and humanitarian beliefs about human nature, some community leaders took the initiative in establishing a few mental hospitals early in the nineteenth century. The most distinguished leader in generating public interest in building state mental hospitals in the United States was Dorothea L. Dix (1802–1887). Although she was not formally educated as a nurse, she devoted her life to public education concerning the needs of the mentally disordered and administered volunteer women nurses during the Civil War.

For three decades, Dix reported to state legislatures the often abominable conditions in the almshouses, jails, and mental hospitals in their states. After making her exposés, she insisted to legislators that the state had moral, humanitarian, and legal obligations toward the mentally disordered. Dix's determination about this single issue gained her a broad base of support, and she was eventually responsible for founding or enlarging over thirty mental hospitals. J. Sanborn Bockoven (1956, p 187), an authority on moral treatment, suggests that Dix's reform movement, with its emphasis on bringing people into asylums without any planning for effective treatment, was responsible at least in part for the downfall of the moral treatment movement in the United States.

From 1825 to 1865, the number of mental hospitals grew from nine to sixty-two. The first state institution that relied on moral treatment was Worcester State Hospital in Massachusetts, opened in 1833. It gained a national reputation for recovery of 80 to 91 percent of its acute patients. *Acute patient* usually meant a person who had been mentally ill for less than six months. Massachusetts became a model for other states. Eventually, institutionalization became an end in itself. As a carryover from the high rate of "cures" effected by moral treatment, people believed that as soon as insane persons were within the walls of an asylum, they were well on their way to recovery. Moral treatment was being replaced by custodial care.

Toward the end of the nineteenth century, approaches to the "mentally ill" began to change again. Insanity was linked to faulty life habits, and separate hospital facilities were advocated for acute patients. New forms of physical therapy—diet, massage, hydrotherapy, and electroshock therapy—were introduced. Family care and the cottage system were initiated, as were training courses for psychiatric nurses and attendants.

As the twentieth century began, a few psychiatrists became interested in research, which led to the founding of the Pathological Institute of New York Hospital in 1895. Adolf Meyer (1866–1950), a Swiss psychiatrist, served on the staff of the institute from 1902 until 1913, when he became director of the newly built psychiatric clinic at Johns Hopkins Hospital. Meyer dedicated himself to improving the situation for psychiatric clients through any approach that seemed sensible and practical. He was opposed to the dualist separation of mind and body. He regarded each person as a biologic unit having unique reactions to social and biologic influences. As his realistic, *commonsense approach* evolved, he became increasingly unwilling to believe that mental disorders were the result solely of brain dysfunction or solely of an overwhelming environment. Both had to be taken into account.

The year 1908 marks another key event in the development of psychiatry. Clifford Beers (1876–1943), a distinguished businessman, published *A Mind That Found Itself,* a book describing intense suffering and mental anguish he experienced while receiving custodial care. This book profoundly affected the social consciousness of the nation and led to the organization of spirited groups that Meyer named the **mental hygiene movement.** Public awareness of the needs of the mentally disordered was responsible for the development of preventive psychiatry and the formation of child guidance clinics.

Era of Psychoanalysis The eighteenth-century emphasis on clinical classification peaked in the work of Emil Kraepelin (1856–1926). This physician, like many of his time, was inclined toward an organic, neurophysiologic explanation of mental disorders. He is best known for bringing the chaotic accumulation of clinical observations into a system of distinct disease entities. He differentiated *bipolar disorder* (which he called *manic-depressive psychosis*) from *schizophrenia* (which he called *dementia praecox*) and theorized that the latter was incurable. A Swiss psychiatrist, Eugene Bleuler (1857–1939), renamed dementia praecox *schizophrenia* and differentiated the disorder into *hebephrenic, catatonic,* and *paranoid* types. Bleuler also expressed a far more optimistic view of the treatment outcome than Kraepelin did.

The psychiatric developments of the late nineteenth century formed the background for the work of one of the most influential figures in the history of psychiatry, Sigmund Freud (1856–1939). He succeeded in explaining human behavior in psychologic terms and demonstrated that behavior can be changed under carefully supervised circumstances. Freud's contributions to psychiatry included his views on the value of catharsis (also recognized in ancient Greek culture), his notion that symptoms represented a compromise between opposing forces (life and death), his interpretations of dreams (also part of ancient traditions), his dynamic explanations of hysteria, and his studies in hypnotism and the character of psychoanalytic technique. For more than thirty years, Freud refrained from constructing a comprehensive theory of personality and instead made detailed observations. Finally, in 1929, he published the first in a series of writings compiled in his *New Introductory Lectures on Psychoanalysis.* In these he explained the logic of psychologic cause and effect. The premises of Freudian psychoanalytic theory are discussed in detail in Chapter 4.

The psychoanalytic concepts of personality and behavior strongly influenced treatment approaches. The aim of psychotherapy became to make the client conscious of formerly unconscious parts of the personality.

Initially, Freud's concepts were met with violent and almost universal rejection. But gradually Freud attracted a handful of followers from Vienna and later from Switzerland, Hungary, and England. This group organized a small professional community devoted to the development of a new discipline, *psychoanalysis.*

• Alfred Adler (1870–1937), known for his pioneering efforts in psychosomatic medicine, held to the notion that the aggressive drive is the strongest influence on personality.

• Carl Jung (1875–1961) developed the notion of a collective unconscious from which universal archetypes emerge regardless of culture and historical periods. He saw the human psyche as a dynamic of persona (social mask), shadow (hidden personal characteristics), anima (feminine identification in man), animus (masculine identification in women), and self (the innermost center of the personality).

• Otto Rank (1884–1939) broke from the psychoanalytic movement and minimized the importance of the Oedipus conflict, theorizing instead that the separation anxiety connected with birth is the most important influence on development and the source of neurosis.

• Ernest Jones (1879–1958), the most faithful pupil of Freud, is best remembered for his biography of Freud (Jones 1953–1957).

• Sandor Ferenczi (1873–1933), among the first to link homosexuality to paranoia, anticipated a later emphasis on *ego psychology* by encouraging clients to unearth unconscious material.

• Helene Deutsch (1884–1982) saw women as being essentially passive and masochistic, as making a transition at puberty from a clitoral to a vaginal orientation, and as possessing an inborn maternal role.

• Karen Horney (1885–1952) anticipated current notions of alienation and believed that cultural factors play a significant part in the development of neurosis.

• Anna Freud (1895–1982), the daughter of Sigmund Freud, devoted herself to the psychoanalytic study of children and is best known for her refinement of ideas about *ego defense mechanisms.*

The Twentieth Century— Contemporary Developments

Dealing with contemporary patterns is difficult, since we do not yet have the historian's hindsight to guide our judgments. Today's ideas, practices, and contributions will be subject to reappraisal in the future.

Ideologic Expansion From the mid-1940s to mid-1950s, psychiatric thought in this country was characterized by a strong rift between *biologic orientation* and *dynamic orientation.*

At the same time that psychiatric thinking was expanding and moving away from psychoanalysis toward a psychiatry emphasizing the importance of the social dimension, drug treatment for mental illness was being developed. By the early 1950s several drugs for the treatment of mental disorder were in common use.

During World War II almost 2,000,000 late adolescent and young adult men were found unfit for military service because of psychiatric and neurologic findings, and large numbers of military personnel and veterans required psychiatric treatment and hospitalization. The great number of psychiatric casualties during World War II directed attention toward the problems of mental and emotional disorders in general. In 1946 the National Institute of Mental Health (NIMH) was opened in Bethesda, Maryland, for the purposes of research, training, and assistance to the states in providing preventive, therapeutic, and rehabilitative psychiatric services.

Dissatisfaction with the theories and methods of psychoanalysis and psychoanalytic ideology has persisted. Psychotherapy has been increasingly influenced by both ego psychology and social psychology. Harry Stack Sullivan (1892–1949), the only American-born psychiatrist to found an independent school during this period, was strongly influenced by social scientists such as Ruth Benedict and Margaret Mead. Central to his thinking is an interpersonal theory of psychiatry that is at variance with the strictly individual emphasis of psychoanalysis. His pioneering psychotherapy was aimed at understanding and correcting the client's disturbed communication process in the context of a client-therapist relationship based on mutual learning.

The American trend emphasizing the social dimension of psychiatry is also seen in the emergence of both group and family psychotherapy. John Bell and Nathan Ackerman were leading proponents of treating a whole family in one place at the same time. Don Jackson, Gregory Bateson, and their colleagues extended this approach to schizophrenic people and their families. By 1960 family therapy had become both a diagnostic tool and a mode of treatment. During this period Erik Erikson formulated his psychosocial theory of development, based on the interplay of biologic and social factors and a progressive unfolding of developmental tasks in an entire life span.

During this period of ideologic expansion, the issue of mental illness received national attention. In the ten years following the end of World War II, the in-patient population of state psychiatric institutions grew from 450,000 to 550,000. New institutions were built, and old ones became more crowded. This had a profound impact on the economic health of many states and drew the attention and concern of politi-cians at local, state, and national levels. They were the moving force behind the National Mental Health Study Act of 1955 that established the Joint Commission on Mental Illness and Health. This group was charged with studying the mental health needs of the nation and making recommendations for a national mental health program.

Psychotropic drugs, especially tranquilizers, were coming into greater use. They helped staff members manage large numbers of clients in crowded conditions. Research into chemotherapy and the etiology of mental illness seemed to promise that an answer or cure could be discovered any time.

Group therapy and short-term (five to six sessions) individual psychotherapy, first used to treat military personnel, began to be used for other segments of the population. Mental health professionals began to consider options other than costly long-term individual psychotherapy or long-term hospitalization.

Milieu therapy, sometimes called sociotherapy, began to develop because of the efforts of Maxwell Jones, who established therapeutic communities in English hospital settings (1953), and Alfred Stanton and Morris Schwartz (1949). Milton Greenblatt, Richard H. York, and Esther Lucille Brown (1955) studied milieus in the United States.

Deinstitutionalization and the Community Mental Health Movement

Psychiatric professionals are fond of calling turning points in psychiatric care "revolutions." The community mental health movement is often called the third revolution in psychiatry (the first was the provision of treatment for, rather than incarceration of, the mentally ill; the second was the emphasis on intrapsychic causes, an outgrowth of psychoanalysis).

By 1961, the Joint Commission on Mental Illness and Health had presented its report, *Action for Mental Health,* to Congress. The report concluded that psychiatric services in this country were woefully inadequate. The landmark recommendations of the group called for:

• A shift from institutional to community-based care

• A more equitable distribution of mental health services

• Preventive services

• Consumer participation in both the planning and delivery of mental health workers

• The hiring and training of citizens in the community as nonprofessional mental health workers

• The education of more mental health professionals

• Public support for research

• Shared federal, state, and local funding for the construction and operation of a system of community mental health centers

President John Kennedy appointed a cabinet-level committee to study the Joint Commission's recommendations, and on February 5, 1963, he delivered the first presidential message about the mental health of the nation. In it Kennedy called for "a bold new approach" in which mental health services would be integrated with community life. Congress responded by passing legislation to implement the president's proposal in the form of the Mental Retardation Facilities and Community Mental Health Centers Construction Act (PL88-164; frequently called the Community Mental Health Centers Act) before the end of the year. This legislation authorized 150 million dollars in federal funds to be matched by state funds over three years for the construction of comprehensive community mental health centers. To qualify for federal funding, centers had to offer the five essential services outlined in Table 1–1.

In 1970, funding for services to children and adolescents was specifically provided in response to the 1969 report of the Joint Commission on the Mental Health of Children, which cited inadequate programs for young people. This amendment to the Community Mental Health Centers Act also provided for services to drug and alcohol abusers, and for mental health consultation.

Unfortunately the Community Mental Health Centers Act program often did not work as planned. Some states and local municipalities could not match federal funds. Some centers, especially those in poor or predominantly rural areas, were unable to generate sufficient revenue through fees. Services that generated little or no income, such as public education and mental health consultation, began to suffer.

The 1975 amendments to the 1963 law (Community Mental Health Center Amendment PL94-63) not only reemphasized the goals of the 1963 legislation but also required that each center provide the seven additional mental health services outlined in Table 1–1. This requirement meant that, to receive funds, a community mental health center might have to provide

---

TABLE 1–1   Essential Community Mental Health Services

1963	1975	1981
In-patient care: 24-hour hospitalization for any person in the community requiring around-the-clock care	Five essential services mandated in 1963 plus:	Outpatient care
Outpatient care: Psychiatric treatment for clients living at home	Follow-up care: Ongoing programs for community residents after discharge from a mental health facility	Partial hospitalization
Partial hospitalization: Treatment programs for clients not requiring around-the-clock care; day treatment programs allowing clients to return home at night; night treatment programs allowing clients to maintain jobs during the day and return to the hospital at night	Transitional services: Living arrangements for persons unable to live on their own but not requiring hospitalization, or newly discharged from a mental health facility and requiring assistance in adjusting to living on their own	24-hour hospitalization and emergency care
Emergency care: 24-hour emergency services	Services for children and adolescents: Mental health diagnostic treatment, liaison, and follow-up services for children and adolescents	Consultation and education
Consultation and education: To professionals or community groups in schools, health clinics, churches, courts, law enforcement agencies, and so on.	Services for elderly: Mental health diagnostic, treatment, liaison, and follow-up services for the elderly	Screening services
	Screening services: Assistance to courts and other agencies to screen persons referred to mental health agencies	
	Alcohol abuse services: Programs geared toward prevention, treatment, and follow-up in alcohol abuse	
	Drug abuse services: Programs geared toward prevention, treatment, and follow-up in drug abuse	

services not necessarily needed by the population it served.

Between 1955 and 1975, the number of resident clients in state mental hospitals decreased from 559,000 to 193,000—almost 66 percent. Proponents of the community mental health and deinstitutionalization movements refer to "a bold new approach," while critics use less enthusiastic terms, such as **dumping,** to characterize modern trends in mental health services. In the latter view, the site of care for the chronically mentally disordered has merely been moved from a single ineffective institution to many ineffective ones.

The next major assessment of the mental health needs of the nation began in 1977 when President Jimmy Carter established a twenty-member President's Commission on Mental Health. *Report to the President of the President's Commission on Mental Health* (1978) focused on the following major areas:

• Providing community-based services as the keystone of the mental health system

• Improving community support systems and networks among families, neighbors, community organizations, and existing service components:

• Establishing national health insurance that would include coverage for mental health care

• Encouraging mental health coverage (including outpatient) in all health insurance plans

• Continuing the phaseout of large public mental hospitals and improving services in the remainder

• Providing funding to increase the number of mental health professionals, especially those working with minorities, children, and the aged

• Establishing a center with a strong emphasis on primary prevention within the National Institute of Mental Health

• Protecting the human rights of persons needing mental health care

• Improving the delivery of services to underserved populations and high-risk populations, such as minorities and the chronically ill, through a new federal program

• Developing an advocacy program for the chronically mentally ill

• Increasing support for research related to mental health and illness

• Providing health education to the public and increasing the public understanding of mental health problems

• Centralizing the evaluation efforts of governmental agencies concerned with mental health

The Community Mental Health Systems Act of 1980 was a major achievement of the outgoing Carter administration. It was designed to implement the recommendations made by the president's commission authorizing the funding of **community mental health centers,** services to high-risk populations, ambulatory mental health care centers, a prevention unit and associate director for minority concerns at NIMH, rape research and services, and recommending a model mental health patient's bill of rights. Its basic task was to coordinate the two-tiered system of mental health care that had evolved since President Kennedy's 1963 efforts. The severely mentally disordered continued to inhabit state institutions, and those with less acute problems used the services of federally funded community mental health centers. Unfortunately, there was little coordination between these two systems. Clients discharged from state institutions often failed to receive follow-up services, and certain populations—the chronically mentally ill, the elderly, and youth—fell between the two systems. This act was intended to coordinate federal and state efforts.

The programs authorized by this legislation were to start in 1982. Before they could get off the ground, the political climate changed, and the role of the federal government in the nation's mental health shrank considerably. The 1980 Community Mental Health Systems Act was essentially repealed in 1981 when the 97th Congress passed the Reagan administration's Omnibus Budget Reconciliation Act (PL97-35). The new budget placed the mental health services programs formerly administered by NIMH into an alcohol, drug abuse, and mental health services block grant, shifting the decision making about allocation of funds to the states and decreasing the federal role in coordination.

The decrease in the federal budget has had and will continue to have far-ranging effects on the community mental health movement. It cuts funding for community mental health centers and other mental health care delivery programs. Community mental health centers were no longer funded after 1984, and funding reductions were felt as early as 1983. Mandated services have been reduced from twelve to five (see Table 1–1), and their continuing existence and quality depend on state support, private funding, and earned revenue.

Some experts conclude that deinstitutionalization and the principles of community psychiatry are a national disgrace and advocate the return of the old state hospital warehouse system. Others, however, prefer to rethink this approach, pointing out that criticism of the deinstitutionalization movement has merely highlighted community psychiatry's lack of true innovation. This group argues not for the return of the old state hospital system, but for the development of alternatives to it that emphasize self-care and self-determination for clients rather than institutionalization (Wilson 1982).

As we move into the 1990s, one of our needs is for sustained life-support systems for certain chronic client groups, not merely transitional ones. Such approaches, however, require sufficient legislation, funding continuity, and coordination to replace the current nonsystem of aftercare left in the wake of the closing of state mental hospitals.

The 1990s: The Decade of the Brain

The psychiatric community has learned some important lessons from its experience with **deinstitutionalization** and the community mental health movement over the last decades. Caregivers have learned to think about the needs of the chronically mentally ill (CMI) in new ways. We have learned:

- The importance of social support

- The need for involving natural or family caregivers

- The importance of planning creative, residential alternatives

- The importance of social skills training

- The importance of self-help

- The potential for nursing to provide a cadre of specialists in psychoeducation, chronic care management, and self-help.

Some view self-help as the bold new approach needed, and nurses are crucial to the implementation of such strategies. Self-help, self-care, and **psychoeducation** are consistent with trends toward realignment of power, control, and responsibility with givers and receivers of health care. Self-help has the potential to meet the increasing demands being placed on formal and institutional mental health services in the next decade.

In addition to the lessons learned from deinstitutionalization, the primary innovation of the 1990s is the so-called biologic revolution: collaboration of science and technology to expand concepts of mental disorder proposed by psychologic, behavioral, and psychoanalytic theories. A report by the National Advisory Health Council calls the gains made in research-based knowledge about the epidemiology, diagnosis, treatment, and prevention of major mental illnesses a "quantum leap in understanding the brain."

Gains made in the understanding of schizophrenia are a good example. Research on brain dysfunction in mental disorders has resulted in a major reconceptualization of the diagnosis and treatment of schizophrenia, which is no longer seen as a unitary or single disorder. As researchers discovered a variety of brain dysfunctions, including ventricular enlargement, cerebral atrophy, and disturbances in neurotransmitters, treatment approaches for schizophrenia became more differentiated. The outcome is less emphasis on providing psychotherapy and more emphasis on achieving social rehabilitation, lowering stress in the client's environment through psychoeducation of families, and managing medication in the clients' best interests. Similar revolutionary discoveries have been made by researchers studying mood disorders, dementias, and substance use disorders.

This up-to-date, research-based knowledge is reflected in contemporary psychiatric and psychiatric nursing literature, including this edition of this text. Research in the twenty-first century will focus on such areas as:

- The effects of various medications on neurotransmitters in the brains of clients with psychiatric disorders

- The role of nutrients in modifying brain function

- The influence on mood and behavior of disruptions of biologic rhythms

- The role of viruses in mental disorders

- The influence of the endocrine system on the brain and behavior

- The effectiveness of exposure to bright light as a treatment for depression, premenstrual syndrome, and sleep problems of the elderly

- The role of the brain in producing physical illnesses

- The development of therapies to prevent the deterioration of mental functions in the aging population

- Biologic markers that might alert clients and clinicians to the onset of a mental disorder

The Reaction of Client Advocacy Groups to New Trends In general, client advocacy groups have welcomed psychiatry's shift in the 1990s toward psychosocial rehabilitation for self-care among clients, social support and psychoeducation for family caregivers, advances in biologic knowledge, and effective biologic treatments. One group, the *National Alliance for the Mentally Ill* (NAMI), has established a separate research foundation to study the biologic basis of major mental illness and vigorously lobby Congress to support brain research at the National Institute of Mental Health. They argue that, without knowledge of the brain, professionals cannot diagnose or treat disorders of the mind. Members of NAMI support the shift away from holding families responsible for creating mental disorders in their offspring. They agree with the view that the mentally disordered are people who suffer from a brain disease that may be treated medically and who experience environmental stress that may be modified through psychoeducation and counseling.

Some criticize the "Decade of the Brain" as a retreat into the past. Proponents counter that instead of a retreat, it is a renaissance of hope. Only research and practice in the next decades will allow us to judge.

Emergence of the Discipline of Psychiatric Nursing

Although nursing functions have existed since ancient times, the profession of nursing, particularly psychiatric nursing, is a product of the late nineteenth and twentieth centuries. Theodor and Friedericke Fliedner founded the first systematic school of nursing in Germany in 1836. It was this school at Kaiserwerth that Florence Nightingale visited in 1851 before organizing a school to educate nurses in England after the Crimean War. Her school, Saint Thomas Hospital in London, stressed the importance of providing an optimum environment for clients. Although it is true that in the context of her time she emphasized the physical environment, Nightingale was among the first to note that the influence of nurses on their clients goes beyond physical care and has psychologic and social components.

Development of Early Psychiatric Nursing Education

In the early 1870s the first three American nursing schools, organized in the pattern of Saint Thomas Hospital, were opened in New York, Boston, and New Haven. Linda Richards, a graduate of the New England Hospital for Women in Boston, spent a significant part of her career developing better nursing care in psychiatric hospitals and is sometimes called "the first American Psychiatric nurse." She echoed Nightingale's earlier observation about the nurse's impact.

The first American school for psychiatric nurses was opened under the direction of Linda Richards at the McLean Psychiatric Asylum in Waverly, Massachusetts, in 1880. Ninety nurses graduated from its two-year course in 1882. By 1890, there were thirty-five such schools in asylums. Unlike graduates of general hospital schools of nursing, these nurses could find employment only in asylums.

By the end of the nineteenth century, trained nurses staffed some mental hospitals in the United States, but they attended mainly to the physical needs of clients and did not pursue systematic interpersonal

work with them. Psychiatric theory in this period emphasized providing a physical environment that would promote recovery. Thus, nurses administered medications such as chloral hydrate and paraldehyde, supervised the use of hydrotherapy, and oversaw the nutrition and physical care of clients. Much of psychiatric nursing practice was custodial, mechanistic, and directed by psychiatrists. A ratio of 1 trained nurse to 140 clients was not unusual, and some large mental hospitals hired no registered nurses at all.

The notion that nurses caring for clients with physical disorders should be trained in a general hospital and that those caring for clients with mental disorders should be trained in a psychiatric hospital dominated nursing education for over half a century. In 1913, the school of nursing at Johns Hopkins Hospital included a psychiatric nursing component in its curriculum, heralding the beginning of a slow but important change in the structure of nursing programs.

The first psychiatric nursing text, *Nursing Mental Diseases,* was written in 1920 by Harriet Bailey, the Assistant Superintendent of Nurses at the psychiatric clinic at Johns Hopkins Hospital. It was for twenty years the standard textbook in psychiatric nursing. Most textbooks were written by psychiatrists who devoted only a few pages to instructing psychiatric nurses in such procedures as tube and rectal feeding and preparing treatment trays.

In the years between the two world wars, mental hospitals were seriously understaffed. In an effort to cope with understaffing, mental hospitals opened schools of nursing at an incredible rate—sixty-seven in 1936 alone.

Movement of Psychiatric Nursing into the Mainstream of Nursing

It was 1937 before the National League for Nursing Education (now the National League for Nursing) recommended, but did not require, that psychiatric nursing content and clinical experience be a part of the curriculum in all basic nursing programs. The league also took over from psychiatrists the tasks of standardizing and accrediting psychiatric nursing education in single-focus schools for psychiatric nurses. The American Psychiatric Association, rather than a nursing organization, had been involved since 1906 in monitoring this aspect of nursing.

Psychiatric nursing moved into the mainstream of nursing in the 1940s, and nurses began to assume increasing responsibility for educating their own and taking over the teaching from physicians. However, the focus of psychiatric nursing activities continued to be the provision of kind, but custodial, nursing care. Nurses supervised or were responsible for providing housekeeping tasks such as scrubbing floors and counting mops and sheets; feeding, clothing, and bathing clients; assisting the physician with treatments; and keeping the keys to locked wards, locked cabinets, even locked toilet tissue containers.

The specialty grew slowly during the 1940s. In one West Coast state seven state hospitals housed 37,000 psychiatric clients but employed only eighteen graduate nurses: one nurse for approximately 2000 clients. In 1944, there were still fourteen states in which no psychiatric nursing course had ever been given (Kalisch and Kalisch 1987).

In the meantime, psychiatric theory expanded to encompass the interpersonal and emotional dimensions of "mental illness." During these years, Sigmund Freud published his works on psychoanalysis, Adolf Meyer had major impact in America and Britain through his *commonsense psychiatry,* and Harry Stack Sullivan, often called "the founder of interpersonal psychiatry," introduced the concept of *milieu therapy* as a new approach to treating hospitalized psychiatric clients. These ideologic changes in psychiatry did not have a noticeable impact on psychiatric nursing care until the early 1950s.

Instead, new modes of physical treatment laid the groundwork for change. To the custodial tasks of psychiatric nurses were added specific medical-surgical procedures as psychiatry developed somatic therapies for the treatment of specific disorders. These included deep sleep therapy in 1930, insulin shock therapy in 1935, psychosurgery in 1935–1936, and electroshock therapy in 1937. Thus, it was through the use of medical-surgical skills that psychiatric nurses gained recognition as significant participants in psychiatric treatment.

Although these somatic treatments controlled dramatically bizarre client behavior and made clients more available for interpersonal interactions, it was not until 1946, with passage of the National Mental Health Act, that any systematic development of psychotherapeutic roles for nurses began. Most psychiatric clients were being cared for in large state mental hospitals where small numbers of staff were expected to manage large numbers of clients living in crowded conditions. Somatic treatments, rather than psychotherapy, were more practical in these settings. Psychotherapy was often reserved for the private clients of psychiatrists in private psychiatric hospitals or in private practice settings.

Confirmation of Psychiatric Nursing as a Specialty

Enactment of the National Mental Health Act was the government's response to growing recognition of mental illness as a national health problem. During World War II, 43 percent of all people discharged from the army were classified as psychiatric disabilities. This created a sharp increase in the demand for psychiatric services. The National Mental Health Act provided for the following:

• Establishment of the National Institute of Mental Health (NIMH)

• Development of programs to train professional psychiatric personnel, including psychiatric nurses

• Support for psychiatric research

• Aid in developing mental health programs

With the establishment of the NIMH in 1946, psychiatric nursing was added to psychiatry, psychology, and social work as a field in which the highest priority became the preparation of clinically capable persons for positions of leadership. Funds administered by the institute facilitated advanced education in psychiatric nursing. Before the 1946 act, fewer than a dozen psychiatric nurses held master's degrees in the United States and fewer than 5 percent of basic nursing education programs were at the baccalaureate level. The psychiatric nursing education given most students consisted of a few weeks of observation on a psychiatric ward. Because of new funding, nine universities received grants to expand and improve graduate programs in 1948. The number increased gradually and steadily. These programs prepared many of the nursing leaders who later developed theoretical frameworks for one-to-one relationship work. Because of its wide-ranging effects, the National Mental Health Act of 1946 is probably the most significant piece of legislation affecting the development of psychiatric nursing.

Nursing leaders began to question the wisdom of single-focus schools of psychiatric nursing. In 1948, a report entitled *Nursing for the Future* (Brown 1948) recommended their elimination. The needs of nursing could best be served, the report indicated, if the psychiatric hospitals conducting schools of nursing made their facilities widely available instead to students in basic schools of nursing. Shortly thereafter, in 1955, the National League for Nursing made the provision of a clinical experience in psychiatric nursing a requirement for the accreditation of nursing schools. Requiring both coursework and hands-on clinical experience further cemented the mainstreaming of psychiatric nursing.

Until the early 1950s, psychiatric nurses formulated only vague concepts about how nurses might participate in one-to-one relationships with clients. Some pressed for trained postgraduate nurses to provide psychotherapy and become functioning members of an interdisciplinary treatment team that would include psychologists and social workers. Ambiguity about professional psychiatric nursing roles characterized this period.

Role Clarification in Psychiatric Nursing

The 1950s and early 1960s were a period of role clarification. Three important milestones in psychiatric nursing occurred in 1952:

• Hildegard Peplau published *Interpersonal Relations in Nursing,* the first systematic theoretic framework in psychiatric nursing. Her framework, grounded in the interpersonal psychiatry of Harry Stack Sullivan and learning theory, is a milestone in the development of psychiatric nursing theory and practice. She delineated several skills, activities, and roles for psychiatric nurses. Peplau emphasized the interpersonal nature of nursing and the need for nurses to understand and use psychodynamic concepts and counseling techniques in their practice. Peplau has had greater impact on psychiatric nursing than any other nursing theoretician to date.

• Gwen Tudor Will published an article in the journal *Psychiatry* demonstrating that nurses can promote emotional growth in clients. She developed a specific nursing intervention with a sociopsychiatric base—a unique contribution, at that time, to psychiatric nursing and to understanding the importance of milieu factors. (Gwen Tudor Will's classic sociopsychiatric nursing approach is discussed in the accompanying Research Note.)

• Frances Sleeper, in an address to the American Psychiatric Association, advocated the use of psychiatric nurses as psychotherapists. Her advocacy ushered in a heated, ten-year controversy over caretaker versus psychotherapist roles for psychiatric nurses.

Over these next ten years, a number of developments further clarified the role of the psychiatric nurse while lending legitimacy to the counselor role. A milestone report published in 1956 (National League for Nursing 1956) introduced the concept of the psychiatric clinical nurse specialist and differentiated functions appropriate to psychiatric nurses with master's level preparation. In this same year, NIMH gave the first grants to integrate mental health concepts into the basic nursing curriculum, and traineeships for graduate students in psychiatric nursing were increased.

In 1957, June Mellow introduced a system of nursing therapy based on her work with schizophrenic clients at Boston State Hospital. Her approach, designed to provide corrective emotional experiences, drew strongly from psychoanalytic theory and provided the theoretic framework for the first doctoral program in nursing in 1960 at Boston University (Mellow 1968). Unlike psychoanalysis, Mellow's nursing therapy did not investigate psychopathologic or interpersonal developmental processes. Peplau, Will, and Mellow demonstrated the effectiveness of psychiatric nurses in the counseling role.

In 1958, the American Nurses' Association (ANA) established the Conference Group on Psychiatric Nursing, now the Council on Psychiatric and Mental Health Nursing Practice, acknowledging the specialty. Ida Jean Orlando's *The Dynamic Nurse-Patient Relationship,* published in 1961, emphasized the importance of the interpersonal relationship in all aspects of nursing care, not only psychiatric nursing. Orlando advocated the involvement of nurses in prevention and in mental health. In that same year, *Action for Mental Health,* the report of the Joint Commission on Mental Illness and Mental Health, encouraged nurses to assume the counselor role. The report recommended that psychiatric nurses become skilled in group and family therapy in addition to individual therapy, nursing's primary counseling mode to this point in time.

But, perhaps the culmination of this ten-year period of role clarification was the publication in 1962 of Peplau's "Interpersonal Techniques: The Crux of Psychiatric Nursing." In this article, Peplau added to and prioritized the psychiatric nursing roles she had identified in her 1952 book. According to Peplau, counseling was the primary role of the psychiatric nurse, and the others were subroles. She also predicted private practice as a legitimate role for the psychiatric nurse before the decade was over.

Confirmation of Specialist Roles

Enactment of the Community Mental Health Centers Act in 1963 further motivated the trend in psychiatric nursing toward expanded and specialized roles, including community mental health and preventive mental health. Psychiatric nurses broadened their practice to include schools, jails, senior citizen centers, outreach clinics, transitional services and alternative treatment settings, and private practice as well as the traditional mental hospital.

The launching in 1963 of *Perspectives in Psychiatric Care,* the journal for psychiatric nurses, was a significant event in psychiatric nursing history. Edited and published by Alice Clarke, a psychiatric nurse, this first psychiatric nursing journal provided a forum for airing issues and sharing psychiatric nursing knowledge. A second journal, the *Journal of Psychiatric Nursing and Mental Health Services* began later that same year and changed its name in 1981 to the *Journal of Psychosocial Nursing and Mental Health Services.* Clinical and research papers by psychiatric nursing leaders in these journals and in the *American Journal of Nursing* further established the counseling role as

RESEARCH NOTE

Citation
Tudor G: A sociopsychiatric nursing approach to intervention in a problem of mutual withdrawal on a mental hospital ward. Psychiatry 1952; 15:174+.

Study Problem/Purpose
The purpose of this study was to demonstrate the effect of nursing intervention on a chronically mentally ill client. Tudor's goal was to document that nurses could not only help clients improve but could also, with less effort, make clients worse.

Methods
Tudor observed the interactional patterns among clients and staff on a busy ward of a private psychiatric hospital. She used sociopsychiatric theory to explain a mutual pattern of avoidance that emerged among the nursing staff, physicians, and one particular female client. Once the pattern had been determined to exist, Tudor determined a nursing intervention designed to disrupt the pattern of avoidance by closing the gap between herself and the client and then engaging her in activities.

To test the reliability of her intervention, Tudor taught her nursing intervention to a nursing student and supervised her in reversing a pattern of mutual withdrawal with another client.

Findings
Tudor demonstrated that:

• Psychiatric nurses can have a profoundly positive or a profoundly negative effect on the client.

• The social milieu of the psychiatric ward can maintain deviant patterns of behavior.

• The psychotherapeutic nursing role can be taught to others.

• Nurses can carry out scholarly research.

Implications
This is the classic scholarly psychiatric nursing research study. This study is significant for its dramatic impact on nursing and its contribution to an understanding of the effects of the milieu. The theoretic principles of Tudor's intervention were adapted by other nurses in other nurse-client interactions. Tudor's work was first published in the medical journal *Psychiatry* because no psychiatric nursing journals existed at the time.

---

the basis of psychiatric nursing, whether it was defined as psychotherapy or not.

Shortly thereafter, the first textbook to address group therapy techniques in nursing practice was written by Shirley Armstrong and Sheila Rouslin (1963), and Shirley Burd and Margaret Marshall (1963) wrote and edited the first compilation of psychiatric nursing papers suitable for graduate students in psychiatric nursing.

A 1967 ANA position paper on psychiatric nursing endorsed the assumption by clinical specialists of the role of therapist in individual, group, family, and milieu work. By 1969, a psychiatric nurse had, as Peplau predicted a few years before, moved into private practice.

The first master's level certification program for advanced psychiatric nursing practice was developed by the New Jersey Nurses' Association in 1971, followed in two years by the New York State Nurses Association. The psychiatric nurses who developed and implemented these early certification programs—

Sheila Rouslin Welt, Carol Ren Kneisl, Marian Pettingill, Marian Krizinofski, and others—recognized the need to acknowledge expertise, distinguish generalist from specialist roles, and safeguard the public. By the mid-1970s, certification at both the generalist and the specialist levels in psychiatric nursing became the responsibility of the ANA.

In 1973, the ANA published the first standards of psychiatric and mental health nursing practice, statements to serve as guidelines for providing the desired quality of care. These standards of practice, revised in 1982, delineate psychiatric nursing roles and functions (see Chapter 2).

The clinical specialist role was further legitimized in 1973 when the ANA formed a specialty subgroup, the Council of Specialists in Psychiatric and Mental Health Nursing. Membership is limited.

Unlike the Joint Commission of 1955, which was dominated by physicians, President Carter's 1977 Commission on Mental Health included a nurse, Martha Mitchell, the chairperson of the ANA Division on Psychiatric and Mental Health Nursing Practice. Three other professional nurses served on adjunct committees. The commission's report had special significance for psychiatric nurses. It was hailed as the first official high-level document to give visibility to the professional competence of nurses in mental health care (Hadley 1978). The document specifically mentioned nurses in sections concerned with staff shortages, training and education for primary care practitioners, and mental health care providers whose services should be reimbursed by insurance companies.

Psychiatric Nursing in the 1980s

According to Osborne (1984), the publication in 1979 of the first edition of this textbook, *Psychiatric Nursing* by Holly Skodol Wilson and Carol Ren Kneisl, signaled a significant change in psychiatric nursing textbooks and psychiatric nursing thinking. This was the first in a new era of comprehensive psychiatric nursing textbooks to provide and consistently use a major conceptual theme based on humanistic interactionism advocating negotiated goals between nurse and client, client advocacy, and political sensitivity, as well as caring and compassion. Since that time, other psychiatric nursing textbooks have followed in the tradition of Wilson and Kneisl. Another psychiatric nursing journal, *Issues in Mental Health Nursing,* also began in 1979.

After decades of apparently unlimited support from the NIMH in the form of money for educational programs and traineeships for psychiatric nurses at the graduate level, funding for psychiatric nursing graduate programs was cut. Programs that educated nurses to meet the needs of unserved and underserved populations (identified by an NIMH task force in 1975 as children and adolescents, the elderly, the chronically mentally ill, women, and minorities) were the only programs that were funded. The passage in 1981 of the federal Omnibus Budget Reconciliation Act further decreased the amount of funding available for even these training programs. Psychiatric nursing found itself on the verge of a period of retrenchment that remains in evidence today.

Recognizing the need for a set of psychiatric nursing diagnoses to supplement those diagnoses identified by the North American Nursing Diagnoses Association (NANDA), the ANA Council of Specialists in Psychiatric and Mental Health Nursing appointed a panel of six nursing leaders (Maxine Loomis, Holly Skodol Wilson, Patricia Pothier, Anita Werner O'Toole, Marie Scott Brown, and Patricia West) to develop a classification system for the phenomena of concern for psychiatric-mental health nurses. This task force began to work on Psychiatric Nursing Diagnosis-I in 1984 and introduced the preliminary taxonomy in 1986 at the biennial ANA convention. In 1987, the

task force began to synthesize its findings with those of NANDA and continues to work on the identification of relevant and useful categories for psychiatric nursing diagnosis.

The newest psychiatric nursing journal, *Archives of Psychiatric Nursing,* made its debut in early 1987. The purpose of this journal is to provide a forum in which psychiatric nurse clinician-scholars can suggest theoretic linkages between diverse areas of practice and shape public policy for the delivery of psychiatric and mental health nursing services.

According to researchers involved in an NIMH study of prevalance of mental disorders in the United States, a mental health crisis is brewing (Kramer 1983). Kramer called this crisis a pandemic of mental disorders and associated chronic and disabling conditions resulting from two phenomena: medical advances that have prolonged the lives of those who have mental disorders and a relative increase in the numbers of young persons at high risk for developing mental disorders (U.S. Department of Health and Human Services 1986). Nationwide, the prevalance of mental disorders in those over 18 is almost 20 percent. According to Kramer, projections into the year 2005 indicate that if only 10 percent of the United States population needs mental health services, 20,000 more psychiatric nurses than were available in 1980 will be needed.

Of major concern to psychiatric nurses is the decrease in the number of nurses selecting psychiatric nursing as a specialty and a shortage of clinical training funds. Ways to encourage recruitment into the specialty are to identify psychiatric-mental health nursing content clearly, to make it highly visible in the curriculum design, and to provide role models in the persons of teaching faculty who are psychiatric nurse experts. To ensure the survival of psychiatric nursing in the year 2000, psychiatric nurses must articulate who they are and what they are about.

Psychiatric Nursing in the 1990s: Toward A Revitalized Identity

This postindustrial decade, characterized by massive social changes, is likely to signal increases in major mental disorders, especially in target populations such as the elderly. As the need for our services increases, psychiatric nurses face many challenges, including the mandate to contain costs and the need to integrate biologic knowledge into our practice. Leaders in our field urge us to use these challenging circumstances as an opportunity to clarify nursing's unique contribution to mental health care—to reverse the sense of psychiatric nursing as a specialty in decline.

A Research-Practice Agenda

McBride (1990) warns that the 1990s will mark a renaissance for the specialty only if psychiatric nurses formulate a contemporary research-practice agenda that involves two major readjustments: (a) stop devaluing biologic knowledge and (b) become fundamentally reassociated with care and caring. In recognition of these needs, the NIMH held the conference "Biological Psychiatry and the Future of Psychiatric Mental Health Nursing" in 1989.

Peplau (1989) makes these additional recommendations:

• To promote political savvy in advocating psychiatric-mental health care resources

• To continue to develop out-of-hospital services, including those offered on a private practice basis

• To pursue evaluation and outcome clinical studies

• To inform the public and others of the work we do

• To keep emphasizing the human aspects of psychiatric work even as psychiatry moves toward remedicalization

She and other leaders believe that the future of psychiatric nursing hinges on our ability to create a new image for ourselves, achieve a new balance of men and women in our profession, foster cultural diversity among psychiatric nurses, and integrate philosophic and theoretic perspectives in our practice and research.

CHAPTER HIGHLIGHTS

• The humanistic interactionist ideology is one response to a need for a framework of values and concepts in psychiatric nursing that views human beings as having purpose and control over their own lives.

• The key premises of interactionism are that people act toward things on the basis of the meanings those things have for them—that the meanings arise out of social interaction with others and are modified through the process of encountering things.

• Implications of interactionism and humanism for the practice of psychiatric nursing include the importance of finding a common ground of negotiated meaning when dealing with clients, of viewing behavior within its social context, of discovering and respecting each client's individual experience and the meaning attached to it, and of viewing physical and mental factors as interrelated.

• The key premises of humanism give rise to a holistic view of mind-body relations, an expanded role for nurses, a collaborative decision-making model, and a general posture of negotiation and advocacy in relation to clients in social, political, and individual arenas.

• In the "Decade of the Brain," we need to synthesize new psychobiologic knowledge and the humanistic interactionist ideology.

• People with mental disorders have been viewed differently at different times in history; at times such persons were perceived as tragic figures to be liberated and at times as dangerous persons to be confined.

• Some contemporary ideas about mental disorders have their origins in earlier centuries.

• Conflicts about the nature of mental dysfunction have always existed; two age-old issues are biologic versus nonbiologic causes and the individual's responsibility or lack of responsibility for actions.

• Landmark recommendations made in 1961 by the Joint Commission on Mental Illness and Health drew the attention and concern of politicians and mental health professionals toward the woefully inadequate psychiatric services in the country.

• Other major studies, such as the 1978 report of the President's Commission on Mental Health, gave visibility to the professional competence of nurses in mental health care and made significant recommendations toward coordinating the two-tiered system of mental health care that had evolved.

• To understand the present and future directions of psychiatric nursing, one needs to understand its historical development as a specialty.

• The profession of psychiatric nursing is a product of the late nineteenth and twentieth centuries and was brought about by ideologic changes, interest in reform, attention to the importance of milieu, and the introduction of physical modes of treatment.

• Nightingale was among the first to note that nursing care has a psychosocial as well as biologic component.

• The focus of psychiatric nursing activities continued to be the provision of kind but custodial nursing care until the early 1950s, when Peplau published the first systematic theoretical framework in psychiatric nursing and emphasized psychotherapeutic roles for nurses.

• In the 1960s and 1970s, psychiatric nurses broadened their roles and functions to include individual, group, family, and milieu work as well as community mental health nursing.

• In the 1980s, psychiatric nursing found itself on the verge of a period of retrenchment that remains in evidence today; fewer funds are available for clinical training programs in the specialty.

• Although there has been a decrease in the number of nurses selecting psychiatric nursing as a specialty, research indicates that the need for psychiatric nurses will be greater than ever in the future.

• Psychiatric nursing's renaissance in the 1990s will require a research-practice agenda that values advances in psychobiologic knowledge of the brain yet maintains the humanistic values of care and caring.

REFERENCES

Alexander FG, Selesnick ST: *The History of Psychiatry: An Evaluation of Psychiatric Thought and Practice from Prehistoric Times to the Present*. Harper & Row, 1966.

American Nurses' Association: *Nursing: A Social Policy Statement*. ANA, 1980.

American Nurses' Association: *Statement on Psychiatric Nursing Practice*. ANA, 1967.

American Psychiatric Association: *Diagnostic and Statistical Manual of Mental Disorders*, ed 3. APA, 1980.

American Psychiatric Association: *Diagnostic and Statistical Manual*, ed 3, revised. APA, 1987.

Armstrong SW, Rouslin S: *Group Psychotherapy in Nursing Practice*. Macmillan, 1963.

Beers CW: *A Mind That Found Itself*, rev ed. Doubleday, 1948.

Blumer H: *Symbolic Interaction: Perspective and Method*. Prentice-Hall, 1969.

Bockoven JS: Moral treatment in American psychiatry. *J Nerv Ment Dis* 1956;125:167–194, 292–321.

Brown EL: *Nursing for the Future*. Russell Sage Foundation, 1948.

Burd S, Marshall M (eds): *Some Clinical Approaches to Psychiatric Nursing*. Macmillan, 1963.

Chamberlain JG: Update on psychiatric-mental health nursing education at the federal level. *Arch Psychiatr Nurs* 1987;1(2):132–138.

Church O: From custody to community in psychiatric nursing. *Nurs Res* 1987;36(1):48–55.

Davis CK: The status of reimbursement policy and future projections, in Williams C (ed): *Nursing Research and Policy Formation: The Case of Prospective Payment*. American Academy of Nursing, 1984.

Deutsch A: *The Mentally Ill in America*, ed 2. Columbia University Press, 1948.

Doona ME: At least as well cared for . . . Linda Richards and the mentally ill. *Image* 1984;16(2):51–56.

Fagin CM: Psychiatric nursing at the crossroads: Quo vadis. *Perspect Psychiatr Care* 1981;14:99–104.

Fagin CM: Concepts for the future: Competition and substitution. *J Psychosoc Nurs* 1983;21(3):36–41.

Foucault M: *Madness and Civilization*. Vintage Books, 1973.

Greenblatt M, York RH, Brown EL: *From Custodial to Therapeutic Care in the Mental Hospital*. Russell Sage Foundation, 1955.

Hadley R: President's commission sets national mental health goals. *Am Nurse* 1978;10:1.

Howells JG: *World History of Psychiatry*. Brunner/Mazel, 1975.

Joint Commission on Mental Health of Children: *Crisis in Child Mental Health: Challenge for the 1970s*. Harper & Row, 1969.

Joint Commission on Mental Illness and Health: *Action for Mental Health*. Basic Books, 1961.

Jones E: *The Life and Work of Sigmund Freud*. 3 volumes. Basic Books, 1953–1957.

Jones M: *The Therapeutic Community*. Basic Books, 1953.

Judd LL: Putting mental health on the nation's health agenda. *Hosp Community Psychiatry* 1990;41:131–134.

Kalisch PA, Kalisch BJ: *The Changing Image of the Nurse*. Addison-Wesley, 1987.

Kennedy JF: Mental illness and mental retardation. Presented at the 88th Congress, 1st Session. House of Representatives Document 58, 1963.

Kramer M: The continuing challenge: The rising prevalence of mental disorders, associated chronic diseases and disabling conditions. *Am J Soc Psychiatry* 1983;3(4):13–23.

Lamont C: *The Philosophy of Humanism*. New York: Frederick Ungar Publishing, 1967.

Liaschenko J: Changing paradigms within psychiatry: Implications for nursing research. *Arch Psychiatr Nurs* 1989;3(3):153–158.

Loomis M et al.: PND-I: A classification of phenomena of concern for psychiatric-mental health nursing. *Arch Psychiatr Nurs* 1987;1(1):16–24.

Mark B: From "lunatic" to "client": 300 years of psychiatric patienthood. *J Psychiatr Nurs Ment Health Serv* 1980;18(3):32–36.

McBride AB: Psychiatric nursing in the 1990s. *Arch Psychiatr Nurs* 1990;4(1):21–27.

McKeon KL: Introduction: A future perspective on psychiatric mental health nursing. *Arch Psychiatr Nurs* 1990;4(1):119–20.

Mellow J: Nursing therapy. *Am J Nurs* 1968;68:2365–2369.

Mora G: History of psychiatry, in Kaplan HI, Sadock BJ (eds): *Comprehensive Textbook of Psychiatry*, ed 4. Williams & Wilkins, 1985, pp 2034–2054.

National Advisory Mental Health Council Report to Congress on the Decade of the Brain. US Department of Health and Human Services, National Institutes of Health, 1988.

National League for Nursing: *The Education of the Clinical Specialist in Psychiatric Nursing: Report of a National Working Conference*. Williamsburg, Virginia, November 26–30, 1956.

Neaman JS: *Suggestion of the Devil: The Origins of Madness*. Anchor Press/Doubleday, 1975.

Orlando IJ: *The Dynamic Nurse-Patient Relationship*. Putnam, 1961.

Osborne OH: Intellectual traditions in psychiatric mental health nursing: A review of selected textbooks. *J Psychosoc Nurs* 1984;22(11):27–32.

Peplau HE: *Interpersonal Relations in Nursing*. Putnam, 1952.

Peplau HE: Interpersonal techniques: The crux of psychiatric nursing. *Am J Nurs* 1962;62:50–54.

Peplau HE: Historical development of psychiatric nursing: A preliminary statement of some facts and trends, in

Smoyak S, Rouslin S (eds): *Collection of Classics in Psychiatric Nursing Literature.* Charles B. Slack, 1982, pp 10–46.

Peplau HE: Future directions in psychiatric nursing from the perspective of history. *J Psychosoc Nurs* 1989;27(2): 18–27.

Report to the President of the President's Commission on Mental Health, vol I. US Government Printing Office, 1978.

Rosen G: *Madness in Society.* Harper & Row, 1968.

Slavinsky A: Psychiatric nursing to the year 2000: From a nonsystem of caring to a caring system. *Image* 1984; 16(1): 17–20.

Strauss A et al.: *Psychiatric Ideologies and Institutions.* The Free Press of Glencoe, 1964.

Stanton A, Schwartz M: The management of a type of institutional participation in mental illness. *Psychiatry* 1949;12:13–26.

Talbott JA: Deinstitutionalization: Avoiding the disasters of the past. *Hosp Community Psychiatry* 1979;30:621–624.

US Department of Health and Human Services, Public Health Service, Alcohol, Drug Abuse, and Mental Health Administration: *Psychiatric-Mental Health Nursing: Proceedings of Two Conferences on Future Directions.* DHHS Publication no. (ADM) 86-1449, 1986, pp 4–6.

Widem P et al.: Prospective payment for psychiatric hospitalization. *Hosp Community Psychiatry* 1984; 35(5):447–451.

Wilson HS: *Deinstitutionalized Residential Alternatives for the Severely Mentally Disordered: The Soteria House Approach.* Grune & Stratton, 1982.

The Psychiatric Nurse and the Interdisciplinary Mental Health Team: Personal Integration and Professional Role

LEARNING OBJECTIVES

- Explore the concept of personal integration as it relates to the self and to psychiatric nursing practice

- Identify problems that influence personal integration

- Relate these problems to some strategies for coping

- Discuss the qualities that enable psychiatric nurses to practice the use of self artfully in therapeutic relationships

- Discuss the use of empathy in psychiatric nursing practice

- Describe the roles of the psychiatric nurse and other members of the mental health team

- Identify how the mental health team achieves collaboration

- Specify three characteristics of excellence exemplars in psychiatric nursing practice

- Explain six qualities associated with power and excellence under real-world conditions

Carol Ren Kneisl
Holly Skodol Wilson

CROSS REFERENCES

Other topics relevant to this content are: Ethics, Chapter 7; Liaison role of the nurse, Chapter 19; Nurses' role with the chronically mentally ill, Chapter 17; Nurses' role in family therapy, Chapter 30; Nurses' role in groups, Chapter 29; Nurses' role in milieu therapy, Chapter 31; Nurses' role in one-to-one relationships, Chapter 26; Relaxation and stress management techniques, Chapter 27; Therapeutic use of self, Chapter 26.

THE VALUE OF SELF-KNOWLEDGE is a recurring theme in both the popular and the professional literature. Libraries are stocked with volumes dealing with the undiscovered self, the expansion of human awareness, values clarification, strategies for self-realization, and the like. A common thread in all these is the idea that the quality and nature of a person's relationship with others are strongly influenced by the person's self-view. Consider the following comments made by students in their psychiatric nursing clinical experience:

I just can't take it. . . . I feel myself getting confused about who is the crazy one. There's such a fine line. Sometimes I think I'll be a patient here.

I hated psych—it just didn't seem like nursing to me. I really like to keep busy. When you change someone's dressing, you really feel like you've helped them. Here it's all so uncertain.

All I kept thinking about was that a lot of the patients had done really weird things. This one guy had lived in an apartment with his dead mother's body for three months before they brought him in. Another had tried to shoot the governor. I never felt safe even turning my back on them.

This chapter helps nursing students and practitioners explore some dimensions of self-knowledge through an examination of the concepts of personal integration and professional role. Specifically, we will examine recurring problems that pertain to the nurse's identity and some strategies for coping with them. Our goal is to enhance the nurse's interactions with persons who may be labeled psychiatric clients.

The Nurse's Personal Integration

Many students and practitioners faced with relating to people whose behavior they view as offensive, frightening, curious, or socially inappropriate find that their personal attitudes, expectations, myths, and values make it difficult for them to fulfill their professional roles. This was the case in the following example:

Penny, a baccalaureate nursing student, had selected a clinical placement at a methadone clinic in the community. Despite her initial interest, she developed a pattern of absences from the clinic. When her faculty adviser discussed this observation with her, she blurted out that, much to her surprise, she was unable to assist with the group meetings for pregnant heroin addicts. The thought of addicting babies before their births—babies who would ultimately suffer because of their mothers' self-indulgence

—horrified Penny. She found herself judging their choices constantly and avoiding interaction with them. "I feel like they should be shot instead of given all this free support and sympathy."

For many nurses, confrontation with **deviance** (behavior outside the social norm of a specific group; should not be construed to mean negative behavior) reinforces a personal sense of stability. Others are threatened by such confrontation.

One psychiatric nurse, in recalling her childhood experiences with community deviants, commented on the intense and sometimes morbid excitement that she and her friends found in taunting "Crazy Helen" to run out on her porch and shout incoherently at the neighborhood children or in telling bizarre stories about a grotesque old man called "Charlie-No-Face," who walked along a road late at night chain smoking from the gaping hole that had once been a mouth.

The interest these characters held for the children, along with "Vince-the-Window-Peeper," "Red-the-Bum," and the other small-town deviants, was reawakened in her as she approached her first psychiatric nursing experience. It was all very frightening, yet seductive and stimulating at the same time. The nursing students gossiped about the bizarre histories of their assigned clients as if to reaffirm their separateness from them—their sense of being normal and OK.

Dealing with people whose personal integration is fragmented, dissolving, divided, or alienated puts the nurse's own identity on the line as well. To respond with both compassion and the critical distance necessary to be effective, psychiatric professionals must confront their own identity; separate it from another's identity, which may indeed be dissolving; and finally integrate different values and behaviors comfortably in the therapeutic relationships they develop with clients.

This personal quality has been called *detached concern*—the ability to distance oneself in order to help others. It is an essential quality not only in avoiding *burnout,* a problem discussed later in this chapter, but also in *values clarification,* in ethical dilemmas, in using appropriate *assertiveness* when collaborating with colleagues, and in maintaining *empathic abilities* in highly stressful situations.

In the conventional focus on the client, the nurse is regarded as the caregiver, the provider of services, the therapist. Little attention is paid to the stresses psychiatric nurses experience attempting to relate fully to clients while maintaining their own personal integration. This chapter is an attempt to explore that aspect of psychiatric nursing.

Negotiated Reality

Nurses often find that encounters with psychiatric clients are distancing experiences. The nurses become acutely aware of their difference and separateness from clients. They reaffirm their own subjective view of reality and rationalize their actions to keep these actions consistent with their sense of self as healthy, normal people.

Since people are all constantly building and protecting their own self-images, they try to get others to see their image of themselves. However, it is impossible to see another's self-image or world view exactly as that person experiences it. Despite this fact, psychiatry has traditionally attempted to get certain people, labeled *crazy,* to assume the perspective of certain other people, called *therapists.*

A more acceptable alternative seems to lie in the creation of some common ground, a mutually understood, **negotiated reality.** Even to this common ground the nurse and the client bring their own conceptions, feelings, and attitudes toward and images of each other and themselves. In many instances, the nurse's image of the client—how the nurse expects the client to act or feel—is not the same as the client's self-image. This is confusing to both client and nurse and hinders the establishment of therapeutic relationships and effective communication.

Feelings: The Affective Self

The ultimate effectiveness of efforts to relate to and communicate with others depends on how well people know themselves and develop the capacity for empathy. **Self-awareness** and empathic caring seem to go hand in hand. At the root of social interaction is people's ability to empathize with each other and to understand each other's attitudes and feelings. Because each human being is unique, empathizing is a difficult and challenging task. One way to develop this ability is to practice it. Learning to be aware of one's responses to expression of feelings from another person is a starting point.

Josh is a middle-aged man who sought out nursing as a career. Although he is highly proficient in technical skills and charming and engaging in relationships with most clients, he discovers a surprising intolerance for some of the tears, complaints, and self-preoccupation of depressed clients. He finds himself responding with admonitions to stop it, to bite the bullet, to grow up. He personally has seldom allowed himself to experience his own sadnesses but jokingly characterizes himself as a firm believer in repression and denial. The need to empathize with people unable to control their feelings evoked such discomfort that he found himself unable to work with such clients.

Self-Awareness of Feelings   Feelings seem like icebergs: only the tips stick up into consciousness, and the deeper parts are submerged. One such feeling is fear (see Figure 2–1). The conscious part may be experienced as dislike, avoidance, or reluctance. At a deeper level, the feeling is reported as anxiety. Even deeper, the person may acknowledge, "I feel scared." Deeper yet, the person may experience genuine panic. Such an iceberg may well explain Josh's attitude toward tearful, depressed clients. His annoyance, irritation, sarcasm, and disdain may represent the tip of the iceberg of Josh's fear of depression.

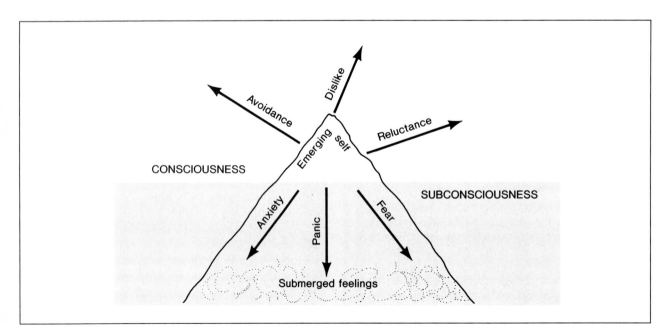

FIGURE 2–1   Self-awareness of feelings.

The iceberg comparison also applies to other feelings, such as love, hurt, and guilt. A person feeling love may be aware only of a liking or attraction for another. Beneath the tip of that iceberg are feelings of warmth and affection. Deeper are feelings of love, and at the deepest level may be feelings of fusion or ecstasy.

Problems with Submerged Feelings

One characteristic of icebergs of feeling is that at the tip the feelings lose their experiental quality and become translated into impulses to act. For example, a person with submerged guilt may express it by frequent worrying and explaining and may be completely unaware of the underlying feelings. The behavior is the only outward manifestation. Snow and Willard (1989) cite the example of a nurse whose need to focus on or take care of others promotes the neglect of self. In this situation, known as codependence, the codependent nurse denies the existence of feelings, especially negative ones. (See Chapter 24 for a discussion of codependence among nurses and other health care workers.) Being out of touch with their feelings lessens people's control over some of their behavior.

People lose touch with their feelings over time as they shape their sense of self. They hear such messages as "boys don't cry" or "girls are too sensitive" and incorporate these injunctions into their emerging self-system, especially into the "me" or "self for others." Not being sufficiently aware of one's feelings has several disadvantages:

- What people don't know *can* hurt them. Repressed feelings may reappear in behaviors that are difficult to alter. For example, hidden anger may emerge in migraine headaches or a tendency to use sarcasm.

- People who are not aware of their feelings find it difficult to make decisions. It is hard to tell a "should" from a wish. Without some awareness of their real wants, they may have trouble saying no or requesting something they need. They are more likely to rely on others—experts, authorities, rules and regulations, and so forth—for guidance.

- People who, like Josh, are "out of touch with" or unaware of their feelings may find it difficult to be really close to and empathic toward others. Intimacy and empathy demand the expression of here-and-now feelings, whether positive or negative.

Most people realize the value of thinking clearly. They understand that it is a learned ability and takes practice. Feeling clearly (authentically) can also be practiced and learned. Most writers acknowledge that feelings are as important as facts, because they shape people's versions of reality as much as facts do. Becoming more aware of feelings begins with the search for one's dominant emotional themes.

Dominant Emotional Themes Nurses need to explore the dominant emotional themes in their personalities. If they find that they respond to many situations with the same feelings, they are probably narrowing their range of potential feelings.

Whatever the occasion, Marge used it to be tired or bored. Fatigue and chronically depressed states were routine for her. Holidays, vacations, dinner engagements all evoked the same predictable response.

Joan was afraid of everything. When she met her brother at the plane, her first question was, "Aren't you afraid of flying?" She was afraid driving home from the airport. The prospect of starting back to school scared her. She was fearful about wearing a bikini to the swimming club.

People who feel the same way in a variety of situations may be missing a lot of what is happening in those situations. They look for and perceive only what will fit a narrowed range of feelings. Becoming aware of limited emotional themes is a way to begin to widen the range of feelings.

Acceptance of Disapproved Feelings Most people have been taught to block off an awareness and expression of certain feelings. Children are taught that being rude or ungrateful or cranky is rarely acceptable to significant others. To retain love and approval, they usually comply, not by stopping the feelings but by acting as if they didn't have them. Nursing students often get similar messages from teachers. It is not acceptable to find a client repulsive, to dislike someone who is sick and dependent, to express anger at or criticism of the teacher. Positive feelings of attraction and love may also seem unacceptable. Failure to recognize these feelings can interfere with interactions.

Recognizing and accepting their own feelings make nurses less vulnerable to other people's ideas about how they should feel. Nurses often feel guilty when they don't feel what others imply they should feel. Instead, nurses need to realize that others merely disapprove of the way they do feel. Nurses who can allow themselves the right to their own feelings can also allow clients the right to have and express feelings.

Beliefs and Values

Beliefs and values take three major forms:

1. Rational beliefs are beliefs supported by available evidence.

2. Blind belief is belief in the absence of evidence.

3. Irrational belief is belief held despite available evidence to the contrary.

Dogmatic belief (opinions or beliefs held as if they were based on the highest authority) includes both blind and irrational belief. Dogmatically held beliefs are not based on personal experience. Operating on the basis of dogmatically held beliefs often causes nurses to distort their personal experiences of the world to fit their preconceptions. The following are examples of strongly held beliefs about behaviors that are labeled "mental illness" and about the people who do and don't engage in those behaviors:

- Most clients in mental hospitals are dangerous.

- People who are mentally disordered let their emotions control them.

- Normal people think things out.

- If parents loved their children more, there would be fewer mental disorders.

- When a person has a worry, it is best not to think about it.

- Many people become mentally disordered just to avoid the problems of life.

- Most psychiatric clients are lazy.

- People would not become mentally disordered if they avoided bad thoughts.

- A woman would be foolish to marry a man who has had a mental disorder.

- Anyone who is in a hospital for a mental disorder should not be allowed to vote.

- To become a psychiatric client is to become a failure in life.

- If a man in a mental hospital attacks someone, he should be punished so that he doesn't do it again.

- Most clients in mental hospitals don't care how they look.

- One of the main causes of mental disorders is a lack of moral strength.

Most research on strongly held beliefs indicates that people usually know more about the things they believe than about those they don't believe. The process works like this: If people let themselves find out about those things they don't believe, they might find some validity in the statements. Then they would have to question the beliefs they already hold. By staying ignorant about anything they don't already agree with, they can avoid changing. This posture cuts off personal growth and learning that could be derived from the unknown. Obviously, clients are better served by nurses who are aware of their own dogmatically held beliefs and then challenge them.

Attitudes and Opinions   A feeling is a transitory experience. A feeling held over a period of time is called an attitude. An attitude linked to an idea or belief becomes an opinion. An opinion, then, involves both thinking and feeling. Research in this area has shown that people are more comfortable when their beliefs are consistent with their attitudes. People do several things to keep their attitudes and beliefs consistent:

- They repress the belief or attitude that seems inconsistent.

- They distract their awareness from conflict either physically (e.g., by leaving the room) or psychologically (e.g., by daydreaming).

- They distort their perceptions to fit an existing attitude or belief.

Similar maneuvers take place to keep actions consistent with attitudes or beliefs. Nurses often justify treating psychiatric clients inhumanely or unkindly by arguing that the clients deserved it or were asking for it.

Nurses need to be careful that their self-image—as people who act intelligently—does not keep them from seeing the world clearly. Some attitudes are inconsistent with beliefs or actions. It is probably preferable to acknowledge this point than to engage in the elaborate self-deceptions necessary to avoid it.

Arriving at Values   Every day, each person meets life situations that call for thought, opinion forming, decision making, and action. At every turn in their personal and professional lives, nurses are faced with choices. Their choices are based on the values they hold, but often those values are not really clear. People actively value something to the degree that they are willing to put energy into doing something about it. Their values are shown in their interests, preferences, decisions, and actions.

In talking with colleagues, Susan, a psychiatric nurse, claims to value interacting with clients more than doing paperwork. Yet a quick assessment of how she spends her time—all excuses taken into account—reveals that she acts on other values.

Mel, a nurse working in a state hospital ward for profoundly retarded children, claims that he believes these clients are human beings, despite their uncommunicative, immobile forms. He demonstrates this value in the hours he spends trying to communicate his presence and concern for them, using acupressure and touch performed slowly and with genuine feeling.

The distinction in the above examples is between *cognitive* and *active values*. Susan verbally subscribes to values but fails to act on them. These are cognitive values. Mel's actions demonstrate that he gives more than lip service to the idea of the dignity of all living beings. He follows active values.

People may learn values in a number of ways:

• Moralizing is a direct, although sometimes subtle, method of inculcating desired values in someone else.

• The laissez-faire approach leaves people alone to forge their own set of values. This may create unnecessary frustration, conflict, and confusion, especially in young people or people being socialized into a profession such as nursing.

• Modeling, in which actions follow professed values, transmits values by setting a living example for a learner to follow.

• Values clarification is a systematic, widely applicable method of teaching the process of valuing rather than the content of any specific values. It uses strategies and exercises (see Wilson and Kneisl 1988) to engage learners in becoming aware of their beliefs and values, choosing among alternatives, and matching stated beliefs with actions.

The small amount of research comparing these four methods of learning values highlights the advantages of the fourth method. People who engage in values clarification are more zestful and energetic, more critical in their thinking, and more likely to follow through on their decisions than those who learn values in other ways. However, values clarification must be undertaken in circumstances that allow for sufficient follow-up with students who may uncover uncomfortable or disturbing values.

Taking Care of the Self

Knowing who they are is just a beginning for nurses. Taking care of others requires that nurses respect and care for themselves. Assertiveness, the need for soli-tude, maintaining physical health, and attending to cues of personal stress are actions crucial to preserving the nurse's personal integration.

Assertiveness

Have you ever had difficulty expressing yourself in a staff meeting? Did you find yourself feeling hopeless, resentful, angry? Were you wishing you had the courage to speak up? Hoping someone else would?

Are you intimidated by the high-pressure tactics of supervisors, physicians, teachers? Do you have trouble standing up to these sacred cows? Do you remain silent but seething? Do you speak up but sound defensive? Do you say yes when you mean no?

Have you ever needed to give someone counseling? Did you avoid the problem, hoping things would change? Did you find yourself beating around the bush? Or did you find yourself being overly harsh when you finally gave the correction?

These questions are from a manual written specifically to help nurses cope with on-the-job stressors (Muff 1984, pp 239–240) by using assertiveness techniques to express themselves more effectively. Often people are either so timid that they do not get what they want or so aggressive and belligerent that they offend and alienate others. Assertiveness is asking for what one wants or acting to get it in a way that respects other people. It is the middle way between timid holding back and inconsiderate, offensive aggression. **Assertiveness training exercises** are designed to teach people to ask for what they want and also to refuse someone without feeling guilty.

Compare the **nonassertive, aggressive,** and **assertive** behaviors listed in Table 2–1 to see which descriptions best characterize your behavior with

TABLE 2–1   **Comparison of Nonassertive, Aggressive, and Assertive Behaviors**

Nonassertive	*Aggressive*	*Assertive*
Denies anger/experiences fear	Denies fear/experiences anger	Recognizes both fear and anger
Does not respect self	Does not respect others	Respects both self and others
Destroys relationships as avoidance and resentment build	Destroys relationships through angry outbursts, self-aggrandizement, and need to control	Builds relationships
Wastes energy by repeating situations that were not adequately resolved	Wastes energy in bluster and argument	Uses energy constructively
Fails to achieve goals	Occasionally achieves goals through intimidation	Achieves goals
Is stressful (low self-esteem, helplessness, hopelessness, depression)	Is stressful (power struggles, painful arguments, need to be ever vigilant)	Is stressful (defying traditional stereotypes; pain of being conscious)

SOURCE: Muff J: Balancing communications: Assertive skills, in Smythe EEM: *Surviving Nursing.* Addison Wesley, 1984, p 248.

others. Fortunately, old behaviors can be unlearned, and new behaviors can be learned.

Nurses need to recognize their rights as nurses before they can assume responsibility for asserting them. The list below (Chenevert 1983) was originally designed to help women health professionals recognize their rights. They are, however, applicable to health professionals of both sexes.

- You have the right to be treated with respect.

- You have the right to a reasonable workload.

- You have the right to an equitable wage.

- You have the right to determine your own priorities.

- You have the right to ask for what you want.

- You have the right to refuse without making excuses or feeling guilty.

- You have the right to make mistakes and be responsible for them.

- You have the right to give and receive information as a professional.

- You have the right to act in the best interest of the client.

- You have the right to be human.

Remembering that you have rights is not enough; you must assert them.

Solitude

Most people need time alone to assimilate what has happened in time spent with other people. They also need it for relief from responding to the demands of others. Aloneness need not mean physical distance. People can be alone in a crowded library. The crucial factors are that they are making no demands on others and that no one is making demands on them. After a sanctioned time away, most people return refreshed to their relationships, work, and usual circumstances. Planning for time alone is highly preferable to reaching a breaking point and then aggressively and irresponsibly running away from others.

Personal Physical Health

An important way of taking care of oneself is to provide for the physical health of the body. A proper diet, adequate rest, and exercise rejuvenate and restore the body. All these activities potentially make nurses more alive and better able to share this quality of aliveness with their clients.

Attending to Internal Stress Signals

Nursing students encountering emotionally disturbed clients commonly begin seeing in themselves all the "symptoms" about which they are learning. This perception is probably due more to heightened awareness of and attention to emotional aspects of their lives than to anything else. However, it is important for nurses to learn to recognize and respond to their own genuine stress signals. All people have times in their lives when they feel a little crazy. They may become very upset at small disturbances or see things out of proportion to their ultimate importance. These feelings are significant warning signals that the person is not coping adequately with stress.

"Crazy" times can be important turning points in people's lives. They are strong messages that change is needed. It is foolish to ignore these messages. British psychiatrist R. D. Laing has found that if people who have "gone crazy" are given supportive and nurturing conditions, they can often work through important matters while they are in this altered state of consciousness.

In their daily lives, nurses are often tempted to handle their own symptoms of stress by suppressing them with tranquilizers or other drugs. They could serve themselves better by really experiencing their feelings and attending to what the signals are saying. Help in managing stress creatively is the subject of Chapter 27. Using the techniques recommended in Chapter 27 will help nurses to gain control of their lives and ease tension before it becomes unmanageable.

Pain and suffering are sources of some of the most intensely experienced stresses in life. Events such as death of loved ones, divorce, illness, separation from loved ones, and failure are all part of the cycle of life's experience. Being told that they deserve it, or that they really don't have it so bad and therefore have no right to feel the way they feel, does not help people cope with pain and suffering. They need to find ways of handling their suffering without being destroyed by it. Classmates, friends, and family members can be great sources of support. Being able to both give and receive support strengthens the individual.

According to an old Buddhist teaching, a third of people's suffering is inevitable but they themselves create the rest of it. Realizing that pain and hardship are part of what it is to be a human being makes the pain a bit gentler. Frequently pain centers around losing or being afraid of losing something or someone valued: a job, mate, money, self-respect. People want to continue what was instead of living with what is. It is important to attend to genuine feelings about the loss or prospective loss. These feelings give messages about what the sufferer needs to do. Some people need to replace what they have lost with something similar. Others need to explore a new dimension in their lives.

The alternative to experiencing pain is to live on the surface, out of touch with the real peak experiences in life as well as the painful ones. A more life-enhancing approach is to experience all of life.

Qualities of Effective Psychiatric Nursing

Psychiatric nursing, according to the American Nurses' Association (ANA) Congress for Nursing Practice, is "a specialized area of nursing emphasizing theories of human behavior as its scientific aspect and purposeful use of self as its art." Self-awareness, empathy, and moral integrity all allow psychiatric nurses to practice the use of self artfully in therapeutic relationships. Some characteristics of artful therapeutic practice are respect for the client, availability, spontaneity, hope, acceptance, sensitivity, vision, and accountability.

Respect for the Client

The behavior of many psychiatric clients indicates their loss of self-respect. Some may appear dirty and disheveled. Others may plead, beg, or cry. Still others may try do to themselves physical harm. A relationship in which they experience a sense of dignity and receive messages of respect is of inestimable value. The nurse can convey respect in relationships with clients by:

- Taking the time and energy to listen

- Not invalidating clients' experience of their world with comments such as, "It's not so bad," "Don't be that way," "Time heals all wounds," or "Keep a stiff upper lip"

- Giving clients as much privacy as possible during examinations and treatments or when they are upset

- Minimizing experiences that humiliate clients and strip them of identity, thus allowing them to make as many of their own choices and be in control of as much of their own lives as possible

- Being honest with clients about medicines, privileges, length of stay, and so on, even when the truth may be difficult to handle

Availability

Of all the members of the psychiatric team, the nurse has the richest opportunity to be available to clients when needed, at any time of day or night. Because they are with clients on a relatively constant basis, nurses have the responsibility for:

- Creating a nurturing, healing milieu in the unit

- Assisting suffering clients to meet their basic human needs

- Collecting and conveying crucial data about clients that will influence decisions around them

Spontaneity

Many nurses have come to believe that therapeutic relationships with psychiatric clients require them to be stiff, stilted robots uttering clichés from a list of unnatural-sounding communication "techniques." Nurses who are comfortable with themselves, aware of therapeutic goals, and flexible about using a repertoire of possible interventions for any particular clinical problem find that being natural and spontaneous is their most effective "technique." Clients experience such nurses as authentic. Each nurse is unique and necessarily brings a different personal style to practice. We have different ways of putting the words together to convey to clients that we accept and care about them. Sometimes we say it with nonverbal behavior: keeping promises, coming on time, touching, and staying with a client who needs someone. We need to trust our own natural styles in working toward therapeutic goals.

Hope

Effective psychiatric nursing practice is characterized by hope and optimism that all clients, no matter how debilitated, have the capacity for growth and change. Even clients whose most marked attributes are chronicity and deterioration can be helped to some optimal level of well-being by a nurse who believes in their possibilities and is willing to search for some strengths to build on. In one locked ward of a huge government psychiatric hospital, a chronic client joined in a partnership with a creative nurse to assist less able clients toward self-care. It is not unusual in such a situation for the healing to become a source of help to the healer-client.

Acceptance

There is a distinction between acceptance and approval. Acceptance means refraining from judging and rejecting a client who may behave in a way the nurse dislikes. Therapeutic work requires that clients be able to examine, explore, and understand their coping mechanisms without feeling the need to cover up or disguise them to avoid negative judgments or punishments. Nurses who tell clients what they should say or do or feel deny these clients the acceptance they need to explore their problems.

Sensitivity

Genuine interest and concern provide the basis for a therapeutic alliance. Clients recognize the falseness of memorized phrases and assumed postures. The nurse conveys general interest and concern by trying to understand the client's perspective, working with the client on mutually formulated goals, and persisting even when breakthroughs and improvements are subtle and slow instead of dramatic and quick.

Vision

Because psychiatric nurses focus their work on enhancing the quality of life for all human beings, they must come to terms with a personal and professional vision of what quality means. Some conditions of life associated with high quality are influence or power, freedom, accountability, self-determinism, openness to gratifying experience, action, mastery, a sense of purpose or meaning, privacy, hope, stability, nonviolence, and intimacy.

Accountability

According to Peplau (1980), the need for personal accountability—professional integrity—is greater in psychiatric practice than in any other type of health care. Clients in mental health settings are usually more vulnerable and defenseless than clients in other health care settings, particularly since their conditions hinder their thinking processes and their relationships with others. Psychiatric nurses are accountable for the nature of the effort they make on behalf of clients and answerable to clients for the quality of their efforts. As Peplau (1980, p 133) puts it, "Personal accountability is an attitude—a quality of the heart and mind of those professionals who are competent and determined that every psychiatric patient will have the best problem-resolving assistance possible."

Psychiatric nurses are also accountable to themselves, their peers, their profession, and the public. Accountability to self involves bringing personal behavior under conscious control so that the nurse becomes the person-as-nurse she or he wants to be. Accountability to peers involves engaging in peer review with nurse colleagues to give and receive feedback intended to improve the quality of care. Accountability to the profession involves clarifying the role of the psychiatric nurse and encouraging self-regulation to protect the public and enhance the quality of care. Accountability to the public requires keeping abreast of the knowledge in the field, becoming credentialed according to level of competence, applying the ANA Standards of Psychiatric-Mental Health Nursing Practice, and protecting the rights of clients and their families.

Empathy

The Value of Empathy in Nursing

Psychiatric nurses are instructed to engage in "therapeutic use of self." They are told that their "relationship" with a client is the primary therapeutic tool, that they should demonstrate qualities of sensitivity and caring. For many beginning students, these instructions are mysterious jargon quite unlike the clear-cut step-by-step procedures they learn for some physical treatments.

I found myself watching the nurses on the unit and my instructors closely when they talked with the clients. Somehow I thought maybe by imitating things that they did or said I'd figure out what "being therapeutic" was supposed to mean. I knew it had something to do with things the nurse said or didn't say when she talked with the clients. But it all got very fuzzy to me beyond that very elementary grasp of it. I used to latch onto ideas like "Agreeing is untherapeutic. So is giving advice or opinions." The only entries I felt safe in putting down in my process-recording were stiff-sounding reflections, like "You sound angry."

Comprehension of and ability to use the process of empathy give the nurse one strategy for responding to the feelings of aloneness often experienced by persons labeled psychiatric clients. Nurses are taught skills of active listening. But listening without empathy is not enough. Empathic understanding not only increases the nurse's grasp of the client's difficulties but also helps the nurse offer feedback on how the client affects others. Perhaps its most important function is to help the nurse to give the client the very precious feeling of being understood and cared about.

Definition of Empathy

Empathy is a pervasive phenomenon in the life experience of all people. It allows a person to feel what others feel and respond to and understand the experience of others on their terms. A nurse who empathizes with a client momentarily abandons the personal self and relives the emotions and responses of someone else. People in everyday life tend to empathize most with those to whom they feel closest. In psychiatric practice, nurses often seek to empathize with persons from whom they feel most separate or whose closeness threatens the nurses' own sense of integration.

Empathy has been defined as a subtle imitation through which people assume an alien personality. They become aware of how it feels to behave in a certain way and then feed back into the other person's consciousness this awareness and sensitivity to what the behavior feels like. Empathy characteristically develops early in an infant's pattern of relating to the parents. Tension or anxiety in the parent, for example, induces anxiety in the baby.

Psychiatric Concepts of Empathy

Intimacy is closely related to empathy. Psychoanalytic theory postulates the development of empathy as a process of "mutual incorporation." The mother compensates for her loss of biologic oneness with the infant at birth by establishing a primitive unity—an emotional bonding—with the child during the first weeks and months of life. Children likewise incorporate the mothering parent into the self. Once children begin to see the mothering parent as a being separate from the self, identification replaces incorporation. At this point, the child experiences the mother as one to imitate in order to secure love and comfort. From identification comes the capacity for empathy. Identification allows human beings to achieve a clear sense of self, to gain another person's point of view, and to establish an intimate association with others.

People have the capacity to identify not only with contemporaries but also with those who have been significant in the past. Adults can empathize through past, present, and future identifications. Psychiatric nurses must be able to shift from one identity to another without losing their own sense of integration.

Social interactionists discuss empathy as **role taking**, a process through which people feel with one another. They are able to sense the feelings of another because they have evoked in themselves the attitude of the person to whom they are relating. Role taking among children is a necessary part of social life. It is a means for developing the sense of self and of learning methods for adjusting to society. Role taking can be likened to learning to play games, in which children not only learn to enact their own roles but also become fully aware of the roles of others.

People form an image of themselves because they have learned to assume the roles of others and have developed the ability to see themselves as others see them. The other, then, is like a mirror in which they see themselves, and that mirror becomes the source of their own image of themselves as persons. Faulty ability to take on roles is the result of limited opportunity for role experimentation. Individuals who have not experimented enough do not develop a clear sense of their own integration and thus cannot shift from the role of participant to that of observer.

The capacity for empathy relies on personal integration. Whether problems with empathy are seen as the loss of primitive instincts for imitation in the psychoanalytic framework or as the result of inadequate opportunities for role experimentation in the social psychologist's view, the conclusion is the same. A firm sense of self is necessary for a person to be a good empathizer. As people continue to interact with others, they learn to be sensitive to others without losing their own integration.

Therapeutic Use of Empathy

From time to time, we hear accounts of dramatic and surprising breakthroughs with psychiatric clients. There are instances in which the usual tools of systematic, logical problem solving and the application of theory seem to be getting nowhere. Instead therapists fall back for a moment on their empathic sensitivity and get an inside comprehension of some complex emotion. This empathic understanding may be a key to establishing trust with a sullen, withdrawn, suspicious adolescent, or beginning verbal interaction with a chronically mute institutionalized person, or controlling the violent flailing rage of an emotionally disturbed child. In all these instances, empathy is used as a therapeutic tool.

The term *empathy* is often mistakenly used synonymously with *sympathy*. Empathy contains no elements of condolence, agreement, or pity. When nurses sympathize, they assume that there is a parallel between their feelings and those of the client. The perceived similarity makes good judgment and objectivity difficult. Empathy also should be differentiated from *identification*. Identification is generally thought to be an unconscious process and only the initial phase of the empathizing process.

Steps in Therapeutic Empathizing

The process of empathic understanding has four phases:

1. *Identification:* Through relaxation of conscious controls, we allow ourselves to become absorbed in contemplating the client and the client's experiences.

2. *Incorporation:* We take in the experiences of the client rather than attribute our own experiences and feelings to the client.

3. *Reverberation:* We interplay the internalized feelings of the client and our own experiences or fantasies. While fully absorbed in the identity of the client, we still experience ourselves as separate personalities.

4. *Detachment:* We withdraw from subjective involvement and totally resume our own identity. We use the insight gained from the reverberation phase as well as reason and objectivity to offer responses that are useful to the client.

Experience in taking on the client role, such as in the simulation designed by Cosgray and associates (1990), can help increase empathy for clients.

Burnout As a Consequence of Empathy

After hours, days, and months of listening to other people's problems, something inside you can go dead and you don't care anymore. That's when you'd rather sit at the desk and do the paperwork than be out talking to clients on the floor.

This nurse verbalizes one of the possible consequences of using empathy when working intensely with troubled people. **Burnout** is the name given this phenomenon, and it happens to poverty lawyers, social workers, clinical psychologists, child-care workers, prison personnel, and others who struggle to retain both their objectivity and their empathic concern for the people with whom they work.

Burnout is a condition in which health professionals lose their concern and feelings for their clients and come to treat them in detached or even dehumanized ways. It is an attempt to cope, by distancing oneself, with the stresses of intense interpersonal work. It hurts not only clients but also psychiatric professionals, in that they become ineffective and dissatisfied.

One nurse noted that her emotions shifted dramatically, first toward cynical feelings, then negative ones about her clients. "I began to despise every one of them and couldn't conceal my contempt for them." Another reported, "I found myself caring less and less and feeling really negative about the clients here." In many cases, burning out involves not only thinking in derogatory terms about the clients but also believing that somehow they deserve any problem they have. Benner and Wrubel (1989) caution us not to make the mistake of thinking that caring is the cause of burnout and thus try to prevent the "disease" of burnout by protecting oneself from caring. According to them, the sickness is the loss of caring, and the return of caring is the recovery.

There is little doubt that burnout plays a major role in the poor delivery of psychiatric care. It is also a key factor in low staff morale, absenteeism, and high job turnover.

Cues to Burnout   Cues to burnout can be found in the language used to depict clients. Burnout victims may refer to their clients as "crocks," "vegetables," "wackos," "brown baggers," and so forth, or they may become highly analytic and abstract: "That's just a manifestation of his primary process thinking."

Another cue is lack of involvement with clients. Some nurses "hide" in the nurses' station or staff conference room to avoid interacting. Some openly reject bids for human contact.

A newly admitted client tearfully pleads at the nurses' desk. "Will you listen to me! Can't you come down to my room to sit with me? I want to lie down. I need somebody." The nurse replies, "No, I'm not going to send somebody to babysit you and hold your hand. Are you an infant?" The client replies, "No, I'm just scared." The nurse retorts, "Then stay out of your room. Doesn't that make sense?"

Another withdrawal technique involves "going by the book" rather than considering the unique factors in a situation. It is a way of minimizing personal involvement with the client. By rigidly applying the rules, the nurse can avoid thinking about the client's specific problems. Burnout can transform an original and creative nurse into a mechanical bureaucrat.

Another cue to burnout is joking put-downs among staff members, which makes their work less frightening and overwhelming.

When the nurse is asked where Mr G is, she laughingly reports that he's taking a shower in preparation for his MMPI test. Everyone in the nurses' station breaks up in gales of laughter.

Staff members on one psychiatric ward referred to their morning meeting as the "laugh-in" show and their discussions of the clients as their sociopathy.

In a discharge conference, the psychiatrist says he'd like to discharge E, a young male client with a history of violent outbursts. The nurse replies, "With or without baseball bat?" and everyone chuckles.

Reducing Burnout   Most research indicates that the causes of professional burnout are rooted not in the permanent psychologic characteristics of individuals but rather in the social context of their work. Most nurses usually expect the presence of negative conditions: large client loads, time pressures, and daily confrontation with suffering, pain, and death. It is the absence of positive factors—a sense of significance, rewarding interpersonal relationships, the appreciation of others, challenge, and variety—that is most distressing. Figure 2–2 illustrates the disequilibrium that burnout creates in the health care system. The strategies listed below can be used to reduce and modify the occurrence of burnout:

- Keep staff-client ratios low. Staff members can then give more attention to each client and have time to focus on the positive, nonproblem aspects of the client's life.

- Provide for sanctioned breaks rather than guilt-provoking escapes from the work situation for staff members.

- Provide some relief from prolonged direct client contact, through shorter work shifts or rotating work responsibilities, so that certain staff members are not always working directly with clients.

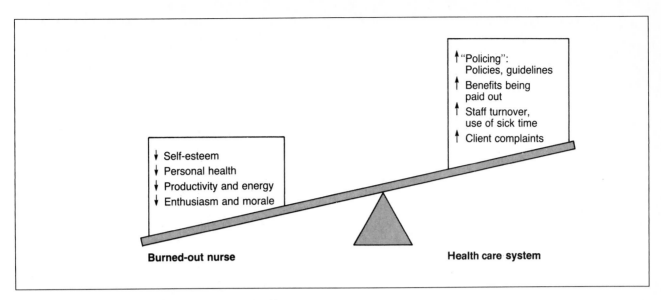

FIGURE 2–2 Burnout toll: disequilibrium in the health care system.
SOURCE: Smythe EEM: *Surviving Nursing.* Addison-Wesley, 1984, p 54.

• Set up formal or informal programs in which staff members can talk over their problems to get advice and support when they need it.

• Encourage staff members to express, analyze, and share their feelings about burning out. This lets them get things off their chest and gives them the chance to get constructive feedback from others and perhaps a new perspective as well.

• Encourage staff members to understand their own motivations in pursuing a psychiatric career and to recognize their expectations for work with clients. Nurses can be on a variety of "ego trips," whose primary purpose is to deal with their own personal problems, not those of the clients.

A nurse's empathic involvement with troubled clients can have a number of stressful consequences in addition to burnout. Problems can arise at any phase in the empathy process. The nurse may overidentify and lapse into sympathy for the client. The nurse may fail to incorporate the client's feelings and instead project personal ones. The nurse may bypass the reverberation phase and substitute gut-level intuitions for rational problem solving. At the detachment phase, the nurse may experience overdistancing or burnout. Each of the common obstacles to achieving an empathic concern for clients can be understood as a failure to cope with one of the four phases of achieving empathy. Burning out has been given particular attention here because it is common and is less psychologic than circumstantial. It therefore is not inevitable and can be prevented with thoughtful planning.

The Nurse's Professional Role

As society and society's needs change, so do the roles and functions of the psychiatric nurse. The role of the **psychiatric nurse** has changed over the years from that of custodian to a multifaceted one that includes the following:

• Providing direct client and family care

• Using the environment constructively

• Teaching self-care

• Coordinating the diverse aspects of care

• Providing continuity of care

• Advocating on the behalf of clients and their families

• Engaging in primary prevention activities

• Rehumanizing psychiatric care

Providing direct client and family care involves using the nursing process in many settings: the community, the in-patient psychiatric setting, walk-in clinics or health maintenance organizations, private practice, schools, industry, general hospital settings, and others. Because nurses are often considered the experts on the environment, helping clients and their families to use the environment constructively is a natural function for the nurse. Psychiatric nurses teach not only the traditional aspects of self-care—e.g., medications and health care—but also those empha-

RESEARCH NOTE

Citation

Warner SL: Humor: A coping response for student nurses. Arch Psychiatr Nurs 1991;5(1): 10–16.

Study Problem/Purpose

The purpose of this study was to answer the following research question: *Under what circumstances do student nurses choose to use humor as a coping method?* This study also identified the cognitive and behavioral efforts of student nurses in managing the emotions engendered by intrapersonal and interpersonal threats in a state psychiatric hospital setting.

Method

Thirty-eight senior student nurses enrolled in a psychiatric-mental health nursing course at a North-Central U.S. university participated anonymously in the volunteer study. They were asked to describe in writing a situation in which they experienced humor during the clinical experience at a state psychiatric hospital. A content analysis of the written narratives was conducted and the situations were categorized by identifying commonalities and differences. Data were examined until all narratives had been placed into mutually exclusive and exhaustive categories. The resulting taxonomy was examined for fit within the tenets of Lazarus's theory of stress and coping.

Findings

Six categories of tension-producing situations that emerged from the data were: (1) novel and bizarre client behaviors, e.g., repetitive behaviors or those that violated conventional social norms; (2) bizarre and novel patient thoughts, e.g., concrete thinking, delusions, neologisms, loose associations, and flights of fancy; (3) threats to self-esteem; (4) perceived role failure from misperceptions, making mistakes, and failing to live up to role expectations; (5) perceived threats to physical safety; and (6) wit (characterized by understanding a double entendre or a play on words). Each of these situations evoked tension expressed as anxiety, anger, bewilderment, boredom, fear, embarrassment, frustration, puzzlement, self-doubt, shame, suspicion, shock, bewilderment, and stunned surprise.

Cognitive coping strategies used to negate these emotions included reframing (from frustrating or frightening to funny), distancing from, rising above, and minimizing the event; escalating of the situation to the absurd; using cognitive shifts; and mastery. Behavioral strategies used to negate these emotions included ignoring, regressing, withdrawing, catharsis by sharing, and laughing.

Implications

Humor allowed the nursing students to regulate stressful emotions and/or alter a stressful person-environment relationship for positive outcomes, thereby qualifying as a coping response according to Lazarus's definition. Providing daily care for mentally disordered clients is draining. Laughing at oneself and one's peers, laughing with one's peers and one's clients, and even laughing at one's clients (assuming it is done in private places) is healthy coping. Delayed gratification (delaying laughter until returning to the dorm or to the classroom) was a recurrent theme in many of the narratives and indicates that the student nurses operated in accord with professional norms. Because learning can be enhanced by humor, such disclosures should be encouraged in clinical debriefings.

sized in psychiatric settings. Among the latter are how to relate to others, solve problems, communicate clearly, and try out new ways of being.

Two crucial roles for the psychiatric nurse are coordinating the diverse aspects of client care and evaluating how the components are functioning. The nurse is often the only professional with a complete appreciation of the client's round-the-clock activities. For this reason, the psychiatric nurse often provides the glue that cements continuity. Psychiatric nurses help to make sure that clients do not fall through the cracks in the health care system and that clients progress toward less restrictive living situations and less restrictive environments for care.

Being an advocate for clients and their families involves more than educating them about their rights and their responsibilities. Nurses must also work to influence local, state, national, and international policy in their dual roles as citizen and mental health professional. It is important to negotiate for mental health services for individuals and the community.

Teaching primary prevention is yet another psychiatric nursing role. Psychiatric nurses can inform the public about available mental health facilities, the nature of psychiatric illness, treatment approaches, and the prevention or reduction of stress.

Finally, rehumanizing psychiatric care involves providing humane care in an increasingly technologic society. It requires a judicious blending of "high touch" with "high tech," a person-to-person human experience.

In 1982, the ANA revised the guidelines for psychiatric nursing and mental health nursing practice. These professional practice and performance standards are given in the Nursing Standards box on page 38.

The Members of the Mental Health Team

Role definitions have become increasingly blurred among mental health workers as various members of the mental health team have taken on tasks traditionally assigned to other disciplines. This blurring of roles is perceived as having positive consequences at times and negative ones at others. It has increased the quantity and raised the quality of care in mental health settings. Some of the role changes have created anxiety among nurses who have become more interpersonally involved, more autonomous, and more responsible for the quality of mental health services delivered to the consumer. Psychiatrists, the traditional heads of mental health teams, have suffered some anxiety as other mental health workers and clients have sought to share in decision making and as other capable professionals have assumed administrative functions. Clinical nurse specialists, social workers, and psychologists, among others, have more direct influence than ever before. Roles are less specifically defined, and in many settings, mental health professionals take on whichever functions they do best.

The descriptions below of the education and tasks of mental health team members reflect traditional distinctions. Students should keep in mind that many of the functions are now shared across disciplines when the team member has been educated for the task and when laws permit the sharing of functions.

The Psychiatric Nursing Generalist

The *psychiatric nursing generalist* may have received basic nursing preparation in a diploma, associate degree, or baccalaureate program. Basically, a generalist who works in a specialized setting, this nurse provides the bulk of the nursing care to clients in in-patient settings. Registered nurses offer direct and indirect care through the nurse-client relationship, although they have received specialized training in psychotherapy. They have major responsibility for the milieu and have contact with clients at all stages of daily life. Nurses at this level may be certified as generalists through the ANA.

Colleagues who are clinical nursing specialists may supervise the registered nurse's therapeutic work and provide consultations.

The Psychiatric Nursing Clinical Specialist

The **clinical specialist in psychiatric nursing** is a graduate of a master's program providing specialization in the clinical area. A number of universities provide graduate study in adult, child, adolescent, and family psychiatric nursing and in community mental health as well. Nurses may also pursue the doctoral degree in two to four more years of study. The National Institute of Mental Health funds some programs, providing stipends and tuition-free study for qualified full-time students.

Clinical specialists may also seek **certification** by a professional nursing body. Certification attests to advanced level competence and is a means of protecting consumers. Certification at the advanced level exists nationally through the ANA.

Clinical specialists in psychiatric settings provide individual, family, and group psychotherapy in in-patient, outpatient, community mental health, and private practice milieus. They also provide indirect services, teach, consult, administer, and do research. The liaison psychiatric nurse provides these services in general hospital settings.

The Psychiatrist

The *psychiatrist* is a physician whose specialty area is mental disorders. Certification in psychiatry by the American Board of Psychiatry and Neurology requires a three-year approved psychiatric residency, two years of clinical psychiatric practice, and successful completion of an examination. Certification in neurology requires further preparation through a two-year neurology residency and an additional examination.

Psychiatrists are responsible for diagnosis and treatment. Some are oriented primarily toward biologic therapies, others are psychotherapeutically oriented, and a few are chiefly interested in community psychiatry. In traditional medical model settings and in many in-patient settings, the psychiatrist is usually the team leader or administrator. This is not so in milieus where role distinctions are less clearly defined.

The Psychoanalyst

In the United States, a person must be a physician in order to become a *psychoanalyst*. Analysts are trained at psychoanalytic institutes that provide training programs in psychoanalysis only. The majority of psycho-

NURSING STANDARDS

1982 ANA Standards of Psychiatric and Mental Health Nursing Practice

Professional Practice Standards

Standard 1 Theory
The nurse applies appropriate theory that is scientifically sound as a basis for decisions regarding nursing practice.

Standard 2 Data Collection
The nurse continuously collects data that are comprehensive, accurate, and systematic.

Standard 3 Diagnosis
The nurse utilizes nursing diagnoses and/or standard classifications of mental disorders to express conclusions supported by recorded assessment data and current scientific premises.

Standard 4 Planning
The nurse develops a nursing care plan with specific goals and interventions delineating nursing actions unique to each client's needs.

Standard 5 Intervention
The nurse intervenes as guided by the nursing care plan to implement nursing actions that promote, maintain, or restore physical and mental health, prevent illness, and effect rehabilitation.

Standard 5A Psychotherapeutic Interventions
The nurse uses psychotherapeutic interventions to assist clients in regaining or improving their previous coping abilities and to prevent further disability.

Standard 5B Health Teaching
The nurse assists clients, families, and groups to achieve satisfying and productive patterns of living through health teaching.

Standard 5C Activities of Daily Living
The nurse uses the activities of daily living in a goal-directed way to foster adequate self-care and physical and mental well-being of clients.

Standard 5D Somatic Therapies
The nurse uses knowledge of somatic therapies and applies related clinical skills in working with clients.

Standard 5E Therapeutic Environment
The nurse provides, structures, and maintains a therapeutic environment in collaboration with the client and other health care providers.

Standard 5F Psychotherapy*
The nurse utilizes advanced clinical expertise in individual, group, and family psychotherapy, child psychotherapy, and other treatment modalities to function as a psychotherapist, and recognizes professional accountability for nursing practice.

Standard 6 Evaluation
The nurse evaluates client responses to nursing action in order to revise the data base, nursing diagnoses, and nursing care plan.

Professional Performance Standards

Standard 7 Peer Review
The nurse participates in peer review and other means of evaluation to assure quality of nursing care provided for clients.

Standard 8 Continuing Education
The nurse assumes responsibility for continuing education and professional development and contributes to the professional growth of others.

Standard 9 Interdisciplinary Collaboration
The nurse collaborates with other health care providers in assessing, planning, implementing, and evaluating programs and other mental health activities.

Standard 10 Utilization of Community Health Systems*
The nurse participates with other members of the community in assessing, planning, implementing, and evaluating mental health services and community systems that include the promotion of the broad continuum of primary, secondary, and tertiary prevention of mental illness.

Standard 11 Research
The nurse contributes to nursing and the mental health field through innovations in theory and practice and participation in research.

*Standards 5F and 10 are specific to clinical specialists with a master's degree in the specialty of psychiatric/mental health nursing.

SOURCE: ANA Standards of Psychiatric and Mental Health Nursing Practice. *Published by the American Nurses' Association and reprinted by permission.*

analysts are in private practice in large urban settings. They may also be certified in the practice of psychiatry, neurology, and/or psychoanalysis. There are nonphysician analysts, called *lay analysts,* who are also trained at psychoanalytic institutes. Some nurses have become lay analysts.

The Clinical Psychologist

The *clinical psychologist* is a psychologist specially educated and trained in the area of mental health. To be certified, the clinical psychologist must hold a doctoral degree from a program approved by the American Psychological Association and must have completed a one-year psychology internship at an approved clinical facility.

Clinical psychologists perform psychotherapy; plan and implement programs of behavior modification; select, administer, and interpret psychologic tests; and carry out research.

The Psychiatric Social Worker

The *psychiatric social worker* is a graduate of a two-year master's program in social work with an emphasis in the field of psychiatry. Social workers deal with the social problems that confront clients and their families. Their goals are to help clients and their families cope more effectively; identify appropriate community resources for clients; help the hospitalized person maintain relationships with family, friends, and the community; and facilitate the client's return to community. With the blurring of traditional mental health roles, social workers have undertaken counseling and psychotherapeutic roles in various settings, including private practice.

The Mental Health/Human Service Worker

The newest addition to the psychiatric team is the *mental health/human service worker.* The growing need for mental health services, the manpower crisis, the widespread popularity and economy of community college programs, and the documented effectiveness of these workers are responsible for the emergence of more than 400 mental health/human service training programs at the certificate, associate, and baccalaureate levels.

The Psychiatric Aide or Attendant

Paraprofessionals provide much of the direct service to hospitalized persons, particularly in large public facilities. These nonprofessional workers are known by a variety of titles, including *psychiatric aide, psychiatric technician,* and *psychiatric attendant.* Most agencies that employ psychiatric aides provide in-service training programs to help them use their interpersonal potential. Because a large number of the personnel who work in in-patient settings are psychiatric aides, it is extremely important that they maintain a therapeutic milieu under the supervision of professional nurses.

The Occupational Therapist

Occupational therapists in mental health settings use manual and creative techniques to elicit desired interpersonal and intrapsychic responses. In some settings they may participate in preparing clients for return to community living by teaching self-help activities or, in sheltered workshop settings, help clients prepare to seek employment. The Occupational Therapist, Registered (OTR) has a baccalaureate degree in occupational therapy or a master's degree in occupational therapy after receiving a baccalaureate in another field. The OTR also supervises Certified Occupational Therapy Assistants (COTA). A COTA is a graduate of an associate degree program and helps clients follow treatment plans.

The Recreational Therapist

The *recreational therapist,* taking into consideration the therapeutic needs of clients, plans and guides recreational activities to provide not only socialization and healthful recreation but also desirable interpersonal and intrapsychic experiences. With increasing frequency, recreational therapists are being prepared in university physical education and health education programs.

The Creative Arts Therapist

Creative arts therapists use art, music, dance, and poetry to facilitate personal experiences and increase social responses and self-esteem. Although creative arts therapists are not found in all settings, they are becoming valued and recognized members of the mental health team. Creative arts therapists have their own programs of study in colleges and universities as well as their own professional organizations, such as the American Art Therapy Association, the American Dance Therapy Association, and the National Association for Music Therapy. Chapter 29 discusses art, music, dance, and poetry therapy groups.

Collaborating On the Mental Health Team

Psychiatric nurses, whether practicing in institutions or in private practice settings, must plan and share with others to deliver maximum mental health services to clients. The purpose of collaboration is to make the best use of the different abilities of mental health team members so that the client receives the most effective service available. Relationship problems among mental health team members must be worked through to avoid distorting the team's efforts in behalf of the client.

Cooperation versus Competition

The key to working together on a common problem for a common purpose is cooperation rather than competition. Cooperation ensures movement toward the common goal, whereas inappropriate competition hinders goal achievement and may be destructive to the competing individuals.

Most of the present understanding of cooperative and competitive behavior has come from the efforts of game theorists, who have researched player behavior. Players have been categorized as:

- Maximizers—those interested only in their own gain

- Rivalists—those interested only in defeating their partners

- Cooperators—those interested in helping both themselves and their partners.

Maximizers and rivalists jeopardize the client's welfare because they put themselves first and the client last. Rivalists direct their energies toward being "one up" through put-downs of others. They are concerned not with the client but with the process of winning. Cooperators are interested in helping both themselves and their colleagues to aid the client. Participants who actively recognize the importance of each individual member of the mental health team can influence maximizers and rivalists to become cooperators.

Respect for the Positions of Others

Most nursing textbooks and nursing instructors emphasize the need to respect and accept the client and to act in ways that demonstrate personal trustworthiness. They less often consider the need to respect, accept, and trust one's colleagues. Yet effective collaboration is based on respect for the position from which another participant acts. Our values and our culture direct our beliefs and the climate in which we operate. Knowing this, we can become aware of the values and culture of others, and, in turn, respect them.

Unfortunately, the process of socialization into a profession may make it difficult for a person to respect, accept, and trust the position of another. As students become committed to a profession through the process of socialization, they tend to view members of other disciplines with suspicion. Nursing is particularly susceptible in this regard because nurses have had to struggle to become colleagues with other health pro-

fessionals. They may not yet have gained the degree of comfort and professional self-esteem that permits nonthreatened respect, acceptance, and trust of others. As lines become blurred and once-sacred tasks and functions are shared, other colleagues may experience anxiety about respecting, accepting, and trusting the psychiatric nurse.

Supervision, support, and self-exploration are recommended for the expansion of nursing roles within and beyond traditional relationships. Clinical supervision of nurses by nurses can help pinpoint times when traditional caretaking roles are appropriate and when they inhibit growth. Administrative and peer support creates an atmosphere in which nurses are free to share their knowledge, skills, and evolving ideas. Such support increases creativity, depth, and perspective in nursing. Self-exploration and self-assessment, through reading and dialogue with other nurses, can help nurses to consider alternatives to traditional stereotypic roles.

Engaging the Client in Collaboration

It is best to include clients in the collaboration of the mental health team whenever possible. This allows clients to participate in their health care and assures nurses that their clients are informed consumers of mental health services.

Clients can also be invited to participate in case conferences. These conferences often have an important place in the functioning of mental health agencies and may have a number of purposes. The client should be invited to participate in case conferences that involve collaboration among a number of agencies or a number of mental health workers moving toward similar goals with the client.

The client should be consulted about the information the nurse shares with other members of the mental health team. It is not always easy for the nurse to determine exactly how much to share and with whom. When the question of confidentiality is not clear, the nurse should also confer with the supervisor or a colleague to determine what should be shared. Decisions should take into consideration what agreement exists between nurse and client about sharing information and how the person or agency receiving information will use that information in the client's best interests.

Excellence and Power in Practice

According to Benner (1984), the *competencies* of a psychiatric nurse can be differentiated from *goals* (how the nurse generally uses psychosocial knowledge to achieve a particular aim or realize an intention in a therapeutic relationship) and from practice *strategies* (how the nurse interacts to help clients move in the direction of growth). Both goals and practice strategies are clearly influenced by the psychiatric nurse's personal and professional philosophies. Benner's exemplars (nurses who served as examples in her study) of excellence revealed that psychiatric nurses:

• Acted as psychologic and cultural mediators to help confused people "carve a path into a more shared, less idiosyncratic world" (p 67)

• Used goals therapeutically in that goals were realistic, workable, and aimed toward improved social and psychologic functioning

• Worked to build and maintain a therapeutic community for working out issues of trust, conflict, and cooperation

Exemplars of excellence in practice challenge nurses to implement their caring power and professional philosophy even under conditions that act as barriers and constraints in the everyday world.

Barriers and Constraints to Excellence

Aspiring toward therapeutic client relationships that are caring, sensitive, holistic, meaningful, and non-judgmental can be stressful. The nurse must work under conditions that are strongly influenced by economics, legislation, multiple levels of bureaucracy and paperwork, competition among members of the interdisciplinary mental health team, increased reliance on psychotropic medication, hasty discharges, limited follow-up care, a revolving-door pattern of hospital use, and short hospital stays.

Toward a New Entitlement

As Benner (1984) concludes, achieving excellence under the constraints described above requires philosophies of commitment and involvement, but it also requires power. She advocates six strategies for balancing professional/philosophic mandates with the constraints of the context in which we practice. At the root of these strategies is the nurse's power to implement change through caring and expertise. In Benner's view, the nurse needs the following:

1. *Transformative power,* by which the nurse helps clients transform their views of self or others

2. *Integrative caring,* through which the nurse helps clients continue with meaningful life activities despite disability and disorders

3. *Advocacy power* to remove obstacles or stand alongside and enable

4. *Healing power* to create a climate that mobilizes hope, to find interpretations of situations that are acceptable and clarifying to clients and families, and to help clients use sources of social, emotional, and spiritual support

5. *Participative/affirmative power,* in which engagement and involvement are sources of energy

6. *Problem-solving expertise* to grasp the problem rapidly, seeing it in relation to similar as well as dissimilar situations encountered in the past, yet not overlooking creative search and cue sensitivity (Benner 1984, pp 210–215)

The chapters that follow in this text offer sources of excellence and power in the practice of humanistic interactionist psychiatric nursing.

CHAPTER HIGHLIGHTS

• The psychiatric nurse's capacity for empathy and ability to collaborate on the mental health team are related to the nurse's consciousness of meaning, use of language, willingness to negotiate, definitions of reality, awareness of feelings, ability to take care of self, and own self-view.

• Psychiatric nurses experience significant stresses in attempting to relate fully to clients and still maintain their own personal integration.

• Burning out is an attempt to cope with the stresses of intense interpersonal work by a form of distancing.

• The causes of professional burnout are most likely rooted in the social context of the work situation, not in the psychologic characteristics of the individual.

• To preserve personal integration nurses can develop assertiveness, recognize the need and plan for some time alone, maintain personal physical health, and attend to cues of personal stress.

• Characteristics of artful therapeutic practice include respect for the client, availability, spontaneity, hope, acceptance, sensitivity, vision, accountability, and empathy.

• Phases in the development of empathic understanding are identification, incorporation, reverberation, and detachment.

• The psychiatric nurse's professional role includes providing direct client and family care, using the environment constructively, teaching self-care, coordinating the diverse aspects of care, providing continuity of care, advocating on behalf of clients and their families, engaging in primary prevention activities, and rehumanizing psychiatric care.

• Members of the mental health team frequently practicing in contemporary United States settings include the psychiatric nursing generalist, the psychiatric nursing clinical specialist, the psychiatrist, the psychoanalyst, the clinical psychologist, the psychiatric social worker, the mental health/human service worker, the psychiatric aide or attendant, the occupational therapist, and the creative arts therapist.

• Quality of mental health services depends on cooperation among health team members and across disciplines, knowledge about each member's contribution, inclusion of the client in decision making, and respect for the position of others.

• Despite barriers and constraints to implementing a professional philosophy in real-world practice, psychiatric nurses can and do find sources of power.

REFERENCES

American Nurses' Association: *Standards of Psychiatric and Mental Health Nursing Practice.* ANA, 1982.

Benfer B: Defining the role and function of the psychiatric nurse as a member of the team. *Perspect Psychiatr Care* 1980;18:166–177.

Benner P: *From Novice to Expert: Excellence and Power in Clinical Nursing Practice.* Addison-Wesley, 1984.

Benner P, Wrubel J: Coping with caregiving, in *The Primacy of Caring: Stress and Coping in Health and Illness.* Addison-Wesley, 1989, 365–406.

Chenevert M: *STAT: Special Techniques in Assertiveness Training for Women in the Health Professions,* ed 2. Mosby, 1983.

Cohen S, McQuade K: Developing empathy with co-workers. *Am J Nurs* 1983;83:1573–1588.

Cosgray RE, et al.: A day in the life of an inpatient: An experiential game to promote empathy for individuals in a psychiatric hospital. *Arch Psychiatr Nurs* 1990; 4(6):354–359.

Cronin-Stubbs D, Brophy EB: Burnout: Can social support save the psychiatric nurse? *J Psychosoc Nurs* 1985; 23(7):8–13.

Edelwich J, Brodsky A: *Burn-out: Stages of Disillusionment in the Helping Professions.* Human Sciences Press, 1980.

Floyd JA: Nursing students' stress levels, attitudes toward drugs, and drug use. *Arch Psychiatr Nurs* 1991; 5(1):46–53.

Foster SW: The pragmatics of culture: The rhetoric of difference in psychiatric nursing. *Arch Psychiatr Nurs* 1990;4(5):292–297.

Henderson FC, McGettigan BO: *Managing Your Career in Nursing.* Addison-Wesley, 1986.

Kalisch P, Kalisch BJ: *The Changing Image of the Nurse.* Addison-Wesley, 1987.

Kilkins SP: Self-assertion and nurses: A different voice. *Nurs Outlook* 1990;38(3):143–145.

Mason DJ, Talbott SW: *Political Action Handbook for Nurses.* Addison-Wesley, 1985.

Mericle BP: The male as psychiatric nurse. *J Psychosoc Nurs* 1983;21(11):28–34.

McBride AB: Psychiatric nursing in the 1990s. *Arch Psychiatr Nurs* 1990;4(1):21–27.

McConnell EA: *Burnout in the Nursing Profession.* Mosby, 1982.

McKeon KL: Introduction: A future perspective on psychiatric mental health nursing. *Arch Psychiatr Nurs* 1990;4(1):119–120.

Muff J: Handmaiden, battle axe, whore: An exploration into the fantasies, myths, and stereotypes about nursing, in Muff J (ed): *Socialization, Sexism and Stereotyping.* Mosby, 1982.

Muff J: Balancing communication, in Smythe EEM: *Surviving Nursing.* Addison-Wesley, 1984.

Peplau HE: The psychiatric nurse—accountable? To whom? For what? *Perspect Psychiatr Care* 1980;18(3):128–134.

Pines AM, Kanner AD: Burnout: Lack of positive conditions and presence of negative conditions as two independent sources of stress. *J Psychiatr Nurs Ment Health Serv* 1982;20(8):30.

Smythe EEM: *Surviving Nursing.* Addison-Wesley, 1984.

Snow C, Willard D: *I'm Dying to Take Care of You.* Professional Counselor Books, 1989.

Thomas S, Witt D: Mental health nursing clinical specialization: Extinction or adaptation? *Issues Ment Health Nurs* 1986;8(1):1–13.

Warner SL: Humor: A coping response for student nurses. *Arch Psychiatr Nurs* 1991;5(1):10–16.

Wilson HS, Kneisl CR: *Learning Activities in Psychiatric Nursing,* ed 3. Addison-Wesley, 1988.

Applying the Nursing Process

Holly Skodol Wilson

LEARNING OBJECTIVES

- Discuss the steps of the nursing process in relation to the 1982 Standards of Psychiatric Mental Health Nursing Practice

- Apply the nursing process to situations involving clients with psychiatric/ mental health diagnoses

CROSS REFERENCES

Other topics relevant to this content are: Assessment, Chapter 9; and Theories, Chapter 4.

How DOES A NURSE approach the following clinical problems? Obviously no quick and easy cookbook formulas are adequate for responding to such genuine human complexities. The 1982 ANA Standards of Psychiatric and Mental Health Nursing Practice reflect the current state of knowledge in the field and offer some guidance in providing nursing care to clients like those described below.

Diane S, a 23-year-old woman, is admitted to a medical unit with severe anorexia nervosa and thoughts of suicide. She is agitated and tearful and says life looks so bad that she just wants to get out of it.

B J. is a 27-year-old man who walked into the hospital emergency room because he sees the walls sparkling and weaving around, he feels like people are laughing at him, and he tastes petroleum in his mouth, which he describes as the "taste of afterbirth." He was on his way to jump off the George Washington Bridge when he saw the hospital and decided to come in for help.

The client is a 52-year-old, disheveled woman dressed in ragged street clothes and wearing a turban on her head. She believes that there are radio waves in her teeth reporting of a plot to have her committed to mental hospitals. She has lived on the streets for the past two years with all her possessions and clothing in four large brown paper bags. She speaks in an uninterrupted monotone and is hostile toward the nurse.

The six standards of psychiatric and mental health nursing presented in the accompanying Nursing Standards box are the focus of this chapter. Together they guide the nurse in the use of the nursing process in the practice of psychiatric-mental health nursing.

Applying the Nursing Process

The word *process* suggests movement toward a goal in phases or stages. The nursing process is the conscious, systematic set of cognitive and behavioral steps that make up the clinical act of nursing practice. It is adapted from the scientific approach to problem solving. The steps include:

1. Assessment of the client's health status from objective and subjective data (collecting and reviewing data)

2. Formulation of a psychiatric nursing diagnosis (identifying problems)

3. Development of a plan for nursing intervention (choosing interventions)

4. Implementation of the planned interventions (putting the plan in action)

5. Evaluation of the nursing care (judging the effectiveness of the plan and changing it when needed)

This chapter describes the ways in which the nursing process approach is applied to psychiatric nursing practice. We urge that the nursing process become the way in which nurses think about clients with the human responses discussed in other chapters of this text. Nursing process is currently used in most nursing curricula and included in most nurse practice acts. The nursing process is flexible and adaptable. It

NURSING STANDARDS

1982 ANA Standards of Psychiatric and Mental Health Nursing

Professional Practice Standards
Standard 1 Theory
The nurse applies appropriate theory that is scientifically sound as a basis for decisions regarding nursing practice.
Standard 2 Data Collection
The nurse continuously collects data that are comprehensive, accurate, and systematic.
Standard 3 Diagnosis
The nurse utilizes nursing diagnoses and standard classification of mental disorders to express conclusions supported by recorded assessment data and current scientific premises.
Standard 4 Planning
The nurse develops a nursing care plan with specific goals and interventions delineating nursing actions unique to each client's needs.
Standard 5 Intervention
The nurse intervenes as guided by the nursing care plan to implement nursing actions that promote, maintain, or restore physical and mental health, prevent illness, and effect rehabilitation.
Standard 6 Evaluation
The nurse evaluates client responses to nursing actions in order to revise the data base, nursing diagnoses, and nursing care plan.

SOURCE: ANA Standards of Psychiatric and Mental Health Nursing Practice. *Published by the American Nurse's Association and reprinted by permission.*

can be applied in a variety of settings with individual clients, families, groups, and aggregates. It requires that the nurse use judgment and creativity in caring for clients in an organized and systematic way.

Assessing

Standard 2 of the 1982 Standards of Psychiatric and Mental Health Nursing Practice states:

The nurse continuously collects data that are comprehensive, accurate, and systematic.

Rationale   The rationale for including assessment among the standards of quality in nursing derives from a belief that effective nursing depends on comprehensive, accurate, systematic, and continuous data collection that enables the nurse to reach sound conclusions about the client's human responses to actual and potential mental health problems. From these data, the nurse plans fitting interventions.

Process Criteria

1. The nurse informs the clients that data collection is their mutual responsibility.

2. The nurse seeks data in at least the following categories:

- Biophysical, developmental, emotional, and mental status

- Spiritual resources and beliefs

- Family, social, cultural, and community systems

- Daily activities, interactions with others, and coping patterns

- Economic, environmental, and political factors affecting the client's health

- Personally significant support systems including those that are available in the community but not yet used

- Knowledge, satisfaction, and motivation for change of health practice and status

- Strengths that can be used in reaching health goals

- Knowledge pertinent to legal rights

- Contribution from the family, significant others, and members of the mental health care team

Outcome Criteria

1. Clients and their significant others participate in and affirm that the data-gathering process was beneficial to them.

2. Data are recorded in a standard format.

RESEARCH NOTE

Citation
Mulhearn S: The nursing process: Improving psychiatric admission assessment? J Adv Nurs 1989;14:808–814.

Study Problem/Purpose
Mulhearn explored whether the current admission assessment procedure in a psychiatric setting assisted in systematic care planning when compared to the introduction of a structured nursing assessment approach.

Methods
Sample. The sample population consisted of 18 qualified staff members working on two wards in two hospitals. These wards, chosen at random, were a psychiatric unit in a large district general hospital and an admissions ward at a local psychiatric hospital in England. The data base comprised the medical records of twenty clients on both wards and comments by the nurses who had admitted them.

Materials and Procedures. The data analyzed were based on the records of clients and staff comments on a "satisfaction indicator" form. (Ten clients were also interviewed to determine how acceptable they found the detailed questioning required by the new structured admission procedure.)

Findings
Results of this exploratory study suggest that structured assessment procedures appeared to assist in the collection of individualized client information and systematic nursing care planning, especially by novice nurses. More experienced staff noted that while the structured approach did assist in systematic care planning, it was time-consuming and would require further modification and study.

Implications
Although the application of artful intuition in psychiatric mental health nursing is valuable, the standard acceptance of nursing assessment procedures, formats, and informatics may enhance clinical credibility, accountability, and communication, especially among novices. Teaching the nursing process continues to be supported by related research.

Data collection requires astute observation, purposeful listening, broad knowledge of human behavior, and understanding of what needs to be known and where to obtain the information. The tools used in psychiatric assessment of individual clients include the following:

- Psychiatric history

- Mental status examination

- Psychosocial assessment

- Neurologic assessment

- Psychologic testing

These assessment tools are discussed in Chapter 9.

Subjective Data Subjective data are reported by the client and significant others in their own words. An example is the **chief complaint** expressed by clients in the course of an intake interview or psychiatric history. Here are some examples of chief complaints:

I was in "warp 5" and pretending to be an undercover cop.

My brother doesn't think I take good enough care of myself.

My husband has been beating me and I think I am losing my mind.

Objective Data Objective data are collected and verified by people other than the client and family. Here are some examples:

- Physical examination findings, e.g., hearing loss

- Neurologic examination findings, e.g., those observed when testing for reflexes or observing for tremors

- Results of psychometric tests, e.g., the Temporal and Personal Orientation Test or the Global Cognitive Function and Language Comprehension Tests used to assess functional status among the elderly

- Scores on rating scales developed to quantify the severity of disabilities among the chronically mentally ill

- Laboratory test results, including complete blood count, sedimentation rate, blood chemistry, thyroid function studies, serum vitamin B_{12}, folate levels, computed tomography brain scan, chest X-ray films, and electrocardiograms

The Nursing History The nursing history is the foremost method of collecting data from the primary source (the client). Nursing histories summarize client information that the nurse can use to individualize care. They differ from medical or psychiatric histories, which are records of previous illness and hospitalizations, in that they focus on the *clients' perceptions and expectations* related to their illness, hospitalization, and care. See the accompanying Assessment box for a sample guide for a holistic nursing history.

The **primary** subjective and objective **data source** is the client. **Secondary data sources** include laboratory and psychologic test results, family members, and other members of the mental health team. Together, these data sources provide a rationale for determining the client's nursing diagnosis and a basis for planning, implementing, and evaluating nursing care. The assessment phase of the nursing process culminates in the formulation of a nursing diagnosis.

Diagnosing

Standard 3 of the 1982 Standards of Psychiatric and Mental Health Nursing Practice states:

The nurse utilizes nursing diagnoses and standard classification of mental disorders to express conclusions supported by recorded assessment data and current scientific premises.

Several definitions of **nursing diagnosis** exist in the nursing literature, including the following one, used in this text: "A nursing diagnosis is the statement of a patient's response which is actually or potentially unhealthful and which nursing intervention can help to change in the direction of health" (Mundinger and Jauron 1975, p 97).

Rationale The rationale for inclusion of Standard 3 is that nurses' logical basis for providing care rests on recognition and identification of actual or potential health problems within the scope of nursing practice. In other words, formulation of nursing diagnoses makes it possible to identify the specific contribution of nurses to the health team. A diagnostic classification system for psychiatric nursing practice that applies diagnoses specific to nursing interventions enhances our ability to define the scope of nursing and answer the question, "What do psychiatric nurses do that is different from what social workers, psychologists, and psychiatrists do?"

Process Criteria

- Peer validation of nursing diagnoses

- Peer exchange, education, and research regarding the scientific and humanistic premises underlying nursing diagnoses

- Nursing diagnoses for psychiatric clients that identify actual or potential health problems in respect to the categories outlined in the Nursing Diagnosis box on page 49.

ASSESSMENT

Psychiatric Nursing History Guide

A. General Information

Client's name, age, medical diagnosis, occupation (client's and spouse), religion, educational level, residence, marital status

B. Guide Questions

1. Family situation
   a. With whom do you live?
   b. How many children do you have, if any?
   c. Who is caring for them while you are here?
   d. How many brothers and sisters do you have?
   e. Do your parents live nearby?
   f. Was there anything that happened to you or your family in the past year other than this illness that was upsetting to you?

2. Work situation (including financial aspect)
   a. What type of work do you do?
   b. How long have you done this type of work?
   c. Are you on sick leave from work?
   d. Do you think your illness will interfere with your work?
   e. Do you have health insurance?

3. Client's activities
   a. What kind of environment and pace are you used to?
   b. What are your feelings concerning your activity schedule in the hospital?
   c. Do you have any special interests or hobbies that you would like to pursue, if feasible, while you are here?
   d. What habits have you had to change here?

4. Eating habits
   a. Are you on a restricted diet?
   b. Are you allergic to any foods?
   c. Are there any particular foods you like or dislike?
   d. Do you eat breakfast?
   e. Do you need an early morning cup of coffee or the like?
   f. How many times do you eat each day?
   g. When do you usually eat your meals?
   h. Has being sick affected your eating habits? How?
   i. Do you foresee any difficulty with hospital food?
   j. Do you prefer plain or ice water?
   k. Are you accustomed to eating snacks? At regular times?

5. Sleeping habits
   a. How long do you usually sleep? Between what hours?
   b. Do you sleep well at home?
   c. Do you nap? Occasionally? Regularly? Rarely?
   d. Are you an early riser?
   e. Do you need medication to sleep?
   f. Do you get up at intervals?
   g. Does light or noise disturb you?
   h. If you are awakened at night, can you go back to sleep?
   i. Do you sleep with a night light on?
   j. Do you like an extra blanket at night?
   k. Do you usually sleep with a window closed or open?
   l. Have you found that strange surroundings decrease your ability to sleep soundly?
   m. How many pillows do you use?

6. Elimination habits
   a. What are your elimination habits at home?
   b. Do you have any difficulty with elimination?
   c. Do you take laxatives? If so, how often?
   d. Do you take any special foods to aid in elimination?

7. Allergies
   a. Do you have any allergies to drugs, food, adhesive tape, etc.?

8. Drugs or special diets
   a. Were you on any medications before you came to the hospital?
   b. Do you routinely take any nonprescription medicines?
   c. Did you bring any of these medications with you?

9. Previous illnesses or hospitalizations
   a. Have you had other experiences when you or members of your family were ill?
      1) What kind of experience was it—good, bad, indifferent?
      2) What problems, if any, did you or they encounter?

▶

ASSESSMENT (continued)

b. Have you ever been sick before?
1) What was wrong?
2) Were you in the hospital?
3) How long were you sick?
4) What do you remember most about being hospitalized?
5) What did you like most about the hospital care, routines, etc.?
c. Do you have any disability, other than your present illness, that may restrict your normal activity?
d. Who cares for you when you are sick at home?
e. What can you do when you are sick at home that makes you feel better?

10. Current illness
a. Why are you in the hospital?
b. What do you think made you ill?
c. How long have you been ill?
d. Can you tell me what you feel about your illness?
e. What kinds of things usually make you feel better when you are sick?
f. Were there other things that happened when you first became ill?
g. What do you feel about the outcome of your illness?
h. What is causing you the most discomfort at this time?

11. Current hospitalization
a. What do you think you need done for you while you are here?
b. What do you feel about being here in the hospital?
c. What do you miss most by being in this hospital?
d. Are there things at home that you would like to have here with you? If so, what?
e. Are there things at home that might bother or worry you while you are here?

12. Personal preferences regarding visitors—family and friends
a. If feasible, would you prefer to be alone or with other clients during the day?
b. Would you like to have visitors?
1) Just family?
2) Just friends?
3) Both family and friends?
4) Just certain individuals? Who?
c. How many visitors would you like at one time and how frequently?

d. Is it possible for your family or friends to visit you if you so desire?
e. Has anyone visited you yet, or did anyone come with you when you were admitted?
f. (For persons with serious illness, or as hospital policy allows) Would you feel better if it was possible for some of your family to stay here with you overnight?

13. Expectations of hospital personnel and physician by client
a. Would you like your doctor and nurses to explain everything that is going on with you?
b. Would you be comfortable enough to ask them questions if they do not explain?
c. Would you like someone to come in frequently during the day just to talk or be with you?
d. Is there anything special you expect or would like me to do for you or see that it gets done, if feasible, while you are here?
e. What do you expect from nurses?
g. What has your doctor told you about your illness and what to expect while you are in the hospital?
h. What do you expect from your doctor?
i. What do you expect from the hospital?
j. What do you expect from hospital policy or routine?
k. Would you like a minister to visit with you, if possible?
l. How best can we help you while you are in the hospital?

C. Visual Observation on General Appearance
1. Immediate general impression of appearance:
2. Overall physical appearance:
3. Motor activity/posture:
4. Build and weight:
5. Prosthesis/limitations/debilitations:
6. Complexion and appearance of skin:
   a. Color   b. Lesions
   c. Abrasions   d. Rash
7. Subjective symptoms:
   a. Watery eyes   b. Running nose
   c. Cough
8. Mouth:
   a. Oral hygiene   b. Dentures

ASSESSMENT (continued)

9. Eyes:
    a. Eye glasses   b. Contact lenses
10. Age group:
11. Clothing:
12. Belongings and objects in environment:
13. Speech:
14. Apparent cultural, educational, and intellectual levels:
15. Other pertinent factors:

D. Nonverbal Behavior Observations
    1. Emotional tone, facial expression, attitude:
    2. Gestures, movements, or activities during interview:

3. Main theme of client's conversation and behavior:
4. Topics the client seemed to avoid:
5. Client's response to interviewer:
6. Interviewer's response to client:
7. Other pertinent factors:

E. Summary

SOURCE: *Lamonica EL:* The Nursing Process: A Humanistic Approach: *Addison-Wesley, 1979. Jones & Bartlett Publishers, Inc., Boston.*

NURSING DIAGNOSIS

Categories of Nursing Diagnoses for Psychiatric Clients According to ANA Standards

- Self-care limitations or impaired functioning with general etiologies, such as mental and emotional distress, deficits in the ways significant systems are functioning, and internal psychic or developmental issues relevant to health

- Emotional stress or crisis components of illness, pain, self-concept changes, and life process changes

- Emotional problems related to daily experiences such as anxiety, aggression, loss, loneliness, and grief

- Physical symptoms, such as altered intestinal functioning or anorexia, which occur simultaneously with altered psychic functioning

- Alterations in thinking, perceiving, symbolizing, communication, and decision-making abilities

- Behaviors and mental states that indicate that the client is a danger to self or others or is gravely disabled

Outcome Criteria The outcome criteria for meeting this standard are that nursing diagnoses are validated by the client or the client's significant others and recorded to facilitate nursing research.

Guidelines recommended by members of the First National Conference on the Classification of Nursing Diagnoses (Gebbie and Lavin 1975) further guide the nurse in this process. They include the following:

- People should be viewed as whole, worthwhile, dignified beings regardless of their degree of dysfunction or level of competence.

- Nursing diagnoses should involve the client and should be validated with the client.

- Nursing diagnoses should be stated in terms of concerns and levels of competence or dysfunction.

- Nursing diagnoses should always be referred to as "nursing" diagnoses to avoid confusion with medical diagnoses.

The Two-Component Statement of Nursing Diagnosis Most authorities propose that the nursing diagnosis statement have two components:

- The client's potential or actual unhealthful response

- The reasons for or possible etiology of the client's unhealthful response

These authorities believe that incorporating both components gives clearer direction to the planning, implementation, and evaluation steps of the nursing process. Others maintain that cause-and-effect relationships are premature given the current state of nursing research and that the etiology component of the diagnosis statement is therefore purely speculative. This text acknowledges the lack of consensus on the issue of etiology and presents nursing diagnosis as a name for a perceived difficulty (ANA 1980, p 11) organized by a classification system. A compromise position is to give the name of a difficulty and add a "related factor" phrase.

Toward a Classification System for Psychiatric Nursing Diagnoses

NANDA The **North American Nursing Diagnosis Association** (NANDA) solicits proposed new nursing diagnoses for review by the association. Such proposed diagnoses undergo a systematic review that concludes with a mail vote by the entire membership. If the proposed diagnosis is accepted, it is included in NANDA's official list of diagnoses. Such acceptance indicates NANDA's view that the diagnosis is ready for use and continuing development.

To assist interested parties in submitting proposed diagnoses, the NANDA Diagnoses Review Committee has prepared a set of guidelines for submission. These guidelines ensure consistency, clarity, and completeness of submissions. Submitted diagnoses that do not meet the guidelines are returned to the person submitting them for revision so that the review process can begin. Proposed diagnoses are reviewed by the Diagnoses Review Committee, the Clinical Technical Review Task Forces, and the NANDA board prior to review and comment by the General Assembly and membership vote. An example of a proposed nursing diagnosis in the required NANDA format appears in the accompanying Nursing Diagnosis box.

The alphabetical list of NANDA nursing diagnoses (in the Nursing Diagnosis box on pp 51–52) is organized into nine "human response patterns." These are:

1. Exchanging—mutual giving and receiving
2. Communicating—sending messages
3. Relating—establishing bonds
4. Valuing—assigning relative worth
5. Choosing—selecting alternatives
6. Moving—activity
7. Perceiving—receiving information
8. Knowing—meaning associated with information
9. Feeling—subjective awareness of information

NANDA nursing diagnoses have the following components:

- Definition
- Etiology
- Defining characteristics

NURSING DIAGNOSIS

NANDA Nursing Diagnosis: Hopelessness

Definition
A subjective state in which an individual sees no alternatives or personal choices available and cannot mobilize energy on own behalf.

Defining Characteristics:
Major: Passivity, decreased verbalization
Minor: Lack of initiative; decreased response to stimuli; decreased affect; verbal cues (hopeless content, "I can't," sighing); turning away from speaker; closing eyes; shrugging in response to speaker; decreased appetite, increased sleep; lack of involvement in care/passively allowing care

Substantiating/Supportive Materials
Eisman, R. (1971). Why did Joe die? *American Journal of Nursing*, March.

Farbertow, N.L.O. (1981). Suicide prevention in the hospital. *Hospital and Community Psychiatry, 32*(2), 99–104.

Jolowiec, A., Powers, M.J. (1981). Stress and coping in hypertensive and ER patients. *Nursing Research*, January–February.

Jourad. (1970). Suicide, an invitation to die. *American Journal of Nursing*, February.

Kritek, P. (1981). Patient power and powerlessness. *Supervisor Nurse, 12*(6), 26–29, 32–34.

Lambert, Lambert. (1981). Role theory and the concept of powerlessness. *Journal of Psychosocial Nursing*, September.

Miller, C., Denner, P., Richardson, V. (1976). Assisting the psychosocial problems of cancer patients: A review of current research. *International Journal of Nursing Studies*.

Related Factors
Prolonged activity restriction creating isolation; failing or deteriorating physiologic condition; long-term stress; abandonment; lost belief in transcendent values/God.

SOURCE: NANDA Diagnosis Review Committee Correspondence.

NURSING DIAGNOSIS

Nursing Diagnoses Accepted by NANDA (Through Ninth Conference, 1990)

Activity intolerance

Activity intolerance: High risk

Adjustment, Impaired

Airway clearance, Ineffective

Anxiety

Aspiration: High risk

Body image disturbance

Body temperature, Altered: High risk

Bowel incontinence

Breast-feeding, Effective (potential for enhanced)

Breast-feeding, Ineffective

Breathing pattern, Ineffective

Cardiac output, Decreased

Communication, Impaired: Verbal

Constipation

Constipation, Colonic

Constipation, Perceived

Coping: Defensive

Coping, Family: Potential for growth

Coping, Ineffective family: Compromised

Coping, Ineffective family: Disabling

Coping, Ineffective individual

Decisional conflict (specify)

Denial, Ineffective

Diarrhea

Disuse syndrome: High risk

Diversional activity deficit

Dysreflexia

Family processes, Altered

Fatigue

Fear

Fluid volume deficit (1)

Fluid volume deficit: High risk

Fluid volume excess

Gas exchange, Impaired

Grieving, Anticipatory

Grieving, Dysfunctional

Growth and development, Altered

Health maintenance, Altered

Health-seeking behaviors (specify)

Home maintenance management, Impaired

Hopelessness

Hyperthermia

Hypothermia

Infection: High risk

Injury: High risk

Knowledge deficit (specify)

Mobility, Impaired physical

Noncompliance (specify)

Nutrition, Altered: High risk for more than body requirements

Nutrition, Altered: Less than body requirements

Nutrition, Altered: More than body requirements

Oral mucous membrane, Altered

Pain

Pain, Chronic

Parental role conflict

Parenting, Altered

Parenting, Altered: High risk

Personal identity disturbance

Poisoning: High risk

Post-trauma response

Powerlessness

Protection, Altered

Rape-trauma syndrome

Rape-trauma syndrome: Compound reaction

Rape-trauma syndrome: Silent reaction

Role performance, Altered

▶

NURSING DIAGNOSIS (continued)

Self-care deficit: Bathing/hygiene
Self-care deficit: Dressing/grooming
Self-care deficit: Feeding
Self-care deficit: Toileting
Self-esteem disturbance
Self-esteem, Low: Chronic
Self-esteem, Low: Situational
Sensory-perceptual alterations: Visual, auditory, kinesthetic, gustatory, tactile, olfactory (specify)
Sexual dysfunction
Sexuality patterns, Altered
Skin integrity, Impaired
Skin integrity, Impaired: High risk
Sleep pattern disturbance
Social interaction, Impaired
Social isolation
Spiritual distress
Suffocation: High risk
Swallowing, Impaired

Thermoregulation, Impaired
Thought processes, Altered
Tissue integrity, Impaired
Tissue perfusion, Altered: Renal, cerebral, cardiopulmonary, gastrointestinal, peripheral (specify type)
Trauma: High risk

Unilateral neglect
Urinary elimination, Altered
Urinary incontinence, Functional
Urinary incontinence, Reflex
Urinary incontinence, Stress
Urinary incontinence, Total
Urinary incontinence, Urge
Urinary retention

Violence, High risk: Self-directed or directed at others

NANDA nursing diagnoses are in the process of being organized into a provisional taxonomy structure. Numeric codes are being established for diagnostic entities and qualifying information. Furthermore, additional diagnoses continue to be proposed for inclusion in the official NANDA classification.

PND-I From its inception in 1973 as the National Group for the Generation and Classification of Nursing Diagnosis, NANDA has taken a strong public position on the incompleteness of its first and even its most recent 1990 list. Nurses have been invited to describe, label, and contribute their phenomena of concern to the collaborative goal of increased scientific growth in the discipline. In such a proactive spirit, the former Division of Psychiatric and Mental Health Nursing Practice of ANA authorized support for a project to identify the phenomena of specific concern for psychiatric-mental health nursing. This action reflected an awareness that such identification was essential for implementing the 1980 ANA Social Policy Statement. The objective was to develop a comprehensive working list of the phenomena of concern for psychiatric-mental health nursing. The strategy was to convene a panel of specialists with expertise in specific age and diagnostic client groups. The outcome of the

first stage of work was a conceptual classification system.

The classification system, called the ANA Classification of Phenomena of Concern to Psychiatric and Mental Health Nursing, is also referred to as **Psychiatric Nursing Diagnoses, First Edition**, or PND-I. PNDs, developed as a possible solution to the incompleteness of the NANDA list, are being incorporated by NANDA. NANDA diagnoses are used in this book.

DSM-III-R and Psychiatric Nursing Diagnoses
The standard interdisciplinary psychiatric diagnosis (DSM-III-R) is used by the whole mental health team. It is a label for a client's psychiatric disorder and thus facilitates communication among team members. The NANDA diagnosis for a psychiatric client is the conceptualization of a client's human response from the unique nursing perspective. Psychiatric nurses must be knowledgeable about both psychiatric diagnostic nomenclature as well as the expanding efforts of nurses to develop our own diagnostic nomenclature. Both are essential for communication with colleagues and for developing an individualized nursing care plan. Table 3–1 compares a sample DSM-III-R diagnosis

TABLE 3–1 Comparision of DSM-III-R and Nursing Diagnoses

DSM-III-R Diagnosis	North American Nursing Diagnosis Association (NANDA)
209.1x Primary degenerative dementia Alzheimer's type, presenile onset	Self-care deficits
	Thought processes, Altered
	Coping, Ineffective individual
	Role performance, Altered
	Social interaction, Impaired

and related psychiatric nursing diagnoses according to NANDA.

Planning

Standard 4 states:

The nurse develops a nursing care plan with specific goals and interventions delineating nursing actions unique to each client's needs.

Rationale The rationale for inclusion of this standard is that the nursing care plan is used to guide therapeutic intervention and to achieve desired goals or outcomes effectively and affirmatively.

Process Criteria Structural criteria for this standard are the following:

• Tools and mechanisms for communicating nursing diagnoses and nursing care plans, progress, and evaluation to colleagues and to the client

• Evidence of a collaborative team effort to plan care so that the client's needs are addressed in a consistent way

The well-developed nursing care plan conforms to the qualities outlined in the accompanying box.

Format of the Plan A nursing care plan usually has at least four components:

• A diagnostic formulation that communicates the phenomena of concern according to nomenclature accepted in the discipline

• Short- and long-term client care goals stated in measurable terms and accompanied by a time deadline

• Nursing orders or interventions that specify what nurses or other mental health team members will do to address clients' diagnosed needs or problems

Properties of an Effective Nursing Care Plan

• Identifies priorities of care

• States realistic goals in measurable terms with an expected date of accomplishment

• Is based on identifiable psychotherapeutic principles

• Indicates which client needs are the primary responsibility of the psychiatric nurse and which will be referred to others with appropriate expertise

• Reflects mutual goal setting and shared responsibility for goal attainment at the level of the client's abilities

• Forms the basis for client care activities done by others under the nurse's supervision

• Outcome criteria, stated in observable terms, on which to base a judgment about the effectiveness of the intervention in achieving client goals

Nursing care plans have various formats depending on the resources and constraints of a setting and the operating conceptual framework or philosophy for practice. A sample nursing care plan is presented on the following page.

Outcome Criteria The ultimate outcome criterion for this standard is evidence that regardless of what format is used for the care plan, it is revised as goals are achieved, changed, or updated. Such goals should be

• Stated in clear, concise, and measurable terms

• Accompanied by a time frame

• Not in conflict with the multidisciplinary team's goals

Planning nursing care requires the setting of both short- and long-term goals for the client. Such goals, however, must reflect the client's own goals, and when the two sets of goals are not compatible, negotiation should occur.

Hints in Negotiating Goals The first step is to determine whether to try to convince the client that the nurse's goals are the right goals or to alter the nurse's goals. One way to do so is to ask clients what their goals are and how the psychiatric professional can help them achieve their goals. Some clients respond that

SAMPLE NURSING CARE PLAN

Client Care Goals	Nursing Planning/ Intervention	Evaluation
Nursing Diagnosis (NANDA): *Social interaction, Impaired*		
Client will be able to tolerate limited interaction with staff (at least 5 minutes 3 times/shift).	Nurse will do the following: Introduce self each shift. Attempt to meet needs despite client's inability to verbalize them. Set up 3 times/shift to be with client. Spend the time in structured ways, e.g., do grooming tasks, go for a walk. Client does not tolerate intense verbal interaction and becomes more inappropriate with direct questions. If client starts to giggle, allow client time to be alone. Help client join activities. Redirect client from situations with too many stimuli. Give encouragement and positive feedback when appropriate. Role model social interaction and use group activities to increase social skills. Use nurse-client relationship to help client learn new social skills.	On discharge, client tolerates limited interaction with others in a structured environment as evidenced by ability to follow schedule.
Nursing Diagnosis: *Self-care deficit: Bathing/hygiene; Dressing/grooming; Toileting*		
Client will: Be up, dressed, and shaved by 9:00 A.M. Make bed and clean area by 9:30 A.M. Do laundry Monday and Thursday P.M. Shower Monday, Wednesday, and Friday P.M.	Nurse will: Arrange hygiene schedule with client. Review schedule early in the shift and give reminders as necessary of tasks to be done. Monitor and give further assistance if needed. Give positive feedback for all tasks accomplished. Allow client to do as much as possible for self. Be alert for progress and allow as much independence as the client tolerates.	At discharge, client performs self-care tasks independently.

they just came along to appease a significant other who is the one with the real problem. Others believe they are there for a "rest" or a "checkup." Some want to be taken care of and protected, and some believe they have been tricked or betrayed and locked up against their will. Having asked, the nurse must *listen*. Sometimes the simple experience of being heard and understood without being invalidated and dismissed out of hand becomes the ground for subsequent negotiations and eventual agreement about mutually determined goals.

Once a nursing diagnosis has been identified and clear, unambiguous goals have been set and listed in order of priority, the nurse can consider possible solutions by using what are known as "predictive principles." Bower (1985) calls predictive principles "guides for developing realistic alternatives of action or action hypotheses that tell the nurse what will promote or inhibit progress toward a desired goal." The nurse selects one intervention from many choices based on a prediction of the likely or probable consequences of each option. The use of predictive principles cuts down on trial-and-error and the rigid use of standard operating procedures.

Intervening

Interventions are the actions to be taken to achieve the stated goals. The actions may be independent, collaborative, or dependent and may include orders from nursing, medicine, and other disciplines. The following are the major categories of nursing intervention with psychiatric clients:

• Psychotherapeutic interventions: individual, family, and group

• Health teaching

• Self-care activities of daily living

• Biologic therapies, including medications

• Therapeutic environment

• Psychobiologic nursing prescriptions regarding diet, nutrition, and exercise

Each of these areas is addressed in depth in a subsequent chapter of this text.

Yura and Walsh (1978) characterize the implementation phase of the nursing process as a time when the nurse continues to collect data about the client's condition, problem, reactions, and feelings. The plan is not carried out blindly as if all decision-making phases have been completed. Changes in identified goals will alter the effectiveness of intervention strategies. Therefore, the nurse must be alert, observant, attentive, thoughtful, and caring, continually using decision-making skills to evaluate and modify intervention strategies and use of available resources.

Evaluating

Standard 6 states:

The nurse evaluates client responses to nursing actions in order to revise the data base, nursing diagnoses, and nursing care plan.

Rationale The rationale for inclusion of this standard is that psychotherapeutic nursing care is a dynamic process whose events sometimes alter previously determined data, diagnoses, or plans.

Structural Criteria Criteria that facilitate achievement of Standard 6 include supervision or consultation with colleagues to help the nurse analyze the effectiveness of care given.

Process Criteria
• The nurse pursues validation, suggestions, and new information, which is subsequently discussed with colleagues.
• The nurse documents results of the evaluation of nursing care.

Outcome Criteria The outcome criteria for this standard are that nursing care plans are revised according to evaluations and that evaluation recordings promote refinement of psychiatric nursing care.

Evaluation is a judgment of merit or worth. It completes the phases of the nursing process by indicating the degree to which the nursing diagnosis and nursing actions have been correct. In evaluation, as in all other phases, clients and their significant others are involved.

Since Isobel Stewart first developed guidelines in 1919 to measure the quality of nursing care, numerous ways of evaluating care have been tested. Some methods simultaneously consider people, activities, and environmental elements, as well as the administrative and organizational structure for delivery of care. Instruments to evaluate client care while the care is in process have been developed and tested. Periodic nursing audits are used increasingly by nurses to inspect or review records and other accounts of nursing transactions. Betts (1978) has related the psychiatric audit to a model for quality assurance in nursing.

Bower (1985) urges nurses to recognize the importance and necessity of structuring evaluation outcome criteria in client-centered behavioral terms. Nurses may have to discard the attitude that nursing care is composed of ethereal, well-meaning qualities or that certain aspects of the clinical act and its art "just can't be evaluated."

Evaluation statements of nursing care plans should include, at the minimum, the following kinds of commentary:

* Client outcomes (changes in the client's behavior as a consequence of the interventions

* Evidence bearing on which interventions were effective and why

* Evidence bearing on which interventions should be altered and why

* Evidence that new planned interventions are necessary

* Evidence that the goals were or were not attained

In short, if interventions are discontinued because of a nursing judgment, documentation is needed. Included in this documentation are changes in client behavior as an outcome of the intervention and as evidence that the goal was attained. Such documentation is essential not only to ensure good quality client care but also to minimize legal liability. Nursing care plans that are updated on working tools such as the Kardex should also be updated in the client's permanent record. New developments in the field of *nursing informatics* that address the use of information and technology by nurses are resulting in computerized systems for care planning and systems of cost accounting.

CHAPTER HIGHLIGHTS

* The nursing process provides a scientific way of planning care for psychiatric clients.

* Phases of the nursing process include assessing, diagnosing, planning, intervening, and evaluating.

* The 1982 ANA Standards for Psychiatric and Mental Health Nursing Practice reflect the current state of knowledge and base practice on theory.

* The nursing process is a conscious, deliberate, yet flexible and adaptable systematic set of cognitive and behavioral steps that describe the clinical act in nursing practice with individuals, families, groups, and aggregates.

* Effective nursing depends on accurate, systematic, and continuous data collection.

* Nursing diagnoses express conclusions about clients' human responses supported by recorded assessment data, current scientific premises, and humanistic principles.

* The nursing care plan is used to guide therapeutic intervention and achieve desired goals; it should reflect agreement between client and professional on short- and long-term goals.

* The implementation phase of nursing process is characterized by continued data collection and observation as well as modification in intervention strategy and timing, if necessary.

* Evaluation completes the phases of the nursing process and occurs so that the data base, nursing diagnosis, and nursing care plan can be revised.

REFERENCES

American Nurses' Association: *A Social Policy Statement.* ANA, 1980.

American Nurses' Association: *Standards of Psychiatric and Mental Health Nursing Practice.* ANA, 1982.

American Psychiatric Association: *Diagnostic and Statistical Manual of Mental Disorders,* ed 3, revised. APA, 1987.

Betts V: Using psychiatric audit as one aspect of a quality assurance program, in Kneisl CR, Wilson HS (eds): *Current Perspectives in Psychiatric Nursing,* vol 2. Mosby, 1978.

Bower F: *The Process of Planning Nursing Care,* ed 4. Mosby, 1985.

Carpenito LJ: *Handbook of Nursing Diagnosis 1989–90.* Lippincott, 1989.

Carroll-Johnson RM: *Classification of Nursing Diagnoses: Proceedings of the Eighth National Conference.* Lippincott, 1989.

Gebbie KM, Lavin MA (eds): *Classification of Nursing Diagnoses.* Mosby, 1975.

Gordon M: *Manual of Nursing Diagnosis.* Mosby, 1989.

Gordon M: *Nursing Diagnosis Process and Application,* ed 2. McGraw-Hill, 1987.

Kim MJ, McFarland GK, McLane AM: *Pocket Guide to Nursing Diagnoses,* ed 3. Mosby, 1989.

Lederer JR et al.: *Care Planning Pocket Guide,* ed 3. Addison-Wesley, 1990.

Loomis M et al.: A classification of phenomena of concern for psychiatric mental health nursing. *Arch Psychiatr Nurs* 1987;1(1):16–24.

McFarland G, Wasli E: *Nursing Diagnoses and Process in Psychiatric Mental Health Nursing.* Lippincott, 1986.

Mundinger M, Jauron GO: Developing a nursing diagnosis. *Nurs Outlook* 1975;23(2):94–97.

Neal MC et al.: *Nursing Care Planning Guides for Psychiatric and Mental Health Care.* Wadsworth, 1980.

Romano CA: Diffusion of technology innovation. *Adv Nurs Sci Nursing Informatics.* 1990:113(2):11–21.

Townsend MC: *Nursing Diagnoses in Psychiatric Nursing,* ed 2. F. A. Davis, 1991.

Yura H, Walsh M: *The Nursing Process.* Appleton-Century-Crofts, 1978.

Theories for Interdisciplinary Psychiatric Care

Holly Skodol Wilson

LEARNING OBJECTIVES

* Identify the assumptions and key ideas of medical-biologic, psychoanalytic, behavioral, social-interpersonal, and nursing theories

* Discuss the implications each theory has for psychiatric nursing practice

* Assess the strengths and weaknesses of each of the theories

* Comprehend and evaluate nursing theories for psychiatric mental health practice.

* Related their own framework to the theories presented

CROSS REFERENCES

Other topics relevant to this content are: Cultural considerations, Chapter 36; Ethics, Chapter 7; Philosophic and historic perspectives, Chapter 1; and Psychobiology, Chapter 6.

To PRACTICE PSYCHIATRIC NURSING humanistically, nurses must devote themselves to understanding what makes people human, how they express their joy of living, their sadness, their desire to love, their hopes for growth. Understanding these phenomena becomes even more crucial when psychiatric nurses must explain how the joy of living suddenly turns to the desire to die, how love of self and others turns to violence and hate, how the hope for growth turns to withdrawal and despair, and how alterations in the brain relate to these human experiences.

In Chapter 1 we described one philosophic framework for understanding the human responses with which psychiatric nurses work. However, the framework presented in Chapter 1 is by no means the only conceptual view nurses use in caring for clients. In this chapter we offer a comparative analysis of the basic assumptions and implications for practice inherent in the dominant models of interdisciplinary psychiatric care. These are the **medical-biologic model,** the **psychoanalytic model,** the **behaviorist model,** the **social-interpersonal model,** and the **models of nursing theory.** Either explicitly or implicitly clinicians choose one or a combination of frameworks from these models in determining what information to assess about clients, what intervention goals and approaches to recommend, and what ultimate evaluation criteria to set. In this chapter, we attempt a critique of these models. By *critique* we mean an inquiry that reveals the hidden assumptions of a model, that grounds it in history, and that involves a systematic appraisal (Wilson 1989). The chapter reflects the humanistic interactionist and psychobiologic perspective outlined in Chapter 1, since it is from that perspective that the authors view the study and practice of psychiatric nursing.

People base their actions on the meaning they attribute to the behavior and situations they confront. Suppose a 20-year-old woman hears and uses a private language and relates more to her paintings than to her peers. If nurses view this woman as having an illness called *schizophrenia* with identifiable symptoms such as hallucinations, it is likely that her treatment program will include the use of phenothiazine medications such as Haldol. The therapeutic emphasis will be on treating and curing a person who has been identified as mentally disordered. If, however, nurses view this woman as "withdrawing into *primary process thinking* to defend against an unconscious conflict rooted in traumatic childhood experiences," the therapeutic approach may emphasize individual psychotherapy designed to bring the conflict to the surface and resolve it. If nurses view this woman's behavior as a learned pattern that has been reinforced by significant others throughout her life, intervention is more likely to follow a behaviorist approach. In this case, the therapist may engage members of the woman's family in planning and learning a new mode of interacting with her, carefully prescribed to extinguish old patterns of behavior and to reinforce new, more functional ones. Some nurses may not view the young woman as having an illness or an exclusively intrapsychic personal problem at all. Rather they may view her as one participant in a network of interpersonal relationships that includes her immediate family and extends to her cultural context. In this case the "client" may include the whole constellation of social variables bearing on the young woman's human responses and the meaning assigned to them by significant others. "Therapy" then may include interventions ranging from family counseling to political action. Yet others may view her as lacking self-care competencies and experiencing stress due to her environment and to her difficulty in adapting. Applying a nursing process approach may require data and ideas that integrate all approaches.

Consider the different actions that a therapist might recommend to this client. She can:

- Take a trip to avoid what is making her anxious

- Take a rest and strengthen her inner defenses

- Yell, scream, cry, and reduce inner pressure

- Have sex if it reassures her

- Avoid having sex if it worsens her anxiety

- Learn sexual techniques that she has avoided out of anxiety, if the sex she is having is unfulfilling and tension producing

- Breathe deeply or try a massage to relieve tension

- Work harder and get a reward, if her narcissism is low

- Fail and get punished, if her guilt is high

- Calm down and try medication

- Leave her family

- Make up with her family

- Enlighten herself, meditate

- Go to an analyst and try to obtain insight into and mastery over her unconscious world

- Eat a special diet

- Enroll in an exercise class

- Join a psychoeducation self-help group

If any of these maneuvers tips the balance so that the woman is better able to deal with destructive forces in her life, it may be called *therapeutic*. However, changes cannot be measured by any absolute standard. They can be measured only by the standards of the individual. One person's inner peace is the inertia of a zombie to another. Integrity to one may be rigidity to another.

What, then, are the predominant theories behind therapy? To answer this question, we must begin by noting that each model is based on a certain view of the human world, a theory of madness and health, a set of practices, qualifications for practitioners, and so forth. Each of the dominant conceptual models for interdisciplinary psychiatric care is discussed in detail below. We will present the basic assumptions of each, its implications for psychiatric nursing, and a summary of our critique of it.

The Medical-Biologic Model

The medical-biologic model in psychiatry originated in the era of classification. The classification of mental disturbances brought the emotional and behavioral aspects of people into the domain of the medical doctor. During this period, the systematic observation, naming, and classification of symptoms were emphasized. Long-standing and somewhat barbaric treatment approaches were all but overlooked. As diagnostic designations became the rage, doctors began to search for the causes of mental illness in an organ or organ system. Emil Kraepelin's monumental descriptive diagnostic classification system is acknowledged as the first comprehensive medical model. It included the notions that the cause of mental illness was organic, that it was located in the central nervous system, that the disease followed a predictable course, and that treatment should be based on accurate diagnosis. Contemporary research findings in the field of psychobiology lend support to some of these early ideas but advance them and make them specific in important ways.

Assumptions and Key Ideas

Proponents of the medical-biologic model, now called the psychobiologic model, view emotional and behavioral disturbances much as they view any physical disease. Thus, abnormal behavior is directly attributable to a disease process, a lesion, a neuropathologic condition, a toxin introduced from outside the human body, or (most recently) a biochemical abnormality of neurotransmitters and enzymes. This position might be summarized as follows:

• The individual suffering from emotional disturbances is sick and has an illness or defect.

• The illness can, at least presumably, be located in some part of the body (usually the brain's limbic system and the central nervous system's synapse receptor sites).

• The illness has characteristic structural, biochemical, and mental symptoms that can be diagnosed, classified, and labeled.

• Mental diseases run a characteristic course and have or haven't a particular prognosis for recovery.

• Mental disorders respond to physical or somatic treatments, e.g., drugs, chemicals, hormones, diet, or surgery.

• The behavioral disorders called "mental illnesses" are properly within the charge of physicians and should be treated according to the principles of general medical practice. In other words, take the client's history, give a general physical exam, conduct laboratory tests, make a diagnosis, and select a treatment method in keeping with the diagnosis.

Implications for Psychiatric Nursing Practice

Nurses who were first involved in the care of psychiatric clients were primarily responsible for the client's physical well-being. Their responsibilities included administering drugs prescribed by the physician and caring for clients undergoing treatments such as insulin shock, electroshock therapy, or hydrotherapy. Although in retrospect the medical model is associated with a comparatively limited view of people and a limited role for nurses, in this era of diagnostic reimbursement groups and cost containment, it is still the major mode of naming phenomena of concern, even among nurses.

The biologic-medical model is the conceptual basis for the continued use of biologic therapies in the care of psychiatric clients, the hospital as the setting for care, research into genetic transmission of mental illness, research on biochemical and metabolic variables among diagnosed psychiatric clients, and dominance of the medical doctor in the psychiatric treatment team. As long as psychiatric clients are admitted to and reimbursed for care according to medical diagnoses, knowledge of this framework is crucial. Furthermore, as long as knowledge expands, psychiatric mental health nurses are responsible for translating that knowledge into care practices.

Understanding Medical Nomenclature   The psychiatric nurse clearly needs to be knowledgeable about current medical nomenclature and emerging psychobiologic research. Before the publication of the third edition of the *Diagnostic and Statistical Manual of Mental Disorders* (DSM-III) and the 1987 revision

(DSM-III-R) by the American Psychiatric Association (APA), the agreement about psychiatric diagnoses was amazingly low (five clinicians examining the same client using the medical model approach tended to reach at least three different diagnoses). Yet the APA's nomenclature predominated. It is still the most frequently used system of classifying behaviorally disturbed people, and its validity and reliability statistics have been considerably improved. Therefore, even psychiatric nurses who disagree with this approach must be generally familiar with it to communicate with peers on the psychiatric team. Knowledge of the system is also needed for identifying human responses associated with disorders so that the nurse can plan care.

Biochemistry Biochemistry is an area of active, biologically oriented psychiatric research. Certain biochemical changes are demonstrably associated with particular behavior disorders. For example, a defect in the metabolism of serotonin is currently being investigated as one possible cause of schizophrenia. Seymour Kety (1959) noted that schizophrenia may result from abnormal transmethylation of catecholamines yielding DMPEA, a compound closely related to mescaline. Wise and Stein (1973) provided evidence that 6-hydroxydopamine (6HD), an aberrant dopamine metabolite, produces schizophrenic symptoms by causing "a prolonged or permanent depletion of brain catecholamine." Evidence of a protein called taraxein in the blood of schizophrenics has also been reported. This agent blocks the action of acetylcholine in the limbic system, resulting in the client's inability to experience pleasure or pain. Carlsson and Lindqvist (1973) noted that central dopaminergic receptors are blocked by all effective antipsychotic drugs, such as chlorpromazine. In sum, it is hypothesized that biochemical neurotransmission may soon explain schizophrenia.

Medical-biologic research has also found relationships between mood disorders and biochemical changes. Some, if not all, depressions are associated with an absolute or relative deficiency of catecholamines, particularly norepinephrine, at functionally important receptor sites in the brain. Conversely, elation may be associated with an excess of such amines. However, the catecholamines have such complex relationships with enzymes and other elements of body chemistry that this hypothesis may be an oversimplification. The most current research findings on advances in psychobiologic knowledge appear in following chapters of this book.

Chronobiology A relatively new avenue of biologic research in psychiatry is the area called **chronobiology.** Implicit in much of this research is the hypothesis that

disturbances in periodic processes (biorhythms) may contribute to psychopathology. These disturbances may not be apparent at the surface level of clinical description and observation. Measurement of such latent periodic processes may therefore be crucial in advancing the psychobiologic understanding of psychiatric illness. Rhythms underlie much of the range of homeostasis (the steady state) in people and in the world. A healthy human being's appearance of stability cloaks an inner symphony of biologic rhythms ranging from microseconds for biochemical reactions, milliseconds for nerve activity, a second for heart rhythm, the twenty-four-hour rest-activity cycle, and the twenty-seven-day menstrual cycle to the entire life span cycle.

Figure 4–1 provides a schematic spectrum of these rhythms, called **bioperiodicities.** Rhythms that are shorter than 24 hours have been designated **ultradian;** those longer than 24 hours, **infradian.** In view of documented **circadian** (daily) fluctuations in human levels of consciousness and liver and kidney function, it is not unreasonable to think that the body also varies cyclically in its ability to tolerate stress or to detoxify and excrete harmful substances. If this line of research continues to yield promising findings, it could provide a new precision in preventive psychiatry, perhaps improving and complementing the traditional retrospective approach of psychoanalysis and the here-and-now emphasis of other therapeutic techniques.

Catherine Norris's (1975) nursing studies on restlessness represent one example of how human rhythmicity can apply to a client problem. (See the Research Note on p 62.) Norris noted that all human life is characterized by rhythmicity. Although some rhythms are learned and others are genetically determined, one of the first indicators of a threat to biologic rhythms may be the feeling of restlessness.

Critique

Perhaps the best known critic of the medical-biologic model was psychiatrist Thomas Szasz (1974), who argued that the concept of mental illness or mental disease, like the explanatory concepts of gods and witches, has outlived its usefulness and now functions merely as a convenient myth. Szasz and others contend that the medical model deals basically with the inner workings of the self, whereas disturbed behavior most often occurs in relationships with others. Since behaviors that are currently referred to as psychiatric symptoms are more likely to be aspects of communication with others, real or illusory, or legal problems about conformity, the medical model overlooks half the data.

Szasz bases his case against the medical model on several central premises:

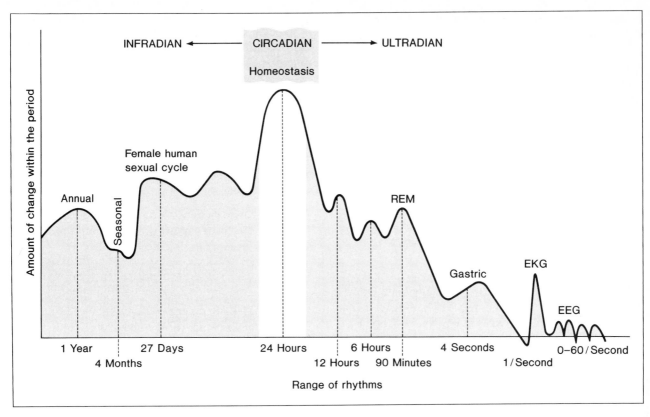

FIGURE 4−1   Schematic spectrum of human biologic rhythms.

• If mental symptoms were manifestations of disease of the central nervous system, they would correspond more to symptoms that result from diseases of the body, such as blindness or paralysis, rather than problems in living or relating to others. Contemporary brain imaging techniques show changes in brain structure and biochemistry not evident in Szasz's time.

• The medical model's view of mental and physical symptoms is not supported by observations. For example, when practitioners speak of physical symptoms, they mean either signs (such as fever) or symptoms (such as pain). When they speak of mental symptoms, they mean clients' communications about themselves, others, and the world. Practitioners have to judge whether a client's statements correspond with their own and society's ideas, concepts, or beliefs. In short, the notion of a mental symptom is inextricably tied to the social and ethical context in which it occurs. Some studies in the past have shown that knowledge about the orientation and education of the clinician is a better predictor of diagnostic outcome than the client's behavior.

• The medical model of mental illness concerns the role of illness in excusing conduct. The idea that serious disease is beyond the control and responsibility of the individual has long been accepted. With the emergence of self-healing practices and evidence that life-style choices, such as diet and exercise, affect physical disease, this notion is coming into question. To relieve people of ethical responsibility for their behavior because they have a disease seems even more questionable. The symptoms of "mental illness" are often behaviors that are associated with the very heart of responsibility—the mind and the character. They are, therefore, quite reasonably beyond excuses.

In his critique of the medical world, Szasz concluded that "mental illness" is a name for problems in living according to certain psychosocial, ethical, and legal norms. The idea, for example, that hostility, vengefulness, or rape is indicative of mental disorder is based on the cultural value attached to love, forgiveness, or consensual sexual relationships. The irony, then, is that a remedy is sought in terms of medical measures, and even the medical diagnostic labels currently in use provide no indication of the specific treatment that will be tried. A diagnosis of schizophrenia may be followed by any one or a combination of treatments, including drugs, electroshock therapy, psychotherapy, group therapy, milieu therapy, or family therapy. The policies of the clinical setting and the client's age, place within the family structure, socioeconomic status, and (often) sex usually have been better predictors of the treatment that will be advised than the diagnosis is.

RESEARCH NOTE

Citation
Norris C: Restlessness: A nursing phenomenon in search of meaning. Nurs Outlook 1975; 23:103–107.

Study Problem/Purpose
In this classic inductive clinical study, Norris set out to observe and describe the clinical phenomenon of human restlessness. Study questions included: What is restlessness? When does it occur? How does one experience restlessness?

Methods
The investigator observed migratory land and sea animals, reviewed related literature, drew on her own practice experience with clients, interviewed nurse colleagues about their experiences, and engaged in purposeful observation under diverse conditions associated with restlessness. These conditions included biologic changes (hemorrhage or toxicity), perception of changes (new or strange experiences), disruption of biologic rhythmicity, fatigue, boredom, and role deprivation. She also observed clients in pain and clients suffering anxiety.

Findings
Although her method was relatively unsystematic, Norris concluded that restlessness may be a person's first response to change, strangeness, or threat.

Implications
If additional research confirms these early findings, restlessness may belong to a group of disturbances in rhythmicity that have a warning function. Although the activity may seem random and without purpose, it may generate the energy needed to cope with a perceived threat. The author urges other clinicians to document and describe such clinical phenomena from their practice to build nursing science.

Human behavior is complex. A change in body structure or body chemistry results in a change in behavior. An organism or toxin can initiate and ultimately alter thought processes. Similarly, a problem in feelings, such as low self-esteem, can produce structural body changes, such as hunched shoulders or muscle contractions. It is likely that there is no single "cause" of the troubled and troublesome behavior called mental illness and the human responses to it. The medical model's attempt to find one is often unnecessarily limiting. It obscures the relevance of interpersonal and cultural factors and challenges nursing to articulate and develop them.

The publication of the American Psychiatric Association's third edition of the *Diagnostic and Statistical Manual of Mental Disorders* (DSM-III) in 1980 and its 1987 revision reflects efforts to respond to these criticisms in several important ways. These responses come even closer to responding to such criticisms in DSM-IV drafts.

• Psychiatric diagnoses according to DSM-III-R are based on specified, empirical criteria not linked to any particular theory of etiology.

• The diagnostic criteria have been field-tested for reliability and validity, with encouraging results.

• A DSM-III-R diagnosis is multifaceted in that it assesses the presence or absence of an individual's biologic, psychologic, and social pathology.

• The diagnosis includes a client's strengths or level of adaptive functioning and contextual stresses.

• The "V-codes" allow the clinician to note the presence of a problem in living that does not represent a psychiatric disorder (Williams and Wilson 1982).

The Psychoanalytic Model

The psychoanalytic model is usually credited to the Viennese physician Sigmund Freud (1962b). Freud's premise was that all psychologic and emotional events, however obscure, were understandable. For the meanings behind behavior he looked to childhood experiences that he believed caused adult neuroses. Therapy in this model consists of clarifying the meaning of events, feelings, and behavior and thereby gaining insight about them. Freud's work shifted the focus of psychiatry from classification to a dynamic view of mental phenomena. Psychoanalytic concepts have so widely permeated the education and practice of psychiatric clinicians that they have come to be regarded as a fundamental part of understanding and approaching emotional disorders. Psychoanalysis has emerged as a method of investigation, as a therapeutic technique, and as a body of scientific concepts and propositions.

Assumptions and Key Ideas

Psychic Determinism A fundamental concept associated with the psychoanalytic model is **psychic determinism.** The psychic determinist believes that no human behavior is accidental. Each psychic event is determined by the ones that preceded it. Events in people's mental lives that seem random or unrelated to what went before are only apparently so. Thus, psychoanalysts never dismiss any mental phenomenon as meaningless or accidental. They always search for what caused it, why it happened. For example, people commonly forget or mislay something. They usually view this as just an accident. Psychoanalysts, on the contrary, seek to demonstrate that the accident was caused by a wish or intent of the person involved. Psychoanalysts also view dreams as subject to the principle of psychic determinism, each dream and each image in each dream bearing some relationship to the rest of the dreamer's life.

Role of the Unconscious   A second fundamental concept in the psychoanalytic model is that significant unconscious mental processes occur frequently in normal as well as abnormal mental functioning. These processes are called simply the **unconscious.** The unconscious is so intimately related to the premise of psychic determinism that it is hard to discuss one without the other. According to psychoanalysts, the fact that much of what goes on in people's minds is unknown to them accounts for the apparent discontinuities in their mental lives. If the unconscious cause or causes of some behavioral symptoms are discovered, then the apparent discontinuities disappear, and the causal sequence becomes clear.

Psychoanalysis   The most powerful and reliable method for studying the unconscious is the technique that Freud evolved over several years, called **psychoanalysis.** The basic logic behind psychoanalysis is as follows:

• The client underwent a *traumatic experience* that stirred up intense and painful emotion.

• The traumatic experience represented to the client some ideas that were incompatible with the dominant ideas constituting the ego. Thus, the client experienced a **neurotic conflict.**

• The incompatible idea and the neurotic conflict associated with it force the ego to bring into action **defense mechanisms** that manifest themselves in the client as neurotic symptoms.

• Therapy is directed toward resolving the conflict by uncovering its roots in the unconscious. If the client is able to release the *repressed feelings* associated with the conflict, the symptoms disappear.

Among the strategies used in psychoanalysis are: (a) hypnosis, (b) the interpretation of dreams, and (c) free association, in which the client is encouraged to express every idea that comes to mind—no matter how insignificant, irrelevant, shameful, or embarrassing—ignoring all self-censorship and suspending all judgment.

In the initial phase of psychoanalysis, the analyst's task is to facilitate establishing a *therapeutic alliance.* In the transition to the middle phase of analysis, **transference** occurs and the analyst uses techniques calculated to induce *regression* in the client. In this stage the analyst remains relatively passive to avoid giving either permissive or authoritarian expressions and to limit observations to interpretations of the client's mental dynamics as heard in the free associations. In the long-range course of analysis, the client undergoes two basic processes—remembering and reliving. *Remembering* refers to the gradual extension of consciousness back to early childhood, when the core of the neurosis was formed. *Reliving* refers to the actual reexperiencing of past events and feelings in the context of the client's relationship with the analyst. The alleviation of symptoms is not usually regarded as the most significant factor for evaluating therapeutic change. Instead the chief basis of evaluation is the client's capacity to attain reasonable happiness, to contribute to the happiness of others, and to deal adequately with the stresses of life. In short, the most important criterion for successful analysis is the extent to which it releases the client's normal potential, which had been blocked by neurotic conflicts.

Topography of the Mind   Freud classified mental operations according to regions or systems of the mind in a body of thought now referred to as *topographic theory.* Any mental event that occurred outside of conscious awareness represented the *unconscious region.* Mental events that could be brought into conscious awareness through an act of attention were said to be *preconscious.* Those that occurred in conscious awareness were regarded as the *conscious surface* of the mind. This topographic model, although still used to classify mental events in terms of the quality and degree of awareness, has been supplanted by the structural model.

Structure of the Mind   With the publication of *The Ego and the Id* (1962a) in 1923, Freud abandoned the topographic model of the mind for the *structural model.* The structural model of the mind contends that there are three distinct entities—the id, the ego, and the superego. The **id** was seen as a completely unorganized reservoir of energy derived from drives and instincts. The **ego** controls action and perception, controls contact with reality, and, through the defense mechanisms, inhibits primary instinctual drives. One of its fundamental functions is also the capacity for developing mutually satisfying relationships with others. The **superego** is concerned with moral behavior. Frequently, the superego allies itself with the ego against the id, imposing demands in the form of conscience or guilt feelings. The id in a child operates according to what Freud called the **pleasure principle:** the tendency to seek pleasure and avoid pain. This is not always possible, so the demands of the pleasure principle have to be modified by the **reality principle.** The reality principle is largely a learned ego function by which people develop the capacity to delay the immediate release of tension or achievement of pleasure.

Drives Freud believed that psychic energy was derived from *drives*. Instincts or drives were genetically determined psychic constituents. He used the word **cathexis** to refer to the attachment of psychic energy to a person or a thing. The greater the cathexis, the greater the psychologic importance of the person or object. Initially Freud postulated a life and death instinct, but by 1920, in *Beyond the Pleasure Principle* (1975), he had revised these ideas to accord with the theory of drives accepted by or modified by analysts today. In the later formulation, Freud accounted for the instinctual aspects of people's mental lives by assuming the existence of two drives—the *sexual drive* and the *aggressive drive*. The former gives rise to the erotic component of mental activity, and the latter gives rise to the destructive component. The two drives can be fused, for example, when an act of intentional cruelty also has some unconscious sexual meaning for the actor and provides a degree of unconscious gratification. The sexual drive has come to be known as the **libido.** See Table 4–1 for the stages of psychosexual development according to Freud.

Implications for Psychiatric Nursing Practice

The psychoanalytic model has historically provided a very limited treatment role for the nurse. Psychoanalytic clients are usually seen in the analyst's office as private clients. With the emergence of psychoanalytically oriented settings such as Chestnut Lodge in Rockville, Maryland, nurses became somewhat more involved, sharing at least in the psychoanalytic language, concepts, and speculations about client dynamics. In the United States a nurse needs a medical degree as well as psychoanalytic training to practice as a psychoanalyst. Some nurses have sought preparation as lay analysts at settings such as the William Alanson White Institute and the Chicago Psychoanalytic Institute. However, the nurse has served more frequently as an adjunct therapist, focusing on here-and-now issues with clients undergoing psychoanalysis or acting in a supportive role to family members.

Acknowledging that the psychoanalytic model has provided few clear-cut therapeutic roles for nurses does not suggest that nurses have failed to do useful work with clients undergoing psychoanalytic treatment or that knowledge of psychoanalytic theory is irrelevant to psychiatric nurses. Concepts derived from the psychoanalytic model, such as the unconscious, pervade not only the field of psychiatry but also the entire culture. These concepts are understood by the educated public and are useful in comprehending fields of human endeavor ranging from public relations to art and literature. Certainly if nurses are to participate as equal members of the psychiatric team, and if they are to be valued as theorists, they must learn the language and ideas of psychodynamics that are the common heritage of many psychiatric professionals.

Critique

We criticize Freudian psychoanalysis somewhat uneasily. As one authority put it, "Who knows, they might be right. All of us hardy souls who persist in our skepticism might be 'resisting'—the very evidence of our sickness." Yet some critical analyses of the psychoanalytic movement have emerged. Several differ with small sections of Freud's work (Adler and Horney, for example, disapproved of psychic determinism, the instinct theory, and the structural approach of id, ego, and superego). Others go so far as to

Stage	Age Span	Task	Key Concept
Oral	0–18 months	Satisfaction and anxiety management from oral activity	Oral activity gives pleasure and is source for learning
Anal	18 months–3 years	Learning muscle control for toilet training	Delayed gratification and rule internalization
Phallic	3–6 years	Gender identification and genital awareness	Repression of attraction to opposite-sex parent leading to same-sex identification
Latency	6–12 years	Repression of sexuality	Oedipal conflict resolved with shift to other interests and friends
Genital	12–young adult years	Channeling sexuality into relationships with opposite sex	Reemerging sexuality to motivate behavior

TABLE 4–1   Freud's Psychosexual Stages

found a whole empirical school of behaviorism in opposition to Freudianism, attacking the "absurdities" of the whole.

Perhaps the most compelling synthesis of critical arguments launched against the psychoanalytic model can be found in the literature of feminism. Feminists have pointed out that

• Psychoanalytic theory's emphasis on early childhood determinism underrates the effects of environmental systems on dynamic processes in people.

• The psychoanalytic model tends to accept as unchangeable the social context in which repression and resulting neurosis must develop.

• Freud's ideas were rooted in the social and political culture of his time (that is, early twentieth-century Viennese society).

These critics have noted further that the psychoanalytic framework is blatantly antifemale. Shulamith Firestone (1971), for instance, comments that Freud's theory about women is limited to analyzing them only as negative males (e.g., the Electra complex is an inverse Oedipus complex). His concept of two types of female orgasms, clitoral and vaginal, was refuted as myth in the research of Masters and Johnson. Widespread acceptance of Freudian theory has promoted social adjustment for women instead of feminist revolt, contends Firestone. Firestone notes examples of analysts' misinterpretations of client interactions based on such notions.

Helene Deutsch, trained in psychoanalysis by Freud and author of a monumental two-volume work on women (1944–1945), expounded the following ideas in her theories of "normal femininity":

• Preadolescent girls have masochistic longings to be raped.

• Women find enjoyment through childbirth, forced intercourse, and lost causes.

• Women with "masculinity complexes," whom Deutsch "unmasked" in therapy, were cases of thwarted femininity, since women cannot compete successfully with men.

• Motherhood is the only true fulfillment for all women.

Deutsch describes truly "feminine" women as the loveliest and most unaggressive of helpmates, women who do not insist on their own rights but are easy to handle in every way if one just loves them. Most critics view such theories of "normal femininity" as representing a traditional perspective that has limited women's choices.

Freud, Deutsch, Erikson, and Reik view the difference in genital apparatus between the sexes as the critical variable affecting personality development in men and women. These theorists posit a separate psychology of women linking all traits, interests, attitudes, emotions, and neuroses to an anatomic "defect." Erik Erikson (1968), a neo-Freudian, makes a valiant attempt to wed cultural relativity with innate biologic differences, but he still ends up with the advocates of "anatomy as destiny." Most feminists argue that, even if an anatomic theory did explain human behavior, birth and breast envy ought to be given equal time with the penis envy so dominant in Freud's essays. Erikson's "Eight Stages of Man" represent a well-known developmental theory (see Table 4–2).

Other feminists writing about psychoanalysis point out that, although adult mental health in American society is masculine centered, most psychoanalytic theory has been written about women. Phyllis Chesler (1972) criticizes Freud's vision of women as essentially "breeders and bearers," potentially warm-hearted creatures, but cranky children with uteruses, forever mourning the loss of male organs and male identity. Freud noted headaches, fatigue, chronic depression, frigidity, paranoia, and overwhelming sense of inferiority in many of his female clients, but he never viewed them as the indirect communications characteristic of slave psychologies. Instead, he saw such symptoms as hysterical and neurotic productions manufactured by spiteful, self-pitying, and generally unpleasant women. Their inability to be happy as women, Freud concluded, stemmed from unresolved penis envy, unresolved Electra complexes, or general mysterious female stubbornness.

Those who do emphasize Freud's psychology of women as the basis for their critique argue that biologic differences between the sexes have been overemphasized and that all mammals show a vast array of bisexual or unisex behaviors. These theorists modify Freud's libido concept to refer to forces in both sexes that lead to experimentation and growth. They conclude that curiosity, aggressiveness, dependence, expressiveness, interest in the body, self-esteem, and the need for growth, security, and creativity are all part of a common human repertoire that transcends anatomy. These givens, however, can be elaborated, drastically altered, or suppressed as each individual comes into contact with his or her immediate family environment and total culture.

The Behaviorist Model

The behaviorist model in psychiatry has its roots in psychology and neurophysiology. To the behaviorist, symptoms associated with neuroses and psychoses are clusters of learned behaviors that persist because they are somehow rewarding to the individual. One of the

TABLE 4–2 Erikson's Eight Stages

Age	Stage of Development	Task/Area of Resolution	Concepts/Basic Attitudes
Birth–18 months	Infancy	Trust versus mistrust	Ability to trust others and a sense of one's own trustworthiness; a sense of hope Withdrawal and estrangement
18 months–3 years	Early childhood	Autonomy versus shame and doubt	Self-control without loss of self-esteem; ability to cooperate and to express oneself Compulsive self-restraint or compliance; defiance, willfulness
3–5 years	Late childhood	Initiative versus guilt	Realistic sense of purpose; some ability to evaluate one's own behavior Self-denial and self-restriction
6–12 years	School age	Industry versus inferiority	Realization of competence, perseverance Feeling that one will never be "any good," withdrawal from school and peers
12–20 years	Adolescence	Identity versus role diffusion	Coherent sense of self; plans to actualize one's abilities Feelings of confusion, indecisiveness, possibly antisocial behavior
18–25 years	Young adulthood	Intimacy versus isolation	Capacity for love as mutual devotion; commitment to work and relationships Impersonal relationships, prejudice
25–65 years	Adulthood	Generativity versus stagnation	Creativity, productivity, concern for others Self-indulgence, impoverishment of self
65 years to death	Old age	Integrity versus despair	Acceptance of the worth and uniqueness of one's life Sense of loss, contempt for others

SOURCE: From Childhood and Society, 2nd ed. by Erik H. Erikson, by W. W. Norton & Company, Inc. Copyright © 1950, 1963. Renewed 1978 by Erik H. Erikson.

most important conceptual contributions to this framework was made by Pavlov (1849–1936), who in 1902 discovered a phenomenon he called the **conditioned reflex** in a famous experiment with a dog and a bell. The basic principle of the conditioned reflex is this:

• A **response** is a reaction to a **stimulus**.

• If a new and different stimulus is presented with or just before the original stimulating event, the same response reaction can be obtained.

• Eventually the new stimulus can replace the original one, so that the response occurs to the new stimulus alone.

The conditioned or learned response has come to be viewed as the basic unit of all learning, the unit on which more complex behavioral patterns are constructed. Such construction occurs through a process called **reinforcement,** in which behaviors are rewarded and persist. Pavlov's theories have continued into the present, valued for their simplicity, concreteness, and objectivity. Some behaviorists see them as the key to understanding and controlling the whole range of undesirable human behavior.

Assumptions and Key Ideas

The fundamental premises of the behaviorist perspective can be summarized as follows:

• Human beings are merely complex animals. The difference between human and animal is one of degree and not kind. Human powers of conceptual thought, propositional language, and abstraction are fully attributable to physiologic complexity rather than some nonmaterial source. Thus the use of animal experience as an analog to human experience is clearly justifiable.

• The self in humans is the sum or repository of past conditionings or simply the behavioral repertoire. Therapists can know clients only by the clients' behavior. The concepts of consciousness and self and the belief in subjective reality are products of human pride rather than scientific discovery. If they are real, they can be inferred only from observable behavior.

• Behavior is what the organism does. It can be observed, described, and recorded.

• There is, properly speaking, no autonomous person. People are what they do and what they are reinforced for doing by conditions in their environment.

The self is a structure of stimulus-response chains or hierarchies of habit. It is possible to know and predict conditions under which behavior will occur.

• The symptoms of a person's disorders are, in fact, the substance of that person's troubles. There is no hidden motive, no underlying cause, no internal pathogenic process. There is only the symptom or the behavior, and the aim of behaviorist therapy is to change the behavior.

• The classification of mental diseases is meaningful only to provide legal labels. It provides little or no assistance in prescribing a treatment program.

• People can control others whether others want to be controlled or not. Control is neither good nor bad in and of itself.

• The therapist determines what behavior should be changed and what plan should be followed. Change is effected by identifying events in the client's life that have been critical stimuli for the behavior and then arranging interventions for *extinguishing* those behaviors. A changed way of acting precedes a changed way of thinking, according to behaviorist theory.

Both Joseph Wolpe (1956) and B. F. Skinner (1953, 1971) are associated with psychiatric treatment approaches that represent one form of *conditioning* and reflect the above assumptions. Wolpe defined *neurotic behavior* as unadaptive behavior acquired in anxiety-generating situations. He based his therapeutics on the introduction of a response that inhibits anxiety when situations occur that ordinarily evoke anxiety. Relaxation, for example, was considered incompatible with anxiety and, therefore, effective in inhibiting it. Thus, Wolpe would direct his intervention to a counter-conditioning technique, usually putting the client under hypnosis and using various techniques for gradual **desensitization.** For example, a man with a fear of dying might gradually attempt to overcome his anxiety at the sight of a coffin, the

attendance of a funeral, and so on, by trying to relax in the face of these situations.

Skinner's approach, called *operant conditioning,* emphasizes discovering why the behavioral response was elicited in the first place and what current variables actively reinforce it. The key concept in operant conditioning is reinforcement. Skinner originally used the term **positive reinforcement** to describe an event that increases the probability that the response will recur—a reward for behavior. A **negative reinforcement** was defined as an event likely to decrease the probability of recurrence because it penalizes the behavior.

Other contemporary behaviorists have redefined Skinner's original terms and introduced some new ones. Positive reinforcement is still an environmental event that rewards and thus increases the probability of a behavioral response. Negative reinforcement can mean removal of an adverse stimulus (e.g., an electric shock to animals or the restriction of people's privileges) to increase the likelihood of a behavior's recurrence. *Positive punishment,* in contrast, is the introduction of aversive stimuli to decrease the likelihood of recurrence of a behavior. *Negative punishment* removes something that has been a prior reinforcer, thus again decreasing the likelihood of such behaviors as smoking, drug abuse, truancy, temper outbursts, and abuse. Table 4–3 contains examples of each of these neobehaviorist concepts.

The frequency with which a response is given is a clear, observable measure of behavior. Most people exhibit aggressive behavior at some time. To say that a client is hostile suggests that this class of response occurs more frequently than usual. The term given to an intervention designed to change a client's behavior is **shaping.** It is a procedure of manipulating reinforcement to bring the person closer to the chosen behavior. There are, according to Skinner, times in a client's life when responses are accidentally reinforced by a coincidental pairing of response and reinforcement. This accidental pairing may play a role in the development

TABLE 4–3   **Examples of Behaviorist Concepts**

Concept	Purpose	Example
Positive reinforcer	Increase recurrence of the behavior through reward	Leave of absence from hospital as per contract with client
Negative reinforcer	Increase recurrence of the behavior by removing aversive consequences	Removal of restrictions on phone calls or visitors as per contract with client
Positive punishment	Decrease behavior by adding aversive consequences	Quiet time
Negative punishment	Decrease behavior by withdrawing a reinforcer or reward	Withdrawal of privileges, such as recreational outings in a residential milieu

of phobias (irrational fears) and other distressing and/or dysfunctional behaviors.

Implications for Psychiatric Nursing Practice

Most psychiatric nurses acknowledge that the application of principles of behavior modification to clients is quite complex, since such interventions are powerful tools with a heavy philosophic overlay. The use of this approach raises issues of control, responsibility for behavior, and the morality of using negative or punitive stimuli in a therapeutic context, to name only a few. Consider the notion of the nurse as "behavioral engineer." Therapists who successfully resolve such basic philosophic issues have designed and implemented successful behavior modification plans with disturbed, overtly aggressive children, developmentally disabled clients, and violently self-destructive people.

In many institutional environments, clients follow prescribed schedules for daily living that include a **token economy.** Clients are rewarded for desired behavior by token reinforcers, such as food, candy, and verbal approval. The movement toward community-based psychiatric treatment has made plain some of the shortcomings and economic realities of therapies aimed toward resolving everyone's intrapsychic conflicts. The movement has instead attempted to replace maladaptive behavior with behavior that allows people to function effectively within their natural environment. When parents or others in the client's environment are taught to implement the behavior change procedures, therapy moves away from the partial and artificial situation of the therapist's office into the client's total environment. It no longer requires the presence of highly trained, often expensive experts and thus makes treatment more affordable.

Psychiatric nurses have had a special role in teaching behaviorist principles to people with little training so that they can act as change agents. Nonprofessional staff on psychiatric wards can be taught effective use of behaviorist principles to eliminate chronic, maladaptive behavior by long-term psychiatric clients. Hyperactive children or children with borderline intelligence can be treated in the home by their parents when nurses teach the parents to use approaches such as frequency counts on specific behaviors to be modified, time-outs (short periods of isolation) for undesired behavior, and the bestowal of attention, praise, and affectionate physical contact as rewards.

In general, behavior modification offers a rapid, efficient, and effective system of intervention congruent both with psychiatric nurses' conventional roles as planners and teachers and with trends in community psychiatry. However, it may not always be in accord with a nurse's personal philosophy.

Critique

Intervention based on the behaviorist model has proved effective in the treatment of persons so alienated from society, functionally incapacitated, or destructive that they are unable to interact with or respond to others. Nonetheless, criticism has been leveled against his model. The criticism fundamentally rests on ethical concerns about people's rights, dignity, and freedom. The model has been criticized for its simplistic explanation of human feelings and behavior and for its authoritarian therapist-client relationship.

Humanistic social scientists contend that ignoring emotions, introspection, and subjective feelings distorts the creative role of people in shaping their environments instead of merely adapting to them. Humanists further argue that these qualities differentiate humans from animals. People are self-aware. They can step outside themselves and reflect on their subjective inner lives. This allows them to talk about themselves and to contemplate their future possibilities. Such self-consciousness is the genius of human individuality. No other animal is burdened with this gift. Crucial to this quality, of course, are the abilities to comprehend meaning and to use language.

If Freud's theories challenged the rationality of human beings, many critics find that behaviorist learning theories reduce humans to little more than cogs in a machine that can be conditioned to do almost anything. Such a conception of human beings ignores uniquely human abilities: the ability to be self-conscious, to act intentionally, to experience reality differently from each other, and to create images, dreams, fantasies, and a private inner life. Many clinicians value certain interventions generated according to principles of stimulus-response learning, but the behaviorists' most basic assumptions about people and their environments contrast harshly with the image of humans and society offered by other theoretic schools. Yet problems such as an abusive parent or spouse, a self-mutilating adolescent, or a fire-setting child urge that we keep an open but ethical mind on this approach.

The Social-Interpersonal Model

The social-interpersonal model of psychiatry grew out of a general dissatisfaction with approaches that account for "mental illness" in terms of either intrapersonal mechanisms (e.g., the symptoms of a disease) or individual personality dynamics such as anxiety, ego strength, and libido. Advocates of this model assert that other models neglect the crucial social processes and cultural variation involved in the development, identification, and resolution of disturbed human responses. It focuses on the larger and more general context of **deviance** and on the processes by which an individual comes to be labeled as deviant. The humanistic interactionist philosophic base for this text represents an extension and refinement of the social-interpersonal model, along with a new synthesis of research-based knowledge in psychobiology.

Assumptions and Key Ideas

Three separate but philosophically congruent schools of thought contribute to the social-interpersonal model. These are the sociocultural, the interpersonal-psychiatric, and the general systems approaches. The assumptions and key ideas of each are discussed below.

The Sociocultural School The sociocultural approach is summarized partially by sociologist Kai Erikson (1962): "Deviance is not a property inherent in certain forms of behavior; it is a property conferred upon these forms by audiences which directly or indirectly witness them." A similar view is proposed by Howard Becker (1963, p 9): "Deviance is not a quality of the act a person commits, but a consequence of the application by others of rules and sanctions to an 'offender.' "

Thus, mental illness is a *label* applied to certain behaviors that violate the rules of conduct imposed by various significant others. The focus for psychiatry is on the interplay between the deviant and the audience—the person and the social context. Sociologically, the critical variable in the study of the forms of deviance labeled "mental illness" is the social audience rather than the individual person, since it is the audience that eventually decides whether any given action will be labeled deviant. Included in the study of "mental illness," then, are various aspects of audience reactions to behavior, the labeling process, the criteria used in labeling, the extent of consensus on such criteria, the consequences for an individual so labeled, etc. The criteria of DSM-III-R represent a move in this direction.

A well-known example of this approach is the research of Thomas Scheff (1966), who concludes that "mental illness" is a label given to diverse forms of deviance that do not fit under any other explicit label, such as delinquency. In this regard, he views mental disorders as a form of **residual deviance**—a label given to nonconforming behavior. The label reinforces and stabilizes that behavior and enters the labeled client into a deviant role of "mental patient." Once a person has been labeled deviant and societal reactions have become organized, Scheff argues, the deviant may incorporate the definitions of others into the self-concept. Recent research establishing brain abnormal-

ities serve as evidence that labeling theory itself is reductionistic.

In the view of the sociologic school, then, behaviors that are often called symptoms acquire meaning only when considered within their social context. This view emphasized the social system consisting of the client, others reacting to the client, and the official agencies of psychiatric control and treatment. It de-emphasizes individual personal dynamics.

The Interpersonal Psychiatric School Psychiatrists Adolf Meyer (1948–1952) and Harry Stack Sullivan (1953) made significant contributions to the social-interpersonal model in the first half of the twentieth century. Sullivan trained with William Alanson White and Adolf Meyer rather than Freud. He is viewed as the least reductionist of psychiatric theorists and emphasizes modes of interaction as the real focus of psychiatric inquiry. Sullivan argues that psychiatry should renounce the futile attempt to define isolated individuals and instead define the significant interpersonal aspects of situations. His main theoretical concern is with the integration of organism and milieu. Sullivan became the theoretic and ideologic leader of the interpersonal school of psychiatry often associated with the William Alanson White Foundation, which sponsors the well-known journal *Psychiatry*. The sociologic theorists differ on some points from those adhering to the interpersonal school of psychiatry (for example, on the relative importance of the self and individual psychology). They are bound together, however, by a number of fundamentally compatible ideas.

One concept that plays a crucial role in the organization of behavior, according to Sullivan, is the **self-system** or *self-dynamism*. The self-system provides tools that allow people to deal with the tasks of avoiding anxiety and establishing security. The self is a construct built from the child's experience. It is made up of **reflected appraisals** the person learns in contacts with other significant people. The self develops in the process of seeking physical satisfaction of bodily needs and security. To feel secure, the self essentially requires feelings of approval and prestige as protection against anxiety. Rewarding appraisals from others yield what Sullivan calls the *good-me* aspect of the self. Anxiety-producing appraisals result in the *bad-me*. The *not-me* occurs normally in dreams and in aspects of experience that are poorly understood and later experienced as dread, horror, and loathing among disturbed people. In summary, Sullivan emphasizes the pervasive interaction between organism and personal environment. He objects in principle to the concept that organized psychologic impulses, drives, and goals belong to the person as an individual. He feels instead that the person cannot be distinguished from the person-in-the-interpersonal-situation.

TABLE 4–4   Sullivan's Stages of Interpersonal Development

Age	Stage	Task/Key Concept
Birth–18 months (to appearance of speech)	Infancy	Experiences anxiety in interaction with mothering one; learns to use maternal tenderness to gain security and avoid anxiety
18 months–6 years (from first speech to need for playmates)	Childhood	Learns to delay gratification in response to interpersonal demands; uses language and action to avoid anxiety
6–9 years	Juvenile	Develops peer relationships and uses environment outside the family to shape self
9–12 years	Preadolescence	Develops caring relationship with same-sex peer, chum relationship
12–14 years	Early adolescence	Develops interest in opposite-sex relationships
14–21 years	Late adolescence	Has satisfying relationships; directs sexual impulses
21 years +	Adulthood	Establishes love relationship

Sullivan uses environmentalist phrasing in many of his key concepts and places a certain emphasis on the effects of cultural configurations on the development and functioning of the personality (see Table 4–4 for Sullivan's stages of development). Nonetheless, Sullivan has comparatively little to say about the impact on behavior of specific variations in the social or cultural scene. Like Sullivan, other advocates of the interpersonal school of psychiatry, such as Karen Horney (1950) and Erich Fromm (1941), stress the general climate in the immediate family. Alfred Adler (1971), however, attempts to understand more of the social and cultural conditions influencing behavior. The interpersonal school of psychiatry in general focuses less on social context than the sociologic perspective and takes basically a developmental-interpersonal view of the self. The **self-actualization** theory of Abraham Maslow (1962) belongs squarely in this school. See Figure 4–2.

The General Systems School General systems theory, when applied to living systems (people), provides a conceptual framework for integrating the biologic and social sciences with the physical sciences. In psychiatry it offers a new resolution of the mind-matter dichotomy, a new integration of biologic and social approaches to the nature of human beings, and a new approach to psycho-

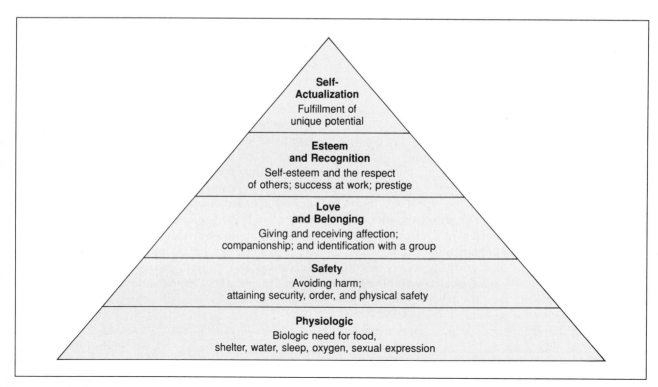

FIGURE 4–2   Maslow's hierarchy of needs.

pathology, diagnosis, and therapy. Karl Menninger (1963) views normal personality functioning and psychopathology in terms of general systems theory. His work addresses four major issues:

1. Adjustment or individual-environment interaction

2. The organization of living systems

3. Psychologic regulation and control, known as *ego theory* in psychoanalysis

4. Motivation, which is often called *instinct* or *drive* in the psychoanalytic framework

A salient point of Menninger's theory is the idea of **homeostasis** (human balance). He asserts that the greater the threat or stress on a system, the greater the number of system components involved in coping with or adapting to it. Therefore, pathology can exist at various levels, from the cell and organ level to the group and community level. An example of the former might be the behavioral changes that follow cellular alterations due to addictive drugs, to a blood clot, or to a tumor. Examples of pathology at the group level include family conflicts. At the community level, overpopulation, pollution, homelessness, and poverty are instances of pathology. In systems theory, all represent abnormalities or stresses on matter-energy processes and would be included within the domain of psychiatric professionals.

In Menninger's view, then, a system's well-being depends on the amount of stress on it and the effectiveness of its coping mechanisms. He asserts that "mental illness" is an impairment of self-regulation in which comfort, growth, and production are surrendered for the sake of survival at the best level possible but at the sacrifice of emergency coping devices (1963, pp 526–527). Psychiatric clients are described as "obliged to make awkward and expensive maneuvers to maintain themselves, somewhat isolated from their fellows, harassed by faulty techniques of living, uncomfortable themselves and often to others" (Menninger 1963, p 5). Therapists using the general systems approach emphasize current conflicts, restoration of impaired systems of functioning, and subsequent reintegration of the restored function into future coping strategies.

Implications for Psychiatric Nursing Practice

The social-interpersonal framework gives independent and collaborative psychiatric nursing clear theoretic direction and support. Nursing roles are associated with shifts in the delivery of psychiatric services variously termed *social psychiatry, community psychiatry, psychoeducation,* and *milieu therapy.* All are associated with efforts to provide psychiatric services more efficiently to large groups of people, particularly those previously neglected, and attempts to counteract the debilitating effects of long-term institutionalization. All are also associated with a political and ideologic movement to address the client's social context in providing psychiatric care. According to these orientations, all social, psychologic, and biologic activity, including research developments in psychobiology, affecting the mental health of the population is of interest to professionals in community psychiatry. Therapeutic interventions may include programs for social change, political involvement, community organization, social planning, family support groups, and education about medications, symptom management, and family environment. Many implications for practice can be derived from this theoretic model.

• Clients are approached in a holistic way, reflecting the interrelation and interaction of the biophysical, psychologic, and socioeconomic-cultural dimensions of human life. This increases the number of factors that the nurse must assess when caring for a client.

• Because of the increased number and diversity of variables to be considered, graduate and undergraduate content in psychiatric nursing education must be revised. Curricula must include concepts, theories, and research findings to support extended and new thinking about mental health, culture, social systems, ethnicity, deviant behavior, social support, psychobiology, and the human condition. These new content areas drawn from the social and natural sciences must then be integrated with conventional psychiatric nursing content to form an internal coherent knowledge base.

• Definitions of the client must include the concept of client system. A family, a couple, an aggregate, or even a community may be the client.

• Intervention strategies include primary prevention achieved through psychoeducation, social change, and research. The goals are to help individuals cope with stresses in their environment, alter environments that contribute to pathology, and conduct research to establish the logical basis for preventive and adaptive measures.

• The yardsticks for measuring "normality" are revised to reflect several notions. First, some deviant behaviors resemble physical illness and others do not. Second, applying psychiatric labels on the basis of selective and flimsy evidence often has destructive consequences. Third, goals for therapy or treatment should not be set without first investigating the client's interpersonal and sociocultural situations.

• Therapy focuses on helping troubled persons to gain a useful perspective on their life-styles and social environments and to develop coping skills and resources, rather than on exclusively repressing and controlling symptoms. Psychiatric nurses need to acknowledge the political and moral implications of involuntary drug therapy and behavior modification therapy.

• The psychiatric nurse must be prepared to function as an autonomous member of the psychiatric team and to assume more responsibilities. There is a shift away from the dominance of the physician in decision making and toward diffusion of roles. Practitioners' roles are based less on background discipline than on availability and interest in helping the client. For example, a cadre of mental health professionals who could become chronic care experts is direly needed, particularly those who can synthesize psychobiologic knowledge with psychosocial rehabilitation skills and psychoeducation.

In short, once clients are viewed as becoming disturbed and/or dysfunctional in the context of unhealthy or problem-filled interpersonal relationships, establishing healthy, constructive interpersonal relationships becomes important in their care. Psychiatric nurses can apply concepts of milieu therapy, primary prevention, social psychiatry, community psychiatry, and psychobiologic interventions to implement this fundamental idea. The following case example illustrates this idea:

Mrs S is a 67-year-old, upper-middle-class woman in good physical health. She has become increasingly untidy, forgetful, reclusive, sad, and suspicious since the death of her aggressive, bank president husband from a heart attach six months ago. She recently sold the large house where she had lived for the past 45 years, and she moved into a two-bedroom apartment in a nearby town. Because of apartment rules, she was unable to take her 12-year-old cat. She sold the house because her husband had told his lawyers that she should do so. (He had made all the family decisions while he lived.) Mrs S has taken to skipping meals except for candy bars, since she must rely on a friend to drive her to the grocery store. (Her husband never felt she needed to learn to drive.) Her younger sister (age 59), seeking advice about Mrs S's behavior, phoned the community mental health center on the suggestion of the family physician.

The social-interpersonal psychiatric nurse assessing this situation would tend not to view Mrs S's symptoms as psychologic conflicts reflecting her ambivalence toward her dead husband or as manifestations of a psychiatric disease, such as major, single-episode depression. Instead, the nurse would focus on the way Mrs S is functioning in her current interpersonal situation and her holistic human responses to it. In this analysis Mrs S is not seen as diseased and therefore in exclusive need of a somatic treatment such as medication. Instead treatment consists of helping Mrs S to develop strategies for coping with her new situation and satisfying her needs. The nurse would seek out the younger sister and other family members in an attempt to enhance Mrs S's social support network. Efforts may be directed toward mobilizing other environmental forces (including the nurse) to provide company, stimulation, and proper nutrition for Mrs S, since the absence of all three contributes to her symptoms and discomfort. The clinical situation would undoubtedly reinforce the psychiatric nurse's political efforts to point out the potential consequences of lifelong passive dependence of some adult women. The nurse may also become involved in community organizations working for better services for the elderly.

Critique

The social-interpersonal model has been criticized on three major fronts: conceptual, philosophic, and practical. Conceptual criticisms are brought most squarely to bear on Sullivan's interpersonal psychiatric theory. Writers such as Ruth Munroe (1955) view interpersonal psychiatric formulations as *word-building*—thinking up new names for old psychoanalytic concepts. Sullivan's theory is perceived as "losing a lot" when contrasted with the richness of Freudian analysis. Sullivan and the other interpersonal theorists, such as Adler, Horney, and Fromm, underplay the role of the biologic demands of the organisms and tend to limit social psychiatry to the immediate family of significant others, neglecting the impact of culture and social structure. Furthermore, according to the critics, if the Freudians have neglected the dynamic importance of the self-system, the self-theories have given the concept too global a role. In sum, the concept does not usually add much to the clinical understanding of any living client. Finally, Munroe proposes that Sullivan's neglect and repudiation of the sexual systems are more a reflection of his era, a reaction against narrow Freudianism, than an intrinsic part of the interpersonal theoretic approach.

Thomas Szasz (1971) emerges as both a proponent and a critic of the social-interpersonal model, at least on a philosophic level. He argues that this model in community psychiatry looks to public health and preventive medicine for both its theoretic model and its moral justification for using the control power of the state. This is an error, says Szasz. If preventive psychiatry is a logical extension of traditional medical practice, psychiatric professionals can justify promoting their own business. Community psychiatry extends the control and power of mental health workers by asserting that psychiatric professionals have responsibility not only for persons who come for help but also for those who do not. Szasz points out the political implications of looking to public health medicine as

TABLE 4–5 A Comparative Analysis of Major Features of Traditional Psychiatric Theories

Theory	Assessment Base	Problem Statement	Goal	Dominant Intervention
Medical-biologic	Individual client symptoms	Disease	Symptom control Cure	Somatotherapies
Psychoanalytic	Intrapsychic Unconscious	Conflict	Insight	Psychoanalysis
Behavioristic	Behavior	Learning deficit	Behavior change	Behavior modification or conditioning
Social-interpersonal	Interactions of individual and social context	Dysfunction	Enhanced awareness and quality of interactions	Group and milieu therapies

the model for community psychiatry. Hypothetically, laws could be passed enacting compulsory mental health measures supposedly designed to protect the community "from psychologic contamination." In summary, Szasz attacks the model for its inclusiveness, its posture of condescending benevolence and righteous paternalism, and its covert potential for political repression.

Finally, criticism is brought to bear on the social-interpersonal model from real-world mental health workers who must cope with the stressful clinical realities, e.g., the window smashing, verbal abuse, and self-destructiveness of a young man brought to the psychiatric ward for threatening to assassinate the governor. To complicate matters further, sociocultural diagnoses are not currently among the categories being considered for psychiatric diagnostic reimbursement groups (DRGs). In our economic reality, they would not qualify a client for financial reimbursement. For these critics, the social-interpersonal model is impractical, idealistic, economically naive, and ill-suited to the realities of psychiatric care—where time is limited, money and supplies are even more so, and immediate problems of symptom control must be solved. A comparison of traditional psychiatric theories appears in Table 4–5.

Overview of Nursing Theories

A **theory of nursing** is a grand general theory that addresses the definition of the domain and scope of nursing. A **theory for practice** is a set of interrelated propositions that specify actions and intended consequences in a situation. In other words, a theory for practice guides the clinician in deciding what to do to achieve certain results.

The concept of nursing as primarily technologic (e.g., hypodermics, bedpans, and other tools of the trade) has been replaced by the idea that nursing is

theory based. Still, nursing remains more divergent than convergent when it comes to identifying the theories to be applied. Most authorities concur that *theoretic pluralism*—that is the simultaneous refinement and testing of numerous contenders for nursing's dominant theory—is highly appropriate for the present early phase in nursing's scientific and intellectual history. Let's briefly examine a few of the best-known contenders and attempt to identify the concepts and principles most relevant to psychiatric nursing. Most of these theorists accept the focal concepts for nursing as *people, nursing, health,* and *society.*

In the early 1950s, Lydia Hall, Virginia Henderson, and Hildegard Peplau had already published precursors to contemporary nursing theories, and Faye Abdellah had begun empiric observations that led to the formulation of her theory by 1955.

Hall Lydia Hall's (1959) theory is best represented by three interlocking circles depicting what she called the "aspects of nursing." Hall's three aspects of nursing were the person (the core), the disease (the cure), and the body (the care). She developed her theory at the Loeb Center for Rehabilitation primarily for the adult client recuperating from a physical illness in a residential treatment center. She showed relationships among the three concepts by varying the size of the three circles to represent the amount or proportion of nursing time focused on each. See Figure 4–3. Most psychiatric nursing practice would focus on the core component of her model.

Henderson Virginia Henderson (1966) contributed the now famous definition of nursing:

Nursing is primarily assisting the individual (sick or well) in the performance of those activities contributing to health or its recovery (or a peaceful death) that he would perform unaided if he had the necessary strength, will, or knowledge.

Henderson identified fourteen activities addressed in basic nursing care. Nurses, she proposed, either help the client with the activities or provide conditions

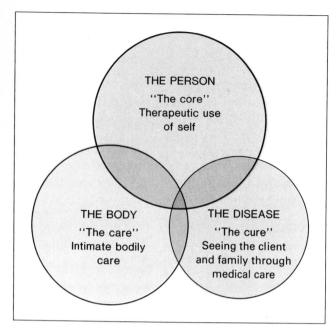

FIGURE 4–3 Hall's three aspects of nursing. *SOURCE: Adapted from Hall L: Nursing—What Is It? Publication of the Virginia State Nurses' Association, Winter 1959.*

under which the client can perform them unaided. These activities are

1. Breathe normally.

2. Eat and drink adequately.

3. Eliminate body wastes.

4. Move and maintain desirable postures.

5. Sleep and rest.

6. Select suitable clothing—dress and undress.

7. Maintain body temperature within normal range by adjusting clothing and modifying the environment.

8. Keep the body clean and well-groomed and protect the integument.

9. Avoid dangers in the environment and avoid injuring others.

10. Communicate with others in expressing emotions, needs, fears, or opinions.

11. Worship according to one's faith.

12. Work in such a way that there is a sense of accomplishment.

13. Play or participate in various forms of recreation.

14. Learn, discover, or satisfy the curiosity that leads to normal development and health and use of the available health facilities.

The first nine activities encompass a version of basic physiologic human needs. The remaining five include needs for communication, spirituality, work, play, and learning—the categories that are emphasized by psychiatric nurses.

Peplau Hildegard Peplau published her nursing theory in the classic book *Interpersonal Relations in Nursing* (1952). She defined nursing as a significant therapeutic interpersonal process, and the core concepts of her theory were the four phases of the nurse-client relationship.

1. Orientation

2. Identification

3. Exploitation (or working)

4. Resolution

Some say that these phases are ancestors of the phases of the nursing process. Psychiatric nurses continue to use Peplau's theory to understand and guide decisions in the one-to-one relationship.

Abdellah Faye Abdellah (1960) presented a list of twenty-one nursing problems that she developed over a five-year period in the late 1950s. The list, presented in the accompanying box, includes physiologic as well as sociopsychologic needs and resembles both Henderson's fourteen nursing care components and Maslow's hierarchy of needs.

Orem Dorothea Orem's (1971) theory of self-care was originally introduced around 1959 and identified ten universal self-care requisites, which are divided into six categories that encompass both physical and psychosocial human needs. Orem also introduced a second order of concepts originally called health deviation self-care demands to refer to care required in the event of illness, injury, or disease. Nursing, a second key component of her scheme, was divided into wholly compensatory, partially compensatory, and supportive-educational systems of care that could be matched to the client's assessed level of self-care functioning in each area (see Figure 4–4). This theory firmly established the notion of a goal of self-care as integral to the discipline of nursing's perspective on the meaning of health. Orem's theory is particularly well adapted to meeting nursing care needs of the severely and chronically mentally disordered.

Rogers Martha Rogers (1970) drew on knowledge from anthropology, sociology, religion, philosophy, mythology, and general systems theory to define nursing as a holistic science of human nature and development. Rogers's key nursing principles are called the principles of homeodynamics. Subprinciples of homeodynamics are:

The Twenty-One Nursing Problems

1. To maintain good hygiene and physical comfort

2. To promote optimal activity: exercise, rest, and sleep

3. To promote safety through the prevention of accidents, injury or other trauma, and infection

4. To maintain good body mechanics and prevent and correct deformities

5. To maintain a supply of oxygen to all body cells

6. To maintain nutrition of all body cells

7. To facilitate elimination

8. To maintain fluid and electrolyte balance

9. To recognize the pathological, physiological, and compensatory responses of the body to disease conditions

10. To maintain regulatory mechanisms and functions

11. To maintain sensory function

12. To identify and accept positive and negative expressions, feelings, and reactions

13. To identify and accept the interrelatedness of emotions and organic illness

14. To maintain effective verbal and nonverbal communication

15. To promote the development of productive interpersonal relationships

16. To facilitate progress toward achievement of personal spiritual goals

17. To create or maintain a therapeutic environment

18. To facilitate awareness of self as an individual with varying physical, emotional, and developmental needs

19. To accept the optimum possible goals in the light of physical and emotional limitations

20. To use community resources in resolving problems arising from illness

21. To understand the role of social problems as influencing factors in the cause of illness

SOURCE: Reprinted with permission of Macmillan Publishing Co., Inc., from Patient-Centered Approaches to Nursing *by Faye G. Abdellah, Almeda Martin, Irene L. Beland, and Ruth V. Matheney. © Copyright, Macmillan Publishing Co., Inc., 1960.*

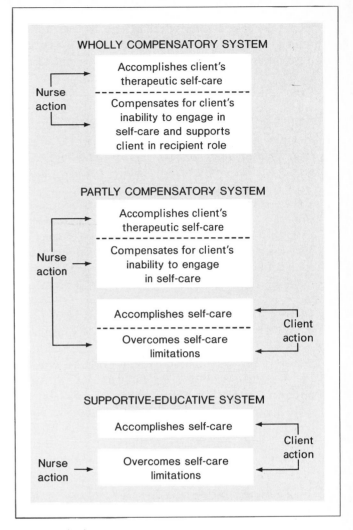

FIGURE 4–4 Orem's self-care deficit theory. *SOURCE: Adapted from Orem DE:* Nursing: Concepts of Practice. *McGraw-Hill, 1971.*

• The principle of complementarity, which refers to the continuous, simultaneous interaction between human and environmental fields

• The principle of resonancy, which refers to the tendency of humans to function according to patterns that can be studied

• The principle of helicy, according to which the nature and direction of human and environmental change are continuous, innovative, probabilistic, and diverse but also evolutionary and goal directed

These three principles are ways of viewing human beings holistically. Changes in life processes are irreversible, nonrepeatable, and rhythmic and indicate patterns of increasing complexity and organization. Most of her concepts have counterparts in general systems theory, but she has added the notions of life processes, change, and human-environmental interaction to the concepts central to nursing. Rogers's work gives psychiatric nurses a mandate to use holistic principles as a guide to practice and to consider physical as well as psychosocial problems and needs.

Roy   Sister Callista Roy's (1976) adaptation theory views people as constantly faced with the need to adapt to focal, contextual, and residual stimuli. She identifies four modes of human adapting: (1) *physiologic needs,* (2) *self-concept,* (3) *role function,* and (4) *interdependence.* Obviously, these adaptive modes again include physiologic, psychologic, and social aspects of people. The notion of coping or adapting to stimuli again relates nursing to people in interaction with their environment. Self-concept, role function, and interdependent areas of coping all lend themselves to the conceptualization of the practice of psychiatric nursing.

Others   The theories presented in the past few pages in no way represent the entire universe of contenders. Ida Jean Orlando (1961) stresses the interaction of meanings between nurse and client. Ernestine Wiedenbach's (1964) work presents an example of a "situation-producing" theory that conceptualizes a goal and a nursing prescription for fulfilling the goal. Myra Levine (1967) uses four conservation principles to conceptualize nursing interventions: (1) *conservation of energy,* (2) *conservation of structural integrity,* (3) *conservation of personal integrity,* and (4) *conservation of social integrity.* Imogene King (1971) discusses concepts of social systems, perceptions, interpersonal relations, and health and their impact on people.

A review of these theories indicates some clear differences in emphasis and perspective and some intriguing similarities. From these theories are emerging the parameters of our discipline. Such parameters provide the beginnings for directing practice, focusing nursing research, and providing a framework of concepts integral to the teaching of professional students.

Critique

Critics challenge us to demonstrate how nursing theory is more than mere restatement of well-known psychologic, physiologic, systems, or medical principles in a special jargon. If all nursing theory exists ultimately for the sake of practice, the theory developed to guide psychiatric nursing practice ought to be clearly distinguishable from mental health practice based on borrowed theories in other disciplines. Colleagues in other disciplines cannot be expected to learn and apply new terms to describe familiar phenomena just because we in nursing choose to use them. Nursing theories must have both intellectual and practical coherence if they are to achieve a foothold in the knowledge base of the mental health team.

The Choice of a Theory for Practice

Psychiatric nurses use one or a combination of theoretic frameworks to guide the application of the nursing process to their practice. In this text, we use the humanistic interactionist philosophic approach in combination with new knowledge in psychobiology discussed in Chapter 1 as the basis for ideas about human responses. As acknowledged earlier, this approach synthesizes strengths derived primarily from the social-interpersonal and the biologic models and allows for the evolution of nursing theories as our body of knowledge grows. In clinical work, however, the selection of a theoretic framework may be influenced by various factors. Among them are the practitioner's education, the philosophy of the setting in which clients are treated, the nature of the client's present problem, the available treatment, the need to be efficient and practical, and even client attributes such as social class and gender. For example, in most cases physicians are inclined to view clients according to the medical model, the approach stressed in their education. This is particularly likely when the client's problem is identified as one of the syndromes for which biologic treatment is readily available and effective in symptom control, such as major depression or bipolar mood disorder, manic type. The former syndrome has been shown to respond to antidepressant medication and electroshock therapy, and the latter to lithium carbonate. The choice of a biologic-medical model is even more likely when the client is from a lower- or lower-middle-class background, or elderly, or not highly intelligent or verbal. These characteristics are often used to rule out candidacy for psychotherapy. If the setting must respond to large numbers of clients on a short-term basis, the decision to label, sort, patch up with medicines, and dispatch back into the community often seems the only realistic alternative.

Social-interpersonal theory is more likely to be the basis for assessment and planning of client care under the following conditions: The clinician is a psychiatric nurse or social worker; the client's problem is one of relating to others or adjusting to a situation in life; the client is relatively verbal, intelligent, young, motivated, and from an upper-middle-class background; and the setting one in which long-term residential milieu therapy or group or individual psychotherapy is possible.

The failure to effect a "cure" according to the principles of any one theory may induce clinicians to recast the problem in different theoretic terms, adopting different treatment options. For example, a psychotic client who does not respond to medication may respond to a well-planned behavior modification program. Approaches associated with two or more different models are often used in combination. For example, bizarre, self-destructive behavior may be controlled with medications so that the client is more available for group or individual therapy. Such a combined or eclectic approach demands that a clinician be capable of functioning according to all theories of care, depending on which is best for the client and best fits the resources and limitations of the situation. If nurses give adequate consideration to the theoretic framework of their psychiatric nursing, they will foster practice-oriented research and clinical judgments that can be articulated and taught to others. Research is a tool for developing psychiatric nursing theory that synthesizes the most useful elements of these theories.

CHAPTER HIGHLIGHTS

• The choice of a theory for psychiatric nursing treatment determines information assessed, goals and interventions recommended, and evaluation criteria set.

• Therapeutic models for interdisciplinary mental health practice traditionally include the medical-biologic model, the psychoanalytic model, the behaviorist model, the social-interpersonal model, and nursing theories.

• In the medical-biologic model, emotional and behavioral disturbances are viewed as diseases. In the past, this view tended to limit the nurse's role to administration of biologic treatments and observation.

• Critics of the medical model of mental illness suggest that (a) social, ethical, interpersonal, and cultural factors are overlooked or obscured; (b) labeling behavior as "illness" relieves people of responsibility for their behavior; (c) mental symptoms correspond more to problems in living and relating to others than to diseases of the body.

• Psychoanalytic theory developed by Freud purports that all psychologic events have meaning and are understandable.

• Psychoanalytic theory states that much of what goes on in people's minds is unknown to them, or unconscious, and accounts for apparent discontinuities in their lives that are due to unresolved conflicts in stages of psychosexual development.

• In the psychoanalytic model, the nurse usually functions in a supportive therapeutic role.

• Criticism of Freudian psychoanalytic theory has come from feminists, behaviorists, and ego psychologists.

• In the behaviorist model, the self and mental symptoms are viewed as learned behaviors that persist because they are rewarding to the individual.

• In the behaviorist model, the nurse's role is expanded to planner, counselor, and educator, but therapeutic goals are limited to symptom control through behavior-modification techniques that raise ethical issues.

• The behaviorist model has been criticized for its ethics, its reductionist explanation of human feelings and behavior, and its controlling, authoritarian therapist-client relationship.

• In the social-interpersonal model, (a) treatment occurs within an interpersonal context; (b) social processes (e.g., labeling by those involved in disturbed behavior) are assessed; (c) the clinician views deviant behavior in its broader context and uses a general systems perspective to integrate biologic and sociocultural data.

• In the social-interpersonal framework treatment is likely to include helping clients develop strategies for coping, mobilizing social support networks, and involving the therapist in community organization and planning.

• The psychiatric nurse's role in the social-interpersonal framework is expanded to include social and political action and community intervention as well as direct intervention with individuals, families, and groups.

• Concepts serving as the focus for contemporary nursing theories are people, nursing, health, and society.

• Research that develops nursing theory can synthesize the most useful ideas from all the dominant theoretic frameworks for psychiatric care.

REFERENCES

Abdellah FG, et al: *Patient-Centered Approaches to Nursing.* Macmillan, 1960.

Adler A: *The Practice and Theory of Individual Psychology.* Translated by P. Radin. 1929; reprint edition, Humanities Press, 1971.

Becker HS: *Outsiders: Studies in the Sociology of Deviance.* Free Press, 1963.

Carlsson A, Lindqvist M: Effects of chlorpromazine or haloperidol on formation of 3-methoxytyramine and normetanephrine in mouse brain. *Acta Pharmacolog Toxicol* 1973;20:140.

Chesler P: *Women and Madness.* Doubleday, 1972.

Chinn PL, Jacobs MK: *Theory and Nursing,* ed 2. Mosby, 1987.

Dasheff CJ: Theory development in psychiatric-mental health nursing: An analysis of Orem's theory. *Arch Psychiatr Nurs* 1988;3(6):366–372.

Deutsch H: *Psychology of Women.* Grune and Stratton, 1944–1945, 2 vols.

Erikson EN: *Identity, Youth and Crisis.* W. W. Norton, 1968.

Erikson K: Notes on the sociology of deviance. *Soc Prob* 1962;9:308.

Fawcett J: *Analysis and Evaluation of Conceptual Models of Nursing.* FA Davis, 1984.

Firestone S: *The Dialectic of Sex.* William Morrow, 1971.

Fitzpatrick J, Whall A, Johnston R, Floyd J: *Nursing Models and Their Psychiatric Mental Health Applications.* Prentice-Hall, 1982.

Fraiberg S: *The Magic Years.* Charles Scribners' Sons, 1959.

Freud S: *Beyond the Pleasure Principle.* W. W. Norton, 1975.

Freud S: *The Ego and the Id.* W. W. Norton, 1962 (a).

Freud S: *The Standard Edition of the Complete Psychological Works of Sigmund Freud.* Hogarth Press, 1962 (b), 24 vols.

Fromm E: *Escape from Freedom.* Irvington Publishers, 1941.

Hall L: *Nursing—What Is It?* Publication of the Virginia State Nurses' Association, Winter 1959.

Henderson V: *The Nature of Nursing.* Macmillan, 1966.

Hollingshead AB, Redlich FC: *Social Class and Mental Illness.* John Wiley, 1958.

Horney K: *Neurosis and Human Growth.* W. W. Norton, 1950.

Kallman FG: *Heredity in Health and Mental Disorder.* W. W. Norton, 1953.

Kety SS: Biochemical theories of schizophrenia. *Science* 1959;129:1528,1590.

King IM: *Toward a Theory of Nursing: General Concepts of Human Behavior.* Wiley, 1971.

Laing RD; *The Politics of Experience.* Ballantine Books, 1967.

Lemert E: *Social Pathology.* McGraw-Hill, 1951.

Levine ME: The four conservation principles of nursing. *Nurs Forum* 1967;6:45–59.

Maslow A: *Toward a Psychology of Being.* D. Van Nostrand, 1962.

Mechanic D: Some factors in identifying and defining mental illness, in Spitzer S, Denzin NK (eds): *The Mental Patient: Studies in the Sociology of Deviance.* McGraw-Hill, 1968.

Meleis A: *Theoretical Nursing: Development and Progress,* 2e. Lippincott, 1991.

Menninger K: *The Vital Balance.* Viking Press, 1963.

Meyer A: *Collected Papers of Adolf Meyer.* Johns Hopkins University Press, 1948–1952, 4 vols.

Munroe RL: *Schools of Psychoanalytic Thought.* Holt, Rinehart and Winston, 1955.

Norris C: Restlessness: A nursing phenomenon in search of meaning. *Nurs Outlook* 1975;23:103–107.

Orem DE; *Nursing: Concepts of Practice.* McGraw-Hill, 1971.

Orlando IJ: *The Dynamic Nurse-Patient Relationship: Function, Process and Principles.* Putnam, 1961.

Peplau HE: *Interpersonal Relations in Nursing.* Putnam, 1952.

Rogers ME: *The Theoretical Basis of Nursing.* FA Davis, 1970.

Roy C: *Introduction to Nursing: An Adaptation Model.* Prentice-Hall, 1976.

Scheff T: *Being Mentally Ill: A Sociological Theory.* Aldine, 1966.

Skinner BF: *Beyond Freedom and Dignity.* Knopf, 1971.

Skinner BF: *Science and Human Behavior.* Macmillan, 1953.

Stevens BJ: *Nursing Theory,* ed 2. Little, Brown, 1984.

Sullivan HS: *The Interpersonal Theory of Psychiatry,* Perry HS, Gawel ML (eds). W. W. Norton, 1953.

Szasz TS (ed): *The Manufacture of Madness.* Dell Publishing, 1971.

Szasz TS: *The Myth of Mental Illness: Foundations of a Theory of Personal Conduct.* Harper and Row, 1974.

Wiedenbach E: *Clinical Nursing, A Helping Art.* Springer, 1964.

Williams JBW, Wilson HS: A psychiatric nursing perspective on DSM-III. *J Psychosoc Nurs* 1982;20:14–20.

Wilson HS: *Research in Nursing,* 2e. Addison-Wesley, 1989.

Wise CD, Stein L: L dopamine beta-hydroxylase deficits in the brains of schizophrenic patients. *Science* 1973; 181:384.

Wolpe J: Learning versus lesions as the basis of neurotic behavior. *Am J Psychiatry* 1956;112:923–931.

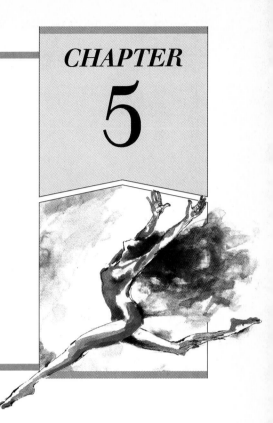

Stress, Anxiety, and Coping

LEARNING OBJECTIVES

- Describe the effects of stress on an individual
- Compare three theories that purport to explain stress
- Discuss the sources of anxiety
- Describe the effects of anxiety on an individual
- Explain everyday methods for coping with stress and anxiety
- Explain the resources that help people resist stress
- Discuss constructive and destructive coping strategies
- Define common defense-oriented behaviors and give examples of them

Carol Ren Kneisl

CROSS REFERENCES

Other topics relevant to this content are: Applying the nursing process to the care of anxious clients, Chapter 14; Assessing the severity of stress according to Axis IV of DSM-III-R, Chapter 9 and Appendix A; Posttraumatic stress disorder, Chapter 14; Psychophysiologic conditions thought to result from stress, Chapter 18; Relaxation and stress-management techniques, Chapter 27.

Health care professionals have long been interested in stress and anxiety and in the ways that healthy and dysfunctional persons cope or fail to cope with them. Stress and anxiety affect the person's well-being. Various behavioral and physiologic disorders have been linked to stress and anxiety. Some behavioral manifestations are discussed here and elaborated in later chapters. The cost of stress and anxiety can be quite high: They can cost a woman her job, a man the love and respect of his family. When sufficiently prolonged, stress can kill.

Stress

Stress is a part of being alive. Standing erect stresses the muscles and bones that must work together to keep the body erect; eating stresses the digestive system, which must produce enzymes and absorb nutrients; and breathing stresses the respiratory system, which must exchange carbon dioxide and oxygen. More broadly and holistically, **stress** designates a broad class of experiences in which a demanding situation taxes a person's resources or coping capabilities, causing a negative effect. This broader definition approximates the humanistic perspective of this textbook. In this view, stress is a person-environment interaction. The source of the stress, the demanding situation, is known as a **stressor.** The internal state the stress produces is one of tension, anxiety, or strain.

There is no universally accepted definition of stress among stress theorists and researchers. An interactional view of stress, such as the one given above, is consistent with how nurses view human experiences. The theories of stress that follow are the perspectives in common use. Although they do tell us a great deal about responses to stressful situations, it is crucial for nurses to recognize that these explanations are not necessarily consistent with nursing's orientation. Such factors as cause, the situational context in which the stressful event occurs, and the psychologic interpretation of the demanding situation must be considered in a holistic, humanistic approach to the client. Axis IV of DSM-III-R offers some general parameters for assessing the severity of stress. (See Chapter 9 and Appendix A for further information.)

The Fight-Flight Response to Stress

Beyond the routine and essential stress of everyday life, humans risk encountering undesirable or excess stress that threatens well-being and may even be life threatening. They cope with such threats through either a **fight** (aggression) or **flight** (withdrawal) response. The

fight-flight response was first discussed by Walter Cannon, a physician, in 1932 when he identified stress as an actual cause of disease. Consider the following situation of extreme stress: A woman is walking down a dark, deserted street when a man with a knife emerges from the shadows just in front of her. Does she try to defend herself? Does she run away? Whichever action she takes is a result of a variety of physiologic responses to extreme danger. According to Mason (1980), when a person faces such a situation

• The heartbeat increases to pump blood throughout the necessary tissues with greater speed, carrying oxygen and nutrients to cells and clearing away waste products more quickly.

• As the heart rate increases, the blood pressure rises.

• Breathing becomes rapid and shallow.

• Epinephrine and other hormones are released into the blood.

• The liver releases stored sugar into the blood to meet the increased energy needs of survival.

• The pupils dilate to let in more light; all the senses are heightened.

• Muscles tense for movement, either for flight or protective actions, particularly the skeletal muscles of the thighs, hips, back, shoulders, arms, jaw, and face.

• Blood flow to the digestive organs is greatly constricted.

• Blood flow increases to the brain and major muscles.

• Blood flow to the extremities is constricted, and the hands and feet become cold. This is protection from bleeding to death quickly if the hands or feet are injured in fight or flight and allows blood to be diverted to more important areas of the body.

• The body perspires to cool itself, because increased metabolism generates more heat.

Although these physiologic responses seem appropriate for the situation described, imagine the wear and tear on the body if humans responded to all stress in these ways.

Selye's Stress-Adaptation Theory

Hans Selye, a Canadian endocrinologist and the most well known and widely recognized stress researcher, developed another framework for understanding how persons respond to stress. According to him, each person has a limited amount of energy to use in dealing with stress. How quickly it is used and, therefore, how quickly one adapts to stress depend on several factors such as heredity, mental attitude, and life-style, among others.

Selye defines stress as the rate of wear and tear on the body. He disputes the idea that only serious disease or injury causes stress. Selye thinks that any emotion or activity requires a response or change in the individual. Stressors can be physical, chemical, physiologic, developmental, or emotional. Playing a game of tennis, going out in the rain without an umbrella, having an argument, or getting a promotion are all examples of stressful events. Life itself is basically stressful, since it involves a process of adaptation to continual change. Though the experience of adaptation is stressful, it is not necessarily harmful. Indeed, it can be exciting and rewarding under certain circumstances, and although we cannot avoid the stress of living, we can learn to minimize its damaging effects.

While a medical student, Selye made an interesting and important observation that became the cornerstone of his stress-adaptation theory. He observed that, regardless of the diagnosis, most clients had certain symptoms in common—they lost their appetite, they lost weight, they felt and looked ill, they were anxious and fatigued, and they had aches and pains in their joints and muscles. A long series of experiments (1956) led to more objective evidence of actual body damage—enlargement of the adrenal glands; shrinkage of the thymus, spleen, and lymph nodes; and the appearance of bleeding gastric ulcers.

Feelings of anxiety, fatigue, or illness are subjective aspects of stress. Though stress itself cannot be perceived, Selye found that it can be objectively measured by the structural and chemical changes that it produces in the body. These changes are called the **general adaptation syndrome** (GAS) because when stress affects the whole person, the whole person must adjust to the changes. The GAS occurs in three stages: alarm, resistance, and exhaustion. An example of the GAS can be found in combat soldiers. These men are exposed to ever-present threats of death and mutilation. They also experience the severe psychologic shock of witnessing the destructiveness of war. Other psychologic and interpersonal factors, such as loss of personal freedom and separation from loved ones, contribute to their overall stress load. The experiences of combat soldiers can be used to illustrate the three stages of the GAS, which are summarized in Table 5–1.

Alarm Reaction When soldiers first encounter the stress of war, they experience the *alarm* reaction. During the alarm reaction, the body undergoes biochemical reactions, such as the production of the adaptive hormones adrenocorticotropic hormone (ACTH), cortisone, and aldosterone. The biochemical

reactions also enlarge the adrenal cortex and lymph nodes. These changes lower the person's overall resistance. For example, soldiers may show such behavioral changes as increased irritability, sleep disturbances, and recurrent nightmares. Soldiers are described as being hypersensitive to minor stimuli. For instance, they will leap up in fright at the sound of a branch cracking. This behavior generally indicates failure to maintain psychologic integration.

Stage of Resistance Many soldiers are able to adjust to combat. As they do so, the next stage, *resistance*, occurs. In the stage of resistance the biologic changes in hormonal levels, adrenal cortex, and lymph nodes are reversed. These soldiers can maintain their psychologic integrity. They may become used to killing and may even take pride in it. They may be able to maintain a fatalistic attitude about their own and their comrades' survival. Soldiers who have made this adjustment may be able to resign themselves to fate and believe that they serve for an important purpose, even though they cannot fully understand it. They may take comfort in the thought that combat will not last long, or that they will soon be rotated out of the combat area to a less stressful role.

The nature of this adaptation seems to depend on many psychologic and social factors. These include the stability of the soldier's personality, the morale of the combat unit, the sense of security and control provided by the leadership, and the friendships the soldier forms with other soldiers, which provide emotional support.

Exhaustion The third stage, *exhaustion*, occurs if stress continues over a prolonged time. It also occurs when multiple stressors are active simultaneously, or when the person undergoes repeated or overwhelming stress. When too many life changes occur within a short time, there is not enough time for the body to accommodate and adjust. Adaptive energy is exhausted, and the body surrenders to stress. The adrenal glands again enlarge and then are depleted. The lymph nodes enlarge, producing a subsequent dysfunction of the lymph system. There is an increase and then a decrease in hormonal levels.

The longer soldiers are in combat, the more vulnerable and anxious they are likely to feel. Prolonged combat lowers stress tolerance. It may produce increased anxiety, depression, tremulousness, and impairment of judgment and self-confidence. This decompensation results in disturbances in interpersonal relationships. The soldier may lose all sense of loyalty to comrades. In some cases, the residual effects of combat exhaustion persist for a long time. Combat experience may continue to disturb former soldiers after they return to civilian life. They may experience guilt about killing and have nightmares about war experiences.

TABLE 5–1   The General Adaptation Syndrome

Stage	Physical Change	Psychosocial Changes
Stage I: Alarm reaction Mobilization of the body's defensive forces and activation of the "fight-or-flight" mechanism	Release of norepinephrine and epinephrine causing vasoconstriction, increased blood pressure, and increased rate and force of cardiac contraction Increased hormone levels Enlargement of adrenal cortex Marked loss of body weight Shrinkage of the thymus, spleen, and lymph nodes Irritation of the gastric mucosa	Increased level of alertness Increased level of anxiety Task-oriented, defense-oriented, inefficient, or maladaptive behavior may occur
Stage II: Stage of resistance Optimal adaptation to stress within the person's capabilities	Hormone levels readjust Reduction in activity and size of adrenal cortex Lymph nodes return to normal size Weight returns to normal	Increased and intensified use of coping mechanisms Tendency to rely on defense-oriented behavior
Stage III: Stage of exhaustion Loss of ability to resist stress because of depletion of body resources	Decreased immune response with suppression of T cells and atrophy of thymus Depletion of adrenal glands and hormone production Weight loss Enlargement of lymph nodes and dysfunction of lymphatic system If exposure to the stressor continues, cardiac failure, renal failure, or death may occur	Defense-oriented behaviors become exaggerated Disorganization of thinking Disorganization of personality Sensory stimuli may be misperceived with appearance of illusions Reality contact may be reduced with appearance of delusions or hallucinations If exposure to the stressor continues, stupor or violence may occur

SOURCE: Kneisl CR, Ames SW; Adult Health Nursing: A Biopsychosocial Approach. Addison-Wesley, 1986, p 20.

Exhaustion may be reversible if the total body is not affected and if the individual is eventually able to eliminate the source of stress. However, if stress is unrelieved, or if the body's defenses are totally involved, the individual may not regain psychologic stability and may become physically ill (see the accompanying Psychobiology box).

Life Changes As Stressful Events

Most people are accustomed to thinking of untoward events as stressful, but they do not realize that desirable events such as job promotions, vacations, or outstanding personal achievements may also prove stressful. Holmes and Rahe (1967) studied life changes as stressful events to learn the amount of social readjustment required to cope with them. These authors believe that the life events that require coping behavior tend to decrease a person's ability to handle illness or subsequent stress.

Their research assigned ratings to forty-three different life changes, called *life change units* (LCUs). They asked subjects to indicate what life changes had occurred in the past year and then add up the points assigned to each identified life event. According to these researchers, a low score indicated that the subject was not likely to have an adverse reaction. A "mild"

score meant that there was a 30 percent chance that the person would manifest the impact of stress through physical symptoms. Persons in the "moderate" category had a 50 percent chance of a change in health status, and a "high" score meant an 80 percent chance of major illness in the next two years. High LCU scores also correlated with an increased probability of accidental injury. The example given below demonstrates how this model could be applied in understanding one individual's situation.

Marcia M, a 22-year-old woman in group therapy, had recently been divorced from her husband (LCU 73) after attempting to achieve a marital reconciliation (LCU 45). Marcia's pregnancy (LCU 40) earlier in the year was uneventful, and the Ms' healthy son was born on June 2 (LCU 39). At 6 weeks of age, the child suddenly and unexpectedly died in his crib (LCU 63). The Ms began to argue frequently (LCU 35) before they made the decision to divorce. After the divorce, Marcia found herself short of funds (LCU 38) and went to work as a waitress in a pizza restaurant (LCU 36). She found it necessary to move to a smaller and less expensive apartment (LCU 20). In the short period of one year, Marcia accumulated an LCU score of 390 and was in the high-risk group.

In the early 1970s, other researchers correlated life stress events and mental health. In a study of 720

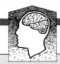

PSYCHOBIOLOGY: THE MIND/BODY CONNECTION

Stress! It's Enough to Make You Sick!

Have you ever noticed that you begin to develop symptoms of a cold, the flu, or allergy exacerbations as the end of the semester or quarter draws near? The symptoms may vary, but the theme is consistent: illness. Recent knowledge gains in the field of immunology indicate that this phenomenon is not surprising. There are three general components of immunity: the surveillance for and destruction of disease-causing microorganism; the rejection of foreign material in the body; and the ongoing process of differentiating self from non-self. The latter category involves autoimmune processes.

In the face of significant or uncontrollable stress, the immune system often reacts with alterations in both humoral and cell-mediated immunity. This process of altered immune function occurs as a result of complex psychobiologic mechanisms involving the endocrine system, particularly the hypothalamic-pituitary-adrenal axis. Stress has been implicated in a variety of conditions, including immunosuppression, dermatologic responses, rheumatoid arthritis, depression, and even cancer.

The relationship between stress, altered immune function, and the emergence of disease states leads us to believe that preventive measures are critical in the prevention of disease. The way in which a person thinks, responds, and reacts will determine the course of his or her own psychobiology. According to Hales (1989), there are several strategies that can be used to bolster immunity. First, vitamin and mineral intake is essential. These substances, especially vitamins B_6, B_{12}, folic acid, iron, and zinc are critical to effective immune functioning. Avoidance of fatty foods, especially those characterized as saturated fats, may also allay cardiovascular disease. It is also important to get enough sleep. Several things occur during sleep; most importantly, the secretion of the hormones essential to the repair and production of immune cells. The final recommendations include no smoking, avoidance of heavy alcohol intake, and participating in a regular exercise program. Smoking diminishes the levels of certain immune cells, as does heavy alcohol intake. Exercise, especially aerobics, not only helps to diffuse stress, but also stimulates the production of immune boosters.

Psychoimmunology is an evolving branch of science that takes a **holistic** approach to the understanding of illness. This specialty holds that one of the major factors in maintaining health and well-being is the modulation and control of stress. This control may be exerted from *within* by learning to respond differently to life events. Additionally, control of the external environment via the modulation of stressful life circumstances will also influence the course of a person's psychobiology.

Many of the concepts inherent in this information are not new. These concepts and ideas, however, have moved into a more objective realm, from speculation to fact. Psychiatric nursing may be in the forefront of psychoimmunologic approaches in care, with the potential for true integration of the art and science of nursing. This may be accomplished through an understanding of the potentially neutralizing impact of spirituality, attitudes, thoughts, and hope on stress and its psychobiologic consequences.

— *Geoffry McEnany*

households in a metropolitan area, J. Meyers and his associates (1972) found a relationship between a high number of life changes and changes in the mental status of individuals. For example, an increase in the number of life changes preceded worsening of psychiatric symptoms, whereas a decrease in life changes brought improvement. The more stressful the life changes, the greater the likelihood of mental ill health. Meyers and his associates also found that entrance-related life events (those involving the addition of a new person into one's social sphere, perhaps through marriage or the birth of a child) produced less symptomatology than did exit-related life events (those associated with the loss of a valued individual or status).

A number of nurse researchers have studied life changes and hospitalization as stressful events. However, nurses applying the Holmes and Rahe model should be aware of the following cautions. This model is based on several assumptions that depict a person as a passive recipient of stress. It assumes that events affect all people in the same way, regardless of how the individuals perceive the event. It also assumes that there is a common threshold beyond which disruption occurs. In addition, it assumes that the same amount of adaptation is required for each event among all persons. Further, it equates "change" with "stress" (Lyon and Werner 1987).

To understand the effects of life changes on health, the nurse needs to identify what each individual perceives as stressful. Only then can the nurse use the Holmes and Rahe model to help people become aware of the stress they face in their lives. It is also useful in planning for the future. To return to the example of Marcia M:

During the course of group therapy, Marcia shared her desire to return to college and complete the junior and senior years of a medical technology program in which she had been enrolled before her marriage. To do so, she would have to make a number of changes—move to an apartment close to the college because she could not afford to own a car, change her working hours or job so that she could attend day classes, change her sleeping habits, change her recreational and social activities, and reduce her other expenses to pay school costs. The changes required would add almost 200 LCUs to her score.

In group, Marcia was able to consider this information and re-evaluate her goals. She decided to delay her return to school until she could get on her feet financially. She chose not to make any other changes in her life for the present time.

Clients can use this information, much as Marcia did, to decide when it is advantageous or disadvantageous to engage in life change. This knowledge helps them make responsible decisions about the directions their lives will take. Nurses can assist clients by incorporating the guidelines below in their practice:

• Help clients to recognize when a life change occurs.

• Encourage clients to think about the meaning of the change and identify some of the feelings experienced.

• Discuss with clients the different ways they might best adjust to the event.

• Encourage them to take time in arriving at decisions.

• If possible, encourage clients to anticipate life changes and plan for them well in advance.

• Encourage clients to pace themselves. It can be done, even if they are in a hurry.

• Encourage clients to look at the accomplishment of a task as a part of daily living and to avoid looking at such an achievement as a stopping point or a time for letting down.

Stress As an Interaction

Richard Lazarus, a pioneering theorist and researcher in stress, coping, and health, is known for his interactional approach to understanding stress. Lazarus (1966, 1976) sees *perceived* threat as the central characteristic of stressful situations, and in particular, threat to a person's most important goals and values. His view is reflected in the definition of stress given at the beginning of this chapter. He believes that stress depends not only on external conditions but also on the constitutional vulnerability of the person and the adequacy of that person's coping styles. He also considers the role of frustration and conflict in producing stress. **Frustration** is the thwarting or the delaying of some important ongoing activity or the attainment of some important goal. **Conflict** is the coexistence of opposing desires, feelings, or goals. Conflict, of necessity, leads to frustration because activity designed to achieve one goal frustrates the attainment of the other. Satisfactory resolution of conflict is impossible as long as the person remains committed to both courses of action or both goals. This imbalance gives rise to the experience of stress.

The major points of Lazarus's theory are discussed below.

Conflict As a Stressor The concept of conflict is useful in identifying the stresses that help cause disturbed coping patterns. Conflict often explains such observable behaviors as hesitation, vacillation, blocking, and fatigue. Conflict is frequently seen in the behavior of psychotic clients, who may have difficulty making even the simplest decisions.

The following conflicts are the most likely to cause stress:

• Conflicts that involve social relations with significant people

• Conflicts that involve ethical standards

• Conflicts that involve meeting unconscious needs

• Conflicts that involve the problems of everyday family living

A conflict proceeds according to the following four steps:

1. The person holds two goals simultaneously.

2. The person moves in relation to both of the goals, using

    a. Approach-avoidance movements, or

    b. Avoidance-avoidance movements.

3. The person shows hesitation, vacillation, blocking, or fatigue.

4. Resolution occurs either temporarily or permanently.

Conflict with Approach-Avoidance Movements

When a person holds two incompatible goals at the same time, the goals usually constitute an either-or situation. If the person chooses one goal, the other goal is rejected or abolished automatically. This situation is called a double approach-avoidance conflict. Here is an example:

Mrs R holds two goals. She wants to talk with the nurse about her fears of going back to work. At the same time, she wants not to be perceived as weak or "a bother." Mrs R makes a movement in relation to her first goal—talking to the nurse—by walking up to her. When the nurse stops and turns toward her, Mrs R asks some superficial question about her supper. In this way she avoids discussing her real concerns. When the nurse offers an opening to talk further, Mrs R avoids the conversation she needs by saying she wants to rest. An hour later, she rings the bell with an apologetic but vague question about her medication.

Vacillation describes Mrs R's behavior.

Principles That Explain Vacillation   To understand how vacillation comes to be the manifest behavior and what is going on during a conflict situation like the one described above, we need to understand four key principles.

1. As you near a desirable goal, the approach tendency is strengthened.

2. As you near an undesirable goal, the avoidance tendency is strengthened.

3. The strength of the avoidance tendency always increases more rapidly with nearness to the goal than does the strength of the approach tendency.

4. The strength of both tendencies varies with the strength of the need basic to the tendencies. That is, an increased need can strengthen both tendencies and intensify the conflict, whereas a decreased need can weaken both tendencies and lessen the conflict.

Avoidance-Avoidance Conflict   In avoidance-avoidance conflict, a person is faced with two undesirable goals at the same time. The person attempts to avoid the nearer of these two goals, but with the retreat from the nearer goal, the tendency to avoid the second goal increases. Unless the tendency to avoid one of the goals overpowers the tendency to avoid the other, or unless there is a third way out of the conflict, the person feels trapped by the conflict.

Robert P, the 35-year-old son of well-to-do parents, was strongly attracted to "the good life." He wanted to live in a creative, esthetic environment, read good books, attend the opera, drink quality wine. Simultaneously he wanted both to avoid working to earn the money for the life-style he desired and not to depend on his parents for support. His life-style became one of waiting to find a resolution to his conflict. He neither worked nor accepted "handouts" from his family, but his preferred life-style became one that he talked about rather than lived.

Anxiety

Anxiety is a state of uneasiness or discomfort experienced to varying degrees. It is frequently coupled with guilt, doubts, fears, and obsessions. Beyond the mild level, anxiety is often described as a feeling of terror or dread; anxiety is believed to be the most uncomfortable feeling a person can experience. In fact, anxiety is so uncomfortable that most persons try to get rid of it as soon as possible.

Anxiety is a potent force, because the energy it provides can be converted into destructive or constructive action. When used destructively, anxiety can immobilize a person with problems. When used constructively, anxiety can stimulate the action necessary to alter the stressful situation, fill a painful need, or arrange a compromise. A client who understands the source of anxiety is best able to use it constructively.

Sources of Anxiety

Anxiety is an inevitable result of the attempt to maintain equilibrium in a changing world. People experience anxiety in many different situations and interpersonal relationships. The stimulus varies with the individual. However, the general causes of anxiety have been classified into two major kinds of threats:

1. Threats to biologic integrity: actual or impending interference with basic human needs, such as the needs for food, drink, or warmth

2. Threats to the security of the self:

    a. Unmet expectations important to self-integrity

    b. Unmet needs for status and prestige

    c. Anticipated disapproval by significant others

    d. Inability to gain or reinforce self-respect or to gain recognition from others

    e. Guilt, or discrepancies between self-view and actual behavior

It is crucial to understand that either actual *or* impending interference may cause anxiety (i.e., actual interference with a biologic or psychosocial need is not a necessary condition). All that is necessary is the *anticipation* of one of these major threats.

Threats to biologic integrity or to the fulfillment of such basic human needs as food, drink, warmth, and shelter are a general cause of anxiety. Threats to the security of self are not as easily categorized. In some instances, they are obvious; in others, they are more obscure because each person's sense of self is unique. To one person, power and prestige may be essential; to another, independence; to a third, being of service to others.

Consider the last category—being of service to others. Suppose that Mrs C, a nurse, is convinced that a client would feel much better if he expressed his fears to her. But no matter how often she provides the opportunity, he insists, "This is not the time to talk about it," and thwarts her attempt. She is not able to help him in a way that is important to her sense of self. In addition, she believes that the unit's head nurse (whose communication skills she admires) expects her to have been successful in this endeavor. When unmet needs or expectations related to essential values (e.g., being of service to the client) are coupled with the actual or anticipated disapproval of others who are important (the head nurse), anxiety is generated.

Anxiety As a Continuum

Many theorists conceptualize anxiety as a continuum. Mild to moderate anxiety can be functionally effective in that it helps us focus our attention and generates energy and motivation. Thus, anxiety is an aspect of problem solving in that it alerts us to the need to concentrate our resources. However, severe anxiety and panic narrow our attention to a crippling degree. Under these conditions alertness is greatly reduced, and learning does not usually take place.

Mild Anxiety Mild anxiety (+) helps one deal constructively with stress. A mildly anxious person has a broad perceptual field because mild anxiety heightens the ability to take in sensory stimuli. Such a person is more alert to what is going on and can make better sense of what is happening with others and the environment. The senses take in more—the person hears better, sees better, and makes logical connections between events (Figure 5–1). The person feels relatively safe and comfortable. Because learning is easier when one is mildly anxious, mild anxiety helps clients learn, for instance, how best to administer their own insulin. Mild anxiety can also help a nursing student review psychiatric-mental health nursing before a final examination.

Moderate Anxiety In moderate anxiety (++), a person remains alert, but the perceptual field narrows (see Figure 5–1). The moderately anxious person shuts out the events on the periphery while focusing on central concerns. For example, the nursing student

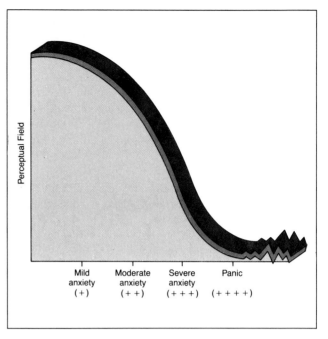

FIGURE 5–1   The effect of anxiety on the perceptual field.
SOURCE: Adapted from Kneisl CR, Ames SW: Adult Health Nursing: A Biopsychosocial Approach. Addison-Wesley, 1986, p 119.

who is moderately anxious about the final examination may be able to focus so intently on studying that she or he is not distracted by an argument between roommates, loud music on the stereo, and a rousing chase scene on television. The student shuts out the chaos in the environment and focuses on what is of central personal importance—preparing for the exam. This process of taking in some sensory stimuli while excluding others is called **selective inattention.**

People also use selective inattention to cope with anxiety-provoking stimuli. This phenomenon may account for the anxious preoperative client who fails to remember what the nurse said about postoperative pain or the need to cough and deep breathe after surgery.

Although the perceptual field is narrowed and the person sees, hears, and grasps less, there is an element of voluntary control. Moderately anxious individuals can, with direction, focus on what they have previously shut out.

Severe Anxiety In severe anxiety (+++), sensory reception is greatly reduced (see Figure 5–1). Severely anxious persons focus on small or scattered details of an experience. They have difficulty in problem solving, and their ability to organize is also reduced. They seldom have the complete picture. Selective inattention may be increased and may be less amenable to voluntary control. The person may be unable to focus on events in the environment. New stimuli may be experienced as overwhelming and may cause the anxiety level to rise even higher.

The sympathetic nervous system is activated in severe anxiety, causing an increase in pulse, blood pressure, and respiration and in increase in epinephrine secretion, vasoconstriction, and even body temperature. A multitude of physiologic changes may be observed, which are described in the section that follows.

Panic   The panic level of anxiety (++++) is characterized by a completely disrupted perceptual field (see Figure 5–1). Panic has been described as a disintegration of the personality experienced as intense terror. Details may be enlarged, scattered, or distorted. Logical thinking and effective decision making may be impossible. The person in panic is unable to initiate or maintain goal-directed action. Behavior may appear purposeless, and communication may be unintelligible.

Not all those in panic behave alike. At the scene of an auto accident in which an elderly couple lost control of the travel trailer they were towing, the husband remained immobile in the driver's seat, hands firmly fixed to the steering wheel, eyes focused on some distant spot despite the threat of explosion from the smoking car. The wife ran around in circles. She lost her shoes in the accident, but, despite numerous bleeding cuts, she was unaware she was running barefoot through the broken glass of the windshield.

Recognizing Anxiety

Anxiety can be assessed in the physiologic, cognitive, and emotional/behavioral dimensions. This observation illustrates the relationship between the mind and the body. Anxiety is a multidimensional phenomenon in that the total person is involved in every aspect of it. Objective data, particularly nursing observations, may be critical because of the nature of anxiety. Selective inattention and dissociation interfere with the client's awareness of anxiety and ability to give accurate reports. Families and friends also can contribute data useful to the assessment of anxiety.

Physiologic Dimension   Observations of the client's physiologic state are likely to indicate autonomic nervous system responses, particularly sympathetic effects. Various organs may be affected, such as the adrenal medulla, heart, blood vessels, lungs, stomach, colon, rectum, salivary glands, liver, pupils of the eyes, and sweat glands (Figure 5–2). Anxious clients may have an increased heart rate, increased blood pressure, difficulty breathing, sweaty palms, trembling, dry mouth, "butterflies in the stomach" or a "lump in the throat," as well as other symptoms.

Laboratory tests are not routinely done to evaluate anxiety because observation is faster and more accurate, but anxiety affects the results of laboratory tests. Blood studies may show increased adrenal function,

elevated levels of glucose and lactic acid, and decreased parathyroid function and oxygen and calcium levels. Urinary studies may indicate increased levels of epinephrine and norepinephrine.

Cognitive Dimension   Assessment of cognitive function may indicate difficulty in logical thinking, narrowed or distorted perceptual field, selective inattention or dissociation, lack of attention to details, difficulty in concentrating, or difficulty in focusing. The level of anxiety determines the extent to which cognitive function is affected. Mild, moderate, severe, or panic level of anxiety is assessed according to the descriptions earlier in this chapter.

Emotional/Behavioral Dimension   In the emotional/behavioral dimension, clients may be irritable, angry, withdrawn, and restless, or they may cry. The affective response can often be assessed through the client's subjective description. Clients may describe themselves as "on edge," "uptight," "jittery," "nervous," "worried," or "tense." They may feel dizzy or faint and may experience a feeling of impending doom as if something terrible were about to happen.

Coping with Stress and Anxiety

Nurses can be helpful if they understand the changes the client is undergoing. Reactions to threatening situations, such as illness and hospitalization, can be divided into two general categories: task-oriented and defense-oriented responses. When we feel competent to deal with stress and the situation is not too threatening to our sense of self, our behavior tends to be task oriented. Task-oriented behavior is geared toward problem solving. A student who is majoring in mathematics fails his courses. If he is not too frightened by the possibility that he may not be suited for a career in this field, he can assess the situation and change his major. This is a task-oriented reaction. It is based on a realistic appraisal of the situation and involves a series of carefully thought-out judgments about what course of behavior would be most effective.

When we feel inadequate to cope with stress and the situation is extremely threatening to our sense of self, we tend to engage in defense-oriented reactions. The diagnosis of a terminal illness, for instance, may be so overwhelming that a person must temporarily defend against acknowledging this reality. Everyone uses defense-oriented behavior from time to time as a protective measure. Such behavior becomes harmful only when it is the predominant means of coping with stress. In such cases, problem-solving and reality-based behavior are continually avoided.

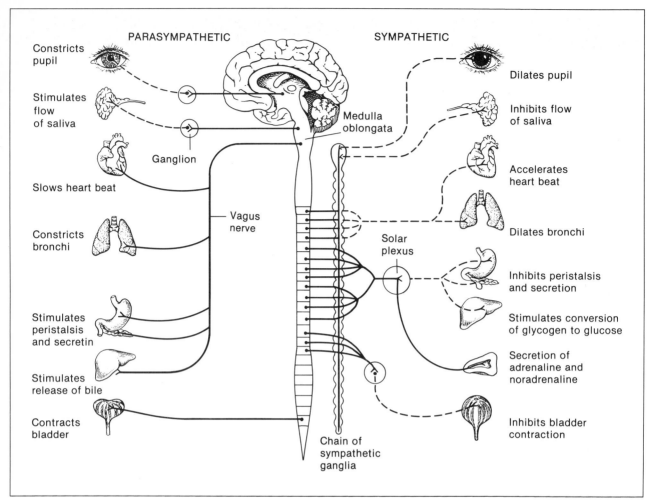

FIGURE 5–2   The autonomic nervous system and some of the organs it innervates. In anxiety, sympathetic nervous system responses are most common.   *SOURCE: Ramsey JM: Basic Pathophysiology: Modern Stress and the Disease Process. Addison-Wesley, 1982, p 46.*

Coping strategies are a set of behaviors persons under stress use in struggling to improve their situations. Coping strategies can be thought of simply as ways of getting along in the world.

Everyday Ways of Coping with Stress

Everyday coping strategies offer an immense repertoire of defenses to maintain control and balance in the face of stress. A person can cope on different levels, including the physical, social, cognitive, and emotional levels. However, the devices people choose to cope with stress depend on many factors. Among them are the external circumstances, the suddenness and intensity of the stress, the resources available to the person, and the person's predisposition to one or another coping pattern. Certain coping patterns are established in the course of one's development. One man who is late for an appointment because he gets caught in a traffic jam may react with a furious outburst of anger. Another may begin to daydream and forget where he is going. A third may use the time to solve some problem.

Most often, individuals use behaviors that have worked well for them in the past. Sometimes they behave in a certain way because it is the only method they have of coping with stress or because other coping strategies failed to work. Some persons learn to turn to others for protection and nurturance; some learn to turn to chemicals or to food; some rely on self-discipline and keeping a stiff upper lip; others feel better after the intense expression of feelings; some withdraw physically and/or emotionally; still others work out or talk the problem out. Common coping methods are discussed below.

Turning to a Comforting Person   No doubt the earliest coping strategy is the familiar method of turning to a nurturing figure for soothing and protecting. To get love is to be reassured that one is lovable. Love from supportive others may take the form of physical touching, rocking, patting, or verbal reassurances of various kinds ("Don't be afraid, I'll stay with you"). This category also includes the function of eating in times of stress and for general support.

RESEARCH NOTE

Citation
Floyd JA: *Nursing students' stress levels, attitude toward drugs, and drug use.* Arch Psychiatr Nurs 1991;5(1):46–53.

Study Problem/Purpose
This study investigated relationships among nursing students' drug use and two variables usually assumed to contribute to the development of chemical dependency, i.e., stress, and positive attitudes about drugs (pharmacologic optimism).

Method
Drug use was defined as the use of any psychoactive substance, including prescription drugs, over-the-counter drugs, recreational drugs, nicotine, and alcohol. Senior nursing students and liberal arts students (selected using a stratified sampling technique to provide a sample comparable to nursing students on gender and race) at an urban university were asked to complete a set of questionnaires. Instruments used were: The SCL-90-R, a self-report system inventory to reflect psychologic symptom status, from which the Depression, Anxiety, and Somatization Scales were used to measure stress; and the Substance Use Questionnaire, a multiple-part questionnaire in development by the investigator, from which the Frequency Scale to measure students' drug use and the Willingness-to-Use Scale to measure pharmacologic optimism were used.

Findings
The first hypothesis, that nursing students would report less drug use than liberal arts students, was not supported. There was no drug category for which nursing students reported significantly less frequent use than their non-nursing peers. However, nursing students did report a significantly greater frequency of using over-the-counter analgesics than liberal arts students

(twice a week for nursing students compared to once every two weeks for liberal arts students). Although the correlations were low, drug use increased with age and men reported greater drug use than women. The second hypothesis, that nursing students and liberal arts students do not differ on symptoms of stress, was supported. There were no significant differences in scores on the Anxiety, Depression, or Somatization Scales of the SCL-90-R.

Nursing students reported more willingness than did liberal arts students to use two of the drug groups listed: depressants, including tranquilizers and barbiturates; and narcotics. For both drug groups, the median score for nursing students was 2 (Only If I Think I Need It) and 1 (Only If Prescribed) for liberal arts students.

Implications
Interpretation of the results of this study must be cautious and tentative for a number of reasons. Because the sample was drawn only from one campus, it is possible that the self-reports are not representative of nursing students and their non-nursing peers on this campus. Furthermore, the SUQ is still under development. The findings of this study provide no support for the idea that stress and resultant substance use are greater problems in the nursing student population than other student populations. In addition, they do not provide support for the belief that the nursing students' knowledge of drugs will lead to less substance use than their peers. Of special concern is the nursing students' pharmacologic optimism about tranquilizers, barbiturates, and narcotics, and future use of these drugs. Nursing students who already report greater use of over-the-counter analgesics may be more willing to use psychoactive drugs to manage symptoms of emotional and physical pain, which may be a factor in the development of chemical dependency.

Alcohol, nicotine, and other chemicals are often used to enhance well-being in the face of stress. Many theorists view these alternatives as substitutes for the dependent comfort of being a baby in the care of a nurturing parent.

Relying on Self-Discipline Whereas some people under stress tend to turn to the comfort of friendly company, food, or alcohol—all of which are reminis-

cent of childhood dependency—others rely on self-discipline. Self-control ranks high in the value system of many cultures and subcultures. This coping style involves pride in the ability to laugh off problems, endure frustrations, and discount anxiety. Keep a stiff upper lip, bite the bullet, and get over it are all admonitions that people address to themselves when self-discipline is their patterned response to stress. These people are unlikely to want the company of supportive others and may even push them away. They are often unresponsive when others seek comfort from them, for they see such dependency as weak.

Intense Expression of Feeling Crying, swearing, and laughing all tend to relieve tension. Swearing loses its usefulness as an escape valve if it becomes a habit. This is less likely true of crying and of laughing. Crying and laughing tend to release energy and exert a soothing effect on a person who is experiencing tension.

Avoidance and Withdrawal While some people find it hard to sleep when they are under tension, others react to worries, bad news, or an argument with somnolence. Still others respond with a form of waking sleep like apathy or emotional withdrawal, which accomplishes the same thing.

Talking It Out Many people relieve tension by talking it out. Talking implies establishing and maintaining a contact of sorts with another human being. In addition, it enables new ideas to emerge and new perspectives to be entertained. Obviously, this device is the medium of most therapeutic intervention.

Privately Thinking It Through Some people believe that the unexamined life is not worth living. When faced with a problem that causes them anxiety, these individuals become introspective about it. The rationalizations that emerge serve as effective tension relievers.

Working It Off Acting to relieve tension may range from pointless activity such as finger tapping, floor pacing, and door slamming to activities purposely designed to alter the tension-producing circumstances. In addition, some tense individuals feel a lot of aggressive energy. Physical exertion in the form of demanding sports, like soccer or tennis, or manual labor, like washing walls or scrubbing the floor, is a way to use this energy constructively.

Using Symbolic Substitutes Stress may be relieved by ascribing symbolic values to acts or objects. These acts or objects may or may not have other meanings. There are symbolic devices for the management of tensions in religious conventions like meditation, confession, prayer, or sacrifice. For some people, the automobile has a symbolic significance; others ascribe symbolic significance to their annual income or their physical appearance.

The list is almost endless, but the principle is always the same. Some people attach a meaning beyond the obvious one to objects, experiences, and people. Through their involvement with these meanings, they find a means to reduce their tensions.

Somatizing Many organs have an expression and communication function. This is sometimes known as *somatizing* or *organ language*. Some organs communicate their messages only to their owner. For example, the heart may communicate by means of palpitation. Other demonstrations are public, e.g., blushing or stuttering. Urination and defecation, increased sweating, and altered sexual activity are other familiar examples of organ language.

Coping Resources

Early classic research on coping was concerned with how individuals respond to specific stresses in a laboratory setting. More recent studies that consider the whole being in interaction with the environment have helped in viewing coping as a dynamic process that involves the demands and restrictions on a client as well as the resources available. For example, according to Antonovsky (1980), persons stay healthy or cope adequately with stress because they possess what he calls *generalized resistance resources* (GRRs). A GRR is any factor in the person, group, or organization that helps in managing tension.

Physical and biochemical GRRs are physiologic characteristics, such as genetic features and levels of immunity. These GRRs also include interaction of the nervous and endocrine systems that help in adaptation (e.g., interactions involving ACTH, thyroid-stimulating hormone or TSH, vasopressin, norepinephrine, and insulin and their influence on human behavior). Not only are individuals different in their genetic and biochemical makeup, but the physiologic effects of illness and stress may also alter the person's ability to use physical and biochemical GRRs positively.

Material goods and relative wealth constitute the *artifactual and material* GRRs; having these attributes makes it easier to cope with illness. Money helps to ensure the best health care available. Effective coping is often interrelated with one's socioeconomic status simply because the higher the socioeconomic status, the greater the resources to help the person cope. For example, household help not only relieves an ill person's worries but also reduces the practical burden.

Cognitive GRRs have to do with intelligence and knowledge. When persons know about stressors, they can avoid them. They can also predict when periods of stress are imminent and thus reduce their impact. Knowing what community services are available is also a cognitive GRR.

People who are self-aware—who know their own capacities and potentials and have a well-developed sense of themselves—possess *emotional* GRRs. Emotional GRRs determine the extent of psychologic hardiness. In general, they have to do with how competent and self-assured one feels.

Valuative and attitudinal GRRs are the products of a person's culture and environment. Persons are apt to respond in learned ways. The attitudinal aspect also is related to how flexible, rational, and farsighted the person is. The more rational or accurate one's appraisal of a threatening situation and the more flexible one is in approaching the situation and envisioning the consequences, the greater one's resources for coping.

Interpersonal-relational GRRs are available social support systems. The greater a person's social contacts, the greater the social resources available to augment the ability to deal with stress. Love, affection, and nurturance are hallmarks of interpersonal-relational GRRs.

Institutional structures that facilitate coping are called *macrosociocultural* GRRs. These resources include governmental programs such as Aid to Dependent Children as well as cultural institutions such as death and funeral rites, religious rituals, and ceremonies.

According to this model, the ability to cope is determined by the extent and effectiveness of each person's generalized resistance resources. Yet the actual process of coping remains unclear. Theorists and researchers still do not fully understand exactly which personal resources should be mobilized and under which conditions.

Little research has been performed on the preferred coping methods of "normal" subjects (those not facing a crisis). Ziemer (1982) found that over 50 percent of the study population reported that their preferred method of coping was to talk to someone. This finding has profound implications for nursing, because nurses are the health care providers who spend the most time with clients. It also has profound implications for clients whose communication is dysfunctional or whose ability to communicate freely is restricted. Psychiatric clients generally fall into these categories.

Defense-Oriented Ways of Coping: Defense Mechanisms

The coping strategies described above are considered normal. They are simply ways of getting along. In some people, however, what passes for a normal adjustment is actually a very tenuous one with few outlets for controlled aggression, few sublimations, few love objects, few opportunities for satisfaction and growth. These people find it more and more difficult to cope with additional stress. Ultimately the external stress that the person is trying unsuccessfully to ward off is matched by a mounting internal stress. The

person suffers both from increased anxiety and from the strain on overworked stabilizers. And, what happens to the client who has no one to talk with, who can't jog five miles, or who can't laugh off the problem?

When a person is unable to ward off stress or reduce tensions in the usual way, anxiety mounts as the person feels increasingly inadequate to cope with the situation. Under these circumstances, the person is more likely to engage in *defense-oriented behavior*. Defense-oriented behavior is not a specific attempt to solve a problem. It consists of using mental mechanisms to lessen uncomfortable feelings of anxiety and to prevent pain regardless of cost. These characteristic mental mechanisms are commonly called **defense mechanisms.** They protect the self by allowing the person to deny or distort a stressful event or to restrict awareness and reduce the sense of emotional involvement. But they can also interfere with rational decision-making. People who use defense mechanisms are excluding some information about the situation they are in. They are also denying their own feelings about it.

Defense mechanisms are primarily unconscious and often inflexible coping patterns that protect a person through intrapsychic (those that come from within) distortions that are really self-deceptions. The person usually has little awareness of what is happening or even less control over events. Although these reactions may help keep the lid on anxiety, they also limit the ability to grow from and savor the experience, they interfere with rational decision making and the ability to work productively, and they impair and erode interpersonal relationships. Even adaptive devices can go wrong.

Because human behavior is so complex and varied, defense mechanisms can be classified in many ways. Often, they are classified according to whether they are simple or complex, whether they are most likely to arise in a specific phase of development, or whether they are commonly associated with a particular form of psychopathology. Definitions of various defense mechanisms overlap, and the same observed behavior may often be explained by more than one type of defense. To make things even more complicated, people do not use one method of defense at a time. Usually they rely on a combination of defenses. For study purposes, the common defense mechanisms discussed here are repression, suppression, dissociation, identification, introjection, projection, denial, fantasy, rationalization, reaction formation, displacement, and intellectualization. They are summarized in Table 5–2.

Repression Repression, the basis of all defense mechanisms, is the dynamic behind much of "forgetting." When persons repress, they unconsciously ex-

TABLE 5–2 **Defense Mechanisms**

Name	Definition	Example
Repression	Unconsciously keeping unacceptable feelings out of awareness	A man is jealous of a good friend's success but is unaware of his feelings.
Suppression	Consciously keeping unacceptable feelings and thoughts out of awareness	A student taking an examination is upset about an argument with her boyfriend but puts it out of her mind so she can finish the test.
Dissociation	Handling emotional conflicts, or internal or external stressors, by a temporary alteration of consciousness or identity	A woman has amnesia for the events surrounding a fatal automobile accident in which she was the speeding driver.
Identification	Unconscious assumption of similarity between oneself and another	After hospitalization for minor surgery, a girl decides to be a nurse.
Introjection	Acceptance of another's values and opinions as one's own	A woman who prefers a simple life-style assumes the materialistic, prestige-oriented values of her husband.
Projection	Attributing one's own unacceptable feelings and thoughts to others	A man who is quite critical of others thinks that people are joking about his appearance.
Denial	Blocking out painful or anxiety-inducing events or feelings	A boss tells an employer he may have to fire him. On the way home the employee shops for a new car.
Fantasy	Symbolic satisfaction of wishes through nonrational thought	A student struggling through graduate school thinks about a prestigious, high-paying job he wants.
Rationalization	Falsification of experience through the construction of logical or socially approved explanations of behavior	A man cheats on his income tax return and tells himself it's all right because everyone does it.
Reaction formation	Unacceptable feelings disguised by repression of the real feeling and by reinforcement of the opposite feeling	A woman who dislikes her mother-in-law is always very nice to her.
Displacement	Discharging of pent-up feelings on persons less dangerous than those who initially aroused the emotion	A student who has received a low grade on a term paper blows up at his girl friend when she asks about his grade.
Intellectualization	Separating an emotion from an idea or thought because the emotional reaction is too painful to be acknowledged	A man learns from his doctor that he has cancer. He studies the physiology and treatment of cancer without experiencing any emotion.

clude distressing emotions, thoughts, or experiences from awareness. It bars access to consciousness of feelings and thoughts that would cause anxiety and disrupt the self-concept. It also affords protection from a sudden trauma until the individual is able to deal with the shock. From the individual's point of view, a repressed memory is "forgotten" and cannot be deliberately brought to awareness. Although the repressed feelings remain out of awareness, they continue to exert pressure for expression. The self tries to maintain the repression but in people experiencing extreme stress or anxiety, or in febrile (feverish) or toxic states, repression may begin to fail. Clients who are intoxicated by alcohol or drugs or who are emerging from anesthesia may verbalize feelings that they usually repress.

Susan was raped. She was brought to an outpatient clinic by her roommate. Susan said she felt very anxious and could not recall the circumstances surrounding the rape or what the rapist looked like. Her use of repression protected her from facing her fears and humiliation.

Nursing intervention in such cases should be supportive and protective of the client's defenses. After the initial shock has lessened and the client's anxiety level has been reduced, the client can be helped to examine the traumatic event.

Suppression Suppression is an intentional act that helps to keep thoughts, feelings, wishes, or actions that cause anxiety out of conscious awareness. Suppression is the conscious form of repression.

A middle-aged male business executive discovers bright red rectal bleeding the day before he is to leave for a visit to his company's international offices in three European countries. Worrying about the bleeding interferes with his concentration and his ability to complete a report about the division he heads. His decision to put off worrying about the bleeding until he returns in three weeks is an example of using suppression to deal with the emotional discomfort of this discovery.

Clients may refuse to consider their difficulties by saying that they "don't want to talk about it" or that they will "think about it some other time." This, too, is suppression. Suppression can be dealt with in the same way as repression. Suppression is generally easier to deal with because the material remains conscious. Nurses can be somewhat more directive in assessing why the client avoids talking about a situation, and they can suggest that the client try to look at the situation because it affects future plans. Offering the executive information about rectal bleeding may help him look at his situation objectively. As he learns more about his condition, it may become less threatening to him.

Dissociation In **dissociation,** the individual handles emotional conflicts, or internal or external stressors, by a temporary alteration of consciousness or identity (see Chapter 14 for specific mental dysfunctions in which dissociation is the major mental mechanism). Dissociation resembles repression, but it has a different origin. The self is formed through the process of disapproval and approval from significant other people. Therefore the self *dissociates* or refuses awareness to the expression of personal qualities and experiences of which significant others disapprove. These feelings come to exist separately from the person's self-concept. A little girl with artistic abilities that are not validated by her parents will not think of herself as artistic. She may deny her abilities even when other people point them out.

People who dissociate do not "notice" what they are doing. This limitation of awareness is maintained because the person experiences anxiety whenever permissible levels for the self are trespassed.

Ms T consciously believes that sexual overtures are wrong, yet she behaves seductively toward men. She cannot understand why men see her behavior as a sexual invitation. The use of repression or dissociation complicates Ms T's problems. She needs to ignore or deny aspects of her situation to feel comfortable in it. Other people notice and point out Ms T's seductive behavior, but she cannot recognize it because it is not a part of her self-concept. If Ms T admitted her sexual feelings she would experience severe anxiety and personality disorganization.

Identification **Identification** is the wish to be like another person and to assume the characteristics of that person's personality. It represents a turning away from our own personality. Identification is unconscious. In this it differs from *imitation,* which is the conscious copying of another person's qualities. Identification with admired persons can serve an important function in maturation by evoking latent qualities. For instance, the little girl who identifies with her mother and sisters thus learns the behavioral characteristics of womanhood.

The most primitive type of identification is seen in the infant's relationship with the mother. Infants seem to perceive no difference between their mothers and themselves and only gradually become aware that their mothers exist apart from them. Small children deal with people in terms of how these people meet their needs. They do not see them as separate persons with needs of their own. Such identifications may persist into adult life in people who have not differentiated themselves psychologically from seemingly powerful parents.

One specific manifestation of identification is passiveness in relationships. People who feel they have no resources of their own will overvalue the resources of others and expect to be taken care of. People who are most identified with their parents tend to be people who were not allowed to develop their own individuality. Part of the process of self-realization occurs in adolescence, when we discard, with much anxiety and insecurity, our identification with the parents on whom we have been so dependent. Some clients may not have achieved a degree of self-identity sufficient to do this. Identification can inhibit our usefulness, because it prevents us from focusing on our own capacities.

Identification can be seen in clients who rely heavily on the nurse's advice and support. They expect that all their needs will be met and that nothing will be expected of them.

Mr L is diabetic. He is not interested in learning about the diet he must follow and the medication he must take. He expects the nurse to take the responsibility for seeing that he gets the right food and medicine. Identification prevents him from being self-reliant.

Nurses who work with clients like Mr L should clarify what the client's expectations of the nurse are and then correct any misperceptions about the nurse's role. It is important to help Mr L increase his own skills and to take responsibility for his own care. Initially, the nurse can offer the client collaboration and interdependence. The long-term goal in dealing with identification is for the client to formulate a self-care plan independently of the nurse.

Introjection **Introjection** is closely related to identification. It is the process of accepting another's values and opinions as one's own if they contradict the values one had previously held. A man whose employer engages in shoddy workmanship may introject his employer's values even though they are contrary to his own moral beliefs because he is afraid of losing his job. Introjection also occurs in severe depression following the death of a loved person. The depressed person may assume many of the deceased person's characteristics and in so doing lose some self-awareness. The nurse can treat introjection like identification, remembering that introjection is more primitive and more intractable. It originates in our experience of being fed as infants. We incorporated people and objects into ourselves in the same way that we swallowed food. We felt a sense of oneness with everything in the external world and could not differentiate ourselves from others. Because thinking processes are not involved in the first experience of introjection, this defense tends to be difficult to explore on the verbal level.

Projection Projection is an unconscious means of dealing with personal difficulties or unacceptable wishes by attributing them to others. We blame other people for our shortcomings or see them as harboring our own unacceptable feelings or thoughts. In the course of development, the child, who needs the parents' approval, will identify with them and will also deny what they seem to condemn or fail to acknowledge. For instance, if her parents do not openly express and recognize angry feelings, a little girl will tend to regard anger as dangerous. She will then deny awareness of her own anger. Anger in others will disturb her, and she will tend to condemn in others the anger she cannot accept in herself. It is common knowledge that people often tend to criticize others for their own unacknowledged inferiorities. The person who fears being taken advantage of is often an opportunist.

In adult life, projection can be destructive if it interferes with our ability to acknowledge our own feelings. The tendency to attribute our own undesired feelings to others also blurs the boundaries between ourselves and others. This, in turn, makes it difficult to understand other people's feelings. People who make excessive use of projection tend to attribute to others hostile or seductive motives that do not actually exist. This prevents them from forming trusting and reciprocal relationships. A tendency to projection may also interfere with problem solving. A young woman who believes she is failing a course because of her teacher will not focus her energies on her studies.

Clients who must deal with the stress of serious illness may shift the blame for their condition onto the nurse. They may complain of poor nursing care to a nurse who is actually very skillful. These clients may actually fear that they have caused their own problems by neglecting their health. They may believe that they are being "paid back" for wrongdoing in the past. If nurses feel that such a client is accusing them falsely, they should not show anger or retaliate but should show, through consistency and attention, that they respect these clients and are concerned about their welfare. As clients feel more secure in the nurse-client relationship, nurses can encourage these clients to explore the realistic aspects of their situation. For example, a man who blames his family for his alcoholism can be helped to explore objectively what is known about the etiology of alcoholism. This may help him come to terms with his feelings of guilt and anger. This type of intervention helps the client to separate his own feelings from the objective facts of the situation.

Denial Denial of reality is one of the simplest of the defense mechanisms. In denial, painful or anxiety-producing aspects of awareness are blocked out of consciousness. The reality of a situation is either completely disregarded or transformed so that it is no longer threatening. Denial is one of the commonest defenses against the stress of diagnosis and illness and is typically present in the first few minutes of adjustment to the death of a loved person. If may be helpful as a temporary protection against the full impact of a traumatic event.

A father reacts with denial when he shouts, "No, it can't be true; there must be a mistake," when told his 8-year-old son has just died in the trauma unit of injuries incurred when his bicycle collided with an automobile.

A young woman admitted to a psychiatric hospital because of acute anxiety and frightening hallucinations says she just "needs a rest."

Sometimes denial is the best solution for the client. In such situations, the defense should be supported. A terminally ill client who believes she will soon recover and who cannot think about her illness should be allowed the protection of denial. Not all clients need to face up to reality. The nurse should recognize that denial may be preventing serious personality disorganization.

Sometimes, however, denial is directly harmful to the client, as when a man refuses to take medication that is crucial to his survival. In such cases, the motivation for the client's behavior should be assessed. After discovering the protective function the denial is serving, the nurse can focus attention on helping the client meet these needs in a way that is not self-destructive. The nurse can also help by taking care not to reinforce patterns of denial but rather to focus on instances when the client seems to be dealing with reality.

Fantasy Fantasy is a form of nonrational mental activity that enables the individual to escape temporarily the demands of the everyday world. Fantasies are not confined by the reality consideration of cause and effect and time and space. Fantasy normally characterizes the thinking of children before they are able to engage in consensually validated communication. Adults revert to fantasy during times of stress to obtain a symbolic satisfaction of wishes.

A businesswoman facing financial difficulties temporarily escapes by daydreaming that she is enjoying a luxurious vacation on a Caribbean island.

Another woman with advanced multiple sclerosis imagines herself a famous ballerina with complete control of her body.

A man whose wife has told him she wants a divorce imagines how much his wife will appreciate him now that he has been diagnosed with cancer.

Fantasy may offer temporary relief from pressures, but people who spend too much time in fantasy may be unable to meet the requirements of reality.

Clients who are very ill may fantasize that when they recover many good things will happen to them. They may imagine that they will receive special recognition in their work or that they will get along better with their families. These fantasies may help such clients deal with the deprivations caused by illness. However, they may also cause unrealistic expectations. Such clients may expect to be paid back for their suffering. They may cherish "suffering hero" fantasies. These fantasies may make one feel good temporarily but interfere with problem solving.

Clients who are engaging in fantasy related to their illness need gradual help in assessing the responses others are likely to make and the achievements they themselves may realistically expect. Clients who fail to adjust to reality will be very disappointed when their grandiose expectations are not met.

A helpful approach that will not devastate clients who need to hold onto some fantasy is to ask them to discuss their specific future plans. Examining the details of work and interpersonal adjustment may help a person to relinquish unrealistic expectations and make more realistic plans. For example, the man who believes that a diagnosis of cancer will improve his marriage because his wife will appreciate him more fully must recognize that this is improbable. He needs to examine the real effects his illness will have on her. He must plan how to make specific improvements in their communication by anticipating problem areas.

Imagination does have a creative aspect, however. Fantasies have a richness and variety that is lacking in the everyday world. Certain artists, such as Dalí and Picasso, enrich their works of art through fantasy. Evidence also exists that insights into scientific discovery do not come about as the result of step-by-step logical thinking. Rather, they are created through fantasy.

Rationalization Rationalization is the attribution of "good" or plausible reasons for questionable behavior to justify it or to deal with disappointment. Rationalizing helps to avoid social disapproval and to bolster flagging self-esteem.

A nurse fails to return to the bedside of the elderly nursing home client despite a promise to do so before leaving work. She feels her behavior is justified because the client has problems with recent memory and probably wouldn't remember anyway.

Many people use rationalization because they wish to prove to themselves or others that their actions are governed by reason and common sense—even though they may not fully understand the reasons for their own behavior. Such explanations may be essential to maintain personal integrity. They are not destructive as long as they do not prevent one from solving everyday problems.

Rationalization becomes more of a hindrance when it prevents us from making necessary changes in our behavior by interfering with our ability to examine that behavior. One sign of rationalization is an active search for reasons to justify our behavior or beliefs. Another is an inability to recognize inconsistencies in our beliefs. A third is being upset when our reasons are questioned, since each questioning threatens our defenses.

Clients may use rationalization to soften the blow of losses caused by illness. For instance, a man who is ill may give up work prematurely after rationalizing that he wouldn't have been successful in that field anyway. Such unnecessary restrictions deprive us of possible achievements.

Nurses must respect their clients' need to rationalize fears and insecurities they cannot face. However, nurses must hold out to clients the possibility for change. Nurse can help clients face the reality of their situation by encouraging them to explore ways they can change to deal with it more effectively. One way is to help them explore in detail past instances in which they did change to cope with a stressful situation. Believing that we have real strengths helps us to face areas of insecurity.

Reaction Formation Reaction formation is a defense whereby we keep an undesirable impulse out of awareness by emphasizing its opposite. To protect ourselves from recognizing dangerous feelings, we develop conscious attitudes and behavior patterns that are just the opposite of those feelings. Hostility may be concealed behind a facade of love and kindness. The desire to be sexually promiscuous may be concealed behind a moralistic demeanor. People who use this defense are not conscious of their true feelings.

People who crusade passionately against alcohol or pornography may have an underlying wish to enjoy these things. Of course, this is not true of everyone who is devoted to a cause. Clues that reaction formation is occurring are an inappropriate intensity of feeling and the inability to consider alternative points of view. The person who is always unnaturally sweet and loving and cannot consider the possibility of being angry is probably using this excess of feeling to counteract an unacceptable anger.

Reaction formation can be useful. It can help us maintain socially approved behavior and avoid awareness of desires that are not socially acceptable. But this defense, too, results in self-deception, because it is not under conscious control. Therefore, it may result in exaggerated or rigid behaviors that leave us ill equipped to deal with crisis. People who feel they can never express annoyance and discomfort may need to be "good" clients, who never question their care or make demands. Such clients may not be able to allow themselves to depend on others. They may not be able to acknowledge their needs and seek fulfillment. This rigid stance is a reaction formation against the unconscious wish to be completely dependent. It is destructive because it masks the individual's needs. It also prevents the person from meeting a crisis with flexibility, because many possible actions are blocked from awareness. People who use this defense may also be excessively harsh in dealing with other people's weaknesses. They may be unable or unwilling to help others because they think people should be able to solve their own problems.

A client manifesting reaction formation requires essentially the same approach as one manifesting repression. The nurse should respect and support the client's defenses while providing a secure relationship in which to explore feelings and new behavioral alternatives. Nurses must also be aware that it is easy to be annoyed at clients who cannot face their true feelings. The rigid and excessive display of what seems to be an insincere emotion can be frustrating. It is important for nurses to remember that these clients are not "lying" or pretending. They are unconsciously protecting themselves against having to recognize threatening feelings.

Displacement **Displacement** is the discharging of pent-up feelings, generally hostility, on an object less dangerous than the object that aroused the feelings. This defense is used when emotions are aroused in a situation where it would be dangerous to express them.

John has just failed an important examination. He believes his failure was the instructor's fault. He cannot express the full extent of his anger, because that would get him into worse trouble with the instructor. John goes quietly back to the dormitory. But when his roommate turns the stereo on too loud, John explodes. He doesn't fear retaliation from his roommate—they are peers and friends.

In some cases, we turn our anger toward another person inward on the self. When this happens, we experience exaggerated self-accusations and guilt.

Clients may express inappropriate anger to the nurse when they are actually angry at someone or something else. The client may feel more secure with the nurse, who offers a safe target for displaced feelings. Displacement differs from projection in that people who use displacement are not distorting their feelings and attributing them to someone else. The feelings are clear, and the person acknowledges them. They are simply being directed at the wrong person. Therefore, it may be easier to help these clients acknowledge the real situation. This may be achieved by remaining calm and accepting during an angry outburst. For example, a nurse can say this after the outburst is over, "You seem so angry. I wonder if you really are angry because your breakfast is cold or if there might be some other reason." Opening up the possibility for a discussion of anger may help these clients to sort out just why and at whom they are angry.

Intellectualization **Intellectualization** is the process of separating the emotion aroused by an event from ideas or opinions about the event because the emotion itself is too painful to acknowledge. The painful emotion is avoided by means of a rational explanation that divests the event of any personal significance. Failures are made less significant by telling oneself that the situation could have been worse. A woman may deal with her husband's death by saying objectively that sudden death is better than chronic illness. A boy who breaks his pelvis skiing seeks consolation by reminding himself that he could have broken his neck.

Clients may use intellectualization to blunt the emotional impact of their problems. This may be difficult for the nurse to perceive, because such clients often seem to know a great deal about their condition. They may be able to discuss in great detail the metabolic processes in diabetes or the psychodynamics of anxiety. At the same time they cannot apply these concepts to their own situation in an emotional sense.

Intellectualization resembles rationalization in that it provides a verbal means of dealing with anxiety. Its use closes off the possibility of accepting and working out problems. Clients often use intellectualization at the onset of a crisis, and the need for this defense may decrease in a supportive nurse-client relationship. The nurse can help the client relate emotionally to a problem by not forcing the expression of feeling. This will only frighten the client further. Asking these clients to explain how their knowledge relates to them personally may encourage them to accept and explore their emotional reactions.

CHAPTER HIGHLIGHTS

• Stressful situations tax a person's resources or coping capabilities, causing a negative effect. The source of the stress is known as a stressor.

• Selye's stress adaptation theory can be used to explain the physiologic effects of stress.

• In the psychobiologic view, stress is a function not only of external conditions but also of the constitutional vulnerability of the person and the adequacy of that person's coping styles.

• Anxiety is an uncomfortable feeling that stems from threats to biologic integrity and the security of the self.

• Nurses can expect clients and their families to become anxious in the face of unknown or potentially painful, dangerous, or disfiguring events.

• Stress, changes, and threats to one's self-concept cause anxiety and place additional coping demands on the individual.

• The choice of coping strategy often depends on external circumstances, the suddenness and intensity of the stress, the resources available to the person, and a predisposition to a certain coping pattern.

• Persons cope with stress in a variety of ways that seem to have worked in the past. Some talk it over with others; some jog; others pray or laugh off the problem.

• When someone is unable to ward off stress or reduce anxiety in the usual way, tension mounts. Persons may have to rely on largely unconscious and inflexible coping patterns that are self-deceptive.

• Anyone may use defense mechanisms to cope with anxiety or stress, but a healthy person tends to use problem-solving methods more often.

• Defense mechanisms include repression, suppression, dissociation, identification, introjection, projection, denial, fantasy, rationalization, reaction formation, displacement, and intellectualization.

REFERENCES

Aldwin C, Revenson TA: Does coping help? A reexamination of the relation between coping and mental health. *J Pers Soc Psychol* 1990;41:131–134.

Antonovsky A: *Health, Stress, and Coping.* Jossey-Bass, 1980.

Benner P, Wrubel J: *The Primacy of Caring: Stress and Coping in Health and Illness.* Addison-Wesley, 1989.

Bolger N, DeLongis A, Kessler R, Schilling E: Effects of daily stress on negative mood. *J Pers Social Psychol* 1989;57(5):808–818.

Borysenko J: *Minding the Body, Mending the Mind.* Addison-Wesley, 1987.

Cousins N: *Head First: The Biology of Hope.* E. P. Dutton, 1989.

Dohrenwend BS, Dohrenwend BP (eds): *Stressful Life Events and Their Contexts.* Rutgers University Press, 1984.

Floyd JA: Nursing students' stress levels, attitude toward drugs, and drug use. *Arch Psychiatr Nurs* 1991;5(1):46–53.

Garber J, Seligman MEP: *Human Helplessness: Theory and Applications.* Academic Press, 1980.

Graydon JE: Measuring patient coping. *Nurs Papers* 1984;16:3–12.

Holmes TH, Rahe RH: The social readjustment rating scale. *J Psychosom Res* 1967;11:213–218.

Kneisl CR, Ames SW; *Adult Health Nursing: A Biopsychosocial Approach.* Addison-Wesley, 1986.

Kobasa SC, Maddi SR, Kan S: Hardiness and health: A prospective study. *J Pers Soc Psychol* 1982;42:168–177.

Lazarus RS: *Patterns of Adjustment.* McGraw-Hill, 1976.

Lazarus RS: *Psychological Stress and the Coping Process.* McGraw-Hill, 1966.

Lazarus RS, Folkman S: An analysis of coping in a middle-aged community sample. *J Health Soc Behav* 1980;21:219–239.

Lazarus RS, Folkman S: *Stress, Appraisal, and Coping.* Springer, 1984.

Lyon BL, Werner J: Stress: Ten years of practice-relevant research, in Werley H, Fitzpatrick J (eds): *Annual Review of Nursing Research.* Springer, 1987.

Mason LJ: *Guide to Stress Reduction.* Peace Press, 1980.

McBride AB: Mental health effects of women's multiple roles. *Am Psychol* 1990;35:381–384.

Meyers J, et al: Life events and mental status. *J Health Human Behav* 1972;1:398–406.

Mishel MH: Perceived uncertainty and stress in illness. *Res Nurs Health* 1984;7:163–171.

Norbeck JS: Modification of life event questionnaires for use with female respondents. *Res Nurs health* 1984;7:61–71.

Pelletier KR: *Healthy People in Unhealthy Places; Stress and Fitness at Work.* Doubleday, 1984.

Perley NZ: Problems in self-consistency: Anxiety, in Roy C: *Introduction to Nursing: An Adaptation Model.* Prentice-Hall, 1984.

Rahe RH: Life change events and mental illness: An overview. *J Human Stress* 1979;5:2–10.

Robinson KM, Bridgewater SC, Molla PM, Wathen CA: Concepts of stress for nursing. *Issues Ment Health Nurs* 1982;4:167–176.

Selye H: *The Stress of Life.* McGraw-Hill, 1956.

Selye H: *The Stress of Life.* McGraw-Hill, 1976.

Selye H: *Stress without Distress.* American Library, 1974.

Sherbourne CD: The role of social support and life stress events in the use of mental health services. *Soc Sci Med* 1988;27(12):1393–1499.

Sutterley DC, Donnelley GF (eds): *Coping with Stress: A Nursing Perspective.* Aspen, 1982.

Tache J, Selye J: On stress and coping mechanisms. *Issues Ment Health Nurs* 1985;7:3–24.

Thomas SP: Gender differences in anger expression: Health implications. *Res Nurs Health* 1989;12:6–12.

Warner SL: Humor: A coping response for student nurses. *Arch Psychiatr Nurs* 1991;5(1):10–16.

Ziemer MM: Coping behavior: A response to stress. *Top Clin Nurs* 1982;2(4):8.

Psychobiology Box References

Hales D: *An Invitation to Health* ed 4. Benjamin/Cummings, 1989.

Restak RM. The brain, depression and the immune system. *J Clin Psychiatr* 1989;50(5) (Suppl):23–25.

Stein M. Stress, depression and the immune system. *J Clin Psychiatr* 1989;50(5) (Suppl):35–40.

Vollhardt LT. Psychoimmunology: A literature review. *Am J Orthopsychiatr* 1991;61(1):35–47.

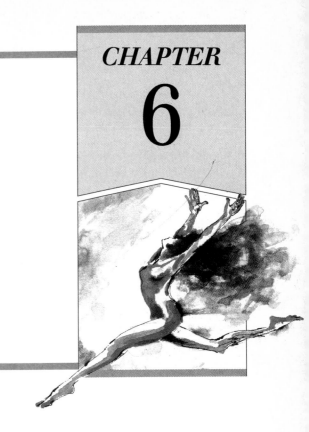

Psychobiology

CHAPTER 6

LEARNING OBJECTIVES

- Identify the historical roots of the psychobiologic tradition
- List and describe gross neuroanatomic structures and their functions
- Discuss the role of neurotransmitters in health and disease
- Discuss one biologic theory of schizophrenia, mood disorders, and anxiety disorders
- Enumerate two basic principles underlying clinical ecology
- Discuss three areas of nursing care for psychiatric clients that are amenable to psychobiologic assessment
- List and describe two psychobiologic nursing interventions

Geoffry McEnany

CROSS REFERENCES

Other topics relevant to this content are: Biologic therapies, Chapter 32; History, Chapter 1, Mood disorders, Chapter 13; Organic mental syndromes and disorders, Chapter 10; Philosophy, Chapter 1; and Schizophrenia, Chapter 12. Also see Appendix B.

PSYCHOBIOLOGY—THE WORD BRINGS to mind some ultramodern, high-tech future. But psychobiology is neither a new concept nor a recent discovery. It has existed since the birth of humankind and has been a subject of discussion for at least the last 2000 years. What *is* new in psychobiology is a broader understanding of the biologic basis of the mind and behavior. Contemporary knowledge of the biologic components of behavior is revolutionizing not only psychiatry but also our view of psychiatric disorders and their treatment.

A comprehensive definition of psychobiology is difficult at best. Psychobiology encompasses an enormous body of information that is growing almost exponentially. For this reason, the conceptual "face" of psychobiology is changing. With these thoughts in mind, we can offer the following definition: **Psychobiology** is the study of the biochemical foundations of thought, mood, emotion, affect, and behavior. It takes into consideration both internal and external influences—e.g., genetics, the effects of other body systems such as the endocrine and immune systems, and the external environment—across the life span of an individual.

When students study the neurologic system in an anatomy and physiology class, they are likely to look at the material through the "lens" of an anatomist or physiologist. Similarly, when they study psychosis in a psychology or psychiatric nursing class, they probably explore the behavioral or psychodynamic aspects of psychosis, not really knowing how they will use the knowledge from an anatomy and physiology class in the psychology classroom or in clinical work. In this chapter we strive to give students an overview of psychobiology and make them aware of how psychobiology principles fit with those of nursing. It is impossible in one chapter to even touch upon all of the facets of psychobiology in any detail; this chapter is an attempt to motivate students to apply psychobiologic principles in professional work.

A Historical Perspective of Psychobiology

Every achievement that people perceive as great or spectacular—the seven wonders of the world, the Roman Empire, the landing of men on the moon, a Mozart concerto, test-tube babies, artificial hearts, computers, telecommunications—is due to the capacity of the human brain. Extraordinarily complex in its composition and functioning, the human brain is the source of all creativity, logic, thought, and emotion.

The brain has been regarded as a mysterious wonder throughout history. Hippocrates (460 B.C.) the "father of medicine," postulated that the brain is the central organ of intellectual functioning and that mental disorders are secondary to brain pathology:

Men ought to know that from the brain, and from the brain only, arise pleasures, joys, laughters, jests, and our sorrows, pains, griefs or fears. . . . It is the same thing that makes us mad or delirious, inspires us with dread or fear, whether by night or by day, brings sleeplessness, inopportune mistakes, aimless anxieties, absent-mindedness, and acts that are contrary to habit.

In light of the Greek belief that mental disorders were of supernatural origin, Hippocrates' biologic model of illness must have seemed shocking. Nonetheless, it established a differentiation between mind and body in the Greek thought of Hippocrates' era.

Plato and Aristotle also influenced the concept of mental illness. Plato (ca. 400 B.C.) was more supportive of what might be termed today as a psychologic rather than biologic notion of "mental" illness. For example, in *The Republic*, Plato discussed three subdivisions of the soul, which have been compared to the id, ego, and superego. In contrast, Aristotle (ca. 350 B.C.) believed that disturbed mental functioning was secondary to an imbalance in the four body humors (blood, phlegm, black bile, and yellow bile) postulated by Hippocrates, thus associating states of the mind with body function.

Ancient Romans furthered the idea that mental illness had a biologic base and was not due to supernatural influences. Asclepiades, founder of a Roman school of medicine, described phrenitis and mania, noting physical aspects of each condition. Additionally, Asclepiades recommended coarse biologic treatments, e.g., placing clients with certain mental conditions in rooms filled with light, rather than in the dark. Today, exposure to light is known to influence the reticular activating system, a part of the brain that controls various states of wakefulness. Additionally, exposure to full spectrum light is used today to treat conditions such as seasonal affective disorder.

During the Dark Ages (400–1200) there was little support for the notion that mental illness has a biologic basis. However, some important ideas emerged about the classification of psychobiopathologic states. Several descriptions of illness, including cyclic patterns of mood, melancholia, mania, psychotic behaviors, epilepsy, and dementia, were written during this period. Treatments of mental disorders were physical, e.g., bloodletting and trepanation. Others were spiritual, as evidenced by the popularity of exorcisms during that period.

The Renaissance contributed a miscellaneous collection of explanations about the cause of mental disorders and varied treatments. One school of thought held closely to the belief that mental disorders were the result of spiritual imbalance or witchcraft. Another group, led mainly by Johann Weyer, viewed psychopathology as the result of interacting physical and spiritual factors. Weyer expanded on the descriptive classifications of mental disorders and emphasized the importance of accurate assessment and close observation during treatment.

During the seventeenth and eighteenth centuries, a marked shift in thought occurred, as the mind-body explanation of illness reemerged. During this era mental disorders came under the domain of medicine, and many physicians believed that doctors should be the sole caretakers of the mentally disordered. During this period great attention was given to the physical manifestations of "hysterical" conditions, which were perhaps the beginnings of what has come to be known as psychosomatics.

Between the nineteenth century and the present, the greatest strides have been made toward understanding mental disorders from a biologic perspective. A clearly biologic model began to emerge. In the latter part of the nineteenth century, physicians began to view psychopathology as a result of changes in the nervous system. Eventually other causes were considered, e.g., genetic predisposition and the role of endocrine dysfunction in various states of mental illness.

Of course, during the late nineteenth and early twentieth centuries, Sigmund Freud developed his theory of psychoanalysis. Prior to becoming interested in emotional conditions, Freud was a neurologist. Unfortunately, he was unable to make the link between psychologic defenses against anxiety and the biologic processes of anxiety. Nonetheless, Freud made significant contributions to the developing, although inexact, science of psychiatry, allowing for the unfolding of new ideas and a reexamination of old beliefs about mental disorders.

A major shift in contemporary Western psychiatry occurred during the 1930s and 1940s with the introduction of solely biologic therapies, e.g., shock treatment and various psychosurgeries. These treatments, with their subsequent successes and failures, kindled a strong interest in the biology of behavior. This trend led to biologic research and new treatments. An important step in the development of a biologic model in psychiatry was the introduction of psychotropic drugs, substances that affect the brain and central nervous system to produce a desired change in behavior. This intervention was revolutionary. Psychotropic medications clearly refuted dualism and gave psychiatry objective evidence for a holistic view of the person. Although the effects of the drugs were clearly visible in the behavior of the people who took them, many mental health professionals continued to deny the existence of a biologic basis of mental disorders.

Despite empiric evidence to the contrary, many today continue to explore solely psychologic explanations for behavior when physical explanations exist. The persistent denial of the physiologic aspects of mental illness possibly constitutes a nemesis. In the words of Illich (1976), a *nemesis* is "the inevitable punishment for attempts to be a hero rather than a human being" (p 35). It is dreadful to think that people bear the "punishment" of continued symptoms of mental disorders because a professional believes that "the harder the client works, the better the cure" (Lickey and Gordon 1983, p 9). Anyone who has ever tried to talk someone out of a hallucination, delusion, major depression, anorexia nervosa, or panic attack knows how ineffective this approach can be. However, because psychiatric illness is not unlike other forms of illness, it responds to varied interventions, depending on its severity. For some unbalanced states of emotion, behavioral intervention may be adequate. For clients with more severe states of disequilibrium, medications may be necessary for a full return to wellness. Psychobiology and its behavioral correlates are undeniable, and nurses need to foster an understanding of psychobiologic principles in practice. Such applied knowledge is likely to lend greater integrity to the practice of psychiatric-mental health nursing, while refuting the ancient tradition of dualism.

Brain, Mind, and Behavior

A Neuroanatomic Review

Volumes have been written about the anatomy of the nervous system. In this chapter it is impossible to examine all of the major neuroanatomic structures. The points of interest here include the structures of the brain believed to be involved in the formation of thought and emotion. The first half of this section focuses on gross neuroanatomy, and the latter explores neuroanatomy and physiology from a cellular perspective.

The brain is defined in various ways. The definition that best suits the perspective of this chapter is that the brain is that part of the central nervous system encapsulated by the skull. The brain is the core of our humanity. Intercommunications of different parts of the brain yield the experiences of love, hate, elation, joy, or madness. The brain provides the underlying biology for will, determination, hopes, and dreams. Without the brain to integrate experience, people would neither enjoy the wonder nor fear the horror of life.

This review explores the following six anatomic structures of the brain: cerebrum, diencephalon, cerebellum, medulla oblongata, pons, and midbrain; the last three make up the brain stem.

Cerebrum The **cerebrum** is the largest part of the human brain. It is divided into two seemingly equal components, the *cerebral hemispheres*. The deep furrow that divides the hemispheres is known as the *longitudinal sulcus*. A small but important piece of tissue, the *corpus callosum*, connects the two hemispheres medially and allows communication between them. In the past, scientists believed that each hemisphere had separate functions, such a logic or creativity and spatial accommodation. With the advent of new technologies such as positive emission tomography, it is now possible to assess metabolic activity in the brain as it occurs. Scientists are able to observe brain activity and have realized that creative as well as logical activities require input from both cerebral hemispheres.

The brain in general, and the cerebral hemispheres in particular, are well protected not only by the skull but also by a protective fluid (cerebrospinal fluid) that circulates around and within the brain. Deep within the brain are three spaces or *ventricles* that aid in the circulation of cerebrospinal fluid.

The cerebral hemispheres are divided into lobes, which are named after the parts of the skull under which they lie, i.e., frontal, temporal, occipital, and parietal (see the accompanying box and Figure 6–1). All of the lobes contain many *gyri* (ridges) and *sulci* (grooves) that maximize brain surface area.

The cerebral hemispheres consist of both white and gray matter. Gray matter consists of myelinated fibers that are referred to as *nerves;* bundle of nerves are called *tracts.* The cerebral cortex consists solely of gray matter with underlying white matter. The cerebral cortex works much as the processing unit of a computer does. The cortex is the part of the brain that makes sense out of the volumes of input. It synthesizes thought, reasoning, will, and choice and is the seat of dreams.

As essential as the cerebral hemispheres are to emotional, intellectual, and biologic functioning, they are only as good as the quality of other interdependent structures in the brain. For example, people need input from and clear communication between different brain structures to produce efficient and purposeful behavior. An example of the intercommunication between brain structures is the activity of the **limbic system.** This system, often referred to as "the emotional brain," is believed to be responsible for the modulation of emotions, memory, and possibly some aspects of attention (Andreasen 1984). The limbic system consists of neuroanatomic structures from the cerebral hemispheres and the **diencephalon,** a part of the brain located between the cerebrum and midbrain (Figure 6–2).

Two limbic structures play an especially important role in the enactment of emotion: the *amygdala* and the *hippocampus.* Begley et al. (1983, p 42) define the

Gross Functions of the Cerebral Lobes

Frontal Lobes

- Responsible for any movements; the right frontal lobe controls left side body movement and vice versa
- Contain the *premotor cortex,* which organizes complicated movement
- Contain *prefrontal fibers,* which produce a "social conscience," inhibiting unacceptable behaviors

Parietal Lobes

- Contain the *sensory cortex,* which interprets contact sensations such as touch
- Facilitate spatial orientation

Temporal Lobes

- Are involved in hearing and memory
- Connect with the limbic system (the "emotional brain") to allow for memory and expression of emotions such as anger, fright, and possibly love

Occipital Lobes

- Contain centers responsible for the complete experience of vision
- Are involved in language formation
- Collaborate with other brain structures in the formation of memory

amygdala as a "bulbous waystation . . . [that] seems to process sensations wrapped in an aura of happiness or sadness and, perhaps, index the memory under the headings such as 'joy' or 'grief.' " It is important to discuss the amygdala in relation to the hippocampus for the purpose of understanding the role both structures play in the formation of memories. Do you remember what you were doing on January 20, 1991? Unless that day had some major significance for you, chances are that you don't remember that day or remember it only vaguely. If, however, you won a million dollars on that day or attended a close friend's wedding or funeral, you are likely to remember it clearly. Emotion and memory are closely linked and are mediated through the structures of the limbic system. Of course, the view presented here is brief and oversimplified. All of the psychobiologic components of emotion, memory, and cognition are not known.

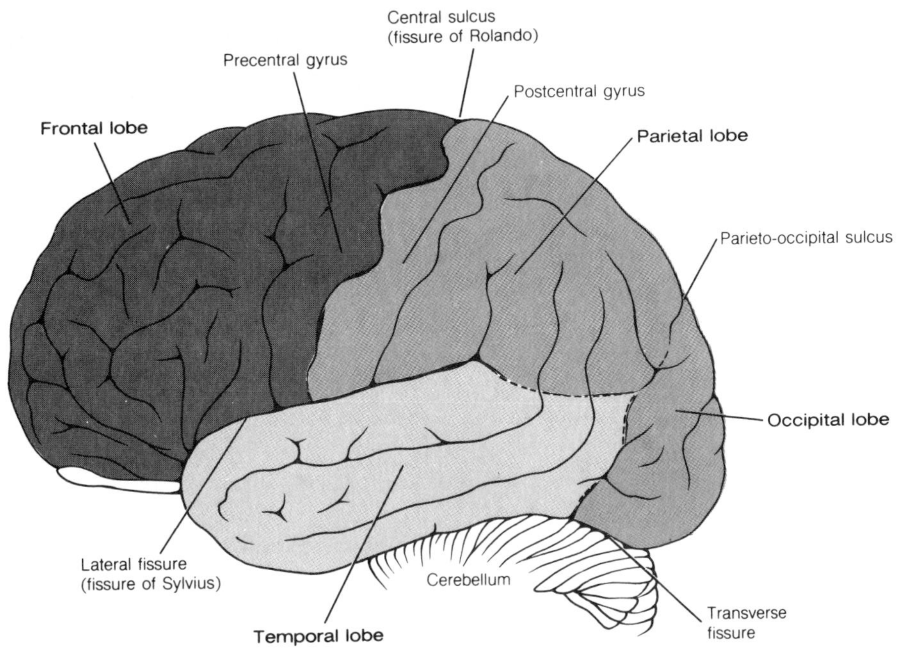

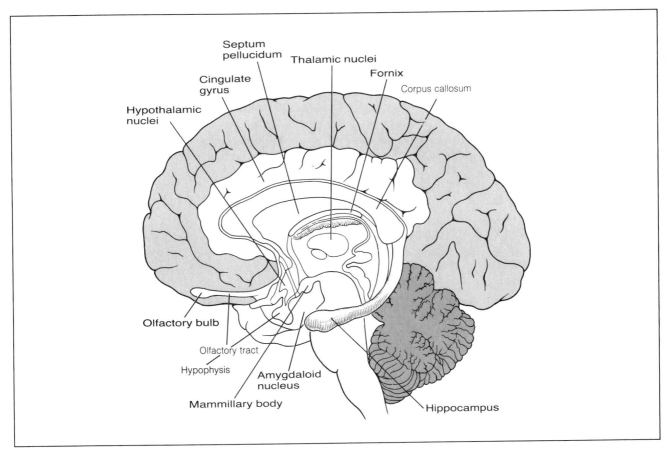

FIGURE 6–1   Delineation of the cerebral lobes.   *Source: Spence AP, Mason EB:* Human Anatomy and Physiology, *ed 3. Benjamin/Cummings, 1987, p 341.*

FIGURE 6–2   Structures of the limbic system.   *SOURCE: Spence AB, Mason EB:* Human Anatomy and Physiology, *ed 3. Benjamin/Cummings, 1987, p 350.*

What is known is that expression of thought or emotion involves the coordination of many different areas of the brain. An important assumption is that the neuroanatomy and physiology underlying thought and emotion must be relatively intact for an individual to think clearly and experience emotion fully. What is not clearly known is the degree of neurophysiologic variability among normal people. The behavioral correlates of neurophysiologic activity are seen in the behaviors of familiar persons and strangers. A bus-driver making change for a rider, a police officer directing traffic, a mentally ill person on the street mumbling and yelling to seemingly nobody—all of these behaviors are the result of some form of activity in the brain. Surely a huge variance exists between illness and wellness behavior, but the finer points of how these differences manifest themselves in the realm of neurobiologic activity are not yet completely known.

Thalamus and Hypothalamus

Other limbic structures are in the diencephalon and include the thalamus and the hypothalamus. The *thalamus* functions as a relay station, receiving many impulses from the spinal cord, brain stem, and cerebellum. With the aid of many connections in the cerebral hemispheres and cortex, the thalamus regulates activity and movement, sensory experience, and emotional behavior.

The *hypothalamus* is a neuroanatomic market-place of sorts, consisting of many structures such as the *supraoptic nuclei,* parts of the *pituitary gland,* and the *mamillary bodies.* The hypothalamus weighs approximately 4 grams and accounts for less than 1 percent of the total brain volume. However, its size is not a good indication of its importance. The hypothalamus is responsible for appetite control, fluid balance within the body, sexual impulse regulation, endocrine function, and temperature modulation. Within the hypothalamus lie the motivation of humankind and an awesome coordination of behaviors accompanying emotional expression. Mahler's frenzy, Frankenstein's monster's rage, and Lady MacBeth's woeful fears are most likely components of hypothalamic activity. Students may be very aware of their hypothalamic activity when they experience fatigue after final examinations, middle-of-the-night munchies, and irritation at an inconsiderate roommate. Currently, some psychobiologists believe that the roots of such disorders as bulimia and anorexia nervosa lie in the hypothalamus.

Cerebellum

The **cerebellum** is that part of the brain that lies below the posterior section of the cerebrum. It is the second-largest structure within the brain (Figure 6–3). Like the cerebral hemispheres, the cerebellum has an outer layer of gray matter and is mainly composed of underlying white matter. The main function of this highly specialized part of the brain is movement and coordination. The hand-eye coordination of a diamond cutter, the fluid movements of a ballerina, and the success of a quarterback's moves all depend on cerebellar functions. As you read this page, you are depending on your cerebellum to send messages to your eyes that allow you to follow the print as you read from one line to the next.

Brain Stem

The final section of this review involves an examination of the brain stem. The brain stem consists of three smaller structures: the medulla oblongata, the pons, and the midbrain (Figure 6–4). The **medulla oblongata** (Latin for oblong marrow) is the connecting piece of tissue between the brain stem and the spinal cord. It is less than 2 inches long but is responsible for many vital functions, including respiration, regulation of blood pressure, and partial regulation of heart rate. It also controls vomiting, swallowing, and some aspects of talking. Incoming fibers from the spinal cord cross over in the medulla, yielding left cerebral hemispheric control of the right side of the body and vice versa.

Pons means *bridge,* and bridging is its function. The pons contains conduction paths between the spinal cord and the brain. It also contains reflex centers that mediate sensations of the face, chewing, abduction of the eyes, facial expressions, balance, and regulation of respiration. Connections with the limbic system allow the pons to modulate expressions that indicate states such as tenderness, anger, fear, or happiness.

The **midbrain** is above the pons and below the cerebral hemispheres. Not unlike the pons, the midbrain (or mesencephalon) is a reflex center for the regulation of eye movement, visual accommodation, and regulation of pupil size. Additionally, the midbrain is essential for relaying impulses to the cerebral cortex and sending behavior-producing messages back to the periphery.

Certain portions of the brain function in concert with other parts to create a system with a given function; the limbic system is a good example. Other systems that are of special interest to psychiatric nurses include the reticular activating system and the extrapyramidal system.

The **reticular activating system** (RAS) consists of nerve pathways that originate in the spinal cord and connect in the reticular formation, a system of neurons that modulates awareness and states of consciousness. The RAS screens stimulation from the environment and allows people to concentrate. Imagine what it would be like to have to pay attention to all sounds, smells, and sights in the environment around you as you read this page. Reading would be impossible, and concentration would suffer greatly. The RAS also permits routine inattention, allowing for sleep. In states of mental illness, there is obviously some

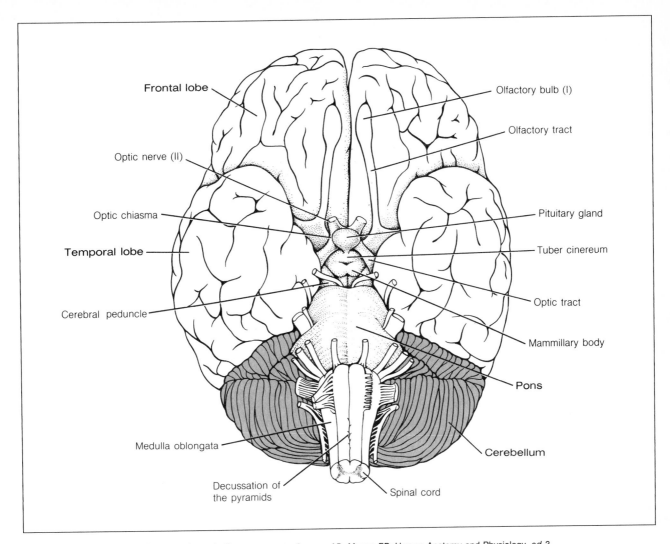

FIGURE 6–3   The cerebrum and cerebellum.   *SOURCE: Spence AP, Mason EB: Human Anatomy and Physiology, ed 3.
Benjamin/Cummings, 1987, p 346.*

biologic disequilibrium of the RAS. However, the details of this imbalance are complex and not well understood at this time.

The **extrapyramidal system** consists of tracts of motor neurons from the brain to parts of the spinal cord. This system has complex relays and connections to areas of the cortex, cerebellum, brain stem, and thalamus. These tracts play an important role in gross movements and responses of emotional tone, e.g., smiling and frowning.

Antipsychotic drugs create side effects that affect the extrapyramidal system, hence extrapyramidal side effects or EPS. The four general classes of extrapyramidal side effects include (a) parkinsonism, (b) dyskinesias and dystonias, (c) akathisias, and (3) tardive dyskinesia.

Central Nervous System Cells   The anatomic structure of the brain is incredibly complex on gross examination; things become even more complex as one looks at the biochemical processes that occur with

every thought, emotion, inspiration, dream, or hope. Thought and feeling are made possible by complex interplays and communications between cells in the central nervous system in relation to the environment. The specialized cells of the nervous system are called **neurons.** Like other cells in the body, each neuron has a cell body that contains the cytoplasm and the nucleus. Unlike other cells, a neuron has at least two other processes: an axon and one or more dendrites (Figure 6–5). An **axon** is that portion of the neuron that conveys electric impulses *from* the cell body to other neurons. Axons are covered with a white myelin sheath and compose the white matter in the brain and spinal cord. **Dendrites** are *not* myelinated but allow for the conduction of electric messages *to* the cell body. There are approximately 100 billion neurons in the brain with nearly an equal number of supporting (glia) cells.

Neurons are classified according to the direction in which they conduct impulses. *Sensory neurons,* also known as afferent neurons, send messages from the

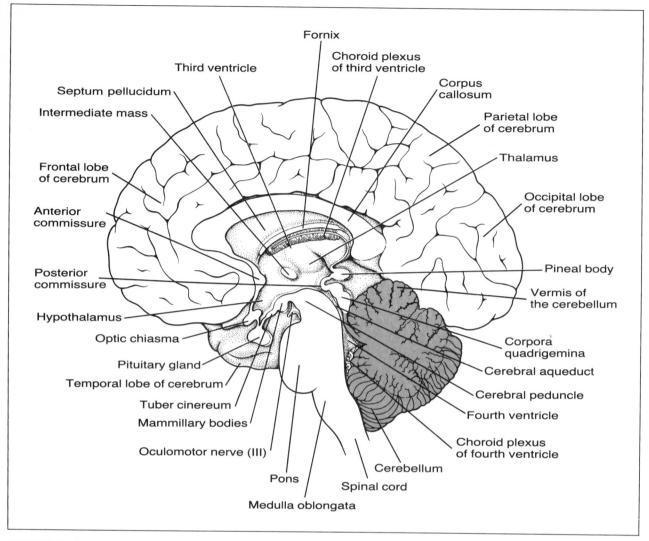

FIGURE 6–4 Structures of the cerebrum and cerebellum. *SOURCE: Spence AP, Mason EB: Human Anatomy and Physiology, ed 3. Benjamin/Cummings, 1987, p 348.*

periphery to the brain. For example, if someone puts a foot into a tub of scalding water, the message that the water is too hot is sent to the brain on sensory neuron pathways. *Motor* or efferent *neurons* carry messages that originate in the brain and yield a behavioral change in the periphery. In the example of the foot in the hot water, the message from the brain is to remove the foot (quickly!) from the hot water; this message travels on motor neuron paths. Sometimes, specialized neurons that communicate between sensory and motor neurons help to produce a given, desirable behavior.

Communication among and between neurons is complex and specific. This communication is believed to be the basis of behavior. Any given neuron is likely to have contact with hundreds or thousands of other neurons, and the actual number of synaptic contacts in the brain alone may number 100 trillion. Interneuron communication is electric and chemical and occurs at the synapses, or points of contact between neurons, as

well as along the neuron itself. The **synapse** is a microscopic gap on the cleft between neurons. Disordered activity can occur in this space, perhaps yielding affective and schizophrenic symptoms. Of course, the belief that disordered synaptic activity alone can yield complex psychiatric symptoms is overly simplistic. It is important to keep in mind that, from a holistic perspective, disordered biologic processes are an important facet of the illness experience.

Neurotransmitters

A closer look at the synapse reveals some fascinating information (Figure 6–5). The membrane of the end point or axon terminal of one neuron contains many saclike projections known as **synaptic vesicles.** The vesicles contain the chemicals that allow the transmission of electric impulses across the synapse. These chemicals are known as **neurotransmitters.** As an

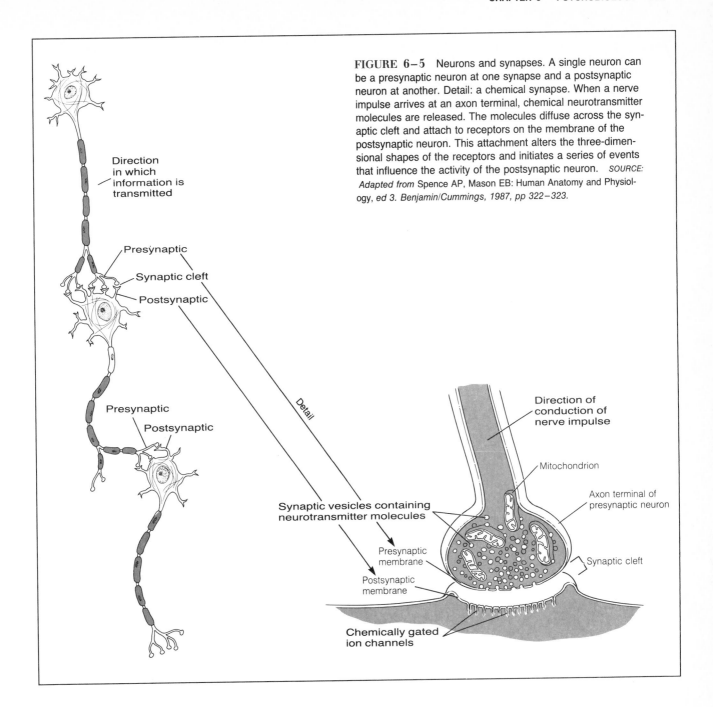

FIGURE 6-5 Neurons and synapses. A single neuron can be a presynaptic neuron at one synapse and a postsynaptic neuron at another. Detail: a chemical synapse. When a nerve impulse arrives at an axon terminal, chemical neurotransmitter molecules are released. The molecules diffuse across the synaptic cleft and attach to receptors on the membrane of the postsynaptic neuron. This attachment alters the three-dimensional shapes of the receptors and initiates a series of events that influence the activity of the postsynaptic neuron.   *SOURCE: Adapted from Spence AP, Mason EB: Human Anatomy and Physiology, ed 3. Benjamin/Cummings, 1987, pp 322-323.*

Direction in which information is transmitted

Presynaptic

Synaptic cleft

Postsynaptic

Presynaptic

Postsynaptic

Detail

Synaptic vesicles containing neurotransmitter molecules

Presynaptic membrane

Postsynaptic membrane

Direction of conduction of nerve impulse

Mitochondrion

Axon terminal of presynaptic neuron

Synaptic cleft

Chemically gated ion channels

impulse travels down an axon toward the synapse, it stimulates a change in the cell membrane and commands the vesicles to release the neurotransmitter into the synaptic cleft. This results in the neurotransmitter chemicals binding to specific receptors on the dendrites of the adjacent neuron, allowing the electric impulse to cross the synapse and continue its course to the next neuron. It takes less than 0.0005 second for the impulse to move from the presynaptic terminal to the postsynaptic receptors (Lickey and Gordon 1983). What happens to the neurotransmitter substance that was released into the synapse *after* the impulse has

passed? One of two things can occur: The neurotransmitter can be dissolved by enzymes in the synapse, or the chemical can be reabsorbed for recycling by the presynaptic neuron (re-uptake). In either case, the synapse and its pre- and postneurons are reset for the next impulse, at which time the process is repeated.

At this time, nobody actually knows how many neurotransmitters exist in the human brain, but there is evidence that the number is likely to exceed sixty. Part of the problem has been in deciding specific criteria to determine what chemicals in the brain can actually be called neurotransmitters. Several other neurochemical substances, known as neuromodulators, neurohormones, and neuroregulators, modify the actions of neurotransmitters but are not neurotransmitters themselves (McEnany 1990). The following sections examine the neurotransmitters and their functions (see the Theory box below).

Biogenic Amine (Monoamine) Neurotransmitters This group of neurotransmitters includes dopamine, norepinephrine, serotonin, and histamine; the first three are implicated in mood disorders and schizophrenia (Brown and Mann 1985). Dopamine is a plentiful neurotransmitter synthesized from the dietary amino acid tyrosine and found in three parts of the brain: the brain's substantia nigra motor center (affecting movement and coordination), the midbrain (involving emotion and memory), and the hypothalamus/pituitary connection (involving emotional responses and stress-coping patterns). Norepinephrine receptors are found in the cerebral cortex (affecting cognitive functions), the limbic system (yielding emotional responses), the hippocampus and thalamus (contributing to emotion, pleasure, and memory), the cerebellum (influencing movement), and the hypothalamus (influencing thirst, body temperature, and appetite). Serotonin pathways are somewhat similar to norepinephrine pathways and have similar effects and influences. Histamine, although of extreme importance in the peripheral nervous system, has not received great attention as a central neurotransmitter.

Acetylcholine The first neurochemical to be identified as a true neurotransmitter, acetylcholine is the "grandparent" of neurotransmitters. It is available practically everywhere in the brain and spinal cord but is especially abundant in the neurons involved with some form of movement (motor neurons). It is considered to be highly significant in neuromuscular transmission.

Amino Acids This group of neurotransmitters is of special interest because they are readily available in the form of proteins in the diet. As ingested proteins, the substances are precursors to neurotransmitters; brain cells convert these proteins into neurotransmitters. For example, there is truth in the folk wisdom that warmed milk with honey helps people sleep. Milk contains the amino acid *tryptophan*. In the presence of a carbohydrate such as honey, the tryptophan molecule binds with the glucose (carbohydrate) from the honey. Since the brain runs on glucose, the glucose-tryptophan combination can cross the blood-brain barrier. Once inside the brain, tryptophan is converted to serotonin and aids in the induction of sleep. Other examples of dietary amino acids include glutamate (also known as monosodium glutamate), choline (available from soybeans), and tyrosine. These amino acids are discussed later in this chapter. Amino acids in the central nervous system seem to be used for fast transmission of impulses in all regions of the brain. Chains of amino acids are believed to have a regulatory effect on central nervous system activity, especially in the area of pain regulation.

Recent interest in the amino acid neurotransmitter gamma-aminobutyric acid (GABA) has led to new information on its function (Fawcett 1989). This information has shed light on the role GABA plays in anxiety, the effect of certain medications on GABA functioning, and the use of these medications to relieve anxiety. Other amino acid neurotransmitters include glycine, aspartate, and glutamate.

Neurotransmitter activity cannot be underestimated in states of both health and illness. If synaptic activity controls events such as thought, emotion, movement, and overall biologic functions, then one can anticipate that attention and research will expand knowledge in this area, eventually offering greater

THEORY

Known Neurotransmitters in the Brain

Amine Neurotransmitters

- Dopamine
- Serotonin (5-HT, 5-hydroxytryptamine)
- Norepinephrine
- Histamine

Amino Acid Neurotransmitters

- Gamma-aminobutyric acid (GABA)
- Glycine
- Aspartate
- Glutamate

Cholinergic Neurotransmitters

- Acetylcholine

Peptides

- Hypothalamic releasing hormones
- Pituitary hormones
  - Anterior lobe hormones
  - Neurohypophyseal hormones

options for intervention in psychiatry and psychiatric nursing.

Psychoendocrinology and Psychoimmunology

This section refutes the concept of dualism by examining the interaction of the brain and two subsystems: the endocrine and immune systems. Grebb and Reus (1984) describe **psychoendocrinology** as a subspecialty of endocrinology that explores the relationship between behavior, biology, and endocrine function. Endocrine action is mediated through chemical substances such as hormones. Three classes of hormones exist: steroids, peptides, and amino acids. The peptides are of special interest to those in psychiatry because these hormones coexist with certain neurotransmitters (monoamines) and affect actions in the synapse. The

peptides function as neurotransmitters, i.e., they assist in neurotransmission but are not solely responsible for the entire biochemical synaptic sequence. The peptides are also involved in the regulation of hormonal axes; recently, the cortisol axis has received significant attention in conjunction with the dexamethasone suppression test for depression. The accompanying Theory box shows the main hormonal axes and conditions that result from disordered peptide functioning. It is important to remember that neuroregulators are influenced by input from the limbic system (the "emotional" brain), the cerebral cortex (the "thinking" brain), and the hypothalamus and pineal gland (involved in hormonal secretion).

In the last few years there has been an upsurge of interest by psychiatrists and psychiatric nurses in the behavioral manifestations of thyroid dysfunction. As Vogel (1986, p 9) points out, clients with thyroid dysfunction present a "mixed bag" of symptoms

THEORY

Behavioral Conditions Related to Hormonal Disruption

Cortisol
Hypercortisolism may lead to:
- Depression
- Mania
- Psychosis
- Confusion

Hypocortisolism may lead to:
- Apathy
- Fatigue
- Depression

Thyroid
Hyperthyroidism may lead to:
- Anxiety
- Restlessness
- Irritability

Hypothyroidism may lead to:
- Depression
- Cognitive impairment
- Confusion
- Psychosis

Autoimmune thyroiditis may produce a variety of concurrent behaviors, including:
- Anxiety
- Depression
- Somatic complaints (common)

Growth Hormone
- May be involved peripherally in the mechanism of Alzheimer's disease
- Causes acromegaly or dwarfism

Prolactin
Hyperactivity of the prolactin regulatory system may lead to:
- Lethargy
- Irritability
- Increased thirst

Other hormones of behavioral interest include endorphins, enkephalins, and cholecystokinin.

SOURCE: From Table 11–3, p 134, "Neurobehavioral Chemistry and Physiology" by JA Grebb, VI Reus. Reproduced with permission from Review of General Psychiatry by HH Goldman (ed). Copyright © 1984 by Lange Medical Publications. Reprinted by permission of Appleton-Lange Publishing Co., Los Altos, CA.

including those that suggest mood disorders, heart disease, organic brain syndrome, and lithium toxicity.

A psychiatric nurse, for instance, might encounter the following scenario. The nurse walks into the room of Rose, a 44-year-old depressed woman.

Nurse: Hello, Rose.

Rose: (Rose is initially silent but rolls over in her bed and looks at the nurse.) Leave me alone . . .

Nurse: It's clear to me that you'd like to be left alone, but it's 8:30 in the morning, and you're expected at breakfast.

Rose: Take a hike, nurse! I'm exhausted, I've got aches and pains. If I eat, I'll just get more constipated. And besides, it's freezing in this place! Don't you people believe in using heat? What day is this anyway? And who *are* you? Did I work with you yesterday? I can't remember your name . . .

Rose's behaviors match the DSM-III-R criteria for major depressive disorder. But what other behaviors is she demonstrating? She complains of fatigue, constipation, and vague pains and aches. She reports feeling cold, and her memory is poor. She is not oriented to the day. One of a thousand things might be going on with Rose, right? Not necessarily. Rose is perhaps demonstrating early signs of hypothyroidism. A quick review of her laboratory tests shows normal thyroid function. Reviewing her admission physical exam, the nurse notices that her thyroid was basically normal, although slightly larger on the left than the right. At this point the nurse might abandon the idea that Rose's behaviors may be linked to thyroid dysfunction. But did the physician check Rose's thyroglobulin and thyroid microsomal antibodies? Some clients who show no clinical signs of thyroid dysfunction actually suffer from *autoimmune thyroiditis*. This condition produces an autoimmune process within the thyroid that eventually leads to atrophy of the gland and subsequent hypothyroidism. The early clinical indices used are those aforementioned thyroid antibody tests.

The nurse's expert clinical skills proved to be correct in Rose's case. It was not just depression that caused Rose to behave as she did. She was suffering from a treatable psychobiologic condition, autoimmune thyroiditis. Because of the nurse's keen assessment and interdisciplinary collaboration, Rose can receive the appropriate treatment and care.

There has been a recent upsurge of interest in autoimmune thyroiditis, Rose's condition. Stein and Uhde (1988, 1989) have investigated the connection between thyroid function and conditions such as panic disorder. In the earlier article, they report no significant differences in the thyroid functions of normal subjects and those with a diagnosis of panic disorder. They do point out, however, that clients with primary thyroid dysfunction may be predisposed to secondary development of anxiety syndromes. In a subsequent article, Stein and Uhde (1989) explore the correlation between autoimmune thyroiditis and the emergence of panic disorder. Although they failed to find a higher prevalence of autoimmune thyroiditis among patients with panic disorder than among healthy control subjects, they make some valuable observations that support the need for close clinical observation of clients who may be at risk for this psychoendocrinologic condition.

Psychoimmunology explores the relationships among the central nervous system, the immune system, and behavior. Nurses, physicians, and others working in the health sciences have long been aware of the relationship between stress and illness. Arthritis, colitis, thyrotoxicosis, asthma, and cancer are a few of the conditions believed to be influenced by inordinate stress and its effect on immune system mediation. In the last decade, the relationship between stress and illness (not solely "physical") has been amply documented in the scientific literature. Of course, to a holistic practitioner, it makes little sense to speak of physical illness as different from mental illness other than as a way to describe the qualities of the presenting symptoms.

The ways stress influences illness and disease are mostly unknown at this time. Most researchers who have examined the effects of stress on disease states conducted animal studies that are difficult to generalize to a human population. The AIDS epidemic has generated new interest in the effect of stress on immune function. Both the professional and lay literature report various methods to reduce the effects of stress with the hope of improving immune function. The consistent difficulty in generalizing such findings to all persons probably reflects differences among individuals, not only in responses to stress but also in responses to stress-reducing measures.

Circadian Rhythms

Life on this planet has evolved by the rhythm of the day-and-night cycle, and humans are no exception. Human life and biology demonstrate cycles of approximately 24 hours. One of the major functions of the circadian timing system is the sequencing of metabolic/physiologic events and compatible coordination of the same. Additionally, certain sleep disorders, endocrine disorders, and bipolar disorders may have circadian bases.

What underlies the human propensity for maintaining this approximate 24-hour cycle? **Circadian rhythms** within the body are believed to be *endogenous,* i.e., diurnal changes are likely to occur even when people are not in the natural environment. In other words, a person placed in a room with a constant amount of light and sound over 24 hours but not exposed to natural events such as sunlight and darkness would still experience predictable shifts in cortisol, body temperature, sleep, and other circadian-dependent variables. The cyclic pattern is likely a response to the environment that evolved over time.

Currently, two circadian pacemakers are believed to exist: One is connected to the eyes and vision, and the location of the other is uncertain (Moore-Ede et al. 1983). Because at least one of the pacemakers is located in a light-sensitive area, it makes great sense to hypothesize that the body learns its rhythms from light-dark cycles. Disorders of rhythmicity are observed in insomnia and affective disorders; some clinicians report seeing clients whose symptoms seem to be seasonally related. The belief is that these clients are very sensitive to changes in the number of hours of exposure to light each day. Also, early morning awakening is a common complaint of depressed people. High serum cortisol levels are common in depressed people. Is the sleep disturbance a part of the depression, a result of high serum cortisol, or an independently disturbed rhythm? Resolution of such a question requires accurate assessment and appropriate intervention.

Defective circadian mechanisms may cause depressed or manic symptoms in vulnerable people. Some people who have affective illnesses demonstrate behavior indicative of faulty circadian pacemaker systems. Additionally, follow-up studies at the National Institute of Mental Health (NIMH) showed that people who respond to antidepressants do so in a fraction of the usual time if they are deprived of sleep for one night. Some people with *bipolar disorder* demonstrate a keen sensitivity to changes in the length of day due to seasonal changes; they experience seasonal depression in the autumn that terminates in hypomania in the spring.

Some disturbances of circadian rhythm are amenable to nursing intervention. For instance, the nurse can help to "reset" a client's circadian clock by regulating that person's sleep pattern. Plumlee (1986), a nurse who has written on the subject of biologic rhythms, offers several helpful suggestions to psychiatric nurses who need to assess client rhythms. Other interventions, prescribed by physicians, include circadian rhythm—altering substances, such as lithium, some steroids, and possibly tricyclic antidepressants (Moore-Ede et al. 1983).

Psychobiology and Mental Disorders

This section examines current theories of the causes of schizophrenia, mood disorders (bipolar disorder, mania, depression), anxiety disorders, dementia, seizure disorders, and disorders of clinical ecology and environmental illness.

Schizophrenia

Schizophrenia continues to be the subject of heated debate among psychiatric professionals. Some maintain that schizophrenia is a single disorder, but others argue that the condition is a complex of disorders that produce symptoms labeled as schizophrenia. Some scientists believe that *if* schizophrenia is a single entity, then a single cause for the condition will be found. As of this writing, no cause is known for schizophrenia, but several psychobiologic hypotheses exist.

The *dopamine hypothesis* is the most probable explanation of schizophrenia to date. This hypothesis is that the amount of dopamine available at certain synapses is significantly altered in persons demonstrating schizophrenic symptoms. A clinical observation that contributed information to the development of this hypothesis was that antipsychotic drugs decrease dopamine at the synapse and lessen schizophrenic symptoms. When *neuroleptics* (substances that act on the autonomic nervous system) are given to clients with Parkinson's disease, a condition of dopamine deficiency, their symptoms become markedly worse. The correlation between dopamine, antipsychotic drugs, and schizophrenic symptoms does not establish a causal relationship. Some psychobiologists suggest that the reason schizophrenic symptoms improve with dopamine blocking agents is that the synaptic biochemistry of schizophrenics is dysfunctional.

The *monoamine oxidase* (MAO) hypothesis of schizophrenia is that a certain type of MAO is lower in chronic schizophrenic clients than in the normal population (Schwartz and Africa 1984). This MAO abnormality may be indicative of an abnormality of neurotransmitter metabolism, especially that of dopamine. As with the dopamine hypothesis, there is no way of knowing the significance of this finding on the source or clinical course of schizophrenia.

The *transmethylation hypothesis* of schizophrenia is interesting but of uncertain clinical significance. The hypothesis is that certain catecholamines (specific neurotransmitters) undergo an abnormal chemical transformation process known as o-methylation. The end result of this chemical transformation is a substance that is very close in chemical structure to mescaline. This substance produces illusions, hallucinations, and other symptoms common to the experience of psychosis. Discussion continues regarding whether the transmethylation process is the result of an endogenous substance or something externally induced, perhaps by diet.

In recent years there has been significant discussion about whether the "human-made" morphines—the enkephalins and endorphins—play a part in the emergence of schizophrenic symptoms. To date, however, there is no empiric basis for such a claim. Several researchers have tagged certain proteins (e.g., immunoglobulins) or electrolytes (e.g., calcium) in an effort to find the cause of schizophrenic symptoms; none of these attempts have met with success. As more psychobiologic research is done to examine the causes of schizophrenia, answers may be found. The findings to date suggest that either the condition has multiple causes or one complex and multifaceted cause.

Mood Disorders

The term *mood disorders* covers a lot of psychiatric turf. Much research is being conducted on mood disorders, and there are several schools of thought about the cause of mood disorders. Some psychobiologists believe that most psychiatric conditions, including anorexia nervosa and bulimia, are simply variants of affectively disordered states, while others maintain more traditional psychiatric nomenclature and classification.

The last several years have seen a great rise in the amount of research conducted on mood disorders. Recent technologic advances allowing more precise assessment of such disorders and shifts in the overall understanding of the psychobiologic foundations of mood have changed clinicians' view of mood disorders substantially. Since Egeland (1988) and her colleagues discovered a genetic mode of transmission of major mood disorders several years ago, our understanding of the biologic components of such conditions has increased greatly.

For instance, recent scientific advances have given us a greater understanding of depression and its biologic mechanisms. A variety of biologic changes

RESEARCH NOTE

Citation
Nasrallah AH, Coryell WH: Dexamethasone nonsuppression predicts the antidepressant effects of sleep deprivation. Psychiatry Res 1982; 6:61–64.

Study Problem/Purpose
Dexamethasone nonsuppression has been linked to disrupted circadian rhythms in depressed persons. Sleep deprivation allegedly exerts a transient antidepressant effect. This study aims to examine dexamethasone nonsuppression as a predictor of antidepressant response to sleep deprivation with clients who are diagnosed as having major depression.

Methods
Twenty-two depressed (by DSM-III-R diagnostic criteria) adults received the dexamethasone suppression test (DST) upon admission to the hospital. Two to three days after the DST, the participating clients were deprived of sleep for 36 hours. Baseline depression severity was rated by a psychiatrist (blind to the DST results) on a valid/reliable scale (Hamilton Depression Scale). Clients also rated their own depression using a visual analog scale. At 8:00 A.M. on the day following sleep deprivation, a psychiatrist and nurse rated the clients' global improvement, and the clients simultaneously rated their own improvement. Improvement was defined as receiving a higher rating from at least one staff member in addition to a higher self-rating by the client or "improved" ratings from both staff members without improved self-rating.

Findings
Four of the dexamethasone nonsuppressors and one suppressor improved with sleep deprivation. Three dexamethasone nonsuppressors and fourteen suppressors remained unimproved after sleep deprivation. The difference between the suppressor/nonsuppressor improvement is significant ($p = 0.02$, Fisher Exact Text).

Implications
This study documents a psychobiologic index of circadian rhythmicity in conjunction with sleep/wake cycles of depressed clients. The authors of the study point out that the antidepressant effects of sleep deprivation are possibly related to a correction of an abnormal diurnal biorhythm in depression. Although few nurses have studied circadian rhythmicity in depressed clients, the opportunity exists for an explanation of such rhythms through a nursing perspective. Such knowledge might allow for the evaluation of specific nursing assessment measures to examine circadian rhythms and to prescribe nursing interventions aimed specifically at correcting imbalance in biorhythm.

seems to underlie each mood disorder. See the accompanying Psychobiology box. The following mood disorders are potentially implicated in depression: bipolar mood disorder, major depression, dysthymia, seasonal mood disorders, and adjustment disorder with depressed mood. Because the biologic mechanisms underlying these depressive disorders probably vary considerably, this discussion can give only a brief overview of some potential mechanisms.

According to Gold and colleagues (1988), much of the research on depression has focused on the role of neurotransmitters. Early research suggested that a defect in the action of one particular neurotransmitter probably accounted for the emergence of symptoms, but this view is now thought simplistic. We still believe that depression is likely the result of neurotransmitter system dysfunction, but we now think that this dysfunction results from a complex interplay

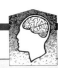

PSYCHOBIOLOGY: THE MIND/BODY CONNECTION

That Mood Indigo: It's Not All in Your Head

Almost everyone has an occasional bout with "the blues," and most people can describe its associated feelings. For some people, however, depression is a disease state. People suffering from the disease of depression may exhibit a variety of symptoms in addition to the obvious feelings of sadness. For example, some people lose weight during a depressive episode, while others gain weight. Many people report feeling so tired that they could sleep all day, while others sleep for brief periods but never feel rested. As the disease progresses, emerging symptoms may include difficulty concentrating, slowed movements, and constipation.

From the psychobiologic perspective, depression is a complex phenomenon. The signs and symptoms may be clear to an objective observer, and even to the depressed person, but the stress on the body systems is not always obvious. For example, the stress that often underlies or precedes an episode of depression can be measured in alterations of the *endocrine system,* evidenced in shifts in cortisol. Such endocrinologic shifts often accompany severe depression.

Humans operate on a series of daily rhythms called **circadian rhythms.** These rhythms are usually about twenty-four hours in duration, and are the result of the environmental cycles of day and night. Some of the most common rhythms control sleep/wake, thermoregulation, and reproductive cycles; however, almost every human function is subject to a rhythm. Depressed people experience disturbed circadian rhythms, as evidenced in disturbed sleep, shifts in appetite, and activity intolerance.

On the microscopic level, depression may be traced to the functioning of neurons in the brain. Neurons contain small gaps called synapses. Synapses have membranes that contain sophisticated mechanisms for creating chemical bridges between the neurons. These bridges are critical to the normal process of neurotransmission. In depression, the mechanism for normal functioning of the chemical bridges goes awry; some theories speculate that depression represents an overall deficit of certain neurochemicals involved in the formation of emotional response. Antidepressant drugs correct this deficit state.

The incorporation of this sophisticated, technical information into nursing practice is a challenge. However, recent work, especially in the area of sleep manipulation, holds great promise for new directions in nursing assessment and intervention. For example, the connection between mood and sleep is becoming more apparent. Nurses have long known about the disabling sleep disturbances that accompany a depressed state. Recent evidence raises the possibility of using a period of sleep deprivation to reduce the painful symptoms of depression (Raymond, 1988). Keeping depressed persons awake for specified periods of time may improve the depressive symptoms. This approach is still in the experimental stage, but it highlights the strong connection between daily rhythms and their impact on mood.

The above example illustrates one of the exciting innovations on the horizon. The collaboration of various new fields of knowledge with that of nursing science will enrich the practice of psychiatric nursing and facilitate its growth into the twenty-first century.

— *Geoffry McEnany*

between neurochemicals, including norepinephrine, dopamine, serotonin acetylcholine, and probably gamma-aminobutyric acid (GABA).

In the past, the catecholamine hypothesis was the most widely accepted explanation of mood disorders. According to this hypothesis, depression is characterized by a marked deficiency of a particular catecholamine neurotransmitter in certain parts of the brain, and mania is likely to be characterized by the opposite. We now realize we must investigate the role of other mechanisms in depression. For example, according to Russ and Ackerman (1989), depression is often associated with hypothyroidism. This finding suggests that neuroendocrine mechanisms may play a role in depression. In addition, there is evidence that other endocrine mechanisms may play a similar role. Examples include cortisol, growth hormone, and luteinizing hormone regulation. For instance, there is a clear relationship between faulty cortisol regulation and exposure to stress. Changes in cortisol regulation yield the **vegetative signs of depression** and include symptoms such as psychomotor retardation, anorexia, constipation, lethargy, diminished libido, poor concentration, and insomnia. The issue of postpartum depression also raises a variety of questions about the role of such hormones as prolactin in the emergence of depression. To understand the complex biochemical foundations of the depressed person's experience, we need further research.

Such information has significant implications for nurses working with psychiatric patients. Nurses cannot assess client behavior fully without an understanding of the underlying psychobiologic dysfunction. This knowledge will have a significant impact on the course of routine nursing practice in psychiatry.

Anxiety Disorders

The clinical arena of anxiety disorders is bustling with activity, especially since 1977 when an actual mammalian neuron cell surface was found to have specific receptors for benzodiazepine drugs (e.g., diazepam). The clinical significance of that finding is that neurotransmitters are involved in the mediation of anxiety, making anxiety a psychobiologic condition with identifiable biologic markers. Braestrup (1982, p 1030) states: "All we can now say is that anxiety occurs when, in the brain, there is a certain activity pattern in certain neurons that are firing in a certain spatial and temporal pattern, and that this structurally complex activity is anxiety." Braestrup believes that anxiety probably involves neurotransmitters from the brain such as GABA, serotonin, norepinephrine, and dopamine. Psychobiologists believe that at least serotonin and norepinephrine are implicated in depression. How then, can one determine with any certainty that anxiety disorders that can be mediated by serotonin

and norepinephrine are not simply variants of depression? At this time, it is impossible to make such a distinction in a reasonable fashion. But the question opens the door to an ongoing discussion among psychobiologists: Since some anxiety disorders respond to antidepressant medications, are they not, in fact, depressions? Relationships exist among panic disorder, generalized anxiety disorder, and major depressive disorder; these relationships need further exploration if we are to discover more specific and effective interventions.

Nurses, especially those working with psychiatric clients, constantly deal with anxious clients. How do nurses differ in their approaches to mildly anxious clients versus clients with moderate, high, or crisis levels of anxiety? Providing that nurses assess the client's anxiety accurately, how *prescriptive* are the interventions, and what *objective* evaluative measures of anxiety control do nurses use? Anxiety is a psychobiologic condition that responds to both behavioral and pharmacologic interventions; it is recognized as amenable to nursing care. Although many nurses have written about or researched anxiety and its related behaviors in clients, we need to use this knowledge in the clinical arena more fully, allowing for more consistent assessment and more prescriptive interventions for anxiety.

Dementia

There are many causes of dementia. The most common is Alzheimer's disease, a psychobiologic process of slow onset and uneven progression leading to death. What happens to the brain of someone with Alzheimer's disease? The destruction of neurons begins in the memory centers in the brain. The destroyed nerves are replaced with nonfunctional fibers, preventing smooth transmission of impulses from neuron to neuron. As memory deteriorates, so does overall brain functioning. The resulting behaviors include disorientation, rambling speech, unstable emotions, and a poor understanding of the environment. Eventually, the affected individual seems to lose personality features and over time seems to become a totally different person. Unfortunately, no cure for Alzheimer's disease exists at this time.

The AIDS epidemic has brought a new perspective to clinicians assessing dementia. According to Hall, Koehler, and Lewis (1989), the most common neurologic disorder in persons with AIDS is the **AIDS dementia complex (ADC)**. Symptoms of ADC range from mild memory loss to severe global confusion, loss of motor skills, depression, mood swings, psychotic symptoms, and hysteric reactions. ADC is believed to be the direct result of invasion of the central nervous system by the AIDS virus. Nurses need to be aware of the subtle cues of early ADC—forgetfulness, changes in routine or affect and changes in personal appearance. By becoming aware of the early indications of ADC, nurses can facilitate early detection and treatment.

Seizure Disorders

Recent advances in neurophysiology and psychoneurobiology have greatly contributed to the understanding of seizures from a cellular perspective. For example, carbamazepine (Tegretol) has become a popular treatment for mood disorders. This shift in practice is due, in part, to an improved understanding of temporal lobe epilepsy via refinements in electroencephalography (EEG) technology. In other words, many of the behaviors that were considered routine manifestations of mood disorder may indeed be symptoms of an underlying seizure disorder in the temporal lobes. As Kessler, Barklage, and Jefferson (1989) point out, temporal lobe epileptic symptomatology may manifest as lability of mood with alternating episodes of anger, dysphoria, anxiety, and changes in thought process patterns.

Of the many types of seizures, the ones of greatest interest to people working in psychiatry are probably those involving the temporal lobe. Psychomotor or complex partial seizures fit into the category of temporal lobe seizures. They involve limbic structures, particularly the amygdala. This type of seizure activity is characterized by movements such as chewing, swallowing, and lip smacking. Such seizure-related behaviors can be easily overlooked because they occur normally. However, close assessment allows nurses to delineate seizure-related behaviors from normal behaviors.

Clinical Ecology and Environmental Illness

Iris Bell (1982), an expert in the field of clinical ecology (CE) describes CE as an interdisciplinary subgroup of environmental medicine. The CE group proposes that chronic exposure to chemicals and inhalants in the environment and in ordinary foods may lead to psychobiologic disorders in people who are susceptible to this form of illness (see the accompanying box). Clinical ecologists emphasize that to understand environmental illness, one must consider the total load of low-dose environmental stressors a person encounters and the frequency of, as well as time between, exposures to substances.

Clinical ecologists observe for reactions in the behavior of the environmentally ill person. Common reactions include psychiatric, central nervous system, and psychophysiologic symptoms. Bell points out that the mechanisms involved in environmental illness are likely to be both immune and nonimmune. No

---

Potential Mechanisms in Environmental Illness

Hypotheses Derived from Clinical Observations

- Specific foods in a susceptible individual can cause multisystem symptoms.
- Symptoms can include emotional, cognitive, behavioral, somatic features—e.g., anxiety, irritability, depression, fatigue, impaired memory, difficulty concentrating, poor coordination, hyperactivity, sleepiness, grand mal seizures—in individual patterns in a given person.
- Different foods can cause the same symptoms in different individuals, i.e., no single food triggers a particular disorder in all individuals with that disorder.
- Multiple foods can provide the same symptoms in a given individual.
- Increased frequency of ingestion leads to increased sensitivity.
- Frequent ingestion can mask the presence of sensitivity; therefore, diagnosis depends on unmasking (avoiding the food) for four or more days before challenging with the food.
- Adverse food reactions often have delayed onset from 1 to 24 hours after the meal and can last up to three to four days.
- Mechanisms for such reactions are unknown, but classical IgE-mediated allergy is unlikely. Postulated mechanisms include IgG, immune complexes, complement, mediators such as neuro/gut peptides, prostaglandins, kinins.
- Behavioral reactions can be biphasic in course, with stimulatory and depressed phases.

SOURCE: *Iris R. Bell, MD PhD: Personal communication, 25 March 1986.*

---

particular abnormality is consistently noted among environmentally ill persons, but trends among this population point to a variety of immune and central nervous system changes.

There are three approaches to the treatment of environmentally ill clients (Bell 1982, p 47):

- Avoidance of offending substances

- Rotation diet of tolerated foods

- Neutralization or prevention of adverse reactions by subcutaneous injections or sublingual drops

Clinical ecology is in its early stages of development. Although many of the assumptions that underlie this science are not yet tested, clinical ecology does illuminate issues that need attention in the arena of psychoneuroimmunology and its related fields.

Psychobiology and Nursing

The idea of applying psychobiologic principles to psychiatric nursing practice seems reasonable, even though they are not commonly applied today. The advances in the understanding of the brain and its functions gives nurses an opportunity for advancements in the areas of nursing assessment, planning, implementation, and evaluation.

There are many unanswered questions about the connections between the brain and behavior. For example, nurses may be able to do psychobiologic assessments of diet, sleep, anxiety, and their effects on other behaviors but may not yet have any interventions *specific to nursing* that address such behaviors.

Nursing science is at a stage that invites exploration of nursing approaches, models, and theories to help nurses function more from a theoretic/empirical base than from intuition. In medical-surgical nursing, many interventions have been researched, refined, and used in practice with empiric backing. For example, a nurse who works in a cardiac intensive care unit has knowledge relevant to cardiac symptomatology and bases nursing intervention on that knowledge. At present, psychiatric nurses have the opportunity to help eliminate a dualistic approach to their work by incorporating psychobiologic principles into their care of clients, thus truly making psychiatric nursing practice a holistic science and art that is theoretically based.

CHAPTER HIGHLIGHTS

• Psychobiology is not a new concept, but we are gaining knowledge about the underlying biologic bases of human behavior.

• From a psychobiologic perspective, the human brain is the source of creativity, logic, thought, and emotion.

• Ancient Greeks who influenced early psychobiologic thought included Hippocrates, Plato, and Aristotle.

• Behavior is the result of a complex interplay of chemical and electric processes within the brain; intercommunication among the various parts of the brain produce behavior.

• The limbic system is commonly referred to as "the emotional brain" and consists of structures from the cerebral hemispheres, the diencephalon, and the midbrain.

• The reticular activating system is a complex of neurons that modulates states of consciousness and awareness.

• The extrapyramidal system consists of tracts of motor neurons from the brain to parts of the spinal cord; this system coordinates coarse automatic movements.

• Psychoendocrinology and psychoimmunology are two subspecialties that explore the relationships between behavior, biology, and endocrine/immunologic functions.

• Thyroid dysfunction is often masked as depression and when due to autoimmune thyroid processes is difficult to assess.

• Human functions demonstrate a 24-hour cycle; these cycles are commonly referred to as circadian rhythms.

• Several biologic explanations of schizophrenia exist, but the most probable is the dopamine hypothesis.

• Several hypotheses attribute a psychobiologic basis to mood disorders, anxiety disorders, and dementia.

• Clinical ecology is a subgroup of environmental medicine that proposes that chronic exposure to chemicals, inhalants, and foods may cause psychobiologic disorders in susceptible individuals.

REFERENCES

Andreasen NC: *The Broken Brain*. Harper & Row, 1984.

Bell IR: *Clinical Ecology*. Common Knowledge Press, 1982.

Binder RL: Organic mental disorders, in Goldman HH (ed): *Review of General Psychiatry*. Lange Medical Publications, 1984.

Braestrup C: Anxiety. *Lancet* 1982;2(Nov 6):1030–1034.

Brown RP, Mann JJ: A clinical perspective on the role of neurotransmitters in mental disorders. *Hosp Community Psychiatry* 1985;36(2):141–150.

Egeland JA: A genetic study of manic-depressive disorder among the old order Amish of Pennsylvania. *Pharmacopsychiatry* 1988;21:74–75.

Fawcett JC: Valproate use in acute mania and bipolar disorder: An international perspective. *J Clin Psychiatry* 1988;50(3):10–12.

Gold PW, Goodwin FK, Chrousos GP: Clinical and biochemical manifestations of depression. *New Engl J Med* 1988;319(6):348–420.

Grebb JA, Reus VI: Neurobehavioral chemistry and physiology, in Goldman HH (ed): *Review of General Psychiatry*. Lange Medical Publications, 1984.

Hall JM, Koehler SL, Lewis A: HIV-related mental health nursing issues. *Semin Oncol Nurs* 1989;5(4):276–283.

Harris E: The dexamethasone suppression test. *Am J Nurs* 1982;82(5):784–785.

Illich I: *Medical Nemesis.* Random House, 1976.

Kaplan HI, Saddock BJ: *Modern Synopsis of Comprehensive Textbooks of Psychiatry,* ed 4. Williams & Wilkins, 1985.

Kessler AJ, Barklage NE, Jefferson JW: Mood disorders in the psychoneurologic borderland: Three cases of responsiveness to carbemazepine. *Am J Psychiatry* 1989;146(1):81–83.

Lickey ME, Gordon B: *Drugs for Mental Illness—A Revolution in Psychiatry.* Freeman, 1983.

McEnany GW: Psychobiological indices of bipolar mood disorder: Future trends in nursing care. *Arch Psychiatr Nurs* 1990;4(1):29–38.

Moore-Ede MC, Czeisler CA, Richardson GS: Circadian timekeeping in health and disease. *N Engl J Med* 1983;309(8):469–476.

Nasrallah HA, Coryell WH: Dexamethasone nonsuppression predicts the antidepressant effects of sleep deprivation. *Psychiatr Res* 1982;6:61–64.

Pincus JH, Tucker GJ: *Behavioral Neurology,* ed 2. Oxford University Press, 1978.

Plumlee AA: Biological rhythms and affective illness. *J Psychosoc Nurs Mental Health Serv* 1986;24(3):12–17.

Russ MJ, Ackerman SH: Antidepressant treatment response in depressed hypothyroid patients. *Hosp Community Psychiatry* 1989;40(9):954–956.

Schwartz SR, Africa B: Schizophrenic disorders, in Goldman HH (ed): *Review of General Psychiatry.* Lange Medical Publications, 1984.

Stein MB, Uhde TW: Thyroid indices in panic disorder. *Am J Psychiatry* 1988;145(6):745–47.

Stein MB, Uhde TW: Lack of efficacy of carbamazepine in the treatment of panic disorder. *Am J Psychiatry* 1988; 145(9):1104–09.

Stein MB, Uhde TW: Autoimmune thyroiditis and panic disorder. *Am J Psychiatry* 1989;146(2):259–260.

Vogel P: Lithium and the thyroid. *J Psychosoc Nurs Mental Health Serv* 1986;24(3):9–14.

Psychobiology Box References

McEnany GW: Psychobiological indices of bipolar disorder: Future trends in nursing care. *Arch Psychiatr Nurs* 1990;4(1):29–38.

Raymond CA: Sleep patterns scrutinized as depression therapy. *JAMA* 1988; February 19.

PART TWO

Processes for Clinical Practice in Psychiatric Nursing

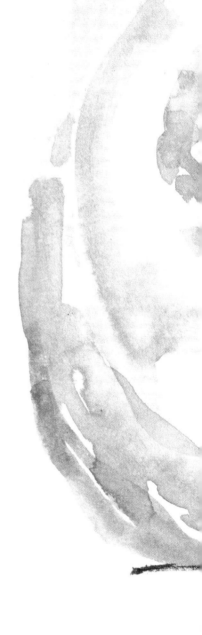

CONTENTS

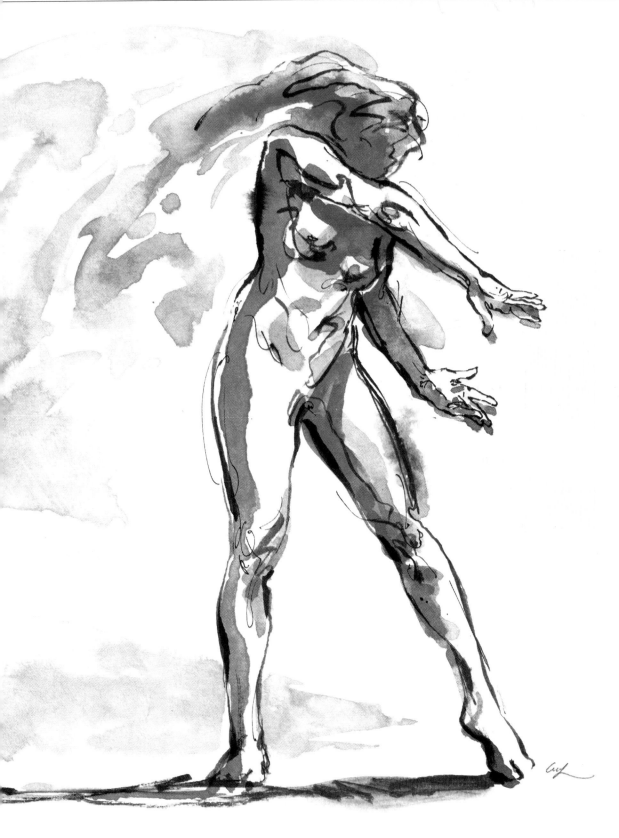

Movement represents the exterior world of structure and the
interior world of feelings, the grace of human experience.

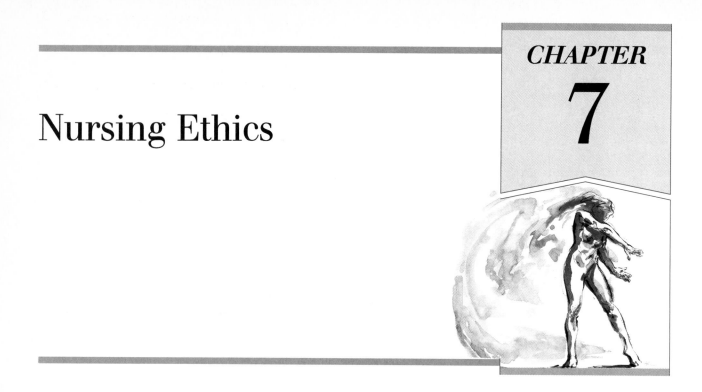

CHAPTER

7

Nursing Ethics

LEARNING OBJECTIVES

- Discuss the process of analyzing an ethical issue
- Compare and contrast dominant ethical perspectives
- Define the six major principles of bioethics
- Identify and discuss ethical dilemmas in psychiatric nursing
- Formulate a personal stand on the ethics and politics of psychiatric nursing practice

Holly Skodol Wilson

CROSS REFERENCES

Other topics relevant to this content are: Cultural considerations, Chapter 36; Elder abuse, Chapter 35; Ethics in milieu therapy, Chapter 31; Legal issues, Chapter 37.

A YOUNG TEACHER OF NURSING ethics and philosophy once said, "Reasoning in ethics means bringing all one's faculties in a balanced way to bear on the sincere concern for human well-being in general and the meaning of human experience. Being reasonable in ethics is more like having integrity than like being smart." This chapter describes a framework for analyzing ethical issues and resolving ethical dilemmas in psychiatric nursing. Reason and reflection have always held an important place in the study of ethics, for ethics is more than a personal or inspirational enterprise used to answer moral questions. Moral judgments are most highly developed when the *process of arriving at them* and the *reasons for believing in them* are clear and convincing. At the heart of ethical judgments are the reasons for them.

Throughout the history of nursing education, teachers and students alike have been concerned with ethical matters. A closer look, however, reveals that the concern has been less with moral principles and ethical dilemmas and more with legal aspects of practice and what psychiatric nurse–bioethicist Anne Davis refers to as "the etiquette of the profession" (Davis and Aroskar 1978). Nursing has made notable advances toward professional autonomy in recent years. Greater autonomy, however, has created a greater need and responsibility to account for and accept the consequences of professional decisions and actions. Autonomy, according to Aroskar (1980) has to do with the right of self-determination, governance without outside control, and the capability to exist independently. Professionals do this by:

• Developing codes of ethics, which provide guidelines for defining professional responsibility

• Setting rigorous qualifications for entry into the profession

• Establishing peer review procedures

• Setting standards for practice, such as the *ANA Standards of Psychiatric and Mental Health Nursing Practice*

Professionals need to balance the goal of more autonomy in nursing with efforts to achieve what providers and consumers determine is the common and the individual "good" in health care. The goal of this chapter is not to preach right and wrong but to help students develop a way of thinking about complex ethical issues and dilemmas in psychiatric nursing.

Analyzing Ethical Issues

One of the major difficulties in ethical analysis is that there are no definite, clear-cut solutions to ethical

---

Framework of Questions for Analyzing an Ethical Issue

• Who are the relevant actors in the situation?

• What is the required action?

• What are the probable and possible consequences of the action?

• What is the range of alternative actions or choices?

• What is the intent or purpose of the action?

• What is the context of the action?

---

dilemmas. For centuries moral philosophers—beginning with Socrates, Plato, and Aristotle—have struggled with two main ethical questions: (a) What is the meaning of right or good? and (b) What should I do? To identify, clarify, define, and defend a stand on an ethical issue, we must engage in a process of reflective thinking about data that can be gathered by using the framework of six critical questions set out in the accompanying box.

Psychiatric nurses must often identify alternative courses of action and decide what to do when there is a conflict of rights and obligations between clients and families, between themselves and other mental health workers, or between the clients' good and the community or social good. For example, if a woman's disturbed functioning or distress is in part a reaction to aspects of her social context, a therapist can alleviate the disturbance either by helping the woman adjust to her situation as it is or by helping her to change her situation. In a sense a psychiatric nurse becomes both an ethicist and a political agent in resolving this choice.

Dominant Ethical Perspectives

Various ethical perspectives provide different ways of structuring the answers to the questions in the accompanying box, thus leading to different decisions about what is the right action. The dominant ethical perspectives include the following traditions:*

• **Egoism.** The egoist answers questions about the morally right thing to do by saying that something is good because "I desire it." The right act, then, is the one that maximizes the pleasure of the person asking the question.

• **Deontology.** The deontologic or formalist approach suggests that rightness or wrongness depends

*Adapted from Davis AJ, Aroskar MA: *Ethical Dilemmas and Nursing Practice*. Appleton-Century-Crofts, 1978.

Principles of Bioethics

- Autonomy—the right to make one's own decisions
- Nonmaleficence—the intention to do no wrong
- Beneficence—the principle of attempting to do things that benefit others
- Justice—the distribution, as fairly as possible, of benefits and burdens
- Veracity—the intention to tell the truth
- Confidentiality—the social contact guaranteeing another's privacy

SOURCE: *Davis AJ: Ethical dilemmas in nursing. Recorded at JONA and Nurse Educator's 1981 Joint Leadership Conference. Available from Teach'em Inc., 160 East Illinois St., Chicago, Ill. 60611.*

---

on the nature or form of the action for moral significance. In this tradition there are both *act deontologists* and *rule deontologists*—i.e., rightness may be based on performing certain morally significant acts properly or adhering to certain preestablished rules or principles. This position requires a commitment to the principle of **universality**—i.e., one will make the same moral judgment in any similar situation regardless of time, place, or persons involved. Many rule deontologists believe in the divine command theory—an act is wrong because it is forbidden by God. The difficulty for both believers and nonbelievers in this theory is that sometimes the rules conflict. In an attempt to get out of the problem of conflicting rules, Immanuel Kant, writing in the late eighteenth century, stated that you should act only on a maxim that you can simultaneously will to be a universal law. Unfortunately, Kant's position doesn't help with moral *conflict.* For example, if returning the institutionalized mentally disturbed to the community was identified as a morally good action, Kant would have us ignore any specifics of a particular situation, even though an individual might end up living in a dingy stairwell and stealing food.

- **Utilitarianism.** In the theory of utility, good is "happiness or pleasure," and right is "the greatest good for the greatest number of people." Implicit in this position is the assumption that one can weigh and measure harm and benefit and come out with the best possible balance of good over evil. Among the questions raised by this position is what happens to

individual justice when the general welfare is emphasized.

- **Theory of obligation.** The basic principles of the theory of obligation are: (a) the principle of beneficence, which requires that we not just *want* good but *do* good rather than evil, and (b) the principle of justice, which requires that we distribute benefits and burdens equally through society. A problem with this position is what to do when the two principles conflict at the public and individual levels.

- **Ideal observer theory.** This perspective outlines the characteristics of ethical reason as consistency, disinterest, dispassion, omnipresence, and omniscience. These are the qualities of an *ideal observer* or *moral judge.* The ideal observer has only general interests, such as the welfare of all, and does not make decisions on practical or emotional grounds. The questions of who should be the moral judge and where the development of this moral consciousness will occur are left unanswered.

- **Justice as fairness.** The principles of justice as fairness are: (a) each person is to have an equal right to the most extensive liberty for all, and (b) social and economic injustices are to be addressed so that the least advantaged receive the greatest benefit. In this system, the first principle of maximizing liberty for all has absolute priority. Five criteria emerge from this tradition for judging the rightness of any ethical principles:

1. Universality. The same principles hold for everyone.

2. Generality. They must not be geared to specific people or situations.

3. Publicity. They must be known and recognized by all.

4. Ordering. They must order conflicting claims.

5. Finality. They may override the demands of law or custom.

Principles of Bioethics

The preceding ethical traditions or a combination of them operate when nurses reflect on ethical dilemmas. Bioethics is a field that applies ethical reasoning to issues and dilemmas in the area of health care.

Taking a stand on an ethical issue involves much more than merely accepting the moral position or personal values of another. Bioethicists (Davis 1981) offer the six principles (see the box above) as important guidelines.

Ethical Dilemmas in Psychiatric Nursing

The nurse must protect the rights of the individual client yet mediate between these rights and the interests of the social group. Sometimes the two are in conflict. To complicate the situation, Kai Erikson (1962) and Thomas Szasz (1974) argue that deviance can sometimes help stabilize society and therefore actually makes a valuable contribution to social life. According to these authors, only by public displays of rule-breaking behavior can the group learn its tolerance ranges for acceptable behavior. This position is a far cry from a view of the psychiatric client as a dangerous enemy of society—an actual or potential aggressor to be controlled by society's designated keepers. Ultimately nurses must reconcile a number of crucial ethical dilemmas with their personal and professional values. Among these issues are:

• The potential stigma of psychiatric diagnostic labels

• Psychiatry's right to control individual freedom

• The justification for involuntary treatment

• The use of restrictive treatment interventions

• The client's right to suicide

• The client's right to privacy

• The politics and ethics of women's mental health

• Psychiatry's responsibility in defending society's dominant life-style

• The psychiatric professional's role in social and political reform

To practice psychiatric nursing requires ethical responsibility. The quality of a nurse's moral commitment is a measure of professional excellence. However, problems arise when there is conflict about the ground rules for behavior, whether the conflict is between client and social group, nurse and profession, or nurse and agency. These problems are phrased in the ethical language of right and wrong. Circumstances likely to give rise to such problems include the following:

• The professional and the client are from different social classes and have different statuses or cultural values.

• The voluntary nature of the client's participation is compromised.

• The client's competence to enter into an agreement about intervention is questionable, or the client does not realize that certain interventions are being implemented.

Every nursing relationship begins with an unusual burden of ethical responsibility. The following pages explore some of these moral issues.

The Stigma of Psychiatric Diagnoses

The list of stereotypes associated with diagnostic categories is well known to most nurses. Equally familiar are the consequences to people with these diagnoses. People labeled as drug addicts, alcoholics, homosexuals, convicts, paranoids, etc. acquire a discredited social identity because of the character flaws often associated with these categories. To much of society, the labels used in psychiatry suggest decadence, immorality, and wanton disregard for society's values. Sociologist Erving Goffman subtitles his monograph on stigma *Notes on the Management of Spoiled Identity* (1963). It is important to consider how and when psychiatric nurses, while advocating humane treatment for clients, indirectly contribute to their spoiled identities by participating in the arbitrary use of oppressive labels.

The Need for Diagnostic Labels Diagnosis has considerable value in psychiatric practice. Putting clients into diagnostic categories makes it easy for health professionals to communicate with each other about the client. The diagnosis often dictates a particular course of treatment and enables the health team to prognosticate about a client's recovery. Diagnostic categories enable nurses to plan comprehensively for client care and to conduct research.

Before the publication of the third edition of American Psychiatric Association's *Diagnostic and Statistical Manual of Mental Disorders* (DSM-III) and its revised edition, diagnostic categories such as schizophrenia, paranoia, or sociopathy were not sufficiently precise to give a clear idea of desirable treatment. A person labeled schizophrenic can be treated with phenothiazines, milieu therapy, or behavior modification techniques. All of these could be justified by one theoretic orientation or another. Nonetheless, the diagnostic label was felt to be the key to subsequent decisions about a client, especially the choice of medication. In some cases when clients failed to respond favorably to the medication indicated by their diagnosis, the diagnosis was changed. Advocates for the criteria-based DSMs believe that their use will greatly improve diagnostic practices.

Drawbacks of the Labeling Process A substantial proportion of "treatment time" in any modern in-patient setting is devoted to piecing together stories about the clients in order to assign diagnostic or legal labels. Staff members trying to uncover information about a client interact with clients trying to hide what they believe are damaging data about themselves. One staff member comments to another, "Have you picked up a little paranoia in David or is it only guardedness?" Clients often sense that they are being evaluated for fateful decisions. They try to learn the scripts that will produce the most positive fates for them. One client asked the nurse, "Does it go against you to be lying down two hours in a row?"

A highly ritualized example of the process of piecing together a story occurs in group intake interviews in most in-patient settings.

Bianca, a newly admitted client, is confronted by a group of eight staff members in an interview room and questioned in a mildly interrogative style. Because of the need to "get to know the client as quickly as possible," her story does not just unfold. Instead she is frequently faced with a barrage of questions. She is standing, barefoot, in a robe, in front of eight strangers. At one point, she pleads: "I just want to go home. I feel like I'm going to be put away for the rest of my life. I don't like it here. I'm sorry, I'm trying to cooperate. I just don't feel I can be close to any of you." She starts to cry. "I'm confused because you ask so many questions. I just don't trust a group of strangers. I'm sorry, but I just need time to think."

Based on this interview and data in the client's chart, the staff pieces together her "story." One staff member summarizes: "I think we've observed a depressed gal with a history of inadequacy and dependency. The pathology is first and foremost depression with her hysterical personality disorder coming out to cover up."

The Self-Fulfilling Label   One of the most common characteristics of psychiatric labeling might be called a *correctness assumption*. Frequently, staff members have already decided that a client will be given medication, even though the client has refused it. Before the start of the precertification observation period, staff members may have decided that the client will be certified for fourteen days. Contacts with the client are then used more to justify the decision than to make a decision in the first place.

Another major characteristic of psychiatric diagnosis is the *invalidation of the client's point of view*. A client's statement that he or she does not want psychiatric help is used as evidence that the person needs it. A client's tears in an interview are viewed as a psychiatric symptom rather than a result of the immediate social context of interrogation, locked ward, involuntary confinement, fatigue, or other stressful circumstances.

Setups—contrived situations—often characterize the information-gathering operations prerequisite to diagnosis. Because diagnostic decisions usually must be made on the basis of limited contacts with clients, setting a situation up to "see how the client reacts" is sometimes used to help establish one diagnosis over

another. The client's response to the setup is considered evidence of illness.

A client's diary had been brought to the hospital by a friend. Some discussion ensued among the psychiatric team members about whether "she knows we have this." The staff members decided to leave the diary on the desk in front of the interviewee to "see how she reacts." Any sign of outrage and anger would be viewed as an indicator of her emotional disorder rather than as a justified response to the circumstances.

Sociocultural Influences on Diagnosis   The diagnostic labels used in Western psychiatry have been of limited value in cross-cultural comparisons. Observations indicate that the behavior called *schizophrenia* differs from one culture to another. Even in Western society, the diagnostic label given to a particular behavior under DSM-III's predecessors was related to the client's position in the class structure. "Neurotic" disorders predominated among the upper classes, and psychoses characterized the lower classes. Repressive attitudes toward women, blacks, and homosexuals influenced diagnoses. In sum, more often than we would like, conventional psychiatric diagnoses may be affected by characteristics of the social situation in which the deviant and the labelers interact. Factors that influence the outcome of deviant acts include (a) whether the act is labeled as symptomatic by a professional outsider, (b) how serious the act itself is, (c) how frequently the act has occurred, and (d) what the social context is. Most of the time families develop elaborate accommodation mechanisms to keep a deviant member within the home setting. These accommodation patterns are disrupted only when the public visibility of deviant behavior is highlighted by a diagnosis. The "V-codes" of DSM-III-R are intended to improve this situation. The V-codes refer to problems in living that are a focus of attention but *do not reflect a mental disorder.*

Diagnostic Stereotypes

The Homosexual   Acts of physical love with a member of the same sex often provoke harsh responses and attitudes in the United States. Society's aversion to homosexuality is demonstrated by the fact that it has been considered both a crime and a disease. Oppression of the homosexual today is maintained primarily by the fear that homosexuality threatens the stability of the society, by the irrational belief that homosexuality implies weakness, and by widespread concern about catching AIDS from homosexuals. Even though the label of homosexuality has been replaced in the psychiatric nomenclature by the more limited **ego-dystonic homosexuality** (meaning that the pattern of homosexual arousal causes distress to the client and is unwanted), some psychiatric professionals continue to view this particular life-style as reflecting immaturity, deep-seated psychologic problems, emotional disturbances, and severe conflicts. This obsolete attitude is being changed in the 1990s.

The Schizophrenic   On the basis of a rather vague concept, thousands of Americans have been labeled and hospitalized as schizophrenics. An individual designated schizophrenic becomes an outcast who is approached with a mixture of distrust and fear. The labeled schizophrenic may be denied employment, particularly in sensitive or important jobs. The pride and self-confidence of diagnosed schizophrenics are often shattered, and they may come to view themselves as incapable of controlling their impulses. Some clients living in agony find reassurance in being told that at least they are not schizophrenic. This diagnosis has become psychiatry's equivalent of cancer in its connotation of hopelessness. Again, DSM-III-R considerably narrows the concept of schizophrenia, and new psychobiologic and psychoeducational approaches for families offer hope.

The Paranoid   The diagnostic term *paranoid* has taken on an almost totally negative meaning. The term is not restricted to those who behave strangely, are overtly suspicious, or tend to blame their failings on others. Professionals apply it to many who take deviant positions on social issues. To accuse an adversary of being paranoid has become a kind of trump card for discrediting any opponent's position.

The Addict   A person who uses alcohol or other drugs to excess may be overwhelmed with all sorts of personal and social difficulties and still maintain a respectable role in society. However, once labeled an alcoholic or addict, the person is often viewed as disgraced rather than as having a disease. Programs like Alcoholics Anonymous work to educate others about addictive disease and enhance the addict's self-esteem. Addicts elicit pity from some, scorn from others. Under some circumstances they can be imprisoned, even though the substances they use are harmful only to themselves. Mandatory drug screening is an emerging social trend.

The Nurse's Moral Stance on Diagnoses   Does labeling with psychiatric diagnoses merely provide psychiatric professionals with some additional sense of control in their dealings with clients? It is true that a diagnosis gives staff members an increased sense of being able to predict client behavior and a way of viewing calmly what might otherwise be upsetting behavior: "That's just her hysterical personality coming out," or "Those complaints are just paranoid delusions." The consequences of psychiatric labels for clients and their families, however, raise moral questions about the legitimacy of their arbitrary use.

Consider the following, adapted from a letter to a newspaper advice columnist.

I am a 12-year-old girl who is left out of all social activities because my father is an alcoholic. I try to be nice and friendly to everyone, but it's no use. The girls at school have told me that their mothers don't want them to associate with me because my father might be dangerous. Is there anything I can do? I am very lonesome because it's no fun to be alone all the time. My mother tries to take me places with her, but I want to be with people my own age. Please give me some advice.

Sincerely,
An Outcast

Nurses have a moral responsibility to question practices that exact a price from clients far in excess of the benefits. Only through involvement in such issues can nurses create a moral environment for health care in which practices truly respond to clients' needs. Every moment of moral injustice takes its toll on nurses as well as clients. Every moment of moral responsibility strengthens their sense of personal integrity.

Control of Individual Freedom

Psychiatric professionals limit and control the freedom of clients through the subtle process of assigning labels to their behavior. Professionals also control individual freedom in more straightforward ways. The most frequent examples of direct controlling interventions are involuntary hospitalization, and use of restrictive treatments, usually when a person is judged to constitute a danger to self or others.

Involuntary hospitalization and treatment of psychiatric clients are usually considered humanitarian efforts to help "the mentally ill." Yet any practice that directly and coercively deprives a person of freedom has political implications. In most states a client who is involuntarily committed to a mental hospital has few of the legal protections that even a criminal offender has. In addition, in some states clients have no guarantee that they will ever be released from this hospital unless they alter their behavior sufficiently to please their keepers. This ethical issue is further complicated by the fact that psychiatric professionals can no longer argue that involuntary hospitalization is necessary to restore mental health. Instead, the confinement must be justified as necessary to protect the client or others from harm.

Violence and Social Control

Violence against Others   Psychiatric nurses are faced with the dilemma of trying to be both healer-helpers and agents of social control. In dealing with violently destructive clients, and some others, the value of life is being balanced against the value of liberty. Thomas Szasz (1974) argues that there is never adequate justification for involuntary commitment under the guise of medical help. He believes that violence toward others is a crime and should be treated as such, not as a mental disease. Szasz argues that contemporary psychiatrists confuse deviance with disease and control with cure and make decisions and policies that constitute grave threats to personal freedom and dignity. Seymour Halleck (1971), another politically oriented psychiatrist-writer, suggests that society needs to make distinctions among the kinds of violence to decide which kinds might legitimately be controlled by civil procedures. His intent is to limit severely the instances that justify psychiatric intervention. Like Halleck, psychiatrists Andrew Skodol and T. B. Karasu (1978) contend that psychiatric professionals can do little to help prevent spontaneous violence.

So many variables contribute to such behavior that it is practically impossible for anyone to predict its occurrence. Because it is so difficult to know precisely who will be violent, it is an unjustifiable violation of civil liberties to lock up someone who behaves peaceably most of the time and has not committed a crime but is only suspected of being prone to impulsive outbursts. In contrast, Halleck identifies a group of people who plan violence and act in irrational, strange, or self-defeating ways even with members of their own subculture. It is reasonable to assume that these people are experiencing emotional difficulty, he feels. In this group would be a woman who talks of killing her children because she is commanded to do so by God, or a person who feels driven to obtain sexual pleasure by mutilating and molesting strangers. These individuals are justifiable candidates for involuntary detention on psychiatric grounds, in Halleck's view. Szasz, on the other hand, prefers the application of legal-criminal controls to this category of people.

Suicide   Suicide is a form of violence to oneself. As such, it raises for psychiatric nurses the moral issue of balancing liberty and life. The extent to which homicide and suicide are equivalent is another basic ethical question that bears on society's right to control suicide. Szasz believes that homicide and suicide bear the same relation to each other as rape and masturbation do. Homicide, according to Szasz, is the gravest crime, while suicide in his opinion is a basic human right.

Traditionally, nurses have felt that they should do everything possible to preserve life. They have relied on this imperative to justify coercive intervention in suicide attempts as well as heroic technical measures to avert impending deaths. Recent reconsideration of euthanasia, however, seems to raise questions about a client's right to suicide. *Euthanasia* has been defined as the intentional termination of a life of such poor quality that it is not worth living. The concept of allowing a person to die without the use of life-prolonging treatment is called **passive euthanasia.** **Active euthanasia,** by contrast, is defined as an act that results in the death of a person. The treatment given to dying clients is often in conflict with the treatment they desire. For example, a physician may disregard a client's protests against treatment. The doctor may assert that the client's medical condition is causing the client to behave irrationally. It is no great logical jump from clients dying of physical deterioration to clients dying of emotional or mental deterioration. Many of the same ethical questions emerge about the suicidal client:

- How is *quality of life* defined?

- Is the definition limited to physical factors?

- Who should have the right to make the definition?

- How is rationality to be measured?

- Are people always in conscious control of their choices?

An individual's right to choose when and how to die is a complex biomedical issue currently receiving more attention than ever before. The thoughtful professional nurse needs to clarify the issues, give them careful consideration, and search for a personal position. There are many ways in which people can deliberately shorten their own lives. They can destroy themselves quickly with a gun, or slowly through the chronic use of drugs such as tobacco or alcohol. When is coercive intervention by psychiatric practitioners justified? Do professionals have the right to restrain people against their will if those people have not committed an illegal act?

Use of Restrictive Treatments   At some time in their lives, all people experience the kind of excessive stress that makes them feel miserable or even desperate. Some people, however, communicate these feelings in ways that are inappropriate, troublesome, unreasonable, or frightening to others. A young woman who in times of stress mutilates her body by burning it repeatedly with cigarettes; a teenager who breaks everything in sight during violent, destructive outbursts; and a belligerent male who initiates physical fights with anyone and everyone without provocation all usually become candidates for *symptomatic treatments*—behavioral control measures often used against the person's will.

Psychosurgery   The most dramatic of restrictive measures is *psychosurgery,* the surgical removal or destruction of brain tissue with the intent of altering behavior even though there may be no direct evidence of structural disease or damage in the brain. Psychosurgery has become the subject of marked controversy on ethical grounds. Advocates claim that it is done to

RESEARCH NOTE

Citation

Akerlund BM, Norberg A: An ethical analysis of double-bind conflicts as experienced by care workers feeding severely demented patients. Int J Nurse Stud 1985;22:207–216.

Study Problem/Purpose

What is the nature of care workers' experiences when they must feed clients with incurable dementia who no longer take food or fluid voluntarily?

Methods

Thirty-nine care workers were interviewed about their thoughts, feelings, and attitudes toward feeding severely demented clients. Sample members were chosen using a stratified random procedure with number of years in the profession as the stratified variable. The interviews were semistructured and covered nine topics that were raised in no consistent sequence. Tape recordings of the interviews were analyzed using phenomenologic strategies, including text interpretation.

Findings

Feeding clients presented ethical conflicts between two principles: "Keep the client alive" and "Don't cause the client suffering." Care workers fell into four categories according to which ethical rule they gave priority to and how they felt about it. Feeding was a source of conflict for most workers. Workers' attitudes about autonomy and paternalism and time in the profession were not sources of significant differences.

Implications

According to this study, the source of anxiety for care workers feeding demented clients was a lack of discussion about ethics. A theory of ethics applicable to urgent nursing problems is needed.

1. The illness being treated is seriously disabling and untreatable by nonsurgical means such as medication or therapy.

2. The treatment is undertaken with some sort of systematic investigative protocol—in short, it is accompanied by evaluation research.

3. The treatment occurs in settings with as many safeguards as possible to arrive at informed consent, if possible, perhaps using a client advocate during the procedure.

Psychotropic Drugs   The discovery that certain drugs can radically alter human emotions has had an enormous impact on psychiatry. The mental hospital is no longer seen as a warehouse for storing society's deviants; it is now a clearinghouse where clients are sorted, renovated, and dispatched back into their communities with symptomatic behavior under control through one or another of the current psychiatric medications.

Psychiatric professionals have associated the advent of psychotropic medications with a new optimism and less fear about working with persons labeled mentally ill. Conceivably, the impact of the drugs on attitudes of nurses may increase the amount of humane contact clients are given while in the hospital. Furthermore, it might be argued that the drugs have helped keep people out of the hospital and have decreased the need for other more dramatic treatments, such as electroshock treatment.

Drugs that make people feel better, however, can lessen their motivation to confront an oppressive situation. This can have serious implications for the political and moral climate of society. Consider, for example, a common clinical problem:

A woman is married to a domineering and insensitive man. She becomes increasingly unhappy, then intensely anxious. When she is on the verge of fighting back to try to alter her oppressed situation, she becomes more agitated and visits a psychiatric clinic. Her therapist prescribes a medicine that alleviates her tension. As a consequence the client has less awareness of her plight and is less inclined to confront her problems. She ultimately continues to submit to her husband's oppressiveness.

It is conceivable that pills could be developed to keep such a woman quietly enslaved throughout her married life. Suppose drugs were coercively given to anyone whose unhappiness was rooted in social oppression. We can even contemplate the possibility that the government might become repressive enough to force all dissidents to take medicine.

Drugs cautiously and judiciously used with the consent of clients can be helpful to people. Used unreflectively, they can close off moral and political confrontations. Decisions about the use of drugs must

restore rather than destroy individual freedom. They argue that before psychosurgery, the client is crippled by mental illness. Individual autonomy is compromised by the client's bizarre behavior or internal psychologic state. After the surgery, clients supposedly are more autonomous than before, by their own and others' criteria. Advocates of selective use of psychosurgery, even when it is against the client's will, outline three conditions that must be met to justify it:

be made in the context of the social situation and environment.

In the in-patient setting, medications are regularly used to reduce symptoms and make client behavior more manageable. Most staff members justify their use of chemical controls by defining violent or bizarre behavior as an indirect request for limits. By assigning this meaning to the use of drugs, practitioners can feel that their actions to suppress symptoms are based on the needs of the client rather than on the staff's management motives.

After pacing angrily up and down the hall in front of the nurses' station for 20 minutes or so, Carlotta kicks over some mops in a bucket. A male staff member shouts to the nurse to get her p.r.n. medication ready and strides into the hall telling the client to stop it. She cries and shouts, and they begin struggling. Several other staff members rush over to assist. They drag and carry her into her room, where she gets Haldol (10 mg). She continues fighting and screaming. The staff members decide to put her in "soft" restraints and continue to wrestle with her in her room. Finally they decide to transfer her to the ward downstairs, where she can be put into a seclusion room. In a report, a staff member describes the incident as, "Carlotta blew up and needed controls." In further discussion of the case, it became apparent that the decision to put her into seclusion was made because restrained clients have to be checked and released every 15 minutes, which is a lot of work for the staff.

It is possible that all these controls would not have been necessary had a nurse behind the glass windows of the nurses' station responded to the nonverbal cues of mounting tension that the client communicated before kicking over the mops.

Structural Controls Even the physical characteristics of psychiatric in-patient settings convey the notion that clients are not expected to be capable of self-control and that staff members have the responsibility for providing it. Many clients view these interventions as forms of abuse, while the staff sees them as "helping people who can't take care of themselves." Consider the following directions on use of restraints:

The acutely psychotic client who is delusional, the angry individual who is testing limits, and the intoxicated client are the types of individuals to whom restrains may be applied for their own protection and that of others. These individuals are nonverbally asking for help to control their potentially inappropriate behavior. When all other techniques have failed and it is quite obvious that the client is out of control, the staff must take action and forcibly apply restraints.

All the judgments that must be made about restraints involve moral decisions. What other techniques have been tried? Is the client obviously out of control? How does the nurse decide? Is the client cognitively compromised? What will be the effects on the client of such a dramatic intervention? What are the effects on others in the milieu? In weighing decisions, nurses must keep in mind that any intervention that removes symptoms without simultaneously increasing the client's awareness of the underlying experience is potentially repressive.

Clients themselves have begun to guard against repressiveness by issuing a bill of rights (see the accompanying box). This issue captured public attention in the notorious case of Joyce Brown, a homeless New York woman forcibly removed from the streets because of her self-neglect and provocative behavior. She was judged competent, however, to refuse medication despite her status as an involuntary patient. Deciding that impairment is sufficient to deprive a client of the right to **informed consent** is yet another controversy in nursing ethics.

Client Privacy and Confidentiality

When people seek psychiatric help, they must usually reveal highly personal, possibly embarrassing, and potentially damaging information about themselves. Almost all modes of therapeutic intervention rely on the client's willingness to talk openly and honestly about personal concerns, feelings, or problems. The solo therapist in private practice with voluntary clients is usually able to avoid compromising the clients' rights to confidentiality. In fact, many private therapists view themselves as vigilant protectors of their clients' privacy. Nurses, however, may encounter a serious ethical conflict in being at the same time the confidant of the client and employee of the organization. These nurses have dual allegiances—to the client and to the agency. Clients usually assume that health professionals have no other purpose than to help them. They lose sight of the fact that nurses often are asked to collect data about them that might be highly influential in determining their medications, their disposition, and even their civil rights. While it is often the psychiatrist who makes final pronouncements about a client's mental health status, diagnosis, prognosis, and the like, such pronouncements rest on information collected and communicated to the doctor by nurses. This information-gathering process merits serious scrutiny.

It is not unusual for a kind of fiction to develop about a hospitalized client, in the staff's eagerness to gather juicy tidbits of information. Data are passed from one nursing shift to another and written on the chart without thought to their validity or reliability. These are then used to make generalizations about the client. The following are typical entries about clients in nurses' notes:

Little socialization

Somewhat seclusive

CHAPTER 7 NURSING ETHICS 129

Mental Patient's Bill of Rights

We are ex-mental patients. We have been subjected to brutalization in mental hospitals and by the psychiatric profession. In almost every state of the union, a mental patient has fewer de facto rights than a murderer condemned to die or to life imprisonment. As a human being, you are entitled to basic human rights that are taken for granted by the general population. You are entitled to protection by and recourse to the law. The purpose of the Mental Patients' Liberation Project is to help those who are still institutionalized. This Bill of Rights was prepared by those at the first meeting of MPLP held on June 13, 1971, at the Washington Square Methodist Church. If you know someone in a mental hospital, give him/her a copy of these rights. If you are in a hospital and need legal help, try to find someone to call the number listed below.

1. You are a human being and are entitled to be treated as such with as much decency and respect as is accorded to any other human being.

2. You are an American citizen and are entitled to every right established by the Declaration of Independence and guaranteed by the Constitution of the United States of America.

3. You have the right to the integrity of your own mind and the integrity of your own body.

4. Treatment and medication can be administered only with your consent and, in the event you give your consent, you have the right to demand to know all relevant information regarding said treatment and/or medication.

5. You have the right to have access to your own legal and medical counsel.

6. You have the right to refuse to work in a mental hospital and/or to choose what work you shall do and you have the right to receive the minimum wage for such work as is set by the state labor laws.

7. You have the right to decent medical attention when you feel you need it just as any other human being has that right.

8. You have the right to uncensored communication by phone, letter, and in person with whomever you wish and at any time you wish.

9. You have the right not to be treated like a criminal; not to be locked up against your will; not to be committed involuntarily; not to be fingerprinted or "mugged" (photographed).

10. You have the right to decent living conditions. You're paying for it and the taxpayers are paying for it.

11. You have the right to retain your own personal property. No one has the right to confiscate what is legally yours, no matter what reason is given. That is commonly known as theft.

12. You have the right to bring grievance against those who have mistreated you and the right to counsel and a court hearing. You are entitled to protection by the law against retaliation.

13. You have the right to refuse to be a guinea pig for experimental drugs and treatments and to refuse to be used as learning material for students. You have the right to demand reimbursement if you are so used.

14. You have the right not to have your character questioned or defamed.

15. You have the right to request an alternative to legal commitment or incarceration in a mental hospital.

The Mental Patients' Liberation Project plans to set up neighborhood crisis centers as alternatives to incarceration and voluntary and involuntary commitment to hospitals. We plan to set up a legal aid society for those whose rights are taken away and/or abused. Although our immediate aim is to help those currently in hospitals, we are also interested in helping those who are suffering from job discrimination, discriminatory school admissions policies and discrimination and abuse at the hands of the psychiatric professions. Call the number listed below if you are interested in our group or if you need assistance.

Mental Patients Alliance of Central New York
P.O. Box 158
Syracuse, N.Y. 13201
(315) 947-5822

SOURCE: *Mental Patients Alliance of Central New York Inc.*

Superficially appropriate

Looks flat

Very poor insight

High as a kite

May be hallucinating

Often the requirement that nurses exchange tidbits such as these with each other becomes the motivation for getting out to talk to the clients so that the nurse will have something to report. Yet it is considered sufficient simply to have a comment to make. Little concern is shown about how representative that comment may be.

The information garnered in this way may be confirmed with repetition in shift reports and daily charting, without additional exploration. This arouses another reaction in some nurses—reluctance to report any observations.

On one occasion a few staff members in an in-patient facility expressed concern about the things people choose to put in reports, because of "the way things get latched onto around here." For example, a client may acquire a reputation as a homosexual or heroin addict because of revealing one experimental experience to a nurse in what the client believed to be a confidential exchange. One nurse said, "Somehow it seems more ethical to write 'I didn't talk to the client today' or 'I don't know what's going on with this person' than to select out of an eight-hour period one or two phrases or behaviors, often expressed in clichés."

Information gathering and sharing are part of the psychiatric nurse's role. When the employer is a federal- or state-supported agency that might have some investment in quelling deviants, however, the nurse is put in a double-agent role. The client's rights to privacy and confidentiality are increasingly threatened by computerized data banks for information storage, certain medical and other insurance procedures, and even the professional standards review organization (PSRO) system in clinical agencies. Thoughtful handling of this dilemma is facilitated by three safeguards:

1. Nurses must convey to clients the limit of confidentiality in their exchanges—that is, what the nurses do with the information a client shares.

2. Nurses must attempt to portray accurately to others the reliability, validity, and representativeness of the data they communicate about a client.

3. Strict confidentiality may have to be violated when an innocent third party is endangered.

The Ethics and Politics of Women's Mental Health

In the past two decades, nurses have become aware of the impact of feminism on the institution of psychotherapy and the sensibilities of those professionals who concern themselves with a special subsection of the client population—women. Brodsky's (1973) review of a decade of feminist influence on psychotherapy cited changes in theories, treatment techniques, and assessment approaches, all reflecting more enlightened attitudes toward women as therapists and clients.

Yet, Phyllis Chesler (1972), the outspoken author of *Women and Madness*, analyzes the status of women in our culture in her own unique, rhetorical style.

Women are submissive. We're altruistic. And especially we're self-sacrificing. Usually our altruism comes from very low self-esteem. We're always guilty. We're losers—trained to be losers in life. We're also mothers or can be mothers and that's another reason why we might be altruistic.

Chesler goes on to identify four premises that run through all the theories of psychiatry and apply to most clinical practices. These premises, in Chesler's view, reflect how the mental health professionals see women and how women have been taught to see themselves.

1. Everybody is crazy.

2. While everybody is crazy, women are crazier. To be mentally healthy is to be male.

3. Male homosexuality is sick, and lesbians don't exist.

4. In order for a woman to be a real woman, she's got to become a mother, and once you've become a mother, everything that goes wrong with your family's mental health is your fault.

Political versus Psychiatric Solutions

Environmental Stress In the complex superstructure of global society, environmental stresses may be generated both directly by the selfishness, apathy, or malice of those in power and indirectly by subtly imposed prejudices, outmoded and inflexible rules, the threat of nuclear war, and an economic system that deprives certain citizens (often the poor and members of minority groups) of basic human needs. African Americans directly exposed to humiliation by bigoted whites have a clear idea who their oppressors are. They are aware of their anger and know toward whom it is directed. African Americans living in a society where racism is institutionalized but not openly expressed may be exposed to repeated indirect aggressions that leave them frustrated and angry, but they have difficulty identifying the source of their sense of oppression. Halleck (1971) asserts that any citizens who believe in the basic benevolence of their society but do not partake of its benefits have similar reactions. It is not unusual for people in these circumstances to express their frustration and anger in alcoholism, drug use, violence, or suicide.

Environmental stress is also generated in immediate families or groups of significant others. A parent may abuse a child. An employer may harass or insult an employee. These are direct sources of stress.

Stress generated in immediate social systems also may be indirect, leaving the individual totally or partially unaware of its source. For example, a domineering husband may send day-to-day demeaning messages that chip away his wife's self-esteem in disguised ways. She may find herself feeling chronically depressed or anxious without knowing why. A domineering wife may do the same to her husband. An AIDS client may be refused care by health professionals because of fear based on misunderstanding. (See Chapter 25.)

The End of Neutrality   For a long time nursing has hidden behind the cloak of political neutrality, arguing that the role of caretakers and healers permits, even demands, a detachment from political, economic, and social issues. Psychiatric nursing services have been defined as client-oriented activities designed to reduce pain and discomfort and to increase the capacity of the individual to adjust satisfactorily. As long as nurses saw their psychiatric work as simply treating illnesses of the mind in the same way they treated illnesses of the body, they could accept the notion that psychologic illness, like physical illness, indicated a defect in the individual, not in the social milieu. Practitioners tended to search for the causes of emotional suffering exclusively in anomalies of the client's biologic or psychologic past. They did not consider the interaction stresses in the client's environment that might account for strange, troublesome, or irrational behavior. This view of the human condition and the nurse's role avoided any critical examination of society and the nurse's relationship to it.

New conceptual frameworks and nursing theories take into consideration not only internal individual perceptions of stress but also the immediate and broader social contexts that contribute to an individual's experience of stress. Nurses are beginning to realize that a person identified as a client may be miserable and not coping at any given moment not only because of personal perceptions of oppression, but also because they are actually being oppressed. As the saying goes, "Even paranoids have real enemies."

The Social Psychiatric Model   A psychiatric nurse who is willing to try to help clients to change the stresses in their environment rather than just adapt to them is engaging in an aspect of social psychiatric practice. Halleck (1971), describing a social psychiatric model for practice, urges psychiatric professionals to abandon the hoax of a politically neutral profession and make their personal political positions explicit. He feels that it is illogical to believe that professional activities designed to change the status quo are political, while those designed to strengthen the status quo are neutral. Halleck emphasizes the important role of psychiatric professionals in social reform. All therapists base their efforts to help clients and society on some idea of the optimum human condition. Therefore, psychiatric professionals must think through the meaning of *optimum human condition* to gain insight into their own ideologies and to sharpen their ethical criteria for intervening in social systems or sustaining the status quo.

Acting to sustain and preserve a desirable social order is by no means immoral or unethical. Society relies on psychiatric professionals as agents of social control to bring a humane and caring perspective to their often difficult and uncertain work with clients. Many of these clients have engaged in behavior patterns believed to be evil, destructive, and burdensome to others. As one somewhat hardened nurse put it:

We are the junk pickers of society—picking up society's casualties and trying to rework them into some useful form.

Balancing the Individual and the Social Good

The judgments that lead people to label someone's experience as paranoid rather than simply unpopular are frequently based on arbitrary and shifting criteria. Behavior that is considered bizarre or unreasonable in one cultural context may be considered desirable in another. The definitions of those who need psychiatric help are constantly changing. Nurses are necessarily guided in therapeutic work by a belief system—by some vision of what kinds of changes would improve a client's life. Nurses are further guided by some moral principles that limit the extent to which they will help a client obtain happiness at the expense of others and the extent to which they will participate in the oppression of an individual in the interests of societal control. Laws represent yet another source of limits.

Nursing is frequently faced with two goals:

• To respond to the therapeutic needs of individuals

• To serve society by preserving some degree of social order

Often these two goals are in conflict, and nurses must face the dilemma of placing one above the other. The only way to resolve the conflict is for them to clarify their own goals and values through a process of ethical reflection.

CHAPTER HIGHLIGHTS

• Ethical reflection is a process for achieving clear and convincing reasons for making moral decisions rather than discovering a singular right or wrong solution for ethical dilemmas.

• An ethical dilemma is a conflict between two obligations.

• Nurses move toward professional autonomy through development of codes of ethics, setting qualifications for practitioners, participating in peer review, setting standards, and accepting consequences for professional decisions.

• Known dominant ethical perspectives include egoism, deontology, utilitarianism, theory of obligation, ideal observer theory, and justice as fairness.

• Principles of bioethics include anatomy, nonmaleficence, beneficence, justice, veracity, and confidentiality.

• Contemporary health-related ethical dilemmas include the effects of psychiatric labeling, control of personal freedom, use of restrictive treatments, and the rights of the client.

• The nurse must protect the rights of the individual yet mediate between these rights and the interests of the social group.

REFERENCES

American Association of Colleges of Nursing: *Essentials of College and University Education for Professional Nursing; Final Report.* 1986, pp. 6–7.

American Psychological Association. Task Force on Sex Bias and Sex Role Stereotyping in Psychotherapeutic Practice: Guidelines for therapy with women. *Am Psychol* 1978;33:1122–1123.

Aroskar MA: Establishing limits to professional autonomy: Whose responsibility? *Nurs Law Ethics* 1980; 1.

Brodsky A: The consciousness-raising group as a model for therapy with women. *Psychother Theory Re Prac* 1973;10:24–29.

Chesler P: *Women and Madness.* Doubleday, 1972.

Colorado Society of Clinical Specialists in Psychiatric Nursing. Ethical guidelines for competence. *J Psychosoc Nurs* 28(5);1990:38–39.

Cournos F: Involuntary medication and the case of Joyce Brown. *Hosp Community Psychiatry* 40;1989:736–740.

Davis AJ: Ethical dilemmas in nursing. Recorded at JONA and Nurse Educator's 1981 Joint Leadership Conference, available from Teach'em, Inc., 160 East Illinois Street, Chicago, Illinois.

Davis AJ: Professional obligations, personal values in conflict. *Am Nurs* May, 1990:7.

Davis AJ, Aroskar MA; *Ethical Dilemmas and Nursing Practice.* Appleton-Century-Crofts, 1978.

Erikson K: Notes on the sociology of deviance. *Soc Probl* 1962;9:308.

Goffman E: *Stigma: Notes on the Management of Spoiled Identity.* Prentice-Hall, 1963.

Halleck SL: *The Politics of Therapy.* Harper and Row, 1971.

Skodol A, Karasu TB: Emergency psychiatry and the assaultive patient. *Am J Psychiatry* 1978;135:202–205.

Spencer E: Psychiatric ethics: Entering the 1990's. *Hosp Community Psychiatry* 41(4);1990:384–386.

Szasz T: *The Myth of Mental Illness,* rev ed. Harper and Row, 1974.

Task Force on Mental Health of Women. *Report to the President's Commission on Mental Health.* U.S. Government Printing Office, 1978.

Viens DC: AIDS ethics. *California Nurs* 1990(Nov/Dec):8.

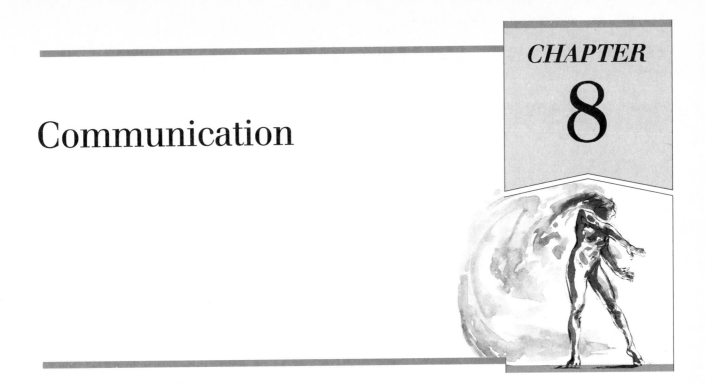

Communication

CHAPTER
8

LEARNING OBJECTIVES

- Describe the process of human communication
- Compare linear, interactional, and transactional models of communication
- Identify the major concepts in a humanistic interactionist approach to communication
- Discuss verbal and nonverbal modes of communication
- Relate three major theories of communication to humanistic psychiatric nursing practice
- Identify concepts of facilitative communication that are essential ingredients of interpersonal relationships
- Apply skills that foster effective communication throughout the nursing process

Carol Ren Kneisl

CROSS REFERENCES

Other topics related to this content are: Culture, Chapter 36; Empathy, Chapter 2; Influence of territoriality and personal space on communication, Chapter 29; and Role of human values in the communication of the nurse, Chapter 2.

WHEN JOHN BOWLBY (1951) discovered that infants in foundling homes were literally dying for lack of contact and affection, the scientific community began to attach new importance to the old saying that *people need people*. We recognize today that the mechanism for establishing, maintaining, and improving human contacts is interpersonal communication. Communication is a very special process and the most significant of human behaviors. Moreover, it is the main method for implementing the nursing process.

The therapeutic interpersonal relationship in humanistic psychiatric nursing practice often develops through a storytelling experience. Telling stories is as natural and human as breathing. When they tell "their story," clients explain themselves, the events of their lives, and the circumstances they face.

The major role of the psychiatric nurse is to help clients tell their stories, explore the circumstances of their lives, and resolve the things that have gone wrong. However, the process of communication is so complex and has so many dimensions that it cannot be reduced to a few simple steps that nurses can memorize and perform.

The Process of Human Communication

Communication is an ongoing, dynamic, and ever-changing series of events, each of which affects and is affected by all the others. The essence of effective communication is *responding with meaning*. Unfortunately, some persons define communication simply as the transfer of information or meaning from one human being to another. However, meaning cannot be transferred from one human being to another but must be mutually negotiated, because meaning is influenced by a number of significant variables.

Variables That Influence Communication

Perception A person's image or perception of the world is an essential element in communicating. The term **perception** refers to the experience of sensing, interpreting, and comprehending the world in which the person lives. This makes perception a highly personal and internal act.

People process through their senses all the information they have about the world around them. However, seeing is not always believing. Contemporary communication specialists have discovered that because of human physiologic limitations, the eye and brain are constantly being tricked into seeing things

that are not really what they seem (**illusions**). Figure 8−1 shows an illusion that reflects physiologic constraints. Before continuing to read, stare at Figure 8−1 for 20 seconds. The illustration will appear to swing back and forth. Verify that the movement is an illusion by checking the visual perception against tactile sensations.

What people "see" or sense is influenced very strongly by a number of factors. Stop reading here and look at Figure 8−2. Past experiences have prepared us to see things, persons, and events in particular ways. When we read the sayings in Figure 8−2, past experience encourages us to see them inaccurately as the familiar sayings "Snake in the grass," "Quick as a flash," and "Paris in the spring." The words actually are "Snake in *the the* grass," "Quick as *a a* flash," and "Paris in *the the* spring."

People tend to observe more carefully when a purpose guides the observation. The purposes or reasons for engaging in an observation also determine what people observe. The nurse in an intensive care unit observes a cardiac surgery client differently than a family member does.

Finally, when understandings differ, people can look at the same object and see different things. Mental set helps determine how and what a person perceives. Before you read any further, look at the picture of the young woman in Figure 8−3. Do you see the silhouette of a young woman? Do you also see the face of an elderly woman? Our use of the phrase "the picture of the young woman in Figure 8−3" encouraged you to perceive the illustration in a particular

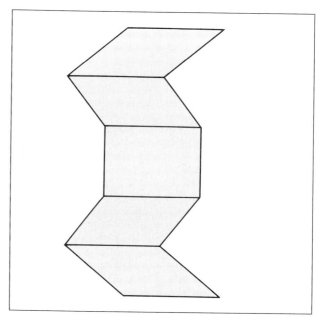

FIGURE 8−1 A perceptual illusion.

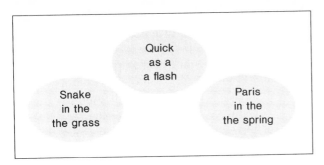

FIGURE 8–2   The influence of past experience on perception.

way. Now you should also be able to see the elderly woman in the illustration.

As the illustrations demonstrate, the old axiom might be better stated: "Believing is seeing." Because people tend to perceive in terms of past experiences, expectations, and goals, perceptions may be a prime obstacle to communication. No two individuals perceive the world in exactly the same way, and the meanings of events differ because people's perceptions

of them differ. Perceptions of other human beings are of particular importance since human communication is inevitably affected by participants' perceptions of one another. To see others at all as they are, people need to know themselves and to know how the self affects the perceptions of others.

Values   Values are concepts of the desirable. People value what is of worth to them. Values influence the process of communication, because people's values, like their perceptions, differ.

Value systems differ for a number of reasons. Age is one. Children's values shift when they become teenagers. The college or work experience generally influences values in yet other directions. Marrying or being a parent or grandparent may cause other value changes or shifts.

Psychiatric nurses must ultimately come to terms with the problem of values, because conflicting value systems among mental health professionals expose clients to uncertainty and confusion. Consider the following examples:

The parents of a 15-year-old girl were upset to find a small plastic bag of marijuana in her dresser drawer. She had been playing hooky from school and wore jeans that her parents considered sloppy. After a series of lengthy, angry discussions with her parents, she was confined to her room. During this period she refused to eat or drink.

When the girl was seen by a mental health treatment team, the members' opinions were divided. Some said that her behavior signaled an emotional disturbance and labeled her antisocial, depressed, and anxious. Others believed her parents were too rigid in attempting to force her to accept their values.

In another instance, a 35-year-old man was firmly committed to prayer. Most of his spare time was connected in some way to church-related activities. Staff members at a mental health clinic where he sought counseling told him that he was resorting to an early infantile attitude about God as the magic worker.

Clearly, these staff members were influenced by their own values.

The daily roles people take also influence their values. In any one day a man may be a student, husband, father, nurse, citizen, speaker, artist, son, and teacher.

Culture   Each culture provides its members with notions about how the world is structured and what it means. These preconceptions, learned at an early age, are so subtle that they often go unrecognized. They nonetheless set limits on communication and interaction with others. Relying on culturally determined generalizations or stereotypes can have profound effects on people's relationships with others.

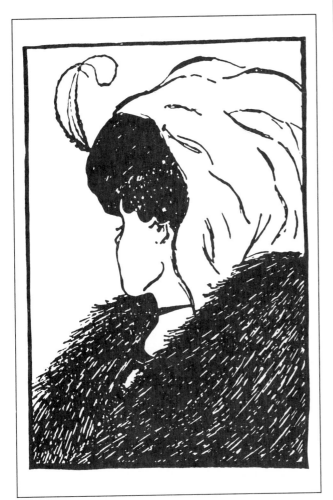

FIGURE 8–3   The influence of mental set on perception.

Communication is culture-bound in a wide variety of ways. The culture and the subculture (the culture within the culture) teach people how to communicate through language, hand gestures, clothing, and even in the ways they use the space around them.

The nurse who does not know that "run it by me" means to explain something, that a "close-knuckle drill" is a fistfight, or that "hit on a broad" means to sweet-talk a female may be confused by conversations with members of certain subcultures—adolescents and street people, for example. The nurse who overhears two clients talking about "angel dust" is likely to come to erroneous conclusions if unaware that the terms refers not to a Christmas decoration but to PCP—an animal tranquilizer. In some cultures, belching after dinner is a compliment to the host and is considered proper etiquette. In other cultures, belching may be thought uncouth or an insult. When Americans make a circle with thumb and forefinger and extend the other fingers, they mean "OK." To Brazilians, the same gesture is an obscene sign of contempt. These examples make it obvious that communicating with meaning requires that the participants take culture well into account. How people communicate with others who do not share similar histories, heritages, or cultures is of critical importance in humanistic psychiatric nursing practice.

Levels of Communication

Communication takes place on at least three different levels—intrapersonal, interpersonal, and public. **Intrapersonal communication** occurs when people communicate within themselves. A nurse who walks into a client's room and thinks, "The first pint of blood is almost finished. I'd better get the next one ready for infusion," is communicating intrapersonally.

Interpersonal communication, which this chapter discusses in depth, takes place between dyads (groups of two persons) and in small groups. This level of person-to-person communication is at the heart of psychiatric nursing.

Public communication is communication between a person and several other people. Its most common form is the presentation of a public speech. Communications through the mass media are other forms of public communication.

Models of Human Communication

One of the easiest ways to illustrate the nature of human communication and the elements of the process is through a model, or visual representation.

People use models frequently for many purposes. They might use a map, which is a visual representation of a territory, to find their way to the community mental health center they plan to visit. Health professionals use EEGs to see a visual representation of the electrical activity in the brain. However, models provide incomplete views—a map does not show all the trees, buildings, or park statues in the territory, and the EEG tracing does not show the color, size, or blood supply of the brain. It is important to keep this in mind when looking at models. They sometimes make a process look simpler than it is.

Communication As an Act

Viewing human communication as an act is to see it as a one-way phenomenon: person A talks to person B. Communicators who follow this concept attempt to transfer the thoughts or ideas in their heads into someone else's head. Communication then becomes something that is done *to* another person.

Two major assumptions behind this view are that skill is all-important, and that meaning is transferable. Such a model fails to take into account the variables discussed earlier—perception, values, and culture. It suggests that the receiver plays a passive role and does not affect the communicator. It places primary emphasis on the selection of "correct" messages. When misunderstandings occur, either the communicator is faulted for failing to send the correct message or the receiver is faulted for having allowed something to interfere with the transmission of a correct message. Both persons become preoccupied with laying blame and the need to construct "perfect messages." These implications and assumptions are evidence that the model of communication as an act is inadequate.

Communication As an Interaction

Communication as an interaction takes into account the process of mutual influence in communication. In this view, when two people interact, they put themselves into each other' shoes. Each tries to perceive the world as the other perceives it, in order to predict how the other will respond. In other words, communication is not a one-way process. It is a circular process in which the participants take turns at being communicator and receiver: person A (communicator) talks to person B (receiver), and person B (communicator) talks to person A (receiver).

Clearly, this model accounts for more factors than the previous one. However, it still oversimplifies human communication, because it treats it as a series of causes and effects, stimuli and responses.

Communication As a Transaction

Mutual Influence between Communicators

a transaction, the participants are both communicators. No one is labeled either as communicator or receiver. Communication is viewed as a process of simultaneous mutual influence rather than as a turn-taking event.

In a transactional perspective, participants are who they are in relationship to the other person with whom they are communicating. For example, in each dyadic (composed of two people) communication event there are at least *six* persons involved: A's A, A's B, A's impression of the way B sees A, B's B, B's A, and B's impression of the way A sees B. Therefore, in addition to the content message, a relationship message also exists. Suppose A passes B in the corridor, and A says "Hi, how are you." B answers, "Just fine, thanks," moving down the corridor and away from A as quickly as possible. B's behavior is a comment on the relationship between A and B. Their subsequent communication will be affected by how A perceives B's response. If A thinks B walked away because B wanted to get home before the thunderstorm that was predicted, A is likely to respond one way to B the next time they meet. If A believes B is angry with A, A is likely to respond quite differently at the next encounter. The symbolic interactionist model described below helps explain what takes place between A and B.

A Symbolic Interactionist Model of Communication

A symbolic interactionist model is based on a transactional perspective. It views human communication on the social, interpersonal level and accounts for the whole persons involved in the process. The participants are products of their social system and integral parts of it. In the communication, some events take place *within* the participants (they are intrapersonal), and some take place *between* the participants (they are interpersonal).

A model constructed by Hulett (1966, p 14) according to symbolic interactionist principles, and adapted for this text, is shown in Figure 8–4. It shows five phases in each person's communication sequence: input, covert rehearsal, message generation, environmental event, and goal response.

During the phase of *input,* the person is motivated through some stimulus, either external or internal, toward some goal that requires engaging in a social relationship with another. Let us say that Jeff is attracted to Sarah and would like to get to know her better.

In the *covert rehearsal* phase, the person moves to make sense of the input received and develops and organizes a message *before* generating it. Figure 8–5 represents the symbolic interactionist model of the covert rehearsal. The individual first scans the information about self and others (Jeff enjoys theater and remembers hearing Sarah tell a friend that she'd really like to see the new musical comedy in town) and then mentally rehearses possible actions to take (role playing) and possible reactions of the other (role taking). This gives Jeff the chance to think of four or five different ways to approach Sarah. This process is represented by the intrapersonal feedback loop.

The covert rehearsal phase is really the core of the communication process. In it, Jeff decides what to say,

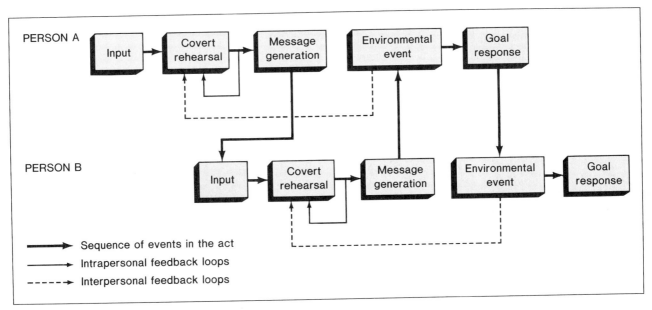

FIGURE 8–4 Symbolic interactionist model of communication   SOURCE: Adapted from Hulett JE Jr:
A symbolic interactionist model of human communication. AV Communication Review 1966;14:14.

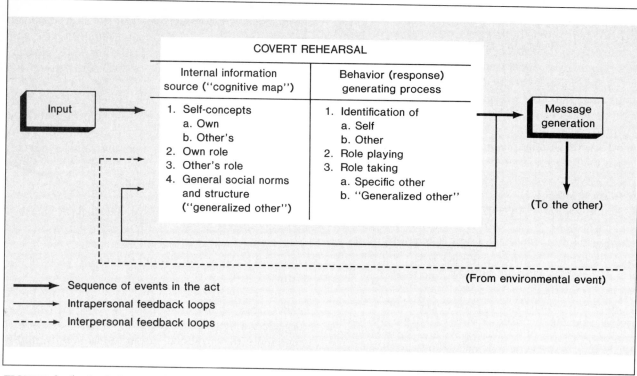

FIGURE 8–5 Symbolic interactionist model of the covert rehearsal phase. *SOURCE: Adapted from Hulett JE Jr: A symbolic interactionist model of human communication. AV Communication Review 1966;14:18.*

how to say it, and even whether to send the message to Sarah at all.

During *message generation,* the third phase, the instrumental act of giving a message is performed. (Jeff asks Sarah to the theater.) A message generated by one person serves as the input or the stimulus for another person. (Sarah thinks about Jeff's invitation, decides whether she wants to go to the theater with him, and considers what response to make to Jeff.) Once the second person completes the covert rehearsal and generates a message, this message becomes an *environmental event* for the first person. In our example, the environmental event is the fourth stage in the sequence for Jeff, whose *goal response* serves as another environmental event for Sarah, and so on.

A second, or interpersonal, feedback loop connects the person's environmental event phase to the covert rehearsal stage. It allows the person an opportunity to determine whether he or she has made an error in the approach to the other and to make appropriate corrections by repeating the covert rehearsal and devising an altered message. (Jeff carefully considers Sarah's response. He listens to what she says and watches her behavior toward him. If her response is less than enthusiastic, he will try to determine what went wrong and how to correct it.)

In summary, the symbolic interactionist view of communication includes the following concepts:

• People run through a series of internal trials in the process of organizing a message.

• People select and transmit the message that will, in their view, have the highest probability of success.

• Success depends on the accuracy and completeness of the cognitive map of the environment and the accuracy and efficiency of the intrapersonal and interpersonal feedback loops.

• Communication is a dynamic (ever-changing) process that is unrepeatable and irreversible.

• Communication is complex.

• The meaning of messages is not transferred, it is mutually negotiated.

Communication is, at the very least, a very complicated process.

Modes of Communication

The Spoken Word

Verbal language, the ability to utter the spoken word, makes people human and distinguishes them from other animals. Yet problems arise as humans discover that words mean different things to different people. That is, *words* do not "mean" something, *people* do.

If communication between nurse and client is to be mutually negotiated, the nurse at least must understand the four concepts discussed next.

Denotation and Connotation   A *denotative meaning* is one that is in general use by most persons who share a common language. A *connotative meaning* usually arises from a person's personal experience. While all Americans are likely to share the same general denotative meaning of the word *pig*, the word may have completely different connotations for a farmer, a butcher, a consumer of meat, a person of the Moslem faith, an orthodox Jew, a college student, a prisoner, and a police officer. These positive and negative connotative meanings can evoke powerful emotions.

Private and Shared Meanings   For communication to take place, meaning must be shared. This bewildering conversation between Alice and Humpty Dumpty shows what happens when meaning is not shared:

". . . There's glory for you!"
"I don't know what you mean by 'glory.' " Alice said.
Humpty Dumpty smiled contemptuously. "Of course you don't—till I tell you. I meant 'there's a nice knock-down argument for you!' "
"But 'glory' doesn't mean 'a nice knock-down argument,' " Alice objected.
"When I use a word," Humpty Dumpty said, in rather a scornful tone, "it means just what I choose it to mean—neither more nor less."

(Carroll 1965, p 93)

By assigning meanings to a word without agreement, Humpty Dumpty essentially created a private language.

People can use private meanings to communicate with others only when the parties agree about what the word means. The private meaning then becomes a shared meaning. It is common for families, two friends, or members of larger social groups (military personnel, drug users, adolescents) to use language in highly personal and private ways. Problems arise when the assumption is made that persons outside of the group share these meanings.

People labeled schizophrenic may use language in an idiosyncratic way or may use a private, unshared language referred to as **neologisms.** Such people are unaware that others don't share this use of language. They expect to be understood and may become upset when they are not.

A young man who was hospitalized on a psychiatric unit complained to other clients and staff that he had been

odenated, and he became increasingly frustrated and anxious when it became apparent that he wasn't being understood. With some help he was able to explain that he was upset about having been moved to a private room. The room was, he said, so dark and dingy that it looked like a cave. Animals live in caves that are called *dens.* In his view he had been *o-den-*ated—put in a cave.

In trying to make private meanings shared, the nurse should make an effort to reach mutual understanding of the client's message. It is insufficient, and quite possibly inaccurate, to attach meaning based solely on the nurse's (or the client's) interpretation of an event, a word or phrase, or a nonverbal gesture.

Nonverbal Messages

Most researchers agree that **nonverbal communication** channels carry more social meaning than verbal channels. Nonverbal cues help us judge the reliability of verbal messages more readily, especially in the presence of a **mixed message** (inconsistency between the verbal and nonverbal components).

There is a wide variety in nonverbal channels—facial expressions; hand gestures; body movements; use of space; pitch, rate, and volume of the voice; touch; body aromas; and so on. The following categories are considered here: body movement, voice quality and nonlanguage sounds, use of personal and social space, touch, and use of cultural artifacts (such as clothing and cosmetics).

Body Movement   The study of body movement as a form of nonverbal communication is called *kinesics.* Facial expressions, gestures, and eye movements are the most commonly used categories.

Facial expressions are the single most important source of nonverbal communication. They generally communicate emotions. The silent film comedians—blank-faced Buster Keaton and comic, endearing Charlie Chaplin—and the great mime Marcel Marceau communicate not only isolated acts but complete sequences of behavior with kinesics alone.

Body movements and gestures provide clues about persons and about how they feel toward others. Hand gestures can communicate anxiety, indifference, and impatience, among other things. Foot shuffling and fidgeting may express the desire to escape. Body position gives cues about how open a person is to another person, or how interesting and attractive one person is to another. People tend to position their bodies according to their feelings about the person with whom they are communicating.

Eye contact is another very important cue in communicating. For example, proper sidewalk behavior among Americans is for passers-by to look at each other until they are about eight feet apart. At this distance, both parties look downward or away so they will not appear to be staring. Erving Goffman (1963, p 84) refers to this phenomenon as a "dimming of our lights." Michael Argyle (1967, pp 105–116) points out several of the unstated rules about eye contact.

• Interaction is invited by staring at another person on the other side of a room. If the other person returns the gaze, the invitation to interact has been accepted. Averting the eyes signals a rejection of the looker's request.

• A looker's frank gaze is widely interpreted as positive regard.

• Greater mutual eye contact occurs among friends.

• Persons who seek eye contact while speaking are usually perceived as believable and earnest.

• If the usual short, intermittent gazes during a conversation are replaced by gazes of longer duration, the person looked at is likely to believe that the person gazing considers the relationship between the two persons as more important than the content of the conversation.

Voice Quality and Nonlanguage Sounds *Paralinguistics* or *paralanguage* refers to something beyond or in addition to language itself. The two principal components are *voice quality*, such as pitch and range, and *nonlanguage vocalizations*, such as sobbing, laughing, or grunting—noises without linguistic structure.

Vocal cues can differentiate emotions. Who hasn't heard the injunction: "Don't speak to me in that tone of voice!" Sometimes people use vocal cues to make inferences about personality traits. For example, persons who increase the loudness, pitch, timbre (overtones), and rate of their speech are often thought to be active and dynamic. Those who use greater intonation and volume and are fluent are thought to be persuasive. Status cues in speech are based on a combination of word choice, pronunciation, grammar, speech fluency, and articulation, among other features.

Use of Personal and Social Space *Proxemics* is the study of space relationships maintained by persons in social interaction. It includes the dimensions of *territoriality* (fixed and permanent territory that is somehow marked off and defended from intrusion) and *personal space* (a portable territory surrounding the self that others are expected not to invade).

Knowing something about proxemics is useful, for example, in planning the physical space in which communication is to occur. Nurses can arrange furniture to increase or decrease interpersonal distance. Nurses should be especially sensitive to the constraints imposed on communication by physical objects. Nurses can use proxemics to decipher verbal communication by paying attention to how others use interpersonal space.

Touch Touching behaviors, because they tend to personalize communication, are extremely important in emotional situations. In American society, the use of touch is governed by strong social norms. Unwritten guidelines control who, when, why, and where people touch.

Most of the taboos against touching seem to stem from the sexual implications of touching behavior. However, although touching is a physical act, it may or may not be sexual in nature. A realization of the importance of touch and an understanding that touching is not necessarily a sexual behavior may make this channel of communication available to more people. It is equally important to be sensitive to the other person's disposition toward touching, so as not to alienate another by infringing on the person's right not to be touched.

Cultural Artifacts Artifacts are items in contact with interacting persons that may act as nonverbal stimuli: clothes, cosmetics, perfume, deodorants, jewelry, eyeglasses, wigs and hairpieces, beards and mustaches, and so on.

Think about what information is communicated through artifacts such as a full-length mink coat, hair that has been dyed purple, a gold band on the third finger of the left hand, a military uniform, or a Phi Beta Kappa key.

Relationships between Verbal and Nonverbal Systems

The verbal and nonverbal elements of human communication are inextricably linked. Six different ways in which verbal and nonverbal systems interrelate are discussed below.

1. A nonverbal cue may say the same thing as a verbal cue but in a different way. The deep-sea fisherman who verbally describes the size of the sailfish he caught may also extend both hands to indicate its length. The gesture serves to *repeat* the idea.

2. Nonverbal behavior may also *contradict* verbal behavior. Consider the woman who meets a college roommate she hasn't seen for quite some time. She says, "You haven't changed a bit," but her tone of voice and facial expression convey sarcasm. When verbal and nonverbal cues contradict one another, it is usually safer to put more faith in the nonverbal cues.

RESEARCH NOTE

Citation

Tommasini NR: The use of touch with the hospitalized psychiatric patient. Arch Psychiatr Nurs 1990;4(4):213–220.

Study Problem/Purpose

The purpose of this descriptive study was to identify and describe how registered nurses use nonprocedural touch in the in-patient psychiatric setting.

Methods

Tommasini spent 27.5 hours observing three in-patient psychiatric units (one adolescent unit and two adult units) of a large northeastern United States university teaching hospital. Assuming the role of a nonparticipant, Tommasini unobtrusively observed the common areas of each unit. Staff were told that the researcher would be observing and recording notes on nurse-patient interactions; nurses were not told of the researcher's specific interest in touch. All nurses who were observed to use touch participated subsequently in an audiotaped interview with the researcher focused on the nurse's decision to use touch and intention in doing so. Content analysis was conducted on the transcripts of interviews.

Findings

Over the 27.5 hours of observation, Tommasini recorded twenty-six incidents of touching. Although they used touch, several nurses alluded to a "touch taboo" in psychiatry. In 92 percent of the interactions, touch was used in a purposeful, therapeutic manner. Nurses used touch to establish contact with the client; enhance communication; communicate caring, interest, and recognition; and provide reassurance and comfort. Touch was more commonly used with clients who were either much younger or much older than the nurses.

Implications

Touch is clearly a part of the repertoire of nurses' interventions with psychiatric in-patients. Results of this study support the need for future research on touch, including study of clients' perceptions of its use. Further study is indicated to examine why a middle-adult client population was not touched.

3. Nonverbal messages that *add to or modify* verbal messages are said to be complementary. When a man says he is a "little" irritated about being kept waiting, his tone of voice and body actions may indicate a more profound anger.

4. Certain nonverbal cues *accent or emphasize* verbal cues. A woman shrugs her shoulders when she says she doesn't really care which movie she and her companion see. A master of ceremonies holds up his hand when he asks for quiet. These gestures and body movements emphasize the words.

5. Cues that *regulate,* such as those that tell people when to start talking or when to stop talking, are usually nonverbal. A woman who keeps opening and closing her mouth briefly while others are talking is indicating that she wants a turn too.

6. Sometimes nonverbal cues are used in place of words. A wave from a friend at a distance *substitutes* for "hello." Applause at the end of a play tells the actors that they have pleased the audience.

Communication in Humanistic Psychiatric Nursing

Ruesch's Theory of Therapeutic Communication

The psychiatrist Jurgen Ruesch (1961) developed a theory of therapeutic communication. In his view, communication includes all the processes by which one human being influences another. Ruesch's theory applies to the humanistic interactionist view because it takes into account the perceptions and interpretations that influence one person's view of the other. Further, Ruesch assumes that, to survive, the individual must communicate successfully.

Basic Concepts The basic concepts of Ruesch's theory are:

• Communication occurs in four different settings: intrapersonal, interpersonal, group, and societal.

• The ability to receive, evaluate, and transmit messages is influenced by perception, evaluation (which involves memory, past experiences, and value systems), and transmission quality of messages (amount, speed, efficacy, and distinctiveness).

• Messages achieve meaning when they are mutually validated or verified between the two parties. (In Ruesch's view, however, it is the psychiatric therapist's reality that verifies a message. The definition is not mutually agreed on by client and therapist.)

• Metacommunicative messages (messages about the message) tell both the sender and receiver how to interpret the message.

• Correction through feedback is basic to adaptive, healthy behavior and successful communication.

Growth and Development in Communication

According to Ruesch, communication is one of the hardest human functions to master. It takes a long time to learn because it occurs in a series of steps, each building on the previous one. To communicate effectively requires decades of continuous practice. It is believed that interference hampers development and leaves an indelible mark.

Characteristics of Successful and Disturbed Communication

The four formal criteria for successful communication are efficiency, appropriateness, flexibility, and feedback. When these criteria are not met, communication is disturbed.

Efficiency Simplicity, clarity, and correct timing are all components of efficient messages. Psychiatric nurses and other mental health professionals may find themselves using complex and scientific words or professional mental health jargon to convey messages. Obscure or clumsy language and irrelevant or useless information may also prevent others from understanding a message.

Clear messages give a sense of order or structure and reduce ambiguity by narrowing the number of possible interpretations of meanings. Emphasizing the important ideas helps.

Proper timing also is important. It is best to give messages when the other person is able to "hear" them, when there are no intervening noises or inputs, and when the other person can interpret them without undue haste. Problems occur if the interval between the messages is either too short or too long.

Appropriateness   Messages are appropriate when they are relevant to the situation at hand and when there is mutual fit of overall patterns and constituent parts. Communication is inappropriate when it does not fit the circumstance, is irrelevant, or is misconstrued.

Communication can also be inappropriate in amount. Since every individual has both high and low tolerance levels for stimulation, a person's ability to cope with ideas, make decisions, and act is affected by the amount and rate of sensory input received. Exceeding a tolerance level is called **overload.** A person who is overloaded by too many messages or by messages too closely spaced cannot handle incoming messages. **Underload** occurs when delay or lack of information

interferes with the person's ability to comprehend the message of another.

The **tangential reply** is another example of inappropriateness. A tangential reply to a statement disregards the content of the message and is directed toward either an incidental aspect of the initial statement, the type of language used, the emotions of the sender, or another facet of the same topic.

Flexibility People cannot always be sure how a message will be received, because each person with whom they communicate is unique and changing. Since they cannot expect constancy from others, people need to be flexible. In communication, lack of flexibility manifests itself as either exaggerated control or exaggerated permissiveness. Both extremes increase the likelihood of frustrating, ungratifying, or disturbed communication.

Maintaining flexibility can be difficult if doing so requires a person to abandon or temporarily lay aside a carefully planned goal. To be flexible, a person must have the ability to set new priorities and to move to meet immediate goals. People who practice humanistic psychiatric nursing work to achieve flexibility in their relationships with clients and colleagues.

Feedback   Feedback is the process by which performance is checked and malfunctions corrected. It performs a regulatory function in the communication process. Feedback allows people to decide which messages have been understood as intended. It requires the cooperation of two persons—one to give it, and one to receive it.

Under certain circumstances of disturbed communication, feedback either fails or functions poorly. When messages do not get through or are distorted, appropriate replies cannot be obtained, and corrective feedback does not occur. Content that elicits anxiety, fear, shame, or any of several other strong emotions is likely to hamper feedback. Feedback is discussed in greater depth later in this chapter.

The Theory of Pragmatics of Human Communication

Watzlawick, Beavin, and Jackson (1967), based their theory of human communication on the assumption that communication is synonymous with interaction. These authors maintain that, in the presence of another, all behavior is communicative. This theory is concerned with the pragmatics, or the behavioral effects, of human interaction. Here, the term *pragmatics* refers to the interpersonal relation between communicators. What makes this theory particularly useful for this book is its conception of human communication as a reciprocal process.

Some Axioms of the Theory   According to this theory, one cannot *not* communicate. Both activity and inactivity, verbalizations and silences, convey messages. This communication occurs on two levels. The *content level* of a communication is the report aspect, in which information is conveyed. The *relationship level* is communication about a communication, a *metacommunication,* which says something about the relationship between the participants.

All interchanges can be viewed as either **symmetrical** (based on equality) or **complementary** (based on difference). In symmetric relationships, the partners usually mirror each other's behavior, thus minimizing difference. Complementary relationships, in contrast, maximize difference.

Disturbances in Human Communication Communication can be disturbed when a person attempts *not* to communicate. In this framework, the basic dilemma in schizophrenia is the schizophrenic person's attempt not to communicate. However, because it is impossible not to communicate, schizophrenics are faced with the need to deny that they are communicating while denying that this denial is a communication.

Another disturbance occurs when a person communicates in a way that invalidates the messages sent to or received from the other person. Such communications, called *disqualifications,* include a wide range of behavior: self-contradictions, inconsistencies, subject switches, incomplete sentences, misunderstandings, obscurities in style, literal interpretations of metaphors, and metaphorical interpretations of literal statements.

A person may communicate in a way that confirms, rejects, or disconfirms the other person's view of self. Confirmation of one person's self-view by another is thought to be the greatest single factor ensuring mental development and stability. Rejection of the other's definition of self essentially conveys this message: "You're wrong." Disconfirmation, by contrast, conveys this message: "You don't exist." Disconfirmation questions the other's authenticity. Disconfirmation leads to alienation and has been found to occur with some regularity in interactions between persons labeled schizophrenic and the members of their families.

Although all relationships are necessarily either symmetric or complementary, *runaways* (exaggerations to the point of disturbance) may occur in either of the patterns. For example, the danger of competitiveness is ever-present in symmetric relationships. Symmetric interactions that lose their stability may enter a spiral in which each individual attempts to be just a little bit "more equal" than the other. Runaways are seen in quarrels between people or wars between nations, behaviors that are relatively open. Rejection of the other's self generally occurs when a symmetric relationship breaks down.

Breakdowns in complementary relationships, however, are generally characterized by disconfirmations of the other. For this reason, they are usually viewed as more serious.

Ego States As Communication Analysis

Eric Berne's (1960) **transactional analysis** is a model of communication analysis proposing that a person may display the self from different psychologic positions. Transactional analysis (TA) is a method of therapy as well as a method of communication analysis. Transactional analysis theory is appropriate to this chapter because it is concerned with the changes in a person's posture, verbalization, voice, attitude, and feeling. Transactional analysis is both quick and easily understood. It is useful in brief contacts with clients or colleagues when there is little time to establish a rewarding relationship. Nurses can use TA concepts in understanding their own behavior as well.

Structural Analysis Each person has three main sources of behavior, or ego states—the Parent, the Adult, and the Child. The **Child** is manifested through archaic modes of communication and relationship as well as by childlike behavior similar to that of a child less than seven years old. Giggling, coyness, naïveté, charm, boisterousness, and whining are characteristics of the Child ego state. So are "I want"; "gosh"; "golly"; "me"; "mine"; "I dunno."

By the time children become adults, they learn that they must adapt the spontaneous and free expression of feelings in their natural state, the Natural Child ego state, to meet the demands and expectations of parents and the culture in which they live. Their adaptive behavior results in the Adapted Child ego state, which has two common manifestations: compliance with parents or other authority figures or rebellion and refusal to follow orders. Most people's Child falls somewhere between the two extremes.

Objective appraisal of reality and the capacity to process data are the domain of the **Adult**. The Adult is manifested in accomplishments beyond those of children, such as accurate analysis of complex realities and realistic manipulation of concepts. Perceptive skill, data processing, sociability, and communicativeness are attributed to the Adult. So are "it appears"; "I think"; "why"; "what"; "where"; "when"; "how."

The **Parent** incorporates the feelings and behaviors learned from parents or authority figures. A Parent ego state can be identified when the person's behavior includes the language, intonations, attitudes, postures, and mannerisms of one or both parents. All-wise, all-knowing, benevolent, prim, critical, or righteous attitudes are some examples. So are "if I were you"; "how many times have I told you"; "poor dear";

"disgusting"; "now what"; "do it this way." The Nurturing Parent ego state cuddles, protects, and cares for, while the Critical Parent ego state corrects or condemns.

Berne postulated that an individual exhibits a Parent or an Adult or a Child ego state, and that shifts can occur from one ego state to another. A nursing student, new to an in-patient unit of a community mental health center, reported her ego state switches in the following situation.

When I walked into the TV room to pick up the pen that I had left there, I saw a man pacing the floor; he was angrily muttering a string of obscenities (Adult ego state). I don't mind telling you that I was plenty scared. I was afraid that he might hurt me (Child ego state). I told myself that I should do something about reducing his anxiety and stress (Parent ego state). But, I felt so helpless and dumb (Child ego state). Then I decided that I really didn't know how to handle this situation and remembered something you said in class—that it's OK to ask for help—and I didn't feel scared or dumb any more. This has really turned into a good learning situation for me (Adult ego state).

In TA theory, structural analysis includes the determination of which ego state controls the executive power at a particular time. Spontaneity, charm, creativity, and enjoyment reside in the Child. The Adult not only is necessary for survival in dealing effectively with the outside world but also regulates and mediates the activities of the Parent and the Child. The Parent enables an individual to act effectively as a parent and makes many automatic responses that free the Adult from routine, trivial decisions. Each of the three ego states serves vital functions.

Ego States in Wellness/Illness Most of the time, persons who are ill or hospitalized are in a Child ego state. A stereotype in the general hospital setting is the "problem client" who is demanding, becomes extremely dependent, or refuses to follow a prescribed medical regimen. These problem clients are using the Adapted Child to cope with unfamiliar or frightening situations. The overly cheerful, overly friendly, or overly helpful client is less often identified as a problem but is also using the Adapted Child ego state to cope with the stress of hospitalization. The Child ego state is also at work in the client who is confused, disoriented, and enraged; who screams or strikes at others; or who withholds information because of fear of retaliation.

Sick people in their Parent ego state may be critical of hospital staff or suspicious of their intentions. Sometimes they nurture and protect other clients or even the staff. People in a Parent ego state are critical of themselves for being ill or unable to cope with the stresses of life. Such people berate themselves for

bothering staff, family, and friends. Some persons even hallucinate figures or voices that criticize them for their real or imagined transgressions.

The client in the Adult ego state contributes to wellness by deciding when to sleep or rest, whether to visit with friends or family, and what steps to take to decrease stress. People in this ego state are able to accept the temporary limitations imposed by illness or stress, to care for themselves within the imposed limitations, and to seek partnership in decisions about the directions of health care.

Obviously, the sick person in the Adult ego state is in the best possible situation under the circumstances. However, other ego states can also contribute to both illness and wellness. For example, persons in the Nurturing Parent ego state can allow themselves to be taken care of by others and may give themselves "permission" to be sick or to feel depressed. They are more likely to return quickly to a state of well-being than those who constantly berate themselves for being ill or succumbing to life's stresses. The Child ego state is helpful in achieving wellness, because it allows for the natural expression of feelings that can then be handled. Figure 8–6 shows these ego states in a wellness/illness relationship.

Transactional Analysis Whereas structural analysis is directed toward the analysis of the individual's personality, transactional analysis is broadened to focus on what occurs between two or more persons.

Complementary Transactions In **complementary transactions,** the transactional stimulus and the transactional response occur on identical ego levels. Transactions are complementary when a message sent to an ego state is responded to from that ego state. Complementary transactions can go on uninterrupted until one or the other of the participants changes ego state. Most of the time, productive communication occurs in complementary transactions, because the participants behave according to the perceived and predicted ego states of one another. However, continuing, or locked, complementary transactions—for instance, from Critical Parent to Adapted Child—result in uninterrupted but uncomfortable, nonfacilitative communication. The Parent-Child transaction of nurse and client in Figure 8–7 limits the client's growth. It encourages dependency and discourages responsibility.

Crossed Transactions **Crossed transactions** result from changes in ego states that terminate the complementary relationship. Figure 8–8 illustrates one such crossed transaction: The client tries to relate to the nurse on an Adult to Adult level, but the nurse responds on a Parent to Child level. In crossed transactions, communication is usually not smooth or satisfactory and is soon terminated. When complemen-

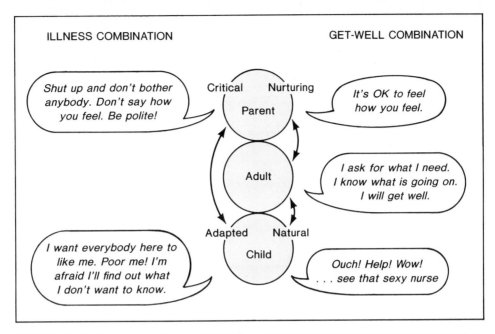

FIGURE 8–6 The wellness/illness relationship. *SOURCE: Elder J: Transactional Analysis in Health Care. Addison-Wesley, 1978, p 19.*

tary transactions become locked (and interpersonally uncomfortable), it may be useful to cross ego states to move the communication forward. For example, if a nurse is aware of having behaved like a Critical Parent to a client who responds from the Adapted Child state, the nurse can alter communication behavior by switching to Adult ego state. The client will probably follow this lead, leaving client and nurse better able to work together effectively.

Ulterior Transactions and Games Ulterior **transactions** are complex phenomena that occur on two levels—social (the surface, or overt one) and psychologic (the hidden, or covert one). **Games** are series of ulterior transactions with concealed motivations. Figure 8–9 shows an ulterior transaction as it occurs in the "Why don't you . . . Yes, but . . ." game. In this game, one person presents a problem to another person or to members of a group, who offer

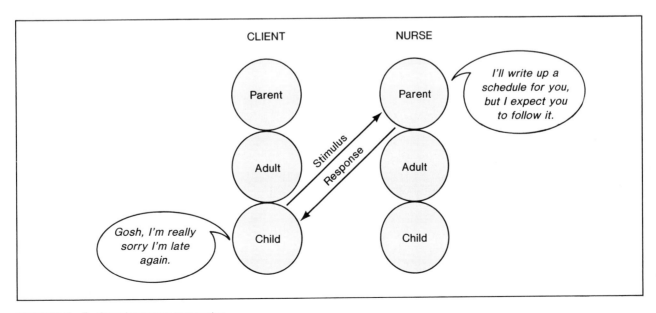

FIGURE 8–7 Complementary transaction.

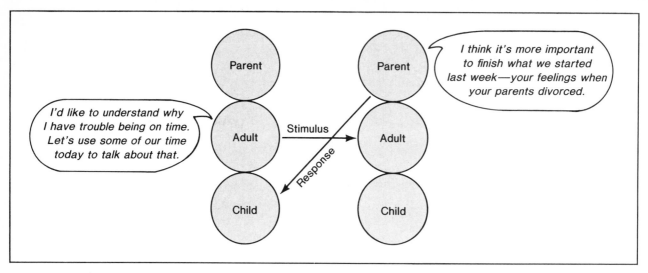

FIGURE 8—8 Crossed transaction.

solutions to the problem. The first player, however, rejects all solutions. The gimmick, or concealed motivation, is that, although this is supposedly an Adult request for information, the psychologic level is Child to Parent. The Child always wins, as the supposedly "wise" Parents are confounded and confused one by one.

Since the interactions are complementary at both social and psychologic levels, the game can be played indefinitely until the Parents give up or a more sophisticated person who recognizes what is happening breaks it up. "Why don't you . . . Yes, but . . ." can also take place in one-to-one relationships, particularly when it is a behavioral pattern of the client and the nurse is unaware of the psychologic level. The following interaction is typical of such a client-nurse situation. The client has been discussing her view of

the problems she has experienced since her mother-in-law moved in.

Nurse: The problem seems to be that you give in to your mother-in-law all the time. How about trying to talk to her?

Client: If I talk to her, it won't do any good. She'll just continue to act the same way.

Nurse: How about getting your husband to help?

Client: I'd ask him to talk to her, but he says that it's my house, so I should give the orders and there should be no problem.

Nurse: You mentioned that she has another son. Do you think that you could talk to him and work out some plan to have her live by herself?

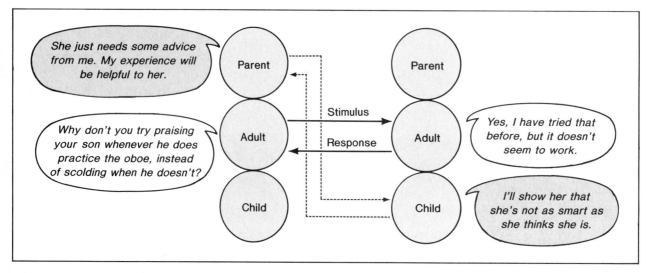

FIGURE 8—9 Ulterior transaction in "Why don't you . . . Yes, but . . ." game.

Client: No. We haven't talked to him in a long while, and anyway she doesn't have enough money to live on her own.

Nurse: How about a nursing home?

Client: We can't afford to send her to a nursing home.

Apparently giving up on finding a solution for the client's "mother-in-law problem," the nurse begins to work on other tangentially related household problems.

Nurse: You said that taking care of six children is quite a job. Do you think you could hire a baby-sitter to watch them in the afternoon?

Client: There's nobody in the neighborhood who I can get to sit. Either they're too young or they don't want to.

Nurse: Do you think you could hire someone to clean the house one day a week?

Client: Well, we could afford it, but my husband says that I don't need anyone to help me and that I could do everything by myself.

After the nurse assessed her own and her client's ego states, the game broke up, and the participants moved on to more productive communication. The nurse did so by moving into her Adult ego state, figuring out the dynamics and her contributions to them, and then changing her responses.

Analysis of Ego States in Clinical Practice

The transactional analysis of ego states helps nurses gain a better understanding of the processes and behaviors that take place in an interpersonal relationship. It is a way of viewing the self-in-process—i.e., the self changing in response to interaction with another self—a way of understanding a person in the process of becoming. It can be used to understand how ego states of participants—nurses as well as clients—help or hinder communication efforts.

Neurolinguistic Programming Theory

Neurolinguistic programming (NLP) is a communication model developed in the early 1970s by Richard Bandler and John Grinder (1975, 1976). The model is derived from theory in linguistics, neurophysiology, psychology, cybernetics, and psychiatry. Relatively new to nursing, NLP first appeared in the nursing literature in 1983 (Brockopp 1983, Knowles 1983).

Bandler and Grinder first observed psychotherapists who were known as expert communicators to discover what made them so effective as therapists. They concluded that people take in, or *access* information in three sensory modalities—the auditory, the

visual, and the kinesthetic modalities. Further, each person prefers one mode over the others. Sounds may facilitate communication with one person, while touch or sight may be more effective with another person. In addition, people also *process* information, or make sense out of it, according to the representational system (the NLP phrase for sensory modality) through which they receive it.

They also found that the expert communicators they observed were able to adapt themselves to match the client's representational system and to imitate the client in a natural and respectful way. Bandler and Grinder theorized that by tuning in to and then using the other person's preferred sensory mode, one could greatly enhance the ability to establish rapport. The most effective communicators, according to NLP theory, are those who can use all three modalities and easily move from one representational system to another.

Determining the Representational System   To determine whether a client's representational system is auditory, visual, or kinesthetic, one identifies the client's:

• Preferred predicates (verbs, adjectives, adverbs that tell something about the subject)

• Eye-accessing cues

• Gross hand movements

• Breathing pattern

• Speech pattern and voice tones

Preferred Predicates   The Assessment box on p 148 categorizes predicates according to the auditory, visual, and kinesthetic modes. A necessary first step before attempting to link words with nonverbal behavior is observing the client to see which set of predicates is preferred.

Eye-Accessing Cues   Eye-accessing cues correlate with an individual's thinking process. Persons who are visualizing generally turn their eyes upward or look straight ahead, focusing on nothing. Someone processing auditory information usually moves the eyes from side to side. A person engaging in intrapersonal communication usually focuses the eyes down in the direction of the nondominant hand. A person in the kinesthetic mode looks down toward the dominant hand when experiencing sensations or emotions.

Gross Hand Movements   Gross hand movements also give clues to the client's sensory mode. People have a tendency to point toward or touch the sense organ that matches their current sensory mode. The person in a visual mode often points toward the eye, and the person in an auditory mode often points toward or touches the ear.

ASSESSMENT

Preferred Predicates

Auditory	Visual	Kinesthetic
Argue	Appear	Attach
Chant	Bright	Breathless
Debate	Colorful	Calm
Eavesdrop	Glimpse	Excite
Hassle	Image	Fondle
Hear	Observe	Hurt
Listen	Pretty	Rough
Overhear	Scan	Sharp
Praise	Sight	Soft
Quiet	Spy	Sore
Scream	Stare	Support
Silent	Ugly	Tension
Tell	View	Throw
Whine	Watch	Touch
Whisper	Wink	Warm

SOURCE: *Adapted from* Neurolinguistic Programming Resource Manual. *American Society for Training and Development,* 1986.

Breathing Pattern   Assessing the breathing pattern helps the observer understand the client's representational model. Shallow, thoracic breathing is often associated with visual accessing. Even breathing or prolonged expiration is associated with auditory accessing, and deep abdominal breathing is associated with kinesthetic accessing.

Speech Pattern and Voice Tones   Visual accessing often correlates with quick bursts of words that are high pitched, strained, or nasal. Auditory accessing is often associated with a clear, midrange voice tone or with a rhythmic tempo and clearly enunciated words. Kinesthetic accessing is associated with a slow voice and a low volume or deep tone, or with a breathy tone and long pauses.

Therapeutic Use of NLP   Using NLP theory in psychiatric nursing practice gives us yet another way to empathize with clients by "trying on" their style. People tend to be less anxious with the familiar. Nurses who mirror the client's sensory mode are likely to be experienced as more comfortable and safer to be with, conditions that facilitate rapport.

Knowles (1983) suggests that nurses can use mirroring to help the client follow the nurse's lead. For example, with an anxious client, the nurse might begin by mirroring the behaviors that indicate the client's anxiety and then shift into a more relaxed posture and

less anxious behaviors. According to Knowles, the nurse can lead the client from a more anxious state to a less anxious state by employing the NLP principles discussed here.

An important benefit of the NLP approach is that it allows nurses to assess the client's style and preferred sensory mode and to communicate more effectively with clients by using both verbal and nonverbal communication in the client's preferred mode. Brockopp gives these examples of how to express the same nursing intervention with different predicates, depending on the client's preferred mode (Brockopp, 1983, p 1014):

Visual—"Yes, I can *see* that you are much better. you *look* good, your eyes are *clear,* your *appearance* has certainly changed."

Auditory—"Yes, I can *hear* from the *sound* of your *voice* that you are better. *Talking* with you today is quite different from yesterday."

Kinesthetic—"Yes, you do seem to be *feeling* much better today, you're *holding* your head up, and your *grasp* is certainly *firmer* than yesterday."

By expanding their abilities to communicate with clients in all three modes, nurses can become more effective communicators. This section is a brief introduction to some of the basic uses of NLP; see the references at the end of this chapter for further information.

Facilitative Communication

Facilitative communication aims at initiating, building, and maintaining fulfilling and trusting relationships with other people. Communicating ideas and feelings with clarity, efficiency, and appropriateness helps a person be interpersonally effective. In reading the rest of this chapter, try to relate the therapeutic communication principles and practices discussed earlier to these ideas about facilitative communication.

Social Superficiality versus Facilitative Intimacy

Most relationships between people begin at the level of social superficiality. In a client-nurse relationship, we try to develop facilitative intimacy, which differs from social intimacy. For example, the interdependence that characterizes the social relationship is greatly reduced. In social relationships participants may "tell their stories" to one another. In facilitative relationships that have therapeutic goals, only the client is engaged in storytelling with the nurse. The progress is specifically focused. Clients not only explain themselves, the events of their lives, and the circumstances they face but also do so with a purpose in mind—understanding the circumstances through exploring them and moving to improve the circumstances of their lives.

The movement toward therapeutic intimacy may be difficult at first. For one thing, such intimacy violates certain social taboos. For example, at a cocktail party it may be socially incorrect to comment on a person's anxiety, stuttering, or facial tic. During facilitative and therapeutic communication, all messages, including these nonverbal ones, are heeded and may be discussed.

Therapeutic intimacy also requires that the participants move beyond social chitchat into meaningful areas of concern for the client. Therapeutic intimacy requires high involvement and commitment.

Essential Ingredients

Several interpersonal principles and practices are essential to the achievement of facilitative intimacy.

Responding with Empathy   Most theorists believe that empathy is the most important dimension in the helping process. Without a high level of empathic understanding, nurses have no real basis for helping. Empathy facilitates interpersonal exploration.

Responding with Respect   Responding with respect demonstrates that the nurse values the integrity of the client and has faith in the client's ability to solve problems, given appropriate help. By encouraging clients to put forward possible plans of action, the nurse conveys respect for their ability to take charge of their own destiny. Giving advice, by contrast, conveys a directly opposite message.

Responding with Genuineness   Genuineness refers to the ability to be real or honest with another. To be effective, genuineness must be timed properly and based on a solid relationship. Honesty is not always the best policy, especially if it is brutal or if the client is not capable of dealing with it.

Clients who can experience the authenticity of the nurse can risk greater genuineness and authenticity themselves. The nurse who is genuine is more likely to deal with and eventually help the client resolve real problems rather than just those that are safe or socially acceptable.

Responding with Immediacy   Responding with immediacy means responding to what is happening between the client and the nurse in the here-and-now. Because this dimension may involve the feelings of the client toward the nurse, it can be one of the most difficult to achieve. For example, the client may confront the nurse with overt or implied criticism of the nurse's role or competence. If the nurse responds in a defensive or evasive way, the relationship may be threatened. If the nurse is open, reasonable, and concerned, the relationship may be strengthened. However, by focusing attention on the relationship too early, the nurse can hinder the formation of an adequate base.

Responding with Warmth   Warmth is so closely linked with empathy and respect that it is seldom communicated as an independent dimension. It is important, however, to note some additional points about the expression of warmth. Effusive, chatty, "buddy-buddy" behavior should not be confused with warmth. Warmth is most often conveyed in communications of respect and empathy.

The nurse should be aware of and accept the client's right to maintain distance. Warmth and intimacy cannot be forced. Initially high levels of warmth can be counterproductive for clients who have received little warmth from others in their lives or have been taken advantage of by others. Warmth alone is insufficient for building a relationship and solving problems.

Facilitative Communication Skills

To present a how-to manual or cookbook of communication skills goes against the thrust of the book. Using a set of communication skills as a sort of relationship "magic" is antihumanistic in many ways. Relationships, and the people in them, are unique and much too complex for the nurse to rely on a formula for facilitative communication. The following skills are therefore presented with many misgivings. It is important to remember that a holistic approach essentially precludes the rigid, inflexible application of communication techniques. Those presented here should be viewed as having the potential to foster effective communication. They must be adapted individually for each human encounter.

Reflecting Content   **Reflecting** is repeating the client's verbal or nonverbal message for the client's benefit. In reflecting the *content* of the message, the nurse basically repeats the client's statement. This gives clients the opportunity to hear and mull over what they have told the nurse.

- "You believe things will be better soon."

- "You think it would be better to take a part-time job."

Content reflection is perhaps one of the most misused and overused methods in mental health counseling. It loses its effectiveness when used for lack of other choices.

Reflecting Feelings Reflecting *feelings* is verbalizing the implied feelings in the client's comment.

- "Sounds like you're really angry at your brother."

- "You're feeling uncomfortable about being discharged from the hospital."

In reflecting feelings, the nurse attempts to identify latent and connotative meanings that may either clarify or distort the content. Reflection is useful because it encourages the client to make additional clarifying comments.

Imparting Information Imparting **information** is helping the client by supplying additional data. This therefore encourages further clarification based on new or additional input.

- "Group therapy will be held on Tuesday evening from 6:30 until 8:00."

- "I am a psychiatric nurse."

It is not constructive to withhold useful information from the client or to reply "What do you think?" to a straightforward, information-seeking question. However, the nurse must be careful not to cross the line between giving information and giving advice or give information as a way of avoiding an area of interpersonal difficulty. Also, the nurse who gives personal, social information may move out of the realm of therapeutic intervention.

Clarifying Clarifying is an attempt to understand the basic nature of a client's statement.

- "I'm confused about. . . . Could you go over that again, please."

- "You say you're feeling anxious now. What's that like for you?"

Asking the client to give an example to clarify a meaning helps the nurse understand the client's intended message better. A person who describes a concrete incident is more likely to see the connections between it and similar occurrences. Illustrations are very useful qualifiers.

Paraphrasing In **paraphrasing,** the nurse assimilates and restates what the client has said.

- "In other words, you're fed up with being treated like a child."

- "I hear you saying that when people compliment you, you feel embarrassed. If they knew the real you, they'd stay away."

Paraphrasing gives nurses the opportunity to test their understanding of what a client is attempting to communicate. It is reflective in nature, in that it lets the client know how another person is understanding the message.

Checking Perceptions Checking perceptions means sharing how one person perceives and hears another. After sharing perceptions of the client's behaviors, thoughts, and feelings, the nurse asks the client to verify the perception.

- "Let me know if this is how you see it too."

- "I get the feeling that you're uncomfortable when we're silent. Does that seem to fit?"

Nurses use perception checks to make sure that they understand a client. An effective perception check conveys the message "I want to understand. . . ." It allows the other person the opportunity to correct inaccurate perceptions. It also allows the nurse to avoid actions based on false assumptions about the client.

Questioning Questioning is a very direct way of speaking with clients. But when used to excess, questioning controls the nature and range of the client's responses. Questions can be useful when the nurse is seeking specific information. When the nurse's intent is to engage the client in meaningful dialogue, however, questions should be limited.

When the nurse is using questions, it is best to make them open-ended rather than closed. An *open-ended question* focuses the topic but allows freedom of response.

- "How were you feeling when your mother said that to you?"

- "What's your opinion about . . . ?"

The *closed question* limits the client's choice of responses, generally to "yes" or "no" ("Were you feeling angry when your mother said that?"). Closed questions limit therapeutic exploration.

"Why" questions usually have the same effect. They often are impossible to answer and rarely lead to a clearer understanding of the situation. However, "who," "what," "when," and "how" questions may be helpful when used judiciously.

Structuring Structuring is an attempt to create order or evolve guidelines. The nurse helps the client to become aware of problems and the order in which the client might deal with them.

- "You've mentioned that you want to improve your relationships with your wife, your sister, and your boss. Let's put them in order of priority."

- "No, I won't be giving you advice, but we can discuss the possible solutions together."

Structuring is particularly useful when clients introduce a number of concerns in a brief period and have little idea of which to begin work on. Nurses use structuring not only to explore content but also to delimit the parameters of the nurse-client relationship and to identify how the nurse will participate with the client in the problem-solving process.

Pinpointing **Pinpointing** calls attention to certain kinds of statements and relationships. For example, the nurse may point to inconsistencies among statements, to similarities and differences in the points of view, feelings, or actions of two or more persons, or to differences between what one says and what one does.

- "So, you and your wife don't agree about how many children you want."

- "You say you're sad, but you're smiling."

Linking In **linking,** the nurse responds to the client in a way that ties together two events, experiences, feelings, or persons. The nurse can use linking to connect past experiences with current behaviors. Another example is linking the tension between two persons with current life stress.

- "You felt depressed after the birth of both your children."

- "So the arguments didn't really begin until after you got your promotion."

Giving Feedback   **Feedback** helps others become aware of how their behavior affects us and how we perceive their actions. Responding with feedback can be therapeutic self-disclosure. It allows the nurse to offer clients constructive information that makes them aware of their effect on others. Total self-disclosure by the nurse is inappropriate in the nurse-client relationship. It places a burden of interdependence on the client and limits the time and energy available to work on the client's concerns. Reciprocal self-disclosure is more appropriate in friend and colleague relationships.

- "When you wring your hands I feel anxious."

- "Sometimes when you turn your head away from me I think you're angry."

It is important to give feedback in a way that does not threaten the client and increase defensiveness. The more defensive the client, the less likely the client will hear and understand the feedback. The Intervention box on page 152 lists some characteristics of helpful, nonthreatening feedback.

Confronting Constructive confrontations often lead to productive change. **Confronting** is a deliberate invitation to examine some aspect of personal behav-

ior that indicates a discrepancy between what the person says and what the person does. Confrontation requires careful attention to nonverbal communication and the discrepancies between nonverbal and verbal messages.

Confrontations may be informational or interpretive, and they may be directed toward both the resources and the limitations of the client. An **informational confrontation** describes the visible behavior of another person. An **interpretive confrontation** expresses thoughts and feelings about the other's behavior and includes drawing inferences about the meaning of the behavior.

- "You say you're 'the dummy in the family,' yet none of your brothers or sisters made the honor roll like you did."

- "Ever since Sally and Joe criticized the way you conducted the meeting, you haven't spoken to them. It looks like you're feeling angry."

Six skills to be incorporated in constructive confrontations are:

1. Use of personal statements with the words *I, my,* and *me*

2. Use of relationship statements expressing what the nurse thinks or feels about the client in the here and now

3. Use of behavior descriptions (statements describing the visible behavior of the client)

4. Use of description of personal feelings, specifying the feeling by name

5. Use of responses aimed at understanding, such as paraphrasing and perception checking

6. Use of constructive feedback skills (see the Intervention box on page 151)

Summarizing   **Summarizing** is the highlighting of the main ideas expressed in an interaction. Both the client and the nurse benefit from this review of the main themes of the conversation. Summarizing is also useful in focusing the client's thinking and aiding conscious learning.

- "The last time we were together you were concerned about. . . ."

- "You had three main concerns today. . . ."

The nurse can use this technique appropriately at different times during an interaction. For example, it is useful to summarize the previous interaction in the first few minutes the nurse and the client spend together. Early summarizing helps the client recall the areas discussed and gives the client the opportunity to see how the nurse has synthesized the content of a

INTERVENTION

Characteristics of Helpful, Nonthreatening Feedback

Strategy	Rationale	Strategy	Rationale
Focus feedback on behavior rather than on client.	Refer to what client actually does rather than how nurse imagines client to be.	Focus feedback on exploration of alternatives rather than answers or solutions.	Focusing on variety of alternatives for accomplishing a particular goal prevents premature acceptance of answers or solutions that may not be appropriate.
Focus feedback on observations rather than inferences.	Refer to what nurse actually sees or hears client do; inferences refer to conclusions or assumptions nurse makes about client.	Focus feedback on its value to client rather than on catharsis it provides nurse.	Feedback should serve needs of client, not needs of nurse.
Focus feedback on description rather than judgment.	Report what occurred rather than evaluating it in terms of good or bad, right or wrong.	Limit feedback to amount of information client is able to use rather than amount nurse has available to give.	Overloading will decrease effectiveness of feedback.
Focus feedback on "more or less" rather than "either/or" descriptions of behavior.	"More or less" descriptions stress quantity rather than quality (which may be value laden).	Limit feedback to appropriate time and place.	Excellent feedback presented at an inappropriate time may be ineffective or harmful.
Focus feedback on here-and-now behavior rather than there-and-then behavior.	The most meaningful feedback is given as soon as it is appropriate to do so.	Focus feedback on what is said rather than why it is said.	Focusing on why things are said or done moves away from observations and toward motive or intent (which can only be assumed, unless verified).
Focus feedback on sharing of information and ideas rather than advice.	Sharing ideas and information helps client make decisions about own well-being; giving advice takes away client's freedom to be self-determining.		

previous session. Summarizing is useful because it keeps the participants directed toward a goal.

Injudicious use of summarizing is a common pitfall. A nurse may rush to summarize despite other, more pressing and immediate client concerns. In this instance, summarizing is likely to meet the nurse's needs for structure but does nothing to address the client's here-and-now concerns.

Processing   **Processing** is a complex and sophisticated technique. Process comments direct attention to the interpersonal dynamics of the nurse-client experience. These dynamics are illustrated in the content, feelings, and behavior expressed.

• "It seems that important things that need to be taken care of come up in the last five minutes we have together in our session."

• "Today is the first day our session has started out with silence. Last week it seemed there wouldn't be enough time."

Processing is most useful when therapeutic intimacy has been achieved.

Ineffective Communication Styles

The three clinical situations presented below are meant to show some unhelpful or even harmful ways of responding to clients (adapted from Gazda 1973, pp 62–65). They illustrate a few of the common response styles that do not facilitate constructive communication. An example of a helpful response is given at the end of each of the situations.

Situation 1
Client: They wouldn't let me join their pinochle game!

Responses that are not helpful:

Detective: Who wouldn't?

Detectives are eager to track down the facts of the case. They grill the client about the details of what happened and respond to this factual content instead of paying attention to feelings. Detectives control the flow of the conversation, often putting the client on the defensive.

Magician: It's time to eat dinner, so it doesn't matter now, does it?

Magicians try to make the problem disappear by telling the client it isn't there. This illusion is not lasting. Denying the existence of a problem denies the validity of the client's own experience and perception.

Manager: Would you help me get everyone together for the picnic?

Managers believe that they can make the client forget the problem by keeping the client too busy to think about it. This conveys the message that the task the manager has assigned is more important than the client's problem. An effective nurse communicates awareness of the magnitude of any particular problem to the client.

Judge: Remember yesterday when you didn't play fair? Of course they wouldn't want to play with you today!

Judges give rational explanations to show that the client's past actions have caused the present situation—that the client is the guilty party. Although such responses may be accurate, they are rarely helpful, because they are premature—they are being given before the client is ready to accept and use them.

Responses that are helpful:

"It hurts to be turned down!" or "That hurt!"

Situation 2

Client: You asked me to chair the community meeting next week, but I can't do that. Please get somebody else. Anybody would be better than me.

Responses that are not helpful:

Drill sergeant: Later tonight figure out what each person should do. Give them assignments and make sure they work on it some each day. Get organized now and it will come out fine.

Drill sergeants give orders and expect them to be obeyed. Because they know just what the client should do, they see no need to give explanations, listen to the client's feelings, or explain their commands to the client.

Guru: You won't find out what you can do if you don't try new things. It's better to try and fail than not to try at all.

Gurus dispense proverbs and clichés on every occasion, as though they were the sole possessors of the accumulated wisdom of the ages. Unfortunately, their words are too impersonal and general to apply to any individual's situation with force or accuracy, and often the sayings are too trite to be noticed at all.

Magician: You don't *really* mean that do you?

Responses that are helpful:

"You're sort of afraid to accept this responsibility. It looks like more than you can handle."

Situation 3

Client: I don't know what to do with my kids! They won't listen!

Responses that are not helpful:

Detective: What's causing the problem?

Florist: With all your ability? I can't believe that! Why, you're such a good parent.

Florists are uncomfortable talking about anything unpleasant, so they gush flowery phrases to keep the client's problem at a safe distance. Florists mistakenly think that the way to be helpful is to hide the problem under bouquets of optimism.

Judge: You know, you got off to a bad start with your kids. You are going to have a hard time changing them.

Sign painter: You're a born pessimist!

Sign painters think that naming a problem solves it. They have an unlimited inventory of labels to affix to persons and their problems.

Drill sergeant: First get them all tested psychologically. Then write up some behavior contracts. Keep your kids busy with simple projects. Then . . .

Guru: Things always look the worst before they get better.

Prophet: If you don't get some results with them pretty soon there will be trouble!

Prophets know and predict exactly what is going to happen. By declaring the forecast, prophets relieve themselves of responsibility. They sit back to let the prophecy come true.

Magician: You're imagining things. They're good kids, and you know it. They're a lot better than you give them credit for!

Responses that are helpful:

"I guess it gets you down when you do all you know how to do and then don't get results."

CHAPTER HIGHLIGHTS

• Communication is an ongoing, dynamic, and ever-changing series of events, each of which affects all others; it is the mechanism by which people establish, maintain, and improve their human contacts.

• Meaning cannot be transferred from one human being to another but must be mutually negotiated between persons. Words and gestures do not "mean" something, people do.

• Communication takes place on intrapersonal, interpersonal, and public levels and includes nonverbal messages that are interrelated with the spoken word.

- Relationships with clients are initiated, built, and maintained through the vehicle of interpersonal communication.

- To help clients deal with problems, nurses need to be aware of how their own perceptions, values, and culture influence the way they process information about the world.

- The symbolic interactionist view of human communication posits that (a) after a series of internal trials people reflect and transmit the message they believe has the highest chance of success; (b) success depends upon the accuracy and completeness of the person's "cognitive map" of the environment and of the intrapersonal and interpersonal feedback loops; (c) communication is a complex, dynamic process in which the meaning of messages is mutually negotiated, not merely transferred.

- Nonverbal communication channels that help us judge the reliability of a message include facial expressions; hand gestures; body movements; use of space, voice, and touch; and body aroma.

- In the development of the client-nurse relationship, a major focus is the development of facilitative intimacy.

- Facilitative intimacy is enhanced when nurses respond with empathy, respect, genuineness, immediacy, and warmth.

- Relationships are unique and too complex for a set of rigid, inflexible communication techniques to be consistent with humanistic psychiatric nursing practice.

- Communication skills that may foster facilitative communication include reflecting content, reflecting feelings, imparting information, clarifying, paraphrasing, checking perceptions, questioning, structuring, pinpointing, linking, giving feedback, confronting, summarizing, and processing.

REFERENCES

American Society for Training and Development: *Neurolinguistic Programming Resource Manual*. The Society, 1986.

Argyle, M: *The Psychology of Interpersonal Behavior*. Penguin, 1967.

Bandler R, Grinder J: *The Structure of Magic*. Science and Behavior Books, 1975, vol 1.

Bandler R, Grinder J: *The Structure of Magic*. Science and Behavior Books, 1976, vol 2.

Berne E: *Games People Play*. Grove Press, 1964.

Berne E: *Transactional Analysis in Psychotherapy*. Grove Press, 1960.

Bowlby J: *Maternal Care and Mental Health,* ed 2, World Health Organization, 1951.

Brockopp D: What is NLP? *Am J Nurs* 1983;83:1012–1014.

Carroll L: *Through the Looking Glass and What Alice Found There*. Random House, 1965.

Davis AJ: *Listening and Responding*. Mosby, 1984.

Duldt B, Griffin K, Patton B: *Interpersonal Communication in Nursing*. F.A. Davis, 1984.

Elder J: *Transactional Analysis in Health Care*. Addison-Wesley, 1978.

Fritz PA et al.: *Interpersonal Communication in Nursing: An Interactionist Approach*. Appleton-Century-Crofts, 1984.

Gazda GM: *Human Relations Development*. Allyn and Bacon, 1973.

Gazda G, Childers W, Walters R: *Interpersonal communication: A Handbook for Health Professionals*. Aspen, 1982.

Goffman E: *Behavior in Public Places*. Free Press, 1963.

Heineken J: Treating the disconfirmed psychiatric client. *J Psychosoc Nurs* 1983;21(1):21–25.

Hulett JE Jr: A symbolic interactionist model of human communication. *A V Communication Review* 1966; 14:5–33.

Kasch C: Interpersonal competence and communication in the delivery of nursing care. *Adv Nurs Sci* 1984; 6(2):71–88.

Knowles RD: Building rapport: Through neuro-linguistic programming. *Am J Nurs* 1983;83:1011–1014.

Nigro A, Maggio J: A neglected need: Health education for the mentally ill. *J Psychosoc Nurs* 1990;28(7):15–19.

Pelletier LR: Interpersonal communications task group. *J Psychosoc Nurs* 1983;21(9):33–36.

Ricci M: An experiment with personal space invasion in the nurse-patient relationship and its effect on anxiety. *Issues Ment Health Nurs* 1981;3(3):203–218.

Rosenberg L: The use of therapeutic correspondence: Creative approaches in psychotherapy. *J Psychosoc Nurs* 1990;28(11):29–33.

Ruesch J: *Therapeutic Communication*. W. W. Norton, 1961.

Ruesch J, Bateson G: *Communication: The Social Matrix of Psychiatry*. W. W. Norton, 1968.

Sluder H: The write way: Using poetry for self-disclosure. *J Psychosoc Nurs* 1990;28(7):26–28.

Stewart CJ, Cash WB: *Interviewing Principles and Practices,* ed 4. William C. Brown, 1985.

Tommasini NR: The use of touch with the hospitalized psychiatric patient. *Arch Psychiatr Nurs* 1990;4(4):213–220.

Watzlawick P, Beavin J, Jackson D: *The Pragmatics of Human Communication*. New York: W. W. Norton, 1967.

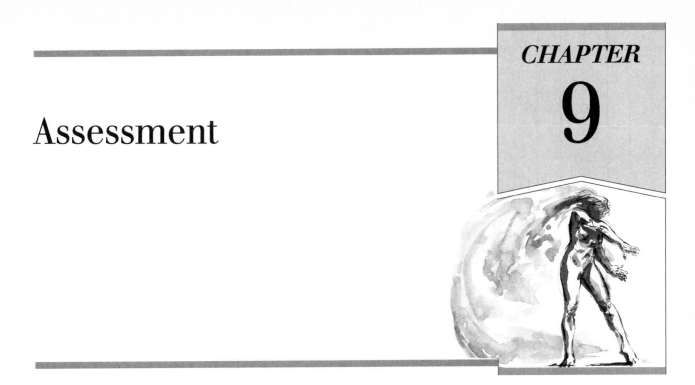

Assessment

Holly Skodol Wilson
Carol Ren Kneisl

LEARNING OBJECTIVES

- Describe the processes of psychiatric history taking, mental status examination, neurologic assessment, and physiologic and psychologic testing

- Discuss the DSM-III-R multiaxial system for making a psychiatric diagnosis

- Evaluate the DSM-III-R's congruence with nursing diagnoses

- Describe the process of individual psychosocial assessment

- Discuss the differences between processes of source-oriented and problem-oriented systems of recording

- Identify methods of recording verbatim nurse-client interactions

- Comprehend the organization and function of the Interaction Process Analysis (IPA)

CROSS REFERENCES

Other topics relevant to this content are: Assessing clients with mood disorders, Chapter 13; Assessing clients with organic mental disorders, Chapter 10; Assessing clients with psychoactive substance use disorders, Chapter 11; Assessing clients with schizophrenic disorders, Chapter 12; Family characteristics and dynamics, Chapter 30; Group process, Chapter 29; Nursing process, Chapter 3; and Suicide assessment, Chapter 23.

THE SYSTEMATIC SCIENTIFIC APPROACH known among nurses as the *nursing process* has evolved as the cornerstone of clinical practice. The nursing process begins with assessment for the purpose of collecting and analyzing objective and subjective data about the clients with whom nurses work. The primary sources of client data in most instances are the clients themselves. Psychologic tests, nurses' notes, physicians' orders, and other secondary data sources can enlarge, clarify, and substantiate data obtained directly from the client.

Collecting, Assessing, and Recording Client Data

The Psychiatric Examination

Systems of collection and assessment vary among mental health agencies. The psychiatric examination consists of two parts: psychiatric history and mental status exam. It is most often done during initial or early interactions with a client. It is often seen as a function of the psychiatrist, because a major goal of the examination is making a psychiatric diagnosis, although in some agencies the psychiatric examination has become the responsibility of the intake worker. The traditional psychiatric examination is discussed in this chapter because it is still used in settings in which psychiatric nurses work and is considered the counterpart of the physical examination and history.

In less traditional settings, the psychiatric history and the mental status examination have given way to the *psychosocial assessment*—an assessment of the social and psychologic data gathered from interaction with the client. The primary goals of a psychosocial assessment are to make a psychiatric diagnosis and assess the client's difficulties in living.

Initial Contact Form   The initial contact form (Figure 9–1) is filled in before the history and mental status exam are done. It provides basic demographic and problem information at the time the client requests service or is referred by another person or agency. This information should provide the clinician with enough data to make some early key decisions.

• How urgent is the situation? (See the accompanying Assessment box.)

• Who is to be assigned responsibility for proceeding with the next step?

• What type of response is indicated as "the next step"?

This form is used chiefly by the member of the mental health team designated to handle all incoming calls and requests for service during a specified period of time.

The Psychiatric History

Data Sources   Not all data gathered during psychiatric history-taking are obtained from the client. There are several other sources. Family, friends, police, mental health personnel, and others may contribute data to the **psychiatric history.** When the sources are varied, the psychiatric history focuses on the perceptions of others: how they see the client and the circumstances of the client's life. The sources of the psychiatric history and their relationship to the client should always be clearly indicated. Information given by these sources should be reviewed and understood in terms of that relationship.

ASSESSMENT

Crisis Rating: How Urgent Is Your Need for Help?

• *Very urgent:* Service request requires an immediate response within minutes; e.g., crisis outreach; medical emergency—requiring an ambulance to be called (overdoses); severe drug reaction; police contacted if situation involves extreme danger or weapons.

• *Urgent:* Response requires rapid but not necessarily immediate response, within a few hours. Example: low/moderate risk of suicide, mild drug reaction.

• *Somewhat urgent:* Response should be made within a day (approximately 24 hours). Example: planning conference in which key persons are not available until the following evening.

• *Slightly urgent:* A response is required within a few days. Example: client's funding runs out within a week, and client needs public assistance.

• *Not urgent:* A situation has existed for a long time and does not warrant immediate intervention; a week or two is unlikely to cause any significant difference. Example: child with a learning disability, certain types of marital counseling.

INITIAL CONTACT SHEET

Today's Date _12-4-91_

Time __9__ AM
    PM

Walk-in _____
Phone ___✓___
Outreach _____
Written _____

ID # _____
SS # _123-45-6789_
Welfare /
Medicaid # _____

SERVICE REQUESTED FOR

Client's NAME __Mary__ __Jane__ __Smith__
         First   Middle   Last

Permanent ___✓___
Temporary _____

Address _1 Success Drive_ __West Egg, N.Y.__ _10101_ _____
     Street   City / Town   Zip   County

Catchment Area _____

Phone # _666-1234_ Means of Transportation _Auto_

Directions to home _____
(if outreach) _____

Sex __ Male _____   Date of Birth _1-14-43_   Age _48 yrs_ _____
    Female __✓__

SERVICE REQUESTED BY

☐ AGENCY   Name _____   Phone # _____
☐ OTHER   Address _____   Time(s) seen by
☑ SELF   If Agency-Contact Person _____   the agency _____

PRESENTING SITUATION / PROBLEM - What made you decide to seek help today?
    (use other side if needed)

Feeling depressed about relationship with husband and life in general. Difficulty sleeping, low energy level, "I need to get help."

Have you talked with anyone about this?   Yes _____ Who? _____
Address _____   No ___✓___   Phone # _____
                    Date of last contact _____

Are you taking ANY medication now?   Yes ___✓___   What? 1. _Valium_
    (If more than 3 begin list on MH-2) No _____   2. _Dalamane_

CRISIS RATING How urgent is your need for help?   3. _Aspirin_
☐ Immediate (within minutes)
☐ Within a few hours
☐ Within 24 hours
☐ Within a few days
☑ Within a week or two

	Comments

DISPOSITION (Check all that apply)
☐ Crisis
☐ Medical Emergency
☐ Assessment (specify) _____
☐ Discharge Planning
☐ Expediting / Advocacy
☐ Other (explain) _____

Intelligent housewife with marital problems — would probably benefit from counseling and perhaps couples group later

☑ Referral made to _Individual Counseling_ _____   Confirmed—Yes _✓_ No _____ Date _12-14-91_
Date of Next Contact _12-15-91_ _____ Assigned to _____
Date of Assignment _____ Request taken by _____

MH-1

FIGURE 9–1   Initial contact sheet.   SOURCE: *Reproduced by permission of the Erie County Department of Mental Health; Mental Health Services, Erie County, Corporation IV, South East Corporation V, and Lakeshore Corporation VI.*

Categories of Data   The psychiatric history generally includes the following information:

• *Complaint*—the main reason the client is having a psychiatric examination. The client may have personally initiated the psychiatric examination, or others (courts, hospital staff, family, referral from school or industry) may have initiated it. The "chief complaint" should be recorded verbatim and indicated as such with quotation marks in the write-up ("I just don't want to live any longer" or "My drug use has become unmanageable").

• *Present symptoms*—the nature of the onset and the development of symptoms. These data are usually traced from the present to the last period of adaptive functioning.

• *Previous hospitalizations and mental health treatment.*

• *Family history*—generally, whether any family members have ever sought or received mental health treatment.

• *Personal history*—the person's birth and development; past and recent illnesses; schooling and educational problems; occupation; sexual development, interests, and practices; marital history; use of alcohol, drugs, and tobacco; and religious practices.

• *Personality*—the client's relationships with others, moods, feelings, interests, and leisure-time activities.

The main purpose of history-taking is to gather information, although it is often effective in establishing rapport with a client. The interviewer can promote rapport by avoiding an interrogative approach and allowing the client's story to unfold naturally.

The Mental Status Examination*

The **mental status examination** is usually a standardized procedure in agencies that use it. Its primary purpose is to help the examiner gather more objective data to be used in determining etiology, diagnosis, prognosis, and treatment. The sections of the mental status examination that deal with *sensorium* and *intellect* are particularly important in determining the existence of organic brain disease. The purpose of this examination differs from that of psychiatric history in that it identifies the person's *present* mental status.

The mental status examiner generally seeks the following categories of information, not necessarily in the sequence presented here.

1. *General behavior, appearance, and attitude*—a complete and accurate description of the client's physical characteristics, apparent age, manner of dress, use of cosmetics, personal hygiene, and responses to the examiner. Postures, gait, gestures, facial expression, and mannerisms are included in the description. The examiner also notes the client's general activity level.

A 35-year-old white male, dressed in torn, disheveled jeans. Presented a blank facial expression, slouched posture, shuffling gait, generally low activity level, and sullen behavior.

---

*Reprinted with permission of Sandoz Pharmaceuticals, Division of Sandoz, Inc. From Small SM: *Outline for Psychiatric Examination,* 1980.

RESEARCH NOTE

Citation
Cox C: *The health self-determination index.* Nurs Res 1985;34:177–183.

Study Problem/Purpose
To conduct a psychometric evaluation of a new measure of motivation in health behavior titled the Health Determinism Index.

Methods
The Health Determinism Index was completed by 202 randomly selected adults via a mail survey. The multidimensionality of the construct basic to this index was examined through factorial isolation for four subscales: self-determined health judgments, self-determined health behaviors, perceived competency in health matters, and internal-external cue responsiveness.

Findings
The four factors accounted for 56 percent of the total variance in the measure. The reliability coefficient for the total scale was 84, the internal consistency of the four subscales was supported by similar alpha reliability coefficients.

Implications
This instrument offers a means of examining nursing's ability to alter clients' motivation in relation to specific health behaviors. It also offers a basis for beginning a study of the role of motivation in health outcomes.

Other descriptors that may be used include "frank," "friendly," "irritable," "dramatic," "evasive," "indifferent," and so forth. Details should be sufficient to identify and characterize the client.

2. *Characteristics of talk*—the form, rather than the content, of the client's speech. The speech is described in terms of loudness, flow, speed, quantity, level of coherence, and logic. A sample of the client's conversation with the examiner may be included in quotation marks. The goal is to describe the quantity and quality of speech to discern difficulties in thought processes. The following patterns, if present, should be particularly noted.

a. *Mutism*—no verbal response despite indications that the client is aware of the examiner's questions.

b. *Circumstantiality*—cumbersome, convoluted, and unnecessary detail in response to answer the interviewer's questions.

c. *Perseveration*—a pattern of repeating the same words or movements despite apparent efforts to make a new response.

d. *Flight of ideas*—rapid, overly productive responses to questions that seem related only by chance associations between one sentence fragment and another. Associated with flight of ideas might be rhyming, clang associations, punning, and evidence of distractibility.

e. *Blocking*—a pattern of sudden silence in the stream of conversation for no obvious reason but often thought to be associated with intrusion of delusional thoughts or hallucinations.

3. *Emotional state*—the person's pervasive or dominant mood or affective reaction. Both subjective and objective data are included. Subjective data are obtained through the use of nonleading questions, for instance, "How are you feeling?" If the client replies with general terms, such as "nervous," the interviewer should ask the client to describe how the nervousness shows itself and its effect, since such words may mean different things to different individuals. The examiner should observe objective signs, such as facial expression, motor behavior, the presence of tears, flushing, sweating, tachycardia, tremors, respiratory irregularities, states of excitement, fear, and depression. The attitude of the client toward the examiner sometimes offers valuable clues. Attitudes of hostility, suspiciousness, or flirtatiousness, a desire for bodily contact, or outspoken criticisms should be noted.

The psychiatric client is apt to have a persistent emotional trend reflective of a particular emotional disorder, such as depression. If this is true, the examiner should probe further to discover the intensity and persistence of this reaction.

It is desirable to record verbatim the replies to questions concerning the client's mood. The relationship between mood and the content of thought is particularly significant. There may be a wide divergence between what clients say or do and their emotional state as expressed by attitudes or facial expressions.

Note whether intense emotional responses accompany discussion of specific topics. *Shallowness* or *flattening of the affect* is indicated by an insufficiently intense emotional display in association with ideas or situations that ordinarily would call for a stronger response.

Dissociation or *disharmony* is often indicated by an inappropriate emotional response, such as smiling or silly behavior, when the attitude should be one of concern, anxiety, or sadness.

It is difficult to evaluate emotional reactions in clients who use *simulation* or play-acting. Clients who are trying to cover up a deep depression may feign cheerfulness and good spirits. The reverse may also be true.

The client's emotional reactions may be constant or may fluctuate during the examination. Try to specify the ease or readiness with which such changes occur in response to pleasant or unpleasant stimuli. Use such terms as the following to indicate intensity of response:

• Composed, complacent, frank, friendly, playful, teasing, silly, cheerful, boastful, elated, grandiose, ecstatic

• Tense, worried, anxious, pessimistic, sad, perplexed, bewildered, gloomy, depressed, frightened

• Aloof, superior, disdainful, distant, defensive, suspicious

• Irritable, resentful, hostile, sarcastic, angry, furious

• Indifferent, resigned, apathetic, dull, affectless

Pay attention to the influence of content on affect, and note especially disharmony between affect and content or thought. Also important is constancy or change in the emotional state.

4. *Content of thought: special preoccupations and experiences*—delusions, illusions, or hallucinations, depersonalizations, obsessions or compulsions, phobias, fantasies, and daydreams. (These terms are defined in the glossary.) You can elicit these data by asking such questions as "Do you have any difficulties?" or "Have you been troubled or ill in any way?"

If the client has delusions of being the object of environmental attention, some of the following questions might reveal them: "Do people like you?" "Have you ever been watched or spied upon or singled out for special attention?" "Do others have it in for you?"

Delusions of *alien control* (passivity) are feelings of being controlled or guided by external forces. If you suspect these delusions, ask the client such questions as "Do you ever feel your thoughts or actions are under any outside influences or control?" "Are you able to influence others, to read their minds, or to put thoughts in their minds?"

A client with *nihilistic* delusions more or less completely denies reality and existence. The client states that nothing exists, or that everything is lost. Statements such as "I have no head, no stomach," "I cannot die," or "I will live to eternity" suggest nihilistic delusions.

Delusions of *self-deprecation* are often seen in connection with severe depressions. The client describes feeling unworthy, sinful, ugly, or foul-smelling.

Delusions of *grandeur* are associated with elated states such as great wealth, strength, power, sexual potency, or identification with a famous person or even God.

Somatic delusions are focused on having cancer, obstructed bowels, leprosy, or some horrible disease. These are to be distinguished from a preoccupation with normal, visceral, or peripheral sensations.

Hallucinations are false sensory impressions with no external basis in fact. Try to elicit the clearness of the projection to the outside world—e.g., the source of the voices (from outside or inside the head), the clarity and distinctness of the perception, and the intensity. Be subtle in approaching the client for evidence of hallucinatory phenomena, unless the client is obviously hallucinating. In the case of obvious hallucinations, it's appropriate to ask about the directly.

Obsessions are insistent thoughts recognized as arising from the self. The client usually regards them as absurd and relatively meaningless, yet they persist despite endeavors to get rid of them.

Compulsions are repetitive acts performed through some inner need or drive and supposedly against the client's wishes. yet not performing them results in tension and anxiety.

Fantasies and *daydreams* are preoccupations that are often difficult to elicit from the client. The difficulty may be that the client misunderstands what the examiner wants, but often people are ashamed to talk about them because of their content.

5. *Sensorium or orientation*—orientation in terms of time, place, person, and self to determine the presence of confusion or clouding of consciousness. You may introduce such questions by asking "Have you kept track of the time?" If so, "What is today's date?" Clients who say they don't know should be asked to estimate approximately or to guess at an answer. Many clinicians begin the mental status exam with these questions because disorientation should cause the examiner to question the validity and reliability of data obtained subsequently.

6. *Memory*—the person's attention span and ability to retain or recall past experiences in both the recent and the remote past. If memory loss exists, determine whether it is constant or variable and whether the loss is limited to a certain time period. The examiner should be alert to *confabulations*—invented memories to take the place of those the client cannot recall. It is useful to introduce questions relating to memory by some general statement such as "Has your memory been good?" or "Have you had difficulty remembering telephone numbers or appointments?"

a. *Recall of remote past experiences.* Ask for a review of the important events in the client's life.

Then compare the response with information obtained from other sources during the history-taking.

b. *Recall of recent past experiences,* such as the events leading to the present seeking of treatment.

c. *Retention and recall of immediate impressions.* The examiner might ask the client to repeat a name, an address, or a set of objects, e.g., car, coin, and telephone, immediately and again after 3 to 5 minutes. Another test is to have the client repeat three-digit numbers at a rate of one per second, or to repeat a complicated sentence.

d. *General grasp and recall.* You might ask the client to read a story and then repeat the gist with as many details as possible. In a concise guide for conducting a psychiatric examination, S. M. Small (1980), includes the following story as an example:

THE COWBOY STORY

A cowboy from Arizona went to San Francisco with his dog, which he left at a friend's while he purchased a new suit of clothes. Dressed in the new suit, he went back to the dog, whistled to him, called him by name, and patted him. The dog would have nothing to do with him in his new hat and coat, but gave a mournful howl. Coaxing had no effect, so the cowboy went away and donned his old garments. Then the dog immediately showed his wild joy on seeing his master as he thought he ought to be.

7. *General intellectual level*—a nonstandardized evaluation of intelligence. The examiner looks for the person's ability to use factual knowledge in a comprehensive way.

a. *General grasp of information.* You may ask the client to name the five largest cities of the United States, the last four presidents, or the governor of the state.

b. *Ability to calculate.* Tests of simple multiplication and addition are useful for this purpose. Another test consists of subtracting from one hundred by sevens until the person can go no further (serial sevens test).

c. *Reasoning and judgment.* A common test of reasoning is to ask clients what they might do with a gift of $10,000. Examiners must be particularly careful to correct for their own biases and values in assessing each client's answer.

8. *Abstract thinking*—the distinctions between such abstractions as poverty and misery or idleness and laziness. It is common to ask the client to interpret simple fables or proverbs, e.g., "Don't cry over spilled milk."

9. *Insight evaluation*—whether clients recognize the significance of the present situation, whether they feel the need for treatment, and how they explain the symptoms. Often it is helpful to ask clients for suggestions for their own treatment.

10. *Summary*—the important psychopathologic findings and a tentative diagnosis. Any pertinent facts from the medical history and/or physical examination should be added to the summary.

Table 9–1 lists some of the mental status examination findings differentiating organic brain syndromes, psychosis, and mood disorders.

Biologic Assessment

As the summary of the mental status examination and Table 9–1 suggest, nurses must carefully consider the possibility that a client's symptoms may have a biologic, particularly neurologic, basis. In some reported instances, clients with brain tumors or bromide intoxication have been hospitalized on psychiatric units and treated exclusively for their seemingly psychiatric symptoms. Such a critical oversight obviously delays and seriously hampers appropriate treatment of an organic or neurologic problem. The value of careful screening for biologic disorders cannot be overemphasized. In many community settings, psychiatric nurses are the only mental health care providers prepared to undertake a biologic and neurologic assessment and interpret the results.

Objectives of Neurologic Assessment

1. Detection of underlying and perhaps unsuspected organic disease that may be responsible for psychiatric symptoms

2. Understanding of disease as a factor in the overall psychiatric disability

3. Appreciation of somatic symptoms that reflect primarily psychologic rather than organic problems

Biologic History-Taking   Of several procedures that enlighten the nurse who is attempting to account for biologic aspects of psychiatric symptoms, the client's history is certainly a major one. The nurse should inquire into two primary aspects of biologic history: (a) facts about known physical diseases and dysfunction, and (b) information about specific physical complaints. Information about previous illnesses may provide essential clues. For example, suppose the presenting symptoms include paranoid delusions and the client has a history of similar episodes. During each previous episode, the client responded to diverse forms of treatment and demonstrated no residual symptoms.

This history suggests a strong possibility of amphetamine- or other drug-related psychosis, and a drug screen laboratory test may be indicated. An occupational history may provide information about exposure to inorganic mercury leading to symptoms of psychosis or exposure to lead resulting in an organic mental disorder.

The second emphasis in history-taking is eliciting information from the client about specific physical complaints. Again, it is crucial for the nurse to consider symptoms in terms of not only psychiatric conditions but also physical diseases. Symptoms that are atypical of psychiatric disorders are particularly revealing clues. For example, suppose a client with hallucinations and delusions also complains of a severe headache at the onset of the symptoms. The symptoms together suggest possible brain disease and call for careful and repeated neurologic assessment. History-taking should also include information about medications the client currently takes. Digitalis intoxication may result in impairment. Reserpine may produce symptoms generally considered psychiatric in nature.

Observation   Observation also yields important data bearing on the possible presence of organic disorders:

• An unsteady gait may suggest diffuse brain disease or alcohol or drug intoxication.

• Asymmetry—dragging a leg or not swinging one arm—might be a sign of a focal brain lesion.

• Although inattention to proper dress and hygiene is common in people with emotional disorders, it is also a hallmark of organic brain disease, particularly lapses such as mismatched socks or shoes.

• Frequent, quick, purposeless movements are characteristic of anxiety, but they are equally characteristic of chorea or hyperthyroidism.

• Tremors accompanied by anxiety may point to Parkinson's disease.

• Recent weight loss, although often encountered in depression and schizophrenia, may be due to gastrointestinal disease, carcinoma, Addison's disease, and many other physical disorders.

The nurse should observe the skin color, pupillary changes, alertness and responsiveness, and quality of speech and word production, keeping in mind the possibility of organic brain dysfunction, substance intoxication, or other diseases.

Neurologic Assessment   A careful neurologic assessment is mandatory for each client suspected of having organic brain dysfunction. Its goal is to

TABLE 9-1   **Differentiation of Mental Status Examination Findings**

| | ORGANIC BRAIN SYNDROME | | PSYCHOTIC DISORDERS | | MOOD DISORDERS |
	Delirium	Dementia	Manic Episode	Schizophrenic Disorder	Depressive Disorder
Appearance and behavior	Fluctuating impairment of consciousness, restlessness	May show deterioration of personal habits but state of consciousness not clouded	Hyperactive, elated, assertive, boisterous, with rapid emphatic speech; may become suddenly angry or argumentative	Variable	Dejected, slowed, slumped, troubled
Mood	Anxiety, fear, lability	Irritability, lability	Elation, sometimes anger and irritability	Blandness, impoverishment or inappropriateness of affect	Depression, hopelessness
Thought processes and perceptions					
Coherence and relevance	May be confused, incoherent	May become confused	Rapid association of ideas that may seem illogical	Often incoherent, disorganized	
Thought content	May have delusions		May have delusions and feelings of persecution	May have feelings of unreality, depersonalization, persecution, influence and reference; delusions that are bizarre and symbolic	May have delusions, often involving guilt, self-deprecation, somatic complaints
Perceptions	May have illusions, hallucinations		May have illusions, rarely hallucinations	May have hallucinations and illusions, often bizarre and symbolic	May have illusions, rarely hallucinations
Cognitive functions					
Orientation	May be disoriented	May be disoriented	Well-oriented	Usually but not always well oriented	Well oriented
Attention and concentration	Poor	Poor	Distractable		
Recent memory	Poor	Poor		Usually well preserved but may be difficult to test because of inattentiveness and indifference	
Remote memory	May become poor	May become poor		Usually well preserved but may be difficult to test because of inattentiveness and indifference	
Information	Preserved until late	Preserved until late			
Vocabulary	Preserved until late	Preserved until late			
Abstract reasoning	Concrete	Concrete		Concrete, may be bizarre	
Judgment	Poor	Poor			
Perception and coordination	May be poor	May be poor			

SOURCE: Adapted from Bates B: A Guide to Physical Examination. ed 3. Lippincott, 1983, pp 312–313. Reprinted by permission of Lippincott/Harper & Row.

| TIME & DATE | PUPILS | | | L.O.C. | S-R | T.R. | MOTOR | | | | TOTAL |
	R	< = >	L				RUE	RLE	LUE	LLE	MAX. 25

Explanation of Codes

Pupils

Reaction time, right (R) and left (L)

(2) Reacts briskly

(1) Reacts slowly

(0) No reaction

Size

(=) Equal

(<) Right lesser than left

(>) Right greater than left

Level of Consciousness (L.O.C.)

(5) Alert and oriented x 3 = awakens easily; oriented to person, place, time

(4) Alert and partially oriented = awakens easily but oriented in only one or two of the three spheres

(3) Lethargic but oriented = slow to arouse, possibly slurred speech, but oriented x 3

(2) Lethargic and disoriented = slow to arouse, oriented in only one or two spheres or completely disoriented

Chart continues on next page

FIGURE 9–2 Neurologic assessment guide. *SOURCE: Copyright © 1977. American Journal of Nursing Company. From* American Journal of Nursing, *September, Vol 77, No 9.*

discover signs pointing to circumscribed, focal cerebral dysfunction or diffuse, bilateral cerebral disease. A guide for evaluating the presence of signs of central nervous system disorders or "neurologic soft signs" is presented in Figure 9–2.

Authorities in mental health practice consistently remind clinicians of the need for thorough biologic assessment of clients seen in psychiatric settings. The psychiatric literature abounds with stories of clients whose symptoms were initially considered exclusively psychiatric but ultimately proved organic, especially neurologic. Assessment errors occurred not because the features did not suggest organic disease but because such features were accorded too little weight or were misinterpreted.

Psychologic Testing

Clinical psychologists administer and interpret a wide variety of psychologic tests. There are two types of psychologic tests: (a) those concerned with intelligence, and (b) those concerned with personality. Both

OR

(2)   Restless/combative (confused) = spontaneously thrashing about in bed; striking out at others; inattentive to commands

(1)   Responds to stimulation only = exhibits only some type of withdrawal or posturing in response to stimulation

(0)   Unresponsive = gives no response of any kind

Stimulus-Response (S-R)

(5)   Responds to commands = gives appropriate responses to orientation questions, complies with instructions on hand grasp, toe wiggling, etc.

(4)   Responds to name = opens eyes to name or gives some indication that he or she hears (nods, moves, etc.), but does not follow all commands

(3)   Responds to shaking = responds only to vigorous physical stimulation

(2)   Responds to pinprick = responds to light pain applied with pin to trunk or extremities to elicit either withdrawal or posturing

(1)   Responds to deep pain = responds only to mandibular pressure, periorbital rub, sternal rub, or pinch

(0)   Unresponsive = gives no response to any stimulus

Type of Response (T.R.)

(3)   Complex withdrawal = withdrawal and attempt to remove stimulus

(2)   Simple withdrawal = withdrawal from stimulus alone

(1)   Posturing = decorticate—head, arms, and hands flexed; decerebrate—head extended, arms extended and pronated, back arched

(0)   Flaccid = no response

Motor

Right Upper Extremity (RUE)

Right Lower Extremity (RLE)

Left Upper Extremity (LUE)

Left Lower Extremity (LLE)

(2)   Full spontaneous use = moves designated extremity or extremities with or *without* any stimulus

(1)   Moves to stimulus only = responds only to touch, pin, or deep pain

(0)   No movement = does not respond to any stimulus

Weakness of an extremity is indicated by writing ''weaker'' under the appropriate column.

FIGURE 9–2   Neurologic assessment guide (continued)

kinds are included in a comprehensive psychologic evaluation.

Intelligence Tests Intelligence tests may be useful particularly in evaluating the presence and degree of mental retardation. Commonly used intelligence tests are the **Stanford-Binet Test,** the **Wechsler Adult Intelligence Scale,** the **Wechsler Intelligence Scale for Children,** the Gesell Developmental Schedules, and the Vineland Social Maturity Scale.

Personality Tests Personality tests are also called **projective tests** because they evoke projection in the responses of the person being tested.

The Rorschach Test Hermann Rorschach, a Swiss psychiatrist, developed the **Rorschach Test** in 1921. It consists of ten standardized inkblots in black and white or color on separate cards, displayed one by one. Clients are asked to respond in terms of their associations, thoughts, and impressions. Because each card contains only inkblots, clients' responses are *projected,* that is, they come from within the clients themselves. People may see persons, animals, insects, objects, anatomic parts, or other things. The examiner scores the response using a system of symbols in relation to the following:

• *Location.* Where on the blot area was the response seen?

• *Content.* What did the client see?

• *Determinant.* What characteristic of the blot prompted the response?

• *Form-level.* How closely did the response correspond to the contour of the blot area used?

• *Originality.* How common a response is it?

Interpretation is based on a complicated system of scoring symbols and analyzing content. The Rorschach is the most highly developed of all the projective tests used to evaluate the personality.

The Thematic Apperception Test (TAT) The **TAT** also consists of a series of cards shown one by one. However, TAT cards are pictures of people in various emotional situations (see Figure 9–3). Clients are asked to describe what seems to be happening in the picture or to tell a story about it. Because the pictures are ambiguous, the responses reveal aspects of the clients' own emotional lives. The psychologist who interprets and scores the TAT looks for themes, threads, and patterns in the response. Some adaptations of the TAT for use with children are available.

The Minnesota Multiphasic Personality Inventory (MMPI) The **MMPI** is a complex and lengthy test consisting of 550 questions. Scoring is done in relation to nine areas: preoccupation about body diseases; depression; hysteria; antisocial personality; masculine or feminine features; paranoid qualities; anxiety, phobias, and psychogenic fatigue states; schizophrenic features; and manic features. A clinical profile of personality structure is drawn from the client's responses in these areas.

Since the MMPI is largely self-administered and can be scored quickly on computers, it has been advocated as a screening measure for colleges and universities, industry and business, and government agencies, among others. The large-scale collection and use of such information are alarming because of the negative labeling that such psychologic testing may lead to.

The Draw-a-Person Test In the Draw-a-Person Test, clients are asked first to draw a human figure and then, usually, to draw a figure of a member of the opposite sex (see Figure 9–4). The drawings may be interpreted to give information about clients' concepts of their own bodies and personality structures; their relationships with persons of the opposite sex, the

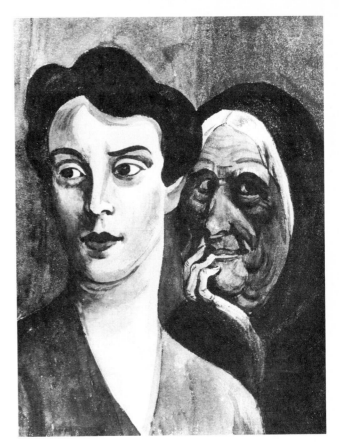

FIGURE 9–3 Card 12 GF of the Thematic Apperception Test. *SOURCE: Reprinted from Murray HA: Thematic Apperception Test. Harvard University Press, 1943. Copyright © 1943 by the President and Fellows of Harvard College; 1971 by Henry A. Murray. Reprinted by permission.*

same sex, and parents; and their views of the roles of men and women.

The Sentence Completion Test The Sentence Completion Test presents an extensive series of incomplete sentences to clients, who are asked to complete the sentences with the first thoughts that come to mind. The sentences are designed to elicit responses concerning fantasies, fears, daydreams, and aspirations, among other things.

The Bender-Gestalt Test The **Bender-Gestalt Test** asks clients to reproduce, as best they can, nine geometric designs that are printed on separate cards. Because this test can be used to evaluate memory, it is believed to be particularly helpful in identifying organic brain damage. It is also used to evaluate the maturation level of children in the coordination of visual, motor, and intellectual functions. For an example of a Bender-Gestalt design series, see Figure 9–5.

These and other instruments commonly used by clinical psychologists are briefly discussed in Table 9–2 on page 167.

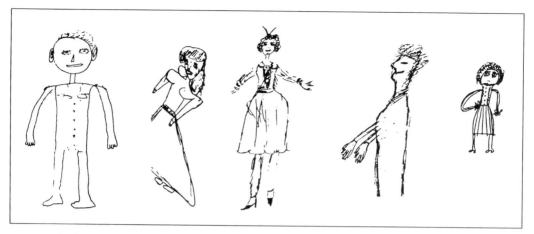

FIGURE 9—4 Examples of the Draw-a-Person Test done by five women who had been hospitalized for two years. *SOURCE: Spire RH: An experimental study of the use of photographic self-image confrontation as a nursing procedure in the care of chronically ill schizophrenic female patients. Project in partial fulfillment of MS degree, State University of New York at Buffalo, 1967, pp 243, 248, 249, 251, 256.*

Psychiatric Diagnostic Practice According to APA's Criteria (DSM-III-R)

The first edition of the DSM was published by the APA in 1952. The second edition, published in 1968, attempted compatibility with the International Classification of Diseases, Injuries, and Causes of Death (ICD-9) published by the World Health Organization. DSM-II was widely criticized for its low reliability and tendency to reflect an individual psychiatrist's philosophy or such client characteristics as social class rather than actual clinical data.

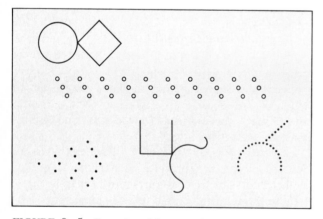

FIGURE 9—5 Examples of figures to be copied on Bender-Gestalt Test. Subjects are asked to copy the figures on a single sheet of paper and then to draw them from memory. The clinician looks for distortion of the figures in terms of incompleteness, rotation, oversimplification, perseveration (giving more than is present in the stimulus). The interpreter also looks at the use of space on the page. The recall drawings also test for memory deficits. *SOURCE: Bender L: A Visual-Motor Gestalt Test and its Clinical Use, Research Monograph no. 3. American Orthopsychiatric Association, 1938.*

The American Psychiatric Association (APA) published a third edition of the **Diagnostic and Statistical Manual of Mental Disorders** in 1980 and a revised edition in 1987. (See Appendix A for an outline of categories for diagnosis and numeric codes.) Important features distinguish DSM-III-R from its predecessors, DSM-II and DSM-I. It uses specified diagnostic criteria to improve the reliability of diagnostic judgments and offers a multiaxial or multidimensional approach to clinical assessment of psychiatric clients in which five different classes of data are collected and assessed.

The DSM-III-R represents the current state of knowledge about diagnosing **mental disorders.** It is composed of a list of all the official numeric codes and terms for all recognized mental disorders, along with a comprehensive description of each and specified diagnostic criteria that must be present in order to make each diagnosis. Work is underway to publish DSM-IV in 1993 and further to refine these advances.

Nurses have historically avoided instruments and tools for client assessment that ignore stressors in a person's social context and emphasize symptoms or illness to the exclusion of strengths, capabilities, and areas of adaptive functioning. In short, nurses have avoided traditional "medical model approaches." Many of our colleagues believe that the DSM-III-R, while not entirely free of controversy, represents the state-of-the-art in the field of psychiatric diagnosis. According to Spitzer, Williams, and Skodol (1980), the DSM-III had been adopted for use in most facilities throughout the United States. The DSM-IV task force, chaired by Allen Frances, M.D., and the thirteen work groups and 50 to 100 advisers are seeking the widest possible participation from the interdisciplinary team.

Basic Principles of the Multiaxial System The multiaxial framework for client assessment provided

TABLE 9–2   Common Psychologic Tests in Clinical Use

Name of Test	Description	Method
Bender-Gestalt Test	A test of visual-motor coordination that is most useful with adults as a screening device to detect the presence of organic impairment. It may also be used to evaluate the level of maturation in the coordination of intellectual, muscular, and visual functions in children.	The client is asked to copy nine separate geometric designs onto plain white paper, one at a time. Sometimes the client is asked to draw the design from memory after an interval of 45 to 60 seconds.
Blacky Test	A projective test used most frequently with children (although it is also designed for adults) to determine the level of psychosexual development.	The client is shown various cartoons about a dog (who may be identified as male or female) and the dog's family and is asked to make up a story about each cartoon.
Draw-a-Person Test	A projective test used with both adults and children to elicit information on the client's body image or perception of self and the client's relationship to the environment. It is also used as a screening device to detect the presence of organic impairment. With children it may be used to compare the age level of expression with the child's chronologic age for a rough approximation of intelligence.	The client is asked first to draw a human figure and later to draw a person of the opposite sex. The test may be expanded by asking the client to draw a picture of a house and a tree as well (called the House-Tree-Person Test), an animal, or a family.
Minnesota Multiphasic Personality Inventory (MMPI)	A self-administered objective (as opposed to projective) personality test designed to yield a broad examination of personality functioning that is amenable to statistical interpretation—such as self-attitudes, certain aspects of ego functioning, and profiles of symptoms or psychopathology.	The client responds to 550 statements, by indicating either "true," "false," or "cannot say." The client's personality profile is sketched in terms of: • Preoccupation with body diseases • Depression • Hysteria • Antisocial personality • Masculine or feminine features • Paranoid qualities • Anxiety, phobias, and psychogenic fatigue • Schizophrenic features • Manic features
Rorschach Test	A projective test that is the most highly developed of the personality tests. It reveals personality features and symptoms and is commonly used as a diagnostic tool.	The client responds to ten cards, one at a time, consisting of black-and-white or colored standardized inkblots. Responses include the impressions, thoughts, and associations that come to mind while the client looks at the inkblot.
Sentence Completion Test	A projective test designed to elicit conscious associations to specific areas of functioning thus illustrating the fears, preoccupations, ambitions, and idiosyncrasies of the client.	The client is asked to complete spontaneously sentences such as: "I feel guilty about . . . ," "Sex is . . . ," "My mother . . . ," "Sometimes I wish. . . ." Both mood and content are noted.
Stanford-Binet Intelligence Test	A general intelligence test based on an age-level concept from 2 years to about 15 years. It is particularly useful to test children and to evaluate mental retardation.	The client is asked to do a graded series of tasks designed to correlate with the abilities of children of a particular age group. Each set is more difficult than the one before it.

by DSM-III and DSM-III-R and retained for DSM-IV is congruent with holistic views of people, recognizes the role of environmental stress in influencing behavior, and requires that the clinician collect data about client adaptive strengths as well as about symptoms or problems. One of the most important features of DSM-III-R is its increased interclinician reliability due to the use of specified observable criteria rather than diverse theories of etiology for mental disorders (Spitzer and Forman 1979). Its multiaxial approach is undoubtedly of equal significance to psychiatric nursing (Williams and Wilson 1982).

TABLE 9-2   *(continued)*

Name of Test	Description	Method
Thematic Apperception Test (TAT)	A projective test offering a standardized set of stimuli for exploring the client's emotional life. Themes and interpersonal problems emerge in the client's responses.	The client is shown a series of ambiguous pictures of people in various emotionally significant situations and is asked to respond by describing what is happening in the picture and telling a story about it. Adaptations have been designed for use with children. In these, the central figure is a child or the pictures are cartoons of animals.
Wechsler Adult Intelligence Scale (WAIS)	A general intelligence test for persons 16 years of age and older. It is the most widely used and best standardized intelligence test.	The client completes eleven subtests, which yield both verbal and performance scores as well as full-scale IQs. Subtest raw scores may also be compared to reveal variability in functioning. The subtests are: information, comprehension, arithmetic, similarities, memory for digits, vocabulary, digit symbol, picture completion, block design, picture arrangement, and object assembly.
Wechsler Intelligence Scale for Children (WISC)	A general intelligence test for children from 5 through 15 years of age.	Similar to the Wechsler Test for adults, this test asks the client to complete ten subtests, which yield separate verbal, performance, and full-scale scores.
Wechsler Memory Scale	A psychologic test for immediate, short-term, and long-term memory.	The client is asked to do seven memory tests, including current information, orientation, mental control, logical memory, digits forward and backward, visual reproduction, and associate learning. A memory quotient (MQ) score is useful in the determination of organic mental syndrome.
Word Association Test	A projective test similar in form and organization to the Sentence Completion test. It is designed to elicit associations to areas of conflict.	The client is asked to respond spontaneously to a series of fifty or more words, presented one at a time. Words presumed to be related to the conflicts of the specific client are mixed with words that generally produce an emotional reaction.

The following example illustrates the principle behind a multiaxial system:

A 35-year-old man came to an outpatient mental health clinic for evaluation. This young man came in for treatment of a severe fear and avoidance of flying that amounted to a phobia. However, he also had a long-term personality disturbance and suffered from eczema. Suppose three different clinicians were asked to evaluate this man. A biologically oriented clinician would certainly diagnose the eczema but might fail to notice the personality disturbance and make little of the phobia. A psychodynamically oriented clinician would be sure to diagnose the personality disorder but might overlook the eczema and the phobia, considering them to be merely manifestations of the underlying personality disturbance. Finally, a clinician who was behaviorally oriented would notice the phobia but might fail to diagnose the personality disturbance and the eczema. It is clear, then, that because of their differing theoretic orientations, these clinicians have a rather high likelihood of diagnostic disagreement.

Now suppose this same man were presented to the same three colleagues, but this time the clinicians were required to evaluate him in each of three different areas of functioning: (a) behavioral or psychologic, (b) personality, and (c) physical functioning. In this case, all three clinicians would be much more likely to diagnose all three conditions and thus agree on the total evaluation of the individual.

In the DSM-III-R multiaxial system, each individual is evaluated on five axes, each dealing with a different class of information about the client. A multiaxial evaluation system provides a much more comprehensive evaluation of an individual and increases the likelihood that clinicians will agree among themselves about the condition of the individual being evaluated.

The DSM-III-R multiaxial system includes the five axes presented in the accompanying box. Axes I and II

DSM-III-R Axes

Axis I: Clinical syndromes
          Conditions not attributable to a mental disorder that are a focus of attention or treatment (V-codes)
          Additional codes
Axis II: Personality disorders
          Developmental disorders
Axis III: Physical disorders
Axis IV: Severity of psychosocial stressors
Axis V: Global assessment of functioning (GAF)

include all the mental disorders in DSM-III-R and so might be said to represent the intrapersonal or *psychologic* area of functioning. Axis III is for recording physical disorders and conditions that are related to the understanding or management of the individual, and thus represents the area of *physical* functioning. Axes IV and V, for psychosocial stressors and a global assessment of functioning, includes an evaluation of the individual's *social* functioning. In this sense, the multiaxial system provides a more comprehensive biopsychosocial approach to assessment.

Description of the Axes To use the multiaxial system effectively, nurses must understand its components.

Axes I and II: Clinical Syndromes, V-Codes, Personality and Developmental Disorders Axes I and II comprise all the "mental disorders and conditions not attributable to a mental disorder that are a focus of attention or treatment" (called V-codes). The easiest way to differentiate between these first two axes is to deal first with Axis II. On Axis II are personality disorders, usually diagnosed in adults, and developmental disorders including mental retardation, diagnosed in children and adolescents. The remaining mental disorders and associated conditions are recorded on Axis I. The classes of disorders on Axis II were given their own axis because their usually mild and chronic symptomatology is often overshadowed by a more florid Axis I condition. DSM-III-R clarifies the conceptual distinction between Axis I and Axis II by noting that Axis II conditions

- Have an early onset

- Have a stable, not episodic, course

V-Codes In addition to the other mental disorders, Axis I includes the V-codes. The V-codes include such conditions as marital problems, occupational problems, and parent-child problems, in which the problem being evaluated or for which clinical care is sought is not due to a mental disorder. *A mental disorder is differentiated from other problems in living as a clinically significant behavioral pattern that occurs and is associated with either a painful symptom (distress) or impairment in functioning (disability).* Further, the distress or disability does not primarily reflect a conflict between an individual and society.

If a man with bipolar disorder that has been in remission for many years develops marital difficulties for reasons unrelated to his psychiatric history or condition (perhaps, for example, because his wife wants to resume a career), both "Marital problem" and "Bipolar disorder in remission" could be recorded on Axis I. If, however, the bipolar disorder is not in complete remission, and marital conflict develops as a result of his changeable moods and other symptoms associated with the mental disorder, the marital problem would not be recorded in addition to the bipolar disorder, since the marital problem in this case is due to the person's mental disorder.

Axis I also includes a code for "Unspecified mental disorder (nonpsychotic)." Clinicians use this code when they determine that there is some (nonpsychotic) Axis I mental disorder but, perhaps due to lack of information, cannot yet be more specific. Finally, there are codes for indicating that a diagnosis or condition is deferred on either Axis I or Axis II, or that there is no mental disorder. Examples of evaluations of individuals using only Axes I and II are presented in the box below.

Axis III: Physical Disorders and Conditions Clinicians use Axis III to record physical disorders and conditions that must be taken into account in planning treatment or are relevant to understanding the etiology or worsening of the mental disorder. A

Examples of DSM-III-R Multiaxial Evaluation on Axes I and II

Example 1
Axis I: 393.93 Alcohol dependence, in remission
Axis II: 301.70 Antisocial personality disorder

Example 2
Axis I: V71.09 No diagnosis
Axis II: 301.22 Schizotypal personality disorder

Example of DSM-III-R Multiaxial Evaluation on Axes I, II, and III

Axis I: V71.09   No diagnosis

Axis II: 312.23   Conduct disorder, social-
                    ized, aggressive

Axis III: Diabetes

clinician might also want to record other significant physical findings, such as "soft" neurologic signs or even a single symptom (e.g., vomiting). An example of an evaluation done through Axis III is presented in the accompanying box.

In this example, the client, a child in this case, will probably not be very compliant with the diabetes treatment regimen because of psychologic problems (conduct disorder, noted on Axis II).

If there is lack of information on Axis III, that fact should be stated: "No information" or "Diagnosis deferred—not evaluated" or "Referred to Dr. Smith for evaluation." In an event, *something* should be noted on this axis; omitting it for lack of information undermines the purpose of a holistic multiaxial system. Of course, recent advances in psychobiologic knowledge make Axis III findings particularly important for psychiatric mental health nursing.

Axis IV: Severity of Psychosocial Stressors
Axis IV provides the rating scale shown in Table 9–3. This scale rates the severity of the psychosocial stressors that helped to bring about, worsened, or account for a recurrence of a mental disorder. In making this judgment, the nurse should generally take into account only stressors that occurred in the year preceding the mental disorder. Changes are expected in the DSM-IV revision of Axis IV.

To standardize the severity ratings across stressors, and to avoid rating an individual's idiosyncratic vulnerabilities, the evaluator should rate the severity of

TABLE 9–3   Axis IV: Severity of Psychosocial Stressors Scale

Code	Term	Examples of Stressors	
Adults		**Acute Events**	**Enduring Circumstances**
1	None	No acute events that may be relevant to the disorder	No enduring circumstances that may be relevant to the disorder
2	Mild	Broke up with boyfriend or girlfriend; started or graduated from school; child left home	Family arguments; job dissatisfaction; residence in high-crime neighborhood
3	Moderate	Marriage; marital separation; loss of job; retirement; miscarriage	Marital discord; serious financial problems; trouble with boss; being a single parent
4	Severe	Divorce; birth of first child	Unemployment; poverty
5	Extreme	Death of spouse; serious physical illness diagnosed; victim of rape	Serious chronic illness in self or child; ongoing physical or sexual abuse
6	Catastrophic	Death of child; suicide of spouse; devastating natural disaster	Captivity as hostage; concentration camp experience
0	Inadequate information, or no change in condition		
Children and Adolescents			
1	None	No acute events that may be relevant to the disorder	No enduring circumstances that may be relevant to the disorder
2	Mild	Broke up with boyfriend or girlfriend; change of school	Overcrowded living quarters; family arguments
3	Moderate	Expelled from school; birth of sibling	Chronic disabling illness in parent; chronic parental discord
4	Severe	Divorce of parents; unwanted pregnancy; arrest	Harsh or rejecting parents; chronic life-threatening illness in parent; multiple foster home placements
5	Extreme	Sexual or physical abuse; death of a parent	Recurrent sexual or physical abuse
6	Catastrophic	Death of both parents	Chronic life-threatening illness
0	Inadequate information, or no change in condition		

SOURCE: *American Psychiatric Association:* Diagnostic and Statistical Manual of Mental Disorders, *ed 3, revised. APA, 1987.*

the stressors with an "average" person in mind. The nurse should take into account the individual client's circumstances and sociocultural background, and rate the severity of the stressors as experienced by the "average" person under these circumstances. For example, an abortion would probably be more stressful for a Catholic than for an atheist.

The nurse should also take into account (a) how many stressors the client recently experienced, (b) how desirable they were and to what extent they were under the client's control (e.g., whether the individual quit a job or was fired), and (c) how much change they caused in the individual's life (e.g., the development of a serious chronic physical illness could be expected to cause a great deal of change in the "average" person's life).

In addition to rating the severity of the stressors, evaluators should also note in their own words the specific stressors that they consider pertinent. Thus, a multiaxial evaluation, up through Axis IV, might look like the example in the box below. Changes in DSM-III-R required stating if stressors were enduring or discrete events. In this example, the client developed panic disorder (recurrent panic attacks) as she began classes in college.

Axis V: Global Assessment of Functioning This axis in DSM-III-R provides the rating scale shown in the box on p 172. One of the most accurate indicators of clinical outcome is the level of premorbid functioning that an individual sustained. For this reason, Axis V provides a **Global Assessment of Function Scale** (GAF) to rate the highest level of psychologic, social, and occupational functioning that an individual was able to sustain for at least a few months during the past year as well as at the time of evaluation.

Overall adaptive functioning was defined in DSM-III (1980) by three areas of functioning: (a) social relations, (b) occupational functioning, and (c) use of leisure time. Changes are expected on Axis V in DSM-IV. The quality of the client's functioning in each of these three areas should be considered, with the breadth and quality of social relationships being given

the greatest weight because of their high prognostic value. Use of leisure time is a serious consideration only in those individuals who have been functioning on a very high level.

DSM's Usefulness to Psychiatric-Mental Health Nursing From the perspective of psychiatric nursing, the DSM-III-R represented some progress toward values that mental health nurses have espoused for decades. For example, as Williams and Wilson (1982) state, DSM-III (and DSM-III-R)

• Provides a framework for interdisciplinary communication

• Based revisions on a series of formative evaluations

• Represents a collaborative achievement

• Represents progress toward a more holistic view of mind-body relations

• Provides for diagnostic uncertainty

• Incorporates, at least in part, biologic, psychologic, and social variables

• Has achieved positive results of extensive field testing for validity and reliability

• Considers adaptive strength as well as problems

• Reflects a descriptive, phenomenologic perspective rather than any theoretic psychiatric orientation

Of the axes represented in DSM-III-R, Axes IV and V, Psychosocial Stressors and Functioning, are the areas in which nursing can make the greatest contribution. The Nursing Adaptation Evaluation (NSGAE) represents one proposed refinement of Axis V useful in planning and determining resources for nursing care (Morrison et al. 1982). See the boxes on pp 173 and 174 for the rating format and the definitions and behavioral criteria. The NSGAE could also become a sixth axis on its own.

Psychosocial Assessment

Psychosocial assessment is a dynamic process. It begins during the initial contact with the client, and it continues throughout the nurse-client experience. Psychosocial assessments may be made of an individual, a family, or a group. In any case, they begin with the identifying characteristics, such as name, sex, age, marital status, and ethnic and cultural origins. Problem identification and definition are also necessary phases in the assessment process. The method for assessment described below has been adapted from the problem-solving model of Compton and Galaway (1979, pp 250–251).

Example of a DSM-III-R Multiaxial Evaluation on Axes I, II, III, and IV

Axis I:	300.01	Panic disorder
Axis II:	301.83	Borderline personality disorder
Axis III:		No diagnosis
Axis IV:		3—Mild (began college)

Axis V: Global Assessment of Functioning Scale (GAF Scale)*

Code

90
|
81

Absent or minimal symptoms (e.g., mild anxiety before an exam), good functioning in all areas, interested and involved in a wide range of activities, socially effective, generally satisfied with life, no more than everyday problems or concerns (e.g., an occasional argument with family members).

80
|
71

If symptoms are present, they are transient and expectable reactions to psychosocial stressors (e.g., difficulty concentrating after family argument); no more than slight impairment in social, occupational, or school functioning (e.g., temporarily falling behind in school work).

70
|
61

Some mild symptoms (e.g., depressed mood and mild insomnia) or some difficulty in social, occupational, or school functioning (e.g., occasional truancy, or theft within the household), but generally functioning pretty well, has some meaningful interpersonal relationships.

60
|
51

Moderate symptoms (e.g., flat affect and circumstantial speech, occasional panic attacks) or moderate difficulty in social, occupational, or school functioning (e.g., few friends, conflicts with coworkers).

50
|
41

Serious symptoms (e.g., suicidal ideation, severe obsessional rituals, frequent shoplifting) or any serious impairment in social, occupational, or school functioning (e.g., no friends, unable to keep a job).

40
|
31

Some impairment in reality testing or communication (e.g., speech is at times illogical, obscure, or irrelevant) or major impairment in several areas, such as work or school, family relations, judgment, thinking, or mood (e.g., depressed man avoids friends, neglects family, and is unable to work; child frequently beats up younger children, is defiant at home, and is failing at school).

30
|
21

Behavior is considerably influenced by delusions or hallucinations or serious impairment in communication or judgment (e.g., sometimes incoherent, acts grossly inappropriately, suicidal preoccupation) or inability to function in almost all areas (e.g., stays in bed all day; no job, home, or friends).

20
|
11

Some danger of hurting self or others (e.g., suicide attempts without clear expectation of death, frequently violent, manic excitement) or occasionally fails to maintain minimal personal hygiene (e.g., smears feces) or gross impairment in communication (e.g., largely incoherent or mute).

10
|
1

Persistent danger of severely hurting self or others (e.g., recurrent violence) or persistent inability to maintain minimal personal hygiene or serious suicidal act with clear expectation of death.

*Consider psychological, social, and occupational functioning on a hypothetical continuum of mental health-illness. Do not include impairment in functioning due to physical (or environmental) limitations.

NOTE: Use intermediate codes when appropriate, e.g., 45, 68, 72.

SOURCE: American Psychiatric Association: Diagnostic and Statistical Manual of Mental Disorders, ed 3, revised. APA, 1987.

Individual Assessment During the individual assessment, the nurse considers the following factors:

1. *Physical and intellectual*

   a. Presence of physical illness and/or disability

   b. Appearance and energy level

   c. Current and potential levels of intellectual functioning

   d. The way the client sees personal world and translates events around self; client's perceptual abilities

   e. Cause-and-effect reasoning, ability to focus

2. *Socioeconomic factors*

   a. Economic factors—level of income, adequacy of subsistence: their effect on life-style, sense of adequacy, and self-worth

Rating Scale for Patient's Current Overall Level of Functioning on NSGAE

Level 1. The patient demonstrates self-care abilities in meeting all the basic biologic needs and consistently uses appropriate resources when difficulties become manifest.

Level 2. The patient demonstrates the ability to independently accomplish specific self-care activities, but limited ability to utilize available resources.

Level 3. The patient is limited in the ability to accomplish self-care and requires either physical assistance or consistent verbal direction to ensure needs being met.

Level 4. The patient is severely limited in the ability to accomplish self-care and requires either physical assistance or consistent verbal direction to ensure needs being met.

SOURCE: Morrison E, et al: NSGAE: a proposed Axis VI of DSM-III. J Psychosoc Nurs Ment Health Serv 1985; 23(8):11.

b. Employment and attitudes about it

c. Racial, cultural, and ethnic identification; sense of identity and belonging

d. Religious identification and link to significant value systems, norms, and practices

3. *Personal values and goals*

    a. Presence or absence of congruence between values and their expression in action; meaning of values to individual

    b. Congruence between individual's values and goals and the immediate systems with which client interacts

    c. Congruence between individual's values and assessor's values; meaning of this for intervention process

4. *Adaptive functioning and response to present involvement*

    a. Manner in which individual presents self to others—grooming, appearance, posture

    b. Emotional tone and change or constancy of levels

    c. Style of communication—verbal and nonverbal; ability to express appropriate emotion, follow train of thought; factors of dissonance, confusion, uncertainty

    d. Symptoms or symptomatic behavior

    e. Quality of relationships individual seeks to establish—direction, purposes, and uses of such relationships for individual

    f. Perception of self

    g. Social roles that are assumed or ascribed; competence in fulfilling these roles

    h. Relational behavior

        (1) Capacity for intimacy

        (2) Dependence-independence balance

        (3) Power and control conflicts

        (4) Exploitiveness

        (5) Openness

5. *Developmental factors*

    a. How role performance is equated with life stage

    b. How developmental experiences have been interpreted and used

    c. How individual has dealt with past conflicts, tasks, and problems

    d. Whether present problem is unique in life experience

The Place of Assessment in Practice Assessment is essential in clinical practice and serves several purposes:

• Identifying problems

• Identifying client motivations, strengths, and resources

• Identifying forces (both internal and external to the client) that may hinder the therapeutic plan

• Setting reasonable goals

• Determining appropriate intervention strategies

• Providing continuous evaluation of the process and indicating when the therapeutic plan should be changed

Assessment is an ongoing, dynamic process that Compton and Galaway (1979, p 287) describe as a

Definitions and Behavioral Criteria for NSGAE

Nutrition Level (N)

1. Is able to maintain nutrition and hydration independently.

2. Needs assistance with culturally accepted table manners.

3. Needs assistance selecting food or staying with meal.

4. Cannot report hunger or thirst.
Inadequate/excessive intake due to fear of food, inability to be with others, medications or physical handicap.

Solitude and Social Interaction Level (S)

1. Is able to use nonhospital support system constructively to meet basic needs.

2. Is able to use nurse-patient relationship to solve problems and validate feelings and perceptions of self and others.

3. Is preoccupied with internal stimuli but responds when approached.
Verbally provocative with peers or staff.

4. Is withdrawn or mute.
Unable to control excitement, intrusiveness, or abusiveness.

Grooming and Personal Hygiene Level (G)

1. Is able to dress and groom self at own initiative according to environmental demands and cultural norms.

2. Is able to use hospital structure to care for own clothes, personal space, and grooming.

3. Needs assistance to prepare and complete hygiene tasks. Has no belongings and needs interventions to obtain basic articles of clothing or grooming tools.

4. Cannot dress self according to environmental demands or cultural norms.
Cannot perform basic hygiene tasks.

Activity and Rest Level (A)

1. Is able to select and participate in activities, able to sleep restfully.

2. May still have sleeping difficulties but able to verbalize solutions.

3. Is over or underactive but has some control over behavior and responds to directions.

4. Cannot sleep for restful periods or sleeps continuously. Is unable to control harmful activity without locked seclusion, restraints, and medications.

Elimination Level (E)

1. Able to regulate elimination pattern independently.

2. Able to ask for help to maintain elimination pattern.

3. Cannot maintain elimination without medication or other active treatment.

4. Cannot report bowel/bladder function.
Antisocially urinates, defecates, or smears feces.

SOURCE: *Adapted from Morrison E, et al.: NSGAE: A proposed Axis VI of DSM-III.* J. Psychosoc Nurs Ment Health Serv 1985;23(8):13. Adapted from Smith S: In Underwood P: Self-Concepts Manual. *University of California, Department of Mental Health and Community Nursing, 1981.*

"squirming, wriggling, alive business." It provides an opportunity for nurse and client to engage in a partnership based on mutual definition of problems and goals.

Systems of Recording

Nurses need to communicate adequately in writing to inform members of the mental health team of the client's patterns of interaction. Recording is an important process; it should provide the basis for

• Altering a treatment plan

• Determining appropriate intervention strategies

• Allowing communication among members of the mental health team or mental health agencies

• Providing around-the-clock data on hospitalized clients

• Evidence in court

• Research

An often unrecognized or disregarded purpose of recording is to provide quality accountability of psychiatric nursing practice. Recorded data can be used to give nurses feedback about their practice, through processes such as the *psychiatric audit* (discussed later in this chapter). Careful recording is also critical to avoiding legal exposure in a law suit. Exactly what system of recording is used depends on the agency.

Essentials in Recording

The most significant events the nurse records are the behavior patterns and interpersonal interactions of the client. It may also be important to record other significant happenings—the client's sleeping, eating, and elimination patterns; physical appearance; somatic treatments and medications; and so on. Certainly any changes in a client's suicide potential should be carefully documented.

The following types of notes should be made:

• *Intake interview and mental status exam results.*

• *Progress over time.* Mental health agencies may require that notes be entered at specific times, e.g., at the end of each eight-hour shift or at the end of each 24-hour period. When events of special significance occur, they should be recorded as soon after the event as possible, not held until the 8 or 24 hours have elapsed. In the case of special observation precautions some form of recording may be necessary every 15 minutes.

• *Nurse-client relationship.* Notes are often made after each session with the client in individual, group, or family therapy. These notes summarize what occurred during the experience.

• *Summary report.* Summary reports are usually made at the termination of contact with the client—i.e., when individual, group, or family therapy has ended. The summary report presents a clear and concise picture of the highlights of the experience.

Behavior and interaction notes should include examples rather than interpretations. Instead of writing "Ms W. is hallucinating," it is preferable to write "Ms W. states she hears Moses telling her not to get dressed today or leave her room."

The mental health field is rich in terms that nurses must learn if they are to speak the language in which mental health professionals converse. However, too much jargon may cloud meaning. The language of mental health, which relies heavily on words and phrases from psychology, has also borrowed from public health, sociology, anthropology, philosophy, and the federal bureaucracy. As Morgan and Moreno put it (1973, p 2): "In staff meetings of some centers, English is hardly spoken at all."

Nurses should use jargon sparingly. The glossary at the end of this book may be particularly useful not only in defining the terms that mental health professionals use but also in identifying the point of view or perspective from which the terms have come into popular use.

Source-Oriented Recording

Source-oriented records are becoming less common as more agencies institute problem-oriented methods of recording. Source-oriented recording usually consists of a clinical record or chart that includes unassembled chronologic notations made by individual health team members. Physicians write orders and progress notes in one place, and nurses chart their notes in another. Other members of the team may not contribute in writing at all. Laboratory findings are kept in a third isolated section of the chart. Source-oriented recording hinders close communication among members of the mental health team. Such systems often duplicate efforts and fail to pull information about the client into a logical whole.

Problem-Oriented Recording

The problem-oriented system of recording is a major improvement over the source-oriented form. It is a way of organizing the same raw data into a comprehensive whole that can be used for assessment, planning, evaluation, research, and health care audits. The process stimulates mental health team members to gather, document, and describe data.

There are four necessary elements in problem-oriented recording systems:

1. *Data base.* The data base consists of all the information gathered at the initial contact with the client. It includes psychiatric history, psychosocial assessment, laboratory and physical findings, and the results of mental status examinations and psychologic tests. Figure 9–6 shows the mental health supplement to the standard defined data base used in one mental health facility.

2. *Problem list.* The problem list emerges from the data base and summarizes the problems of the client. It should also include the client's assets. It is continually updated to present an accurate picture of the client's current situation.

3. *Initial plans.* A section of the record delineates the therapeutic plans for the client. Plans are formulated in terms of the problems to which they relate.

MEDICAL RECORD	SUPPLEMENT DEFINED DATA BASE

SUPPLEMENT TO *(Check only one)* PART ☑ I ☐ II ☐ III ☐ IV ☐ V ☐ VI

PREPARED BY *(Signature & Title)*	SERVICE	DATE
I. Knight, R.N. Clinical Specialist	Emergency	12-23-91

CHIEF COMPLAINT: In patient's own words and your impressions.

Gaunt, disheveled man in mid-thirties complains, "I have no purpose in life."

HISTORY AND DEVELOPMENT OF COMPLAINT

A. Date of onset and circumstances under which complaint developed.

Since resigning responsible position as electronics engineer 10 years ago, client has been drifting aimlessly, living at minimal level of subsistence. Brought in by police who found him living in his car in a school parking lot.

B. Previous hospitalizations and treatment-response to psychotropic drugs.

Unknown

C. Previous history of violent behavior, suicidal behavior, alcohol and drug abuse, previous arrests, and treatment by alcohol, drug and forensic program.

Experimentation with LSD and marijuana for 10 years at least 3x per week ... often once per day, with related impairment of social & occupational function. (No job, no dating relationships or social life)

MENTAL STATUS EXAMINATION

A. Overall general appearance. *Thin, unshaven dirty man in mid-thirties with poor nutrition, hygiene and tearful expression.*

B. Attitude and degree of cooperativeness.

Generally despondent but passively cooperative

C. Thought content and process—what patient thinks about—how patient thinks over and underproductive, spontaneous, circumstantial.

Thought content focuses on discovering solution to life's mysteries ... finding the key or answer.
Thought processes are vague and disconnected. Long periods of silence between verbalizations.

SUPPLEMENT

DEFINED

DATA BASE

VA FORM 10-7978g

FIGURE 9–6   Example of supplement to data base.   SOURCE: *Veterans Administration Hospital, Buffalo, NY.*

D. Motoric behavior—overactive, underactive, inappropriate.

Slow, underactive bordering on catatonic low energy level

AFFECT

A. How the patient feels—shallow, anxious, depressed appropriate, inappropriate.

Depressed and discouraged — feelings of inadequacy

SENSORIUM MENTAL GRASP AND CAPACITY

A. Orientation/memory

Oriented to time, place + person

B. Abstract thinking

Can interpret proverbs but ponderously

C. Judgment/insight, adequate, complete, incomplete, distorted

Questionable

D. Cognitive disorder—hallucinations and delusions

No data available at this time

E. Estimate of intelligence

Average or above

DIAGNOSTIC IMPRESSION

Substance use disorder, Dysthymic Disorder (or Depressive Neurosis), Possible Avoidant Personality

TREATMENT PLAN

PROBLEMS	GOALS	TREATMENT
Poor nutritional status	*Improve status*	*Offer balanced, high cal diet suited to his vegetarian preference.*
Poor hygiene status	*Improve status*	*Encourage daily bathing. Refer to Dentist*
Dependence on Cannabis	*Decrease usage*	*Refer to Group Therapy*
Depression	*Control Sx*	*Prescribe anti-depress. medication. Refer to Psych. Therapist for individual counseling*

FIGURE 9–6 (continued)

4. *Progress note.* Progress notes parallel items in the problem list. They are used to monitor the plans, identify the need for modification, and provide a follow-up. The progress notes include narrative notes, flow sheets, and a discharge summary.

    a. Narrative notes are written in SOAP style, an acronym for *subjective* (the problem as perceived by the client), *objective* (clinical findings or observations), *assessment* (what is suggested by an analysis and synthesis of the subjective and objective data), and *plan* (proposed solutions for the identified problems).

    b. Flow sheets are used to tabulate information in graphic form. They are useful when some factor must be monitored frequently.

    c. The discharge summary is a summary of each problem area and the level of resolution reached. It provides the essential data for community follow-up services.

Figure 9–7 demonstrates how one mental health facility uses problem-oriented progress notes.

Nursing Care Plans

Nursing care plans are a means of providing nursing personnel with information about the needs and therapeutic plans for each client. They are of major importance when an agency uses source-oriented recording methods, because they provide an ongoing, up-to-date record of goal-directed, individualized nursing care. When problem-oriented recording methods are used, nursing care plans may be an outgrowth of the record.

Algorithms

Algorithms are behavioral steps, or step-by-step procedures, for the management of common problems. Algorithms have proved useful protocols, particularly in settings that employ large numbers of paraprofessionals. At intake points in community mental health settings, such as walk-in neighborhood clinics, mental health workers often make the initial psychosocial assessment and may plan and implement treatment strategies. Clinical algorithms for common mental health problems would provide the nonprofessional with structured, standardized guidelines for decision making.

Professional nurses in nonpsychiatric settings find clinical algorithms particularly useful. Algorithms for depression and suicidal lethality have been found reliable and valid in these circumstances.

Psychiatric Audits

The psychiatric audit is one way to evaluate the quality of mental health services received by consumers. The client's chart is reviewed to compare criteria for quality care with actual practice. Problem-oriented recording systems provide the descriptive documentation necessary for such a program. Although documentation may not always accurately indicate the quality of the care given, it is an important part of the process of keeping mental health workers accountable to consumers of their services.

The Interaction Process Analysis (IPA)

The **interaction process analysis** is a verbatim and progressive recording of the verbal and nonverbal interactions between client and nurse within a given time. It is an important means of communication between nurses or nursing students and their clinical supervisors, consultants, or instructors about their client relationships. To learn the function of therapeutic intervention, nurses must study and review with objectivity the verbal and nonverbal components of the interaction to learn their potential significance. These components may express the existence of problems or attempts at resolution of these problems.

Purposes The IPA serves a number of purposes:

• It helps nurses sharpen their skills of observation and listening by providing an opportunity to find clues that were not recognized during the face-to-face encounter.

• It promotes the communication skills of nurses. By examining their words, gestures, and nonverbal communication, nurses can reduce their use of clichés, double messages, and stereotyped automatic comments.

• It gives the nurse a tool for assessing nurse-client interactions and gives the instructor, clinical supervisor, or consultant a tool for assessing and guiding the nurse in clinical work. It supplements memory, facilitates evaluation, and acquaints the student with rudimentary applied research skills. It also asks the nurse to produce written comments grounded in theory.

• It provides data from which nurses can assess their own behavior in interactions with clients. By encouraging nurses to examine their personal reactions to client behavior, the IPA enriches their self-understanding and experience. An added advantage of the IPA is that it allows nurses to look at the dynamics of nurse-client behavior when they are away from the

MEDICAL RECORD	PROBLEM-ORIENTED PROGRESS NOTES

PROBLEM
DATE | NO.

Format—Problem title (Do not abbreviate) S-Subjective O-Objective A-Assessment P-Plans. (All notes must have signature and title of person making entry.) Continue on reverse.

12-4-91 | 3

Problem Title: Angry and agitated.

Subjective: "I can't take anymore of this— I have to get out!"

Objective: Client is pacing, crying, waving his hands, yelling at nursing staff and other patients. Looks very upset.

Assessment: Client has just completed interview with his private therapist, who told him his wife has filed for divorce, and won't talk to him about it.

Plan:
1. Give client time and space to decrease agitation
2. Offer him use of quiet room
3. Keep him in eye contact but do not engage him at this time
4. If he is not quieter in 1 hr offer PRN medication.

J. Knight, RN
Clinical Specialist

PROBLEM-ORIENTED
PROGRESS NOTES

EXISTING STOCK OF VA FORM 10-7978i,
OCT 1974, WILL BE USED.

VA FORM 10-7978i

FIGURE 9–7   Sample form for problem-oriented progress notes.   SOURCE: Veterans Administration Hospital, Buffalo, NY.

interpersonal situation. They can often gain some objectivity through distance.

• It helps nurses plan nursing interventions. By evaluating the effectiveness of therapeutic strategies in actual clinical situations and linking their observations to theory, nurses can identify additional or alternative nursing interventions.

Methods There are several ways to structure IPAs. Two-, three-, or four-column styles may be used. Regardless of the organizational style, however, the IPA should include these components:

• The verbal and nonverbal communication of the client

• The verbal and nonverbal communication of the nurse

• Analysis or interpretation of the possible significance of the communication

• Identification of the nurse's own feelings

• Identification of the possible intent of the nurse's communication

• Identification of the nurse's perception of the client's emotions and the intent of the client's communication

• Evaluation of the effectiveness of the approach, based on the above data

• The nursing alternatives used and the rationale for their use

The raw data or verbatim recording can be obtained in a number of ways.

On-the-Spot Recording The nurse may make brief notes on the spot, perhaps using some shorthand code of symbols and abbreviations, in a stenographer's notebook. There are several advantages to this form of recording. Notes on verbal communication can be made easily, it is a more accurate technique than attempting to recall after the experience, and it prevents the nurse from unwittingly omitting important material. It also demonstrates that the nurse is paying close attention to what the client says and does. However, the nurse usually interacts less freely and becomes less spontaneous when recording on the spot, because of the need to attend to the note-taking task. It may also limit observation of the nonverbal components of the client's communication.

After-the-Fact Recording When the nurse gathers data by recall, it is important to record them as soon as possible after the interaction with the client. The most successful method is for nurses to structure their time so that they can begin writing in a quiet area immediately. The longer the time between interaction and recording, the less able nurses are to remember words and actions and their sequence. If it is difficult to set aside enough time, the nurse should record only raw data at once and delay analysis. A delay may actually improve analysis. It may allow a more objective interpretation, because time and distance make nurses less protective of their original behavior.

The advantage of this method is that it does not require the nurse to take notes while paying close attention to the client. It thus does not curtail the nurse's spontaneity. The major disadvantage is that the nurse may not remember completely and thus distort the interaction. Nurses using this method of recording tend to omit or shorten important details.

Tape Recording The most common form of mechanical recording is by audiotape. Tape recorders are now smaller, less expensive, and less obtrusive than earlier models were. Videotape recordings may also be used. Although now available in portable form, they are costly and are less commonly used.

Tape-recorded data can be transcribed at the nurse's leisure and provide a more accurate record of verbal interactions than notes do. The recording avoids unintentional editing or condensation of important content. Nurses who use a tape recorder can reexperience tones of voice, pauses, silences, speaking rates, actual words, and sequences of responses. Because tapes force nurses to listen to themselves as they actually are rather than as they would like to be, using a tape recorder may cause anxiety. Clients may fear being "on tape" and refuse to give the nurse permission to tape the session. Other disadvantages are that tape recording does not pick up visual cues, and transcribing the tape can be costly and/or time-consuming.

Confidentiality and Comprehensiveness of IPAs The nurse who records client data has the responsibility to protect the client from unwarranted exposure. The client's name should not appear on the IPA, and the record should not be treated carelessly or left lying about. The nurse's respect for the client's self-disclosures is one way for the client to gauge the nurse's trustworthiness.

Cutting corners in preparing an IPA is inadvisable, because meaningful exchanges may be bypassed. To be an effective learning tool, the IPA should be comprehensive.

Chapter Highlights

• The nursing process begins with assessment, and the primary source of client data in most instances is the client.

• Correct problem identification and intervention strategies often depend on the quality of information sharing.

• Psychiatric client information is gathered and assessed through psychiatric history-taking, mental status examination, physiologic assessment, psychologic testing, psychosocial assessments, and interaction process analysis.

• Traditionally, history-taking has followed a medical model and is most concerned with gathering information about a client's psychiatric problem.

• The mental status examination is used to identify a person's general behavior and appearance, characteristics of talk, emotional state, special preoccupations and experiences, sensorium or orientation, memory, general intelligence, abstract thinking, and insight; its primary purpose is to gather data to formulate a psychiatric diagnosis, prognosis, and treatment plan.

• Psychologic tests are tests concerned with measuring intelligence or personality.

• It is particularly important for the nurse to rule out a physiologic or neurologic basis for mental symptoms by conducting a thorough history, directly observing the client, and completing a neurologic assessment.

• The DSM-III-R is the APA's most recent system for diagnosing and classifying mental disorders and is more congruent with holistic views of people than were DSM-II or DSM-I.

• Axes IV (Severity of Psychosocial Stressors) and V (Global Assessment of Functioning in the past year) of DSM-III-R best represent the practice domain of nursing and are the areas in which nursing's greatest contribution may lie.

• In conducting a psychosocial assessment to determine a client's problems, the nurse should include physical, intellectual, socioeconomic and developmental factors, personal values and goals, adaptive functioning, and response to present involvements.

• Recording provides the basis for altering the treatment plan, determining intervention, linking health team members, gaining around-the-clock data on hospitalized clients, evidence in court, and research.

• The most significant events the psychiatric nurse records are the behavior patterns and interpersonal interactions of the client.

• The psychosocial nurse uses psychiatric jargon sparingly, recognizing its inadequacies for understanding the depth and variety of human problems.

• Problem-oriented systems of recording are comprehensive and logically structured; they can be used in performing the psychiatric audit, developing nursing care plans, and devising algorithms.

REFERENCES

Carpenito L: *Nursing Diagnoses: Applications to Clinical Practice.* Lippincott, 1983.

Compton BR, Galaway B: *Social Work Processes,* ed 2. Dorsey Press, 1979.

Diagnostic and Statistical Manual of Mental Disorders, III-R. American Psychiatric Association, 1987.

Frances A et al.: An introduction to DSM-IV. *Hosp Community Psychiatry* May 1990;41(5):493–494.

Hagerty B: *Psychiatric-Mental Health Assessment.* Mosby, 1984.

Kaplan HI, Sadock BJ: *Modern Synopsis of Comprehensive Textbook of Psychiatry,* ed 4. Williams & Wilkins, 1985.

McFarland GK, Wasli EL: *Nursing Diagnosis and Process in Psychiatric Mental Health Nursing.* Lippincott, 1986.

Morgan AJ, Moreno JW: *The Practice of Mental Health Nursing: A Community Approach.* Lippincott, 1973.

Morrison E, et al.: The NSGAE. *J Psychosoc Nurs Ment Health Serv* 1985;23(8):10–13.

Patient assessment: Neurological examination. (Programmed instruction.) *Am J Nurs* 1975;75 (Part I, September): PI, pp 1–24. 1975;75 (Part II, November): PI, pp 1–24. 1976;76 (Part III, April): PI, pp 1–25.

Small SM: *Outline for Psychiatric Examination.* Sandoz, 1980.

Spitzer RL, Forman JBW: DSM-III field trials: II. Initial experience with the multiaxial system. *Am J Psychiatry* 1979;136:818–820.

Spitzer RL, Williams JBW, Skodol AE: DSM-III: The major achievements and an overview. *Am J Psychiatry* 1980;137:151–164.

Williams JBW: DSM-IIIR preview: Psychotic and mood disorders. *Hosp Community Psychiatry* 1987;38(1):13–14.

Williams JBW, Wilson HS: A psychiatric nursing perspective on DSM-III. *J Psychosoc Nurs Ment Health Serv* 1982;20:14–20.

Wilson HS, Skodol AE: Introduction and overview of changes in DSM-III-R. *Arch Psychiatr Nurs* 1988;1(2):87–94.

PART THREE

Human Responses to Distress and Disorder

CONTENTS

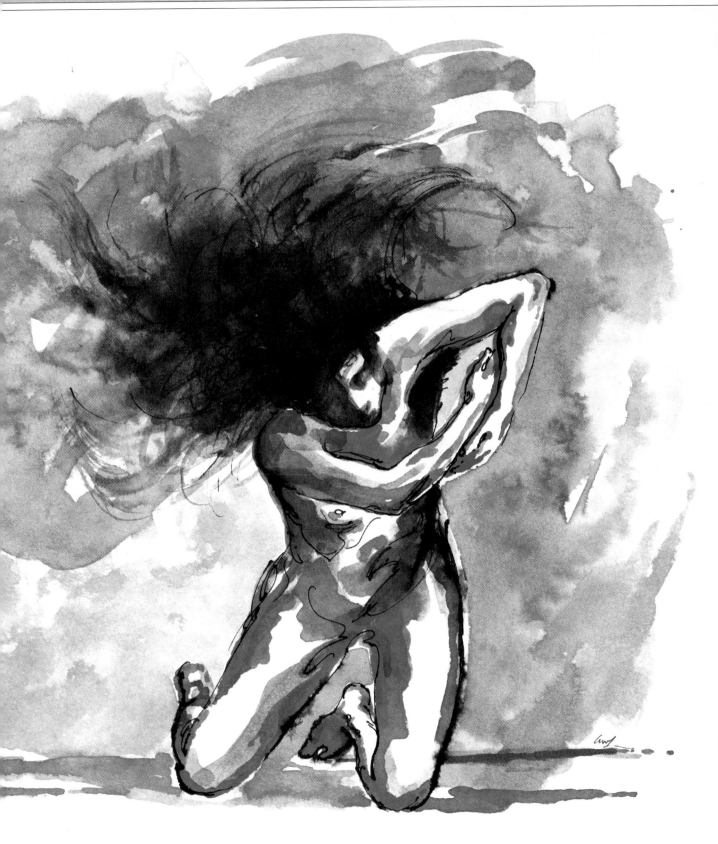

Movement gives visible substance to things felt. Out of emotion comes form—powerful, jagged, tense, or soft, fluid, vulnerable.

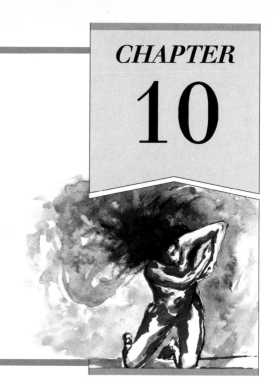

Applying the Nursing Process for Clients with Organic Mental Syndromes and Disorders

LEARNING OBJECTIVES

- Understand theories that explain organic mental syndromes and organic brain disease

- Differentiate among types of dementias and delirium

- Specify diagnostic criteria for dementia and delirium

- Apply the nursing process with clients who have organic mental syndromes and organic brain disease

- Assess relevant subjective and objective data for clients with organic mental syndromes and organic brain disease

- Formulate nursing diagnoses for clients who have organic mental syndromes and organic brain disease

- Plan and implement nursing interventions for clients who have organic mental syndromes and organic brain disease

- Identify outcome criteria to evaluate nursing interventions for clients with organic mental syndromes and organic brain disease

Gloria Kuhlman
Gail DeBoer
Holly Skodol Wilson

CROSS REFERENCES

Other topics relevant to this content are: Elderly, Chapter 35; Families, Chapter 30; Neuropsychiatric complications of AIDS, Chapter 25; Substance abuse–related organic brain syndrome and organic mental disorder, Chapter 11.

UNTIL RECENTLY PSYCHIATRIC NURSING has for the most part ignored mental disorders due to cerebral dysfunction. The psychobiologic revolution has changed the focus, and interest is growing in the organic mental syndromes and disorders. Cook-Deegan et al. (1988) and Dickson and Ranseen (1990) identify the following factors contributing to this shift:

• Aging of the population

• Rapid advances in medical technology, such as brain imaging and electrophysiology

• Increasingly specific neuropsychologic testing

Ms L was a 57-year-old widowed schoolteacher who had begun experiencing difficulties with her memory for the past year. She complained that she was having problems selecting the words she wanted to use and putting her thoughts on paper. She began to miss appointments and scheduled workdays. Gradually, handling her own financial affairs became impossible.

Over three years, Ms L was forced to quit her job and become more and more dependent on her family. Her eldest daughter moved into her home, and other friends and family took turns sitting with her. Ms L became incontinent as she wandered confusedly about the house, unable to find the bathroom. Increasingly anxious and paranoid, she began to see things crawling on the walls and mistook her own reflection in a mirror for a painting. When agitated she was just as likely to walk out into the street as to become belligerent with her daughter.

Ms L was admitted to a long-term care facility when she became increasingly belligerent and aggressive with her daughter, wandered the house at night, and slept sporadically. After two years, Ms L was bedridden and unable to speak. She had to be tube fed. Ms L finally succumbed to pneumonia.

Historical and Theoretic Foundations

Before the twentieth century, all organic brain disorders of the aged were categorized as **senile dementia.** Beginning at the turn of the century, neuropathologists doing autopsy work distinguished senile dementia from arteriosclerotic conditions and neurosyphilis (Butler and Lewis 1982). Arteriosclerotic brain disease was then considered the primary cause of confusional states in the elderly. It was believed to be the result of diseased cerebral vessels (Wolanin and Fraelich-Philips 1981). By the middle of this century, a new category, **organic brain disease (OBD),** was added. This category was broader, allowing for both a defect in the vessels and in the brain itself. The category **organic brain**

syndrome (OBS) then followed, which recognized the need for a diagnosis that included symptoms without a known cause. Today, the term **organic mental syndrome (OMS)** refers to a group of psychologic or behavioral signs of unknown or unclear etiology. **Organic mental disorder (OMD)** refers to a particular syndrome whose etiology is known or presumed. The knowledge explosion regarding these disorders is likely to result in a major reconceptualization in DSM-IV, planned for publication in1993.

Factors in Pathology

Dementia

In the United States today, approximately 1.5 million people over age 65 suffer from dementia to the extent that they cannot care for themselves, and 1–5 million suffer from milder forms (Cook-Deegan, et al. 1988). This number is ten times greater than at the turn of the century. Over 60 percent of people in nursing homes have been diagnosed with dementia (Brody et al. 1984). A now common clinical syndrome, **dementia** is marked by the following:

• Global cognitive impairment extending to the areas of abstract thinking, judgment, complex capabilities (language, tasks, recognition), and personality change.

• Memory impairment

• Decline in intellectual function

• Altered judgment, in awake and alert states

• Altered affect

Dementia is an organic mental disorder in which a client's previous functioning declines in multiple cognitive areas, including memory (Dickson and Ranseen 1990). Symptoms related to specific areas of brain damage are shown in Figure 10–1. The DSM-III-R further differentiates *dementia* as "a disturbance severe enough to interfere significantly with work or usual social activities or relationships with others" (DSM-III-R, p 103). (See the box on page 187 for the DSM-III-R diagnostic criteria.)

Dementias are classified according to causal agent or area of neurologic damage. The latter scheme distinguishes between cortical and subcortical dementias. Alzheimer's disease is the classic cortical dementia, whereas Huntington's disease and Parkinson's disease are common subcortical types. These categories are quite similar. People with subcortical dementias, however, have a higher order of functioning.

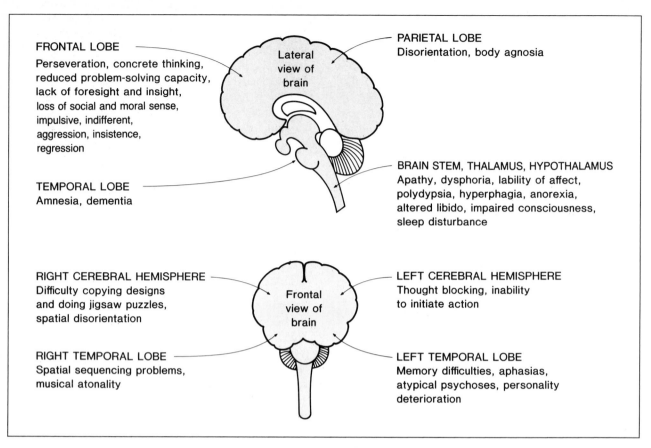

FIGURE 10—1   Behavior changes related to specific areas of brain damage.

Alzheimer's Disease   Alzheimer's disease, an OMD, is the most common form of dementia seen in the elderly. It accounts for over 50 percent of the dementias of old age (Buckwalter et al. 1988). Alois Alzheimer first recognized it in 1907 while conducting an autopsy on a 51-year-old woman with a 4½-year history of dementia. He discovered **senile plaques** and other pathologic lesions that he called **neurofibrillary tangles.** These are now referred to as Alzheimer-type changes. This disease may also destroy those neurons that secrete the neurotransmitter acetylcholine, which plays a role in the memory and learning (Jarvik and Greenson 1987).

Alzheimer's disease is defined as a chronic, progressive disorder that is the major cause of degenerative dementia in the United States (Cook-Deegan et al. 1988). The clinical course may vary from one to more than ten years (Burns and Buckwalter 1988).

Signs of Alzheimer's Disease   Signs of this disease include:

• **Aphasia** (loss of language ability). Initially, the person experiences difficulty in finding words. Eventually this condition progresses to loss of all verbal ability (Dawson et al. 1986).

• **Apraxia** (loss of purposeful movement without loss of muscle power or coordination in general). The ability to conceptualize or perform motor tasks deteriorates. People with apraxia may display difficulty in pursuing complex tasks or become so obsessed with an aspect of an act that they cannot complete it (Buckwalter 1988).

• **Agnosia** (loss of sensory ability to recognize objects). Initially, the person has difficulty recognizing everyday objects. In the later stages, people with agnosia recognize neither loved ones nor their own body parts.

• **Mnemonic disturbances** (memory loss). The inability to remember recent events, especially in new or changing environments, extends to profound memory loss of both recent and past events (Petrie 1985).

Progression of Alzheimer's Disease   Stages of the progression of Alzheimer's disease have been variously described in the literature. In the early stage, the person has difficulty remembering names and appointments and may forget where things were placed. The person may also have problems with spatial orientation, show affect changes, and seem emotionally unstable at times. Epileptiform seizures may occur, along with muscle twitching (Johnson and Keller 1989).

The second stage presents with apparent cognitive deficits. This stage may last from two to twelve years.

Memory for past events may still exist, but the person has no recall of recent ones. Orientation and concentration are now affected, and the person has increasing difficulty comprehending everyday events. The client manifests restlessness at night and increased aphasia, agnosia, and apraxia. Activities of daily living must be supervised, and former social habits are forgotten. The client has hypertonia and an unsteady gait, along with perseveration phenomena, hyperorality, and an insatiable appetite without weight gain (Johnson and Keller 1989).

The final stage is terminal, usually lasting from several months to 5 years. Severe disorientation, psychotic symptoms (e.g., delusions, hallucinations, and paranoid ideation), and severe agitation are present. A **Kluver-Bucy-like syndrome** occurs, which includes hyperorality, blunting of emotions, bulimia, and attempts to touch every object in sight. The individual eventually becomes bedridden, emaciated, and helpless. Death usually results from pneumonia or other infection, malnutrition, and dehydration (Johnson and Keller 1989).

Causes of Alzheimer's Disease The actual cause of Alzheimer's disease remains unknown, but several factors are believed to play a role. Alzheimer's disease has been correlated with loss of specific groups of nerve cells and disruption of communication between nerve cells (depressed acetylcholine and serotonin). Genetics may play a role in 10–20 percent of cases as evidenced by the occurrence in members of the same family; the incidence is from 50 percent to 100 percent (Farrer et al. 1989). An autosomal dominant

DSM-III-R Diagnostic Criteria for Dementia

1. Demonstrable evidence of impairment in short- and long-term memory. Impairment in short-term memory (inability to learn new information) may be indicated by inability to remember three objects after five minutes. Long-term memory impairment (inability to remember information that was known in the past) may be indicated by inability to remember past personal information (e.g., what happened yesterday, birthplace, occupation) or facts of common knowledge (e.g., past presidents, well-known dates).

2. At least one of the following:
   a. Impairment in abstract thinking, as indicated by inability to find similarities and differences between related words, difficulty in defining words and concepts, and other similar tasks.
   b. Impaired judgment, as indicated by inability to make reasonable plans to deal with interpersonal, family, and job-related problems and issues.
   c. Other disturbances of higher cortical function, such as aphasia (disorder of language), apraxia (inability to carry out motor activities despite intact comprehension and motor function), agnosia (failure to recognize or identify objects despite intact sensory function), and "constructional difficulty" (e.g., inability to copy three-dimensional figures, assemble blocks, or arrange sticks in specific designs).
   d. Personality change, i.e., alteration or accentuation of premorbid traits.

3. The disturbance in a and b significantly interferes with work or usual social activities or relationships with others.

4. Not occurring exclusively during the course of delirium.

5. Either a or b:
   a. There is evidence from the history, physical examination, or laboratory tests of a specific organic factor (or factors) judged to be etiologically related to the disturbance.
   b. In the absence of such evidence, an etiologic organic factor can be presumed if the disturbance cannot be accounted for by any nonorganic mental disorder, e.g., Major Depression accounting for cognitive impairment.

Criteria for Severity of Dementia
Mild: Although work or social activities are significantly impaired, the capacity for independent living remains, with adequate personal hygiene and relatively intact judgment.

Moderate: Independent living is hazardous, and some degree of supervision is necessary.

Severe: Activities of daily living are so impaired that continual supervision is required, e.g., unable to maintain minimal personal hygiene; largely incoherent or mute.

SOURCE: American Psychiatric Association: Diagnostic and Statistical Manual of Mental Disorders, *ed 3, revised. APA, 1987, p 107.*

trait is believed to cause high incidences. Work is also being done to discover a slow-acting viruslike causal agent. This work has been prompted by the findings of just such an agent in Creutzfeldt-Jakob disease (Cook-Deegan et al. 1988). Aluminum has also been implicated, since it can cause dementia in animals and has been found with silicon in significantly higher than normal concentration on autopsy in people with Alzheimer's disease (Cook-Deegan et al. 1988). Vitamin B_{12} deficiency has been identified as a condition that mimics Alzheimer's disease, according to the accompanying Nutrition box. Alzheimer's disease may also be related to a specific chromosome or genotype. People with Down syndrome who survive to adulthood eventually develop Alzheimer lesions in the brain (Cook-Deegan et al. 1988). A possible defect in the immune system, as evidenced by decreased levels of supressor lymphocytes in people with Alzheimer's disease, is under investigation (Cook-Deegan et al. 1988). Several investigators have reported disrupted biochemical pathways and other metabolic (glucose) abnormalities.

Multi-Infarct Dementia

Multi-infarct dementia (MID), the second most common cause, accounts for about 17 percent of the dementias. Unlike Alzheimer's disease, which is slowly progressive, MID is usually abrupt in onset and episodic, with multiple remissions (Cook-Deegan et al. 1988). The client also demonstrates focal neurologic signs, such as one-sided weakness, emotional outbursts when frustrated, a stepwise rather than progressive decline in intellectual functioning, and a history of hypertension, diabetes, or cardiovascular disease affecting other organs (Duthrie and Glatt 1988).

In MID, brain tissue is destroyed by intermittent emboli that can range from a few to over a dozen. Individual infarcts may vary by 1 centimeter in diameter, symptoms are commonly absent until 100 to 200 cubic centimeters of brain tissue have been destroyed (Kase 1986).

Parkinson's Disease

Only recently has the OMD, **Parkinson's disease,** been associated with dementia. A minority of clients with dementia have Parkinson's disease. There is a subset of clients showing both Parkinson's disease and Alzheimer's disease, and this diagnosis may be difficult. There are several different varieties of Parkinson's disease. The cause of classic Parkinson's disease is unknown. Another type, postencephalitic, has been linked to previous viral infection in the brain. An interesting feature of this type is the presence of neurofibrillary tangles in the substantia nigra. These tangles are similar to those found in clients with Alzheimer's disease (Cook-Deegan et al. 1988).

Huntington's Disease

Huntington's disease is a genetic disorder characterized by both motor and cognitive changes. This OMD usually begins between the ages of 30 to 50 years. The movement disorder is thought to be caused by a loss of nerve cells in the brain. The motor dysfunction is characterized by **chorea:** quick, jerky, purposeless, involuntary movements. **Subcortical dementia** is seen, with personality and cognitive changes ranging from apathy to violent emotional outbursts, inability to solve problems and process information quickly, and poor concept formation (Cook-Deegan et al. 1988). Average life span after an initial diagnosis is fifteen years.

Pick's Disease

Pick's disease is a rare disorder clinically similar to Alzheimer's disease, but senile plaques and neurofibrillary tangles are not found on autopsy; instead there are pale, swollen nerve cells containing globules of protein called "Pick's bodies" (Cook-Deegan et al. 1988). Cerebral atrophy is confined to the frontal and temporal cortex (Masliah et al. 1989).

Early signs of Pick's disease include emotional blunting, lack of inhibitions, and lack of insight and social awareness. As the disease progresses, the deterioration becomes more global, affecting memory and language. The expected life span after the original diagnosis is seven years. A higher incidence is seen in some families, pointing toward a genetic predisposition (Cook-Deegan et al. 1988).

Creutzfeldt-Jakob Disease

Creutzfeldt-Jakob disease is a transmissible degenerative dementia. This OMD affects the cerebral cortex through cell destruction and overgrowth. It is marked clinically by a very rapid onset. Creutzfeldt-Jakob disease was a concern for individuals receiving human growth hormone until 1985. From that point a genetically engineered bacteria has been used to prevent transmission of the disease. There is also concern in connection with blood transfusions, so donations of blood by demented individuals is being discouraged. Handling of fluids and tissues from affected individuals requires special precautions (Cook-Deegan et al. 1988).

Normal Pressure Hydrocephalus

First recognized in 1965, **normal pressure hydrocephalus** is a relatively uncommon cause of dementia. Its importance is not frequency, but potential for correction. The classic description of findings is a combination of dementia with urinary incontinence; a slow, hesitant gait; and dilation of the fluid-filled spaces of the brain (Cook-Deegan et al. 1988). A history of head trauma or bleeding in the brain may suggest normal pressure hydrocephalus.

Treatment is to implant a shunt to drain fluid from the brain to another body cavity (usually the abdo-

Is It Alzheimer's Disease or Vitamin B₁₂ Deficiency?

A deficiency of cobalamin, or vitamin B_{12}, can easily be mistaken for the dementia of Alzheimer's disease. Clinicians' ability to detect this common dietary disorder can prevent a great deal of misery among geriatric clients.

Vitamin B_{12} depletion is common among older adults because of age-induced changes in the gastrointestinal tract. More specifically, the elderly are prone to atrophic gastritis (Berkow 1987), which in turn reduces acid production and secretion of digestive enzymes. Both are needed to separate B_{12} from other food components, thus freeing it for intestinal absorption (Herbert 1988). With time, gastric atrophy also reduces levels of intrinsic factor, a third substance required for cobalamin absorption.

Many nursing and medical textbooks state that a lack of vitamin B_{12} first causes pernicious anemia, and clinicians look for a drop in hemoglobin and a variety of other hematologic markers. The same texts explain that, with time, anemia is accompanied by neurologic signs and symptoms, including diminished vibration and position senses and dementia.

Unfortunately, it is rare for a clinician to suspect B_{12}-induced dementia when a client's complete blood count is normal. Recent research has shown that many older clients suffer the psychiatric effects of vitamin B_{12} deficiency *without* developing anemia.

For instance, Carmel (1988) found that among seventy patients with clear-cut vitamin B_{12} deficiency, 19 percent had no anemia and 33 percent had no evidence of macrocytosis: abnormally large red blood cells seen in pernicious anemia. Despite the normal blood profile, several clients had neurologic problems, including confusion, belligerence, disorientation, bizarre behavior, and numbness and weakness in the hands and feet. Sadly, many of these clients did not respond to vitamin therapy because irreversible nerve damage had already taken place. One way to prevent such needless tragedies is to perform routine serum B_{12} screening on all geriatric clients, thus increasing the likelihood of detecting a deficiency in an early, easily reversible stage.

A few words of caution, however, are in order about B_{12} screening: Recognizing a deficiency in its early stage is possible but requires astute assessment skills and a willingness to act as a strong client advocate, even in the face of resistance from other health professionals. Special effort is needed because some primary care physicians may not know how to interpret the diagnostic markers used to pinpoint the disorder.

Most reference works say serum B_{12} levels below 100–110 ng/L are consistent with B_{12} depletion. Thus, many clinicians ignore readings above that cutoff (Tietz 1985). Carmel (1988), however, has detected the disorder in clients with neuropsychiatric complaints and serum B_{12} readings between 100 and 299 ng/L. Others (Lindenbaum et al. 1988) have found similar symptoms in clients with readings of 100–200 ng/L. Of course, readings in this "subnormal" range—in the face of normal hematologic findings—do not prove conclusively that a client has B_{12} deficiency; some clients with "subnormal" serum levels have adequate cobalamin tissue levels. This finding should nevertheless prompt clinicians to investigate B_{12} status more thoroughly by performing either a Schilling test, which determines the ability to secrete intrinsic factor, or a deoxyuridine suppression test (Carmel 1985), which can detect a subtle B_{12} deficit when the interpretation of serum B_{12} readings is questionable.

Once a B_{12} deficit is found, its origin must be determined. As mentioned earlier, older adults with this disorder are more likely than most to have gastric atrophy and poor absorption of the nutrient. Clients who have had a total gastrectomy and about 20 percent of those with partial gastrectomy will also develop a deficiency (Herbert and Colman 1988). Similarly, any disease or condition that severely damages the ileum—the site of B_{12} absorption—may induce a deficit. Among these are gluten intolerance, Crohn's disease, intestinal resection, and cancers of the small intestine. Likewise, certain drugs, including para-aminosalicylic acid, colchicine, and neomycin, can inhibit B_{12} absorption.

A B_{12} deficiency can result from poor eating habits alone, although this cause is less common among geriatric clients. Those at greatest risk are strict vegetarians who avoid milk, eggs, and meats, virtually the only sources of the vitamin.

To correct a B_{12} deficiency, a clinician must first address the cause. In many malabsorption syndromes, including atrophic gastritis, the nutrient must be given intramuscularly, often for life. Among vegetarians, an oral supplement is adequate.

—Paul L. Cerrato

men). Successful relief of symptoms occurs in 40 percent of cases and brings rapid clinical improvement (Cook-Deegan et al. 1988).

Neurosyphilis Neurosyphilis or *dementia paralytica* is the direct result of untreated primary syphilis. The infecting organism (*Treponema pallidum*, a spirochete) produces cerebral atrophy in the frontal and anterior temporal lobes. Symptoms of this OMD may appear two to thirty years following the primary lesion (Wolanin and Fraelich-Philips 1981). The usual symptoms are paranoia, poor memory, faulty judgment, and disturbed emotional displays. Neurologic signs include fine and coarse tremors, abnormal reflexes, **dysarthria** (difficulty in speaking), and convulsions. Untreated, the disease is usually fatal within three years of onset.

Progressive Supranuclear Palsy **Progressive supranuclear palsy (PSP)** is a disorder similar to Parkinson's disease. PSP results from cell atrophy in the midbrain. Although PSP was not clinically distinguished from Parkinson's disease until 1964, it accounts for 4 percent of all Parkinson's diagnoses.

Chemical imbalances in PSP involve dopamine and possibly acetylcholine. The disorder differs from Parkinson's disease in that clients lose the ability to gaze up or down, and usually there is no tremor (Cook-Deegan et al. 1988).

Pseudodementia Affective disorders, particularly depression, can be masked by symptoms suggestive of dementia. Clinical symptoms may include impaired attention and memory, apathy, self-neglect, and no complaints of depression. It is essential to detect these pseudodemented clients because, with appropriate treatment, they can recover. **Pseudodementia** should be suspected when the onset is abrupt, the clinical course is rapid, and the client complains about cognitive failures. Clients with dementia often fail to perceive or attempt to cover up their deficits (Stern and Bernick 1987).

Delirium

Mr R, an 80-year-old bachelor with bilateral cataracts, lived alone in a small midwestern town with his pet cat, Suzy. With help from family and friends, he lived a full, active life. He walked a mile daily, did his own cooking, and attended church services regularly.

Mr R was admitted to the community hospital for a hernia repair that he had been putting off for several months. Never hospitalized before, he was extremely anxious on admission and became more so with each preoperative procedure that day. By ten o'clock that evening, Mr R was found wandering in the hallway looking and calling for Suzy. The nurse gave him a barbitu-

rate sleeping preparation and returned him to his room. Three hours later he was again found wandering, this time nude and more disoriented than before. He was again sedated and confined to bed with a vest and soft wrist restraints. By morning, Mr R was so disoriented and agitated that the surgery was canceled. Mr R's physician then ordered Valium for sedation and the client remained confined to bed. Within one week, Mr R's behavior had deteriorated to the extent that he was felt to need institutionalization. He was transferred to a local nursing home for permanent care.

The elderly, especially the demented, are prone to transient cognitive disorders, usually referred to as either *delirium* or *acute confusional states*. It is estimated that 30 to 50 percent of elderly medical/surgical clients will experience a life-threatening acute confusional state. One-fourth of these delirious elderly die within one month of admission (Foreman 1986). In spite of these and other compelling statistics, research in this area continues to be grossly neglected (Lipowski 1983).

Delirium has been called senile delirium, acute confusional states, acute brain syndrome, acute brain failure, pseudosenility, and clouded states. **Delirium** is defined as an "organic brain syndrome, characterized by global cognitive impairment of abrupt onset and relatively brief duration (usually less than 1 month) and by concurrent disturbances of attention, sleep-wake cycle, and psychomotor behavior" (Lipowski 1983, p 1427). (See the accompanying box for DSM-III-R diagnostic criteria.)

Signs of Delirium

Cognition The three components of cognition—perception, thinking, and memory—are all disrupted in delirium:

• *Perception.* The person shows reduced ability to distinguish and integrate sensory information and to discriminate it from hallucinations, dreams, illusions, and imagery.

• *Thinking.* This process is fragmented and disorganized to the extent that the elderly person is unable to reason, judge, abstract, or solve problems.

• *Memory.* Memory is impaired in all three spheres; the elderly person is unable to register, retain, or recall information.

Attention and Wakefulness Attention is impaired in all three spheres. The person has difficulty with

• Alertness or the maintaining of vigilance

• Selectiveness, or the ability to focus on and selectively attend to stimuli at will

DSM-III-R Diagnostic Criteria for Delirium

1. Reduced ability to maintain attention to external stimuli (e.g., questions must be repeated because attention wanders) and to appropriately shift attention to new external stimuli (e.g., perseverates answer to a previous question).

2. Disorganized thinking, as indicated by rambling, irrelevant, or incoherent speech.

3. At least two of the following:
   a. Reduced level of consciousness, e.g., difficulty keeping awake during examination
   b. Perceptual disturbances: misinterpretations, illusions, or hallucinations
   c. Disturbance of sleep-wake cycle with insomnia or daytime sleepiness
   d. Increased or decreased psychomotor activity
   e. Disorientation to time, place, or person
   f. Memory impairment, e.g., inability to learn new material, such as the names of several unrelated objects after five minutes, or to remember past events, such as history of current episodes of illness

4. Clinical features develop over a short period of time (usually hours to days) and tend to fluctuate over the course of a day.

5. Either a or b:
   a. Evidence from the history, physical examination, or laboratory tests of a specific organic factor (or factors) judged to be etiologically related to the disturbance.
   b. In the absence of such evidence, an etiologic organic factor can be presumed if the disturbance cannot be accounted for by any nonorganic mental disorder, e.g., Manic Episode accounting for agitation and sleep disturbance.

SOURCE: *American Psychiatric Association:* Diagnostic and Statistical Manual of Mental Disorders, *ed 3, revised. APA, 1987, p 103.*

• Directiveness, or the ability to direct and focus one's mental processes

Wakefulness is usually reduced during the day, and the person experiences sleeplessness, restlessness, and agitation at night. Interestingly, delirium and dreaming are characterized by the same electroencephalographic (EEG) changes. The elderly person is then caught between dreaming and hallucinating, sleep and wakefulness.

Psychomotor Behavior The delirious client is either hyperactive or hypoactive, often alternating between. Speech may be slurred and disjointed, with aimless vocalizations and repetitions. Tremors and irregular spasmodic (*choreiform*) movements may be present.

Miscellaneous Features The delirious person may manifest rage, depression, fear, and apathy. Incontinence of urine and feces is common.

Delirium is common among the elderly, particularly among those with acute CNS injury. Because delirium is usually caused by an underlying systemic illness, a prompt search is essential for treatable conditions like dehydration, diabetes, hyponatremia, hypercalcemia, thyroid crisis, infection, silent myocardial infarction, drug intoxication, or liver or renal failure. If the cause is removed, complete recovery can be achieved (Stern and Bernick 1987).

Differentiating Delirium from Dementia

Several criteria distinguish delirium from dementia (Cook-Deegan et al. 1988).

• *State of consciousness.* Persons with delirium have fluctuating consciousness, whereas demented individuals are as attentive as they can be.

• *Stability.* In clients with delirium, the ability to pay attention and respond varies, whereas in clients with dementia it is relatively stable.

• *Duration.* Delirium is short-lived; dementia is prolonged.

• *Rate of onset.* Delirium develops rapidly, whereas dementia is insidious.

• *Cause.* Delirium may be traced to a recent source, whereas dementia cannot be linked to another cause.

See Table 10–1.

Pseudodelirium In 5 to 20 percent of the cases of delirium, no organic cause can be identified. As in pseudodementia, the presence of inconsistencies in cognitive functioning (e.g., the client does not know where he or she is but can find the bathroom, bed, etc.) should raise the suspicion of a **pseudodelirium.** If the client also has a history of psychiatric illnesses, is grossly and consistently delusional, has marked manic or depressive features, or is unmotivated during cognitive testing, the diagnosis of this OMS may be appropriate (Lipowski 1983).

Amnestic Syndrome **Amnestic syndrome,** a relatively uncommon OMS, is characterized by short- and

TABLE 10-1 Impaired Cognitive Function

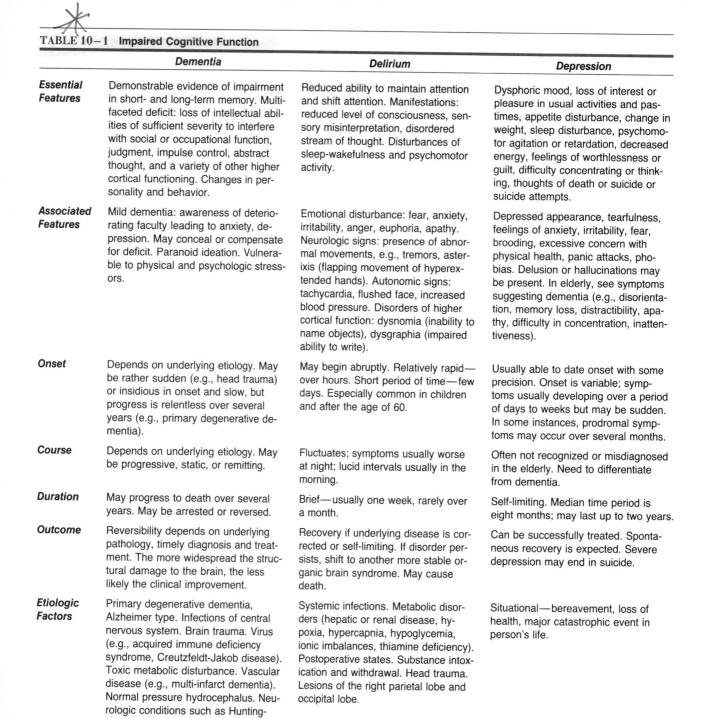

	Dementia	Delirium	Depression
Essential Features	Demonstrable evidence of impairment in short- and long-term memory. Multifaceted deficit: loss of intellectual abilities of sufficient severity to interfere with social or occupational function, judgment, impulse control, abstract thought, and a variety of other higher cortical functioning. Changes in personality and behavior.	Reduced ability to maintain attention and shift attention. Manifestations: reduced level of consciousness, sensory misinterpretation, disordered stream of thought. Disturbances of sleep-wakefulness and psychomotor activity.	Dysphoric mood, loss of interest or pleasure in usual activities and pastimes, appetite disturbance, change in weight, sleep disturbance, psychomotor agitation or retardation, decreased energy, feelings of worthlessness or guilt, difficulty concentrating or thinking, thoughts of death or suicide or suicide attempts.
Associated Features	Mild dementia: awareness of deteriorating faculty leading to anxiety, depression. May conceal or compensate for deficit. Paranoid ideation. Vulnerable to physical and psychologic stressors.	Emotional disturbance: fear, anxiety, irritability, anger, euphoria, apathy. Neurologic signs: presence of abnormal movements, e.g., tremors, asterixis (flapping movement of hyperextended hands). Autonomic signs: tachycardia, flushed face, increased blood pressure. Disorders of higher cortical function: dysnomia (inability to name objects), dysgraphia (impaired ability to write).	Depressed appearance, tearfulness, feelings of anxiety, irritability, fear, brooding, excessive concern with physical health, panic attacks, phobias. Delusion or hallucinations may be present. In elderly, see symptoms suggesting dementia (e.g., disorientation, memory loss, distractibility, apathy, difficulty in concentration, inattentiveness).
Onset	Depends on underlying etiology. May be rather sudden (e.g., head trauma) or insidious in onset and slow, but progress is relentless over several years (e.g., primary degenerative dementia).	May begin abruptly. Relatively rapid—over hours. Short period of time—few days. Especially common in children and after the age of 60.	Usually able to date onset with some precision. Onset is variable; symptoms usually developing over a period of days to weeks but may be sudden. In some instances, prodromal symptoms may occur over several months.
Course	Depends on underlying etiology. May be progressive, static, or remitting.	Fluctuates; symptoms usually worse at night; lucid intervals usually in the morning.	Often not recognized or misdiagnosed in the elderly. Need to differentiate from dementia.
Duration	May progress to death over several years. May be arrested or reversed.	Brief—usually one week, rarely over a month.	Self-limiting. Median time period is eight months; may last up to two years.
Outcome	Reversibility depends on underlying pathology, timely diagnosis and treatment. The more widespread the structural damage to the brain, the less likely the clinical improvement.	Recovery if underlying disease is corrected or self-limiting. If disorder persists, shift to another more stable organic brain syndrome. May cause death.	Can be successfully treated. Spontaneous recovery is expected. Severe depression may end in suicide.
Etiologic Factors	Primary degenerative dementia, Alzheimer type. Infections of central nervous system. Brain trauma. Virus (e.g., acquired immune deficiency syndrome, Creutzfeldt-Jakob disease). Toxic metabolic disturbance. Vascular disease (e.g., multi-infarct dementia). Normal pressure hydrocephalus. Neurologic conditions such as Huntington's disease, multiple sclerosis, Parkinson's disease. Postanoxic or posthypoglycemic states.	Systemic infections. Metabolic disorders (hepatic or renal disease, hypoxia, hypercapnia, hypoglycemia, ionic imbalances, thiamine deficiency). Postoperative states. Substance intoxication and withdrawal. Head trauma. Lesions of the right parietal lobe and occipital lobe.	Situational—bereavement, loss of health, major catastrophic event in person's life.

SOURCES: *American Psychiatric Association: Diagnostic and Statistical Manual of Mental Disorders, ed 3, rev. APA, 1987. Blazer DG: Epidemiology of late life depression. J Am Geriatr Soc 1982;30:587–592. Raskind MA, Storrie MC: The organic mental disorders, in Busse EW, Blazer DG (eds): Handbook of Geriatric Psychiatry. Van Houten, 1980, pp 305–328.*

long-term memory deficits, an inability to learn new material, confabulation, apathy, and a bland affect. Impairment may be moderate to severe. Possible causes include head trauma, hypoxia, herpes-simplex encephalitis, thiamine deficiency, and chronic use of ethanol (Varcarolis 1990).

Organic Hallucinosis In **organic hallucinosis,** persistent hallucinations range from pleasant to terrifying. The person may be aware that the hallucinations are not real. Degree of impairment depends on how the person responds to the hallucination. Possible causes include long-term ethanol use, use of hallucinogens, sensory deprivation, and temporal or occipital lesions (Varcarolis 1990).

Organic Anxiety Syndrome The essential feature of **organic anxiety syndrome** is recurrent panic attacks or overwhelming anxiety that has organic bases. The attacks range from mild to severe, with cognitive impairment especially in the ability to sustain attention. Possible causes include hyper- or hypothyroidism; hypoglycemia; withdrawal from CNS depressants, ethanol, or sedatives; use of psychoactive substances such as cocaine, caffeine, or amphetamines; pulmonary embolis; and chronic obstructive pulmonary disease.

Organic Delusional Syndrome In **organic delusional syndrome,** both paranoid and schizophrenia-like symptoms are present. Although delusions are the dominant symptom, hallucinations, mild cognitive impairment, rambling or incoherent speech, hyperactivity or immobility, or stereotypic behavior may be present (Varcarolis 1990). This OMS is believed to be a result of cerebral disorders that involve the temporal lobe, e.g., epilepsy, encephalitis, or cocaine and amphetamine intoxication.

Organic Mood Syndrome Organic mood syndrome is characterized by an abnormal mood (depressive or manic) that is the result of a cerebral disorder only. There is mild cognitive impairment. Possible causal agents of this OMS include acute viral infections, Cushing syndrome, pernicious anemia, hyperthyroidism or hypothyroidism, Parkinson's disease, and hallucinogens and reserpine (DSM-III-R 1987).

Organic Personality Syndrome The distinguishing symptoms of **organic personality syndrome** include unstable affect, recurrent outbursts of rage, marked apathy, and indifference. Cognitive functions are intact, even though social judgment is not. Possible causes include: neoplasms, temporal lobe epilepsy, and multiple sclerosis (Varcarolis 1990).

The Nursing Process and Clients with OMS and OMD

Assessing

It is often difficult to gather data about clients with organic mental syndromes and disorders. Such clients are sometimes anxious and defensive; confused clients give unreliable histories; and often there is no reliable secondary source of information. All data should be gathered in a milieu that is free of distraction. The nurse should pace the questions slowly to allow the client time to answer comfortably. Aging people can normally process information after receiving it but may have difficulty taking in information. Placing the client in a situation that interferes with an already compromised sensory apparatus only heightens the client's anxiety and seriously compromises the nurse's attempts to evaluate effectively.

Health History When completing the client's health history, include all past and present medical conditions, paying special attention to chronic conditions for which the client is being treated and any recent changes in health status. The Theory box on page 194 indicates the significant number of medical syndromes that may result in cognitive changes. Ask the client, "Are you seeing a physician at this time?" "Why did you seek medical help?" "What does the doctor say is the problem?" Keep in mind that infections may present as confusion and other symptoms of dementia before any change in temperature, pulse, and respirations is noted.

Sensory Impairment The elderly are particularly sensitive to the confusion associated with sensory deprivation. Physiologic changes in their sensory apparatus may be directly related to aging or to pathologic processes. Both diminish sensory receptive ability. The sensory changes, however, are not clear-cut. The person may have difficulty hearing high-frequency sounds, such as consonants. Turning up the volume on the radio may help the person hear one range of sounds but produce sensory overload because the rest of the sounds are too loud. The result is deprivation and distortion.

Try to ascertain any possible sensory problems, especially in hearing and vision. To test hearing, stand so that the client can see your face and ask a question in a normal tone of voice. The question should require more than a yes/no answer. Test vision with pictures that the client will easily recognize.

Dietary History When possible, obtain an estimate of the client's food intake. "What do you eat for breakfast? lunch? dinner?" Make special note of protein and vitamin intake. Avitaminosis, pellagra, anemia, and hypoglycemia have all been associated with reversible brain syndromes (Butler and Lewis 1982). Hydration is also an important factor, easily noted in the client's physical state (e.g., saliva pool below the tongue). Dehydration can also cause confusion.

Head Trauma Falls are common among the elderly. Cerebral contusions, midbrain hemorrhage, and subdural hematoma should all be considered. Confusion may be the primary result of such trauma.

Medication The elderly are prone to adverse drug reactions as a result of age-related bodily changes. These factors are compounded by high

Physiologic, Psychologic, and Environmental Etiologies of Acute Confusional States in the Hospitalized Elderly

I. Physiologic
   A. Primary cerebral disease
      1. Nonstructural factors
         a. Vascular insufficiency—transient ischemic attacks, cerebral vascular accidents, thrombosis
         b. Central nervous system infection—acute and chronic meningitis, neurosyphilis, brain abscess
      2. Structural factors
         a. Trauma—subdural hematoma, concussion, contusion, intracranial hemorrhage
         b. Tumors—primary and metastatic
         c. Normal pressure hydrocephalus
   B. Extracranial disease
      1. Cardiovascular abnormalities
         a. Decreased cardiac output states—myocardial infarction, arrhythmias, congestive heart failure, cardiogenic shock
         b. Alterations in peripheral vascular resistance—increased and decreased states
         c. Vascular occlusion—disseminated intravascular coagulopathy, emboli
      2. Pulmonary abnormalities
         a. Inadequate gas exchange states—pulmonary disease, alveolar hypoventilation
         b. Infection—pneumonias
      3. Systemic infective processes—acute and chronic
         a. Viral
         b. Bacterial—endocarditis, pyelonephritis, cystitis
      4. Metabolic disturbances
         a. Electrolyte abnormalities—hypercalcemia, hyponatremia and hypernatremia, hypokalemia and hyperkalemia, hypochloremia and hyperchloremia, hyperphosphatemia
         b. Acidosis/alkalosis
         c. Hypoglycemia and hyperglycemia
         d. Acute and chronic renal failure
         e. Volume depletion—hemorrhage, inadequate fluid intake, diuretics
         f. Hepatic failure
         g. Porphyria
      5. Drug intoxication—therapeutic and substance abuse
         a. Misuse of prescribed medications
         b. Side-effects of therapeutic medications
         c. Drug-drug interactions
         d. Improper use of over-the-counter medications
         e. Ingestion of heavy metals and industrial poisons
      6. Endocrine disturbance
         a. Hypothyroidism and hyperthyroidism
         b. Diabetes mellitus
         c. Hypopituitarism
         d. Hypoparathyroidism and hyperparathyroidism
      7. Nutritional deficiencies
         a. B vitamins
         b. Vitamin C
         c. Hypoproteinemia
      8. Physiologic stress—pain, surgery
      9. Alterations in temperature regulation—hypothermia and hyperthermia
      10. Unknown physiologic abnormality—sometimes defined as pseudodelirium

II. Physiologic
   A. Severe emotional stress—postoperative states, relocation, hospitalization
   B. Depression
   C. Anxiety
   D. Pain—acute and chronic
   E. Fatigue
   F. Grief
   G. Sensory/perceptual deficits—noise, alteration in functioning of senses
   H. Mania
   I. Paranoia
   J. Situational disturbances

III. Environmental
   A. Unfamiliar environment creating a lack of meaning in the environment
   B. Sensory deprivation/environmental monotony creating a lack of meaning in the environment
   C. Sensory overload
   D. Immobilization—therapeutic, physical, pharmacologic
   E. Sleep deprivation
   F. Lack of temperospatial reference points

consumption of many different drugs: 45 percent of all prescriptions are written for elderly clients. The aged are particularly susceptible to drugs with anticholinergic properties (major tranquilizers, antidepressants, barbiturates, adrenal steroids, atropine, antiparkinsonians, antihistamines, antihypertensives, and diuretics). Question the client about both prescription and over-the-counter drugs: "Are you now taking any medicines that your doctor prescribed?" "Do you take laxatives, cold pills, or other medicines that you buy at your drug store without a prescription?"

Alcohol Consumption   Ask the client about alcohol consumption. Alcohol is a central nervous system depressant, and intoxication may mimic symptoms of OMD. Alcohol also compromises nutritional status and may cause withdrawal effects. Ask questions such as "How much alcohol do you drink in one day/week?" and "Have you ever had periods of not remembering after drinking?"

Cognitive Functioning   Cognitive functioning includes memory, reasoning, abstraction, calculations, and judgment. Clients will not respond effectively unless they feel that the information requested is relevant, they see some purpose in the interview, and they are interested in the material. Choose testing materials carefully, and keep the endurance of the client in mind at all times.

Appearance   Clients who appear disheveled, dirty, or unkempt may be experiencing problems with poor memory or a shortened attention span. This deficit may not be apparent if the client has a caregiver who helps with grooming.

Manner   Some clients may exaggerate mannerisms to compensate for a perceived decline in functioning. For example, compulsive clients may become more set in their ways.

Attitude   An attitude of defensiveness, withdrawal, or paranoia may be a response to increasing anxiety about diminished abilities.

Communication   The nurse assesses communication in the areas of speech, gestures, facial expression, and writing (Ninos and Makohon 1985). Difficulty in finding words and naming objects may suggest **expressive aphasia**. Difficulty grasping complex concepts may suggest **receptive aphasia**. Assess the client's ability to use gestures and facial expressions to compensate for verbal aphasia. Not using facial expressions and gestures and speaking in a monotone may indicate depression. Written communication and reading ability are also tested.

Assess the client's ability to follow verbal instructions, increasing the number of sequential commands. ("Please pick up the paper, fold it in half lengthwise, and place it on the other side of the table.") This knowledge helps the nurse intervene appropriately. Overly difficult communications confuse the client, but

infantile communications rob the client of dignity. Also assess the individual's language ability. Elderly individuals whose primary language is not English may revert to their first language.

Perception   Perception is the client's ability to recognize and integrate sensory information. It also includes the conscious recognition of oneself in relation to the environment. Clients with asymmetric brain involvement of Alzheimer's disease may neglect one side of their body. These clients may also have difficulty recognizing objects (**agnosia**).

Clients with perceptual difficulty may distort sensory information, with resulting hallucinations and delusions. Auditory hallucinations are the most common; visual hallucinations usually indicate an acute toxic state. When listening to a client describe a delusional system, note the underlying feelings and theme, e.g., fear, sorrow. Also keep in mind that the isolation and fear that are the usual causative agents may be as much a product of hearing loss as of the imagination.

Attention and Wakefulness   Attention refers to alertness and the ability to attend selectively to stimuli and to direct one's focus. Can the client sustain or pay attention to the interview process, or is he or she easily distracted by the environment? Attention can be assessed by asking the client to spell a word such as *movie* backward. Wakeful states range from hyperalertness to stupor. Stupor can be the result of medication intoxication or an acute systemic disease, e.g., a brain abscess or pneumonia.

Motor Activity   Lethargy often is a symptom of depression but can also be the result of such medications as tranquilizers, antihypertensives, antidepressants, and antihistamines. Lethargy can also be caused by a number of disease processes, e.g., urinary tract infection, anemia, and meningitis. A shift between hypermotor and hypomotor activity is a sign of delirium. Agitation and physical striking out are occasionally demonstrated.

Mood and Affect   Depression may accompany the earlier stages of dementia. The more demented the client, however, the less depressed he or she is. Clients with organic disease of the cerebral area are emotionally labile. Ask the client about any changes in eating or sleeping habits. Also inquire about a recent loss of energy and interest in usual activities. If depression is suspected, evaluate the client for risk of suicide: "Have you felt like life is not worth living?" "Do you think you would take your own life?" Ask all questions about suicide matter of factly and without hesitation and record the findings carefully in the assessment notes.

Orientation   Disorientation to time, place, and person must be measured in an environment where the client has easy access to the information. Days in a hospital are all the same to many of us. Acute disorientation in all spheres is commonly found in toxic states and traumatic brain disease. Disorientation to place and person usually indicates a degenerative disorder.

Memory At present there is no set of tests that can adequately measure the memory capacity of demented clients (Tariot et al. 1985). (See Table 10–2.) Most tests measure **episodic memory**—the processing and storage of information, e.g., recalling the events of the day. This type of memory is impaired in most clients with OMD, depression, and drug or alcohol intoxication. **Semantic memory,** or knowledge memory, allows people to synthesize and think about events. It is used in language, abstraction, and logical operations. People with Alzheimer's disease have difficulty with semantic memory; however, depressed clients do not. Test episodic memory by asking the client to repeat a series of words or to recall a recent event, such as a meal. Test semantic memory by asking the client to develop a scenario, such as describing the events from dinner until bedtime.

Episodic memory is also tested in relation to time and usually divided into three spheres: recent, remote, and past. It was previously believed that recent memory is lost before remote, and remote before past. No research validates this theory. Rather, past memory is now believed to be irrefutable, and its accuracy is thus not readily assessed. People with dementias have difficulty in recent memory acquisition or learning; this symptom may be a key to early detection of dementia.

Abstract Reasoning Proverbs are the most common way of testing abstract reasoning. "What does it mean when we say, 'People who live in glass houses shouldn't throw stones'?" "What does 'A stitch in time saves nine' mean to you?" Clients with Alzheimer's disease often interpret these proverbs quite literally.

Calculations The most common test of calculation ability is the serial sevens test: The person counts back from 100 in decrements of 7. This is a difficult process for the demented or delirious client. The test measures the client's ability to concentrate and focus thought. It may also be a measure of educational level.

Judgment The test for judgment should predict whether a person will behave in a socially accepted manner, including the planning and carrying out of activities that call for the client to discriminate reality from unrealistic situations. You might ask the client, "If you needed help during the night, how would you get it?" "If you had lost your wallet while on errands, what would you do?"

Psychosocial History The psychosocial history should include an assessment of the client, the client's family, and their joint coping styles and level of intimacy. Some assessment of the client's function in the community should be included. Unlike cognitive testing, this assessment shows what clients are doing rather than what they might do.

Family History The families of impaired older persons can be a major source of information and support. In the United States, almost 90 percent of the elderly have seen one or more relatives the previous week, and more than 75 percent live within 30 minutes of their nearest child. Common living arrangements for the elderly include living with a spouse, child, or sibling (Reifler and Eisdorfer 1980). The family assessment includes the following:

- Living arrangements

- Care arrangements for the elderly, e.g., shopping assistance, daily visits, telephone calls

- Family knowledge of the current illness

- Family expectations for the future

- Special family concerns about client care

- Family style of coping with stress, e.g., death of a relative, illness

- The identified spokesperson for the family

- The family's perception of the client's coping abilities

Throughout the interview, note the interactions between the family and the client. Do they support the client and respect what the client says? Do people listen to one another? What is the atmosphere in the group? What is the level of intimacy between family members?

Activities of Daily Living Assess the client carefully for level of self-care. This is often called a **functional assessment.** What can the client do without help? For which activities is help required? What type of help is needed? As cognitive deficits increase, the client becomes more dependent on others for assistance.

Community Functioning The Comprehensive Functional Assessment (CFA) tool measures ability to sustain oneself in the community (Besdine 1983). Assess not only ability to live independently in the community but also degree of social involvement. Does the client belong to any clubs or groups? Do friends visit the client at home? Does the client belong to a particular church or temple?

Objective Data Larson et al. (1984) have developed a three-step process for evaluating the elderly with mental impairment.

Step 1: Physical assessment. The client is given a thorough medical workup, including a complete neurologic exam (including evaluation of cranial nerves, motor and sensory systems, and reflexes) and a psychiatric consultation for possible functional illness.

RESEARCH NOTE

Citation

Chiverton P, Caine ED: Education to assist spouses in coping with Alzheimer's disease—A controlled trial. J Am Geriatr Soc 1989; 37(7):593–598.

Study Problem/Purpose

This study investigates whether a brief educational program provided to spouses of clients with Alzheimer's disease improved the caregiver's coping skills and also questions whether the gender of the spouse has an effect on coping ability.

Methods

The sample consisted of forty spouses who were in-home caregivers: twenty participated in the educational program and twenty acted as controls. The participants were solicited from families attending an Alzheimer's memory clinic, the local ADRDA, and a long-term care program.

Procedure

The researchers conducted a quantitative assessment of overall family coping with both potential and actual health problems in the psychosocial and physical domains of health. They used the Health-Specific Family Coping Index (HSFCI) prior to the educational intervention and at the end of the four-week intervention period.

Findings

Paired *t*-tests were done to compare demographic variables of the two groups. The results were statistically significant, but the investigators indicated this should not affect the results of the study. A *t*-test on the change between pre- and postintervention total coping score showed a significant difference. No significant effect was found between gender of spouse and change in coping. Limitations of the study included a lack of participants from lower socioeconomic classes and nonwhite ethnic groups. No data were collected regarding support systems and previous relationships.

Implications

The results of the study suggest an educational program can improve one's ability to deal with the daily demands of having a spouse with Alzheimer's disease. The pilot project indicates a need for further study with a larger, ethnically and socioeconomically diverse population.

Because elderly people with organic illness frequently manifest confusion and depression, one works from the assumption that reversible organic illness is present. Chest X-ray films and an electrocardiogram are taken.

Step 2: Laboratory assessment. The following tests are routinely ordered for the elderly.

- Complete blood count, including folic acid and vitamin B_{12} levels to detect anemia

- Erythrocyte sedimentation rate to detect infection

- SMA-12 to detect electrolyte imbalances

- Syphilis tests (VDRL)

- Thyroid function studies

- Serum levels of barbiturates, bromides, and digitalis

- Liver function studies

Step 3: Computed axial tomographic brain scan (CT scan). This test is ordered for those clients at high risk, e.g., those having acute deterioration in cognitive functioning of recent onset. This deterioration is often associated with focal lesions and hydrocephalus.

A number of elective procedures can also be used. Their use should be limited unless indicated, due to their cost to the family and client. These are:

- Skull X-ray films

- Lumbar puncture

- Electroencephalography

- Positron emission tomography (PET)

- Single-photon emission computed tomography (SPECT)

- Magnetic resonance imaging (MRI)

- Cerebral angiography

- Isotope cisternography

There are a number of brief rating scales for testing cognitive impairment (see Table 10–2). None

TABLE 10–2 **Brief Rating Scales for Assessing Organic Mental Impairment**

Title	Items Measured
Cognitive Capacity Screening Examination (CCSE)	Orientation, memory, recall Calculation, language
Mental Status Questionnaire (MSQ)	Orientation, memory, general knowledge
Short Portable Mental Status Questionnaire (SPMSQ)	Orientation, memory, general knowledge, subtraction
Mini-Mental State (MMS)	Orientation, registration, recall, calculation, language, graphomotor function
Cognitive Assessment Scale (CAS)	Orientation, general knowledge, mental ability, psychomotor function
Global Deterioration Scale (GDS)	Assessment of primary degenerative dementia and its stages, including orientation, memory, neurologic exams
Functional Dementia Scale (FDS)	Activities of daily living, orientation, affect
SET Test	Alertness, concentration, short-term memory, problem solving
Nurse's Mental Status Exam (NMSE)	Consciousness, mood, orientation, memory, language, judgment
Extended Mental Status Questionnaire (EMSQ)	Orientation, remote memory, lower/higher levels of cognitive functioning
Philadelphia Geriatric Center (PGC)	Recent memory (story recall)

SOURCE: Adapted from Cooper B, Bickel H: Population screening and the early detection of dementing disorders in old age: A review, Psychol Med 1984;14:81–95. Cambridge University Press, England.

of these is perfect, and most need to be augmented by another test. The SET Test, developed in Scotland, is a tool for effective and quick nursing assessment (Hays and Borger 1985). The test measures mental function as a whole rather than its individual components. The test requires the person to count, name, and remember items, demonstrating motivation, alertness, concentration, short-term memory, and problem-solving ability.

The test takes less than five minutes to administer. The client is asked to list ten items from each of four groups: fruits, animals, colors, and towns/cities (FACT). The maximum score is 40; a score of 15 or below is positively correlated with dementia. Scores between 15 and 24 may not indicate dementia but may indicate some early mental changes due to other factors. The mood disorders do not affect the results of this test as much as they do those of so many others.

Diagnosing

A list of nursing diagnoses common to clients with organic mental syndromes and disorders follows. These have been developed by NANDA, The North American Nursing Diagnosis Association.

Impaired Physical Mobility   Gait changes due to neurologic involvement are seen in a number of the dementias. These include Alzheimer's disease, Huntington's disease, Parkinson's disease, Creutzfeldt-Jakob disease, normal pressure hydrocephalus, and progressive supranuclear palsy. Restlessness in the delirious client is reflected in hyperactive behavior. The client usually alternates between hyperactivity and hypoactivity.

Self-Care Deficit: Bathing/Hygiene, Dressing/Grooming, Feeding, Toileting   Delirious clients are unable to perceive, organize, or carry out the activities of daily living. They are far too distracted by stimuli and unable to focus. The Alzheimer client has a distinct problem: *apraxia*, or the loss of ability to perform formerly known skills. In the late stages of all the dementias, total care is a necessity as the client moves toward brain failure.

Sleep Pattern Disturbance   Sundowning—confused behavior at night when environmental stimulation is low—is commonly seen in delirious clients. The client catnaps during the day and wanders at night. Poor sensory processing can also be seen in demented clients who also wander at night. The client with Alzheimer's disease may not sleep for several days, moving about in a confused state.

Altered Thought Process (Agnosia)   Agnosia, the failure to recognize familiar objects, is a progressive problem that eventually leaves the person without knowledge of loved ones. Overall, in both delirium and dementia, the client's ability to use information in making judgments may be seriously impaired.

Altered Thought Processes (Memory)   Episodic short-term memory is affected by delirium, dementia, and the affective illnesses. Long-term memory is diminished in the later stages of Alzheimer's disease and acute delirium.

Altered Thought Processes (Orientation)   Disorientation is seen in both demented and delirious clients. In the former it is related to progressive cerebral changes; in the latter, to an acute, usually identifiable causal agent.

Altered Thought Processes (Delusions)   Delusions may be present in delirium and dementia. The client is prone to these cognitive processes as a result of reduced ability to distinguish and integrate sensory information. The problem is compounded by short- and long-term memory loss.

Impaired Verbal Communication   Aphasia, both receptive and expressive, is one of the hallmarks of Alzheimer's disease. In the late stage of this illness, the client is completely mute. Confabulation is a common defense used by clients who cannot remember required information and therefore use fantasy to fill in the memory gaps.

High Risk for Violence: Self-Directed or Directed at Others In clients with Alzheimer's disease and the majority of the other dementias, there is a gradual decline in social acceptability of behavior. Hyperorality and touching all objects seen are a few of these impulsive and unpredictable behaviors. The client may also strike out at others while hallucinating or in a hyperactive phase. These behaviors are also seen in delirious clients, who are similarly unpredictable.

Altered Role Performance As the result of decreasing intellectual competence, the demented client moves from role of spouse, parent, employee, and community member to that of a dependent, regressed family member. The role loss and role change are anxiety-provoking and at times overwhelming for the client and family. Characteristically the family members experience a period of acute grief after receiving the diagnosis. Their level of depression should be assessed. Feelings of isolation and being overwhelmed are common (Kuale 1986).

Sensory/Perceptual Alterations The inability to attend and focus concentration is a hallmark of delirium. Decreased attention is also seen in the later stages of the dementias when the client loses the ability to encode. Delirium alters perception by reducing the client's ability to distinguish and integrate sensory information. As a result, the client has difficulty in discriminating reality from hallucinations, dreams, illusions, and imagery. In the later stages of dementia, clients also experience hallucinations and delusions, which complicate delivery of care.

Self-Esteem Disturbance During the first stage of Alzheimer's disease and other dementias, the client is acutely aware of cognitive failure. This awareness and the resulting anxiety can be damaging to the self-esteem of a person living in a culture that does not tolerate or provide for dependence.

Functional Urinary Incontinence, Bowel Incontinence Incontinence of urine or feces is usually the result of confusion and failure to use the facilities. In the later stages of dementia, clients lose cortical control, but physiologic function remains. Incontinence of urine may also be an indication of normal pressure hydrocephalus.

Altered Nutrition, Less/More Than Body Requirements Poor nutrition and some metabolic disorders can be the direct cause of confusion in the elderly. The reverse can also be true; confusion and cerebral change can cause nutritional deficits. Without supervision, many clients are not able to provide for or ingest adequate amounts of food. Clients in the later stages of Alzheimer's disease have symptoms of bulimia followed by total loss of appetite.

Planning and Implementing Interventions

Nursing interventions for clients with organic mental syndromes and disorders can be divided into two broad groups: interventions for demented clients and those for delirious clients. Sample nursing care plans for these are presented on pages 205–211. With few exceptions, the interventions are similar, although the overall goals are different. The goal with the demented client is to minimize the loss of self-care capacity. Although functional loss is progressive, at every stage of the illness the nurse needs to assess and support the client's self-care capacity. With the delirious client the overall goal for nursing intervention is to support existing sensory perception until the client's cognition stage can return to previous levels of functioning.

Promote Normal Motor Behavior Because of the demented client's impaired coordination, falls become a safety concern. Living areas need to be well lit and furniture left in the same place. Evaluate the client for visual and balance disturbances. Safety bars should be installed near toilets, showers, and tubs. Teach clients who need assistance the safe use of walkers and wheelchairs (Burnside 1981). Evaluate all clients using tranquilizers and antidepressants for postural hypotension. Blood pressure taken supine and standing is an indication. Restlessness and wandering can be dealt with by allowing the demented client to wander in a closed milieu. Avoid crowds or large open spaces without boundaries.

With the delirious client, hyperactivity can be decreased by controlling environmental stimuli. If this does not help, medications can be used judiciously. Take vital signs one hour before and after the administration of any medication, and observe the client carefully for signs of stupor. Interrupt prolonged periods of client hypoactivity with range-of-motion exercises, frequent turning, and having the client stand up at bedside, as tolerated. During periods of fluctuating motor behavior, there is always concern for the client's safety. Staff should be present at all times, keep the bed lowered, and the side rails should be up.

Maintain Self-Care Allow the client to do as much as possible unassisted. The more the client can effectively control the daily routine, the less anxiety the client will experience. Remind the client about daily grooming and personal hygiene and repeat instructions. If the client resists oral hygiene, use mouth swabs with dilute hydrogen peroxide. If the client resists this as well, having the client eat an apple may help to clean the mouth. If the client resists any routine procedures, wait a few moments and try again. The client often forgets to offer new resistance. Clients who are acutely delirious or in the last stages of dementia need total bed care.

Promote Adequate Sleep Clients with dementia and delirium respond poorly to hypnotics, which increase confusion and aggravate sundowning in the elderly. A small amount of beer or wine at bedtime may produce enough relaxation without side-effects. The most helpful measure may be to allow sleepless clients to wander in a confined area until they are tired. If the client is disorganized at night, make sure the room is light and without shadows. Possibly leave a radio on to provide more stimulation. Low doses of haloperidol or an antianxiety agent may be prescribed. (These medications should be used with caution and not on a nightly basis.) A Posey vest and soft restraints may have to be used if a staff member cannot sit with the delirious client or if the client attempts to remove IV tubing or bandages. (Use these according to established policy.) Reassure restrained clients that they are safe and that the restraints are there to protect and help.

Support Knowledge Processes The same interventions that are used to support memory and orientation are applied to the support of knowledge processes. Family education is imperative and can take the form of professional help or self-help groups.

Support Optimal Memory Function Gently orient the client. To allay anxiety, do not argue with the client about verbal discrepancies. Rather, direct the client toward areas of interest that are familiar and pleasurable. The environment needs to support whatever memory functions are still intact. Do not test the client for episodic memory unless it is absolutely necessary. If the client uses confabulation to fill in the memory gap, do not argue; rather note it as an ego-protective mechanism.

Because of their episodic memory loss, the Alzheimer clients do not respond well to reality orientation classes. The nurse, however, can trigger semantic memory by initiating a procedure that the client can then complete. In this leading technique, a combination of words and nonverbal cues are used. For instance, while handing the client a toothbrush and pointing toward the mouth with a brushing motion, say, "Brush your teeth." Constant repetition in a kind, firm manner is often necessary. Music therapy may also trigger past associations, aid the client's long-term memory, and help a normally aphasic client to participate in a group (Dietsche and Pollman 1982).

Drug therapy has also been proposed to assist the client in the early stages of Alzheimer's disease to maintain memory and orientation. **Tetrahydroaminoacridine (THA)**, a potent anticholinesterase, is currently being studied in human trials. A clinical trial of THA with ten Alzheimer clients showed no results after three weeks. Three of the six patients who continued the trial long term showed measurable cognitive improvement. THA is not proposed as a cure but rather as an approach that may make early stages of Alzheimer's disease more bearable (Fitten, Perryman, Gross, Fine, Cummins, Marshall 1990).

The family caregivers of clients experiencing advanced agnosia need support when their loved one no longer recognizes them.

Promote Optimal Orientation Structure the client's environment to support cognitive functions. The client should be wearing whatever aids (hearing, vision) are necessary to prevent sensory loss or distortion. Familiar objects from home, such as slippers, robe, and photographs, also help to orient the client. Easily read clocks, orientation boards, and a consistent daily routine that includes physical activity and socialization without sensory overload also help to orient the client (Wolanin and Fraelich-Philips 1981). Verbally orient the client during conversation. Do not quiz the client.

Support Optimal Verbal Expression As communication skills decrease, the client's nonverbal communications become more important. Clients respond physically to the environment, especially if they feel threatened. Call the client by name, approach in clear view, and give simple directions.

Support Appropriate Conduct/Impulse Control All measures used to support perception and orientation are imperative here. The client may strike out in response to hallucinations or delusions. The client functions best in an environment where stimulation is controlled and sensory overload prevented. All changes, whether environmental or personal, need to be made slowly. Always approach the client in full view, calling his or her name, and refrain from touching the client. Requests should be simple and nondemanding. A client with short-term memory loss can often be distracted. Restraints may be used to protect the client and others. They are, however, a last resort when the presence of staff members is no longer effective.

Support Optimal Role Performance To continue functioning in the family, the client must be viewed as an active member. Most demented clients remain at home with their families until the caregiver is exhausted and can no longer manage the client's round-the-clock needs. The family needs support throughout this time. Formal support includes home visits, day care, respite care, and family support groups.

After the client is institutionalized, the family should be made an integral part of the client's daily routine. The family needs extra emotional support as the client no longer recognizes them and the rewards for maintaining involvement diminish. For the delirious client, role maintenance involves supporting the client's ongoing need to be oriented and helping the family through the acute period.

Maintain Optimal Attention Span Repeat requests as needed. Speak in simple phrases, loud enough to be heard, and reinforce meaning with nonverbal gestures. To decrease distractability and hyperalertness, keep environmental stimulation at a minimum. Every effort should be made to lower the client's anxiety level by moving slowly, speaking clearly, and providing new information slowly.

Promoting Optimal Self-Concept/Self-Esteem
During the early stages of dementia, every effort should be made to maintain clients' self-esteem as they struggle with the personal awareness of cognitive loss. Encourage clients to express fears and concerns and listen attentively. Allow for the expression of anger and sadness.

Manipulate the environment to help the client with a failing memory. Helpful measures include labeling the bathroom and bedroom, posting notes to remind the client to turn off the stove and lock the door, and labeling the contents of drawers. Gently remind the client of forgotten events, and do not confront confabulations. Encourage the family to maintain the client as a productive member of this important group.

Support Optimal Perceptual Functioning A quiet environment with soft music prevents the client from experiencing sensory overload. When speaking with the client, stand or sit so that you are in direct view. First giving a verbal warning, touch the client's shoulder or hand, and slowly and clearly explain all procedures. Use touch with caution. Sometimes a very soothing touch can overexcite the client, who may respond by striking out. Make sure that the client is wearing hearing aids and eyeglasses if necessary.

In responding to hallucinations, simply state that you understand that these thoughts seem very real but that you do not experience the same thoughts. Do not argue or ask the client to elaborate. Give reassurance that these thoughts will go away. Say, "You are in a safe place." Do not leave the client alone or in an isolated room without some stimulation to help the client block out the hallucinations and support reality testing. The room should be well lit without shadows

or glare. If the client becomes combative, use physical restraints, but for as brief a period as possible. Then attempt to distract, reassuring the client "You are in a safe place." Do not use restraints unless the client is a threat to others or self; restraints only frighten and aggravate perceptual problems.

Promote Optimal Patterns of Elimination A regular toileting schedule helps the delirious client control bowel and urine incontinence. Clients are often not able to let the nurse know when they have to use the toilet or have soiled themselves.

During the early stage of dementia, a toileting routine is essential. As the disease progresses, the client no longer recognizes a toilet or its purpose. Such a client may resist sitting on the toilet. Forcing the client will only produce agitation and combativeness. Distract and try again. If all efforts at maintaining a routine fail, use disposable pants or diapers. The use of catheters and external drains is not recommended because of the possibility of infection and their certain removal by a confused client.

Promote Optimal Nutritional Status Monitor the client's food and fluid intake. Give hyperactive clients a diet high in protein and carbohydrates, in finger-food form. Some clients may need double portions. Clients who chew constantly need to be reminded to swallow. Depending on the client's level of perception and motor activity, supervision and assistance at mealtimes may be necessary. Weigh the client routinely and increase caloric intake as needed. In the final stages of the disease, the client loses all interest in food and must receive nasogastric, gastrostomy, or intravenous feedings (Dietsche and Pollman 1982).

Evaluating/Outcome Criteria

Specific outcomes for clients experiencing the organic mental syndromes and disorders are listed in the care plans.

Dementia Evaluation Criteria Dementia entails progressive intellectual, behavioral, and physiologic deterioration. The goal of nursing care is not to effect a cure but rather to sustain the client at the optimal level of self-care. The nurse also helps the family sustain a personally rewarding relationship with their loved one throughout this terminal process.

Delirium Evaluation Criteria The evaluation of nursing care for delirious clients is based on the premise that clients are capable of returning to their previous level of functioning. During that process, the goal is to help the client maintain optimal levels of sensory perception, participate in activities of daily living, and maintain physiologic homeostasis.

A Client with Organic Mental Disease*

Identifying Information

Rosie W is an 83-year-old white Jewish woman, living alone in an apartment in the city; she was widowed two years ago. She was referred by her brother, who states, "She has been extremely forgetful recently." She lives off her husband's retirement and also receives Social Security. She completed nine years of school and has no current therapist.

Client's Definition of Present Problem, Precipitating Stressors, Coping Strategies, Goals for Care

Rosie comes to the clinic this morning at the request of her brother, stating, "I had nothing to do with it. My brother's daughter must have a friend here." She states that she has been feeling "confused" and cannot remember things "from one moment to the next." She cannot remember how long this has been going on. She attributes this to getting old.

History of Present Problem

Rosie states that nothing unusual has happened over the past year. She is able to provide limited information about her present problem. Her brother was contacted to provide the necessary details. According to Rosie's 72-year-old brother, she has become increasingly disoriented over the last six months. On his own initiative, he brought her to her doctor who was unable to find anything physically wrong. Her brother describes her as "forgetful and just not herself. She doesn't even remember my name sometimes." On occasion, when he has gone to visit her, he has found her door unlocked, and the burner on the stove left on. He says he now manages her finances, since she can no longer balance the household budget herself. She has become increasingly withdrawn and no longer spends time with her friends. When he does take her out, she will often act in an embarrassing manner and say inappropriate and rude things. She is easily distracted, and he finds her mumbling to herself frequently. He states, "She will often start to do something, and right in the middle of doing it, she will go and start something else." He feels she is not reliable enough to prepare her own meals and is concerned that if he or his daughter does not bring her food, she will not eat. He is concerned that something will happen to her living alone and feels that she should have somebody live with her. She has refused to live with her brother, and because it is becoming increasingly difficult for him to get around, he cannot visit her as frequently as he would like. He thinks that Rosie's memory has gotten even worse over the past two to three months, although he cannot recall precisely when it all started.

Rosie has lived in her apartment for thirty-five years with her husband and for the past two years alone following his death. She states that she likes being "left alone." Her daily routine consists of "cleaning the apartment and shopping." She says she keeps her apartment "very orderly," so that she knows exactly where everything is. Recently, she has found it helpful to write things down so that she does not forget anything. When asked what she had for breakfast, she responded, "I don't remember, exactly." She states that she has difficulty sleeping because of all the noise and awakens frequently during the night.

Rosie describes her brother as her "right hand." She states that she has "a few friends" who live in the apartment building where she lives, but she does not socialize with them anymore because "There just isn't enough time in the day." She says that she has been surrounded by people all her life but now prefers to be left alone. She has a 52-year-old married daughter, who lives about 300 miles away and with whom she speaks once a week. When asked when she saw her daughter last, she responded "last Thanksgiving . . . she ruined my grandson; now he's into dope!"

*This case study was provided by Kathleen Tomaselli while a graduate student in psychiatric nusing at University of California, San Francisco.

Psychiatric History No previous hospitalizations and no previous therapists or treatments.

Family History According to Rosie, her husband of sixty years "dropped dead two years ago while watching TV." She was unable to recall exactly when her parents died. however, she says that it was "many years ago." Rosie has one brother, 72 years old, who is married with one daughter and who also lives in the city, and a daughter, 52 years old, who is married with three children and lives "in another state." Her older sister died ten years ago. Her son died "quite young" of a brain tumor. The client says that she is close to her brother. During the interview, she repeatedly interjects, "I love my brother, but I wish he'd get off my back! I am I, as I am, not who he wants me to be!"

Social History Rosie appears to have had a normal adulthood, passing through developmental milestones—such as marriage, parenting, grandparenting, retirement, widowhood—without any problems. Rosie states that she was forced to quit high school because of a nose condition. Her brother states that she completed nine years of school, but was not aware of Rosie's being forced to quit school. Rosie has no formal occupational training. She reminisces at length and with great detail about her work at the theater as a dresser. She quit the theater when she was offered a job as business agent for the wardrobe union. She does not remember for how long she worked at either job nor at what age she retired. She recalls that "It was a very happy time for me. I was very well received." Her recollection of the events that have taken place between the time she retired from the wardrobe union and the present is sketchy.

Rosie was married when she was 21 years old. When asked how long she had been married before her husband died, she replied, "too many years." Her brother was able to report that she had been married for sixty years before her husband's death. Rosie described their relationship as "not very good. He had no use for me, and I never knew what he wanted from me." She continued, "Oh, he fooled around all right, but that never bothered me. I had gorgeous red hair that every man admired. All the attention I received made my husband jealous."

Rosie never smoked and denies any history of drugs and alcohol.

Rosie spends most of her days in her apartment. She leaves the apartment only to go to the YWHA for her lunch and dinner. "I know my way there because it's only a stone's throw from my apartment."

Significant Health History No history of major illness or injuries. Has had cataract surgery on both eyes. According to her brother, surgery on her left eye was done three months ago and her right eye was operated on two weeks ago. Currently, her right eye is patched. She states that she has hypertension and takes medication for it, but is unable to recall when it was first diagnosed. According to Rosie's brother, she has no other medical problems. When asked if she has enough energy, she responded, "at my age, it's not too bad."

The client appears well nourished. She says her appetite is "so-so" but thinks she may have gained weight. When asked if she had any difficulty bathing, she responded defensively, "I don't smell! I don't need to bathe any more often than anybody else!" She states that she has no difficulty "getting around," except at night since her vision at night is poor and she cannot find her flashlight. Sometimes it is difficult for her to see objects clearly and she is unable to read most things. She states, "It doesn't matter, since I don't remember anything I read anyway."

Current Mental Status Rosie is a cooperative, white-haired, elderly woman who appears somewhat unkempt with uncombed hair, wrinkled dress, and smelling of strong perfume.

▶

CASE STUDY (continued)

Current Mental Status (continued)

She sits leaning forward, clutching her pocketbook in her lap. She is oriented to person and place, knows the year, but is unsure of the month and date. Her fund of general knowledge is poor and she is unable to name the last five presidents. When asked if she knew who the president of the United States is, she responded, "Do I *know* that so-and-so? I don't like him!" When asked if she knew who the current mayor is, she replied, "Of course I know who he is! Don't you?" Her memory and recall are poor; she performs digit span ×4 forward and ×2 backward. She is unable to repeat the names of three objects after five minutes and unable to name objects (keys, quarter) on sight and feel.

Her calculations are poor (unable to perform simple addition and subtraction and serial 7s). Client states, "It's frustrating for me since I used to be a bookkeeper and I was very good at math." Her judgment is poor. When asked what she would do if she found a stamped, addressed letter on the street, she replied, "I would read it and then, maybe mail it."

Rosie is alert, labile, superficial, sporadically anxious, and irritable. She appeared depressed when talking about her grandson but cheerful and elated when describing her work in the theater. She states that she has no thoughts or plans of suicide. Her voice is soft, speech fluent. She becomes slightly pressured when trying to remember.

She denies having illusions, hallucinations, or delusions. She shows loose associations but can be redirected easily. Her ability for abstract thought is impaired. She provides concrete interpretations of proverbs. Her thoughts are tangentially related and responses to questions are irrelevant and circumstantial at times. She seems distractible and appears to have difficulty concentrating. She answers "I just don't know" frequently.

Rosie becomes anxious and attempts to minimize cognitive defects. She tries to conceal them by circumstantiality, perseveration, and changing the topic. She has little insight into current situation. She states, "I wish people would just leave me alone and get off my back. I don't know why everyone is so excited. I'm just getting old."

Diagnostic Impression

Nursing Diagnoses

Social isolation
Sleep pattern disturbance
Ineffective individual coping
Altered thought processes
Sensory/perceptual alteration

DSM-III-R Multiaxial Diagnosis

Axis I: 290 Primary degenerative dementia of the Alzheimer type, senile onset with depression
Axis II: V71.09 (No diagnosis or condition; obsessive compulsive traits)
Axis III: Poor vision, high blood pressure, Alzheimer's disease
Axis IV: 2 Mild (cognitive impairment: enduring)
          4 High (psychosocial stressors resulting from severe loss of memory. These include inability to balance finances; isolation from community, family, and friends; inability to maintain independence and self-care functioning; acute)
Axis V: Current GAF: 50 Serious symptoms (social and cognitive impairment)
          Highest GAF in past year: 60

Nursing Care Plan

See the nursing care plan for a client with dementia on pages 205–208.

▶

NURSING CARE PLAN

A Client with Dementia

Client Care Goals	Nursing Planning/ Intervention	Evaluation
Nursing Diagnosis: *Impaired physical mobility*		
Client will demonstrate normal motor behavior.	Evaluate the environment for hazards that may cause falls, e.g., throw rugs, poorly lit rooms; lack of safety bars in bathroom; teach client use of walkers and wheelchairs. Client using tranquilizers needs standing and supine blood pressures taken to check for hypotension. Allow wandering in a prescribed area.	Maintains full physical activity.
Nursing Diagnosis: *Self-care deficit*		
Client will perform self-care.	Encourage independence in self-care; use verbal and nonverbal communication when making requests; repeat requests as needed. Use clothing with elastic, eliminating buttons and zippers if possible. Label clothing items and important rooms. Provide mouth swabs and fresh fruit if client refuses oral hygiene. Repeat self-care requests at a later time if client is resistant. Total physical care during last stages.	Functions at highest possible level of self-care.
Nursing Diagnosis: *Sleep pattern disturbance*		
Client will maintain adequate sleep.	Offer beer or wine at bedtime; allow client to wander in a prescribed area till tired; if restraints used, remove them when client has fallen asleep. Active daily schedule.	Is able to sleep at regular intervals in amount necessary to maintain health.
Nursing Diagnosis: *Altered thought processes (Agnosia)*		
Client will maintain optimal cognitive functioning.	Use the same interventions prescribed for altered memory. Label objects, supervise client when warranted. Support family as they care for a loved one who no longer recognizes them as individuals.	Participates in self-care and family environment at optimal level.

▶

NURSING CARE PLAN (continued)

A Client with Dementia

Client Care Goals	Nursing Planning/ Intervention	Evaluation
Client will maintain optimal memory function.	Structure ward environment to enhance memory, e.g., clocks, calendars, orientation board. Use verbal and nonverbal communication to emphasize requests, repeating as necessary. Have client attend music therapy and other "reminiscing" groups; place familiar objects in room; allow open visiting with family.	Participates in self-care and groups at optimal level.
Client will maintain optimal orientation.	Provide easily read clocks and orientation boards, consistent daily routine, socialization that does not produce sensory overload. Maintain physical activity; avoid use of tranquilizers. Client should wear aids (hearing/vision) as needed.	Is oriented to time, place, and person if possible.
Client will demonstrate clear thought processes.	Structure ward environment to enhance memory and orientation. Do not argue with validity of delusions, rather try to understand the feelings being indirectly expressed. Low-dose haloperidol may be prescribed.	Does not verbally express delusional material.

Nursing Diagnosis: *Impaired verbal communication*

Client will demonstrate optimal verbal expression.	Call client by name, approach in clear view, and give simple commands. Substitute pictures if client experiencing aphasia. Attempt to attach meaning to nonverbal communications, checking interpretations with client or family.	Is able to communicate needs.

Nursing Diagnosis: *High risk for violence*

Client will demonstrate appropriate conduct/impulse control.	Decrease environmental stimuli; make all changes slowly; make nondemanding requests; refrain from touching. Always approach in full view calling client by name. Distract as necessary; low dose of antipsychotic p.r.n.	Participates in daily living situation without striking out at self or others.

▶

NURSING CARE PLAN (continued)

A Client with Dementia

Client Care Goals	Nursing Planning/ Intervention	Evaluation
Nursing Diagnosis: *Altered role performance*		
Client will demonstrate optimal role performance.	Use community resources to support family and client in home, e.g., day care, home visits, respite care, family support groups. Encourage family to participate in client's daily activities once institutionalized and include client in family functions. Support family through their own grieving as their loved one becomes more confused and withdrawn.	Functions at highest possible level within the community and family.
Nursing Diagnosis: *Sensory/perceptual alterations*		
Client will demonstrate optimal attention span.	Decrease environmental stimuli that agitate client. Repeat requests in a clear, simple manner, using gestures to supplement.	Focuses long enough to participate in simple tasks.
Nursing Diagnosis: *Self-esteem disturbance*		
Client will demonstrate optimal self-concept/self-esteem.	Encourage client to express feelings in a nonjudgmental environment; allow for expression of anger and sadness. Encourage family to include client in social activities. Gently remind client of forgotten events. Organize the environment to enhance memory, e.g., label rooms and contents of drawers, write notes to remind to do some things.	Participates in self-care as much as possible; able to express both positive and negative comments about personal level of functioning.
Nursing Diagnosis: *Sensory/perceptual alterations*		
Client will demonstrate optimal perceptual functioning.	Decrease environmental stimuli; provide soft music, slower-paced unit, eyeglasses and hearing aids as needed. Restrain client if combative; distract if agitated; give reassurance that client is safe and will not be harmed; postpone procedures if client is agitated.	Perceives environment with a minimum of distortion.

▶

NURSING CARE PLAN (continued)

A Client with Dementia

Client Care Goals	Nursing Planning/ Intervention	Evaluation
Nursing Diagnoses: *Functional urinary incontinence; Bowel incontinence*		
Client will demonstrate optimal patterns of elimination.	Establish regular toileting schedule; use disposable diapers/ pants if client will not participate willingly in toileting; do not use catheters or condoms if possible.	Is continent of urine and feces; elimination controlled by other safe means.
Nursing Diagnosis: *Altered nutrition: less than body requirements*		
Client will demonstrate optimal nutritional status.	Monitor food and fluid intake, 24-hour intake; output documented as necessary. Supervise at mealtimes and assist as necessary. Give diet high in protein and carbohydrates in finger-food form with double portions. Weigh client frequently; increase caloric intake p.r.n.; if client refuses to eat, administer nasogastric, gastrotomy, or IV feedings.	Takes in adequate daily amounts of food and fluids; does not lose weight; assists self as much as possible.

NURSING CARE PLAN

A Client with Delirium

Client Care Goals	Nursing Planning/ Intervention	Evaluation
Nursing Diagnosis: *Impaired physical mobility*		
Client will demonstrate normal motor behavior	Decrease environmental stimuli if client is hyperactive, a low dose of antipsychotic medication (haloperidol) may be necessary; check vital signs one hour before and after administration. If client is hypoactive, use range-of-motion exercises, up at beside. Fluctuating hypoactivity to hyperactivity: staff should be present to ensure safety; side rails up, bed lowered.	Exhibits normal motor behavior in response to stimuli.
Nursing Diagnosis: *Self-care deficit*		
Client will perform self-care.	Encourage client to do as much for self as possible; assist as necessary. Explain all procedures simply and clearly.	Performs activities of daily living (ADL) without assistance.
Nursing Diagnosis: *Sleep pattern disturbance*		
Client will maintain adequate sleep.	Prevent nighttime confusion by increasing stimulation, e.g., light in room, radio; give low dose of antipsychotics or antianxiety agents. Restrain only if absolutely necessary. Reassure client that the environment is safe. Discourage daytime napping.	Sleeps at regular intervals in the pattern normal to the client prior to delirium.
Nursing Diagnosis: *Altered thought processes*		
Client will demonstrate optimal cognitive functioning.	Present new information as client is able to accept without confusion; keep requests that require judgment to a minimum. Support the orientation and memory of the client.	Participates in daily decision making.
Client will demonstrate optimal memory function.	Speak to client about mutual areas of interest. Do not dispute memory discrepancies, this will only increase anxiety. Gently orient the client. Surround client with familiar objects from home, clocks, calendars, etc.	Remembers recent and remote experiences.

▶

NURSING CARE PLAN *(continued)*

A Client with Delirium

Client Care goals	Nursing Planning/ Intervention	Evaluation
Client will demonstrate optimal orientation.	Client should be wearing aids (visual/hearing) as needed. Familiar objects from home along with clocks, calendars, etc. Orient client during conversation; do not quiz.	Is oriented to time, place, and person.
Client will express clear thought processes.	Structure ward/environment to enhance memory and orientation. Do not agree with delusional material; however, do not argue. Respond to feelings being indirectly expressed.	No longer verbally expresses delusional material.

Nursing Diagnosis: *High risk for violence*

Client will maintain appropriate conduct/impulse control.	Use the measures to support orientation and perception. Medicate with a low dose of an antipsychotic (e.g., haloperidol). Restrain to protect self/others only if an emergency or when staff presence is no longer effective. Move slowly in the room, speak clearly, and explain all procedures.	Manifests socially appropriate behavior; verbalizes fears/concerns without striking out.

Nursing Diagnosis: *Altered role performance*

Client will maintain optimal role performance.	Encourage family to participate in client's care. Support family emotionally as they work with a loved one whose behavior may be very bizarre.	Client's role within the family is not jeopardized by the period of delirium.

Nursing Diagnosis: *Sensory/perceptual alterations*

Client will demonstrate optimal attention span.	Reduce environmental stimuli; all procedures should be reduced to only those absolutely necessary. While working with client, move slowly, speak clearly, and provide information slowly; reduce the number of different people having contact with client.	Sustains a normal attention span to participate in ADLs.

NURSING CARE PLAN *(continued)*

A Client with Delirium

Client Care goals	Nursing Planning/ Intervention	Evaluation
Client will demonstrate optimal perceptual functioning.	When speaking to the client, stand or sit so client can clearly see you, touch to hold his or her attention, and slowly explain all procedures. Respond to hallucinations by orienting without arguing; do not ask for elaboration. Reassure client that these perceptions will go away. Do not isolate; maintain stimulation, e.g., adequate lighting, another person present to speak to. Restrain only as a last resort.	Perceives environment as it is without distortion; is not frightened by environmental changes.

Nursing Diagnoses: *Functional urinary incontinence; Bowel incontinence*

Client will maintain optimal patterns of elimination.	Maintain regular toileting schedule; check frequently for incontinence to prevent skin breakdown. Supervise food and fluid intake to prevent constipation; administer stool softeners p.r.n.	Is continent of urine and feces; has routine bowel movements.

Nursing Diagnosis: *Altered nutrition: Less than body requirements*

Client will maintain optimal nutritional status.	Monitor food and fluid intake; document 24-hour intake-output as necessary; supervise at mealtimes, assisting as needed. Note condition of skin for hydration. Weigh frequently.	Takes in adequate daily amounts of food and fluids; does not lose weight; can feed self.

CHAPTER HIGHLIGHTS

• Dementia is a condition marked by a loss of intellectual abilities of sufficient severity to interfere with social and occupational functioning.

• Dementias are classified as cortical and subcortical; clients with the latter retain higher levels of functioning than those with cortical dementias.

• Alzheimer's disease, the most common form of dementia among the elderly, is a progressive, age-related chronic dysfunction marked by phases: early phases of forgetfulness, more advanced phases of

disorientation and diminished concentration, and later and terminal phases of severe agitation, disorientation, psychosis, and complete helplessness.

• Decreased levels of acetylcholine and serotonin, genetic factors, viruslike substances, aluminum intoxication, immune dysfunctions, and metabolic dysfunction are all under consideration as possible causes of Alzheimer's disease.

• Pseudodementia, progressive supranuclear palsy, neurosyphilis, normal pressure hydrocephalus, Creutzfeldt-Jakob disease, Pick's disease, Huntington's disease, Parkinson's disease, and multi-infarct dementia are among the other dementias seen in psychiatric nursing practice.

• Delirium is an organic brain syndrome characterized by global cognitive impairment of abrupt onset and relatively brief duration in which perception, thinking, and memory are all disrupted.

• Delirium, common in the elderly, is usually caused by an underlying systemic illness.

• Criteria to distinguish delirium from dementia include the individual's state of consciousness, stability of attention, duration of symptoms, rate of onset, and course.

• Assessment for OMS and OBS is particularly challenging because confused clients are often poor historians; furthermore, the interview environment and procedure may increase the client's anxiety and seriously compromise the nurse's attempts to assess.

• Areas of subjective assessment include health history (including psychosocial life-style patterns), sensory impairment, dietary history, possibility of head trauma, medication use, cognitive functioning, and overall mental status.

• Objective data are obtained from physical examination, assessment of routine laboratory tests and scans, and objective rating scales of cognitive functioning.

• Nursing diagnoses and interventions targeted toward them include mobility, self-care, thought processes, communication, role performance, and sensory/perceptual alterations.

• The overall goal of nursing interventions for clients with dementia is minimizing the loss of self-care capacity.

• The overall goal of nursing interventions for delirious clients is to support existing sensory perception until the client returns to previous levels of cognitive function.

REFERENCES

American Psychiatric Association: *Diagnostic and Statistical Manual of Mental Disorders,* ed 3, revised. APA, 1987.

Besdine RW: The educational utility of comprehensive functional assessment in the elderly. *J Am Geriatr Soc* 1983;31:651–656.

Brody E, Lawton M, Liebowitz B: Senile dementia: Public policy and adequate institutional care. *Am J Public Health* 1984;74:1381–1383.

Buckwalter KC, Abraham IL, Neundorfer MM: Alzheimer's disease: Involving nursing in the development and implementation of health care for patients and families. *Nurs Clin North Am* 1988;23(1):1–9.

Burns EM, Buckwalter KC: Pathophysiology and etiology of Alzheimer's disease. *Nurs Clin North Am* 1988; 23(1):11–29.

Burnside IM: Psychosocial issues in nursing care of the aged. *J Gerontol Nurs* 1981;7:689–694.

Butler RN, Lewis MI: *Aging and Mental Health,* ed 3. Mosby, 1982.

Cook-Deegan RM, Mace N, Baily MA, Chavkin D, Hawes C: Confronting Alzheimer's disease and other dementias, in *Science Information Resource Center.* Philadelphia: Lippincott, 1988.

Dawson P, Kline K, Wianco DC, and Wells D: Preventing excess disability in patients with Alzheimer's disease. *Geriatric Nursing* 1986:(Nov/Dec.):298–301.

Dickson LR, Ranseen JD: An update on selected organic mental syndromes. *Hosp Community Psychiatry* 1990; 41(3):290–300.

Dietsche LM, Pollman JN: Alzheimer's disease: Advances in clinical nursing. *J Gerontol Nurs* 1982;8:97–100.

Duthrie EH, Glatt SL: Understanding and treating multi-infarct dementia. *Clin Geriatr Med* 1988;4(4):749–766.

Fitten LJ, Perryman KM, Gross PL, Fine H, Cummins J, Marshall C: Treatment of Alzheimer's disease with short- and long-term oral THA and THA and lecithin: A double-blind study. *Am J Psychiatry* 1990;147(2):239–242.

Foreman MD: Acute confusional states in hospitalized elderly: A research dilemma. *Nurs Res* 1986;35:37–38.

Hanley IG, McGuire RJ, Boyd WD: Reality orientation and dementia: A controlled trial of two approaches. *Br J Psychiatry* 1981;138:10–14.

Hays A, Borger F: A test in time. *Am J Nurs* 1985;85:1107–1111.

Jarvick L, Greenson H: About a peculiar disease of the cerebral cortex. *Alzheimer Dis Assoc Disord* 1987; 1(1):7–8.

Johnson L, Keller KL: Staging Alzheimer's disease. *Geriatr Nurs* 1989;10(4):196–197.

Kase CS: Multi-infarct dementia: A real entity? *J Am Geriatr Soc* 1986;34:482–484.

Kuale JN: Alzheimer's disease. *Ann Fam Pract* 1986; 34:103–110.

Larson E, Reifler B, Canfield C, Cohen G: Evaluating elderly outpatients with symptoms of dementia. *Hosp Community Psychiatry* 1984;35:405–428.

Lipowski ZJ: Transient cognitive disorders (delirium, acute confusional states) in the elderly. *Am J Psychiatry* 1983;140:1426–1436.

Masliah E, Terry RD, DeTeresa RM, Hansen LA: Immunohistochemical quantification of the synapse-related protein synaptophysin in Alzheimer's disease. *Neurosci Lett* 1989;103(2):234–239.

Ninos M, Makohon R: Functional assessment of the patient. *Geriatr Nurs* 1985;6:139–142.

Petrie WM: Alzheimer's disease. *Compr Ther* 1985;11(7): 38–43.

Reifler B, Eisdorfer C: A clinic for the impaired elderly and their families. *Am J Psychiatry* 1980;137:1399–1403.

Reifler B, Larson E, Hanley R: Coexistence of cognitive impairment and depression in geriatric outpatients. *Am J Psychiatry* 1982;139:623–626.

Stern LZ, Bernick C: Mental disorders in the elderly. *Compr Ther* 1987;13(5):43–50.

Tariot P, Sunderland T, Murphy D, Cohen R, Weingartner H, Makohon R: How memory fails: A theoretical model. *Geriatr Nurs* 1985;6:144–147.

Task Force Sponsored by the National Institute on Aging. Senility reconsidered: Treatment possibilities for mental impairment in the elderly. *JAMA* 1980;244:259–263.

Varcarolis EM: *Foundations of Psychiatric Nursing.* Saunders, 1990.

Wells CE: Chronic brain disease: An update on alcoholism, Parkinson's disease, and dementia. *Hosp Community Psychiatry* 1982;33:111–126.

Whelihan WM, Lesher EL, Kleban MH, Granick S: Mental status and memory assessment as predictors of dementia. *J Gerontol* 1984;39:572–576.

Wolanin MO, Fraelich-Philips LR: *Confusion, Prevention and Care.* Mosby, 1981.

Wright AF, Whaley LJ: Genetics, aging and dementia. *Br J Psychiatry* 1984;145:20–38.

Zarit S, Reever K, Bach-Peterson J: Relatives of the impaired elderly: Correlates of feelings of burden. *Gerontologist* 1980;20:649–655.

Nutrition Box References

Berkow R (ed): *Merck Manual of Diagnosis and Therapy,* ed 15. Rahway, N.J.: Merck and Co, 1987, pp. 738–739.

Carmel R: The deoxyuridine suppression test identifies subtle cobalamin deficiency in patients without typical megaloblastic anemia. *JAMA* 1985;253(9):1284–1287.

Carmel R: Pernicious anemia: The expected findings of very low serum cobalamin levels, anemia, and macrocytosis are often lacking. *Arch Intern Med* 1988;148(8):1712–1714.

Herbert V: Don't ignore low serum cobalamin (vitamin B_{12}) levels. *Arch Intern Med* 1988;148(8):1705–1707.

Herbert V, Colman N: Vitamin B_{12} and folic acid, in Shils M, Young V (eds): *Modern Nutrition in Health and Disease.* Philadelphia: Lea and Febiger, 1988, pp. 394–395.

Lindenbaum J et al.: Neuropsychiatric disorders caused by cobalamin deficiency in the absence of anemia or macrocytosis. *N Engl J Med* 1988;318(26):1720–1728.

Tietz N: Reference ranges and laboratory values of clinical importance, in Wyngaarden J, Smith L (eds): *Cecil Textbook of Medicine,* ed 17. Philadelphia: Saunders, 1985, p. 2337.

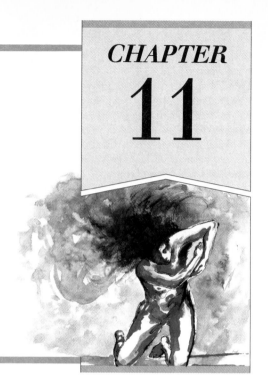

Applying the Nursing Process for Clients with Psychoactive Substance Use Disorders

LEARNING OBJECTIVES

- Contrast the different definitions of substance abuse

- List key legislation in the history of substance abuse

- Analyze major theoretic explanations for substance abuse

- Compare and contrast the major categories of substance use

- Identify the groups at risk for substance abuse

- Assess the physical, psychologic, and withdrawal effects of the major categories of substance use

- Apply the nursing process with clients with psychoactive substance use disorders

- Identify questions that are integral to a nursing assessment of clients who are substance abusers

- Compare and contrast nursing diagnoses from NANDA with diagnoses from DSM-III-R

- Discuss a variety of nursing intervention strategies for clients demonstrating various types of substance abuse

- Identify evaluation/outcome criteria for clients who are substance abusers

Sally A. Hutchinson

CROSS REFERENCES

Other topics related to this chapter are: Adolescents, Chapter 34; Depression, Chapter 13; Organic mental disorders, Chapter 10; Poly-drug use among the elderly, Chapter 35; Psychobiology, Chapter 6; Risk of AIDS for intravenous drug users, Chapter 25.

The assistance of Karen Hogan, MSN, in preparing this revision is greatly appreciated.

DRUG AND ALCOHOL ABUSE, already a widespread problem, is rapidly escalating. Substance abuse is a psychosocial and a biologic problem. In the United States and Europe, television and radio advertisements entice viewers with the hope of relief from pain and problems. The cultural values portrayed are clear: Discomfort should be erased; drinking is vital to a stress-free life; drugs are acceptable mediators of emotions.

Substance abuse is a major public health issue of grave ramifications. It increases the crime rate, auto accident deaths, number of teenage pregnancies, and the suicide rate. Individuals and families are destroyed. Every part of a substance abuser's life—social life, family life, work productivity and relationships, physical health—is affected. Substance abuse in the work environment increases accidents, workers' compensation claims, absenteeism, and theft.

This chapter is an in-depth biopsychosocial exploration of the substance abuse issues relevant to the practicing nurse.

Historical Foundations

From the beginning of recorded history, humans have experimented with drugs and drink in an effort to feel good or to experience an altered state of consciousness. Drugs first touted for their healing effects often become, with time, problems to society. William James, a brilliant American psychologist, wrote of a "tremendously exciting sense of an intense metaphysical illumination" after using nitrous oxide (Klein 1985, p 40). Freud believed cocaine to be a new wonder drug because of its euphoric effects. William Halstead, a surgeon, used cocaine for regional anesthesia. Others found it useful for alcohol and morphine addiction, asthma, colds, corns, eczema, neuralgia, and even spiritual awakening (Rottenberg 1980). In the 1960s, Timothy Leary, a Harvard psychologist, was an avid supporter of the use of LSD for the purpose of achieving heightened awareness. Over time, each of these drugs has left a wake of horror in people's lives. Deaths, brain damage, violence, and ruined lives are the result of abuse.

Efforts at Controlling Substance Abuse

While one segment of the population experiments with drugs and alcohol, another segment attempts to set limits. By examining events over the last eighty years, we can trace changing perspectives on substance abuse and efforts to control it. This significant legislation mirrors changing trends:

- The Harrison Narcotics Act of 1914 was the first United States legislation that attempted to control narcotics.

- In 1920, the Volstead Act prohibited alcohol.

- From 1919–1923, addicts were able to obtain heroin from clinics.

- In 1924, Congress passed the Narcotics Drugs Import and Export Act and the Marijuana Tax Act.

- In 1933, the Volstead Act was repealed.

- In 1946, the Mental Health Act brought increased attention to substance abuse.

- In 1946, the United Nations and World Health Organization became involved in the control of illicit drugs.

- In the 1960s, President Kennedy declared drug education a national priority, and federal monies were allocated to substance abuse programs.

- In 1968, the Bureau of Narcotics and Dangerous Drugs (formerly under the Food and Drug Administration) was transferred to the Department of Justice. Today, it is the Bureau of Narcotics and Dangerous Drugs and Customs.

- In 1970, the Harrison Narcotics Act was repealed. A new act, the Comprehensive Drug Abuse Prevention and Control Act (also known as the Controlled Substance Act) regulated the availability and use of controlled substances.

- In 1972, regulations for the handling and distribution of methadone were planned.

- In the 1980s, federal drug and alcohol funds were rechanneled into alcohol, drug abuse, and mental health block grants (ADAMH).

- In 1985, Congress pursued legislation attached to a foreign aid bill that required the Drug Enforcement Administration and the State Department to share information on international narcotics traffickers.

- By 1986, programs for nurses who are substance abusers were in effect in twenty-one states and were being developed in most other states.

Beliefs about Causes

Beliefs about the causes of substance abuse changed over the years. In the early 1900s, alcoholics and drug addicts were considered morally weak people who yielded easily to temptation. In 1956, the American Medical Association declared alcoholism a disease; this relabeling had important ramifications for diagnosis and treatment. The following year, the American Hospital Association accepted alcoholism as an illness appropriate for treatment in general hospitals. At this time, insurance companies offer financial coverage.

Gradually, as substance abuse became redefined as a psychiatric disorder, researchers found the topic worthy of study. Initial research was conducted in the 1950s at the Yale University Center of Alcohol Studies. The Controlled Substance Act of 1970 provided Department of Health, Education, and Welfare grants for treatment, rehabilitation, and educational programs related to drug abuse. Today, substance abuse is a major public health issue and, consequently, research monies from federal and private agencies are plentiful.

As substance abuse was redefined, the writings about substance abuse gradually changed in quantity and quality. Initially confined to psychiatric nursing journals and medical journals, literature on alcoholism and drug addiction began to appear in the general nursing literature (Naegle 1983). At the present time, psychiatric nursing has yet to develop adequate theories to guide the care of clients who are substance abusers. Research is in the early phase of development. Theories are being generated and also borrowed from other disciplines and applied to nursing. Nursing research on the assessment, diagnosis, and intervention with the substance-abusing client is increasing and should soon have some effects on nursing practice.

Theoretic Foundations

Before examining the theories that attempt to account for the "why" of substance abuse, we should define the term. According to the National Council on Alcoholism, a **substance abuser** is a person who experiences problems with health, work, family, and social relations as a result of drug or alcohol use.

According to Dr. G. Douglas Talbott, a pioneer in the study of addiction, **abuse** is the misuse of a drug that can be discontinued at will; addiction occurs when misuse is uncontrollable. Addiction, a *disease,* occurs when a person with a genetic predisposition to addiction abuses a drug (Gallagher 1986, pp 7–8).

In 1964, the World Health Organization (WHO) Expert Committee on Addiction-Producing Drugs voted to substitute the term *drug dependence* for *addiction* and *habituation.* In 1980, the American Psychiatric Association's *Diagnostic and Statistical Manual of Mental Disorders,* third edition (DSM-III), divided substance use disorders into two major categories: substance abuse and substance dependence. The DSM-III-R proposes two major categories: psychoactive substance–induced organic mental disorders and psychoactive substance use disorders (American Psychiatric Association 1987). These various definitions and categories demonstrate the changing terminology of substance abuse.

In this chapter, *substance* refers to alcohol, prescription drugs, over-the-counter medications, and illicit drugs. Contemporary explanations of substance abuse derive from biologic, psychologic, sociocultural, and family systems theories.

Biologic Perspectives

The biologic explanation, especially of alcoholism, has assumed a greater importance in the last few years. Research to determine genetic predispositions to alcoholism continues. The following are examples of research that is gaining respect in the scientific community:

- Classic research by Jellinek in the 1940s and 1950s revealed that alcoholics proceed through phases, including the prealcoholic symptomatic phase, the prodromal phase, the crucial phase, and the chronic phase (Jellinek 1946). He recognized "loss of control" in addictive alcoholics and conjectured that it may have a biochemical basis.

- Cultural differences may affect alcoholism rates. For example, Asians frequently experience adverse reactions to alcohol, including palpitations and a flush of the skin. These responses are genetic and probably account for the lower rate of alcoholism in the Orient.

- Alcoholics have been noted to have a type of color blindness. A study of relatives of alcoholics indicates possible transmission by sex-linked recessive genes (Cruz-Coke and Varela 1966, Varela et al. 1969).

- In the late 1950s, researchers studied Scandinavian twins to determine if alcoholism was inherited. The scientists studied twins of alcoholic parents who were reared by (a) their own parents, (b) foster parents, and (c) different foster families. After twenty-five years, the records reveal that the degree of alcoholism in all three groups is almost identical. This finding suggests that a genetic factor predisposes to alcoholism (Mann 1983).

- Some people are born with a faulty hepatic enzyme system that may predispose them to alcohol addiction.

- Researchers have found that alcoholics metabolize ethanol more efficiently than nonalcoholics through the creation of alternative pathways and in response to chronic high blood alcohol levels. This phenomenon suggests an explanation for the abnormal increase in ethanol tolerance noted in the alcoholic population (Lieber and DeCarli 1970, Ugarte et al. 1972).

- P-450, an enzyme with opiatelike characteristics, has been found to develop in alcoholics, possibly creating the craving and compulsion to drink addictively (Koop et al. 1982).

• In animals, alcohol is metabolized into tetrahydroisoquinolones (TIQs), opiatelike compounds that affect nerve receptors much as morphine and endorphins (the body's naturally produced opiates) do. TIQ from alcohol has an opiate effect. In response, the body decreases or stops endorphin production. When the alcohol wears off, the endorphin levels remain low, and the alcoholic cannot feel good without drinking. Some researchers believe alcoholics may be born with an endorphin deficiency, creating a low tolerance to pain and stress (Franks 1985).

• Animal research advances the notion that alcoholics have a metabolic anomaly that causes them to derive more pleasure from alcohol than other people do. When alcohol is absent from the body, the absence of this pleasure is felt as a deficiency (Franks 1985).

• Alcoholics may have neurophysiologic defects. They may be vulnerable to intense sensory input and use alcohol as a protection from this heightened sensitivity.

• Research demonstrates that children of alcoholics are at fourfold risk of becoming alcoholics. Even if they are adopted by different families at birth, identical twins of alcoholic parents have more than a 60 percent chance of becoming alcoholics; fraternal twins have less than a 30 percent chance. Children of nonalcoholics reared by alcoholics are not at increased risk of alcoholism (Schuckit 1985).

• When a control group of sons of nonalcoholics (a low-risk population) and an experimental group of sons of alcoholics (a high-risk population) were compared, three differences were found (Schuckit 1985):

1. Sons of alcoholics appear to show less intense responses to modest ethanol dosages, demonstrate lower amplitudes of a brain wave that might measure selective attention, and may have different brain alpha rhythms.

2. Subjective and objective tests showed that sons of alcoholics were less affected by ethanol than sons of nonalcoholics.

3. When both groups were given the same dosage of ethanol, controls showed poor performance on a number of cognitive and psychomotor tests and more intense changes in cortisol and prolactin, two hormones known to be affected by injection of ethanol.

Schuckit (1985) concludes "there is consistent evidence that those in the high-risk group demonstrate significantly less intense reactions to modest doses of ethanol than those in the low-risk group. It may be that they are feeling less ethanol effect at the blood alcohol concentrations at which most people make a decision to stop drinking."

Scientists now are working on computerized methods of analyzing blood chemistries. These techniques may help in diagnosing early alcoholism. Another blood test will detect liver changes that warn of cirrhosis (Franks 1985). When these tests are perfected, their use will raise difficult ethical and legal issues for employers, as the use of urinalysis to detect drug abuse does now. One such issue is the employee's right to privacy. A second is the possibility of error. The error rate in urine tests is 50 to 100 percent (often due to technical errors and poor quality control), giving an unjustly accused employee a cause for legal action. Another problem with urine tests is that they cannot detect when a person used a drug or whether a person is an addict, a habitual user, or an occasional user. Also, test results do not indicate job performance. There remain the difficult questions of whom to test, when to test, how to test, and what steps to take if the test is positive. In spite of these questions, one-third of the nation's largest companies are doing urinalysis on their employees.

Psychologic Perspectives

From the psychologic perspective, the substance abuser is viewed as regressed and fixated at pregenital, oral levels of psychosexual development. Some writers relate the pattern of drug taking to parental inconsistency, self-centeredness, and inner dishonesty. The following personality traits are often associated with disruptive drug use:

• Dominant and critical behavior with underlying self-doubts and passivity

• Tendency to describe own parents as self-reliant and efficient but not emotionally warm

• Personal insecurity

• Problems with sexual identification

• Rebellious attitudes toward authority

• Tendency to use defense mechanisms that are primarily escapist

• Difficulty with intimacy

• Absence of a strong and efficient superego

• Marked narcissistic trends

There is no real agreement about whether certain personality traits are sufficient to account for drug dependence, because the personality traits in question are studied after the diagnosis of substance abuse. Clients diagnosed with primary affective disorders, sociopathy, and certain personality disorders, however, often abuse alcohol and drugs. In such cases, initial assessment, after the client has undergone withdrawal, should focus on accurate diagnoses so that both conditions may be treated simultaneously.

Richard Marohn (1983), the president of the American Society for Adolescent Psychiatry, offers an interesting and plausible psychologic explanation for adolescent, and ultimately adult, substance abuse. Adopting a developmental perspective, Marohn views the alcohol or drugs as having a self-healing or self-medicating function. Adolescents who successfully separate from their parents do so by transferring their object attachment from their parents to idealized others, including peers. With time, adolescents learn how to master a variety of strong emotions—anger, guilt, joy, pain, sexual attraction, love—and recognize that these emotions emanate from themselves and are part of themselves. Such adolescents can then care for themselves by living with and experiencing the powerful emotions that are part of being alive.

Adolescents who are substance abusers, Marohn believes, have severe problems with tension regulation. They have not been able to separate and individuate from significant others. They view their emotions as emanating from the other or from the external world, as children do. The expectation, then, is that the parents are responsible for the teenager's life and feelings. When this expectation is not met and when they experience strong emotions, adolescents resort to substance abuse to manage these emotions. Drugs and alcohol are an escape from powerful and often painful emotions, an attempt at self-soothing and self-care.

Sociocultural Perspectives

Life's harsh realities come in many forms: the hopelessness and defeat of urban slum dwellers, the academic and social pressures generated by upper middle class families, the adolescent's feeling of impotence and alienation, the peer group pressure to join in and share experiences, the social vacuum of unloving families, where meaningful attachments are dissolved or dissolving. All of these social conditions and contexts help create and sustain substance abuse. In addition, however, people who become addicts or alcoholics tend to live in environments where access to chemicals is easy and initiation into their use is widespread. Substance abusers describe in interviews how they learned to drink or use drugs at high school and college parties or at home by watching their families. They recognized chemicals as a remedy for psychic and physical pain.

Deviant subcultures encourage their members to adopt a drug-dependent life-style. The sociologist Howard Becker (1963) studied the process by which a person becomes a marijuana user. In this classic study, Becker emphasizes the role the subculture plays in teaching people to disengage from conventional social controls. The subculture also teaches them how to think about the experience and the techniques that ensure that they will enjoy using the drug. Another sociologist, Alfred Lindesmith (1965), observes that people recognize that they are addicted at the moment when the appearance of withdrawal symptoms makes voluntary abstinence impossible. At this point, they are ready to be assimilated into a genuine drug-dependent life-style, because they must begin planning how to make sure they have a future supply. They must learn the sources, devices, and customs they will use to solve their problems.

Deviant subcultures are not the only cultures that foster substance abuse. The dominant middle class is bombarded by advertising that encourages the taking of pills for pain relief, sleep, constipation, and sinus problems. Acceptance of cigarettes and alcohol use can lead to experimentation with marijuana and other drugs. A 1985 study reported that use of cocaine was strongly correlated with marijuana use and the early use of cigarettes and alcohol (Drug Abuse Update 1989).

Studies clearly show that substance abuse is present in all cultures; however, which substance people abuse is often culturally determined. In Western culture, alcohol is the drug of choice. In Moslem countries marijuana use is a problem because Islam prohibits alcohol use. Opium is used in China and other Eastern countries, whereas people in India and Africa use native herbs and chemicals. Native Americans use peyote and alcohol more than other drugs.

Family Systems Perspectives

A family systems explanation for substance abuse has gained increasing acceptance among health care professionals. Stanton and Todd's (1982) work is particularly useful because it proposes a theoretic framework, a treatment method, and evaluation methods based on family systems theory. Unlike social theorists who stress the power of the peer group, Stanton and Todd view adolescent drug abuse primarily as a family phenomenon. Adolescent drug addicts, they believe, are too close to their parents and consequently feel dependent, inadequate, and fearful of separation. The family is overly *enmeshed* or *entangled*.

Contrary to what one might expect, the adolescent drug abuser is striving to preserve the stability of the entangled family. The adolescent keeps the family in crisis and focused on the problems brought about by drug abuse. If the addict improves and begins to individuate and separate from the family, the underlying familial problems emerge. Thus, the entire family has a stake in maintaining the addiction. The drug use allows the addict to pseudoindividuate—to be both in and out of the family.

Another family systems approach to substance abuse implicates paternal lack of emotional warmth and paternal rejection as factors closely associated with substance abuse. Emmelkamp and Heeres (1989) found that, when compared with controls, addicts felt more rejected by their parents and had experienced less emotional warmth. Addicts also rated parents as more overprotective than controls.

The family systems perspective also includes the phenomenon of codependency, an emotional dysfunction that was first identified in families with an alcoholic member (Friel et al. 1984). Initially, the cause of codependency was thought to be the stress of living with an alcoholic individual. As alcoholics recovered, however, a separate disorder was identified in the family members of the alcoholic (Guy 1990).

Codependents are people who allow another's behavior to affect them while being obsessed with controlling that individual's behavior. Codependents try to control events and people around them because they feel that everything around them and inside them is out of their control (Guy 1990). A codependent is the family member who alternately rescues and blames (persecutes) the addict. Certain behaviors are characteristic of the codependent, also called the coalcoholic. This person is a highly organized achiever who works continuously, attempting to maintain stability in the present situation. The codependent may be married to the addict, and the children in the family are at high risk for becoming substance abusers and emotionally unstable. Survival patterns are usually different for each child. One may become a substance abuser, while another may become the family caretaker ("hero") at an early age. This young child actively "parents" the parents and siblings, covers up for them, and works to promote harmony (placator role) in a volatile, dysfunctional family. Another child may be a "scapegoat," behaving in negative ways so as to deflect blame from the addicted parent. Emotional and behavioral problems are common. This child is at high risk for becoming a substance abuser. "The lost child" escapes into fantasy and also is at high risk for addiction; the "mascot" plays the role of the clown, thereby diverting attention from the parents.

Families with members who are addicted to drugs or alcohol suffer guilt, remorse, and alienation. Conflict is inevitable, and violence is common. The dysfunctional family patterns involve all family members and tend to be transmitted through the generations, making family systems intervention necessary for change.

Although **Alcoholics Anonymous** (AA), a support group for alcoholics, does not openly endorse the family systems theory, they do recognize clearly that alcoholism is a family disease. **Al-Anon** and **Al-Ateen** are groups for spouses, parents, and teenage children of alcoholics. The focus is on helping these nonalcoholics learn to live and work effectively with alcoholics. The underlying belief is that family members often assume the role of **enablers**, or coalcoholics, perpetuating the alcoholic's drinking patterns. As the family attempts to adjust to the alcoholic's life-style, they develop behavioral and emotional problems (*The Family Enablers*, p 3).

A cycle begins when the enablers do what they think is best in the situation. They begin to cover for the addict, e.g., by saying that he or she has a cold, is bruised because of stumbling in the dark, is asleep because of fatigue. Protected by the enabler, the addict is spared the consequences of his or her behavior and continues drinking or using drugs. The enabler, believing that the addict is coping with family, marital, or work problems "the best way he can," denies the disease of addiction. The addict blames the enabler; the enabler feels guilty and then attempts to control family life and the behaviors of the alcoholic/addict, e.g., throwing out liquor, taking the car keys. Of course, this behavior does not work. The enabler has tried the roles of protector, rescuer, controller, and blamer, but none is effective in altering the course of the disease. Consequently, enablers feel worthless and helpless because they are unsuccessful in terminating the addiction. Intervention and confrontation are necessary to break the cycle.

All of these theories—biologic, psychologic, sociocultural, family systems—offer perspectives on the problem of substance abuse. Research that tests hypotheses derived from these theories is necessary to advance our knowledge and to contribute to further theory development.

Factors in Pathology

The DSM-III (American Psychiatric Association 1980, p 163) includes the diagnostic class "substance use disorders," which is concerned with

. . . Behavioral changes associated with more or less regular use of substances that affect the central nervous system. Examples of such behavioral changes include impairment in social or occupational functioning as a consequence of substance use, inability to control use of or to stop taking the substance, and the development of serious withdrawal symptoms after cessation of or reduction in substance use.

The DSM-III-R (American Psychiatric Association 1987) has two categories entitled psychoactive substance-induced organic mental disorders and psychoactive substance use disorders (see the boxes on pages 220 and 221). Psychoactive substance-induced organic mental disorders result in intoxications, withdrawal, delirium, hallucinosis, and delusional disorders, among others. Psychoactive substance use disorders result in dependence or abuse. (See the box on page 222 for the diagnostic criteria for dependence and abuse.)

Psychoactive Substance-Induced Organic Mental Disorders (DSM-III-R)

Alcohol
303.00 Intoxication
291.40 Idiosyncratic intoxication
291.80 Uncomplicated alcohol withdrawal
291.00 Withdrawal delirium
291.30 Hallucinosis
291.10 Amnestic disorder
291.20 Dementia associated with alcoholism

Amphetamine or Similarly Acting Sympathomimetic
305.70 Intoxication
292.00 Withdrawal
292.81 Delirium
292.11 Delusional disorder

Caffeine
305.90 Intoxication

Cannabis
305.20 Intoxication
292.11 Delusional disorder

Cocaine
305.60 Intoxication
292.00 Withdrawal
292.81 Delirium
292.11 Delusional disorder

Hallucinogen
305.30 Hallucinosis
292.11 Delusional disorder
292.84 Mood disorder
292.89 Posthallucinogen perception disorder

Inhalant
305.90 Intoxication

Nicotine
292.00 Withdrawal

Opioid
305.50 Intoxication
292.00 Withdrawal

Phencyclidine (PCP) or Similarly Acting Arylcyclohexylamine
305.90 Intoxication
292.81 Delirium
292.11 Delusional disorder
292.84 Mood disorder
292.90 Organic mental disorder NOS

Sedative, Hypnotic, or Anxiolytic
305.40 Intoxication
292.00 Uncomplicated sedative, hypnotic, or anxiolytic withdrawal
292.00 Withdrawal delirium
292.83 Amnestic disorder

Other or Unspecified Psychoactive Substance
305.90 Intoxication
292.00 Withdrawal
292.81 Delirium
292.82 Dementia
292.83 Amnestic disorder
292.11 Delusional disorder
292.12 Hallucinosis
292.84 Mood disorder
292.89 Anxiety disorder
292.89 Personality disorder
292.90 Organic mental disorder NOS

SOURCE: *American Psychiatric Association:* Diagnostic and Statistical Manual of Mental Disorders, *ed 3, revised APA, 1987, p 51.*

Psychoactive Substance Use Disorders (DSM-III-R)

Alcohol
303.90   Dependence
305.00   Abuse

Amphetamine or Similarly Acting Sympathomimetic
304.40   Dependence
305.70   Abuse

Cannabis
304.30   Dependence
305.70   Abuse

Cocaine
304.20   Dependence
305.60   Abuse

Hallucinogen
304.50   Dependence
305.30   Abuse

Inhalant
304.60   Dependence
305.90   Abuse

Nicotine
305.10   Dependence

Opioid
304.00   Dependence
305.50   Abuse

Phencyclidine (PCP) or Similarly Acting Arylcyclohexylamine
304.50   Dependence
305.90   Abuse

Sedative, Hypnotic, or Anxiolytic
304.10   Dependence
305.40   Abuse
304.90   Polysubstance dependence
304.90   Psychoactive substance dependence NOS
305.90   Psychoactive substance abuse NOS

SOURCE: *American Psychiatric Association:* Diagnostic and Statistical Manual of Mental Disorders, *ed 3, revised. APA, 1987, p 6.*

Alcohol

Josie B, a 62-year-old woman, arrived at the hospital to be admitted for the fifth time. Her gait was unsteady and her speech slurred. Even though drunk, she avoided eye contact, appeared embarrassed, and apologized profusely for "getting into this mess again." She said "I really don't need to be here. I can handle this problem."

The box on page 223 presents the key facts about alcohol abuse. Several years ago alcoholism was considered a neglected disease. Recently, because of its increasing incidence and the highway carnage attributed to alcohol use, alcoholism has been the focus of magazine articles and radio and television programs. Perhaps this media blitz is in part a response to heightened awareness of the devastating effects of chronic alcoholism, e.g., depression; loss of self-respect; alienation from family, friends, and coworkers; malnutrition; infections; and damaging physiologic effects to most body systems (see the box on page 224). Although alcoholism historically was viewed as a moral problem, this increased awareness played a part in the redefinition of alcoholism as a disease. As research about its biochemical aspects became known, earlier beliefs were challenged. The social stigma attached to alcoholism is decreasing, and more people are seeking help. Professionals, laypeople, alcoholics, and nonalcoholics are attending workshops and seminars on alcoholism; college courses at the graduate and undergraduate levels are offered. Recovery programs are reported widely in the popular media.

Effects of Alcohol

A sedative anesthetic, alcohol is absorbed in the small intestine. Approximately 95 percent is broken down by the liver; the rest is excreted through the lungs, kidneys, and skin. Generally, a person can metabolize 10 mL of alcohol or 1 ounce of whiskey every ninety minutes. If taken in exceedingly high doses, alcohol can depress respiration and cause death. Intoxication occurs when a person's blood alcohol level is 0.10 percent or more. This blood alcohol level is the legal definition of inebriation in most states, although there is a trend toward lowering the level to 0.08 in some

Diagnostic Criteria for Psychoactive Substance Dependence (DSM-III-R)

A. At least three of the following:

1. Substance often taken in larger amounts or over a longer period than the person intended

2. Persistent desire or one or more unsuccessful efforts to cut down or control substance use

3. A great deal of time spent in activities necessary to get the substance (e.g., theft), taking the substance (e.g., chain smoking), or recovering from its effects

4. Frequent intoxication or withdrawal symptoms when expected to fulfill major role obligations at work, school, or home (e.g., does not go to work because hung over, goes to school or work "high," is intoxicated while taking care of children), or when substance use is physically hazardous (e.g., drives when intoxicated)

5. Important social, occupational, or recreational activities given up or reduced because of substance use

6. Continued substance use despite knowledge of having a persistent or recurrent social, psychologic, or physical problem that is caused or exacerbated by the use of the substance (e.g., keeps using heroin despite family arguments about it, cocaine-induced depression, or having an ulcer made worse by drinking)

7. Marked tolerance: need for markedly increased amounts of the substance (i.e., at least a 50 percent increase) in order to achieve intoxication or desired effect, or markedly diminished effect with continued use of the same amount

Note: The following items may not apply to cannabis, hallucinogens, or phencyclidine (PCP):

8. Characteristic withdrawal symptoms

9. Substance often taken to relieve or avoid withdrawal symptoms

B. Some symptoms of the disturbance have persisted for at least 1 month, or have occurred repeatedly over a longer period of time.

Criteria for Severity of Psychoactive Substance Dependence

Mild: Few, if any, symptoms in excess of those required to make the diagnosis, and the symptoms result in no more than mild impairment in occupational functioning or in usual social activities or relationships with others.

Moderate: Symptoms of functional impairment between "mild" and "severe."

Severe: Many symptoms in excess of those required to make the diagnosis, and the symptoms markedly interfere with occupational functioning or with usual social activities or relationships with others.

In partial remission: During the past six months, some use of the substance and some symptoms of dependence.

In full remission: During the past six months, either no use of the substance, or use of the substance and no symptoms of dependence.

Diagnostic Criteria for Psychoactive Substance Abuse

A. A maladaptive pattern of psychoactive substance use indicated by at least one of the following:

1. Continued use despite knowledge of having a persistent or recurrent social, occupational, psychologic, or physical problem that is caused or exacerbated by use of the psychoactive substance

2. Recurrent use in situations in which use is physically hazardous (e.g., driving while intoxicated)

B. Some symptoms of the disturbance have persisted for at least 1 month or have occurred repeatedly over a longer period of time.

C. Never met the criteria for psychoactive substance dependence for this substance.

SOURCE: *Adapted from American Psychiatric Association:* Diagnostic and Statistical Manual of Mental Disorders, *ed 3, revised. 1987, pp 167–169.*

Key Facts about Alcohol

Examples
Liquor, wine, beer

Slang Terms
Hooch, booze, moonshine, sauce

Route of Administration
Oral (liquid)

Psychologic Symptoms
Irritability*
Mood swings*
Short attention span*
Talks a lot and loudly*
Decreased judgment
Decreased inhibitions
Interference with memory

Physical Symptoms
Slurred speech*
Lack of coordination*
Unsteady gait*
Blackouts
Decreased REM sleep
Nystagmus*
Flushed face*
Decreased psychomotor functions

Withdrawal Symptoms
Nausea or vomiting
Anxiety

Depressed mood or irritability
Malaise or weakness
Autonomic hyperactivity
Tachycardia
Sweating, elevated blood pressure
Orthostatic hypotension
Coarse tremor of hands, tongue, eyelids

Time Frame for Withdrawal Symptoms
Mild withdrawal may begin within 12–24 hours following last drink. Symptoms may last from 48–72 hours. Major withdrawal symptoms appear within 2–3 days following last drink and may last 3–5 days.

Dangers
Car accidents
Physical injury
Malnutrition
Hepatitis
Cirrhosis
Gastritis
Suicide
FAS (fetal alcohol syndrome)

Typical Users
Teenagers
Adults

Symptoms of intoxication noted in DSM-III-R.

states. Simple intoxication lasts less than twelve hours and is usually followed by a hangover. A *hangover* is the unpleasant symptoms occurring approximately four to six hours after alcohol ingestion. These symptoms include nausea and vomiting, gastritis, headache, fatigue, sweating, thirst, and vasomotor instability. The cause of the symptoms is uncertain, but they are attributed to hypoglycemia and the accumulation of lactic acid and acetaldehyde in the blood.

Alcoholic hallucinosis refers to auditory hallucinations reported by clients with alcohol dependence. The hallucinations occur approximately forty-eight hours after heavy drinking.

Alcohol withdrawal syndrome refers to withdrawal symptoms unaccompanied by delirium. These include tremulousness and hallucinations. Tremulousness may occur during the drinking period or up to two hours afterward, whereas hallucinations begin twelve to forty-eight hours after the person stops drinking. Grand mal seizures ("rum fits") may occur two to three days after the person stops drinking. **Delirium tremens (DTs)**, a rare symptom of withdrawal, is a condition of severe memory disturbance, agitation, anorexia, and hallucinations. Generally, the DTs begin a few days after drinking stops and end within one to five days. Frequently, additional medical illnesses are present and may include pneumonia, pancreatitis, and hepatic decompensation (Kaplan and Sadock 1989). (See the boxes on key facts and physical effects for additional information.)

Physical Effects of Chronic Alcoholism

Hepatic System
Alcoholic fatty liver syndrome
Alcoholic hepatitis
Laënnec's cirrhosis

Neurologic System
Wernicke-Korsakoff syndrome (related to thiamine deficiency)
Peripheral neuropathy (related to vitamin B deficiency)
Marchiafava disease*
Central pontine myelinosis*
Cerebellar degeneration*
Alcoholic amblyopia*

Cardiovascular System
Alcoholic cardiomyopathy
Hypokalemia
Hypomagnesemia
Hyperlipidemia
Altered fluid balance
Beriberi heart disease (related to thiamine deficiency)
Hematologic abnormalities

Musculoskeletal System
Acute alcoholic myopathy
Subclinical alcoholic myopathy
Chronic alcoholic myopathy

Gastrointestinal System
Gastritis
Esophagitis
Mallory-Weiss syndrome
Boerhaave's syndrome
Pancreatitis
Nutritional deficiency diseases
Nausea
Abdominal pain
Erratic bowel function (constipation and diarrhea)
Gastrointestinal hemorrhage
Jaundice
High incidence of digestive tract cancers
Glucose intolerance

Reproductive System
Impotence
Sterility
Gynecomastia
Anorgasmic (women)
Fetal alcohol syndrome (FAS)

Very rare.

SOURCE: *Adapted from Kneisl CR, Ames SA:* Adult Health Nursing. *Addison-Wesley, 1986.*

Medical Treatment

Medical treatment of alcoholism involves management of withdrawal symptoms and the use of medication to deter the alcoholic from drinking. The alcohol withdrawal syndrome occurs after the addicted individual stops drinking. This syndrome is composed of a constellation of physiologic and behavioral symptoms that occur when the alcohol level drops. In the early 1950s, **the alcohol withdrawal** syndrome was divided into four stages: tremor, hallucinations, seizures, and delirium tremens. Today, the syndrome is divided into two categories according to time of onset and severity of symptoms: early or minor withdrawal and late or major withdrawal (Kirk and Bradford 1987).

Minor withdrawal occurs within six to twelve hours after the alcoholic's last drink. Early symptoms include anxiety, agitation, and irritability. As the syndrome progresses, other symptoms occur. These include tremor, tachycardia, hypertension, diaphoresis, and hallucinations. Gastrointestinal symptoms of nausea, vomiting, diarrhea, and anorexia may also be present. The appearance of hallucinations (visual, auditory, olfactory, or tactile) and seizures marks the onset of major withdrawal.

Major withdrawal or delirium tremens is the most advanced, potentially life-threatening stage of alcohol withdrawal. Symptoms associated with delirium tremens usually develop seventy-two hours after the last drink. Physical symptoms of impending DTs include elevated temperature, severe diaphoresis, hypertension, and tachycardia. Behavioral symptoms include confusion and disorientation, agitation, tremors, and alterations in sensory perception (auditory and visual hallucinations).

The best treatment for major alcohol withdrawal is prevention or early detection and treatment of minor withdrawal. Medical treatment for withdrawal includes monitoring the client's fluid status. Although some clients are overhydrated, many are dehydrated or have the potential for developing a fluid volume deficit. Therefore, fluids should be encouraged, up to 3000 mL/day if no evidence exists to contraindicate this. If the client is unable to take fluids by mouth, fluids may be administered intravenously. Many alcoholics suffer from a magnesium deficiency. Administration of magnesium sulfate decreases the central nervous system irritability caused by low magnesium levels and thus prevents seizures. Because alcohol interferes with the absorption of B vitamins, clients often receive vitamins, especially thiamine (vitamin B_1). Benzodiazepines, such as diazepam (Valium) or chlordiazepoxide (Librium) may be given to help prevent DTs. Seizures may be treated with I.V. diazepam, and the client may be placed on phenytoin (Dilantin).

Disulfiram (**Antabuse**) may be prescribed for alcoholic clients. Disulfiram inhibits acetaldehyde dehydrogenase, which normally metabolizes acetaldehyde. As a result, acetaldehyde accumulates if alcohol is consumed. Acetaldehyde is highly toxic, producing nausea and hypotension. Hypotension leads to shock and may be fatal. The dosage of disulfiram is usually 250 mg daily. Often, clients stop taking the drug, and it may be useful to dispense the drug every four days during client visits to a clinic. If the client uses alcohol, a powerful disulfiram reaction may occur and last for up to two weeks. Reaction symptoms include nausea, vomiting, flushing, dizziness, and tachycardia.

Because of the potential danger of disulfiram, the client must be instructed orally and in writing not to use alcohol in any form, including alcohol-based cough syrups or cold remedies. Clients with myocardial disease or taking metronidazole (Flagyl) should not take Antabuse; in the latter case, a disulfiram reaction is possible.

Patterns of Use

According to the DSM-III-R (p 173), alcoholics manifest one of three patterns of use: (a) regular daily intake of large amounts of alcohol, (b) regular heavy drinking limited to weekends, and (c) long periods of sobriety interspersed with binges of heavy drinking lasting for weeks or months. Regardless of the preferred pattern, people who drink excessively experience numerous negative physiologic and psychologic effects (see the earlier boxes on key facts and physical effects). For more information about the physical effects of alcoholism, see Bittle et al. (1986).

Blackouts

Having **blackouts** is frequently confused with passing out. In fact, passing out refers to unconsciousness, whereas a blackout is **anterograde amnesia**: loss of short-term memories with retention of remote memories. A person can function effectively for up to several days—talking on the telephone, working, and shopping—yet have absolutely no memory of doing so. To others, the alcoholic may appear normal or "high." Interestingly, alcoholics appear unconcerned by the blackouts and eventually learn to cover them up. This appearance of unconcern may, in part, be due to *euphoric recall:* The alcoholic recalls only feeling good but not behavior. Reality is distorted. Some clients, however, find blackouts very disturbing; if so they can seek treatment.

Blackouts appearing later in the disease process may be indicative of physical dependence and are not related to the amount of alcohol consumed. They are unpredictable, and exactly how or why they occur is not clear. Some authorities believe blackouts are an acute syndrome due to dehydration of the brain tissue. When assessing an alcoholic client, psychiatric nurses need to determine if blackouts are part of the symptoms.

Fetal Alcohol Syndrome

Nurses also need to be aware of the harmful effects of alcohol on pregnant women and unborn children. **Fetal alcohol syndrome** (FAS) is found in children of alcoholic women. Physical and mental defects include severe growth deficiency, heart defects, malformed facial features, mental retardation, low birth weight, learning problems, and hyperactivity. If a child has one or two of these characteristics, the condition is called *fetal alcohol effects.* FAS affects 1 of every 750 babies born in the United States. A baby born to an alcoholic mother may need to be withdrawn gradually from alcohol.

Suicide

Nurses must be alert to the possibility of suicide attempts by alcoholics. One percent of the general population attempt suicide, but 15 percent of alcoholics do so. The nurse should watch for self-destructive behavior and for events in a client's life that represent a loss, e.g., work, family, health, or legal problems. Such behavior and events put people in a high-risk category (Trenk 1986).

Barbiturates or Similarly Acting Sedatives or Hypnotics

Elizabeth W, a 45-year-old housewife, has been depressed and irritable over an impending divorce. Her physician prescribed Valium (5 mg) for sleep and for anxiety (every six hours as needed). Because this dosage was not helping decrease her anxiety as much as she wanted, Ms W increased her dosage and began taking from 50–100 mg a day over a period of a few weeks. This evening Ms W's estranged husband found her mumbling incoherently. Her speech was slurred, she was bumping into furniture, and she was quite drowsy.

The box on page 227 presents the major facts about barbiturates. Barbiturates are highly addictive drugs that cause people to feel euphoric yet relaxed. They are frequently prescribed to relieve pain, reduce anxiety (sedative effects), and induce sleep (hypnotic effects). In party situations, teenagers and young adults take high doses, often in combination with alcohol, to get "high." The resultant central nervous system (CNS) depression makes this practice especially dangerous. *"Speed freaks"* (amphetamine abusers) use barbiturates to "come down" from a high. Dependence, tolerance, and cross-tolerance to other depressant drugs develop rapidly.

Barbiturates are metabolized in phases by the liver. Initially they are absorbed if taken orally and are partially metabolized. However, the unmetabolized parts become active metabolites that are stored in the fatty tissues. Consequently, taking these drugs over a period of time results in a cumulative effect, unsuspected dependence, and possible overdose.

More Americans die from barbiturate overdose than from opioid addiction. Many take alcohol and barbiturates together. While judgment is impaired, they take more pills, thereby unintentionally overdosing. Because alcohol and barbiturates are synergistic, an overdose can occur quickly. Barbiturates are often used in suicide attempts.

Barbiturate withdrawal is unpleasant and life threatening. A deep sleep is followed by respiration depression, coma, and sometimes death. Babies born to mothers addicted to barbiturates are physically dependent and need to be helped through withdrawal.

Barbiturates were the first drugs used to treat anxiety and insomnia. They were considered dangerous because of their ability to cause significant CNS depression and their lethality if used to overdose. A new class of drugs, the benzodiazepines (BZDS), began to be widely used because of their ability to reduce anxiety without causing significant CNS depression. However, they also have the drawbacks of producing dependence and withdrawal syndromes in some clients (DeVane 1990).

BZDs include many widely prescribed drugs, including diazepam (Valium), clorazepate (Tranxene), lorazepam (Ativan), and alprazolam (Xanax). These drugs are thought to modify anxiety by altering the balance of neurotransmitters, especially norepinephrine and gamma-aminobutyric acid (GABA) in the limbic system. These drugs have a high risk for abuse and physical dependence (Perry et al. 1988).

Withdrawal from benzodiazepines may produce symptoms similar to those of barbiturate withdrawal. The onset of withdrawal symptoms may occur within 24–72 hours of the last dose, depending on the half-life of the drug used. Symptoms include autonomic hyperactivity (alterations in vital signs and diaphoresis) and seizures (Vance 1985).

Opioids

Steven Y, a 20-year-old male, arrived at the hospital in an ambulance. He was unconscious. His respiration was slow, and his pupils were pinpoints. "Tracks" were visible on his arms and behind his knees. A source said Steven had just "shot up" heroin.

The opioids include heroin and morphine, derived from the poppy plant, and synthetic drugs, such as meperidine (Demerol), codeine, methadone, and others. Opioids have analgesic qualities and are prescribed after surgery. Depending on the person, the drugs may produce a euphoric high, as in drug addicts, but generally cause people to feel drowsy and out of touch with the world. Most opiate users are in their twenties or younger. See the box on page 228 for more facts about opioids.

In 1898 heroin became available and initially was not believed to be addictive. Within a short time, its addictive properties became known, and the government intervened (Harrison Narcotics Act of 1914). Addiction to opiates has increased through the years. Because most opioid abusers take the drugs intravenously, they are at high risk for acquired immune deficiency syndrome (AIDS) and hepatitis. Overdose, malnutrition, and infections spread by dirty drugs and needles are dangers. Dealers often add impurities to "cut" heroin, thus increasing the quantity and their own profit. The impurities may cause poisoning and other problems.

Because opioids are physically addicting, withdrawal is a threat. People who use high doses of a drug and who "shoot up" or "mainline" (use the drug intravenously) are at high risk for severe withdrawal symptoms. Withdrawal symptoms are usually evident within twelve hours after the last dose. The person experiences the most severe withdrawal within thirty-six to forty-eight hours, with the symptoms decreasing gradually over two weeks. During this stressful time,

Key Facts about Barbiturates or Similarly Acting Sedative or Hypnotics

Examples
Lorazepam (Ativan), alprazolam (Xanax), diazepam (Valium), chlordiazepoxide (Librium), chloral hydrate, methaqualone (Quaalude), secobarbital (Seconal), phenobarbital, pentobarbital (Nembutal)

Slang Terms
Downers, ludes, sopors, 714s, yellow jackets, reds, blues, rainbows, trenks

Route of Administration
Oral (pills or capsules), intravenous

Psychologic Symptoms
Euphoria
Mood lability*
Intoxication
Loquacity (talkativeness)*
Impaired attention and memory*
Irritability*
Anxiety
Sexual aggressiveness*

Physical Symptoms
Drowsiness
Slurred speech*
Long periods of sleep
Fever
Vomiting
Postural hypotension
Lack of coordination*
Unsteady gait

Withdrawal Symptoms
Nausea and vomiting
Malaise or weakness
Autonomic hyperactivity
Tachycardia
Sweating, elevated blood pressure
Anxiety
Depression or irritability
Orthostatic hypotension
Coarse tremor of hands, tongue, eyelids
Painful muscle contractions
Seizures
Status epilepticus (major epileptic attacks succeeding each other with little or no intermission)
Hallucinations

Time Frame for Withdrawal Symptoms
Short-acting barbiturates and benzodiazepines are associated with withdrawal symptoms within the first 24 hrs after discontinuation. Longer-acting barbiturates and benzodiazepines are associated with withdrawal symptoms within 48–72 hrs of discontinuation. Seizures may occur for up to two weeks after withdrawal.

Dangers
CNS depression
Possible overdose and death, especially if mixed with alcohol

Typical Users
Middle-class, middle-aged females
Teenagers
Young adults

Symptoms of intoxication noted in DSM-III-R.

---

the person craves the drug. Babies born to addicted mothers must be treated for opioid withdrawal. The babies present with irritability, high-pitched crying, increased respirations, fever, sneezing, yawning, and tremors.

In 1964, Dole and Nyswander began to treat opiate addiction with methadone. By the late 1960s and early 1970s, when the federal government allocated money for treatment, methadone maintenance programs mushroomed all over the United States.

Methadone, a synthetic narcotic, was dispensed daily at clinics to narcotic addicts. Although addictive, methadone does not produce the "rush" (ecstatic feeling) associated with heroin. Methadone alleviates the addicts' craving for narcotics and, therefore, was expected to decrease illicit drug trafficking, theft, prostitution, and crime necessary to obtain money for drugs, thereby allowing addicts to lead productive lives. Also, methadone therapy is far less expensive ($2000 annually) than residential programs ($5000) or

Key Facts about Opioids

Examples
Heroin, morphine, hydromorphone (Dilaudid), codeine, methadone

Slang Terms
H, smack, junk, M, Miss Emma, Little D, School Boy, Horse

Route of Administration
Intravenous, oral, intramuscular, subcutaneous ("skin popping")

Psychologic Symptoms
Impaired attention/memory*
Euphoria*
Appears sedated ("nodding out")
Psychomotor retardation*
Insensitivity to pain
Agitation
Apathy*
Dysphoria*

Physical Symptoms
Pinpoint pupils
Drowsiness*
Slurred speech*
Nausea and vomiting
Hypothermia

Withdrawal Symptoms
(Presents much as influenza does)
Dilated pupils
Tearing
Runny nose
Piloerection
Sweating
Diarrhea
Fever
Yawning
Mild hypotension
Tachycardia
Insomnia
Restlessness and irritability
Muscle and joint pains
Increased respiration
Gastrointestinal symptoms
Loss of appetite

Time Frame for Withdrawal Symptoms
Withdrawal symptoms may appear within a few hours after the last dose of a short-acting opiate such as heroin. With longer acting opiates such as methadone, withdrawal symptoms may not appear for 2–3 days and may persist for 1–2 weeks.

Dangers
Death (especially if combined with barbiturates)
Pulmonary edema
Opioid poisoning (coma, shock, respiratory depression)
Malnutrition
Hepatitis/infections
AIDS

Typical Users
Teenagers
Young Adults

Symptoms of intoxication noted in DSM-III-R.

jail ($23,000). Today, methadone maintenance programs remain a major treatment for opioid addicts.

Presently, clonidine hydrochloride (Catapres), a nonopiate hypotensive drug, is being investigated for use during the acute states of opiate withdrawal. Clients who are assessed not to be at risk for complications of the drug are first stabilized on methadone (three to five days), the usual drug of choice for withdrawal. Within one to three days after the methadone is discontinued, opiate withdrawal symptoms often appear. At this time, clonidine is begun and is given in increasing doses, until withdrawal symptoms are alleviated (up to 14 days). Clonidine blocks the withdrawal symptoms, making the detoxification process less painful and more rapid than with methadone. Psychologically, the client feels less anxious and depressed. Side effects of clonidine include insomnia, dry mouth, generalized weakness, and postural hypotension (Schloemer and Skidmore 1983).

Opioid intoxication is indicated by constricted pupils, euphoria, psychomotor retardation, slurred speech, and/or drowsiness. If a client has overdoses, naloxone (Narcan) (0.4 mg– 0.8 mg IV repeated in five to fifteen minutes) is given. It is a fast-acting narcotic antagonist that counteracts respiratory depression. Abdominal cramps, rhinorrhea, and lacrimation may be treated with belladona alkaloids or with phenobarbital.

Amphetamines or Similarly Acting Sympathomimetics

Laura S, a 16-year-old high school girl, was on a diet so she could get into a favorite bathing suit. Her friend's brother, a pharmacist, gave her some Dexedrine "just until you lose the weight." Laura's mother initially noticed her rather unusual hyperactivity, her euphoria, and the fact that she refused dinner. Over a period of a few weeks Laura's behavior changed. She appeared suspicious and irritable and continued to speak and move rapidly.

The amphetamines/sympathomimetics include groups of synthetic drugs derived from ephedrine that stimulate the release of adrenaline. In small doses, they cause a person to feel energetic, euphoric, and "turned on" to life. Users take these central nervous system stimulants to feel good. A growing number of people, who do uppers and downers in a cyclic fashion, take amphetamines to counteract the effects of barbiturates. Amphetamines are dangerous because they alter judgment and obscure feelings. Taken in high doses or intravenously, amphetamines can have dangerous side effects (see the box on page 230).

In the 1950s and 1960s, amphetamines were heralded as wonder drugs for depression and lassitude. By the 1970s, their dangers became known, and physicians today prescribe them less frequently. Amphetamines are still used to control appetite and to treat depression, narcolepsy, minimal brain dysfunctions, and attention-deficit disorders in children. Abusers are usually teenagers or people in their early twenties who are looking for a good time. Truck drivers may use amphetamines to stay awake on long trips, and students may use them to study for exams. Athletes, hoping to improve their performance, may use amphetamines. Tolerance develops rapidly, and chronic abusers may suffer a toxic psychosis presenting with the symptoms of paranoid schizophrenia. Delusions, hallucinations, stereotypic compulsive behavior, increased libido, panic, and violence may occur (Kneisl and Ames 1986). However, unlike a chronic schizophrenic, a person who abuses amphetamines does not present with a thought disorder or a flat affect. Instead, these clients are agitated and extremely anxious. Clients who are chronic amphetamine abusers begin to crave the drugs and require higher and higher dosages. They are rowdy, paranoid, and irritable. A "crash" (depression), often with suicidal symptoms, may last for several weeks. Cyclical patterns of abuse and crashing may occur.

Chlorpromazine (Thorazine) may be ordered to combat the physiologic effects of amphetamines. Diazepam (Valium), given intravenously, decreases tachycardia and the chance of convulsions.

Cannabis

Joe P, a 35-year-old captain of a rescue squad, was having trouble at his job. He paid less and less attention to the accuracy of his patient reports; he was often late for work; he forgot to repair and replace his equipment, causing his unit to be unsafe and ill equipped. Joe told an emergency room nurse that he felt all the marijuana he was smoking was beginning to affect him. He revealed that he'd been a daily smoker for five years. At first, he felt there were no long-term effects, but lately he was concerned because "I never feel like doing anything."

Marijuana arrived in the United States in the early 1900s. Although it has been illegal in the United States since 1937, marijuana is used more than any other chemical except tobacco, alcohol, and caffeine (see the box on page 231). Derived from an Indian hemp plant (*Cannabis sativa),* marijuana contains the psychoactive substance delta 6-3,4-tetrahydrocannabinol (THC). THC is found in the sticky yellow resin secreted by the tops and leaves of the ripe plants (Kneisl and Ames 1986).

THC is transformed into metabolites in the body. Unlike alcohol, which is water soluble and leaves the body through urine, breath, and perspiration, THC is stored in the fatty tissues (especially the brain and reproductive system). Consequently, it can be detected in the body for up to six weeks. From 1984 to 1986, marijuana has increased in potency ten times. Although marijuana contains over 400 chemicals, the THC content determines the potency. With an increase in potency comes an increase in health problems.

Researchers have found marijuana effective in treating epilepsy, glaucoma, asthma, hypertension, and the nausea and vomiting associated with chemotherapy. Researchers presently are studying the effects of marijuana smoking by the pregnant woman on her fetus. The cannabinoids of marijuana cross the placental barrier and are distributed to fetal tissues. The risk of fetal death and abnormalities—CNS disturbances, low birth weight, decreased length, and smaller head circumference—increases when the mother uses marijuana. A suppressed prolactin level in the mother makes nursing impossible. If people with a history of

Key Facts about Amphetamines

Examples
Dexedrine, methamphetamine

Slang Terms
Bennies, dexies, uppers, black beauties, pep pills, crank, speed, diet pills

Route of Administration
Oral, intravenous

Psychologic Symptoms
  Hypervigilance*
  Irritability
  Grandiosity*
  Loquacity (talkativeness)*
  Elation
  Impaired judgment
  Psychomotor agitation*
  Aggressive, violent behavior
  Paranoia
  Hallucinations, delusions
  Disorientation
  Increased libido
  Stereotypical compulsive behavior
  Visual/auditory hallucinations

Physical Symptoms
  Tachycardia*
  Increased blood pressure*
  Dilated pupils*
  Perspiration or chills*
  Nausea or vomiting*
  Diarrhea
  Headache
  Dizziness
  Cardiac arrhythmias
  Hyperthermia
  Decreased appetite
  Delirium

Withdrawal Symptoms
  Depression
  Fatigue
  Disturbed sleep
  Dreaming
  Restlessness
  Disorientation

Dangers
  Malnutrition
  Cerebrovascular accident
  Depression
  Suicide
  Hyperpyrexia
  Convulsions

Typical Users
  Teenagers
  Young adults

————
*Symptoms of intoxication noted in DSM-III-R.

schizophrenia or mood disorders use marijuana, they may have a relapse or their symptoms may worsen.

The National Federation of Drug Free Youth has published the following facts indicating the dangers of marijuana:

• Marijuana appears to lower testosterone levels in boys.

• In girls, hormone levels remain normal, but marijuana's chemicals possibly accumulate in the ovaries.

• Marijuana smoke has 50 percent more tar than regular cigarette smoke.

• Marijuana tar contains 70 percent more benzopyrene, a major cancer-causing chemical.

• Marijuana smoke produces greater cellular changes in the lungs than does tobacco smoke.

• Smoking two "joints" (marijuana cigarettes) can reduce lung capacity more than smoking one pack of tobacco cigarettes.

• Marijuana may cause emphysema twenty times faster than tobacco.

• Marijuana smoke increases airway resistance 25 percent under laboratory conditions in which a similar

Key Facts about Cannabis

Examples
Marijuana, hashish, THC

Slang Terms
Pot, grass, bhang, hashish, ganja, joint, reefer, weed, "shit"

Route of Administration
Smoked in a pipe or cigarette, oral (e.g., mixed in food)

Psychologic Symptoms

Initial anxiety, then euphoria

Altered perceptions

Sensation of slowed time

Decreased concentration

Lack of motivation

Loss of short-term memory

Passivity

Abrupt mood changes

Paranoid ideation

Impaired judgment

Physical Symptoms

Dry mouth

Increased heart rate

Conjunctival irritation

Dilated pupils

Decreased coordination

Increased appetite, thirst

Craving for sweets

Fatigue

Impaired ovulation, impaired sperm count and motility, increase in abnormal sperm cells

Dangers

Lung damage

Psychologic dependence

Panic reaction

Impaired driving ability

Typical Users

Teenagers

Young Adults

amount of tobacco smoke produces no significant increase in airway resistance.

• Brain wave tests show that teenagers who get high twice a week or more often have evidence of diffuse brain impairment for up to two months after the last time they use the drug.

• After a person smokes marijuana, THC can be found in the blood and urine for up to two weeks; if the THC is radioactively labeled, it can be detected for up to one month.

Because marijuana smoking is so prevalent among teenagers and because its dangers are becoming increasingly known, some health professionals advocate a urine screen when teenagers have a checkup by a family doctor. In 1985, the American Academy of Pediatrics was challenged to confront the problem of substance abuse among teenagers. A key point was that chemical dependency takes ten to fifteen years to develop in adults and only a few years to develop in a child. Only 25 percent of kids in drug rehabilitation succeed, compared with 75 percent of adults who succeed. Because substance abuse is a "neglected disease," pediatricians should initiate educational and treatment programs on drug and alcohol abuse (Cherskov 1985). Likewise, psychiatric nurses need to respond to this vital public health issue.

Marijuana use is endemic in the teenage culture. Therefore nurses who work with teenagers must be knowledgeable about marijuana and its effects. When admitting a teenager to a psychiatric unit or interviewing a teenager as an outpatient, be aware of a variety of indicators of marijuana use. Parents should know these facts about marijuana and indications of its use:

• Marijuana smells like hemp or burning rope.

• Teenagers often burn incense or use perfumed sprays to mask its pungent odor.

• Teenagers may use eye drops (e.g., Murine) so that their eyes will not be red, and they may cough a lot.

• A teenager who uses marijuana may have smoking paraphernalia, e.g., plastic baggies filled with dried leaves, rolling paper, and "roach" clips—a clip that holds the marijuana cigarette once it becomes too small to handle.

Cocaine

Will R, a 32-year-old male, was brought to the hospital by his father. Talkative and jumpy, his eyes darted around the examining room, and he repeatedly wiped his nose with his finger and rubbed the bottom of his face. He acted suspicious and kept saying someone was after him. His family stated he had a $400 a day cocaine habit.

Each year, twenty tons of cocaine enter the United States. After the cocaine is adulterated with sugar, quinine, amphetamine, ephedrine, or procaine, 80 to 160 tons are available on the streets (Cocaine: Some Questions and Answers 1983). Since cocaine abuse has been recognized as a widespread problem, government agencies have spent much money trying to block cocaine shipments from South America. Planes, boats, and "mules" (people who transport cocaine) have been seized, and tons of cocaine have been confiscated and destroyed. Yet it still is plentiful and is purer today than ever before. The cocaine industry is a multibillion dollar enterprise involving bribery, corruption, and murder (Cocaine: Some Questions and Answers 1983).

Cocaine is a stimulant derived from the coca plant found in Bolivia and Peru. It has long been known and used. For hundreds of years, South American Indians have chewed coca leaves, enjoying the effects of decreased appetite and increased ability to work at high altitudes. Slaves became more productive when given cocaine. Freud experimented with cocaine. It was an ingredient in Coca Cola before federal regulations prohibited it in 1903. Today, cocaine is used as a local anesthetic in ear, nose, and throat surgery.

Cocaine is no longer just the chic, expensive drug of choice (the champagne of drugs) of young upwardly mobile professionals and stars. Cocaine is now available to all cultural and socioeconomic groups; today, 50 percent of users are women. For some years cocaine was believed to produce euphoria without addictive potential and without negative side-effects. Lately the horrors of cocaine abuse have been described in both lay and professional literature. (See the box on page 233.)

It has not been proved that cocaine is physically addictive, but its ability to cause psychologic dependency is clear. Cocaine users crave the drug. After a brief postuse euphoria (lasting approximately five to ten minutes), they experience a strong desire to repeat the high. This high is followed by a "crashing," a terrible letdown called the "postcoke blues," or cocaine abstinence syndrome. Anxiety, depression, and fatigue are part of this syndrome (Rottenberg 1980). The cocaine crash, lasting for approximately 30–60 minutes, results from depletion of dopamine, a neurotransmitter responsible for feelings of pleasure and well-being. The addict responds to the crash by feeling irritable, depressed, and tired. Although the brain needs to synthesize more dopamine, due to chemical misprogramming from the addiction, it craves more cocaine which offers immediate relief. The crash intensity appears related to the amount of cocaine used. Addicts often use other drugs, such as alcohol, marijuana, or sleeping pills, during the crash (Washton 1989).

One addict described these postcoke blues as "pure hell, the most painful depression I have ever felt. I wanted to die from the pain." This painful depression, along with the memory of the cocaine high, causes people to want to use cocaine again and again to recapture the momentary ecstasy. The period of agitation, anxiety, and insomnia usually ceases within two weeks.

Cocaine addicts develop a tolerance to the drug and use amounts that would have been lethal to them earlier. The euphoria diminishes. The development of new dendrites (branches to the nerve cells) to aid in the uptake of the increased amount of dopamine accounts for the tolerance. Ultimately, the cocaine no longer produces pleasure, but not taking it feels even worse. Dopamine eventually becomes depleted and the user becomes chronically fatigued, irritable, and anxious, even mentally confused, paranoid. Suicide attempts, accidents, and overdoses are common (Washton 1989). Nurses need to assess clients carefully to differentiate cocaine use from manic-depression and chronic anxiety. Figure 11–1 on page 234 illustrates the cocaine use cycle.

Detoxification for cocaine abusers is still in the experimental phase and may depend on the client's symptoms. Some hospitals use nothing; others administer diazepam (Valium) intravenously 1–20 mg at a slow rate (not more than 5 mg/minute). In some hospitals, cocaine abusers are treated with a Valium protocol that lasts approximately four days; Valium is decreased from 10 mg q 4 hours p.o./I.M. to 5 mg q 8 hours p.o./I.M. with additional doses as needed if the client has withdrawal symptoms. Other hospitals have p.r.n. Valium orders only. Another protocol involves the use of phenobarbital in decreasing doses and imipramine hydrochloride (Tofranil). Since the depression is so great, Tofranil or other tricyclic antidepressants may be given for several weeks after detoxification. Tricyclics build up existing levels of neurotransmitters and make them available for transmission. Beta-adrenergic blockers such as propranolol (Inderal) may be used to counteract the tachycardia and hypertension that accompany acute cocaine intoxication (Rappolt 1977), but their use may result in paroxysmal hypertension due to unopposed alpha-adrenergic stimulation. Therefore, they should be used cautiously and with constant blood pressure monitoring (Ramoska and Sacchetti 1985).

Use of tricyclic antidepressants to increase the number of neurotransmitters in the synapse is called *synaptic treatment*. Postsynaptic treatment for cocaine withdrawal and dependence includes the use of drugs such as bromocriptine (Parlodel) or amantadine (Amantidine), which increase dopaminergic activity in the synapse and enhance the effects of dopamine on the postsynaptic receptors. Presynaptic treatment with amino acids such as tryptophan was used until 1989, when tryptophan was removed from the market

Key Facts about Cocaine

Slang Terms
Coke, lady, blow, snow, rabbits, C, powder

Route of Administration
Intranasal (flakes or powder sniffed), subcutaneous or intravenous, smoked in a pipe (freebasing)

Psychologic Symptoms
Psychomotor agitation*

Anxiety

Elation

Talkativeness*

Grandiosity*

Hypervigilance*

Impaired judgment

Ideas of reference/paranoia

Hallucinations

Formication (sensation of insects crawling on the skin)

Euphoria followed by depression and let-down feeling

Violence

Insomnia

Anorexia

Physical Symptoms
Dilated pupils*

Tachycardia*

Elevated blood pressure*

Perspiration or chills*

Nausea or vomiting*

Anorexia

Dry mouth (characteristic bad breath)

Weight loss

Stuffy/runny nose

Burns and sores of nasal membranes

Tremors

Muscle cramping

Seizures

Withdrawal Symptoms
Severe craving

Fatigue

Psychomotor agitation

Hypersomnia

Irritability

Time Frame for Withdrawal Symptoms
Symptoms may appear within 24 hrs after use; peak in 2–4 days. Depression may persist for months.

Dangers
Syncope

Fever

Chest Pain

Depression

Death from convulsions

Cardiac/respiratory arrest

Typical Users
Teenagers

College students

Young urban professionals (yuppies)

Rock and movie stars

Executives

_____

Symptoms of intoxication noted in DSM-III-R.

because of several deaths associated with its use. These amino acids were prescribed because the body converted them into neurotransmitters, which had been depleted by cocaine abuse.

Interestingly, low-level cocaine intoxication presents with symptoms similar to alcohol withdrawal—sweating, dilated pupils, psychomotor agitation, and increased blood pressure/heart rate. With higher doses of cocaine, a person becomes increasingly intoxicated. Symptoms include high fevers, cardiac arrhythmia, seizures, hallucinations, and a paranoid schizophrenic syndrome. Hallucinations typically involve "cocaine bugs," which feel like bugs under the skin. The client may scratch furiously in an attempt to get rid of them. Haloperidol (Haldol) is used to combat the psychotic symptoms; phenothiazines should not be used because they may decrease the seizure threshold.

The strength of the physiologic effects of cocaine are revealed by animal research. Monkeys work harder by pressing a bar to receive cocaine intravenously than to get any other drug. Even when starving to death or when confronted with a sexually receptive female,

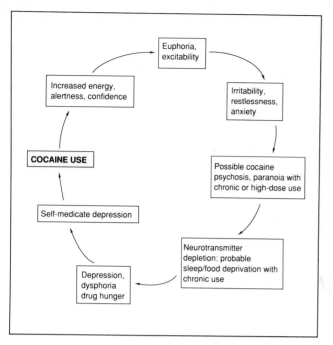

FIGURE 11–1 Cocaine use cycle. *(SOURCE: Landry, M, Smith, DE: Crack: Anatomy of addiction. Calif Nurs 1987; March/April:13.)*

monkeys continue pressing the bar. Receiving an electric shock every time they touch the bar does not alter their behavior. Research with cocaine users indicates that the drug bromocriptine mesylate (Parlodel), a dopamine (DA) receptor agonist, eliminates the craving users feel after they stop using cocaine.

Cocaine initially increases DA neurotransmission. Over time, however, cocaine abuse depletes DA in the brain, and this depletion may be the basis for craving. In a preliminary study, bromocriptine proved successful in decreasing cocaine craving. The researchers suggest doing more studies that are placebo controlled and double-blind. They also suggest that doses of bromocriptine be varied for acute and long-term cocaine abstinence and craving (Bromocriptine as Treatment of Cocaine Abuse 1985, pp 1151–1152).

Crack

"Crack" or "rock" cocaine, recently labeled "the most addictive drug known to man," is "a potent form of hydrochloride cocaine that is mixed with baking soda and water, heated, allowed to harden, and then broken or 'cracked' into little pieces and smoked in cigarettes or glass water pipes" (Gianelli 1986, p 2). Crack is more insidious, addictive, and toxic than cocaine. One user said, "I am worse in three weeks of using crack than in six years of using cocaine."

Crack is cheap and easily bought on the street or in special crack houses where people congregate to smoke. A crack high has a rapid onset and is intensely euphoric, followed by a dramatic crash. Within seconds after "coming down," users feel compelled to smoke more crack. Because addiction is so rapid, many people are "hooked" and seek help when they can no longer support their habit. In New York City in 1985, 55 percent of the cocaine arrests were due to crack. Crack users are flooding treatment centers, many of which have long waiting lists. Recidivism is estimated by some experts at 90 percent.

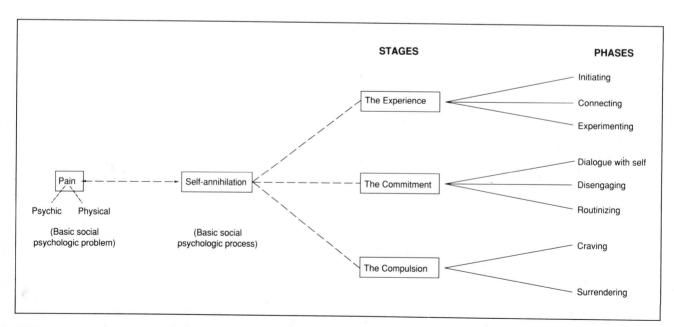

FIGURE 11–2 Chemically dependent nurses: the trajectory toward self-annihilation. *(SOURCE: Hutchinson S: Chemically dependent nurses: The trajectory towards self-annihilation. Nurs Res 1986;34(4):196–201. Copyright © 1986, The American Journal of Nursing Company.)*

Key Facts about Crack (Hydrochloride Cocaine)

Slang Terms

Rock, crack

Route of Administration

Smoked

Psychologic Symptoms

Paranoia

Depression

Insomnia

Irritability

Deterioration of mental function

"Schizophrenic-like" psychosis

Appetite suppression

Physical Symptoms

Wheezing, shortness of breath

Black phlegm

Coughing blood

Parched throat and lips

Singed eyebrows and lashes

Increased heart rate and blood pressure

Weight loss

Withdrawal Symptoms

Severe craving

Depression

Fatigue

Hypersomnia

Irritability

Time Frame for Withdrawal Symptoms

Severe craving within minutes–hours. Depression appears within 3–7 days, may persist for weeks.

Dangers

Seizures

Cardiac arrhythmias

Respiratory paralysis

Paranoid psychoses

Pulmonary dysfunction

Typical Users

Teenagers

Young adults

All socioeconomic and cultural groups

Symptoms of crack use (see the box above) include irritability, paranoia, depression, and physical symptoms that go along with the smoking of a toxic chemical, e.g., wheezing and coughing blood and black phlegm. Cardiac arrhythmias caused by crack use may lead to death. There is an increase in the number of babies being born to mothers who use crack. These babies are more likely to be premature or have low birth weights. They present with irritability, tremors, and muscle rigidity. A related issue is the increasing number of children who are neglected or abused by crack-using parents. Drug needs seem to prevail over child care in many cases (Gianelli 1986, p 18).

Phencyclidine (PCP)

Pete O, an 18-year-old college student, was offered marijuana at a fraternity party. After smoking several joints he was driving home with a friend when he became severely agitated. He insisted his friend stop the car near a pay phone; he jumped out and attempted to call the police, believing someone was trying to kill him. When the police arrived because of the disturbance he was causing (by then he was shouting and hallucinating), he rushed them, kicking at passersby and shooting at them as if he had a gun. During an assessment interview, the friend confessed to putting PCP in the marijuana.

PCP was originally used as an anesthetic for humans and as a tranquilizer for animals. Because of its dangerous side effects (see the box on page 236), it was removed from the market, except for veterinary use. However, by the mid-1960s, PCP was readily available as a street drug. PCP is inexpensive and easily synthesized by home chemists, making a supply always available.

People who use PCP frequently arrive at the emergency room in a psychotic, violent, and agitated state. Some fluctuate between coma and violence. Hallucinations are common. A differential diagnosis is important but difficult because the symptoms are similar to those of schizophrenia. It is believed that

Key Facts about Phencyclidine (PCP)

Slang Terms

PCP, angel dust, crystal, superjoint, hog, elephant tranquilizer, THC, rocket fuel, peace pill

Route of Administration

Oral, intravenous, smoked, inhaled

Psychologic Symptoms

Euphoria*
Psychomotor agitation*
Anxiety*
Grandiosity*
Disorientation swings
Emotional lability*
Sensation of slowed time*
Synesthesias (e.g., seeing colors when a loud sound occurs)*
Facial grimacing
Muscle rigidity
Hallucinations
Paranoid ideation
Violent or bizarre behavior
Hostility, apathy
Depersonalization, isolation

Physical Symptoms

Vertical and horizontal nystagmus*
Increased blood pressure/heart rate*
Insensitivity to pain*
Dysarthria*
Ataxia*
Perspiration
Salivation
Vomiting

Dangers

Violence
Hypertension
Respiratory depression/arrest
Stupor
Coma
Convulsions
Death
Suicide

Typical Users

Adolescents
Young Adults

———
Symptoms of intoxication noted in DSM-III-R.

---

schizophrenics are particularly sensitive to PCP and that PCP may aggravate schizophrenic symptoms.

A PCP high appears about five minutes after a person takes the drug and lasts four to six hours. Effects may last up to forty-eight hours. PCP may be recovered from the blood and urine for seven to ten days. While using PCP, a person experiences a wide variety of feelings ranging from euphoria and utter peace to violence, confusion, and disorganization. Distorted sensory perceptions are common. In a bad "trip," anxiety, fear, and paranoia predominate. The dramatic physical and emotional effects of PCP may last for several weeks. Users may suffer from depression, fatigue, memory loss, difficulty in concentration, and poor impulse control.

Treatment of acute PCP intoxication may include the use of diazepam for muscle spasms, seizures, and agitation. Haloperidol may be used for severe psy-

chotic behavior, but phenothiazines should not be used since PCP is anticholinergic. Calcium channel blockers such as verapamil may be given. These drugs are thought to prevent or reverse PCP-induced vasospasm, thereby decreasing the hallucinogenic effects of PCP (Price 1986). This treatment is controversial, however, because some clinicians feel that the use of verapamil may potentiate the effects of PCP (McCann 1986). Nursing care during this period centers around protecting the client from injury and reorienting the person to reality. Providing a quiet, safe environment and addressing the person in a calm, reassuring manner are important.

A vital problem with PCP is the question of its purity and its concentration. Because it is generally manufactured illegally, users never really know what they are buying. Adulterants are often toxic to humans, causing a wide variety of responses, including death. Originally called the "peace pill," PCP is now recognized for its potential to cause violence, especially when the drug is taken in high dosages.

Hallucinogens

Two seniors in high school decided to take LSD. After eight hours, one student was enjoying music, describing the varied colors he saw as the music changed in tempo. The other student was sweating profusely. His pupils were dilated, and he was trembling. He saw brightly colored dogs with huge teeth and claws changing into cats, snakes, and lions. He said he felt his gallbladder working with his liver and stomach. He eventually became so out of control that the other student took him to the emergency room.

Hallucinogens are synthetic and natural drugs that cause hallucinations and unusual sensory experiences. Developed in 1938 for scientific research, LSD became popular in the 1960s when Timothy Leary, a Harvard psychologist, described how it stimulated great insight and increased awareness. In the 1960s and 1970s, the United States Army secretly experimented with LSD by giving it to unsuspecting army employees. One dramatic and much publicized event concerned the army officer who leapt to his death from a window after unknowingly ingesting LSD. At this time the danger of LSD became publicized, as did the unethical research. Physician researchers also were interested in experimenting with the uses of LSD in the treatment of a variety of diseases; however, in 1966, LSD became illegal and could no longer be used in human research. Peyote, however, is still an integral part of religious rituals of Indians in the Southwest and Mexico.

After a lull in use, LSD ("acid") is again being used by teenagers because it is cheap ($2.00–$5.00 a "hit") and causes an intense high that lasts six to twelve hours. Teenagers today are unacquainted with the horror stories of the 1960s. Today, people use LSD predominantly to get high rather than to expand consciousness. See the accompanying box for additional information.

The dangers of hallucinogens include "bad trips" and flashbacks. Users who experience bad trips may appear psychotic and extremely fearful. Reassuring the person and pointing out reality are helpful; occasionally, tranquilizers or antipsychotics are given. The symptoms usually disappear within twelve hours but may persist for months. People who are mentally ill or emotionally conflicted are more likely to have bad trips and flashbacks and to require hospitalization than ordinary users are.

Flashbacks are a spontaneous reliving of the experiences the person felt while under the influence of

Key Facts about Hallucinogens

Examples
LSD, psilocybin, DMT, psilocin, mescaline, peyote, MDA

Slang Terms
Acid

Route of Administration
Oral

Psychologic Symptoms

Intensification of perceptions

Depersonalization

Derealization

Illusions, pseudohallucinations

Synesthesias (e.g., seeing sound or hearing colors)

Anxiety

Depression

Intense emotions

Body image changes

Ideas of reference

Paranoid ideation

Impaired judgment

Mood swings

Physical Symptoms

Dilated pupils

Tachycardia

Sweating

Palpitations

Blurred vision

Tremors

Lack of coordination

Dangers

Unpredictable behavior, resulting in harm to self or others

"Flashback" hallucinations

Typical Users

Adolescents

Young adults

the drug, although the person is drug free. The experience may involve perceptual distortions, a variety of physical feelings, and strong emotions, e.g., fear or pleasure. Flashbacks are generally brief, and they occur less frequently over time. Flashbacks may be induced by stress, fatigue, and drug or alcohol ingestion.

Some authorities believe hallucinogens pose a particular danger to adolescents in that they may precipitate a psychosis. Because teenagers' egos and defenses are weak, they may be especially susceptible to the effects of hallucinogens.

Psychologic and physical dependence are unlikely because each experience with a hallucinogen is different. At the present time, researchers have demonstrated no relationship between hallucinogens and birth defects. Likewise, increased creativity and brilliant personality revelations, presumed effects of the drugs, are short-lived at best.

Polydrug Use

Most substance abusers today are polydrug users. This fact complicates diagnosis and treatment and increases the hazards associated with abuse. *Synergistic* or potentiating effects are possible. In other words, the effects of two or more drugs taken together are greater than the singular effects of each drug. The whole is greater than the sum of its parts, e.g., alcohol and barbiturates taken together. *Additive effects* occur when two drugs that have similar effects are used together. *Paradoxical effects* occur if a drug causes a reaction opposite to that expected. Paradoxical effects may occur when only one drug is taken or when several drugs are taken. A *pathologic reaction,* too, may result from ingestion of only one or several drugs: It is an unexpected and dramatic response to the drug. For example, the combination of alcohol and marijuana is especially dangerous because THC suppresses the nausea that results from an overdose of alcohol. Consequently, the person may continue to drink, risking respiratory depression, coma, and even death. Cocaine and alcohol are frequently used together; the cocaine gives the user a brief high, and the alcohol masks the ensuring depression. When the cocaine wears off, the person is intoxicated and unable to drive safely. Prescription drugs and alcohol are also a common combination.

Designer Drugs

Designer drugs, a new threat on the drug scene, are chemical derivatives of controlled drugs. They are called analog drugs because they retain properties of controlled drugs, but one molecule is changed, making them initially not classifiable as controlled. According to the Controlled Substance Act of 1970, controlled substances (i.e., federally regulated substances) are classified from I (most regulated) through V, according to the potential for abuse and the current accepted medical use. As new information is made available, drugs may be reclassified.

Produced by underground chemists, analog drugs are initially legal until analyzed and researched by chemists. Once a dangerous pattern of use is determined (often three to six months after police discover the drug), the drug may be classified as a controlled substance. Fentanyl citrate (Sublimaze), a synthetic anesthetic used as an anesthetic agent, is similar chemically to some designer drugs. Fentanyl is 100 times as strong as morphine and 20 to 40 times as strong as heroin. It provides a fast rush and an extraordinary high. A person can become addicted after one shot of fentanyl (Gallagher 1986, p 7). Ecstasy (MDMA, Adam) was a designer drug; it has recently been classified as a Schedule I narcotic because research demonstrates that it causes structural damage to the brain. MTPT (China white), an analog of meperidine (Demerol), has an adverse reaction similar to the rigidity caused by Parkinson's disease.

Groups at Risk for Substance Abuse

Teenagers

Drug abuse among teenagers is pervasive in our society. Although many adolescents experiment with drugs for only a brief time, many more who do so become addicted. Susceptibility to addiction seems to depend on several variables: the form and potency of the drug, the dosage, the frequency, and the pattern of use, stress, the personality and genetic makeup of the user, and the family culture. Straight, Inc., views drug abuse as a primary disease: an incurable chronic disease that is progressive and terminal. Newton (1981) describes drug use as a disease of feelings. Newton believes that psychoactive drugs affect the "old brain," the limbic system and center of feeling, and not "the new brain" (neocortex), the center of conceptualization (p 33). Consequently, a teenager's moods are affected not only at the moment of use but also over time. People use drugs that initially produce good feelings to escape from the stress and strain of life. A teenager who relies on a quick "fix" (a drug) to ease mental pain does not learn healthy coping processes. If teenagers do not learn healthy coping mechanisms or work through the pains and mood swings associated with living, they never complete a necessary developmental stage. As a consequence, they remain fixated at a dependent level of development.

They enter a dangerous cycle that is unlikely to be interrupted without professional intervention. Drug use, regardless of what drug is used, inevitably affects all areas of a teenager's life: school, work, social and family relationships, and sense of self-worth (see the accompanying Assessment box).

Adolescent drug users manifest more psychopathologic conditions that nonusers do. Symptoms include feelings of depression, inadequacy, frustration, helplessness, and self-alienation. These teenagers also have ego structure deficiencies and poor impulse control (Pallikkathayil and Tweed 1983, p 314). Note the behavioral changes in the Assessment box. The earlier a child begins using a dependency-producing drug, the more likely the child is to use other dependency-producing drugs. Alcohol and marijuana are "gateway" drugs; their use often leads to the use of narcotics, cocaine, or more dangerous drugs. There is a progression of drug use: alcohol, marijuana, tranquilizers, analgesics, hypnotics, cocaine, heroin, PCP (least commonly used). Teenagers who use alcohol and drugs are likely to continue to use them in adulthood.

Psychiatric Clients

Nurses need to be alert to possible substance abuse by psychiatric clients in a hospital setting. Problems may occur if clients take a combination of substances, and treatment is hindered if clients are under the influence of drugs or alcohol. Close observation of teenagers and their visitors is useful, and the nurse often needs to ask clients directly if they are taking drugs. In most psychiatric hospitals urine is routinely tested for the presence of drugs, if there are any indications of use. Drug screening is usually done on admission and when the client returns from a pass.

Women

Although alcoholism is a greater stigma for women than men, more women are drinking today. Many of these women are also using other drugs. Women respond to alcohol somewhat differently than men do. Finley (1982, pp 15–16) reviewed the available literature on alcoholism and women and found the following:

• Most women with drinking problems are from 35–49 years of age.

• Depression often precedes alcoholism in women.

• Women are at greater risk of developing liver disease with a shorter duration of drinking at a lower level and at a younger age than men are.

• Women with acute liver disorders have a higher mortality than men with such disorders.

• Estrogen appears to affect alcohol intoxication and metabolism, e.g., a woman taking oral contraceptives of synthetic estrogens gets more intoxicated and remains intoxicated longer than a man who drinks the same amount.

• Women tend to drink in secret and drink continuously rather than binge.

• Women drink before stressful events and report increased drinking before their menstrual periods.

• Women describe personality changes from drinking.

Other researchers reach these conclusions:

• Premenstrual tension is related to alcohol abuse (Belfer et al. 1971).

ASSESSMENT

Behavioral Changes Associated with Teenage Drug Abuse

• Unexplained periods or reactions of moodiness, depression, anxiety, irritability, oversensitivity, or hostility

• Strongly inappropriate overreaction to mild criticism or simple requests

• Lessening in accustomed family warmth— avoids interaction and communication with parents, withdraws from family activities

• Preoccupation with self, less concern for the feelings of others

• Loss of interest in previously important hobbies, sports, activities

• Loss of motivation and enthusiasm (amotivational syndrome)

• Lethargy, lack of energy and vitality

• Loss of ability for self-discipline and assuming responsibility

• Need for instant gratification

• Change in values, ideals, beliefs

• Changes in friends, unwillingness to introduce friends

• Secretive phone calls—callers refuse to identify themselves or hang up when you answer

• Unexplained absences from home

• Disappearance of money or items of value from home; handling of money becomes secretive

• Desire for increased sensory stimuli

• When given the same dose of ethanol (adjusted for body weight), women have higher peak blood alcohol levels than men do (Jones and Jones 1976).

• Women have higher blood alcohol levels premenstrually than at other times in their menstrual cycle (Jones, Jones, and Paredes 1976).

• High alcohol intake can cause infertility, amenorrhea, and failure to ovulate (Pratt 1981).

• Women describe using alcohol and drugs in response to obstetric/gynecologic problems (Busch et al. 1986).

After reviewing existing research on women and alcohol, Blume (1986) suggests that treatment programs should be geared to women's needs. Such programs might include women-only groups, female therapists, meetings with recovered women alcoholics, and help for the clients' families.

General Hospital Clients

Nurses who work in the general hospital need to be alert to the possibility that clients presenting with other illnesses may be substance abusers and may be in danger of withdrawal. Chychula (1984, p 18) suggests that nurses be suspicious if physical assessment reveals any of these:

• Debilitation out of proportion to the presenting health problem

• Physical findings that do not correlate to the chief complaint

• Unsteady gait, slurring of speech, dilated pupils, night sweats, chills, blackouts, tremors, skin tracks, abscesses, nasal septum perforation, jaundice

• Weight loss, poor hygiene, and poor nutrition

The nurse may want to alert the physician and suggest appropriate laboratory studies (e.g., liver function tests). A nursing assessment may include questions about a client's drinking habits. If alcoholism is suspected, a confrontive but nonjudgmental stance facilitates the client's acceptance of treatment for possible withdrawal symptoms.

The Elderly

Elderly clients who often are being treated for several chronic illnesses by different physicians are at risk for drug problems from drug interactions and/or for drug dependence. For this reason, nurses need to obtain a good history from the client, including a list of all the drugs taken, frequency of use, dosage, and duration of use. It is often useful to ask the family of an elderly client to bring all drugs to the hospital for review rather than relying on memory. Frequently the confu-

sion seen in elderly clients is a direct consequence of drug interaction or malabsorption.

In addition, substance abuse (especially alcoholism) is less likely to be detected and treated in the elderly than in younger clients. It often goes unrecognized because the signs of substance abuse are difficult to distinguish from the changes associated with normal aging or degenerative brain disease (Abrams and Alexopoulous 1987). After reviewing the literature on drug abuse and the elderly, Caroselli-Karinja (1985, pp 25–27) presents the following critical facts:

• People 65 years old represent 11 percent of the United States population, yet they take 25 percent of all prescribed drugs.

• Older people often see a variety of physicians who prescribe medication without assessing the other drugs the client is taking.

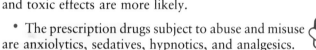

• The physiologic and psychologic changes of aging may affect the way medication is metabolized. Adverse and toxic effects are more likely.

• The prescription drugs subject to abuse and misuse are anxiolytics, sedatives, hypnotics, and analgesics.

• Problems of the elderly—retirement, loss of independence, illness, loss of family/friends, decreased income—are likely to cause depression, anxiety, and loneliness. Such feeling states may cause clients to take over-the-counter drugs and physicians to prescribe drugs.

• The elderly often hoard unused drugs and share them with friends.

Adult Children of Alcoholics

Adult children of alcoholics are at great risk of becoming alcoholics. If both parents are alcoholics, a child has a 70 percent chance of becoming an alcoholic; if one parent is an alcoholic, a child has a 40 percent chance. This type of alcoholism has been labeled *familial*. Research on familial alcoholism has shown that (a) a family history of alcoholism is present, (b) alcoholism develops early, usually by the time the person is in his or her late twenties, (c) the alcoholism is generally severe and usually requires treatment, (d) the risk of alcoholism is increased but not the risk of other psychiatric disorders (Kaplan and Sadock 1989).

Nurses

The issue of chemically dependent nurses has received attention in professional journals and lay literature. Note the following facts:

• Chemical dependency is the number one health problem affecting nurses.

NURSING SELF-AWARENESS

Warning Signs of Chemically Dependent Nurses

- Frequent absenteeism before and after days off; always working (for supply)
- Irritability
- Abrupt mood changes; inappropriate affect
- Sloppy charting and client care
- Problems with drugs (missing drugs, frequent "wasting" of drugs, inaccurate records)
- Frequent errors of judgment

- Alcohol (stale or fresh) on breath
- Frequent disappearance from the unit
- Offering to give medication to other nurses' clients
- Frequent night shift work
- The nurse's clients complain of little or no pain relief

- In 1984, 5 percent of 2.4 million nurses were chemical abusers; 8%–10% were chemically dependent (ANA 1984).

- The incidence of narcotic addiction is estimated to be thirty times greater among nurses than the general population (Caroselli-Karinja and Zboray, 1987)

- Sixty-seven percent of disciplinary cases brought by U.S. boards of nursing are drug related (Creighton 1988)

- The majority of state nursing associations have passed resolutions about the problem.

Many factors place nurses at risk for developing chemical dependency. A primary risk factor is codependency. Many codependents, whether adult children of substance abusers or products of other dysfunctional family systems, choose careers in the helping professions, such as nursing (Beattie 1987). Codependent nurses often give more of themselves than is necessary for effective client care, seek perfection, and tend to ignore or repress problems and difficulties. Codependent nurses are superb caretakers of everyone but themselves (Hall and Wray 1989). Nurses also work under a great deal of stress and have easy access to drugs. Every day, they give people medication to decrease pain. It is an easy leap to begin to self-medicate (Figure 11–2). However, such behavior is a violation of the state nurse practice act and, depending on the drug and method of obtaining it, may be a criminal offense. Colleagues of chemically dependent nurses need to be alert to behavior that is suspicious (see the accompanying Nursing Self-Awareness box) and to document and report such behavior to the head nurse or supervisor. It is very common to cover up such behavior. Shielding such a nurse puts the clients, the nurse, and the nursing profession at risk and violates the nurse practice act, the nurse code of ethics, and the law in many states. Nurses need to understand that their chemically dependent colleagues suffer from

a disease, not a moral problem. This understanding enables nurses to work together to help each other.

Only recently has nursing administration begun to confront the problem by writing policies and developing programs for the chemically dependent professional. Nurse self-help groups are springing up all over, and some hospitals are working closely with recovering nurses on intervention strategies and requirements for treatment. State boards of nursing are usually involved and in some cases hire a person to work with chemically dependent nurses all over the state. Peer assistance programs are available in some states; Florida's Nurse Intervention Program is an example.

Depending on the circumstances, a chemically dependent nurse may need to be terminated or transferred. Voluntary surrender of the nursing license may be suggested. Each nurse is entitled to confidential medical treatment, freedom from stigma, and the opportunity to return to work upon recovering (Naegle 1985, p 24). Intervention with nurse substance abusers follows the pattern presented in the section, "Using Confrontation Strategies," later in this chapter. While in the process of recovery, chemically dependent nurses need regular drug screenings. Their work performance should be monitored, along with their attendance at a treatment program or group for a period of up to two years. With early intervention and continued support and treatment, chemically dependent nurses have a good prognosis.

Research in the area of chemically dependent nurses is just beginning. Hutchinson's (1986) study describes the process by which nurses become chemically dependent. Researchers need to continue studying substance abusers and specific groups at risk. Questions for research can address successful and unsuccessful intervention strategies, successful and unsuccessful treatment programs, the self-help group process, the relationships of environmental and personal factors to chemical dependency, and successful coping strategies of people who, although extremely stressed, do not use chemicals.

NURSING SELF-AWARENESS

Guide to Analyzing Personal Responses toward Substance Abusers

Analyze your responses to the following questions:

- What thoughts and feelings does the term *alcoholic* evoke in me?
- What thoughts and feelings does the term *addict* evoke in me?
- Do I believe that substance dependence occurs out of moral weakness?
- Do I believe that substance dependence is an illness that can be treated?
- Are people who abuse substances deliberately destroying their own lives and the lives of significant others?
- Who in my personal life has abused drugs, alcohol, or other chemicals?
- How does my experience with relatives,

friends, colleagues, or clients who have abused substances affect my attitude toward caring for a substance-abusing client?

- Is substance abuse a social problem, an emotional-psychologic problem, or a physical abnormality?
- How do I view the family, spouse, or friends of the substance abuser? Do they encourage the abuse, or otherwise "enable" the person to continue their abuse? Or are they victims?
- How does my own personal use of nicotine, caffeine, drugs, or alcohol affect my attitude toward clients?

SOURCE: *Bittle S, Feignbaum JS, Kneisl CR: Substance abuse, in Adult Health Nursing: A Biopsychosocial Approach. Addison-Wesley, 1986, p 254.*

A Humanist-Interactionist Perspective

Substance abuse needs to be viewed as a disease and not as a moral problem. A moralistic attitude always alienates the client. Recognizing and accepting that the disease is chronic, often with remissions and exacerbations, should keep the nurse from succumbing to the frustration felt by many who treat substance abusers. Even in cases of regression, there is hope if the client learns something and alters behavior in some positive way. At certain stressful times in life, anyone may develop a dependency on drugs or alcohol; however, certain people seem to be predisposed to the illness. Nurses' expertise in the stages of the nursing process is vital to the care of the client with substance abuse problems. Chychula (1984) suggests that nurses focus on helping the client work toward self-awareness, good health, and good interpersonal relationships. With improvements in these areas and the development of alternative life-styles, these people can lead productive, fulfilling, happy lives.

The Nursing Process and Clients Who Are Substance Abusers

As substance abuse becomes an increasing problem in society, more clients will be admitted to hospitals and clinics for help with intoxication and withdrawal.

Drugs change rapidly, and nurses must keep up with "the drug scene" to assess and treat clients. Along with the knowledge acquired from reading, continuing education programs, and seminars, nurses need self-knowledge to be good therapists with substance abusers. Ongoing critical self-analysis of feelings, attitudes, and behavior toward clients is useful. See the accompanying Nursing Self-Awareness box for a list of useful questions to guide this self-analysis.

Assessing

Physical Findings   Nurses should be alert to the possibility of substance abuse in a client who presents with an assortment of bruises, burns, or other minor injuries. The presence of needle marks may indicate IV drug use, and destruction of the nasal septum may signal intranasal cocaine use.

Substance Abuse Assessment Questions   Part of the assessment process includes a systematic inquiry regarding the client's drug use patterns. It is important to obtain information about which drugs the client uses, in what amounts, and with what frequency. It is also important to know when the client last used drugs or alcohol and what prior experiences with withdrawal have been like (e.g., has the client ever had DTs?). Note any history of drug or alcohol use and deterioration in social or professional functioning. In a rushed situation, as in an emergency room, a nurse need ask only a few key questions:

• What did you take?

• How much did you take?

• When did you take it?

• What have you taken in the last twenty-four hours? the last week?

Of course, in an emergency situation, the client may be unable to given coherent answers and a friend may not have accurate information. In these cases, the presenting symptoms are treated, and the assessment is done when the client is alert and oriented. The kind and number of questions asked in a nursing assessment depend on the setting and the client's behavior. When assessing drug or alcohol use, remember that chemically dependent individuals tend to minimize their use of drugs or alcohol. It is better to ask, "How much do you drink?" or "What drugs do you use?" than "Do you drink or use drugs?" Some drug users, however, overstate their drug use to receive higher doses in a detoxification regimen.

Motivation for Treatment

Nurses need to consider some important psychosocial issues when clients come for treatment. Clients may enter a treatment program voluntarily. This situation is best, because they are internally motivated and therefore have a better chance of success. Clients, however, may be coerced by family, friends, physicians, or the police to undergo treatment. Coerced treatment inevitably causes anger and resentment. These clients may lash out at people, blame them (including the nurse), and demonstrate resistant or arrogant behavior. In these difficult situations, the nurse must remain detached and nonjudgmental to avoid both power struggles and taking the role of persecutor or rescuer. At this time, the nurse functions as a data gatherer: "I know you are (uncomfortable, anxious, afraid, angry) now. To help you feel better, I need to ask you some questions about your drug use." In contrast, a judgmental question is, "Don't you know that if you don't get help now you will only get worse?" Such questions prevent rapport and alienate the client from the therapeutic process.

The Importance of Language

Knowing the language of the drug world is important in obtaining an accurate nursing assessment of a substance abuser. Drug users have a language all their own; to understand them and the extent and nature of their habit, a nurse needs to learn this language. For example, "basing and balling" refer to freebasing (using ether to purify cocaine and make it more potent), and speed-balling (combining heroin and cocaine); "copping an eight-ball" means acquiring one eighth ounce of cocaine; a "mission" is several days' use of crack; "drug of choice" is the client's favorite drug. Often the clients themselves or a recovering addict can teach the nurse.

Rationale for Assessment

The nurse must make an accurate assessment of the substances used and abused to anticipate potential toxic and withdrawal effects and to make nursing care plans as specific and relevant as possible. For example, a chronic alcoholic who is malnourished, exhausted, and depressed needs immediate diet regulation, rest, and gradual involvement in a treatment program. Cocaine or crack abusers are likely to be resistant to treatment and need active staff intervention and a structured program to involve them in treatment. They should not be left alone or purposefully isolated, as might be done with an alcoholic.

Common Defense Mechanisms

Denial and projection are two defense mechanisms common to substance abusers. These mechanisms, along with other behaviors—conning, bargaining, feigning—complicate all phases of the nursing process. Alcoholics and other drug abusers tend to deny they have a problem or minimize the problem: "I drink/use every day but it rarely interferes with my work." Rationalization is common: "I know I shouldn't drink, and I'll stop as soon as I get through this problem. Drinking keeps me calm enough to function." A detailed assessment, along with family/coworker interviews, reveals that the problem is generally worse than the client says. Cocaine users tend to project and blame their difficulties on others, often a spouse. For instance, a man may bring up the issue of his wife's drinking and give a dozen reasons why he does not need treatment.

Substance abusers "con" (manipulate) people to get drugs. *DSB,* a term used in some treatment centers, refers to *drug-seeking behaviors,* e.g., feigning illness or an injury to get a drug. These people also bargain with themselves and staff to get what they want. For example, an alcoholic/drug abuser is likely to think, "I know I shouldn't hang out with B and P since we all get loaded together, but I like them. I'll just be with them, but I won't drink/use." Later on, the person may think, "I'll only use a gram of cocaine"; later, "I'll just do an eight-ball." This client might tell the nurse, "I'll be glad to go to group therapy next week; just let me rest for a few days. I'm really tired." Of course, substance abusers always con themselves first.

Useful Nursing Responses

Recognizing common defense mechanisms and behaviors should help nurses in their client interviews and later in intervention. Coleman (1985, p 74) suggests what nurses can do to refuse to "play the game":

• Recognize and pay attention if you think something is not right.

• Recognize when your feelings of sympathy or compassion are excusing bad behavior and letting someone off the hook.

- Stop and think before you act; check with others for their reactions.

- Decide on a course of action and stick to it; do not argue or explain.

- Do not assume the client's responsibility.

- Talk to the involved staff and agree on a unified course of action. Avoid sending contradicting messages to the client.

- Insist the client follow the rules.

- Negotiate, but do not change agreements.

- Do not scold, blame, or preach. Remain objective.

- Control your temper through the use of humor or detachment.

Substance abusers are frequently demanding (they are used to immediate gratification), frightened, dependent, and grandiose. They need consistency and firmness. Savvy, not naiveté, is required for accurate client assessment and successful interventions.

Nursing assessment requires observation of subjective and objective behaviors. Examples of subjective comments are: "I have a $3000 a week coke habit and I have no more money." "I took all the pills in my medicine cabinet (Tylenol, Valium, Darvocet)." "I've drunk a quart a day for the last three weeks." Objective data relevant to each substance used are given in earlier boxes.

Diagnosing

DSM-III-R and NANDA diagnoses are compared in Table 11-1.

Planning and Implementing

Program Interventions Nurses may hold positions in any of the following settings. Their roles may be slightly different in each setting, depending on the client's stage of illness and presenting symptoms.

Solari-Twadell (1983) describes five types of treatment programs:

General Hospital Care   Substance abusers who are suicidal or acutely ill with delirium tremens, hepatic coma, respiratory depression, or cardiac arrhythmias are often treated in a medical-surgical unit of a general hospital. Life-threatening physiologic symptoms are attended to first. When the client is out of danger, the alcoholism or drug addiction issues are addressed.

In this setting, nurses monitor vital signs and respiratory and cardiovascular support and administer prescribed medications. Ice packs may be used for fever, e.g., fever caused by amphetamine intoxication. If the client is hallucinating and very fearful, as with delirium tremens, the nurse decreases stimulation by providing a darkened room in a quiet area. The nurse points out reality: "I know you are seeing things, and I know you are frightened. You are in the hospital, and we are caring for you. There are no bugs (monsters, etc.) here. You are safe and will feel better soon."

Clients who have taken overdoses of amphetamines, LSD, PCP, or cocaine may be frantic, angry, paranoid, or irrational. Reassuring the client may be ineffective; often, the symptoms subside only with time. Occasionally, restraints are necessary. The nurse makes sure that clients get adequate nutrition and fluids; they are disoriented and generally forget to eat and drink. The nurse plays a critical role in assessing why the client took an overdose.

Specialty Hospital Care   Specialty hospital care is given in in-patient hospital units that are geared specifically for substance abusers. If the hospital is equipped with trained personnel and appropriate resources, acutely ill clients may be admitted. The physical environment is modified to handle problems with substance abusers. For example, padded seclusion rooms devoid of all but a mattress offer a quiet, unstimulating environment that prevents convulsions and decreases anxiety. A primary nurse may be assigned to decrease confusion and stimulation. The staff are experts in detoxification, education, and treatment. Clients also receive treatment for coexisting medical and psychiatric problems. Staff efforts are geared toward stabilization.

Residential Rehabilitation   Residential rehabilitation facilities offer in-patients expert care for substance abuse, but staff are not skilled in treating medical or psychiatric problems.

Extended Residential Care   Extended care facilities provide services for people with physical impairments and provide a home for recovering alcoholics or drug addicts who have been rejected by their families. Apartments for independent living, a relatively new concept, are useful for these clients.

Outpatient Care   Outpatient care may consist of daily, weekly, or monthly individual, group, or

---

TABLE 11-1 Comparison of a DSM-III-R Diagnosis and Nursing Diagnoses

DSM-III-R Diagnosis	NANDA Diagnoses
305.30 Hallucinogen abuse	Self-care deficits
	Sleep pattern disturbance
	Sensory/perceptual alterations
	Altered thought processes
	Impaired thermoregulation
	Ineffective individual coping
	High risk for violence: Self-directed or directed at others

family treatment in a variety of treatment centers. Daily care is usually given only in intensive programs of limited duration, usually one month. Employee assistance programs (EAP) are now common in many industries and are one example of outpatient care given not in a clinic but in the workplace. Substance abuse outreach counselors work with chemically dependent employees.

Nurses who work with substance abusers in any of these settings need to recognize that addiction is a chronic, progressive disease. Each work setting calls for different skills. For example, in general or specialty hospitals, nurses need psychosocial skills along with technical skills to assess and monitor the physiologic components of abuse and withdrawal. In residential rehabilitation and extended residential care centers, the nurse may educate clients about the disease, help clients reenter the community as much as possible, and facilitate or lead support groups. In an outpatient treatment center, the nurse functions as a counselor/therapist. In all cases, the nurse needs psychosocial skills. Such skills may include interviewing, teaching clients about the disease process and alternative coping strategies, referring clients to appropriate sources and community support systems, and knowing how to conduct individual, group, or family therapy. In all situations, the nurse cannot give quality care without an in-depth understanding of the disease process, from the varying theoretic explanations to the varying methods of treatment at different stages.

Self-Help Groups

Twelve-Step Programs: AA and NA In contrast to the previously described treatment programs, **Alcoholics Anonymous (AA)** and **Narcotics Anonymous (NA)** are not specifically treatment programs, but AA/NA community groups do hold meetings at various treatment facilities. Both are successful self-help groups that meet daily in different parts of large cities and weekly in smaller towns. Anyone who has a desire to stop drinking or taking drugs is welcome. This belief pervades both organizations: "Once an alcoholic/addict, always an alcoholic/addict." Members admit they are powerless over chemicals, live "one day at a time," pray the serenity prayer, and believe in "a power greater than man." The members learn to turn their problems over to "the God of my understanding." Their philosophy is revealed in part through their key slogans, "First things first," "Easy does it," and "Let go and let God." Alcoholics learn the "Twelve Steps of AA" (see the accompanying box). Through AA/NA, people learn to change negative attitudes and behaviors into positive ones. A key concept of AA/NA is that total abstinence is essential to recovery. As members become sober or drug-free, they begin "sponsoring" (helping) other substance

---

Twelve Steps of Alcoholics Anonymous

1. We admitted we were powerless over alcohol—that our lives had become unmanageable.

2. Came to believe that a Power greater than ourselves could restore us to sanity.

3. Made a decision to turn our will and our lives over to the care of God, as we understood Him.

4. Made a searching and fearless moral inventory of ourselves.

5. Admitted to God, to ourselves, and to another human being the exact nature of our wrongs.

6. Were entirely ready to have God remove all these defects of character.

7. Humbly asked Him to remove our shortcomings.

8. Made a list of all persons we had harmed, and became willing to make amends to them all.

9. Made direct amends to such people wherever possible, except when to do so would injure them or others.

10. Continued to take personal inventory and when we were wrong promptly admitted it.

11. Sought through prayer and meditation to improve our conscious contact with God, as we understood Him, praying only for knowledge of His will for us and the power to carry that out.

12. Having had a spiritual awakening as the result of these steps, we tried to carry this message to alcoholics, and to practice these principles in all our affairs.

SOURCE: *"The Twelve Steps" from* Twelve Steps and Twelve Traditions *reprinted with permission of Alcoholics Anonymous World Services, Inc.*

---

abusers. This offering of support is believed to be vital to recovery, as is regular attendance at AA/NA meetings.

Women for Sobriety Women for Sobriety (WFS) is another self-help group. Unlike AA/NA, WFS is not based on a spiritual philosophy; instead, the program is based on abstinence. WFS's thirteen acceptance statements focus members on new ways of thinking. The women learn to cope and, over time, to change their daily lives. The group recognizes the differences in male and female alcoholism.

Treatment Models   Contradictory beliefs exist about the correct treatment of substance abusers. In the AA/NA model of treatment, alcoholism and drug addiction are viewed as a primary disease process. Other psychiatric symptoms are seen as resulting from addiction. Certain residential treatment centers and in-patient programs use the AA approach exclusively, to the dismay of many psychiatric professionals. This latter group believes that many alcoholics and drug abusers have fundamental psychiatric problems, such as depression, personality disorders (especially antisocial personality disorders or borderline personality disorders). Such disorders are viewed as primary and substance abuse as secondary. Treatment, they believe, should reflect this reality. Drugs and traditional psychotherapy are often prescribed for these clients. The concept of dual diagnosis may help to reconcile these contradictory beliefs. Some clients may suffer from chemical dependency as well as a coexisting psychiatric disturbance. Professionals treating these individuals need to address both components of the illness rather than using an "either-or" model to guide treatment.

Research has not yet shown which, if any, treatment or combination of treatments yields the best results. At the present time, a variety of theories and treatment modes should be used and studied, including biofeedback, relaxation techniques, group and individual therapy, and education about chemical dependency. The client's particular problems and circumstances should guide the treatment plan.

Relapse is common among substance abusers. This phenomenon complicates treatment greatly. Authorities in the field of alcoholism estimate that 60 to 75 percent of those who complete treatment programs drink again within the first 90 days. Data suggest that only 10 to 20 percent of alcoholics remain abstinent for one year following treatment and that only 35 percent of these are abstinent five years later (Chiauzzi 1987). In fact, recidivism rates are notoriously high across the spectrum of addictive behaviors (Marlatt and Gordon 1985).

Several attempts have been made to identify the various stages of the relapse process. Each proposed model of the relapse process has at least one stage in which commitment to recovery and motivation for abstinence are central. This is followed by stages of initiating change and then maintaining change (Brownell et al. 1986). As a result of a successful initial change, the individual experiences perceived control while remaining abstinent. This feeling of perceived control continues until the individual encounters a high-risk situation involving negative emotional states, interpersonal conflict, or social pressure. The individual can avoid relapse by using effective coping responses in the high-risk situation. If, however, the individual cannot cope successfully, an initial "lapse" occurs in which the individual resorts to the use of a chemical to control stress. The individual then feels less able to exert control and develops a tendency to "give in" to the situation ("It's no use, I can't handle this"). In subsequent high-risk situations, the individual again resorts to the use of chemicals to relieve stress. Repeated lapses set the stage for a return to uncontrolled use (relapse) (Marlatt and Gordon 1985). Many treatment centers are now incorporating the concept of relapse prevention into their treatment program. This is a program designed to teach clients how to anticipate and cope with the problem of relapse. By learning skills to use in high-risk situations, the individual gains confidence and the expectation of being able to cope successfully, thus decreasing the probability of relapse (Marlatt and George 1984).

Research indicates that participation in a twelve-step program, such as AA, can be useful in preventing relapse (Sheeren 1988). These programs focus on the individual being "in recovery" and maintaining sobriety, as opposed to having recovered or being cured.

Nursing Interventions

Using Confrontation Strategies   For many years, it was believed that alcoholics and drug abusers needed to "hit bottom" before they could accept their problem and request help. Today, most people believe that intervention can occur as soon as the problem is identified. Group intervention/confrontation is one strategy that aims to break down the substance abuser's denial. Nurses are often "intervention specialists" and leaders in the process.

Several family members, friends, employers, coworkers, and an alcohol/drug intervention specialist confront the substance abuser in a private meeting. They list the evidence by going around the group, one by one. For example,

> "You had slurred speech and didn't even respond when I told you I had to be hospitalized for surgery."

> "You have not made your daughter's dinner all week. And you forgot to pick her up from school."

> "You missed work for three days, and you have been late eight days in the past month."

> "You have alcohol on your breath (or needle marks on your arms)."

> "I found two bottles (a syringe and empty vial) hidden in the bathroom."

The people, following the leader's cues, speak calmly and slowly with minimal emotion. They are presenting the facts, the objective evidence. Yelling, blaming, and haranguing are avoided because the alcoholic/drug abuser will inevitably respond by denying the behavior or making excuses. However, confrontation by several people who really care and who persistently present the facts breaks through the denial. The next step requires the family/friends/employer to make clear and direct statements about consequences:

> "Either you get help now or you will have to leave your job."

> "Either you enter a treatment program now or I will move out with the kids."

If the client agrees to treatment, the caring people agree to remain involved.

Avoiding Nontherapeutic Intervention

Michael Elkin (1984, pp 81–84), a family therapist, reviews the typical moves in the relationship between an alcoholic and a nurse/therapist. He draws on Eric Berne's belief that the alcoholic plays the part of a victim and the therapist moves from being a rescuer to a persecutor. An inexperienced nurse/therapist is likely to perpetuate this dysfunctional pattern in a long-term "therapeutic" relationship. These are the typical steps:

1. The alcoholic (victim) deceives the nurse/therapist (rescuer) into believing that she or he is an unusually perceptive therapist and that the two of them have a close relationship.

2. The victim does not cut down on drinking, but the rescuer avoids mention of this (becomes a patsy) because such confrontation may endanger the relationship.

3. The victim gets drunk and calls the rescuer.

4. The rescuer becomes furious and moves to the position of persecutor.

5. The victim realizes the rescuer is like everyone else and never really cared. The victim feels rejected and abandoned.

6. The rescuer feels guilty about getting angry and engages in self-blame.

7. The victim, feeling guilty and repentant, returns to see the rescuer. A pattern has begun.

Treatment strategies are designed to help the nurse avoid "taking the bait." The nurse/therapist should avoid the role of rescuer, patsy, and persecutor and function in the role of a nonjudgmental problem solver who points out the consequences of behavior. A focus on reality (e.g., "when you drink you seem to have severe physical, emotional, and family problems") and on strategies to achieve realistic goals is useful. The nurse should avoid collusion with the alcoholic or the family but rather should focus on helping them restructure their relationships to avoid the roles of rescuer and persecutor. Successfully working with substance abusing families is a demanding task that requires education and skill, but it can be a wonder-fully rewarding experience. As in all active therapeutic relationships, both the clients and the therapists learn and share and grow.

Educating

Education is a useful nursing intervention. Videotapes and talks by recovered substance abusers or experts in the effects of substance abuse are helpful. Education may take place in or out of the hospital, in one comprehensive session or several sessions over time. Nurse educators should focus on the types of abused substances and their physical, psychologic, and social effects. Families are often involved in these sessions because substance abuse is a family problem. The belief underlying such education is that knowledge and awareness may be useful in decreasing self-destructive behavior. Knowledge alone, however, is never enough.

Referral and Self-Help Groups

Support and self-help groups are extremely useful in helping clients to feel better about themselves and to acquire new attitudes and behaviors. Merely being with many people who are suffering in similar ways is beneficial. By observing people who have been sober or drug free for long periods, clients can begin to model similar behaviors. They can see that there is hope and that recovery is possible. Self-help groups also provide new friends, generally with healthy life-styles. Clients may choose to attend support groups for the rest of their lives. Some clients who experiment with drugs or alcohol during one period of their lives and who succeed in stopping may attend only during the crisis.

Support groups with cocaine abusers should initially (one to two weeks) be homogeneous and not include other substance abusers. Cocaine and crack are rapidly addicting and give an exhilarating high, and cocaine users are often aggressive, domineering people. For these reasons, some experts believe that initial group efforts should focus only on understanding cocaine addiction. After the two weeks, cocaine users are gradually incorporated into general chemical dependency education programs and AA/NA groups. Nurses often are facilitators in support groups.

Life-Style Change

An emphasis on the requirement for a total life-style change is necessary. Nurses can help clients discuss ways to alter their destructive habits by suggesting different coping strategies and by encouraging clients to discover new interests and capabilities within themselves (see the Research Note on page 248). Nurses and clients can role play new responses to old situations. Recognizing that relapse is always a threat, nurses may set up contracts with clients. For example, clients may agree to contact the nurse or an AA/NA sponsor if and when they feel the urge to drink or do drugs. This agreement represents new behaviors that are necessary for a life-style change.

Clients must realize that spending time with friends who are substance abusers or hanging out at

RESEARCH NOTE

Citation
Banonis B: The lived experience of recovering from addiction. Nurs Sci Q 1989;2(1):37–43.

Study Problem/Purpose
The phenomenologic method was used to evolve a structural description of the experience of recovering from addiction through analysis of the lived experiences of individuals in recovery.

Methods
The three subjects wrote descriptions of a situation in which they were aware of themselves as recovering from their addiction. They were then asked to elaborate on certain portions of the description during an interview. Banonis identified natural meaning units, themes, and focal meanings and then synthesized situated personal structural descriptions and a general structural description.

Findings
For the informants, the experience of recovery involves a choice to struggle to pull oneself out of the darkness of despair into the comfort of light. The individual experiences profound shifts in ways of being. The process of recovery involves a choice to live and to engage in the process of becoming.

Implications
This research supports the focus of nursing practice on illuminating meaning in a situation and mobilizing transcendence so that clients can make choices toward becoming.

in intervention include confrontation strategies, therapeutic strategies, education, long-term self-help groups, and emphasis on a total life-style change.

Helping the Family   Substance abuse affects not only the client but also the entire family system. Family members often engage in behaviors that "enable" clients by protecting them from the consequences of their substance abuse. Helping family members involves clarifying the problem and presenting possible solutions (e.g., treatment) and creating a support system for family members. Referring family members to Al-Anon can be a very helpful strategy (Kaufman 1985).

In dysfunctional families, the substance abuser often becomes the "identified patient," focusing attention on that individual and away from the other problems in the family (Krwanek 1988). Treatment for the substance abuser may need to include some type of family therapy. Family members may need treatment for codependency through group or individual therapy or involvement in a twelve-step program such as Al-Anon or Codependents Anonymous. The Adult Children of Alcoholics (ACOA) support groups are also helpful.

Evaluating

Outcome criteria for substance abusers include sobriety (abstinence from drugs and alcohol, "being clean") and improvement of work, family, and social relationships. Clients become more effective in using new attitudes and behaviors. Better feelings about themselves result. Although the fear of relapse is always present, over time the craving for chemicals diminishes, and the client establishes a new, healthy lifestyle. Chychula (1984, p 24) lists ten criteria that are useful in evaluating the recovery process:

1. Is the client beginning to take responsibility for his or her own actions?

2. Is the abuse pattern decreasing without a dependence on other substances?

3. Is there any indication of increased job stability?

4. Is there improvement in interpersonal relationships with others?

5. Are problem-solving techniques improving?

6. Is the client setting goals and following through?

7. Is the client less impulsive and compulsive?

8. Is the client able to delay gratification?

9. Are stress and anxiety decreasing without the use of chemicals?

10. Is there evidence of increased assertiveness?

Text continues on p. 256

places where they used to do drugs/alcohol is not helpful. The mere sight or smell of paraphernalia or alcohol/drugs is often enough to trigger a relapse. Old ties must be broken; new friends and activities must be pursued.

Nursing Care Plans   The accompanying case studies and nursing care plans focus on cocaine and alcohol because they are such commonly abused drugs. Short- and long-term interventions are quite different, as the nursing care plans show. Nursing interventions with other types of substance abuse have differences and similarities. Differences in intervention tend to be medical (e.g., clonidine for opiates; haloperidol for PCP) and symptomatic (e.g., if a client hallucinates, decrease stimulation and point out reality). Similarities

CASE STUDY

A Client with Cocaine Intoxication

Identifying Information

Leigh S is a 25-year-old married woman who lives at 2205 Long Street. She was brought into the hospital by her husband. Leigh is an advertising executive with a large firm (Weeks, Bedde, and Law). She has a BA in business and an MBA in marketing. She is not and has never been under the care of a therapist.

Client's Definition of Present Problem, Precipitating Stressors, Coping Strategies, Goals for Care

Leigh states she does not need to be in the hospital but rather needs to get back to work on her ideas for ads. She states that she is extremely creative and productive and needs "to get my ideas down on paper." She is incoherent occasionally during the interview. She does state that she is perspiring and "feels sick to my stomach." Leigh admits to "working very hard," but does not feel she needs care right now. She feels she can handle this herself

History of Present Problem

Leigh states she has been using cocaine intranasally for one year. She admits to spending the majority of her salary on cocaine and states that she has used cocaine four to five times a day for the last five days. Prior to this, she generally used cocaine once or twice a week. She has increased her use because "it helps me work harder and faster. I feel more productive." She is having trouble sitting still and sleeping. Leigh thinks that she has not slept more than an hour or two for several days. Leigh's husband and one woman colleague are her main support system.

Psychiatric History

No prior psychiatric history.

Family History

Leigh's parents are living and work in their own business, a shoe store. Leigh has one brother, 21 years old, a senior in college. She feels emotionally close to her family and brother, but because they live 2000 miles away, sees them only on holidays. Leigh's father has a history of alcoholism, which has been under control for five years.

Social History

Leigh has always excelled, both in her academic work and in her job. She is competitive and likes "being number one." She has a few close friends and socializes with numerous "acquaintances from work." She has smoked since age 17, drinks "moderately," but occasionally gets drunk on weekends. She has experimented with a variety of drugs but finds cocaine to be "what works for me." She describes herself as a "workaholic" but enjoys reading and tennis when time permits.

Significant Health History

Leigh has no current or past medical problems. She states that she is in good health, but "feels horrible now." Assessment reveals a blood pressure reading of 140/90 and pulse rate of 110.

Current Mental Status

Leigh is attractive, yet disheveled, agitated, hyperalert, alternately compliant and hostile, and occasionally incoherent. Her sensorium is impaired. She is oriented to time, place, and person; judgment is impaired. Her affect is labile (alternately hostile and compliant); mood swings are evident. She moves rapidly and frequently. Her thought content is grandiose. Delusions and illusions are present. She states that she wants to open her own advertising company very soon and says she is more efficient, intelligent, and productive than her boss. She reports seeing "signs" at work that are messages to her that she should "move onward and upward." Her thought processes reveal a thought disorder; she is occasionally incoherent and tangential. She is easily distracted and has difficulty concentrating. Presently she denies her problem and has little insight, stating, "I can take care of myself. I know what I'm doing."

Other Subjective or Objective Clinical Data	Not on any medications; suicide/violence potential minimal.
Diagnostic Impression	
Nursing Diagnoses	Ineffective individual coping Sleep pattern disturbance Impaired social interaction Altered nutrition: Less than body requirements Altered thought processes
DSM-III-R Multiaxial Diagnosis	Axis I: 305.60 Cocaine intoxication (primary diagnosis) 304.20 Cocaine dependence Axis II: V71.09 (no diagnosis; denial and rationalization) Axis III: Hypertension Axis IV: 3 Moderate (unable to function at work: acute) Axis V: Current GAF: 40 Serious impairment in judgment Highest GAF in past year: 60

NURSING CARE PLAN

Client Care Goals	Nursing Planning/ Intervention	Evaluation
Nursing Diagnosis: *Ineffective individual coping*		
Leigh will agree to become free from cocaine within 48 hours. Leigh will complete detox program.	Meet individually with client to discuss consequences of drug-using behavior, e.g., "You are having trouble at work, at home, and with friends. We will work with you on these problems."	Urine "clean" 72 hrs after last use.
	Assign client to daily group therapy and to an individual counselor.	Meets with counselor and attends group according to schedule without prompting.
	Observe client every half hour; expect drug-seeking behavior. When you notice this, talk about client's feelings, explaining the anxiety and craving will, over time, disappear.	Talks about her feelings, including her anxiety and craving for cocaine. Discusses the problems cocaine has created for her.
Nursing Diagnosis: *Sleep pattern disturbance*		
Leigh will sleep 5–6 hours a night after 1 week.	Record sleep activity every 24 hours. Administer medication as ordered. Teach relaxation skills.	Sleeps 5–6 hours a night. Indicates satisfaction with sleep pattern.
Nursing Diagnosis: *Impaired social interaction*		
Leigh will attend group without leaving the room after 1 week.	Record group attendance and behavior.	Attends group therapy as scheduled and remains seated throughout. If agitated, discusses her feelings.

▶

NURSING CARE PLAN (continued)

Client Care Goals	Nursing Planning/ Intervention	Evaluation
Nursing Diagnosis: *Altered nutrition: Less than body requirements*		
Leigh will become physiologically stable and have no evidence of gastrointestinal upset.	Offer antacids p.r.n.	Is physiologically stable. No GI upset.
	Encourage diet as tolerated; monitor food intake.	Eats three meals a day.
	Weigh each week.	Maintains stable weight or gains weight.
Nursing Diagnosis: *Altered thought processes*		
Leigh will speak clearly and sensibly within 72 hours. She will not mention how wonderful she is, how she will start her own company, or other signs of grandiosity. She will not evidence extreme anger or euphoria when in group or individual treatment or in conversations with others on the unit.	When client is incoherent, ask her to slow down and to repeat again what she was saying. Ask her to discuss some of the problems in her life that she feels are a result of cocaine. When she blames others, get her to focus on herself. When she is angry and agitated, you may say, "I know you have an idea that cocaine could help you now and I know you are suffering, but with hard work on your part, you will get better."	Repeats her statements when requested to do so by nurse. Discusses her own feelings and anxieties and fears. Conversation relevant, goal-directed.

CASE STUDY

A Client with Chronic Alcoholism

Identifying Information

John Mills of 6950 Warden Road is a 54-year-old married civil servant. He is Catholic; has a high school education; and was referred from the Care Unit (a specialty hospital), where he has been for the last thirty days. His therapist's name is J. P. Allen, C.A.C.

Client's Definition of Present Problem, Precipitating Stressors, Coping Strategies, Goals for Care

"I've had a drinking problem for 15 years. My wife and boss told me if I don't shape up, they'll kick me out of my home and my job. I want to feel better. It's been a living hell. But, I'm not sure I can stop drinking. I've tried before." John describes drinking "to cope with my problems for most of my life." Wants to "stay dry."

History of Present Problem

Fifteen years ago, John's social drinking escalated, and he began binging on the weekends and, later, drinking throughout the week. He drank daily for most of the last three years. He drank "enough to keep a buzz on" and occasionally enough "to pass out." John has long-term problems with work (showing up late, absenteeism, errors on the job). He also has long-term problems with his wife, who "either yells at me or takes care of me." John describes years of her pouring out his hidden liquor and her calling his boss to say John had the flu when he really was "hung over."

Psychiatric History

John has been in and out of AA groups and has seen three different psychiatrists. He has been hospitalized three times for car accidents and injuries due to drinking (a broken leg, ribs, contusions, and a concussion). After the last general hospital admission, he was admitted to the Care Unit for a thirty-day alcohol treatment program.

Family History

Both of John's parents are deceased, and both were alcoholics. One female sibling, age 58, is a recovering alcoholic (has been "dry" for ten years). The family has never been close. John feels he was never really "allowed to be a normal, active child." He reports that his sister cared for him when he was young and was "like my mother."

Social History

John developed normally but always "felt different." He worked every summer and took a full-time job after high school graduation. He enjoyed "drinking buddies" from work, but has never had a close friend he could depend on. John smokes one pack of cigarettes daily and uses no other drugs. He spends his leisure time watching TV and at bars with friends.

Significant Health History

Cirrhosis of the liver. Malnourished from history of chronic alcoholism. Long history of insomnia.

Current Mental Status

John is well-groomed, clean, and alert. Sensorium is within normal limits. Affect is appropriate, yet apathetic. He appears depressed, and he expresses feelings of self-reproach and guilt for his years of drinking and their effect on others. He speaks slowly yet spontaneously. Motor behavior, thought content, and thought processes are within normal limits. Defenses are down in that client recognizes his alcoholism and expresses his fear of not being able to stop drinking. Insight is questionable. He recognizes his problem but is only beginning to be knowledgeable about alcoholism as a disease and about the stresses that cause him to drink.

▶

CASE STUDY *(continued)*

Other Significant Subjective or Objective Clinical Data	Client is on multivitamins qd and Antabuse qd; no indication of suicide or violence potential.
Nursing Diagnoses	Altered nutrition: Less than body requirements Sleep pattern disturbance Altered thought processes Anxiety Spiritual distress Social isolation Ineffective family coping: Disabling

DSM-III-R Multiaxial Diagnosis	Axis I: 303.90 Alcohol dependence
	Axis II: No diagnosis
	Axis III: Malnourished, chronic insomnia, alcoholic cirrhosis of liver
	Axis IV: Psychosocial stressors: attempting to combat alcoholism
	    Conjugal: severe marital discord
	    Occupational: threats of losing job
	    Financial: threat of losing job
	    Interpersonal: social isolation
	    Severity: 5 extreme (a combination of predominantly enduring and acute circumstances)
	Axis V: Current GAF: 50
	    Highest GAF past year: 30

NURSING CARE PLAN

Client Care Goals	Nursing Planning/ Intervention	Evaluation
Nursing Diagnosis: *Altered nutrition: Less than body requirements*		
John will eat three meals a day, plus snacks, and take vitamins as ordered.	Monitor intake of meals and snacks. Offer food/drink q 2 hours; initiate dietary consult to learn food preferences. During individual sessions, offer food or drink. In individual meetings and in orientation seminar, discuss the relationship between alcoholism and malnutrition; discuss resultant problems; discuss a well-balanced diet.	Gains 1 or more pounds a week; discusses relationship of alcoholism and malnutrition; discusses a well-balanced diet.

▶

NURSING CARE PLAN (continued)

Client Care Goals	Nursing Planning/ Intervention	Evaluation

Nursing Diagnosis: Sleep pattern disturbance

| John will sleep a total of 6 hours a night. | Assess client's typical sleep pattern and what strategies aid sleep, e.g., if client awakens after 2–3 hours of sleep, does reading or warm milk help client return to sleep? Once useful strategies are determined, have client put them into effect. | Sleeps 6 hours per night; uses sleep-inducing strategies nightly. Reports satisfaction with quality of sleep. |

Nursing Diagnosis: Altered thought processes

John will not use alcohol. He will attend individual counseling sessions and take Antabuse as ordered. He will attend daily AA meetings. He will call counselor whenever he is anxious, fearful, depressed, or craving a drink.	Draw up a contract with the client and have client agree to it and sign it. In the contract, client should agree to: attend AA meetings every night, see individual counselor from inpatient unit every week for the first month, and take Antabuse and return to physician as scheduled for refill.	Remains alcohol and drug free; attends treatment program as contracted; takes Antabuse as prescribed; feels proud for each day of sobriety; feels proud for sticking to contract. Repeats information learned about alcoholism as disease.
	Discuss with client that ambivalent feelings are normal but to counteract them he must call assigned counselor and/or sponsor from AA *whenever* he feels the urge to drink. Client may also write down feelings and experiences that increase the desire to drink.	
	Plan with client other stress-reducing activities, e.g., daily exercise, reading AA books, etc.	
	Help condition client to call counselor and to execute strategies when feeling stressed.	
	Teach client about the biochemical basis of alcoholism.	

Nursing Diagnosis: Anxiety and Spiritual Distress

| John will discuss feelings at AA meeting and with counselor or sponsor. | Explain to client that all alcoholics experience these feelings and that they are worked on at the AA meetings, where clients learn to surrender their problems to "a God of my under- | Works the twelve-step program of AA; guilt and self-reproach decrease over time; client takes moral inventory and makes amends to selected people. |

▶

NURSING CARE PLAN *(continued)*

Client Care Goals	Nursing Planning/ Intervention	Evaluation
	standing" and to confess their guilt and pray for help. They also learn to make amends to people after a rigorous moral inventory.	
	Go over the 12-step AA program with client; encourage client to participate in AA and to read AA books. Help client obtain copies of books.	
	Each week, ask client if and how guilt and self-reproach have changed.	

Nursing Diagnosis: *Social isolation*

Client Care Goals	Nursing Planning/ Intervention	Evaluation
John will go to work. At work, he will eat lunch with one or more people. He will call a friend or acquaintance who does not drink at least once a week.	Discuss with client that it is important to stay away from people, places, and things that are associated with drinking: New friends can come from AA, and alcohol should not be available at new activities.	Makes new friends who are in the AA program; feels better about socializing with people at work; begins to attend and enjoy social events with nondrinkers.
	Make it clear to the client that he must develop an entirely new life-style and that this will be difficult and will take time. Encourage client to attend AA activities and educational programs.	

Nursing Diagnosis: *Ineffective family coping: Disabling*

Client Care Goals	Nursing Planning/ Intervention	Evaluation
Understand alcoholism as a family disease	Refer to family therapist or, if educationally prepared, work with alcoholic and wife and educate them about the typical alcoholic game (victim, rescuer/persecutor).	Wife attends Al-Anon; client attends family therapy if prescribed; correctly recalls information about alcoholism as a family disease; begins to change coping mechanisms (e.g., avoids role of victim, decreases conning and manipulating behaviors); accepts responsibility for self.
	Help client and wife see what games they have played and how these games serve only to perpetuate a dysfunctional family system.	
	Teach client new coping strategies such as honesty about self and disease. Help client learn to accept that life is difficult and painful and there is no "quick fix."	

These two additional questions are useful:

11. Is the client using community support systems?

12. Is the client engaging in social activities with people who are not substance abusers?

Improvement in these areas is a good indication that the client is well on the road to recovery.

CHAPTER HIGHLIGHTS

• Drug and alcohol abuse are serious problems in most industrialized countries.

• One segment of the population experiments with drugs or alcohol while another segment attempts to set limits.

• Contemporary explanations of substance abuse derive from biologic, psychologic, sociocultural, and family systems theories.

• Major DSM-III-R categories of substance use include psychoactive substance–induced organic mental disorders and psychoactive substance use disorders.

• Groups at risk for substance abuse include teenagers, psychiatric clients, women, the elderly, adult children of alcoholics, general hospital clients, and nurses.

• Substance abusers suffer from intoxication and physical and psychologic withdrawal effects.

• To arrive at an accurate nursing diagnosis and design effective nursing interventions, the nurse must make a comprehensive assessment of the substance abuser, focusing on types and amount of substances used and frequency of use.

• Nursing diagnoses for substance abusing clients are gradually being generated.

• After the client is detoxified, effective nursing intervention strategies include education, support groups, writing a contract, and ultimately a change in life-style.

• Evaluation/outcome criteria include improvement in the areas of work, family, and social relationships; increased ability to solve problems and delay gratification; abstinence from all chemicals; increased feeling of well-being; and the use of community services.

REFERENCES

Abrams R, Alexopoulous G: Substance abuse in the elderly: Alcohol and prescription drugs. *Hosp Community Psychiatry* 1987;38:1285–1287.

American Nurses' Association: *Addictions and Psychological Dysfunctions in Nursing.* ANA, 1984.

American Psychiatric Association: *Diagnostic and Statistical Manual of Mental Disorders,* ed 3. AP A, 1980.

American Psychiatric Association: *Diagnostic and Statistical Manual of Mental Disorders,* ed 3, revised. APA, 1987.

Beattie M: *Codependent No More.* Harper/Hazelden, 1987.

Becker H: *The Outsiders.* Free Press, 1963.

Belfer M, Strader R, Carroll M et al: Alcoholism in women. *Arch Gen Psychiatry* 1971;25:540–544.

Bittle S, Feiginbaum J, Kneisl CR: Substance abuse, in Kneisl CR, Ames SA: *Adult Health Nursing: A Biopsychosocial Approach.* Addison-Wesley, 1986, pp 231–268.

Blume S: Women and alcohol. *JAMA* 1986;256,11:1467–1470.

Booth PG: Managing alcohol and drug abuse in the nursing profession. *J Adv Nurs* 1987;12:625–630.

Bromocriptine as treatment of cocaine abuse. *Lancet* 1985; May 18:1151–1152.

Brownell K, Marlatt G, Lichtenstein E, Wilson G: Under standing and preventing relapse. *Am Psychol* 1986; 41:765–782.

Busch D, McBride A, Benaventure L: Chemical dependency in women: The link to Ob/Gyn problems. *J Psychosoc Nurs* 1986;24:26–30.

Caroselli-Karinja M: Drug abuse and the elderly. *J Psychosoc Nurs* 1985;23:25–30.

Caroselli-Karinja, MF, Zboray SD: The impaired nurse. *J Psychosoc Nurs* 1987;24(6):14–19.

Cherskov M: Chemical dependency a major problem for youths. *American Medical News* 1985; Nov. 8;29–30.

Chiauzzi E; Working with relapse patients. *Alcohol Addict* 1987; July–Aug:43.

Chychula N: Screening for substance abuse in a primary-care setting. *Nurse Pract* 1984;9:15–24.

Cocaine: Some questions and answers. The American Council for Drug Education, 1983.

Coleman N: Check . . . Checkmate, Countering the con-games of drug abusers. *Drug Abusers* 1985;77(Feb. 1):68–74.

Creighton H: Legal implications of the impaired nurse— Part 1 *Nurs Management* 1988;19(1):21–23.

Cruz-Coke R, Varela A: Inheritance of alcoholism: Its association with color blindness. *Lancet* 1966;2:1282–1284.

DeVane C: *Fundamentals of Monitoring Psychoactive Drug Therapy.* Williams & Wilkins, 1990.

Elkin M: *Families under the Influence.* Norton, 1984.

Emmelkamp P, Heeres H: Drug addiction and parental rearing style. *Brown University Digest of Addiction Theory and Application* 1989;8(1):7.

Excerpts from surgeon general C. Everett Koop's press conference on drunk driving. *Drug Abuse Update* 1989;30 (Sept):3.

The Family Enablers. Johnson Institute, 1982.

Finley B: Primary and secondary prevention of substance abuse in nurses. *Occup Health Nurs* 1982;30:14–18.

Franks L: A new attack on alcoholism. *The New York Times Magazine* 1985; November:47–69.

Friel J, Sebby R, Friel L: Co-dependency and the search for identity: A paradoxical crisis. Health Communications, 1984.

Gallagher W: Pandora's pharmacy. *This World.* August 31, 1986;7–9.

Gianelli D: Very addictive, appealing to youth, crack poses major health worries. *Am Med News* 1986; September 12, 1986.

Green P: The impaired nurse: Chemical dependency. *J Emerg Nurs* 1984;10(1):23–26.

Gunby P: Nation's expenditures for alcohol, other drugs . . . now exceed $1.6 billion. *JAMA* 1987;258:2023.

Guy D: Co-Dependence. *Vim & Vigor* 1990;4(June):22–26.

Hall S, Wray L: Codependency: Nurses who give too much. *Am J Nurs* 1989;89:1456–1460.

Hutchinson S: Chemically dependent nurses: The trajectory towards self-annihilation. *Nurs Res* 1986;35:196–201.

Increasing use of cocaine correlates with increased problems among users. *Drug Abuse Update* 1989;29(June):12–13.

Jellinek E: *Phases in the Drinking History of Alcoholics.* Hillhouse Press, 1946.

Jones B, Jones M: Male and female intoxication levels for three alcohol dosages, or do women really get higher than men? *Alcohol Technical Report* 1976;5:11–14.

Jones B, Jones M, Paredes A: Oral contraceptives and ethanol metabolism. *Alcohol Technical Report* 1976; 5:28–32.

Kaplan H, Sadock B (eds): *Comprehensive Textbook of Psychiatry,* ed 5. Williams and Wilkins, 1989.

Kaufman E: *Substance Abuse and Family Therapy.* Grune and Stratton, 1985.

Kirk E, Bradford L: Effects of alcohol on the central nervous system. *J Neurosci Nurs* 1987;19:326–335.

Klein J: The new drug they call "ecstasy." *New York* 1985; May 20:38–43.

Kneisl CR, Ames SA; *Adult Health Nursing.* Addison-Wesley, 1986.

Koop D, Morgan E, Taer G, Coon M: Purification and characterization of a unique isozyme of cytochrome P-450 from liver microsomes of ethanol-treated rabbits. *J Biol Chem* 1982;257:8472–8480.

Krwanek J: *Addictions.* Allen and Irwin, 1988.

Landry M, Smith DE: Crack: Anatomy of an addiction. *California Nursing Review.* 1987; March/April:8–36.

Lieber C, DeCarli L: Hepatic microsomal ethanol oxidizing system. In vitro characteristics and adaptive properties in vivo. *J Biol Chem* 1970;245:2505–2512.

Lindesmith A: *Opiate Addiction:* University of Indiana Press, 1965.

Mann G: *The Dynamics of Addiction.* Johnson Institute, 1983.

Marlatt G, George W: Relapse prevention: Introduction and overview of the model. *Br J Addict* 1984;79:261–273.

Marlatt G, Gordon J: *Relapse Prevention.* Guilford Press, 1985.

Marohn R: Adolescent substance abuse: A problem of self-soothing. *Adolesc Psychiatry* 1983;1:2–11.

McCann B: A caution against the use of verapamil in PCP intoxication. *Am J Psychiatry* 1986;143:679.

Naegle M: The nurse and the alcoholic: Redefining a historically ambivalent relationship. *J Psychiatr Nurs* 1983;21:17–24.

Naegle M: Creative management of impaired nursing practice. *Nurs Adm Q* 1985;9:16–26.

Newton M: *Gone Way Down.* American Studies Press, 1981.

Pallikkathayil L, Tweed S: Substance abuse: Alcohol and drugs during adolescence. *Nurs Clin North Am* 1983; 18:313–321.

Perry P, Alexander B, Liskow B: *Psychotropic Drug Handbook,* ed 5. Harvey Whitney, 1988.

Pratt O: Alcohol and the women of childbearing age: A public health problem. *Br J Addict* 1981;76:383–390.

Price W: Management of acute PCP intoxication with verapamil. *J Toxicol Clin Toxicol* 1986;24:85–87.

Ramoska E, Sacchetti A: Propranolol-induced hypertension in treatment of cocaine intoxication. *Ann Emerg Med* 1985;14:1112–1113.

Rappolt R: Propranolol: A specific antagonist to cocaine. *Clin Toxicol* 1977;10:265–271.

Rottenberg R: Cocaine: chic, costly, and what else? *The Care Medic* 1980;1–8.

Royce, JE: *Alcohol Problems and Alcoholism: A Comprehensive Survey.* Free Press, 1981.

Schloemer N, Skidmore J: Opiate withdrawal with clonidine. *J Psychiatr Nurs* 1983;21:9–14.

Schuckit M: Genetics and the risk for alcoholism. *JAMA* 1985;254:2614–2617.

Sheeren M: The relationship between relapse and involvement in Alcoholics Anonymous. *J Stud Alcohol* 1988; 49:104–106.

Solari-Twadell P: *The Multiple Roles of a Nurse in a Comprehensive Level of Care System for Alcoholic Patients.* Gateway Community Services, 1983.

Stanton M, Todd T: *Family Therapy of Drug Abuse and Addiction.* Guilford Press, 1982.

Tennant F, Sagherian A; Double-blind comparison of amantadine and bromocriptine for ambulatory withdrawal from cocaine dependence. *Ann Intern Med* 1987; 147:109–112.

Trenk B: Biochemical abnormalities can be linked to suicide. *Am Med News* 1986; Jan 17:11.

Ugarte G, Perida I, Pino M, Iturriaga H: Influence of alcohol intake, length of abstinence and meprobomate on the rate of ethanol metabolism in men. *Q J Stud Alcohol* 1972;33:698–705.

Vance M: Drug withdrawal syndromes. *Top Emerg Med* 1985;7(3):63–68.

Varela A, Rivera L, Mardones J, Cruz-Coke R: Color vision defects in nonalcoholic relatives of alcoholic parents. *Br J Addict* 1969;64:67.

Washton A: *Cocaine Addiction.* Norton, 1989.

What parents must learn about teens and alcohol. National Federation of Parents for Drug Free Youths.

Applying the Nursing Process for Clients with Schizophrenia and Other Psychotic Disorders

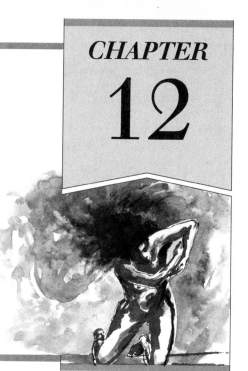

CHAPTER 12

LEARNING OBJECTIVES

- Describe historical antecedents to the current treatment of schizophrenia
- Describe several competing theoretic explanations of schizophrenia
- Recognize the DSM-III-R criteria for the diagnosis of schizophrenia
- Recognize key criteria that differentiate the schizophrenic disorders from other psychotic disorders
- Assess individual and family problems of clients diagnosed with schizophrenia
- Identify nursing diagnoses for clients who have schizophrenic disorders
- Construct nursing interventions appropriate for clients who have schizophrenic disorders and are treated in in-patient settings
- Evaluate the effectiveness of nursing interventions with the individual schizophrenic client and the family

Catherine Chesla

CROSS REFERENCES

Other topics related to this chapter are: Biologic therapies, Chapter 32; Chronically mentally ill, Chapter 17; Communication, Chapter 8; Community mental health, Chapter 38; Family, Chapter 30; Psychobiology, Chapter 6.

Persons with schizophrenia are often feared and misunderstood, both by the general public and by health care professionals. Fear is generated by inaccurate and sensationalized depictions of schizophrenics as violent, aggressive, and evil. Misunderstandings arise because schizophrenia is confused with a rare yet dramatic dissociative disorder called multiple personality disorder, which has been presented in stories like *Sybil* and *The Three Faces of Eve* in the popular media. Persons with schizophrenia may be further misunderstood because the symptoms of the disorder, while varied, generally set them apart from the general public. Schizophrenics' physical presentation, emotional responses to situations, unusual or bizarre thoughts, or altered capacity to relate with others may cause even health care professionals to distance themselves and fail to try to understand the schizophrenic's experience and difficulties.

Persons with schizophrenia are *persons* who suffer from a complex, multifaceted, biologically based, environmentally sensitive disease that affects all areas of their life and functioning. Psychiatric nurses who work with schizophrenics are doubly challenged. The first challenge is to learn the spectrum of problems and combinations of problems that comprise the broad diagnostic category, schizophrenia. The second challenge is to understand and work with the broad variation in human responses to living with this difficult, chronic illness.

Historical and Theoretic Foundations

Descriptive Psychiatry

The work of Kraepelin and Bleuler advanced the understanding of schizophrenia as a disease entity. Kraepelin began to describe the syndrome of schizophrenia, which he labeled **dementia praecox**, or early senility. He believed the syndrome was caused by an organic abnormality, was degenerative, and always ended in a state of disorganization that today would be called *psychosis*. Bleuler, who used the term *schizophrenia*, refined Kraepelin's descriptive picture of the illness. Bleuler attempted a psychologic explanation of schizophrenic symptoms but remained undecided whether the illness was organic or psychologic. Unlike Kraepelin, Bleuler believed that there were many possible courses and outcomes of the disease.

Psychoanalytic Therapies

Successful analytic work with schizophrenics by Sullivan and Fromm-Reichmann challenged earlier beliefs that schizophrenia could not be treated. By focusing on interpersonal relations, particularly from early childhood, these therapists attempted to understand and interpret the schizophrenic's symptoms. Their work represented a departure from Freud's belief that schizophrenics could not form a therapeutic relationship and therefore could not be treated using analytic techniques. They claimed, as do their followers, that schizophrenic symptoms can be diminished through careful in-depth interpretive work. The effectiveness of insight-oriented therapies with schizophrenics continues to be debated today.

Somatic Therapies   Somatic treatments—e.g., insulin coma; drug or electrically induced shock treatments; and psychosurgery, including prefrontal lobotomies—were used in the 1930s. Many hoped these treatments were the long sought-after cure for schizophrenia because they were relatively quick and inexpensive treatments when compared with the analytic therapies. This hope was not realized.

Psychopharmacologic Treatments   The introduction of psychoactive drugs in the 1950s provided new alternatives for the treatment of schizophrenia. Psychotropic medications, which influence the thoughts, mood, and behavior of clients, made previously uncontrolled symptoms manageable. In the period following the introduction of psychotropic medications, the use of seclusion and restraints declined dramatically, as did the duration of hospital stays and numbers of clients in state hospitals.

A new optimism arose regarding the possible outcomes of mental illness. Because they controlled the most difficult symptoms of psychosis, psychotropic medications made psychosocial or behavioral treatments possible for a much greater percentage of psychiatric clients. The major tranquilizers did not live up to their promise of providing a cure for schizophrenia and other chronic psychiatric illnesses. However, these drugs relieved the most debilitating symptoms for many clients and were the beginning step toward recovery or a higher level of functioning.

Community Mental Health   Following the recommendations of the Joint Commission on Mental Health in 1961, Congress enacted legislation to establish a system of community-based mental health centers devoted to treating and preventing mental illness. New services established were community-based outpatient, day treatment, and crisis programs.

In the mid-1970s priority was given to the care of the chronically mentally ill in a federally funded Community Support Program. The aim of this program was to supplement natural helping networks in supporting the chronically mentally ill in the community. In addition to the traditional mental health services, psychosocial rehabilitation, residential services, assistance in securing medical and financial support, and backup support for families were called for.

Biologic Theories of Schizophrenia

It is unlikely that schizophrenia is caused by a specific biologic abnormality. Scientists have searched unsuccessfully for a unique biologic marker consistently found in schizophrenics and not in healthy persons. At the same time, scientific evidence suggests that the disorder is not merely psychologic and that biologic alterations are present. Particularly convincing is the fact that the symptoms associated with schizophrenia, such as delusions or hallucinations, are found in normal persons only when they are in a state of metabolic imbalance or suffer from organic diseases. Persons with brain tumors, or who have ingested certain drugs, for example, may experience hallucinations (Schulz and Tamminga 1989).

Genetic Theories Schizophrenics inherit a genetic vulnerability for the disease rather than the disease itself. Evidence supporting this thesis is the fact that relatives of schizophrenics have a greater chance of developing the disease than the general population do. One percent of the population develops schizophrenia, while 10 percent of the first-degree relatives (parents, siblings, children) of schizophrenics are diagnosed with the disease during their lifetimes. The risk of developing schizophrenia increases with the closeness of relation with a diagnosed schizophrenic. Siblings of schizophrenics have a greater risk of developing the disease than do half-siblings or grandchildren, and these have a greater risk than more distant relatives, such as cousins.

Twin studies indicate that both environmental and genetic factors are important in schizophrenia. Concordance rates (both twins either express or do not express the trait) for schizophrenia are consistently higher for monozygotic twins than for dizygotic twins. This finding supports the hypothesis of genetic transmission. However, concordance rates for monozygotic twins are in the range of 35 to 58 percent, indicating that environment plays a large part in the expression of the illness. If the disease were solely genetically determined, the concordance rates in this group would be close to 100 percent.

Biochemical Theories Investigators believed that the biochemical basis of schizophrenia might be uncovered by studying the biochemical actions of drugs that reduce schizophrenic symptoms. The **dopamine (DA) hypothesis** is the most widely held and extensively studied biochemical mechanism thought to underlie schizophrenia. An alternate biochemical mechanism that links nutrition and psychosis is discussed in the accompanying Nutrition box.

In simplified form, the DA hypothesis is that schizophrenia may be related to overactive neuronal activity that is dependent on DA. The hypothesis is supported by pharmacologic research demonstrating that drugs that increase DA activity worsen schizophrenic symptoms and drugs that decrease DA activity alleviate symptoms. Two classes of drugs used most frequently in the treatment of schizophrenia, the phenothiazines (e.g., Thorazine) and the butyrophenones (e.g., Haldol), have been extensively studied. Although these drugs are chemically quite different, both block DA receptors. The extent to which they block DA is related to their clinical effectiveness in alleviating the positive symptoms of schizophrenia. In addition, drugs in each of these classes that are chemically similar, yet do not block DA receptors, have little effect on schizophrenic symptoms (Schulz and Tamminga 1989).

The cause of excessive DA activity in schizophrenics is not yet known, nor can we conclude that schizophrenia is caused by DA excesses. Biochemical states are influenced by the individual's genetic makeup and by such environmental factors as stress, nutrition, and exposure to viruses. There are many theories about the biologic mechanisms that lead to excessive DA, but none has been adequately tested to receive widespread approval.

Brain Structure Alterations in Schizophrenia Ventricular size has been found to be significantly larger in chronic schizophrenic clients than in control groups. Computed tomography (CT), safer and less invasive than prior tests, has allowed researchers to study this abnormality. It is now believed that schizophrenics with enlarged ventricles may be a subgroup of all schizophrenics, who have similar biologic abnormalities and clinical pictures (Schulz and Tamminga 1989). For example, schizophrenics with enlarged ventricles have a poorer therapeutic response to antipsychotic drugs than those in a matched group of schizophrenics who do not show enlarged ventricles. Enlarged ventricles are also associated with poor performance on psychologic tests.

One theory suggests that there are two types of schizophrenia, each with unique biologic abnormalities and clinical courses. **Type I schizophrenia** is characterized by **positive symptoms** of schizophrenia: hallucinations, delusions, and thought disorder. Type I

NUTRITION AND MENTAL HEALTH

Can Food Intolerance Cause Schizophrenia?

Researchers have spent decades collecting the kind of data needed to establish a cause-and-effect relationship between food and psychosis. To date, there is persuasive epidemiologic and clinical evidence for such a link.

Among 65,000 inland inhabitants of three Pacific islands who consumed little or no cereal grains, only two cases of overt schizophrenia were observed. A comparable survey of European populations—who rely heavily on grains such as wheat, oats, and rye—revealed a prevalence rate of 2 per 1000 adults. Similarly, among Pacific island peoples in more westernized coastal towns, in contrast to the inland groups, the number of cases of schizophrenia was sharply higher, as was the percentage of grain in the diet (Dohan et al. 1984).

Even stronger evidence comes from intervention trials in which gluten, the protein found in the above grains, was removed from the diets of psychotic clients. Of six controlled studies, three have found a significant improvement in those on a gluten-free regimen; three have not. However, the negative studies had a statistical power rating between 0.23 and 0.54. In practical terms, that means they could not rule out significant symptomatic improvement among those on a gluten-free diet because the studies contained too few subjects (King 1985).

A seventh double-blind trial in which twenty-four chronic schizophrenics received either gluten or a placebo demonstrated clear-cut benefits in two subjects. A 34-year-old psychotic with an 18-year history of the disease, for instance, improved markedly, showing less excitability, perceptual disorganization, grandiosity, and depressive mood. Investigators report that they were "impressed to see this almost continuously disturbed patient serving meals, helping staff with various jobs and talking much more rationally." Several psychiatric parameters deteriorated when gluten was reintroduced into the diet (Vlissides et al. 1986).

Although these reports point to food intolerances as a contributing cause of schizophrenia—at least for some clients—they do not shed any light on how to pinpoint the existence of an intolerance in individual clients. Unfortunately, there are no foolproof methods of doing so.

Standard diagnostic procedures, such as the radioallergosorbent (RAST) or interdermal tests, detect the presence of only IgE antibodies, those produced during a true allergic reaction. But several researchers have found that many food sensitivities, although immunologic in nature, do not generate an IgE response. For instance, some food sensitivities are accompanied by abnormal serum levels of IgA, IgG, or a series of proteins referred to collectively as complement (Breneman 1984, Crayton 1984).

Given this complex situation, the most practical way to detect a food intolerance, short of performing an array of expensive, highly sophisticated laboratory tests, is by either taking a careful food history or starting the client on an elimination diet. Clinical experience suggests that certain food-sensitive clients crave the very foods they cannot tolerate, much as drug addicts crave the substance that causes their symptoms. If that's the case, then a food history is likely to turn up a lopsided diet that relies too heavily on the offending food. Thus, someone who is sensitive to milk protein may consume large amounts of cheese, yogurt, and ice cream.

Because there are no controlled studies to confirm this addiction/allergy hypothesis, many clinicians turn to an elimination diet. The beginning diet consists of hypoallergenic foods, such as lamb, cabbage, cauliflower, apple, banana, rice, tapioca, sunflower oil, and milk-free margarine. To prevent nutritional deficiencies, vitamin and mineral supplements are added to the diet. See Krause and Mahan (1986) for a detailed description of this technique.

Although food sensitivities may contribute to schizophrenia, clinicians should also keep in mind that the disease, as well as other psychiatric disorders, can also affect the way clients view food, causing some to invent food allergies as an explanation for symptoms that may have strictly interpersonal or intrapsychic roots. One research team, for instance, was unable to confirm the presence of allergy-induced depression, anxiety, mood swings, sleep disturbance, and poor concentration in nineteen subjects who were tested by means of double-blind food challenges (Pearson and Rix 1983). A psychiatric evaluation, however, found that the subjects had neurotic

---

NUTRITION AND MENTAL HEALTH *(continued)*

depression, hypochondriacal neurosis, phobia, and several other conditions.

There is one other possibility to consider in clients who complain of psychiatric reactions to food: stress-induced food sensitivity. The physiologic stress induced by exercise, for instance, can precipitate anaphylaxis to foods in susceptible clients (Bell 1987). The stress generated by

mental dysfunction may likewise generate an immune response, as is borne out by experiments that have found diminished lymphocyte function after the death of a loved one (Crayton 1986). Put another way, it seems likely that some clients become more allergy-prone when exposed to stress. The resulting food sensitivity in turn may trigger psychiatric symptoms.

—Paul M. Cerrato

---

schizophrenia is thought to be associated with the biologic abnormality of increased dopamine receptors. Its onset is acute, and it responds well to psychotropic medications. **Type II schizophrenia** is characterized by the **negative symptoms** of the disease: flattening of affect, loss of motivation, and poverty of speech. Type II schizophrenia shows little response to treatment with drugs.

Psychologic Theories of Schizophrenia

Information Processing   Many schizophrenic clients have information-processing deficits. Two central types of information processing have been identified: (a) automatic and (b) controlled or effortful processing. Automatic processing is the taking in of information unintentionally. Automatic processing can occur without the individual's being aware of it, and it does not interfere with conscious thought processes occurring at the same time. Examples of automatic information processing are the initial awareness of physical features of a new environment.

Schizophrenics are deficient in controlled information processing. Their ability to perform directed, conscious, sequential thinking—e.g., making comparisons between two stimuli or organizing a set of stimuli—is consistently inferior to that of nonschizophrenics.

We do not know whether the schizophrenic's inability to sustain conscious, directed thought is the primary problem or the result of a primary deficit in automatic thinking. If the primary deficit is in automatic processes, then the schizophrenic is forced to complete automatic tasks at the conscious level, inhibiting and slowing controlled information processing. Sufficient evidence to resolve this question is not yet available.

Attention and Arousal   Physiologic studies of attention and arousal in schizophrenics show promise of identifying clinically significant subgroups. Arousal and attention are measured by physiologic states and alterations, e.g., galvanic skin response, heart rate, blood pressure, skin temperature, or pupillary response. One subgroup of clients exhibits abnormally low response levels to novel stimuli. This finding suggests that these clients are less adept than normal persons at attending and responding to novel situations. Liberman et al. (1984) note that the 40 to 50 percent of schizophrenics who demonstrate this attention abnormality present clinical symptoms similar to those identified as type II schizophrenia.

A second group of schizophrenics demonstrates a state of hyperarousal evidenced by elevated electrodermal activity, heart rate, and blood pressure. Hyperarousal has been noted in schizophrenics during both symptomatic and nonsymptomatic periods. Clinically, this subgroup has characteristics of type I schizophrenia. They demonstrate symptoms of irritability, excitement, and anxiety rather than apathy and withdrawal.

Family Theories of Schizophrenia

Numerous theories have been put forth implicating family interaction as a cause of schizophrenia (Chesla 1989). Terms that represent these theories include schizophrenogenic mothers, double-binds, and pseudomutuality. Research has failed to support the theory that dysfunctional family interaction causes the illness.

One theory suggests that disordered family communication causes schizophrenia only in the presence of a genetic vulnerability to the disease. A communication problem evident in some families of schizophrenics is the inability to focus on and clearly share an observation or thought. Living with this pattern of family communication during early development is thought to impair the schizophrenic's ability to perceive the environment and communicate with others about it.

A second theory is that the family's emotional tone can influence the course of schizophrenia over time. Researchers found that schizophrenics who come from families who are highly critical, hostile, or overinvolved tend to relapse more often than those from families who do not demonstrate these characteristics. Families who demonstrate these characteristics have been described as having high **expressed emotion.** There is some evidence that family expressed emotion may be an influence on, rather than a response to, the illness, but this evidence is not definitive.

Humanist-Interactional Understandings of Schizophrenia

An interactional model of schizophrenia integrates many of the biologic and social theories already discussed. In this view, schizophrenia is due to the interaction of a biologic vulnerability, stress or change in the environment, and the individual's social skills and supports (Liberman et al. 1984). In an interactional model, the influences are multidimensional.

Great biologic vulnerability may inhibit the individual's capacity to cope with even minor stressors. Loss of a primary source of support might trigger decreased functioning in the schizophrenic. Similarly, schizophrenics might grow worse upon entering an environment that demands coping skills they have not developed.

Figure 12–1 is a schematic representation of an interactional model. This model depicts the biologic, behavioral, and environmental domains of variables that influence the disorder. For each domain, three time dimensions are also depicted: enduring vulnerability characteristics, more transient states, and outcomes.

Enduring vulnerability characteristics in the biologic realm include the genetic and biochemical defects already described. Enduring behavioral deficits include poor relationship skills, lack of motivation, and inability to perform productively at work or school. It is theorized that the environment of schizophrenics characteristically provides poor opportunities for learning. An example of a poor learning environment is the family milieu in which parents provide inaccurate or incomplete descriptors of the world, as described in the communication deviance theories.

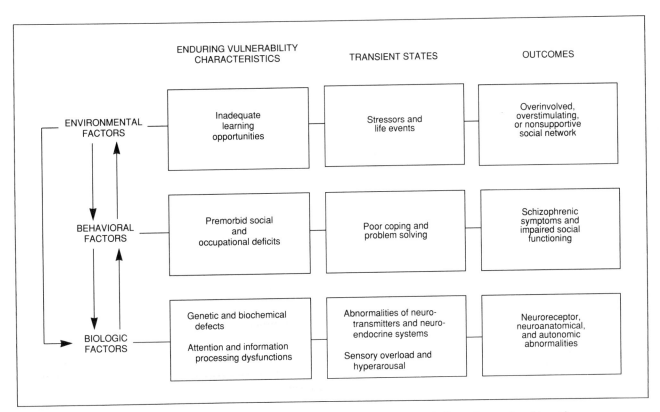

FIGURE 12–1   An interactional model for schizophrenia.   *(Source: Liberman RP, et al.: The nature and problem of schizophrenia, in Bellack AS (ed): Schizophrenia, Treatment, Management and Rehabilitation. Grune & Stratton, 1984, p 4.*

According to the interactional theory, events in the schizophrenic's life are played out on this biologic, behavioral, and environmental stage. Disability is the result of a balance or imbalance that develops as changes occur in each of the three domains. Stressors and life events constitute the changes in the schizophrenic's environment. Fluctuations in the schizophrenic's coping skills and problem-solving abilities constitute the behavioral changes. Neurotransmitter and neuroendocrine abnormalities as well as alterations in arousal and attention are the biologic changes thought to affect the schizophrenic's level of functioning.

The interactional theorists propose that disability may develop because of changes in any domain interacting with response or lack of response in any other domain. The two following examples illustrate this multidirectionality of causation.

Daryl, a 26-year-old with a diagnosis of paranoid schizophrenia, decided to stop taking his Haldol because it made him feel heavy and too tired to get up in the morning. Within a few days of stopping the medication, he was unable to leave the house for fear of someone harming him. Although he liked his unpaid job at the local cannery and knew that he had the chance to earn money in the near future, he refused to go to work for fear that he would be hit by a bus on his way there. He was eventually fired because of poor attendance. In this instance, a decrease in medication increased biologic vulnerability with marked behavioral and eventually environmental consequences.

Jean, 22, had lived with her divorced mother and younger sister Mary since her release from the hospital after her second psychotic episode. She found living alone too frightening and was more comfortable staying in her old room at home. When Mary began preparing to leave home for college, Jean became increasingly anxious, demanding to sleep in Mary's room at night and hiding Mary's belongings. As Mary's departure grew near, Jean began actively hallucinating and withdrew to her room, refusing to talk to her mother or sister. In this case, the client did not have sufficient coping skills to deal with her sister's departure from the household, and the client retreated into psychosis.

Biopsychosocial Factors in Pathology

Diagnostic Criteria for Schizophrenia

The behavioral indicators that must be present to justify a diagnosis of schizophrenia are identified in DSM-III-R. The criteria are specified in the accompanying box.

Five types of schizophrenia are specified in DSM-III-R. Each type of schizophrenia is characterized by a set of predominant symptoms. These are the types of schizophrenia:

- Paranoid
- Catatonic
- Disorganized
- Undifferentiated
- Residual

See the box on page 266 for the clinical features of each subtype of the disorder.

The course of the illness varies from client to client, and thus the American Psychiatric Association (APA) has specified five courses of the illness: chronic, subchronic, chronic with acute exacerbation, subchronic with acute exacerbation, or in remission. The DSM-III-R indicators of the illness course are found in the box on page 267.

Distinguishing Schizophrenia from Other Disorders

Planning care for individual clients requires diagnostic precision because interventions for clients with schizophrenic disorders differ from those for persons with other psychotic disorders. Two categories of psychotic disorders other than schizophrenia are specified in DSM-III-R: delusional disorders, and psychotic disorders not elsewhere classified.

Delusional Disorders Clients with **delusional disorders** are similar to schizophrenic clients because they hold unusual or bizarre beliefs and cannot be reasoned with regarding these beliefs. Unlike schizophrenic clients, delusional clients do not have persistent hallucinations and exhibit few or any of the other features of schizophrenia—e.g., flat or inappropriate affect, social withdrawal or isolation, and inability to care for themselves. The content of the delusions varies. For example, some delusional clients believe that they are being persecuted. Others may think they have special knowledge or powers, have a physical disorder, or are loved by a famous public figure.

Psychotic Disorders Not Elsewhere Classified **Psychotic disorders not elsewhere classified** is a category of diagnoses for clients who present with psychotic features yet do not fully exhibit characteristics of the schizophrenic, delusional, or major mood disorders. Four disorders that fall in this category are

1. Schizophreniform disorder
2. Schizoaffective disorder
3. Brief reactive psychosis
4. Induced psychotic disorder

DSM-III-R Diagnostic Criteria for Schizophrenia

A. Presence of characteristic psychotic symptoms in the active phase: either (1), (2), or (3) for at least one week (unless the symptoms are successfully treated):

1. Two of the following:
   a. Delusions
   b. Prominent hallucinations (throughout the day for several days or several times a week for several weeks, each hallucinatory experience not being limited to a few brief moments)
   c. Incoherence or marked loosening of associations
   d. Catatonic behavior
   e. Flat or grossly inappropriate affect
2. Bizarre delusions (i.e., involving a phenomenon that the person's culture would regard as totally implausible, e.g., thought broadcasting, being controlled by a dead person)
3. Prominent hallucinations [as defined in 1.b above] of a voice with content having no apparent relation to depression or elation, or a voice keeping up a running commentary on the person's behavior or thoughts, or two or more voices conversing with each other

B. During the course of the disturbance, functioning in such areas as work, social relations, and self-care is markedly below the highest level achieved before onset of the disturbance (or, when the onset is in childhood or adolescence, failure to achieve expected level of social development).

C. Schizoaffective disorder and mood disorder with psychotic features have been ruled out, i.e., if a major depressive or manic syndrome has ever been present during an active phase of the disturbance, the total duration of all episodes of a mood syndrome has been brief relative to the total duration of the active and residual phases of the disturbance.

D. Continuous signs of the disturbance for at least six months. The six-month period must include an active phase (of at least one week or less if symptoms have been successfully treated) during which there were psychotic symptoms characteristic of schizophrenia (symptoms in A), with or without a prodromal or residual phase, as defined below.

Prodromal phase: A clear deterioration in functioning before the active phase of the disturbance that is not due to a disturbance in mood or to a psychoactive substance use disorder and that involves at least two of the symptoms listed below.

Residual Phase: Following the active phase of the disturbance, persistence of at least two of the symptoms noted below, these not being due to a disturbance in mood or to a psychoactive substance use disorder.

Prodromal or Residual Symptoms:

1. Marked social isolation or withdrawal
2. Marked impairment in role functioning as wage-earner, student, or homemaker
3. Markedly peculiar behavior (e.g., collecting garbage, talking to self in public, hoarding food)
4. Marked impairment in personal hygiene and grooming
5. Blunted or inappropriate affect
6. Digressive, vague, overelaborate, or circumstantial speech, or poverty of speech, or poverty of content of speech
7. Odd beliefs or magical thinking, influencing behavior and inconsistent with cultural norms, e.g., superstitiousness, belief in clairvoyance, telepathy, "sixth sense," "others can feel my feelings," overvalued ideas, ideas of reference
8. Unusual perceptual experiences, e.g., recurrent illusions, sensing the presence of a force or person not actually present
9. Marked lack of initiative, interests, or energy

Examples: Six months of prodromal symptoms with one week of symptoms from A; no prodromal symptoms with six months of symptoms from A; no prodromal symptoms with one week of symptoms from A and six months of residual symptoms.

E. It cannot be established that an organic factor initiated and maintained the disturbance.

F. If there is a history of autistic disorder, the additional diagnosis of schizophrenia is made only if prominent delusions or hallucinations are also present.

SOURCE: *American Psychiatric Association.* Diagnostic and Statistical Manual of Mental Disorders, *ed 3, revised. APA, 1987.*

DSM-III-R Diagnostic Criteria for Five Types of Schizophrenia

Catatonic Type

1. Catatonic stupor (marked decrease in reactivity to the environment and/or reduction in spontaneous movements and activity) or mutism.

2. Catatonic negativism (an apparently motiveless resistance to all instructions or attempts to be moved).

3. Catatonic rigidity (maintenance of a rigid posture against efforts to be moved).

4. Catatonic excitement (excited motor activity, apparently purposeless and not influenced by external stimuli).

5. Catatonic posturing (voluntary assumption of inappropriate or bizarre postures).

Disorganized Type

1. Incoherence, marked loosening of associations, or grossly disorganized behavior.

2. Flat or grossly inappropriate affect.

3. Does not meet the criteria for catatonic type.

Paranoid Type

1. Preoccupation with one or more systematized delusions or with frequent auditory hallucinations related to a single theme.

2. None of the following: incoherence, marked loosening of associations, flat or grossly inappropriate affect, catatonic behavior, grossly disorganized behavior.

Undifferentiated Type

1. Prominent delusions, hallucinations, incoherence, or grossly disorganized behavior.

2. Does not meet the criteria for paranoid, catatonic, or disorganized type.

Residual Type

1. Absence of prominent delusions, hallucinations, incoherence, or grossly disorganized behavior.

2. Continuing evidence of the disturbance, as indicated by two or more of the residual symptoms listed in criterion D of schizophrenia (see the box "DSM-III-R Diagnostic Criteria for Schizophrenia").

SOURCE: *American Psychiatric Association:* Diagnostic and Statistical Manual of Mental Disorders, *ed 3, revised. APA, 1987.*

See the second box on page 267 for the general clinical features that differentiate delusional disorders and other psychotic disorders from schizophrenia. The nurse should consult DSM-III-R for a description of criteria used to differentiate these disorders.

The Nursing Process and Clients with Schizophrenia

Assessing

Assessment of clients who have schizophrenia occurs at the individual, family, and environmental level. The nurse must be aware of the client's status and of changes in the client's personal life, family situation, and environment to plan care and intervene effectively. Additionally, care that addresses multiple levels of the client's life is consistent with the interactional theory of schizophrenia because it is assumed that changes in any aspect of the schizophrenic's person or environment influence all other aspects of the personal environmental balance.

Perceptual Changes The perceptions of clients with schizophrenia may be either heightened or blunted. These changes may occur in all the senses, or in just one or two. For example, a client may see colors as brighter than normal or may be acutely sensitive to sounds. Another may have a heightened sense of touch and therefore be extremely sensitive to any physical contact.

Illusions occur when the client misperceives or exaggerates stimuli in the external environment. A schizophrenic client may mistake a chair for a person or perceive that the walls of a hallway are closing in. The perceptual changes are sufficient to cause the client to mistake the stimulus for something that it is not.

Hallucinations are the most extreme and yet the most common perceptual disturbance in schizophrenia. A hallucination is a subjective perception of something that does not exist in the external environment. Hallucinations can be visual, olfactory (smell), gustatory (taste), tactile (feel), or auditory. Auditory hallucinations are the most common. Although hallucinations are a hallmark of schizophrenia, their presence alone does not establish the presence of the

DSM-III-R Criteria for Classification of the Course of Schizophrenia

1—Subchronic   The time from the beginning of the disturbance, when the person first began to show signs of the disturbance (including prodromal, active, and residual phases) more or less continuously, is less than two years, but at least six months.

2—Chronic   Same as above, but more than two years.

3—Subchronic with Acute Exacerbation   Re-emergence of prominent psychotic symptoms in a person with a subchronic course who has been in the residual phase of the disturbance.

4—Chronic with Acute Exacerbation   Reemergence of prominent psychotic symptoms in a person with a chronic course who has been in the residual phase of the disturbance.

5—In Remission   When a person with a history of schizophrenia is free of all signs of the disturbance (whether or not on medication), "in remission" should be coded. Differentiating "schizophrenia in remission" from no mental disorder requires consideration of overall level of functioning, length of time since the last episode of disturbance, total duration of the disturbance, and whether prophylactic treatment is being given.

0—Unspecified

SOURCE: *American Psychiatric Association:* Diagnostic and Statistical Manual of Mental Disorders, *ed 3, revised. APA, 1987.*

---

tions are inappropriate laughing or smiling, difficulty following a conversation, or difficulty attending to what is happening at the moment. Fleeting, rapid changes of expression that are not precipitated by events in the real world can be a further sign. Finally, clients may talk to themselves, presumably in answer to the voices they hear. See the Assessment box on page 268.

DSM-III-R Criteria for Delusional and Other Psychotic Disorders

Delusional Disorders

Clinically similar to schizophrenia only because of the presence of delusions. Differences include:

- Delusions have a basis in reality.
- Hallucinations are not a dominant feature.
- Behavior is within normal range except in relation to the delusion.
- Behavior does not meet the criteria for schizophrenia, i.e., catatonia, affective abnormalities, and loosening of associations are not present.

Other Psychotic Disorders Not Elsewhere Classified

Clinical picture is very similar to schizophrenia, but one or more of the essential diagnostic criteria are not met. For example:

- Schizophreniform disorder: The duration of all symptoms (acute and residual) is less than six months and a return to normal functioning is possible.
- Schizoaffective disorder: Dominant schizophrenic symptoms are accompanied at some, but not all times by a major depressive or manic syndrome.
- Brief reactive psychosis: Psychotic symptoms appear shortly after a stressful event or series of events. Duration of symptoms is one month or less, with recovery to normal level of function.
- Induced psychotic disorder: A delusional system develops because of a close relationship with a person who already has a psychotic disorder with delusions. The second person to develop delusions receives this diagnosis.

SOURCE: *Adapted from American Psychiatric Association:* Diagnostic and Statistical Manual of Mental Disorders, *ed 3, revised. APA, 1987.*

---

disorder. Table 12–1 on page 268 lists various types of hallucinations along with a disease process commonly associated with the symptom.

Assess perceptual disturbances by asking the client about the experience and by observing for behaviors that indicate the client is frightened or attending to internal stimuli. Ask the client, "What are you seeing and hearing?" Note the degree to which this description differs from your perceptions of the environment.

Clients may be reluctant to discuss the extreme perceptual disturbance of hallucinations. A classic sign of auditory hallucinations is placing the hands over the ears. The client is frightened by the perception and tries to block it out. Less obvious signs of hallucina-

TABLE 12–1 Disturbances in Perception

Type of Hallucination	Commonly Associated Disease Process	Example
Auditory	Schizophrenia	Hearing voices of family members who aren't present
Visual	Acute organic brain syndrome	Seeing animals walking across the walls of the room
Tactile	Acute alcohol withdrawal	Feeling bugs crawl on the skin
Olfactory	Seizure disorders	Smelling foods that aren't present
Gustatory	Seizure disorders	Tasting a sharp sweet taste on the tongue, in the absence of food
Somatic	Schizophrenia	Sensing that one's head has a tunnel running through it

Disturbances in Thought Clients with schizophrenia find their thinking is muddled or unclear. Their thoughts are disconnected or disjointed, and the connections between one thought and another are vague, a characteristic called **loosening of associations.** When the associations between thoughts are based on the sounds of words rather than their meanings, the client is making **clang associations**, e.g., "I'm great (grate) like in the sewer (sue her), and I'll see you in court."

Schizophrenic clients also have difficulty thinking abstractly. Their responses may be inappropriate because they interpret words literally rather than abstractly. For example, when told to prepare to have his blood drawn, a young man readied some paper and marking pens. Assess abstract thinking by asking clients the meaning of proverbs, a test requiring the client to abstract a general meaning from a specific or metaphysical statement, e.g., "People who live in glass houses shouldn't throw stones."

A disturbance in the content rather than the form of thought is a delusion. **Delusions** are fixed false beliefs about oneself, one's environment, or events occurring in it. A belief is delusional when it cannot be consensually validated. That is, persons who surround the delusional person cannot agree with or validate the belief.

Delusions vary in type and complexity. Table 12–2 describes several types of delusions, including persecution, somatic, and control delusions, that schizophrenics often experience. Delusions can be simple beliefs, relating to only a small part of the person's daily life, or highly complex systems of belief.

Changes in Communication Clients with schizophrenia frequently have difficulty responding appropriately to events and people they encounter. The difficulties arise because of the schizophrenic's distorted perceptions, impaired ability to sort and assimilate these perceptions, and difficulty communicating responses clearly.

The clarity of the client's communication often reflects the level of **thought disorganization.** Client's responses may be simply inappropriate to the situation or conversation. They may have difficulties articulating a response or stop mid-sentence, as if they are stuck, a sign of **thought blocking.**

Note the rate and quality of client's speech. Is it unusually loud, insistent, and continuous? Does the

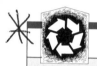

ASSESSMENT

Hallucinations

A complete assessment of hallucinations (Williams 1989) should identify the following:

- Whether the hallucinations are solely auditory or include other senses
- How long the client has experienced the hallucinations, what the initial hallucinations were like, and whether they have changed
- Which situations are most likely to trigger hallucinations, and which times of day they occur most frequently
- What the hallucinations are about (For example are they just sounds, or voices? If the client hears voices, what do they say?)
- How strongly the client believes in the reality of the hallucinations
- Whether the hallucinations command the client to do something, and if so, how potentially destructive the commands are
- Whether the client hears other voices contradicting commands received in hallucinations
- How the client feels about the hallucinations
- Which strategies the client has used to cope with the hallucinations and how effective the strategies were

client wander from topic to topic (tangential communication) or bring up details that are irrelevant to the topic at hand (circumstantial communication)? Are the client's responses slow and hesitant, reflecting difficulty in taking in stimuli and responding?

Disruptions in Emotional Responses   Tone of voice, rate of speech, content of speech, expressions, postures, and body movements indicate emotional tone. Disturbances in emotions commonly seen in schizophrenia are restricted or inappropriate expression of emotions. Assess the congruence between the content of the client's communication and the displayed emotion. For example, does the client laugh when describing a frightening or sad incident? Additionally, lack of emotion is often indicative of schizophrenia.

Motor Behavior Changes   Disruptions seen in schizophrenia include disorganized behavior and **catatonia.** Disorganized behavior lacks a coherent goal, is aimless, or is disruptive. Catatonic behavior is manifested by unusual body movement or lack of movement. This activity disturbance includes **catatonic excitement** (the client moves excitedly but not in response to environmental influences), **catatonic posturing** (the client holds bizarre postures for periods of time), and **stupor** (the client holds the body still and is unresponsive to the environment).

Changes in Role Functioning   An important factor in predicting the course of schizophrenia is the client's level of functioning before the symptoms of the disease became pronounced. Assessment should therefore include a complete history of the client's success at completing developmental tasks. The prognosis is best if the client functioned at a high level prior to the onset of schizophrenic disturbance. Assess how well the client fulfilled role responsibilities in the family, in school, in relation to peers, and in work. Obtain a history of the rate of decline in these various roles. The onset of schizophrenia may be relatively acute, or degeneration may be slow.

Drug Use   Clients with drug toxicity or withdrawal may present with behavior disturbances similar to those seen in schizophrenics. These clients may have auditory or visual hallucinations and may be confused, illogical, and highly anxious. For this reason, it is essential to obtain a detailed drug history. Assess both long-term and recent use of chemical substances. If the client is not a reliable historian, interview family or friends. In addition, both blood and urine should be tested for drugs if reliable information cannot be obtained.

Family Health History   Part of assessment is noting any history of mental illness in the client's family. Of particular interest is a history of schizophrenia or any thought disorder, mood disorders (e.g., cyclical highs or depressions), or alcoholism in any family member. Note any report that family members had "nervous breakdowns" or any other colloquial descriptions of mental or emotional disorders.

Family Cohesion and Emotion   A moderate level of family cohesion is optimal according to many family theorists. The two extremes—lack of cohesion (**disengagement**) and too much cohesion (**enmeshment**)—signify problems in family functioning. In families of schizophrenics, enmeshment, combined with a negative emotional tone, is thought to be detrimental to the ill member's well-being. Schizophrenics from overinvolved families who criticize the client have a high relapse rate (Chesla 1989).

Much of the nursing assessment of families can be carried out unobtrusively. Assess levels of cohesion by noting who accompanies the client during admission. Is it the whole family or just one member? Does the client come in alone? Visits from family are a rich

---

TABLE 12–2   Disturbances in Thought

Type	Definition	Example
Delusions of persecution	Belief that others are hostile or trying to harm the individual	A woman notices a man looking at her and believes that he is trying to follow her.
Delusions of reference	False belief that public events or people are directly related to the individual	A man hears a story on the evening news and believes it is about him.
Somatic delusions	Belief that one's body is altered from normal structure or function	An elderly woman believes that her bowel is filled with cement and refuses to eat.
Thought broadcasting	Belief that one's unspoken thoughts can be heard	A young client believes that everyone around him knows he's attracted to a nurse although he has said nothing.
Delusions of control	Belief that one's actions or thoughts are controlled by an external person or force	A woman believes that her neighbor controls her thoughts by means of his home computer.

source of information. Who visits, how often, and for how long? How do family visitors behave with the client? Do the members spend time interacting and sharing activities, do they sit quietly together, or do they maintain physical and emotional distance from one another? Document these patterns of family interactions and additionally monitor the effect of family visits on the client.

Formal family assessment interviews can be arranged by the nursing staff, in conjunction with the interdisciplinary team. In this forum, family history and current functioning can be completely assessed. Do not overlook natural opportunities to assess families and their needs. During visits, join the family for a few minutes to learn their understanding of the program, their concerns, and their questions. A trusting relationship with key members of the client's family is essential for establishing a flow of information and planning care.

Family Communication Problems Unclear or incomplete communication is frequent in families of schizophrenics. This area requires nursing assessment. Unclear communication may result from continual interaction with the ill member or may contribute to the illness. Although research on this issue is inconclusive, clinicians evaluate how effectively the family communicates to determine the potential need for intervention.

Assess these aspects of family communication: (a) ability to focus on a topic, (b) ability to discuss a topic in a meaningful way with other members, (c) ability to maintain the discussion without wandering from the subject or becoming distracted, and (d) use of language and explanations that are generally understandable, i.e., not peculiar to that family alone. In addition, note who in the family seems to do the talking, who talks to whom, and whether members talk for or interrupt one another.

Family Burden Most families of schizophrenics report that caring for the ill member places a burden on the family unit. Burdens reported most often are financial strains, disruption in family routines, worry about the future, and feeling overwhelmed or unable to cope. Additionally, families report these needs:

• Information about the disorder

• Information about how to manage day-to-day problems due to schizophrenic symptoms

• Support for family members in their roles as caregivers

See the accompanying Research Note.

Environmental Assessment Assess the availability of support and services beyond the bounds of the family, including extended family and friends, as well as community groups and organizations that support schizophrenic clients. Mental health programs that address the specific needs of schizophrenic clients should be sought.

Diagnosing

Nursing diagnoses with schizophrenic clients focus on alterations in the patterns of activity, cognition, emotion processes, interpersonal processes, and perception. Alterations in ecologic, physiologic, and valuation processes are assessed as well, but the central nursing problems relate to the former five processes.

Impaired Communication

Verbal Schizophrenic clients communicate in a disorganized, sometimes incomprehensible fashion. Clients with less severe disorganization skip from topic to topic, making few if any logical links. When more severe thought disorganization is present, the client's statements may be totally incoherent. Some clients manifest thought disorganization by speaking very little, a characteristic labeled **poverty of speech.** Also note poverty of content in speech, in which the client converses but says very little.

Often clients with schizophrenia communicate in ways that are overly concrete (a sign of an inability to think and communicate abstractly) or overly symbolic (a sign of preoccupation with unreal or delusional material). The symbols are usually difficult to decipher because their meanings are idiosyncratic.

Nonverbal In schizophrenic clients, facial and body expressions that accompany verbal communication frequently do not match the content of the verbal message. This lack of congruence is primarily due to the blunting of emotions found in schizophrenia. Expected facial expressions—e.g., smiles, looks of concern or disgust—may not accompany the schizophrenic's statements. In addition, clients with motor or behavioral abnormalities—e.g., posturing, unusual movements, or grimacing—convey a confusing mix of verbal and nonverbal messages.

Self-Care Deficits Persons with schizophrenia frequently appear indifferent to their personal appearance. They may neglect to bathe, change clothes, or attend to minor grooming tasks such as combing their hair. Some show little awareness of current fashion styles, wearing clothing that makes them look out of place. Of greater concern are those who wear clothing that is inappropriate to the current season and weather conditions.

Lack of attention to grooming might be a simple annoyance to those who must live in close proximity to the schizophrenic. Health risks related to prolonged

RESEARCH NOTE

Citation
Chafetz L, Barnes LE: Issues in psychiatric caregiving. Arch Psychiatr Nurs 1989;3:61–68.

Study Problem/Purpose
Because of the trend toward deinstitutionalization and the concomitant failure to develop adequate community support services for the chronically mentally ill, the family has become the primary caregiver for many adults with serious mental disorders. Ill family members often cannot meet the challenges of life in the community, and families find themselves providing housing, help with activities of daily living, and assistance with medical and social services. Family caregivers were surveyed about the problems that arose in care and the resources available to help with care.

Methods
Twenty caregivers of adults with schizophrenic (19) or bipolar (1) disorders were interviewed regarding: (a) the three most important problems they experienced in caregiving, (b) twenty-one problems in caregiving identified in the literature and (c) their ratings of the severity of the problems identified. The interview ended with an extended discussion of the three (of the twenty-four) problems caregivers rated as most severe. The sample consisted predominantly of parents of adult children with schizophrenia, although spouses and sibling caregivers were also represented. The convenience sample was recruited from community organizations and clinical services.

Findings
Most stressful to caregivers were problems having to do with the emotional or mental state of the family member. This included problems with ill members' symptoms as well as their depression and anger about the illness. It is noteworthy that caregivers were most concerned about the status of the ill member, rather than the tasks and time involved in giving care. Caregivers also rated these problems as highly stressful: fears about the future, the unpredictability of the person's illness, and relationship between the caregiver and the ill member.

Caregivers expressed a sense of loneliness or lack of understanding from others about their situation. Most frequently caregivers turned to family for support. Contact with other families who shared the experience of caring for a psychiatrically disabled member was also helpful. Despite support from these others, caregivers emphasized the need for self-reliance.

Implications
Working in mental health systems that are poor in resources, professionals often allocate the fewest resources to individuals with families or informal caregivers. This practice places at risk the caregiver who tries to support the psychiatrically disabled family member but feels isolated and misunderstood. By advocating for treatment programs that support the caregivers of the mentally ill, nurses can promote the well-being of both the psychiatrically disabled individual and the primary caregiver.

---

poor hygiene also arise. Assess immediate problems, e.g., inadequate nutrition, fluid intake, and elimination, as well as long-term problems, e.g., dental caries and increased susceptibility to infections.

Disregard for appearance and hygiene may extend to the schizophrenic's environment. The client may fail to maintain a clean and safe living space. The schizophrenic may not take good care of personal belongings and may misplace them. Self-care deficiencies may result from consistently disturbed thought and perceptual processes. For example, a young man whose chronic hallucinations are only partly relieved by medication has difficulty concentrating for long periods and therefore demonstrates variable attention to grooming.

Activity Intolerance   The emotional disturbances of ambivalence and apathy, common in schizophrenic disorders, can result in lack of interest and inactivity. Inactivity induced by ambivalence is associated with higher levels of emotion. Anxious about choosing one course of action and rejecting another, the client is immobilized. Jim, for example, is ambivalent about taking a pass out alone for the first time. He is undecided about taking the risk of leaving the hospital ward without a staff member yet yearns for the freedom of walking the streets alone. Indecision leaves him standing, immobilized, by the doorway to the unit.

Extreme ambivalence can manifest itself in even the most automatic of behaviors. Mary cannot eat because of ambivalence about where to sit or what to eat. She stands in the center of the dining room, turning first to one chair and then another, unable to choose and thus begin eating.

Clients who are inactive because of apathy demonstrate little emotional tone. Such a client may spend long hours lying in bed staring into space or listening to music. Often, but not always, apathetic individuals prefer isolation. The nurse might find several clients sitting in the same room, engaged in no apparent activities and interacting with one another only when absolutely necessary.

Social Isolation

Extreme anxiety about relating to others often leads schizophrenics to withdraw from interaction and to isolate themselves. Some clients tolerate only a few moments of direct communication, whereas others can manage extended periods of contact. Assess the client's tolerance of brief periods of contact with nurses and other clients. Document patterns of relating and withdrawal, also noting which activities the client engages in when in contact with others and when alone.

Decisional Conflict

Decisional conflict in schizophrenics is probably due to biochemical alterations in the brain that make it difficult for clients to take in, synthesize, and respond to information. Decisional conflict may be evident both in the mundane activities of daily life (e.g., selecting one's diet) and in major life decisions. One example is Murray, who refuses to take medications, even though not taking them means that he will be evicted from the residential treatment program he likes.

Sensory/Perceptual Alterations

Hallucinations   Hallucinations are both a clinical diagnostic sign of schizophrenia and a focus for nursing care. Nurses need to know the extent and nature of clients' hallucinations. Monitoring a client's hallucinations over time provides information on stressors that precipitate hallucinations, the client's response to psychotropic medications, and nursing actions that may diminish this symptom.

The nurse needs to document many aspects of the client's hallucinatory experience. Make note of situations or times of day that seem to trigger hallucinatory experiences. Record all sensory modes affected in the hallucination. The history of hallucinations and changes over time are important. Look for major

themes in the content of the hallucinations, particularly whether the hallucinations command the client to do something. The degree to which the client believes the experience is real and ability to verify the reality of the experience by checking with others have important implications for interventions. Note the client's emotional response to hallucinations; some clients experience depression or despair about the continued presence of voices. Clients' coping strategies, and their effectiveness or ineffectiveness, are also an important aspect of the diagnosis.

Illusions   Illusions—misperceptions of the environment—make the client vulnerable to emotional and physical injury. The level of misperception may vary from day to day and even throughout the day. Misperceptions of the social environment make the client vulnerable to inappropriate responses and therefore ridicule. Misperceptions of the physical environment, e.g., misjudging the speed of an oncoming car, may lead to physical harm.

Body Image Disturbance

A body image disturbance is common in schizophrenics. Clients may lose the sense of where their bodies leave off and where inanimate objects begin. They may become dissociated from various body parts and believe, for example, that their arms and legs belong to someone else. Schizophrenics may worry about the normalcy of their sexual organs. Clients often verbalize this altered sense of self straightforwardly, e.g., "I don't feel like myself" or "I feel like I am looking at my body from somewhere else in the room."

Altered Thought Processes

Delusions   Clients express delusional thinking in direct interactions and, to a lesser extent, through behaviors. When asked, many clients willingly describe their delusional beliefs in detail. They seldom withhold this information because they believe firmly in the validity of the delusion, no matter how bizarre it seems to others. Clients' actions reflect the fixedness of their beliefs.

Jerry has the somatic delusion that her body is riddled with holes. She flatly refuses to drink, convinced that the fluid will flow directly out of the holes and soil her dress.

The content of delusions varies, e.g., delusions of persecution, reference, and so on. (Review Table 12–2, earlier.) Reality-based delusions may seem plausible because they could, under some circumstances, actually occur. Bizarre delusions, more common among schizophrenics, have no possible basis in reality. The false belief that one's husband is having an affair with a neighbor is a reality-based delusion. In contrast, the belief that one's thoughts are directed by a television announcer or that one's unspoken thoughts can be heard by others are bizarre delusions.

Delusions often reflect the client's fears, particularly about personal inadequacies. For example, a man's grandiose delusion that he is the mayor of New York City is a defense against feelings of inferiority. Similarly, persecutory delusions defend against the person's own feelings of aggression. Aggressive feelings are projected onto a person or organization, e.g., the police, whom the client then fears.

Magical Thinking **Magical thinking** is the belief that events can happen simply because one wishes them to. Some schizophrenics claim they can exert will to make people take certain actions or make specific events occur, e.g., winning the lottery.

Thought Insertion, Withdrawal, and Broadcasting Hallmarks of schizophrenic thought are the beliefs that others can put ideas into one's head (**thought insertion**) or take thoughts out of one's head (**thought withdrawal**). In addition, some clients believe that their thoughts are transmitted to others via radio, television, or other means but not directly by the client. This belief is known as **thought broadcasting.**

Altered Emotional Responses*

Inappropriate Emotions Many schizophrenics demonstrate inappropriate affect—emotional responses that are inappropriate to the situation. For example, a client may smile or laugh while relating a history of having been abused as a child. Or, the client may become angry and anxious when asked to join a group of other clients for dinner. The degree to which a client's emotions are inappropriate is a prognostic indicator. Clients whose emotional response is preserved and generally appropriate have a more favorable prognosis than clients who demonstrate inappropriate affect.

A marked decrease in the variation or intensity of emotional expression is called **blunted affect.** The client may express joy, sorrow, or anger, but with little intensity. **Flat affect** is a total lack of emotional expression in verbal and nonverbal behavior. The client's face is impassive, and voice rate and tone are regular and monotonous.

Anhedonia **Anhedonia** is the inability to experience pleasure or to imagine a pleasurable emotion. This inability is very distressing to clients, who are aware of how they differ from other people. One young man lamented, "How can it be possible to feel so many awful things and *never* feel happy?"

Family Overinvolvement and Negativity*   At present there are no clear-cut clinical markers of what

constitutes overinvolvement and negative emotions in families. Research criteria, which are too complex to apply in clinical settings, have been developed to determine families at risk. Nurses should note families who seem excessively bonded emotionally. Family members' inability to maintain emotional, social, or physical separateness is a clear sign of this problem. Also assess a high level of criticism among family members. Discuss families that seem seriously enmeshed or hypercritical with the treatment team.

Altered Family Functioning*   Families burdened with the long-term responsibility of caring for a schizophrenic relative may suffer disruptions in their household routine, work, social interactions, and physical well-being. The household may be disrupted by the client's insistence that the family act on and accommodate delusional beliefs. The family may bend to the client's wish, fearing an increase in the client's anxiety and possible fighting or shouting if they do not comply. For example, one family built an extra bathroom rather than fight their schizophrenic son, who spends hours in the bath completing elaborate washing rituals. Another family must eat out several times each week because their schizophrenic daughter refuses to allow anyone in the room when she eats.

The family social life may be disrupted. For instance, the family may fear leaving the schizophrenic home alone or embarrassing the schizophrenic or visitors if friends are invited in. Some families are willing to be open about the adjustments they make in living with a schizophrenic, whereas others choose to live isolated lives.

Family members' work can suffer because of the emotional strain of living with a schizophrenic. Additionally, they must take time off to accompany the schizophrenic to doctors' appointments, make hospital visits, and help during interviews with social agencies or the police. Family health may suffer because of general inattention or because of prolonged stresses within the home.

Planning

When planning care for any client with a chronic illness, nurses must be careful to set realistic goals for client change. Particular care must be taken with schizophrenics because such clients are extremely sensitive to change and failure. Deterioration in all aspects of functioning is characteristic of the disease. Nurses must focus upon the most troublesome areas of client functioning and set incremental, short-term goals that pave the way for successes in achieving long-term goals.

---

*Not a currently approved NANDA diagnosis.

Text continues on p. 278

CASE STUDY

A Client with Schizophrenia, Paranoid Type

Identifying Information

Jim March is a 24-year-old single male who currently lives with his mother. He is unemployed and supports himself with SSI payments. Jim was brought up as a Catholic and attended Catholic schools through high school. He has sporadically attended the local community college, where he is attempting to complete an AA degree. He has not regularly attended school for two years. He currently attends a day treatment work program five times a week.

Dr. Taylor, Jim's private psychiatrist, referred Jim for admission. The evaluation is based upon the initial interview with Jim and his mother. Additional information is gained from a telephone call with Dr. Taylor and from a copy of Jim's day treatment record.

Client's Definition of Present Problem, Precipitating Stressors, Coping Strategies, Goals for Care

The client states, "My mom and the cops said I had to come here. She's the crazy one. I just want her to leave me alone!"

History of Present Problem

Jim's mother reports that for the past three weeks Jim has been increasingly isolated at home, refusing to come out of his room, to eat, or to talk. She hears him mumbling to himself in his room and knows he runs into the kitchen to eat when she is not around.

Jim's behavior is quite erratic. He unexpectedly leaves the house any time, including the middle of the night, to go to the nearby community college computer center. There, he insists on using a computer terminal to work on his "plan." Lacking an access number, he cannot get the terminal to work, and the staff at the center call the security guard to have him removed. Jim has been unwilling to discuss the "plan" with anyone except to imply that it will protect him from someone who is trying to attack him. This episode of attempting to use the community college computer has been repeated six times in the last few weeks. The police are threatening to cite Jim if he does not agree to in-patient treatment at this time.

Two stressors probably precipitated this episode. First, Jim got a notice from his work program that he would be let go if he was late for work three additional times. He immediately stopped attending the work program. At first, he spent his free time walking the streets in the neighborhood and eventually went out less and less.

Prior to this episode, Jim had established a year-long pattern of fairly regular attendance at work program, which demanded six hours of work in a local restaurant, washing dishes for the breakfast and lunch trade. He worked from 10:00 A.M. to 4:30 P.M. five days a week. When not at work, he spent time in his room listening to rock music or watching television. He had few friends, although he did stay in contact with a few members of the bimonthly medication group conducted at the community mental health center.

A second stressor was Jim's father's announcement of his plan to remarry. When Jim first heard the news, he offered congratulations. He has subsequently refused to talk with his father.

▶

CASE STUDY (continued)

Psychiatric History

At age 20, Jim was hospitalized at Saint Mary's Hospital for six weeks for evaluations of extreme withdrawal and talking to himself. His diagnosis was schizophreniform disorder. Jim was treated with fluphenazine (Prolixin), which had a positive effect on symptoms. The precipitating factor was probably his parents' separation.

At age 22, Jim was rehospitalized at Saint Mary's for evaluation of acting out behavior. Jim had failed all his course work in the community college and was making threatening statements toward his instructors. Hospitalization lasted four weeks. Jim was treated with thiothixene (Navane), with positive effects. He returned home and began attending the local day treatment program.

For the past two years, Jim has been seeing a private psychiatrist for medication management and has attended programs at the community mental health center. He regularly attended day treatment for one year.

Family History

Jim's parents are both living and well. They were separated four years ago and divorced within nine months of the separation. Jim's father is an attorney, and his mother works part time in a stationery store. There are no other children. Jim lives with his mother, and this arrangement is acceptable to both of them. He sees his father once a month and on holidays and special celebrations, such as birthdays.

Social History

Developmental History

Pregnancy, delivery, childhood, and early adolescence were unremarkable, with developmental tasks completed at the expected times. Jim's mother recalls that Jim was always physically active and skilled. Although he was never extremely popular, he always had one or two good friends, both male and female. He dated casually but never developed an intimate relationship with a woman.

Jim began to pull away from friends when he started community college. He claimed to have difficulty keeping up with course work and thus dropped out of most evening and weekend activities. Since his first hospitalization, he has vehemently refused to contact any of his old high school friends. The only people he sees socially are those whom he's met in day treatment or the work program.

Education

Jim's high school performance was average or above average. He went on to community college, intending to get a degree in computer science. Beginning with his first quarter, he received barely passing grades and was asked to leave the program in his second year.

Habits

Jim smokes one pack of cigarettes per day and drinks occasionally, primarily beer. He denies any drug use, past or present, and his mother confirms this report.

Hobbies

Jim has always had a keen interest in computers. In high school, he took elective courses that introduced him to computer uses. Other hobbies in high school were co-rec basketball and track. He never tried out for a competitive team. As his interest in friends has waned, Jim has become increasingly intent on music and on increasing his music library. For the past two years, he has spent nearly all his free time listening to records or watching television rock video programs.

▶

CASE STUDY (continued)

Significant Health History

Jim has no notable medical problems. He has no known allergies, and he has never had a negative reaction to psychotropic medications.

Current Mental Status

General Appearance

Jim is a young-looking, 24-year-old white male who is quite anxious and guarded but cooperative during the interview. He is dressed in jeans and sweatshirt, and his hair is slightly unkempt.

Sensorium

Jim is alert and oriented to person, time, and place. He demonstrates an adequate fund of knowledge and can name past presidents through Kennedy. Memory and recall are good. He calculates serial sevens slowly but correctly to 58. His judgment is marginally impaired: He reports that if he found a signed blank check on the street he would put it in the church collection.

Feelings

Jim's affect is anxious, and his mood is angry.

Speech

Jim's speech is rapid, pressured, and tangential. He frequently interrupts the interviewer to ask questions about the hospital rules and treatment.

Motor Behavior

Jim sits holding himself rigidly in the chair, kicking his foot continuously throughout the interview. He gets up to examine things in the room and to ask about them as well as to peer suspiciously out the window.

Thought Content

Jim describes delusions of persecution and has a grandiose belief that his "plan" will ward off danger. He will not elaborate about the plan but insists that he needs access to a computer terminal while in the hospital. He admits to hearing voices for the past several weeks. It is through the hallucinations that he has become convinced that someone is trying to harm him. Occasionally he hears his father's voice, which is extremely frightening to him. He denies suicidal or homicidal ideation.

Thought Process

Some loosening of associations is evident. When asked about special eating habits, he relates a story about a religious sister he had run into recently. Abstractions are concrete and self-referential. When asked the meaning of "People who live in glass houses shouldn't throw stones," he responds, "If I threw a rock through that window, I'd get cut."

Insight

Jim believes that this hospitalization is a ruse by the police and his mother to keep him out of his room for a week. In this way, progress on his "plan" will be held up, and his mother will be able to clean his room. He is cooperative with admission but insists on a private room.

Diagnostic Impression

Nursing Diagnoses

Anxiety
Altered thought process
Noncompliance (with hospitalization)
Self-care deficit: Feeding
Impaired social interaction
Diversional activity deficit

▶

CASE STUDY *(continued)*

DSM-III-R Multiaxial Diagnosis	Axis I: 295.34 Schizophrenia, paranoid type, chronic with acute exacerbation Axis II: 799.90 Deferred Axis III: No physical disorder at this time Axis IV: Psychosocial stressors: 3, Moderate, acute (fired from part-time job that he held for the past year); 3, Moderate, enduring (father announced plans to remarry) Axis V: Current GAF: 30 Highest GAF in the past year: 40

NURSING CARE PLAN

Client Care Goals	Nursing Planning/ Intervention	Evaluation
Nursing Diagnosis: *Anxiety*		
Jim will be comfortable in the milieu.	Give Jim a private room. Approach Jim with clear warning. Make brief (ten-minute) contacts with Jim. Provide private time in room to decrease anxiety.	Jim reports feeling safe in the milieu.
Nursing Diagnosis: *Altered thought processes*		
Jim will show less preoccupation with threats to his safety.	Reassure Jim of safety on the unit. Avoid contradicting Jim's delusions. Redirect Jim to discussion of other topics, e.g., music. Give Jim prescribed medication.	Jim is able to carry on a conversation with the nurse without bringing up topic of threats.
Nursing Diagnosis: *Noncompliance (with hospitalization)*		
Jim will not escape from the unit and will abide by unit rules regarding the use of passes.	Establish a contract to remain on unit with Jim. Observe Jim closely during periods of increased stress. Help Jim engage in quiet activity when he feels less in control of his impulse to leave. Use p.r.n. medications as needed. Secure unit as needed.	Jim stays on unit except for planned outings with staff.

▶

NURSING CARE PLAN *(continued)*

Client Care Goals	Nursing Planning/ Intervention	Evaluation
Nursing Diagnosis: *Self-care deficit: Feeding*		
Jim will maintain adequate intake of food and fluids.	Allow Jim maximum control over his choice of foods.	Jim eats at least one-half of all meals and drinks a minimum of 2000 mL per day.
	Have Jim eat in a private area to decrease anxiety.	
	Serve foods in their original containers to decrease Jim's fears of tampering.	
	Provide fluids frequently throughout the day.	
Nursing Diagnosis: *Impaired social interaction*		
Jim will participate in all unit activities.	Establish a schedule of daily activities.	Jim participates in all daily activity included in his schedule.
	Allow quiet time alone in room.	
	Prompt Jim to attend activities at scheduled times.	
	Praise Jim's attempts to follow through with schedule.	
Nursing Diagnosis: *Diversional activity deficit*		
Jim will use free time constructively.	Explore Jim's preferred hobbies.	Jim works on hobbies or socializes with other clients during free time.
	Help Jim gain access to materials needed, e.g., records.	
	Work with Jim during unstructured times to begin hobby or interaction.	
	Observe Jim's ability to pursue the activity and provide continued guidance if needed.	

Jean May is a 50-year-old single woman diagnosed with schizophrenia, undifferentiated type. For the past seven years she has lived in a skilled nursing facility because of her extreme regression and inability to care for herself. The nursing home is changing acceptance criteria and will no longer care for clients with a primary psychiatric diagnosis. She is admitted for evaluation of her medications and for alternative placement.

Jean manages none of her own personal cares. Aides in the nursing home have bathed and dressed her, asking only that Jean brush her own teeth. She hasn't made her bed or cleaned up her own living space for years. She can, however, feed herself.

- Short-term goals: Jean will participate in her own care by helping the nurse decide what Jean will wear and by helping the nurse draw the bath. Jean will help the nurse clean up the bedroom.
- Intermediate goal: Jean will manage her personal care needs and clean her room with only verbal direction from the nurse.
- Long-term goal: Jean will independently manage her personal grooming and cleaning responsibilities in the unit.

Client goals are tailored to each person's specific needs and strengths. As the client's status changes during the course of treatment, nursing goals are altered to reflect these changes. The accompanying Intervention boxes list a sampling of nursing goals appropriate to specific problems of schizophrenic clients.

Implementing Interventions

Promoting Adequate Communication   Clients with schizophrenia try to communicate, even though their statements may be hard to understand. Close attention to what the client is saying and honest attempts to understand the real and symbolic aspects of the message are important. The client perceives nuances of the nurse's behavior. Therefore, one of the most direct and successful ways to demonstrate caring and respect is to attend seriously to the client.

Clients make valid observations about their environment, needs, and concerns. A client may make observations about events or situations that are beyond the nurse's awareness. For example, take seriously a client's communications about another client's drug use or suicidal threats. If a client complains of a physical symptom such as stomach distress, consider the symptom as real until there is evidence otherwise. It is easy to dismiss a client's statements, particularly those of a delusional client. Doing so, however, shows

INTERVENTION

Planning Care for the Client with Disorganized Behavior

Goal	Intervention
Will participate in goal-directed activity	Approach client in a calm manner.
Will complete tasks that are begun	Discuss basic behavioral expectations.
	Assess the client's preferred activities.
	Verbally guide clients step by step through essential activities.
	Provide prescribed psychotropic medication.
	Move client to a quiet environment.

INTERVENTION

Planning Care for the Client with Hallucinations

Goal	Intervention
Will demonstrate no signs of attending to internal stimuli	Monitor client for signs of attending to internal stimuli and observe for precipitating stressors.
Will identify stressors that precipitate hallucinations	Discuss your observations with the client: "You appear to be listening to something."
	Make brief, frequent contacts with the client to interrupt the hallucinatory cycle and to maintain trust.
	Encourage the client to attend to stimuli in the environment, such as conversations, rather than to internal stimuli.
	Help the client in activities that require cognitive or verbal involvement, e.g., playing cards, walking and talking with nurse.
	Support coping strategies that the client has identified as personally effective in reducing hallucinations.
	If needed, teach the client that the hallucinations are part of the disease process.
	Help the client monitor events or interactions that increase the hallucinations.
	Protect the client and others who might be harmed by the client's acting on hallucinated commands.

lack of respect for the client's intact capacities to see and respond to what is happening in the environment.

Promoting Compliance with Medical Regimen   Psychotropic medications play an important part in the treatment of schizophrenic disorders. Drugs

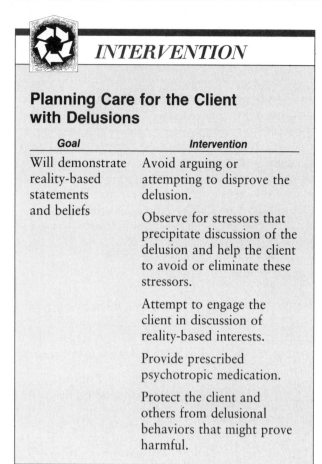

INTERVENTION

Planning Care for the Client with Delusions

Goal	Intervention
Will demonstrate reality-based statements and beliefs	Avoid arguing or attempting to disprove the delusion.
	Observe for stressors that precipitate discussion of the delusion and help the client to avoid or eliminate these stressors.
	Attempt to engage the client in discussion of reality-based interests.
	Provide prescribed psychotropic medication.
	Protect the client and others from delusional behaviors that might prove harmful.

that diminish focal symptoms (e.g., hallucinations and delusions) and yet produce relatively few untoward effects are now available. The nurse must recognize, however, that each individual responds to medications differently.

These interventions are nursing responsibilities:

• Administer prescribed medication.

• Observe client behavior for therapeutic effects.

• Monitor side effects of the medications.

• Teach the client about the therapeutic and possible untoward effects of the medications prescribed.

• Help the client take action to prevent untoward effects, e.g., maintaining fluid intake to avoid postural hypotension.

• Evaluate the client's subjective response to the medication and attitude toward continued use.

Consistent compliance in taking medications as prescribed is not common among this client population. Researchers estimate that as few as 68 percent of psychiatric clients adhere to medication regimens while in the hospital. When these clients return to the community, 37 percent or fewer adhere to drug regimens. Clients may stop taking their medications for these reasons:

• They don't understand the administration instructions.

• They are too disorganized to follow the instructions.

• The side effects of major tranquilizers are too uncomfortable.

• They do not wish to be stigmatized as having schizophrenia and therefore reject treatment.

Schizophrenics who do not take medications are more vulnerable to stressors and risk more frequent relapse of symptoms than those who comply with medication regimens. Efforts to educate clients about their medications and to have them practice self-medication prior to discharge have increased the rate of compliance only marginally. Clearly, such factors as clients' attitudes toward the medications prescribed also influence their willingness to take medications. The nurse is an active participant in assessing compliance and fostering a positive attitude toward medications.

Clients are often ambivalent about taking medications. Maintaining adequate blood levels of therapeutic medications is important for the schizophrenic. To help clients overcome ambivalence, give them time to think about taking the medications. If the client is unable to act within a few minutes, setting a time limit may spur the client to decide to take it. If not, leave and come back later to offer the medications. Two useful strategies are reminding clients of the positive effects of the medication and framing the action as a way for clients to help themselves get better.

Assisting with Grooming and Hygiene Helping clients to establish and maintain personal care habits is a complex process. If the client clearly lacks the skills, then the emphasis is on teaching these skills. If, however, the client has learned grooming skills but does not practice them, the nurse focuses on ways to motivate the client. Intervention begins by establishing clear expectations in regard to essential grooming habits. The frequency and timing of all aspects of grooming—including bathing, dressing, hair care, oral hygiene, and room care—should be specified in writing.

Formal training programs for helping chronically mentally ill clients improve their grooming skills can be applied in in-patient settings. These programs are well developed and tested (Wong et al. 1988). These programs take a systematic approach to helping clients in all steps of personal grooming. These steps include collecting grooming supplies, moving to the grooming area (a bathroom or bedroom with sink and mirror), completing each grooming step, completing appropriate dressing, and storing grooming materials. Nursing interventions at each step can progress from simple verbal coaching, to modeling, to gentle physical guidance. Client efforts during each phase and successful completion of each phase of grooming should be praised. The success of these programs probably depends on daily staff attention to the client's training, and consistent, meaningful rewards.

Avoid power struggles regarding completion of tasks. If initial prompts don't work, leave the client alone for a short period. Praise any effort by the client to meet personal care needs.

Promoting Organized Behavior   Clients whose behavior is disorganized require direction and limits to make their actions more effective and goal directed. The first rule of working with a disorganized client is to go slowly and keep calm. The client's perception of the environment may be distorted, but the nurse's calmness can help to calm the client. The nurse tries to direct the client in simple, safe activities.

Examples of nursing goals and interventions for a disorganized client are given in the Intervention box on page 279. A case example of one such intervention follows.

George is moving quickly yet aimlessly from the refrigerator to the cupboard. He pulls a box of cereal from the cupboard, opens it, and then wanders away. Next he goes to the refrigerator, opens the door, peers in, and closes the door. Rummaging through all his pockets, he locates a cigarette, lights it, places it in an ashtray, and wanders back to the cupboard. This effortful yet unproductive behavior continues for several minutes when the nurse enters.

Nurse: George, are you trying to get yourself some cereal?

George: Sort of. I was going to . . . smoke . . . no . . . eat something. Yeah, I wanted something to eat.

Nurse: Try to concentrate on one thing. First put out the cigarette. (He does so.) Now, come over here and get the cereal box. Here's a bowl. Here's a spoon. (She hands him the utensils.) Why don't you sit right here? (She seats him so that he has his back to the rest of the activity in the room.) Can you sit still for a bit?

George: I think so.

Nurse: Pour yourself some cereal. I'll get the milk for you. (She does so.)

George begins to eat his cereal quietly. The nurse stays with him for a few minutes and directs him to continue eating when he becomes distracted by others who come into the room.

Promoting Social Interaction and Activity   The client's efforts to withdraw from social contact stem from past relationship failures and fear of rejection.

Clients often find their internal world less risky and therefore more attractive than a world that requires interpersonal relating. When making efforts to help the client become less withdrawn, the nurse must respect the client's overwhelming anxiety about human contact.

After establishing a basic level of trust, encourage the client to try out new behaviors within the relationship. The goal is to have the client experience success, and thus small increments of change should be encouraged. If, for example, the client has difficulty initiating conversation, encourage the client to practice this skill once a day. Similarly, if the client avoids any activity in the milieu because of fear of relating to groups, structure an activity involving the client, the nurse, and one other client.

Social Skills Training **Social skills training** is well accomplished in groups of clients (Plante 1989). Small groups provide structure and support as the nurse coaches clients in simple yet essential social interactions. It is best to form groups of clients who function at similar levels. Provide structure by clearly setting times for group meetings, beginning and ending each session with a statement of goals, and recapping what the group has accomplished. Address social skills that are essential to functioning in the milieu: introducing oneself, starting a conversation, ending a conversation, saying no, asking for assistance, and listening. Staff can model these skills and help clients to role play each skill. Focus discussion on situations in which clients might need the skill. If they see its applicability to dilemmas in their personal lives, they will be motivated to learn the skill. Praise and, if available, material rewards can also motivate clients.

Schizophrenia can disturb the person's will and capacity to accomplish meaningful activity. Clients with distorted perceptions and thinking expend considerable energy merely taking in and interpreting their immediate worlds. In addition, major tranquilizers, which control the positive symptoms of the disease, can further inhibit a client's active involvement and interest in activities. Nurses must be aware of how much work it takes to cope with schizophrenic symptoms. Do not assume periods of quiet or inactivity are due to laziness or lack of interest. Rather, assess each individual's need for quiet periods in which to organize perceptions and thoughts.

At the same time, clients with schizophrenia live in a culture in which action and accomplishment are highly prized and rewarded. They are not immune to the press for personal productivity as a measure of personal worth. For this reason, they feel better about themselves when they are involved in meaningful activities. The nurse's task is to help clients find activities that are intrinsically rewarding or bring some social or tangible reward yet are within their capacities.

Learning clients' personal interests is a first step. Providing opportunities for the client to actively engage in an activity of interest, e.g., by providing records, books, craft materials, or access to newspapers and television, is the next intervention. In addition, activities within the milieu, such as attending groups and completing unit "jobs," can provide the external rewards of praise from staff and peers. These activities give clients confidence and develop their work habits. Success in these activities can lead to success in volunteer or paid work in the community after discharge.

Promoting Reality-Based Perceptions   Illusions or hallucinations often frighten clients. Nurses can intervene by

- Reassuring clients of their safety

- Protecting them from physical harm as they respond to their altered perceptions

- Validating reality

- Helping clients to distinguish reality from the hallucinatory experience

Some specific nursing actions to help clients who are actively hallucinating are listed in the Intervention box on page 279. General approaches to working with clients with altered perceptions are highlighted below.

Hallucinations are especially frightening if the client has never experienced them before or if their content is threatening or angry. Attempt to alleviate this anxiety by describing your perception of the frightened behavior and asking clients to discuss what they are experiencing. Make simple reassuring remarks, e.g., "I know the voices are real to you, but no one else can hear them. No one means to harm you."

Protect the client from harm and reassure the client about safety. The client may take impulsive action to escape the frightening experience or to obey voices in the hallucination. Prevent this by:

- Closely observing client behavior during active hallucinations

- Intervening quickly by giving additional doses of psychotropic medications or placing the client in a quiet room

- If necessary, securing the unit so that the client cannot leave and take self-destructive or impulsive action

Make every effort to help the client attend to real rather than internal stimuli, orient the client to the real situation, and encourage the client to focus on the nurse rather than on the hallucination. "George, listen to me rather than to the sounds you say you hear.

Remember, you are in the hospital and I am your nurse. I will help you find your shoes. Come with me." Active involvement in some activity, e.g., finding shoes, helps the client to maintain a focus on real events and perceptions.

Intervening with Delusions   General guidelines for working with delusional individuals are not to argue with their false beliefs, to focus on the reality-based aspects of their communications, and to protect them from acting on their delusions in a way that might harm themselves or others. See the Intervention box on page 280 for suggested nursing interventions with delusional clients.

Promoting Congruent Emotional Responses
Working with clients who display blunted or flat affect can be confusing for nurses who are accustomed to reading emotional responses that fall within a more normal range. Be aware that these clients have feelings about events around them, including their interaction with the nurse, yet have difficulty expressing them.

Note lack of congruence between the person's affect and the content of the message. If the relationship between the nurse and client is well established, then the nurse might comment on the incongruity and explore it with the client. ("George, what you are telling me is sad but you are laughing. What shall I pay attention to?") Modeling clear, congruent communications is helpful. Little can be done to change the client's anhedonia, yet empathic listening might comfort the client.

Ambivalence, the simultaneous experience of contradictory feelings about a person, object, or action, can trouble schizophrenic clients. Ambivalence can become great enough to immobilize the client. Such clients cannot express one emotion or the other, or choose one action over the other. The nurse may partially alleviate the client's unease by identifying aloud the emotions the client may be experiencing. ("John, I think you might be feeling both very happy to see your father and at the same time very angry.") Naming the conflicting emotions gives the client the opportunity to talk about them, although many times he or she may not be able to do so.

Immobility due to ambivalence is extremely uncomfortable. One way of intervening is to limit the number of choices that the indecisive client has to make. For example, a man may be immobilized by his inability to decide whether to go out alone for the first time. The nurse can help by telling him that it seems too soon for him to go out alone and that, for today, he must be accompanied. Another example is a young woman who is undecided about where to sit. The nurse can remove extra chairs at the table in the dining room so that she has only one choice.

Promoting Family Understanding and Involvement When a schizophrenic is hospitalized, the nurse should encourage the family and help them to remain involved in the client's care. Except in unusual circumstances, share information on the client's status, treatment program, and future treatment plans, including discharge plans. Of course, nurses need to comply with the client's wishes and with the laws governing disclosure of information, which vary by state and by institution.

Some mental health professionals have a bias against family involvement. This bias is a remnant of now-discredited theories that family interaction patterns cause schizophrenia. Nurses may need to be active advocates for families' rights to information about, and involvement in, the care of the schizophrenic member. This question is a useful way to check one's bias against the family's rights: Am I responding to this family any differently than I would to the family of a client with a medical condition? The family who has cared for the client with schizophrenia over a period of years has in-depth understandings of the client's illness, history, and ability to function in the community. Include the family's insights in the assessment phase, and, if appropriate, use them in the planning of care, particularly care after discharge (Chesla 1989).

If assessment suggests the family needs information about the disease and treatment, refer the family to education programs, if they are available. Family psychoeducation programs are preferable to direct teaching because they often combine education with mutual support. In such groups, families can meet others who share their life difficulties. These peers can provide informal support and information to help the family deal with the tasks that lie ahead. Nurses can reinforce the formal teaching that occurs in such programs when they meet with individual families.

Without exception, families should know about a national family support group with many local and state affiliates. The **Alliance for the Mentally Ill** serves families through educational programs, local support groups, and political activism. Most local organizations are listed in telephone directories or can be reached through the local community mental health agency responsible for information and referral.

Promoting Community Contacts Awareness of clients' community supports and potential treatment programs guides nurses in preparing clients for discharge. For example, the client's most important peer support group might be the clientele at a local day treatment program. If so, several visits to the program prior to discharge will help the client make the transition back to the community.

Preparing clients for the residence they will enter after hospital discharge is a central nursing task.

Often, placement depends on how the client functions in the hospital. If the client is able to manage medications, participate in a variety of groups, and live cooperatively with other clients, then placement in a residential care facility that supports independent functioning is appropriate. In contrast, clients who need assistance with structuring free time, resist taking medications, or cannot take on responsibilities for self-care require a more structured environment.

Nurses work with clients to help them achieve their highest level of functioning. They document clients' abilities to perform various tasks and make recommendations to the treatment team about appropriate placements.

Evaluating/Outcome Criteria

To complete the nursing process, nurses evaluate changes in client status and behavior in response to nursing interventions. Evaluation criteria are linked to nursing goals and reflect an understanding of the limitations of schizophrenic clients.

Communication: Outcome Criteria Clients will, with greater regularity, express their thoughts clearly and congruently. They will feel sufficient trust to talk to the nurse about troublesome symptoms or experiences.

Self Care: Outcome Criteria Clients will consistently appear clean and well groomed and will independently manage personal grooming and hygiene. Clients will have clean and reasonably appropriate clothes, both in terms of fashion and season.

Activity Intolerances: Outcome Criteria Clients will participate in goal-directed activities with minimal intervention. Clients will complete the activities they begin.

Social Isolation: Outcome Criteria Clients will demonstrate the capacity to interact, for at least brief periods, with nursing staff, with other clients, and in small groups. They will consistently demonstrate socially required interactions, such as greeting and starting a conversation with a stranger, asking for assistance, saying no, and listening to another's conversation. Clients will be inactive for shorter periods and spend more time engaged in interesting or meaningful activity.

Sensory/Perceptual Alterations: Outcome Criteria Clients will have fewer episodes of attending to internal stimuli. If hallucinations persist, clients will begin to identify stressors or situations that precipitate them. Clients will identify and practice personal coping strategies that decrease the hallucination or its effects, e.g., going to a quiet room, engaging in social activities, and performing activities that demand concentration.

Thought Processes: Outcome Criteria   Clients will engage in reality-based discussions. If delusions persist, clients will not act on delusions in ways that are harmful or detrimental to themselves or others.

Emotional Responses: Outcome Criteria   Clients will have increased awareness that their emotional expressions at times do not match their verbal communications. Clients will experience fewer episodes of extreme discomfort due to ambivalence about people, events, or actions.

Family Functioning: Outcome Criteria   Families will be involved in all aspects of the clients' care, including assessment, planning interventions, in-patient treatment choices, and planning for discharge. Families' personal understandings of the illness trajectory and the clients' capacities and limits will improve. The families' difficulties with caring for clients will be considered in treatment and discharge planning, and adequate resources will be identified to support family needs.

Chapter Highlights

• Persons with schizophrenia experience disturbances in perception, thought, affect, and activity.

• The biologic, psychologic, and family theories of schizophrenia can be largely incorporated into one interactional model of the disorder.

• Care of schizophrenic clients requires an awareness of the client's multiple functional deficits and of the nurse's personal response to working with this population.

• Nursing assessment of individual problems in schizophrenia focuses on changes in clients' perceptions, thoughts, expressions, and role functioning.

• Nursing assessment of family problems in schizophrenia focuses on family communication, cohesiveness, emotions, and burdens.

• Nursing diagnoses for clients with schizophrenia identify the communication, conduct, judgment, perceptual, and emotional alterations commonly found in this disorder.

• Nursing planning for clients with schizophrenia involves setting realistic goals and continually reevaluating expectations based on clients' current status.

• Nursing interventions promote adequate communication, compliance with medical regimen, activity, social interaction, grooming, and perception in clients with schizophrenia.

• Nurses evaluate the effectiveness of their interventions with individual schizophrenic clients and their families.

References

Chesla CA: Mental illness and the family, in Gilliss CL et al. (eds): *Toward a Science of Family Nursing*. Addison-Wesley, 1989.

Gerace L: Schizophrenia and the family: Nursing implications. *Arch Psychiatr Nurs* 1988;2:141–145.

Liberman RP et al.: The nature and problem of schizophrenia, in Bellak AS (ed): *Schizophrenia: Treatment Management and Rehabilitation*. Grune & Stratton, 1984.

Plante TG: Social skills training: A program to help schizophrenic clients cope. *J Psychosoc Nurs* 1989; 27:7–10.

Schulz SC, Tamminga CA (eds): *Schizophrenia: Scientific Progress*. Oxford University Press, 1989.

Selzer MA et al.: *Working with Persons with Schizophrenia: The Treatment Alliance*. New York University Press, 1989.

Strome TM: Schizophrenia in the elderly: What nurses need to know. *Arch Psychiatr Nurs* 1989;3:47–52.

Walsh ME: *Schizophrenia, Straight Talk for Families and Friends*. Warner, 1985.

Wilson CA: Perspectives on the hallucinatory process. *Issues Ment Health Nurs* 1989;10:99–119.

Wong SE et al.: Training chronic mental patients to independently practice personal grooming skills. *Hosp Community Psychiatry* 1988;39:874–879.

Nutrition Box References

Bell I: Effects of food allergy on the central nervous system, in Brostoff J, Challacombe S: *Food Allergy and Intolerance*. London: Bailliere Tindall, 1987, p. 710.

Breneman JC: *Basics of Food Allergy*, ed 2. Springfield, Ill.: Charles C. Thomas, 1984, pp. 212–255.

Crayton JW: Adverse reactions to foods: Relevance to psychiatric disorders. *J Allergy Clin Immunol* 1986;78(Suppl 1, Pt 2):244.

Crayton JW: Effects of food challenges on complement in "food sensitive" psychiatric patients. *J Allergy Clin Immunol* 1984;73(Suppl Pt 2):134.

Dohan F et al.: Is schizophrenia rare if grain is rare? *Biol Psychiatry* 1984;19(3):385–399.

King D: Statistical power of the controlled research on wheat gluten and schizophrenia. *Biol Psychiatry* 1985;20: 785–787.

Krause M, Mahan L: *Food, Nutrition, and Diet Therapy*. Philadelphia: Saunders, 1984.

Pearson DJ, Rix KJ: Food allergy: How much in the mind? A clinical and psychiatric study of suspected food hypersensitivity. *Lancet* 1983;2:1259–1261.

Vlissides D et al.: A double-blind gluten-free/gluten-load controlled trial in a secure ward population. *Br J Psychiatry* 1986;148:447–452.

Applying the Nursing Process for Clients with Mood Disorders

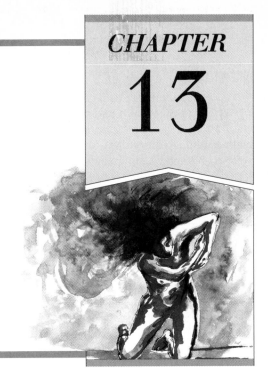

CHAPTER

13

Maxine E. Loomis

LEARNING OBJECTIVES

- Identify and discuss the early development and personality characteristics of persons with mood disorders

- Compare and contrast the behavioral manifestations of a manic episode, a major depressive episode, and dysthymia

- Describe and discuss application of the nursing process in working with persons with mood disorders

- Identify key elements in the human response patterns of persons with mood disorders

- Plan, implement, and evaluate nursing intervention designed specifically for persons with mood disorders

CROSS REFERENCES

Other topics related to this chapter are: Biologic therapies, Chapter 32; Psychobiology, Chapter 6; Suicide, Chapter 23.

THE MOOD DISORDERS ARE a group of psychiatric diagnoses characterized by disturbances in emotional and behavioral response patterns. These patterns range from extreme elation and agitation to extreme depression and a serious potential for suicide. Accurate assessment, diagnosis, intervention, and evaluation by psychiatric nurses are essential in helping clients with mood disorders attain a more comfortable, safe, and productive life.

Ron is a 47-year-old high school football coach whose wife brought him to the emergency room because he was unable to sleep, had not eaten in a week, and was keeping their family awake nights playing game films on their VCR at full volume. He had spent the previous day shouting obscenities from his bedroom window at passersby. He was combative and argumentative with the emergency room staff and had to be restrained prior to admission to the in-patient psychiatric unit.

Marcia is a very bright, poised, articulate, and engaging executive in the pharmaceutical industry whose mood has vacillated between excitement and total lack of energy since she was passed over for promotion six months ago. Marcia, age 32, decided to seek help from a private psychiatric outpatient clinic because she feared "losing control" of her behavior and emotions.

Ann, a 45-year-old secretary, asked for help at a community crisis clinic because she had been preoccupied with thoughts of killing herself. She said she had no friends and no time for fun because of the demands of her job.

Historical and Theoretic Foundations

Bipolar Disorders

The bipolar disorders are mood disorders characterized by episodes of **mania** and **depression.** Either mania or depression may be evident at any given time, elements of both may be present simultaneously, or symptoms of one may alternate with symptoms of the other. The manic phase is characterized by hyperactivity, excitement, agitation, euphoria, excessive energy, decreased need for sleep, and impaired ability to concentrate or complete a single train of thought. The depressive phase is characterized by underactivity, marked apathy, profound sadness, guilt, and lowered self-esteem. Bipolar disorders are referred to as **manic-depressive disorders** in some clinical settings.

Early Development   In clinical practice, the nurse sees a fair number of manic-depressive people who have been exposed to inconsistent or abusive parenting. Such parenting often takes the form of alternating periods of nurturing and unpredictable periods of anger or neglect that seem unrelated to the child's behavior. The youngster reacts to the unpredictable nurturing with elation and to the periodic abandonment and abuse with withdrawal and depression. In adult life, these extremes are repeated as the person experiences "unexplainable" cyclic highs and lows.

Arieti (1974) describes another common parenting experience that leads to development of bipolar personality. Initially, the parents accept and care for the child, and the child is receptive to parenting. At some point, however (and usually between 3 months to 5 years of age), a withdrawal of nurturance occurs. This withdrawal can be either physical—e.g., the sudden departure, illness, or death of a parent—or psychologic—e.g., preoccupation with a family problem, the mother's return to work, or the birth of a sibling who draws attention away from the older child. This sudden withdrawal of nurturance can lead to one of the three following responses.

Overadapted Response   Arieti (1974, p 465) describes the first type of bipolar adaptation to this type of parenting as that of "finding security by accepting parental expectations, no matter how onerous they are." The result is a well-behaved child and, later, a dedicated adult motivated by responsibility and with a high level of investment in doing things well. The important activities of life and the criteria for success are externally defined. The person later relives the experience of a withholding or depriving parent by attaching to a "dominant other" or by dedication to a profession, social cause, church, or some other social institution. The promise of nurturing and the disappointment of deprivation are repeatedly reenacted in these attachments.

Passive-Dependent Response   A second type of bipolar adaptation is more directly and obviously passive-dependent. Instead of adapting by doing things well, the youngster attempts to reengage parents and, later, parent figures by being a helpless baby. At times, people who adopt this response present themselves as inept and incapable of managing their lives. They demand attention and expect to be taken care of by others. They often empower others as responsible for their happiness or unhappiness, success, or failure.

Characterologic Response   Arieti's third bipolar personality type establishes characterologic defenses as a result of deciding not to incorporate or identify with the original parents. The youngster may attempt to identify with other adults or childhood heroes but forms no meaningful attachments. The result is an adult who has difficulty establishing permanent relationships and has few internalized values. This person is actively involved in doing things and may move from one successful, shady business to another. The purpose of all this activity is to escape from self-examination and to avoid closeness with others.

Personality Structure   The personality structure of persons with bipolar disorders is built on this foundation:

- A grandiose approach to thinking, feeling, and behaving

- Development of a fantasized nurturing parent

Regardless of the specific details of their early development, people with bipolar disorders appear to share a common set of personality characteristics.

Grandiosity   Grandiosity with respect to feeling, thinking, and behaving is a hallmark of the bipolar personality structure. Because of the competitive frame of reference and the emphasis on doing things within the parent-infant interaction, nurturing is not experienced as safe or comforting. Within the competitive frame of reference, the parent must win and do things right, resulting in a style of caretaking in which the parent sets the pace and discounts or defines the child's feelings and needs. Holding and feeding are the earliest parent-infant contacts, and here the competition begins about who will set the pace and win control. As a result, the infant experiences agitation or a lack of synchrony during nurturing as parent and child compete to get their needs met.

Parents in these families model inconsistency and agitation. The child experiences parenting that is alternately very good and very bad. Thus, the child must develop a structure that allows for drastic swings, and the self is experienced as either very good or very bad. Denial is the defense that allows the child to tolerate this discrepancy. The child uses denial to separate the experiences of being either very good or very bad and never integrates or realistically resolves the "good" and "bad" selves. A great deal of energy is needed to maintain the denial that keeps the two experiences separate. Denial allows a grandiose or exaggerated approach to feelings. For example, when these people are manic, they may deny ever having been depressed. When they are depressed, they report never having done anything worthwhile. Apparent inconsistencies or contradictions are not experienced as internal conflict.

Because feelings cause competition and agitation in the family, the child associates them with a grandiosity that leads the youngster to conclude that feelings are overwhelming. In families that demonstrate a high level of competition for specific feelings, the youngster may decide not to experience a feeling that "belongs" to the father (e.g., anger) or that "belongs" to the mother (e.g., fear). This system can be maintained only through extensive use of denial.

Within the competitive frame of reference, problems cannot be solved; instead, struggles can only be won or lost. In fact, the competition is more important than arriving at solutions. Because problems are perceived as overwhelming and insoluble, the youngster must learn to discount the significance of external stimuli or regard them as overwhelming. Either approach leads to a very grandiose approach to thinking.

Likewise, the grandiose parent message, "You can do anything," and the punitive parent message, "But you'll never do it well enough," are isolated as separate manic and depressive experiences. Manic persons evidence grandiosity about doing things as a need to be in constant motion. At times they may be involved in a dozen or more major projects at home and at work. Depressed persons who claim that they can do nothing right or have no energy make an equally unrealistic assessment of their capabilities.

Fantasized Nurturing Parent   The fantasized nurturing parent is an internal construct reported by many persons with bipolar disorders. The child develops this internal fantasy of the loving, kind, nurturing parent as a way to deal with the experience of inconsistent or abusive parenting. "If I just work hard enough or do well enough, then they will love me" is the child's way of attempting to control an unpredictable environment. Since the child develops and maintains this construct internally and never tests it against reality, the construct can persist into adulthood. Adults then operate from the assumption that someday they will obtain the fantasized nurturing. They are not prepared for the realistic requirements of caring for themselves in a world that is at times hostile and at times benevolent. Their response to the normal successes and setbacks of life is either unrealistic elation or depression.

The expression of bipolar personality in adulthood varies a great deal. For example, some people are successful at working hard, doing things well, and finding a family and work environment that supports their success while not expecting intimacy. Many successful administrators and business executives find social and professional reinforcement for this personality structure. Others admire their success and constant energy. They may have infrequent episodes of physical illness or fatigue from overwork, but basically they thrive on doing things and are seldom or never depressed.

In contrast, some just cannot seem to get their lives together. They have difficulty focusing their energy or sustaining any goal-directed effort. They may alternate between periods of hypomanic activity and moderate depression, or they may just suffer from chronic fatigue and depression. It is important to realize that the basic personality structures of these people are similar, even though they are acted out differently. People with bipolar personality structures can be viewed on a continuum ranging from functional to dysfunctional. Their placement on this continuum is determined to a large extent by how comfortable or uncomfortable they are with themselves and how comfortable or accepting people around them are with this behavior.

Psychobiology Research on bipolar mood disorder focuses on these four areas (McEnany 1990):

• *Biologic rhythms:* This research explores the role of disturbed circadian rhythms in psychobiologic illness or disorder. Areas of interest include sleep disturbance in bipolar states (Plumlee 1986), effect of light on mood pattern (Rosenthal et al. 1987), and psychobiologic influences (e.g., of melatonin) on mood modulation (Rosenthal et al. 1988).

• *Chemical brain function:* Investigation centers on two areas: (a) influence of diet on neurotransmitter activity (Wurtman 1988) and thus mood-related illness and (b) effects of medications on neurotransmitter synthesis and release (Honig et al. 1988).

• *Biologic influences:* Areas of research include limbic seizure activity in bipolar states (Levy et al. 1988), neuroendocrine dysfunction in mood disordered states (Nemeroff 1989), and "organic" basis of bipolar symptoms (Shukla et al. 1987).

• *Genetics:* Egeland (1988) reports finding DNA markers on the short arm of chromosome 11 that are linked to bipolar disorder.

Clearly, new research is changing the way clinicians look at this disorder and assess, treat, and care for people who have it. See the accompanying Psychobiology box.

Depressive Disorders

The **depressive disorders** are characterized by exaggerated feelings of sadness, melancholy, dejection, worthlessness, emptiness, and hopelessness that are not warranted by reality. Depressive disorders may be expressed in a wide range of biologic, emotional, cognitive, and motor human responses. They should be differentiated from the normal sadness and grief resulting from some personal loss or tragedy. The complex relationship of biology and emotion is reflected in the Nutrition box on page 290.

Early Development   There are several theories about the development of depressive disorders, some of which are similar to theories of the causes of bipolar disorders. Three theories specific to depression—

anger turned inward, object loss, and learned helplessness—are discussed in this section.

Anger Turned Inward Anger turned inward is central to the theory developed by Freud (1957) to explain the neurotic depression he observed in his patients. Freud believes that the loss of a significant object or person precipitates both a loving and an angry response in people, whether adults or children. Since the mixed reaction of love and anger is either emotionally confusing or socially unacceptable, the person deals with the lost object by loving and grieving its loss and turns the anger against the self. For example, a young husband may find it unacceptable to be angry with his wife who died in childbirth, leaving him alone to care for a baby. He therefore turns his anger inward and blames himself for not loving his spouse enough or perhaps even assumes that he was in some way responsible for her death. This man might remain depressed indefinitely, withdraw socially, and never consider marriage again unless he receives help in expressing his anger toward the wife who deserted him.

Object Loss   Object loss is the forced, often traumatic separation of a person from a significant object of attachment. Bowlby (1960) proposes that such a significant loss during infancy or childhood establishes a pattern of anxiety, grief, and helplessness/hopelessness. The person uses this pattern to deal with all subsequent losses. Since it is impossible to go through life without experiencing at least minor losses, separations, or blows to one's self-esteem, the person establishes a lifelong pattern of depression. The person feels helpless to cope with the ups and downs of life effectively and assumes a hopeless, depressed attitude toward existence.

Learned Helplessness   **Learned helplessness** is one of several theories that focus on depression as a learned response to life events that are or were originally outside one's control. Some clinicians propose that depression is caused not by the trauma or loss alone but by the belief that one cannot control the important events in one's life. Others propose that depression is caused by a cognitive mind set. An extremely negative opinion of self, learned in youth, is later converted into absolutes: "No one could ever love me" or "I can't do anything right."

Personality Structure Arieti and Bemporad (1980) describe three types of depressive personality structures. The *dominant other* type of depression is experienced by persons who rely on dominant or significant others for their self-esteem. Their sense of worth is determined externally, and rewards and values are offered by dominant persons or organizations. These people lack personal goals and direction, tend to focus on problems, and are seen as passive, manipulative, and clinging. They avoid anger and

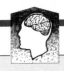

PSYCHOBIOLOGY: THE MIND/BODY CONNECTION

Lighten Up! A Look at the Connection between Light and Mood

Most people are awake during the day and asleep during the night. Anyone who follows this schedule and then is required to work during the night and sleep during the day experiences several unpleasant phenomena. First, it is almost impossible to sleep during the day, even when the fatigue quotient is high and the capacity to stay fully awake is low. Other complaints may include an inability to think clearly, irritability, and chronic mild depression for the duration of the inverted schedule. These facts are significant, especially because a large proportion of the American population works during evening, night, or rotating shifts. According to Tinkleberg (1991), short- and long-term concerns develop with shift work. Short-term issues include safety; the Chernobyl nuclear plant accident may have been the result of poor functioning of night shift workers. The long-term effects concern larger issues such as the overall health of the worker. The previously discussed complaints of the sleep-disturbed individual impact his or her internal experience, as well as social, family, and occupational functioning.

The phenomenon of jet lag may cause similar manifestations. Many travelers experience insomnia, irritability, diminished concentration capacities, and a need for food at very odd hours. After a few days the symptoms begin to abate, depending on the distance traveled. The traveler faces a return of symptoms upon returning home.

Other people may suffer a strange twist of psychobiologic fate on a yearly basis, in that their mood changes as the seasons change. This mood trend can take several directions. For example, some people are depressed in the short days of winter, and elated in the long days of summer, whereas other people experience the opposite pattern. This season-related mood pattern has been long recognized, as evidenced in the writings of Hippocrates. Florence Nightingale also wrote about the importance of light in the modulation of a healing environment.

The connection between the shift-worker, the traveler, and the person suffering from seasonal mood changes may be related to natural light. Frequently taken for granted, light is a powerful force that influences the course of human experience in ways in which most people are not aware. In the three examples above, all the people experience mood shifts and changes in their capacity to function as a result of changes in exposure to natural light. The light in the natural environment may help modulate daily rhythms, which then influence behavioral attributes such as sleep, activity, neuroendocrine functions, and even brain chemical (neurotransmitter and neuroregulator) systems.

For every variation of the change pattern in mood, there are equally as many therapeutic approaches. Some of the research underway explores the application of light. For example, is it better to apply light to the skin or to the eyes, the latter being connected to a circadian rhythm pacemaker. Is it more effective to use light therapy in the morning, afternoon, or evening in an effort to work with the body's natural circadian rhythms? These questions need further research before definitive recommendations for the use of light are applied to clinical work. However, given recent advances, such clinical applications are on the horizon. The environment has always been the domain of nursing, and the modulation of light to reshape circadian rhythms and expedite healing may also be imminent.

— *Geoffry McEnany*

confrontation so as not to anger those in charge of determining rewards. The *dominant goal* type of depression occurs in people who invest all of their energies and self-worth in the attainment of some inflated goal. Whether the goal is realistic or not, the problem is that the person's self-esteem is determined by goal attainment rather than an internal sense of worth. If the goal is blocked, the person's lack of self-esteem becomes evident as depression.

The *depressive character* structure is exemplified by people who cannot form either dominant other or dominant goal attachments. Their lives are empty,

NUTRITION AND MENTAL HEALTH

How Poor Diet Contributes to Clinical Depression

Mounting research strongly suggests that many psychiatric disorders are partially caused by biochemical defects, so it is easy to assume that diet plays a role in these conditions. After all, what is food but a collection of complex chemicals, many of which serve as precursors for neurotransmitters and other psychoactive compounds.

A deficiency of vitamin B_1, for instance, depletes the nervous system of a coenzyme essential for glucose utilization and acetylcholine synthesis. These abnormalities probably contribute to mental depression, apathy, and irritability. Those at greatest risk include alcoholics and clients who consume little or no whole grains or fortified carbohydrates but instead rely heavily on refined starches and sugars (Krause and Mahan 1984).

In its early stage, thiamine depletion may be easily overlooked because clients don't have symptoms of beri-beri, the classical deficiency disease. Thus polyneuritis, pitting edema, or heart failure are also unlikely. Clients do complain, however, of poor appetite and inability to concentrate, in addition to depression and irritability. At least one research team has found these signs and symptoms among 20 "healthy" subjects; that is, without clear-cut organic disease. These symptoms occurred despite the fact that all 20 subjects seemed well-fed. Apparently a marginal B_1 deficit developed because subjects ate too many sugar-laden foods and beverages (Lonsdale and Shamberger 1980).

Pyridoxine, or vitamin B_6, is another nutrient that can affect the brain function. This vitamin is required to convert the amino acid tryptophan to serotonin, a lack of which has been implicated in depression. Low blood pyridoxine levels have been found in a random survey of depressed outpatients, and experimental B_6 depletion has been shown to induce depression (McLaren 1988).

Alcoholics are among the prime candidates for a pyridoxine deficit, as are clients with malabsorption syndromes. Certain drugs, including isoniazid, hydralzine, corticosteroids, cycloserine, and penicillamine, can induce a deficit as well. Several older studies have reported a deficiency among oral contraceptive users, but the recent introduction of low-estrogen preparations has reduced that likelihood.

Physical findings that may accompany a B_6 deficit include cheilosis (fissures on the lips and at the corners of the mouth), glossitis, an abnormal EEG, poor resistance to infection, and seizures.

Folic acid, another B vitamin, has likewise been linked to certain neuropsychiatric disorders, probably because it is involved with the metabolism of serotonin and dopamine. Among 34 patients with folate deficiency-induced megaloblastic anemia, more than half suffered from an affective disorder, most commonly depression. Similarly, surveys of psychiatric in-patients have revealed that as many as 30% have low serum folate levels.

The most convincing evidence to support a link between folic acid and psychiatric disease, however, comes from a recent double blind trial in which folic acid-deficient patients with either major depression or schizophrenia were given either methylfolate—a form of the vitamin that crosses the blood brain barrier readily—or placebo. Among 41 subjects with either disorder, folate was clearly associated with symptomatic improvement and social recovery (Godfrey et al. 1990).

Who is at risk for folic acid deficiency? The indigent—especially those who don't consume enough fresh, green, leafy vegetables, whole grain breads, lean beef, and beans—are most vulnerable. Impoverished pregnant women are even more susceptible because pregnancy increases their need for the vitamin.

A lack of magnesium in the diet, or a metabolic disorder that robs tissue reserves of the mineral can precipitate depression. Among the most likely too ingest too little magnesium are geriatric clients, alcoholics, and those on magnesium-free parenteral feeding. However, there are several other ways to develop a shortfall. Danish investigators reported the case of a woman who had a bowel resection that left her with only 80 cm of ileum, one of the prime absorption sites for magnesium. The resulting depression was mistakenly treated with imipramine until a nutritional workup revealed low serum and urinary magnesium. Within days of replacement therapy, the depression had lifted (Rasmussen et al.

▶

NUTRITION AND MENTAL HEALTH *(continued)*

1989). Other gastrointestinal conditions that may trigger a deficit include gluten intolerance (an inability to digest the protein in wheat, oats, rye, and barley), ulcerative colitis, and Crohn disease.

Any condition that promotes urinary magnesium can likewise bring on psychologic problems. Prolonged use of loop diuretics is a well-documented culprit. So are hyperthyroidism, uncontrolled diabetes mellitus, and aldosteronism. Anorexia, muscle spasms, facial tics, tremor, and ataxia are among the physical findings that may accompany the neuropsychologic symptoms.

Inadequate zinc affects behavior in several ways. A mild deficiency can make clients very lethargic. In time, however, lethargy gives way to irritability and depression. As a rule, certain warning signs precede the irritability and depression: Anorexia, poor growth in children, and impaired taste and smell. In severe zinc deficiency, certain physical signs usually accompany the behavioral changes: Rash around the mouth, eyes, under the arms, and on elbows and knees. Other symptoms include poor wound healing, sexual impotence in males, and nightblindness.

Zinc deficiency can result from poor diet or it may result from various metabolic conditions, but it is uncommon for an imbalanced diet alone to deplete tissue reserves enough to produce depression. The exception is the client who suffers from full-scale protein-calorie malnutrition, in which case there are probably several additional dietary deficits contributing to abnormal behavior.

Nondietary problems that may contribute to severe zinc depletion include ulcerative colitis, pancreatic insufficiency, parasitic diseases such as giardiasis, chronic renal failure, alcoholic cirrhosis, and gluten intolerance. Drugs that deplete the body of zinc include penicillamine, corticosteroids, chlorthalidone, and furosemide.

—Paul L. Cerrato

---

their relationships are petty and shallow, and they have a harsh, critical attitude toward themselves and others. They generally have many physical complaints and are unpleasant companions. Depression is a way of life for these people.

Like persons with bipolar disorders, people with depressive disorders can be viewed on a continuum ranging from functional to dysfunctional. Their level of functioning is often determined by how comfortable they are with themselves and how accepting and comfortable people around them are with the behavior. The nurse has no reliable way to determine the seriousness of the stressor that precipitates depression. Only the person whose self-esteem is affected can determine the significance of the loss or stress in relation to depression.

Psychobiology Chapter 6 covers some of the theories supporting biologic indices of depression. This section highlights recent advances in locating biologic markers of the disorder.

Several studies document biologic shifts related to depression. Although these influences may not be *causative,* they can be clinically assessed in clients with depression. The following list gives only a few of the areas currently under investigation:

- *Neuronal receptors:* It is widely believed that depression is associated with alterations in the sensitivity of the membranes of neuronal receptors. Furthermore, it is likely that alterations in different receptors lead to different behavioral symptoms. The change in receptor function accounts for the efficacy of certain drugs, such as antidepressants.

- *Metabolism of serotonin:* Serotonin is a neurotransmitter commonly found in the central nervous system, particularly in the limbic system. Dysfunction of certain serotonergic neurons has been linked with depression. For this reason, drugs that influence serotonin metabolism, such as fluoxetine (Prozac), have found wide use in the treatment of depression.

- *Measures of the hypothalamic-pituitary-adrenal axis:* **Psychoendocrinology** is the study of the relationship between endocrine function and mood. Over the last ten years, the relationship between hormones and mood disturbances has been actively pursued through examinations such as the **dexamethasone suppression test,** which measures cortisol levels. Many depressed clients demonstrate cortisol hypersecretion. Cortisol levels can be easily assessed with the 24-hour urinary free cortisol test as well.

• *Measures of the hypothalamic-pituitary-thyroid axis:* The relationship between thyroid function and mood states has been long established. Recently, it has become common for physicians to prescribe a low dose of triiodothyronine to potentiate tricyclic antidepressants. The **thyrotropin-releasing hormone (TRH) infusion test** is now being used in the assessment of depression. This test challenges the stimulation of thyroid-stimulating hormone (TSH) with an infusion of TRH. Many depressed clients show a blunted TSH response to TRH, despite otherwise normal thyroid function. The TRH infusion test, while not specific for depression, may be useful in the diagnosis of depression.

The *hypothalamic-pituitary-growth hormone axis* and *hypothalamic-pituitary-prolactin axis* are also being investigated, but their relationship to depression is less evident.

Biopsychosocial Factors in Pathology

DSM-III-R categorizes the mood (affective) disorders as follows (see the box above):

1. Bipolar disorders

   a. Bipolar disorders (mixed, manic, depressed)

   b. Cyclothymia

2. Depressive disorders

   a. Major depression (single episode, recurrent)

   b. Dysthymia

With the exception of dysthymia, the diagnosis of bipolar disorders or depressive disorders is based on the past or present incidence of manic and depressive episodes. These episodes and their symptoms are defined in the boxes on pages 293 and 294.

Bipolar Disorders

Bipolar disorders are of three different types: manic, mixed, and depressed. Generally, clients are first hospitalized because of a manic episode. Both manic and depressive episodes occur more frequently than those falling under the category of major depressive episodes (described later). Often one type of bipolar episode is immediately followed by a short bipolar episode of another kind. Thus, a client might experience a manic episode and appear to recover only to develop symptoms of depression.

Bipolar Disorder, Manic   In bipolar disorder, manic, the most recent or current episode must meet the full criteria for a manic episode. The full criteria

---

> ## Mood (Affective) Disorders (DSM-III-R)
>
> ### Bipolar Disorders
> 296.6x   Bipolar disorder, mixed
> 296.4x   Bipolar disorder, manic
> 296.5x   Bipolar disorder, depressed
> 301.13   Cyclothymia
> 296.70   Bipolar disorder NOS (not otherwise specified)
>
> ### Depressive Disorders
> 296.2x   Major depression, single episode
> 296.3x   Major depression, recurrent
> 300.40   Dysthymia
> 311.00   Depressive disorder NOS
>
> SOURCE: *American Psychiatric Association.* Diagnostic and Statistical Manual of Mental Disorders, ed 3, *revised. APA,* 1987, p. 217.

---

need not be met, however, if the client has had a previous manic episode.

Bipolar Disorder, Mixed   In bipolar disorder, mixed, the most recent or current episode is characterized by symptoms of both manic and major depressive episodes. There is rapid intermingling and alternation of symptoms. Depressive symptoms are prominent and last at least a full day.

Bipolar Disorder, Depressed   In bipolar disorder, depressed, the current or most recent episode is a major depressive one. The client has had one or more manic episodes, and the full criteria need not be met if there has been a previous major depressive episode.

Cyclothymia

In **cyclothymia,** the client alternates periods of abnormally elevated, expansive, or irritable moods with periods of depression and loss of interest or pleasure. The illness is not considered cyclothymia unless periods of both kinds have been numerous during the past two years. Also, it is not cyclothymia if either the expansive or depressed periods meet the symptom criteria for manic or major depressed episodes, respectively. Last, during the previous two years, there cannot have been a period without hypomanic or depressive symptoms lasting longer than two months. According to DSM-III-R (1987) the following are seen in hypomanic episodes:

DSM-III-R Diagnostic Criteria for Manic Episode

Note: A "manic syndrome" is defined as including criteria A, B, and C below. A "hypomanic syndrome" is defined as including criteria A and B, but not C, i.e., no marked impairment.

A. A distinct period of abnormally and persistently elevated, expansive, or irritable mood.

B. During the period of mood disturbance, at least three of the following symptoms have persisted (four if the mood is only irritable) and have been present to a significant degree:
1. Inflated self-esteem or grandiosity
2. Decreased need for sleep, e.g., feels rested after only three hours of sleep
3. More talkative than usual or pressure to keep talking
4. Flight of ideas or subjective experience that thoughts are racing
5. Distractability, i.e., attention too easily drawn to unimportant or irrelevant external stimuli
6. Increase in goal-directed activity (either socially, at work or school, or sexually) or psychomotor agitation
7. Excessive involvement in pleasurable activities that have a high potential for painful consequences, e.g., the person engages in unrestrained buying sprees, sexual indiscretions, or foolish business investments

C. Mood disturbance sufficiently severe to cause marked impairment in occupational functioning or in usual social activities or relationships with others, or to necessitate hospitalization to prevent harm to self or others.

D. At no time during the disturbance have there been delusions or hallucinations for as long as two weeks in the absence of prominent mood symptoms (i.e., before the mood symptoms developed or after they have remitted).

E. Not superimposed on schizophrenia, schizophreniform disorder, delusional disorder, or psychotic disorder NOS.

F. It cannot be established that an organic factor initiated and maintained the disturbance. Note: Somatic antidepressant treatment (e.g., drugs, ECT) that apparently precipitates a mood disturbance should not be considered an etiologic organic factor.

SOURCE: *American Psychiatric Association.* Diagnostic and Statistical Manual of Mental Disorders, *ed 3, revised. APA, 1987, p 217.*

---

1. For a distinct period, moods that are abnormally and persistently elevated, expansive, or irritable.

2. During the period when mood changes occur, at least three of the following symptoms have persisted to a significant degree. There will be four if the mood disturbance has been only irritable.

a. Inflated self-esteem or grandiosity

b. Decreased need for sleep, e.g., feels rested after only three hours of sleep

c. Talkativeness to a greater extent than usual and under pressure to keep talking

d. Flight of ideas or subjective experience that thoughts are racing

e. Distractibility, i.e., attention too easily drawn to unimportant or irrelevant external stimuli

f. Increase in goal-directed activity (either socially, at work or school, or sexually) or psychomotor agitation

g. Excessive involvement in pleasurable activities that have a high potential for painful consequences, e.g., the person engages in unrestrained buying sprees, sexual indiscretion, or foolish business investments

Major Depression

Major depression may occur as a single episode or as a recurrent episode, but the diagnosis is used when there is no history of a manic or hypomanic episode. The illness may be further classified according to the severity of the episode (mild, moderate, or severe) and the presence or absence of psychotic symptoms. It is believed that over 50 percent of those experiencing major depression, single episode, ultimately experience the illness again. Those with the diagnosis of major depression, recurrent, are at higher risk for developing a bipolar disorder.

Major Depression, Single Episode Some individuals experience only one episode of major depression in a lifetime. As opposed to bipolar disorder, which occurs in men as frequently as women, major depression, single episode, occurs twice as often among women.

DSM-III-R Diagnostic Criteria for Major Depressive Episode

Note: A "major depressive syndrome" is defined as criterion A below.

A. At least five of the following symptoms have been present during the same two-week period and represent a change from previous functioning; at least one of the symptoms is either (1) depressed mood, or (2) loss of interest or pleasure. (Do not include symptoms that are clearly due to a physical condition, mood-incongruent delusions or hallucinations, incoherence, or marked loosening of associations.)

1. Depressed mood (or can be irritable mood in children and adolescents) most of the day, nearly every day, as indicated either by subjective account or observation by others
2. Markedly diminished interest or pleasure in all, or almost all, activities most of the day, nearly every day (as indicated either by subjective account or observation by others of apathy most of the time)
3. Significant weight loss or weight gain when not dieting (e.g., more than 5 percent of body weight in a month), or decrease or increase in appetite nearly every day (in children, consider failure to make expected weight gains)
4. Insomnia or hypersomnia nearly every day
5. Psychomotor agitation or retardation nearly every day (observable by others, not merely subjective feelings of restlessness or being slowed down)
6. Fatigue or loss of energy nearly every day
7. Feelings of worthlessness or excessive or inappropriate guilt (which may be delu-

sional) nearly every day (not merely self-reproach or guilt about being sick)

8. Diminished ability to think or concentrate, or indecisiveness, nearly every day (either by subjective account or as observed by others)
9. Recurrent thoughts of death (not just fear of dying), recurrent suicidal ideation without a specific plan, or a suicide attempt or a specific plan for committing suicide

B. 1. It cannot be established that an organic factor initiated and maintained the disturbance.
   2. The disturbance is not a normal reaction to the death of a loved one (uncomplicated bereavement).
   Note: Morbid preoccupation with worthlessness, suicidal ideation, marked functional impairment, or psychomotor retardation of prolonged duration suggest bereavement complicated by major depression.

C. At no time during the disturbance have there been delusions or hallucinations for as long as two weeks in the absence of prominent mood symptoms (i.e., before the mood symptoms developed or after they have remitted).

D. Not superimposed on schizophrenia, schizophreniform disorder, delusional disorder, or psychotic disorder NOS.

SOURCE: American Psychiatric Association: Diagnostic and Statistical Manual of Mental Disorders, ed 3, revised. APA, 1987, pp 222–223.

Major Depression, Recurrent Major depression, recurrent, is diagnosed when there is no history of manic or hypomanic episodes. Recurrent depressive episodes may be separated by many years, may occur in clusters, or may increase with age. Between episodes, functioning is generally at the premorbid level. For some clients, however, this is a chronic condition that causes considerable impairment.

Dysthymia Dysthymia is marked by chronic depressive mood disturbances lasting for extended periods. The diagnosis is made when the individual is never without symptoms for more than two months over a two-year period (one year for children and adolescents). The diagnosis is not made in the presence

of a major depressive episode or when symptoms coexist with some chronic psychotic or organic condition. This includes periods when certain medications, such as antihypertensives, are in use. According to DSM-III-R these symptoms characterize dysthymia:

- Poor appetite or overeating
- Insomnia or hypersomnia
- Low energy or fatigue
- Low self-esteem
- Poor concentration or difficulty making decisions
- Feelings of hopelessness

The Nursing Process and Clients with Mood Disorders

"Nursing is the diagnosis and treatment of human responses to actual or potential health problems" (ANA 1980, p 9). A diagnosis is a predictable cluster or configuration of human responses. For example, a medical/psychiatric diagnosis of the various bipolar disorders is made when a client demonstrates behavior meeting the criteria for a manic episode and a major depressive episode. The medical and nursing diagnoses are therefore very closely related, as the following sections demonstrate.

Assessing

The nurse should obtain assessment data from the client and significant others. Clients who are extremely upset or are using denial as a defense mechanism may not provide accurate information because they cannot remember details of past events. In these cases, a relative or close friend may be the primary source of assessment data. Nursing assessment data include

- Demographic information
- Client's definition of the problem
- Psychiatric history
- Family history
- Social history
- Health history
- Current mental status

A variety of assessment tools are available to assist the nurse with data collection. **Beck's Depression Inventory** (Beck 1967) is a twenty-one-item multiple-choice questionnaire clients can use to rate themselves on variables related to depression, e.g., sadness, pessimism, guilt, suicidal ideas, social withdrawal, insomnia, weight loss, and fatigue. **Zung's Self-Rating Depression Scale** (Zung 1965) contains twenty descriptors of depression—e.g., "I feel downhearted and blue"—on which clients rate themselves on a four-point scale ranging from "a little of the time" to "most of the time." This scale is helpful in determining the depth or intensity of the client's depression. The dexamethasone suppression test is used in some interdisciplinary and in-patient settings to assess the presence of endogenous depression.

Another assessment tool useful for determining the presence and acuity of depression is the **Algorithm for Depression** (Orsolits and Morphy 1982). There are four sections consisting of yes-or-no response sets that yield a total score indicating the level of depression and risk factors involved (see Figure 13–1). The tool focuses on recent losses, behavioral and feeling states, suicidal ideation, lethality, social supports, and judgment of the clinician. It is simple to use and helpful in guiding the client and clinician decisions.

Diagnosing

After collecting and analyzing assessment data, the nurse can formulate multiple diagnoses. The purpose of a nursing diagnosis is to guide nursing interventions. The nursing diagnosis is a general label for a cluster of human responses. Not all nursing diagnoses will apply to every client, and the nurse needs to decide which diagnoses have priority with each client at a given time.

The case studies on pages 304 and 307 demonstrate how assessment data are used to arrive at nursing diagnoses with two very different clients. The nursing care plan illustrates how nursing diagnoses guide nursing interventions. The Nursing Diagnosis box on page 300 contains nursing diagnoses that potentially apply to persons with any of the mood disorders.

Planning and Implementing Interventions

General Relationship Principles The psychiatric nurse treating persons with mood disorders must keep four general principles in mind:

1. Relating from a noncompetitive frame of reference

2. Emphasizing being rather than doing

3. Adopting a reality-oriented approach to thinking, feeling, and behaving

4. Developing realistic adult relationships and contracts for change

Regardless of clients' manic or depressive presentation and their specific human responses, psychiatric nurses must keep these underlying principles in mind while planning and delivering nursing care.

Relating from a Noncompetitive Frame of Reference A noncompetitive frame of reference is essential for dealing with people who have been taught to experience themselves, their relationships, and their environments as competitive. These people tend to polarize issues and argue that such normal functions as thinking and feeling cannot be done simultaneously. They attempt to redefine treatment expectations in competitive terms with such statements as "But you told me not to work so hard" as justification for not completing a project at work and thereby jeopardizing a promotion. The nurse and client must confront this self-destructive process and explore the purpose for the

Text continues on p. 299

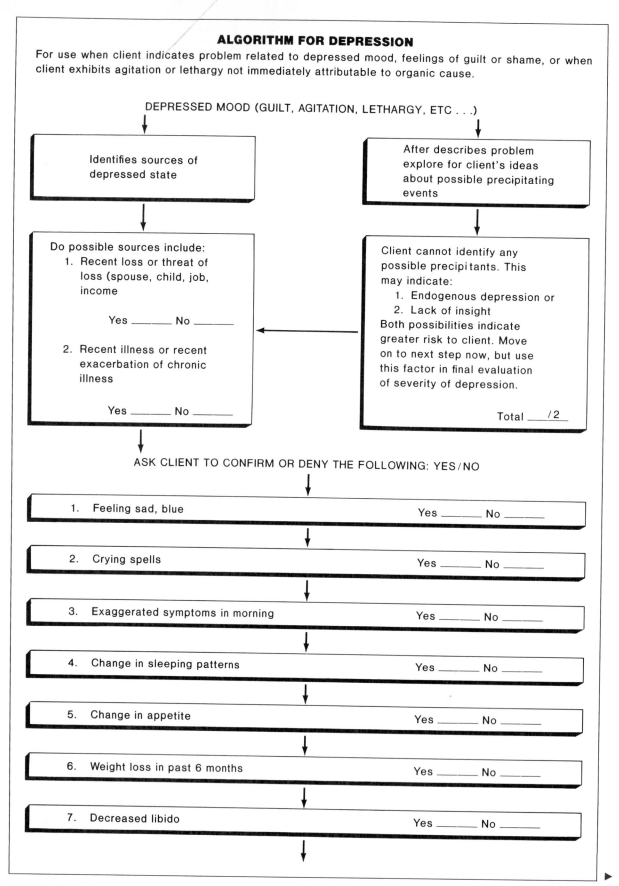

FIGURE 13–1 Depression algorithm. *(SOURCE: Orsolotis M, Morphy M: A depression algorithm for psychiatric emergencies. J Psychiatr Treatment Eval 1982;4:137–135. Reprinted with permission from Journal of Psychiatric Treatment and Evaluation, Pergamon Press, Ltd.)*

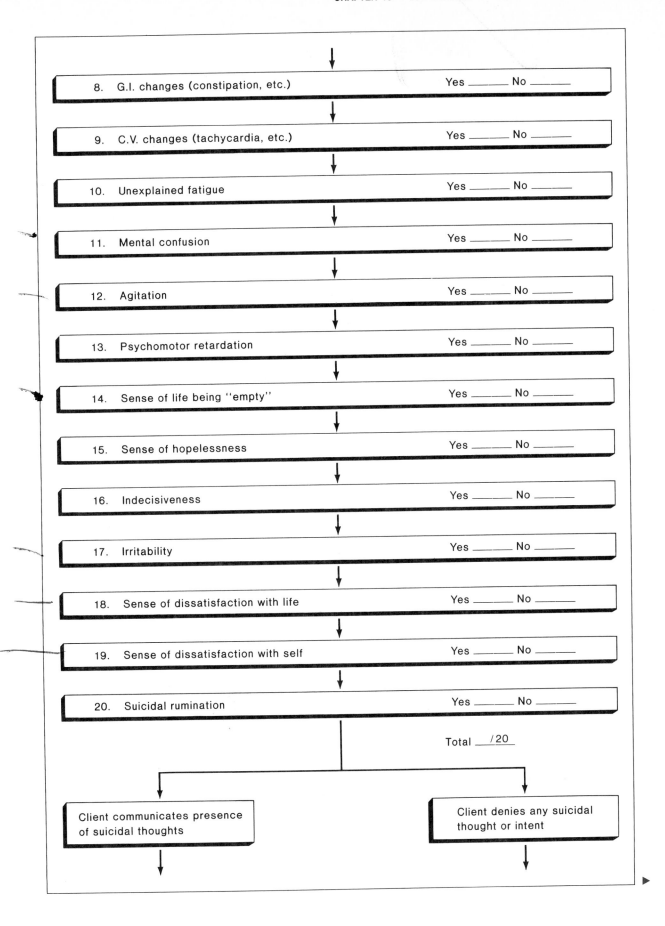

8. G.I. changes (constipation, etc.)   Yes _____ No _____

9. C.V. changes (tachycardia, etc.)   Yes _____ No _____

10. Unexplained fatigue   Yes _____ No _____

11. Mental confusion   Yes _____ No _____

12. Agitation   Yes _____ No _____

13. Psychomotor retardation   Yes _____ No _____

14. Sense of life being ''empty''   Yes _____ No _____

15. Sense of hopelessness   Yes _____ No _____

16. Indecisiveness   Yes _____ No _____

17. Irritability   Yes _____ No _____

18. Sense of dissatisfaction with life   Yes _____ No _____

19. Sense of dissatisfaction with self   Yes _____ No _____

20. Suicidal rumination   Yes _____ No _____

Total ___/20

Client communicates presence of suicidal thoughts

Client denies any suicidal thought or intent

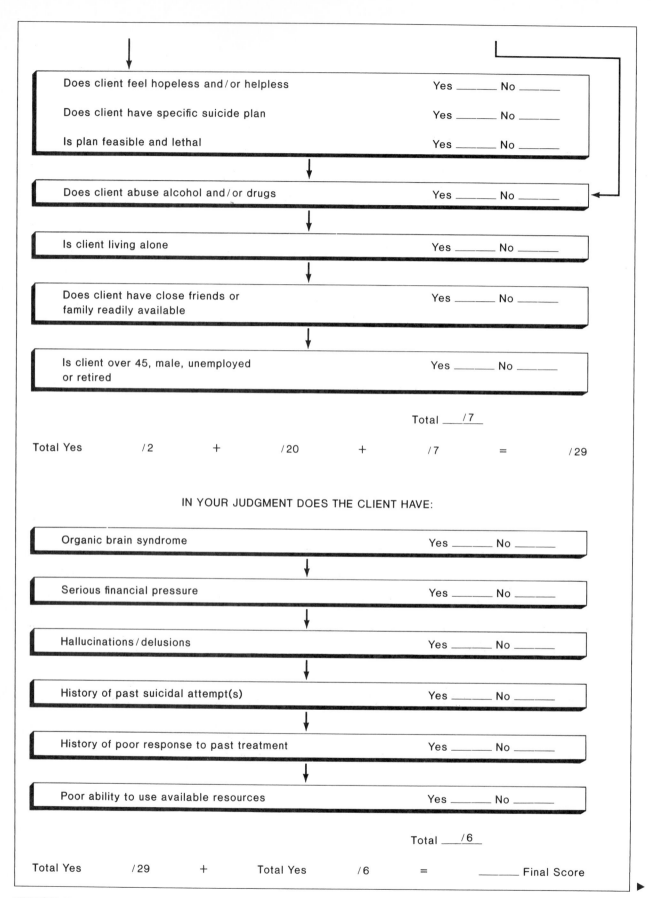

FIGURE 13-1 Depression algorithm. *(continued)*

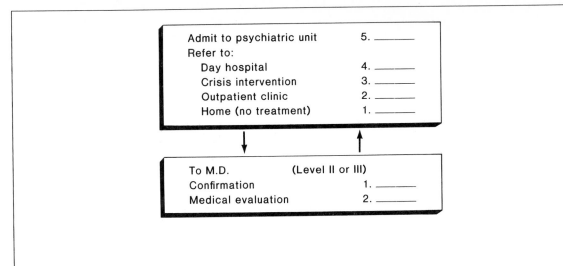

ALGORITHM SCORING

Add the number of "Yes" responses in each subsection to provide a final score. Scoring has been included in the algorithm's construction from the outset in order to facilitate future analysis of data. Correlations of disposition decisions, and possibly other outcome measures, with these subtotal and total scores can be completed.

redefinition of alternatives. Avoid competition for who will win or who is in charge of the therapy. These clients are masters at winning or losing competitive battles, and neither outcome is beneficial.

Emphasis on Being Rather Than Doing   An emphasis on being rather than doing is an important strategy in working with clients who present with so many behaviors that must be managed. As mentioned previously, the early competition with parents is eventually acted out by doing or not doing things successfully, and the person's worth and place in the world are externally defined by their accomplishments or lack thereof. Once this pattern is established, people with mood disorders attempt to repeat the pattern and elicit a predictable response from significant others, including therapists. The nurse must get this message across: "I care about you, no matter who you are, or what you do or don't accomplish." Then the nurse must also deal with the behavioral manifestations of persons with affective disorders.

Reality-Oriented Approach   A reality-oriented approach to thinking, feeling, and behaving is the only way to ensure the safety and successful treatment of persons with affective disorders. Considerable time and energy must be spent confronting grandiosity, and clients must gradually learn to think about the consequences of their behavior. These clients need to internalize the message "You are capable of solving problems" as they confront their manic-depressive grandiosity. These clients commonly have fears of never getting enough, always being depressed,

driving people away, or not being able to "stand it." Such grandiosity is the justification for thinking, feeling, or doing certain things. Therefore, a great deal of time and attention are devoted to reality testing and obtaining information from other people about their experience of reality.

Developing Realistic Adult Relationships and Contracts for Change   The nurse models the development of realistic adult relationships in nurse-client interactions with the hope that the client will generalize the pattern to others in the environment. The goal is to revise the original construct of a fantasized nurturing parent into a more realistic, adult approach to caring, nurturing, and relating to other people. Contracting within relationships is one way to accomplish this objective. A contract is a mutually agreed-on set of expectations between two or more people about what each will contribute to the relationship. If conditions change, as they often do, the contract can be renegotiated. However, it always serves as a clear statement of what people can expect from each other at any given time.

Safe treatment of persons with mood disorders involves the use of several important contracts. The timing and significance of these nurse-client contracts vary according to the issues presented by the client, but all should be considered potentially useful.

Social Control Contract   Social control contracts provide a good way to assess the client's ability to make and keep contracts. Because persons with mood disorders often present with problems of doing

NURSING DIAGNOSIS

Mood Disorders

The following list details a variety of nursing diagnoses that *potentially* apply to the person suffering any of the forms of mood disorder. In no way does this mean that persons with mood disturbances will present *all* of the following behaviors. To diagnose the human response appropriately, the assessing nurse must evaluate the person's presenting symptoms thoroughly.

Activity intolerance

Anxiety (specify level)

Coping, Ineffective individual

Decisional conflict

Denial, Ineffective

Diversional activity deficit

Family processes, Altered

Fear

Grieving, dysfunctional

Health maintenance, Altered

Home maintenance management, Impaired

Injury: High risk

Knowledge deficit (specify)

Noncompliance (specify)

Nutrition, Altered: Less than body requirements

Powerlessness

Self-care deficit

Self-esteem disturbance

Sensory-perceptual alterations: Auditory, visual

Sexual patterns, Altered

Sleep pattern disturbance

Social interaction, Impaired

Thought processes, Altered

Violence, High risk: Self-directed or directed at others

interview for three jobs in one week. The ability to make and keep contracts is essential for therapy, and this expectation should be shared from the outset. Clients who are unwilling to make contracts do not usually stay in treatment. Clients who are unable to keep contracts may require hospitalization for their own protection and safety.

No-Running Contract The no-running contract is a direct way to address the personality structure of persons with mood disorders. This contract is essentially an agreement to deal with issues and not to run away or withdraw, either physically or psychologically. The importance of this contract is evidenced by the great anxiety most clients experience while making it. Some are reluctant to make the commitment and say they feel trapped. The fact is that treatment work with these clients is not likely to succeed unless they agree to stay engaged with the nurse and confront uncomfortable issues previously ignored. The complementary messages delivered by the nurse are:

- Your problems can be solved

- Your feelings are not so overwhelming that you must run away

- You can stay and deal with issues

In this way, the nurse and client establish an alternative to grandiosity and discounting.

No-Secrets/No-Lies Contract The no-secrets/no-lies contract is closely related to the no-running contract. Lies are active misinterpretations of reality, and secrets are the withholding of important information. Both are primary mechanisms that persons with mood disorders use to maintain distance from other people. Because of their extensive use of denial, these clients are often unaware of how greatly they distort reality. For example, they may deny being angry because they are out of touch with their own rage. One manic client denied ever having been depressed, even though she later reported having tried to kill herself on two occasions. The expectation that accompanies the no-lies/no-secrets contract is that it is possible to be aware of thoughts, feelings, and behaviors simultaneously, and that no aspect of oneself should be ignored or excluded.

No-Suicide/No-Homicide Contract   A no-suicide/no-homicide contract gives clients the protection necessary to work on significant underlying issues. The nurse can ask a client to state, "I will not hurt or kill myself or anyone else, accidentally or on purpose, no matter what." Watch and listen for any hesitation, changes in wording, or incongruence between what is said and how it is said. Ask the client to look directly at you while making the contract. Once the client has made a clear and congruent commitment, say that you accept the decision and are willing to help the client keep the contract.

or not doing things, the nurse can begin by addressing practical problems related to time structuring. For example, a client may need help cutting back on an eighty-hour work week filled with overlapping committee meetings. The agreement may be to find ten free hours per week. Another client may require help obtaining employment, and the agreement may be to

Bipolar clients often deny the need for a no-suicide/no-homicide contract. They may not understand why it is so important, but they are usually willing to make the contract. They usually agree because their extensive use of denial has put them out of touch with the homicidal rage within the manic structure and the struggle for existence within the depressive structure. Even though bipolar clients may be willing to make the initial contract, you may need to repeat the contract when they are more in touch with the feelings and thoughts of wanting to hurt themselves or someone else.

Clients with depressive disorders are usually aware of their own suicidal thoughts and depressed feelings and therefore appreciate the need for a no-suicide contract. They are, however, reluctant to give up the option of suicide as a solution to their pain and despair. It may take a number of discussions before they can believably commit to the contract. For these people the process of making the contract is a very important aspect of the treatment and is well worth the time and energy it takes to accomplish. See also Chapter 23.

Specific Intervention Techniques Specific intervention techniques vary significantly according to the individual characteristics of the client and nurse, the setting in which the treatment is conducted, and the social supports available to the client and the therapeutic support available to the nurse (see the nursing care plan on page 309). For example, in some settings all clients with bipolar disorders are routinely treated with lithium, and clients with depressive disorders are routinely treated with antidepressants. The role of the nurse—a very limited role indeed—is to administer medications, encourage compliance, and monitor their side effects.

In other settings, the nurse is one of several mental health professionals who work with clients and their families in community treatment centers. The nurse's role may be that of primary therapist conducting family groups and helping clients return to normal work, social, and family functioning. Nurses in inpatient settings may have little or no contact with the client's family, but may instead be responsible for ensuring the client's safety during episodes of acute illness.

Because of this variation, the intervention techniques presented here are designed to provide a beginning list of considerations for nurses responsible for developing specific therapeutic interventions for clients with mood disorders. The accompanying Intervention box contains nursing diagnoses and related nursing interventions frequently used with clients with mood disorders.

Providing for Safety Safety interventions are of primary importance for clients with mood disor-

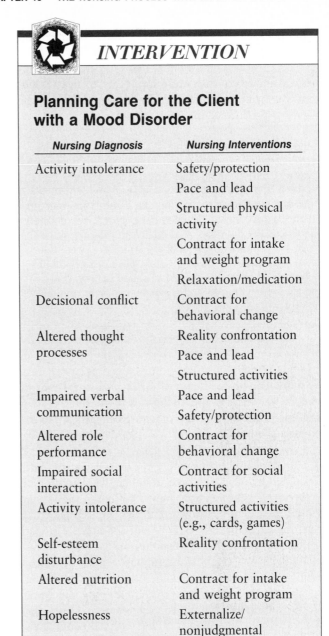

INTERVENTION

Planning Care for the Client with a Mood Disorder

Nursing Diagnosis	Nursing Interventions
Activity intolerance	Safety/protection
	Pace and lead
	Structured physical activity
	Contract for intake and weight program
	Relaxation/medication
Decisional conflict	Contract for behavioral change
Altered thought processes	Reality confrontation
	Pace and lead
	Structured activities
Impaired verbal communication	Pace and lead
	Safety/protection
Altered role performance	Contract for behavioral change
Impaired social interaction	Contract for social activities
Activity intolerance	Structured activities (e.g., cards, games)
Self-esteem disturbance	Reality confrontation
Altered nutrition	Contract for intake and weight program
Hopelessness	Externalize/nonjudgmental approach

ders. As mentioned earlier, suicide is only one of many ways in which these clients can hurt themselves. Accidents, loss of jobs, and destructive relationships are often ways of acting out the same problem. When these clients demonstrate significant alterations in conduct/impulse control, motor behavior, or self-care activities, they may need to be hospitalized for their own safety and protection. Medication may also be used to alter behavior that is either too manic or too depressed. Clients who are actively suicidal must be protected in an environment that is free of all means of harming oneself. They may also require constant observation during certain periods. Hospitals should have policies and procedures for protecting clients who are actively suicidal. It is usually the responsibility of the nursing staff to provide this protection.

No-suicide contracts and other limit-setting, social control contracts are also useful in providing safety and protection. Once a client demonstrates a willingness to make contracts and an ability to keep them, social control contracts can be made specific to the needs of the individual.

One hypomanic woman said she was "picking up energy" from the car engine and radio while driving and had received four speeding tickets during the previous six months. She agreed to drive no faster than 55 miles per hour and contracted to walk or take a cab if she was too "high" to drive safely. To keep her contract, she decided not to use the car radio or to pull off to the side of the road and breathe deeply until she was calm enough to drive. This contract saw her safely through a period of hypomanic agitation. The slower speed actually had a calming effect on her, and she now has a car with cruise control.

Once a client has demonstrated a willingness and ability to make and keep contracts, any alteration in conduct/impulse control, motor behavior, or self-care activities can be dealt with by means of a social control contract to ensure the client's physical safety. Then treatment can expand into other areas important to the client and nurse.

Providing for Understanding Pace and lead is a general intervention that the nurse can use with any client who has an excess or deficit of an emotion or behavior. *To pace* simply means to match the rate at which the client is moving, talking, or feeling. Once that match or pace is established, the nurse can lead the client to a slower or faster pace, as required. For example, when establishing rapport with a depressed client who sits, stares, and shows no interest in talking, sit down near the client and "pace" the quietness. Begin leading by saying just a few words: "Quiet day, isn't it?" or "It's good to be with someone who appreciates peace and quiet." Before leaving, say something like, "I assume that when you want something, you will tell me," thus creating the expectation that the client will be able to talk when the need arises. You may need to repeat this approach several different times or for several days in a row before the client begins to respond, but the client will eventually respond. Once the client begins talking, slowly and carefully increase the rate of speech and the level of emotion expressed. In successive sessions, lead the client to a new rate of speech and expression of affect.

Pacing and leading is also useful with manic clients who need to be slowed down. Their rapid, manic pace is obvious from their rate of communication, the pressure they feel to keep talking, their apparent need to keep moving and doing things, and their inability to sit still or rest. The pace-and-lead intervention is similar to that used with depressed clients. Begin by matching the client's behavior. If the client is walking,

walk fast and gradually slow the pace. If the client is talking, talk, laugh, and be very expressive before gradually diminishing the tone and affect so that a normal or serious discussion can take place.

One potential problem in pacing and leading people engaged in manic behavior is that others in their environment may wish to keep them animated. Manics who are not out of control can be entertaining and fun to be around socially, and others readily pick up the energy they transmit. The high level of energy and activity helps these clients and those around them to avoid their feelings and problems. Nurses may therefore have to make an extra effort to convince others to stop encouraging manic behavior. At times, manic clients are best treated in an isolated area or room where pacing and leading can be done more effectively.

Providing for Structure Structured activities and contracts can be used to address a wide range of client problems. Motor behavior, role performance, self-care, sleep patterns, sexuality, emotional experience and expression, and even thought processes can all be altered by structured interventions. Clients who want to change and work with the nurse to make and alter behavioral contracts are good candidates for structured activities and goal-directed contracts. Remember that these clients tend to act out their difficulties by doing or not doing things, and the structured activities and behavioral contracts may become the stage on which they are able to act out and work through earlier unresolved issues.

Time structuring is often a good way to begin work with clients experiencing mood disorders because their difficulty with doing or not doing things is reflected in how they structure their days and spend their time. One can begin by asking these clients to keep an exact record of all their activities for one week and then thoroughly examine the written record together. This process usually makes clients much more aware of their use of time, the people with whom they spend time, and their feelings about the activities in which they are engaged. The record gives the nurse a wealth of quantitative and qualitative data about these clients and their lives. What are their regular physical activities? What are their usual work, social, and family role-related activities? What are their activity/rest patterns? Are they spending the necessary time for eating and sleeping? Do they have any regular sexual activity? Once both client and nurse have a common data base, they can discuss what they each feel and think about the information and begin to develop specific contracts for change.

Providing Emotional Confrontation and Cognitive Restructuring Emotional confrontation and cognitive restructuring are intervention techniques for dealing with difficulties in feeling and thinking. Alterations in emotional response patterns

RESEARCH NOTE

Citation

Perry PJ, Garvey MJ, Kelly MW, Cook BL, Dunner FJ, Winokur G: A comparative trial of fluoxetine versus trazodone in outpatients with major depression. J Clin Psychiatry 1989;50 (8):290–294.

Study Problem/Purpose

The purpose of this study was to compare the clinical efficacy of two inhibitors of serotonin reuptake (fluoxetine and trazodone) in the treatment of clients diagnosed with major depression.

Methods

Forty voluntary male and female outpatients participated in this double-blind, randomized, parallel-design clinical trial to compare the efficacy of fluoxetine and trazodone in the treatment of major depression. There were two study periods. During the first, lasting one week, all participants received a placebo. The second, lasting six weeks, was a double-blind test of the two drugs. All participants were older than 18 years of age and met diagnostic criteria for major depression, with a symptom presentation of more than one month. The admission score on the Hamilton Rating Scale for Depression (HAM-D) for study participants had to be at least 20. Subjects participating in the study had to maintain a HAM-D score of at least 20 after the one-week placebo period. Clients receiving fluoxetine took doses of between 20 and 60 mg/day, and those receiving trazodone took doses of between 100 and 400 mg/day. Analysis of continuous data included parametric tests, including the paired *t*-test for matched data and the two sample *t*-tests for unmatched data. Analysis of noncontinuous data included contingency table analyses and ranking tests.

Findings

The findings indicate that fluoxetine is as effective an antidepressant as trazodone. Although the authors report the possibility that a fluoxetine dose of 20 mg/day may be ineffective, other data suggest that this drug may be slower to take effect than trazodone. In regard to adverse effects, participants tolerated both drugs well. The authors point out that fluoxetine does not cause weight gain, which may improve compliance with the medication regimen.

Implications

This study demonstrates the complex nature of the psychobiologic treatment of conditions such as depression. Additionally, it suggests that nurses may need to teach patients about biologic substrates of illness, possibly reducing the stigma associated with the disorder.

---

and perceptual/cognitive response patterns are interrelated in clients with mood disorders. For this reason, both emotional confrontation and cognitive restructuring interventions are often done simultaneously. Emotional confrontation is a safe and structured way to let the client deal with emotions previously denied or considered overwhelming. At the same time, cognitive restructuring involves giving the client a new way to think about or understand the emotional experience. For example, a man who thinks that his anger is overwhelming may be asked to obtain feedback from other people about how they experience and deal with their own anger. The man can then compare that information with his own thoughts and feelings. At the same time, this client may also engage in a structured activity, e.g., racquetball, to express his anger safely and increase his range of emotional experiences.

In recent years, **cognitive therapy** has been used more widely with those who suffer from mood disorders. The underlying principle of this approach is that one's thought process can affect feelings. The goal of this therapy is to help the person recognize patterns of thought that lead to maladaptive thought patterns and dysphoric feelings. Cognitive therapy is an active process; clients must assert themselves for the therapy to be effective. The nurse who assists a person with cognitive therapy usually follows certain general guidelines:

• Help the person identify periods during which they experience painful or uncomfortable feelings.

• Have the person rate the severity of the discomfort.

• Identify *automatic thoughts* that accompany the discomfort. For example, a depressed person who feels immobilized in social situations might have these

Text continues on p. 311

A Client with a Bipolar Disorder, Manic

Identifying Information

Ron G is a 47-year-old man brought to the emergency room by his wife. He is a coach at Columbia High School, and his wife is a teacher at Tangerine Elementary. They live at 101 Pressure Drive. Ron has an MS in education and is a practicing Baptist.

Client's Definition of Present Problem, Precipitating Stressors, Coping Strategies, Goals for Care

Ron angrily maintains that there is no problem. "If every one would just leave me alone so I can get ready for the big game, I'd be fine."

Emily, Ron's wife, reports that he has become increasingly agitated over the past two weeks while preparing for the local high school football championship game. "It's like he's possessed by a demon!" She reports that he has not eaten or slept for the past week and has become increasingly abusive to her and the children. Yesterday he spent an entire day watching game films and shouting obscenities at people walking down their street.

History of Present Problem

Ron is the very competitive and successful head coach of the Columbia High Falcons. Since moving to Columbia in 1984, Ron has gained national visibility by turning the Falcons football team from losers into winners. Next Friday's regional championship game is the culmination of the Falcon's first undefeated season. His wife reports that Ron began having difficulty two weeks ago after he was interviewed by *Sports Illustrated*. He got into an argument with his two assistant coaches, who said they thought he was working the team too hard in practice. He became verbally abusive and threatened to have the principal fire them if they interfered with his championship training plan.

Although Ron never went to the principal, he began to work harder himself to prepare for the championship game. He designed new plays and watched game films in his spare time, refusing to talk with his assistants. At practice he began shouting at the players and would tell them to do two or three things at once. This new approach confused everyone, and then he would throw equipment around when they didn't follow his orders. "He acted like a stranger—a madman who frightened everyone." During the past week, Ron became more driven by his desire to win and his fear of losing. He isolated himself from his friends, wife, and children, returning home after midnight to watch game films. He refused to eat, called obscenities out the window at passersby, and became combative when friends and family expressed their concern. When he threatened his children with a baseball bat this afternoon, his wife called the police, who had to restrain him physically and brought him to the ER.

Psychiatric History

Ron was hospitalized for one week for "physical exhaustion" four years ago. He saw a psychiatrist off and on during the following two years to help him deal with stress and pressures in his job. (He was coaching and selling real estate at the time.) He has not sought professional help since moving to Columbia. His wife reports two or three episodes of extreme energy and creativity during the past three years. For instance, last summer Ron and two friends worked night and day to build their new house in three months. "He was on top of the world and did a beautiful job. But then he was too exhausted to enjoy it."

Family History

Parents

Ron's father, a 70-year-old retired postal worker currently living in Fayetteville, Arkansas, is described by Ron's wife as a hard-working, stern man whose major goal in life was to have his children do better than he did. He often worked two jobs while the children were young to earn enough to send his children to college. He continues to be very interested in Ron's success, and talks with him twice a week to give him advice. His mother is 69 years old and lives with her husband in Fayetteville, where she makes and sells quilts to supplement their retirement income. Both parents are in good health.

Siblings — Ron's younger brother (age 45) is a successful used car dealer in Columbus, Ohio, where he lives with his wife and two daughters. He reportedly shares Ron's drive to work hard. His younger sister (age 43) is a homemaker who lives with her husband and two children in Fayetteville, near her parents. She has assumed responsibility for attending to her parents, and Ron regularly sends her money to help out.

Extended Family — Ron sees his uncle, a bank manager in Columbia, regularly. His wife's parents and several aunts, uncles, and cousins live in Columbia, and Ron and Emily see a lot of her family. "They are all so proud of what Ron has accomplished."

Children — Ron and Emily have two sons, Ben (19 years old) and Alan (17 years old), and one daughter, Beth (14 years old). Emily reports that the children are happy and healthy, doing well in school and socially.

Social History

Development — Ron's wife reports that he had a "normal childhood" and was loved by his parents, who are not demonstrative people. "They were tough, but they have always wanted the best for their children."

Education/Work — Ron was a goal-directed, excellent student. Has always wanted to teach and coach high school students. Ron is an excellent athlete who made the all-state teams in football, basketball, and baseball while getting all A's in high school. He played varsity football at Baylor and worked his way through graduate school as an assistant coach at Baylor. He is currently head coach at Columbia High and has begun receiving inquiries about coaching college football. His wife reports that Ron "likes what he is doing and is uncertain about coaching at the collegiate level." However, his father is encouraging him to continue climbing the ladder of success.

Relationships/Support System — The family support system is extensive (see "Family History"). Ron and his family have numerous friends and colleagues in Columbia, many of whom have expressed concern about Ron's behavior in the past month.

Substance Use — None reported. Ron has begun drinking three or four beers per day over the past month.

Hobbies/Leisure Time — Ron works twelve to eighteen hours each day during the football season. He takes great interest in his sons and attends all of their sporting events. Ron enjoys fishing and hunting with his colleagues when he can get away.

Significant Health History — In good health. Only known medical problem is high-normal blood pressure (140/90), which is being treated with a low-cholesterol diet.

Current Mental Status

General Appearance — Unshaven, disheveled, dressed in dirty flannel shirt and blue jeans with socks but no shoes. Combative and wild-eyed, frantic appearance. Struggling to get free of restraints. Very agitated and snarling at ER staff. Shouting obscenities at the door.

CASE STUDY (continued)

Sensorium	Incoherent responses to questions about time, place, and person. Knowledge, memory, and recall questionable. Judgment extremely impaired.
Emotions	Angry and extremely agitated. Alternately swearing and crying uncontrollably. Frantically scanning environment and appears frightened.
Moods	Rapid mood swings from excitement to anger to sadness to fear.
Voice and Speech	Loud swearing, growling, and snarling like an animal. Mostly incoherent, then sobbing, "I'm sorry, Daddy."
Motor Behavior	Kicking and thrashing about. Struggling against the restraints.
Thought Content	Incoherent.
Thought Process	Disorganized and easily distracted.
Other Significant Subjective or Objective Clinical Data	
Medications	No prescription medications. Given 400 mg Thorazine IM in ER.
Suicide or Violence Potential	High potential for violence. Restraints will be continued and 300 mg Thorazine will be given IM every four hours until Ron is calm.
Summary	Ron is clearly experiencing a major manic episode that appears related to his increasing success as a coach, his recent interview with *Sports Illustrated,* and the pressure he feels to win the state football championship. His need to succeed and his fear of failure have resulted in a manic escalation over the past two to four weeks. Ron has history of a previous manic episode four years ago, and he has had several hypomanic episodes since.

Diagnostic Impression

Nursing Diagnoses	Activity intolerance Ineffective individual coping Knowledge deficit (Mood disorder and related care/treatment) Altered nutrition: Less than body requirements Self-care deficit Self-esteem disturbance Sleep pattern disturbance Impaired social interaction
DSM-III-R Multiaxial Diagnoses	Axis I: 296.44 Bipolar disorder, manic with psychotic features Axis II: 301.00 Paranoid personality Axis III: Borderline hypertension Axis IV: Severity: 3— moderate (psychosocial stressors) Axis V: Current GAF: 10 Highest GAF past year: 85

CASE STUDY

A Client with a Bipolar Disorder, Depressed

Identifying Information	Marcia M is a 32-year-old Caucasian, Christian woman who presents for help in controlling her emotions. Marcia is a bright and motivated person, functioning as the executive of a large pharmaceutical company. Her past successes include a summa cum laude graduation from Harvard University with an MBA.
Client's Definition of Present Problem, Precipitating Stressors, Coping Strategies, Goals for Care	Marcia states she is "afraid of losing control" of her behavior and emotions. She vacillates between "excitement and total lack of energy" since she was passed over for promotion six months ago, and has no energy for her friends or social activities. Unable to sleep through the night (only three to four hours sleep) for the month. Says she wants to "get back to normal," i.e., able to be happy and productive without worrying about unpredictable swings.
History of Present Problem	At age 32, Marcia was on the fast track within her corporation, having been promoted every two to three years to positions of increasing responsibility and authority. The next promotion Marcia expected was to associate vice-president for international sales, but she did not receive it. The reasons given to her for being passed over made no sense to Marcia. "We need new blood from outside the corporation." "You're too good at what you're doing; we couldn't afford to lose you from the new projects we're committed to." "You're young. There will be plenty of time for you to advance."

To Marcia, they all seemed like shallow excuses. On one level, she could agree with this logic. It certainly was not the end of the road for her. Yet, another part of her was convinced that she had not performed well enough to warrant the promotion. Yes, she had worked hard, giving eagerly of her time and energy to the corporation and enjoying the success that was personal and collective. But she could not shake the thought that they were not pleased with her work, that there was something wrong with her. And another part of her was furious, convinced that she had been sabotaged by her competitive male colleagues who could not tolerate one more reward for the woman who was more successful than those who played the game straight within the old boy network.

Marcia knew she had potential grounds for a sex discrimination case, yet she could not focus the energy that should have been available from her anger. She half-heartedly pursued opportunities with other companies, yet wound up turning down a lucrative advancement offer from the top corporation in the industry. Marcia was aware that her enthusiasm for work was dwindling. She was unable to convince herself that working evenings and weekends was worth it. But she could think of no better way to spend her free time. She also had no energy for friends, parties, concerts, plays, or cocktail parties. She thought to herself, "Others would kill for your position and success at this stage of your career. You have no right to feel bad." Yet she did feel bad, and she finally decided to find someone to help her sort out her thoughts and feelings.

Psychiatric History	No prior hospitalizations. Reports obtaining tranquilizers from her general practitioner twice in past two years for what sound like hypomanic episodes of overwork and extreme agitation.

CASE STUDY *(continued)*

Family History

Parents

Marcia's mother was a university professor of economics who died of cancer in 1987 at the age of 62. Her father was a neurosurgeon in private practice in Boston. He died of a heart attack in 1990, at the age of 67.

Siblings

None.

Extended Family

Marcia reports being close to one uncle (her mother's brother) who visits her two times each year while traveling on business.

Social History

Development

Marcia reports normal growth and development as the only child of career-oriented parents. She was always the brightest child in the class and had to pretend she wasn't so smart so that the other kids would like her. She never lacked material things but describes a rather lonely childhood with respect to peer and social relationships.

Education/Work

Excellent student. BA, Radcliffe 1978; MBA, Harvard University, 1980. Graduated with honors and received numerous offers from top corporations. Accepted management position with Cure-All Pharmaceuticals because of the possibilities for rapid upward mobility.

Relationships/Support System

Although Marcia has no close friends or relationships, she reports numerous work and social contacts. She has decreased her social activities (concerts, plays, parties) in past four to six months.

Substance Use

Marcia engages in social drinking in moderation and has never smoked or used drugs. In the last month, she has been drinking more (2–3 oz) alone in the evenings.

Hobbies/Leisure Time

Marcia works twelve to eighteen hours/day. Although she used to socialize with her colleagues, she has been refusing invitations for the last two or three months. Prior to that, she attended about three work-related social events per week. In college, she enjoyed playing bridge and going to plays and concerts.

Significant Health History

No known medical problems. Marcia has lost 10 pounds in past three months without dieting. Though thin, she reports excellent physical health. She jogs once or twice a week.

Current Mental Status

General Appearance

Bright, poised, articulate, business executive. "Power dressed" in tailored suit and ruffled blouse. Carries herself like a confident woman who is used to being in charge.

Sensorium

Oriented to time, place, and person. Knowledge, memory, recall, and judgment intact.

Emotions

Flat affect except when excited (e.g., when talking about work). Denies anger or depression.

Moods

Rapid mood swings between hypomanic and depressed affect.

CASE STUDY (continued)

Voice and Speech	Pressured to keep talking.
Motor Behavior	Very proper and controlled movements.
Thought Content	Normal. Denies thoughts of suicide or anger.
Thought Process	Presents herself and her ideas in a very controlled, organized manner, at times without affect. Appears pressured to keep talking. Reports increased difficulty concentrating on her work over the past month. Is working on three large marketing projects simultaneously. Demonstrates little insight into her current situation. Has difficulty reflecting on her own thoughts and feelings.
Other Significant Subjective or Objective Clinical Data	
Medications	No prescription medications. Uses aspirin three or four times a week for tension headaches.
Suicide or Violence Potential	Not at this time. Will monitor as she gets in touch with her anger and sadness.
Summary	Bright, attractive career woman who is having difficulty dealing with perceived rejection and loss over recently not being promoted. Also, she has never dealt with grief over deaths of her mother (1982) and father (1985). She denies anger, guilt, or sadness.
Diagnostic Impression	
Nursing Diagnoses	Activity intolerance Impaired social interaction Ineffective individual coping Self-care deficit Sleep pattern disturbance Diversional activity deficit
DSM-III-R Multiaxial Diagnoses	Axis I: 396.53 Bipolar disorder, depressed with melancholia Axis II: 301.81 Narcissistic personality Axis III: Recent weight loss without dieting Axis IV: Severity: 3-Moderate stressors Axis V: Current GAF: 65 Highest GAF last year: 87

NURSING CARE PLAN

Client Care Goals	Nursing Planning/ Intervention	Evaluation
Nursing Diagnosis: *Activity intolerance*		
Will improve effectiveness/productivity at work.	Set daily and weekly goals to help client with realistic time structuring (e.g., What can she	Client sets and accomplishes work goals three of five days a week.

▶

NURSING CARE PLAN (continued)

Client Care Goals	Nursing Planning/ Intervention	Evaluation
	realistically accomplish each day of the week?). Help client plan to negotiate revised expectations with immediate supervisor if necessary.	
Will be less restless and participate in structured physical activity.	Help client plan to jog five mornings/week. Explore possibility of physical activity (tennis, racquetball, or health club) with friends.	Jogs five mornings per week. Reports being comfortable and in touch with her body.

Nursing Diagnosis: *Impaired social interaction*

Client Care Goals	Nursing Planning/ Intervention	Evaluation
Will restore interest/pleasure in usual social activities.	Plan with client for two social activities per week. Help her select the people and activities that will make her most comfortable and during which she will receive positive strokes.	Plans and attends two social activities per week.

Nursing Diagnosis: *Ineffective individual coping*

Client Care Goals	Nursing Planning/ Intervention	Evaluation
Will improve concentration at work.	Talk with client about what is going on internally when she is having difficulty concentrating. (It is likely she is feeling agitated or pressuring herself to perform.) Help client set realistic expectations of herself. Encourage breaks and more contact with people to increase self-esteem and positive strokes.	Is able to concentrate on work for realistic periods of time. Takes morning and afternoon breaks and lunch with a friend or colleague.

Nursing Diagnosis: *Self-care deficit*

Client Care Goals	Nursing Planning/ Intervention	Evaluation
Will eat more and reverse recent weight loss.	As client expresses feelings and deals with depression, her appetite will probably return. In the meantime, help her structure plans for three meals/day (2200 kcal) to regain weight. Help her select foods she enjoys and pleasant experiences (e.g., lunch with a friend) to support positive eating experiences. Give message that eating properly is one means of taking care of herself.	Eats three meals/day (2200 cal). Gains ten pounds. Reports improved appetite and enjoyment of food.

NURSING CARE PLAN (continued)

Client Care Goals	Nursing Planning/ Intervention	Evaluation
Nursing Diagnosis: *Sleep pattern disturbance*		
Will sleep peacefully through the night.	Teach deep breathing and progressive relaxation techniques. Explore what client is thinking, feeling, and doing while unable to sleep. Help her express her denied feelings (should improve ability to sleep) and problem solve ways to be relaxed and quiet at night.	Gets six or seven hours of uninterrupted sleep each night. Reports sleeping comfortably.
Nursing Diagnosis: *Diversional activity deficit*		
Will participate in structured physical activity and social activities with friends.	Explore possibility of physical activities (e.g., tennis, racquetball, or health club) with friends. Plan ways to meet people with common interests in music and theater.	Plans and attends two social activities per week. Reports enjoyment from social activities.

---

automatic thoughts: "You can't do anything right." "You are socially incompetent." "Nobody likes you anyway."

• To counteract the automatic thoughts, offer rational explanations.

A potential outcome is a heightened awareness of the effect of thought on feeling states. Burns (1980) has been a leading proponent of this approach to dealing with depression.

Evaluating/Outcome Criteria

Nursing diagnosis and treatment are intended to produce beneficial effects in the human responses to actual or potential health problems, which are the phenomena of concern for nurses. "It is the results of the evaluation of outcomes of nursing actions that suggest whether or not those actions have been effective in improving or resolving the conditions to which they were directed" (ANA 1980, p 12).

Nurses, clients, and significant others all participate in determining the treatment goals and outcomes for persons with mood disorders. Table 13–1 shows the nursing diagnoses, treatment goals, and outcome criteria developed during the initial month of treat-

TABLE 13–1   Selected Nursing Diagnoses, Treatment Goals, and Outcome Criteria: Manic Episode

Goals	Outcome Criteria
Nursing Diagnosis: Impaired Verbal Communication	
To decrease quantity of speech	Engages in normal conversation
To decrease rate of speech	Engages in normal conversation
To decrease internal pressure to keep talking	Reports feeling comfortable talking normally with others
Nursing Diagnosis: Altered role performance	
To respond congruently within work and social situations	Jokes less and makes fewer puns
	Sits quietly in serious situations
	Listens to others when they are talking
Nursing Diagnosis: Self-esteem disturbance	
To decrease grandiosity	Makes reasonable appraisal of reality as confirmed by four other people
	Makes realistic statements about his or her own abilities

ment of a client experiencing a manic episode. Outcomes are measured in terms of beneficial changes in human responses: biologic, emotional, cognitive, and motor behaviors.

CHAPTER HIGHLIGHTS

• People with mood disorders range from functional to dysfunctional depending on how comfortable they are with themselves and how comfortable others are with their behavior.

• The DSM-III-R psychiatric diagnosis helps nurses formulate a nursing diagnosis and treatment plan for clients with mood disorders.

• Psychiatric nursing treatment of persons with mood disorders must be delivered from a noncompetitive frame of reference; with an emphasis on being rather than doing; with a reality-oriented approach to thinking, feeling, and behaving; and with the goal of developing adult relationships and contracts for change.

• A contract is a mutually agreed-on set of expectations between two or more people about what each will contribute to the relationship.

• Specific intervention techniques for working with mood disordered clients vary significantly according to the individual characteristics of the client and nurse, the setting in which the treatment is conducted, the social support available to the client, and the therapeutic support available to the nurse.

• Studies have been made in psychobiologic research of mood disorders, and many psychobiologic interventions show great promise.

REFERENCES

American Nurses' Association: *Nursing: A Social Policy Statement.* ANA, 1980.

American Psychiatric Association: *Diagnostic and Statistical Manual of Mental Disorders,* ed 3, revised. APA, 1987.

Arieti S: Manic-depressive psychosis and psychotic depression, in Arieti S (ed): *American Handbook of Psychiatry,* ed 2. Basic Books, 1974, pp 449–490.

Arieti S, Bemporad J: Psychological organization of depression. *Am J Psychiatry* 1980;137(11):1260–1365.

Beardslee WR, Bemporad J, Keller MB, Klerman GL: Children of parents with major affective disorder: A review. *Am J Psychiatry* 1983;140(7):825–832.

Beck AT: *Depression: Causes and Treatment.* University of Pennsylvania Press, 1967.

Bowlby J: Grief and mourning in infancy and early childhood. *Psychoanalytic Study Child* 1960;15:9.

Burns DD: *Feeling Good: The New Mood Therapy.* Signet Books, 1980.

Chaisson M, Beutler L, Yost E, Allender J: Treating the depressed elderly. *J Psychosoc Nurs* 1984;22(5):25–30.

Coryell W, Endicott J, Keller M, Andreasen N, Grove W, Hirschfeld RMA, Scheftner W: Bipolar affective disorder and high achievement: A familial association. *Am J Psychiatry* 1989;146(8):983–988.

Davison GC, Neal JM: *Abnormal Psychology.* Wiley, 1978.

Egeland JA: A genetic study of manic depressive disorder among the older Amish of Pennsylvania. *Pharmacopsychiatry* 1988;21:74–75.

Freud S: *Mourning and Melancholia. Standard Edition of the Complete Psychological Works of Sigmund Freud,* vol 14. Hogarth Press, 1957.

Honig A, Bartlett JR, Bridges PK: Amino acid levels in depression: A preliminary investigation. *J Psychiatr Res* 1988;22(3):159–164.

Levy AB, Drake ME, Shy KE: EEG evidence of epileptiform paroxysms in rapid cycling bipolar patients. *J Clin Psychiatry* 1988;49(6):232–234.

Loomis ME, Landsman SG: Manic-depressive structure: Treatment strategies. *Transactional Analysis J* 1981; 11(4):346–351.

McEnany GW: Psychobiological indices of bipolar mood disorder: Future trends in nursing care. *Arch Psychiatr Nurs* 1990;4(1):29–38.

Meisenhelder JB: Self-esteem: A closer look at clinical intervention. *Int J Nurs Stud* 1985;22(2):127–135.

Nemeroff CB: Clinical significance of psychoendocrinology in psychiatry: Focus on the thyroid and the adrenal. *J Clin Psychiatry* 1989;50(5) [Suppl]:13–20.

NIMH/NIH Consensus Development Plan: Mood disorders: Pharmacologic prevention of recurrences. *Am J Psychiatry* 1985;142(4):469–476.

Orsolits M, Morphy M: A depression algorithm for psychiatric emergencies. *J Psychiatr Diagn Eval* 1982;4:137–145.

Plumlee A: Biological rhythms and affective illness. *J Psychosoc Nurs Ment Health Services* 1986;24(3):12–17.

Rosenthal NE, Jacobsen FM, Sack DA, Arendt J, James SP, Parry BL, Wehr TA: Atenolol in seasonal affective disorder: A test of the melatonin hypothesis. *Am J Psychiatry* 1988;145(1):52–56.

Rosenthal NE, Skwerer G, Sack DA, Duncan CC, Jacobsen FM, Tamarkin L, Wehr TA: Biologic effects of morning plus evening bright light treatment of seasonal affective disorder. *Psychopharmacol Bull* 1987;23(3):364–369.

Shukla S, Cook BL, Mukerjee S, Goodwin C, Miller MG: Mania following head trauma. *Am J Psychiatry* 1987;144(1):93–96.

Wurtman RJ: Effects of dietary amino acids, carbohydrates and choline on neurotransmitter synthesis. *Mt Sinai J Med* 1988;55(1):75–86.

Zung W: A self-rating depressive scale. *Arch Gen Psychiatry* 1965;12:63.

Psychobiology Box References

Hensley M, Rogers S: Shedding light on "SAD"ness. *Arch Psychiatr Nurs* 1987;1(4):230–235.

Rosenthal NE, Jacobsen FM, Sack DA, Arendt J, James SP, Parry BL, Wehr TA: Atenolol in seasonal affective disorder: A test of the melatonin hypothesis. *Am J Psychiatry* 1988;145(1):52–56.

Tinkleberg M: Shift work and circadian rhythm. *Health-watch: The Nurse's Newspaper,* January 7, 1991.

Wehr TA, Rosenthal NE: Seasonality and affective illness. *Am J Psychiatry* 1989;146(7):829–839.

Nutrition Box References

Bernstein A: Vitamin B$_6$ in clinical neurology. *Ann NY Acad Sci* 1990;585:250–260.

Godfrey P et al: Enhancement of recovery from psychiatric illness by methylfolate. *Lancet* 1990;336:392–395.

Krause M, Mahan L: *Food, Nutrition, and Diet Therapy.* Philadelphia: Saunders, 1984.

Lonsdale D, Shamberger R: Red cell transketolase as an indicator of nutritional deficiency. *Am J Clin Nutr* 1980;33(2):205–211.

McLaren D: Clinical manifestations of nutritional disorders, in Shils M, Young V (eds): *Modern Nutrition in Health and Disease,* ed 7. Philadelphia: Lea and Febiger, 1988.

Rasmussen H et al: Depression and magnesium deficiency. *Int J Psychiatry Med* 1989;19(1):57–63.

Reynolds EH: Folic acid, S-adenosylmethionine and affective disorder. *Psychological Medicine* 1983;13(4):705–710.

Applying the Nursing Process for Clients with Anxiety, Somatoform, and Dissociative Disorders

LEARNING OBJECTIVES

- Describe the historical and theoretic foundations pertinent to the understanding of anxiety disorders, somatoform disorders, and dissociative disorders

- Compare and contrast clinical features characteristic to each of these disorders as delineated in DSM-III-R

- Apply the nursing process with clients with these disorders and their families

- Assess clients who have symptoms of disabling anxiety, somatization, or dissociation

- Formulate nursing diagnoses for clients experiencing an anxiety disorder, somatoform disorder, or dissociative disorder

- Develop individualized nursing care plans for clients with these disorders, and their families

- Implement appropriate nursing interventions for clients with these disorders and their families

- Evaluate the effectiveness of nursing interventions for clients with these disorders and their families

Marilynn Petit

CROSS REFERENCES

Other topics relevant to this content are: Basics related to anxiety, stress, and coping, Chapter 5; Crisis intervention for the acute stage of post-traumatic stress disorder, Chapter 28; Dissociative problems in victims of childhood sexual abuse, Chapter 22; Guidelines for teaching clients and families about antianxiety agents, Chapter 32; Psychopharmacologic treatment of anxiety (the anti-anxiety drugs), Chapter 32; Relaxation and stress-management techniques, Chapter 27.

THE TWENTIETH CENTURY HAS been called the "age of anxiety" (Auden 1947). Auden clearly saw the impact of anxiety in the modern era and its influence on day-to-day function. Though recognized as a separate psychologic entity only in relatively recent times, anxiety has influenced human behavior since the beginning of civilization. Only in the past fifty years, however, has anxiety been understood as central to the etiology of many types of emotional disorders. According to DSM-III-R, an estimated 2 to 4 percent of the population has at some time suffered from some type of anxiety disorder (DSM-III-R, p 225).

Anxiety exerts a powerful influence on the maturational process of individuals as they modify behaviors to be accepted in a given society. How people experience anxiety and what precipitates and relieves it are thought to be conditioned by the values and customs of a culture. In a sociologic context, then, the cultural milieu is central to the anxiety experience and must be considered in formulating a diagnosis and in developing treatment approaches and interventions.

A wide variety of problems face individuals today. These include adjustment to an increasingly technological environment in which the individual may be undervalued or overlooked. Standardization, centralization, and mechanization in business and personal life threaten individual identity and create anxiety. These phenomena need to be recognized as significant factors associated with the experience of anxiety.

Although anxiety is a universal experience, people vary in their ability to tolerate anxiety and anxiety-producing situations. This chapter explores the experience of individuals with anxiety disorders, somatoform disorders, or dissociative disorders. Although anxiety may be expressed in different ways, two factors are basic to the experience of all these persons:

1. The anxiety is sufficiently disabling and severe to cause major dysfunction in their lives.

2. A psychologic route of escape is used.

Historical and Theoretic Foundations

Anxiety Disorders

In the late nineteenth and early twentieth centuries, individuals with symptoms of anxiety were generally viewed as suffering from a primary physical illness. In America, for example, people in military hospitals during the American Civil War who suffered acute anxiety symptoms were diagnosed as having a functional disease of the heart, called "irritable heart."

Anxiety disorders are characterized by a mixture of physical and psychologic symptoms, which are discussed later in this chapter. A rapid pulse, pounding heart, chest pain or tightness, and labored breathing are a few of the typical physical symptoms of anxiety. Psychologic symptoms include nervousness, apprehension, hyperalertness, and excessive vigilance. This diversity of symptoms leads to a diversity of theoretic and treatment approaches.

Though psychiatrists and neurologists in Europe and America recognized anxiety as a symptom for several decades prior to the twentieth century, it was not viewed as a separate diagnostic entity. Instead, anxiety symptoms were grouped with other psychoneurotic symptoms such as depression and exhaustion under the label neurasthenia (Nemiah 1985a).

Psychologic Approaches In the past, attempts to understand anxiety disturbances were grounded in Freudian psychoanalytic theory and based nearly exclusively on the study of psychologic factors. Sigmund Freud first conceptualized anxiety neurosis as a discrete clinical syndrome and came to regard anxiety as the fundamental problem in neurotic symptom formation, i.e., that physical symptoms are experienced as a result of anxiety (Freud 1936). In addition, Freud believed that understanding anxiety was essential to the development of a comprehensive theory of human behavior. Most anxiety, he reported, reflected unconscious signals of early childhood dangers. Neurotic behavior was the result of unconscious conflict—an attempt to find a compromise between the impulses of the id and the reality strivings of the ego. In other words, Freud saw anxiety as a sign of psychologic conflict resulting from the threatened emergence into consciousness of forbidden repressed ideas or emotions.

In psychoanalytic approaches, anxiety is seen as a sign of psychologic conflict resulting from the threatened emergence into consciousness of forbidden or repressed ideas or emotions. The individual fears expressing and discharging the forbidden impulses, which occur in four forms, according to the nature of their consequences:

1. Superego anxiety, in which individuals suffer from anxious expectation of guilt should they break their inner code of ethics and standards.

2. Castration anxiety, or fear of fantasized danger or injuries to the body or genitals.

3. Separation anxiety, or fear of losing the love, esteem, and caring of significant people.

4. Id or impulse anxiety, or fear of the complete annihilation of self.

Other analytic views, sometimes referred to as neo-Freudian, evolved from the work of Freud and differ about the nature of anxiety. Rank (1952) believed that anxiety can be traced back to birth trauma. Sullivan (1953) stressed the importance of the early relationship between the mother and the child and the transmission of the mother's anxiety to the child. Existential analysts viewed anxiety as the central feature of the human condition, and the fear of nonbeing as a primary human fear.

Proponents of psychologic frameworks for the understanding of anxiety note that although certain anxiety symptoms may often be related to neural and biochemical processes, the appearance and manifestations of anxiety syndromes cannot be traced to discrete neuropathologic lesions. According to this model, the unconscious conflict must be brought into consciousness so that the real source of anxiety can be discovered and dealt with. Treatment takes the form of analysis or the less time-consuming psychodynamic psychotherapy.

Behavioral Approaches

Behaviorists (learning theorists) view anxiety as a learned response that can be unlearned. For example, behaviorists believe that the cause of phobias is traumatic exposure to the avoided object, situation, or activity. According to learning theory on the development of obsessions, an original neutral obsessive thought evokes anxiety because it becomes associated with an anxiety-provoking stimulus. In compulsions, a person discovers that a certain action relieves anxiety associated with the obsessive thought. The person repeats the action to achieve relief until eventually the act becomes fixed into a learned pattern of behavior.

Behavior modification is the common name for the behavioral treatment that teaches clients new ways to modify their behavior. "Conditioning" techniques—using positive and negative reinforcements—are examples of modification techniques. Another usual method of treatment is **systematic desensitization** in which a client builds up tolerance to anxiety through exposure to a series of anxiety-provoking stimuli.

Behavioral approaches have been most effective in treating behavior disorders and disorders of impulse control such as overeating, excessive alcohol use, and nicotine dependence. However, behavioral approaches are also frequently effective in the treatment of anxiety and are widely used for modifying symptoms in phobic and obsessive-compulsive disorders.

The behavioral therapist believes that it is unnecessary to use analysis to induce the client to struggle with the anxiety. Instead, the client need only face the anxiety repeatedly until it becomes manageable. Many clinicians today consider behavioral psychotherapies the treatment of choice for most phobic disorders (Marks 1985). They are more efficient, less costly, and less time-consuming than other forms of insight-oriented psychotherapy treatment. Like some psychodynamically and psychoanalytically oriented therapists, behavioral therapists tend to avoid the use of medication because they believe that it may interfere with the client's ability to learn behaviors.

Humanistic Interactionist and Psychobiologic Foundations

Recent research in the function of the peripheral autonomic nervous system, the limbic system, and the hypothalamus has led researchers to advance a physiologic basis for anxiety. Much new knowledge has been gained from this increased interest in possible physical-biologic explanations of anxiety disorders. At present, however, the relation of biologic processes to the experience of anxiety has not been completely explained (Teicher 1988).

In the biologic approach to anxiety, treatment frequently revolves around drug therapy. (Drug therapy for anxiety is discussed later in this chapter.) Antianxiety drugs are among the most widely prescribed. These drugs may have serious long-term side effects however, and it is important to monitor their use carefully.

The framework that is adopted in this text implies that the nurse must consider the external situation, the brain, and the mind when assessing, diagnosing, and planning interventions. This nursing perspective identifies biologic, social, cultural, and intrapersonal factors as important.

This perspective is particularly important in understanding the anxiety disorders, somatoform disorders, and dissociative disorders. Environmental stress—the "reality" concerns of the individual—biologic factors, and intrapsychic fears or conflicts cannot be adequately dealt with separately but only as they interact with one another. For example, clients suffering from a phobic disorder experience shame and helplessness as they attempt to cope with fears of annihilation in the presence of the dreaded object or situation. The result may be interpersonal and functional withdrawal, creating long-lasting disability.

This recognition has given rise to a multifaceted approach to the care of clients with these conditions. Humanistic treatment approaches are integrative and may include the range of psychotherapeutic interventions, including psychotherapy (cognitive, behavioral, and/or dynamic), measures to develop or ensure effective social support systems, measures to reduce environmental stress, and psychopharmacologic treatment.

Somatoform Disorders

In **somatoform disorders**, physical symptoms are present but evidence of physiologic disorder is not. The symptoms are thought to be linked to psychologic factors or emotional conflict. Conversion disorders, previously termed hysteric conversion reactions, were among the earliest disturbed coping patterns Sigmund Freud described. They were often associated with the repressive sexual conventions and passive-dependent women's role of the Victorian period.

One of Freud's most famous patients was Anna O., an intelligent, strong-minded woman of 21. After her father's illness and death, she had developed a set of symptoms including paralysis of the limbs, contractures, paresthesias, visual disturbances, disturbances of speech, anorexia, and a nervous cough. Anna had been very close to and fond of her father. She had nursed him on his deathbed.

Using hypnosis as a primary tool, Freud's associate Josef Breuer made the connection between inhibited sexuality and the production of symptoms such as Anna's that have no organic basis. Breuer and Freud outlined a "theory of hysteria" that placed early repressed traumatic sexual experiences, such as seductions, at the root of hysterical symptoms. Later Freud was to modify this hypothesis by abandoning the notion of actual physical seduction and placing a new emphasis on the inner fantasy life of the child.

The point of view advocated in this book leads us to search beyond repressed infantile sexuality for the meaning of conversion disorder. Some communication theorists believe that manifestations are really nonverbal body language intended to communicate a message to significant others. Sometimes the message is as general as "pay attention to me" or "take care of me." At other times the *conversion of anxiety* actually symbolizes the nature of the specific underlying conflict. For example, a woman who wants to strike her children may develop a paralysis of her arm. A girl who feels guilty about reading erotic books may become blind. Both realize the primary gain of protection from their anxiety-provoking impulses, and both get secondary gains of attention and sympathy as well. These patterns are most likely to occur among clients who do not have more aggressive alternatives.

Clients who deal with anxiety by converting it into physical symptoms usually show no other psychologic symptoms, e.g., disturbed thoughts or depressed moods. However, they are often said to exhibit subtler behavior patterns. Characteristics that have come to be associated with conversion disorder clients are self-dramatization, exhibitionism, narcissism, emotionalism, seductiveness, dependency, manipulativeness, childishness, and suggestibility. It is interesting to note, however, that these characteristics have usually been attributed to female clients by male psychiatrists.

Pain is associated with a great many disease processes, including many of the organ-specific somatoform disorders. Pain can be an adaptive or a maladaptive response. It often indicates real danger to the organism, but sometimes it interferes with functioning.

Consciousness, attention, perception, and cognition are all necessary for the experience of pain. According to modern theories of pain perception, humans have a control system over pain that operates as a "gate." Pain stimuli can be "allowed in" to or "shut out" from the cerebral cortex, depending essentially on the meaning the person attaches to the stimulus. This underscores the importance of meaning, symbol, and affect in the experience of pain sensation.

Figure 14-1 shows the basic mechanism for so-called idiopathic pain (pain of unknown origin). In psychoanalytic concepts, the unconscious conflicts are a result of traumatic or frustrating childhood experiences that are reawakened in adult life by a similar stress or frustration. According to this theory, the person cannot express the evoked affect because of feelings of guilt, fear of loss of love, or fear of retribution. The affect is therefore repressed and transformed into physiologic correlates such as pain.

Dissociative Disorders

The **dissociative disorders** encompass a large group of interesting, uncommon, and sometimes bizarre conditions. In each of these disorders, there is a sudden, temporary change in consciousness, identity, or motor behavior so that some part of these functions is lost.

Though awareness of the existence of dissociative phenomena extends far back in history, little was understood about their nature or cause. The phenomena were cloaked in superstition or mysticism during the Middle Ages or associated with "spells" or witchcraft. Because of the increasing scientific attention to the technique of hypnosis in the latter half of the nineteenth century, interest increased in the phenomena of dissociation. Hypnotic techniques were employed in exploring dissociative reactions.

Pierre Janet (1859-1947) was the first to develop the concept of the "splitting off" or dissociation of a part of consciousness. He believed that the individual needed to have a normal amount of "mental energy" to maintain integrative mental processes. When the level of energy was high, integration was maintained. When it became low, however, the personality might cease to function as a unit and split or dissociate.

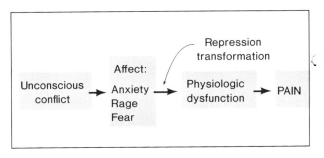

FIGURE 14-1   Basic mechanism of idiopathic pain.

Nearly any type of emotional illness could result, he thought.

Freud, in contrast, proposed the concept of repression to explain the loss of conscious awareness in dissociation. He then introduced the notion of the *dynamic unconscious,* a part of the mind in which affects or ideas that were unacceptable to a person were pushed from awareness or recall. Freud and other early analytic theorists accepted the basic concept of psychologic dissociation. Conceptions and theories of the phenomena of dissociation have continued to evolve during the twentieth century.

Current explanations of dissociation are based on Freud's dynamic concepts. The repression of ideas that leads to amnesia and other forms of dissociation is conceived as a way of protecting the individual from emotional pain arising either from disturbing external circumstances or internal psychologic conflicts. A dissociative reaction may be viewed as a flight from crisis or danger—a major psychologic route of escape from anxiety. Sometimes, as in states of fugue and multiple personality, the dissociated area takes over temporary direction and control of the entire personality. During such times, the individual may even appear to be functioning well to the observer.

Additional specific dynamic considerations relevant to dissociative disorders include the following ideas. In psychogenic amnesia, the pattern is similar to conversion reactions except that the individual does not avoid some unpleasant situations by getting sick. Instead, the person does so by forgetting (repressing or suppressing) certain traumatic events or stresses. In multiple personality disorder there appears to be a deep-seated conflict between contradictory impulses and beliefs. A resolution is achieved by separating the conflicting parts and developing each into an autonomous personality.

Biopsychosocial Factors

Anxiety Disorders

In this group of disorders, anxiety is either the predominant disturbance—as in generalized anxiety disorder—or anxiety is experienced as avoidance behavior when the individual attempts to master the symptoms—as in confronting the dreaded object or situation in a phobic disorder. When anxiety is not tied to a specific stimulus, it may be called *free-floating anxiety.* The accompanying box describes anxiety disorders.

People in anxiety states experience anxiety both as a subjective emotion and as a variety of physical symptoms resulting from muscular tension and autonomic nervous system activity. See Chapter 5 for a discussion of the levels of anxiety. When acute, the

Characteristics of Anxiety Disorders (DSM-III-R)

Panic Disorder (with or without agoraphobia)
Recurrent panic attacks that may be unpredictable or may be associated with specific situations; symptoms such as dyspnea, sweating, palpitations, and chest pain or discomfort; often associated with agoraphobia

Generalized Anxiety Disorder
Generalized persistent anxiety without specific symptoms that characterize other anxiety disorders; symptoms generally involve motor tension, autonomic hyperactivity, and apprehensive expectation

Obsessive-Compulsive Disorder
Recurrent obsessions (persistent ideas, thoughts, images, or impulses that are ego-dystonic) or compulsions (repetitive and seemingly purposeful behaviors performed according to certain rules or in a stereotyped fashion and generally experienced as senseless and ego-alien)

Agoraphobia (without history of panic disorder)
Marked fear of being alone or in public places from which escape might be difficult or in which help might not be available; usually the person is afraid of having a limited symptom attack (a single or small number of symptoms)

Social Phobia
Persistent irrational fear of situations in which an individual may be exposed to scrutiny by others and fear that the individual may behave in a humiliating or embarrassing manner

Simple Phobia
Isolated fears focused on one situation or object

Post-Traumatic Stress Disorder
The experience of a significant recognizable stressor or trauma followed by recurrent subjective reexperiencing of the trauma, a general numbing of responsiveness or reduced involvement with the external world, and two or more of several cognitive and somatic symptoms

anxiety rapidly drives the individual to seek help. When subacute or chronic, anxiety can lead to a number of somatic discomforts or disabilities. Heartburn, epigastric distress, diarrhea, and constipation may occur. Chronic muscular tension can lead to a variety of musculoskeletal aches and pains, e.g., backache, shoulder and neck pain, and headache.

Onset may be sudden or gradual. Some individuals experience an unexpected, incapacitating outbreak of acute anxiety, as in panic disorder. In others, anxiety may express itself through relatively mild somatic symptoms in which the existence of basic anxiety is missed unless specifically inquired about, as in generalized anxiety disorder.

Panic Disorder An apparently common disorder, panic disorder is characterized by recurrent attacks of severe anxiety lasting a few moments to an hour. These attacks are not associated with a stimulus but instead seem to occur spontaneously or out of the blue. They may, however, become associated with certain situations, e.g., going into a shopping mall or driving a car. The person usually experiences physical symptoms such as palpitations, rapid pulse, nausea, diarrhea, dyspnea, and a feeling of choking or suffocation. The pupils are dilated, and the face is flushed. The person may feel dizzy or faint and often has a sense of impending doom or death. Restlessness is acute, and the person may make pleading, apprehensive appeals for help.

In its most advanced state, panic creates a symptom constellation totally mimicking myocardial infarction and mitral valve prolapse. This symptom complex, seen most frequently in young adults, is called *cardiac neurosis*. Symptoms include palpitations, tachycardia, chest pain, dyspnea, easy fatigability, dizziness, sweating, irritability, faintness, and a feeling of impending doom.

Panic attacks may occur on occasion in normal, healthy individuals, leaving little or no residual disability. When the attacks occur frequently and when they interfere with the individual's social functioning at work, school, or in the family, the condition is called panic disorder. The accompanying Assessment box lists psychic and somatic features characteristic of a panic or anxiety attack.

Anticipatory fear of helplessness or of losing control during a panic attack is a common complication of the disorder. The individual frequently avoids situations that induce the fear, sometimes developing a phobic avoidance reaction. The DSM-III-R states that a diagnosis of **panic disorder with agoraphobia** is appropriate for an individual who experiences panic attacks and has phobic avoidance. In the absence of phobic avoidance, the condition is termed **panic disorder without agoraphobia**. This change reflects the fact that many investigators now believe that agora-

ASSESSMENT

Common Features of Panic Attack

Psychic	Somatic
Sudden onset of:	Sudden onset of:
Intense nervousness or apprehension	Tachycardia or palpitations
Feeling of impending doom or death	Chest discomfort
Mental confusion	Dyspnea
Feelings of unreality	Unsteadiness, dizziness, vertigo
Fear of going crazy or doing something uncontrolled during an attack	Sweating
	Choking or smothering sensations
	Faintness
	Hot and cold flashes
	Paresthesias
	Trembling or shaking

phobia (the marked fear of being alone or in public places from which escape might be difficult or in which help might not be available) is secondary to panic attacks and that agoraphobia without panic attacks is uncommon (Spitzer and Williams 1984). This suggests that the cause of agoraphobia is different from the cause of simple or social phobia. In addition, they note that agoraphobia with symptoms of panic attack is now treatable with some drugs. In contrast, simple or social phobias are not.

Panic disorder is often first noted in late adolescence or early adulthood. It may be limited to a single brief period lasting several weeks or months, recur several times, or become chronic. Though it is rarely incapacitating, the disorder can be severe. When complicated by agoraphobia, it can interfere greatly with individual functioning. Panic disorder is diagnosed much more frequently in women than in men, and some clinicians believe that sudden object loss and separation anxiety in childhood predispose to its development. Such physical disorders as hypoglycemia, hyperthyroidism, and amphetamine or caffeine intoxication must be ruled out before a diagnosis of panic disorder can be made. The ways in which hypoglycemia mimics a panic attack are discussed in the Nutrition box on page 320.

Generalized Anxiety Disorder Generalized anxiety disorder is considered less specific and less debili-

NUTRITION AND MENTAL HEALTH

Can Hypoglycemia Mimic an Anxiety Attack?

Much has been written in the lay press about the dangers of low blood sugar. Some popular authors claim it is a major scourge that afflicts millions of Americans, causing severe psychologic harm. Although there is little controlled clinical research to support that view, psychiatric nurses should not dismiss hypoglycemia as a hypochondriac's invention.

Postprandial hypoglycemia is a drop in plasma glucose following a carbohydrate load. It can occur after gastric surgery or in the very early stages of diabetes. However, when it has no clear-cut organic cause, it is called functional hypoglycemia.

Reactive low blood sugar presents in two major ways: Epinephrinelike signs and symptoms include nervousness, faintness, weakness, tremulousness, palpitations, sweating, and hunger. Central nervous system signs and symptoms include headache, confusion, visual disturbances, muscle weakness, ataxia, and marked personality changes (Berkow 1987).

No one challenges the existence of the syndrome or its signs and symptoms. Its prevalence, however, is open to debate. Studies suggest that between 3 and 23 percent of subjects complaining of hypoglycemialike problems actually meet standard diagnostic criteria (Betteridge 1987, Foster and Rubenstein 1985).

Most clinicians use the five-hour glucose tolerance test to detect the condition. The three diagnostic markers are a drop in blood glucose to below 50–60 mg/dL, symptoms of hypoglycemia during the test, and symptomatic relief upon eating sugar. Although it is reasonable to conclude that clients who meet all three criteria have hypoglycemia, one cannot always rule out the condition among those who do not.

Researchers have found that clients with blood glucose readings above 60 mg/dL may still have functional hypoglycemia, apparently because their normal blood glucose range is significantly higher than that of the population mean (Chalew et al. 1986). Clients with blood glucose readings below 50 mg/dL who experience no symptoms during the test most probably do not have hypoglycemia. Apparently their normal range is *below* the average.

The five-hour glucose tolerance test may not be the gold standard for detecting functional hypoglycemia. Some specialists have challenged its validity on the grounds that it does not simulate everyday eating patterns. Very few people consume 75 or 100 grams of pure glucose at one sitting, and clients' glycemic and symptomatic response to that much sugar may not reflect real-world conditions. With that in mind, some clinicians recommend that clients consume a normal diet and that blood glucose levels be measured throughout the day with a portable glucose monitor. A drop in readings during a hypoglycemialike episode strongly suggests the presence of the disorder (Palardy et al. 1989).

If a client does meet the criteria for hypoglycemia, and the possibility of an insulin-secreting tumor of the pancreas has been ruled out as the cause of hypoglycemic symptoms, how should they be managed? Before recommending or adopting a dietary regimen, both nurse and client must understand its rationale. Functional hypoglycemia is brought on by an oversensitivity to carbohydrates. Whereas a normal person secretes just enough insulin in response to a heavy carbohydrate meal to lower blood glucose levels to physiologic levels, someone with functional hypoglycemia secretes too much, causing blood glucose levels to drop too low and depleting the brain of its primary fuel.

To compensate for this abnormality, the diet must allow a slow, steady absorption of sugars, thus preventing the pancreas from overreacting. That is accomplished by reducing intake of simple carbohydrates such as table sugar (sucrose), jams, honey, and corn syrup, replacing them with starches (complex carbohydrates) and proteins. Complex carbohydrates include breads, cereals, potatoes, rice, and corn. Whole-grain versions of these foods are preferable because the fiber they contain helps moderate intestinal absorption. These foods are then combined with protein-rich foods such as meat, fish, beans, and milk to further control sugar utilization. As a rule, between-meal snacks are also encouraged to prevent blood glucose levels from dropping too low two to three hours after main meals.

—Paul L. Cerrato

tating than panic disorder. It is characterized by pervasive, persistent anxiety of at least six months' duration but without phobias, panic attacks, or obsessions and compulsions. The person experiences chronic feelings of nervousness and apprehension "for no reason." Autonomic symptoms may be less frequent or less severe than in panic attacks.

There is little generally accepted information about age of onset, predisposing factors, cause of illness, prevalence, sex ratio, or familial pattern. Some authors note that there appears to be a more equal sex ratio than in panic disorder. Also, generalized anxiety disorder apparently develops more gradually than panic disorder (Anderson, Noyes, and Crowe 1984). Associated mild depressive symptoms are not uncommon in individuals with generalized anxiety disorder. Although impairment in social or occupational functioning is rarely more than mild, abuse of alcohol or other drugs may be a serious complication and may interfere with effective motivation.

Obsessive-Compulsive Disorder Obsessive-compulsive disorder is classified with the anxiety disorders because of the anxiety symptoms that develop when an individual tries to resist an obsession or compulsion. Although compulsions are attempts to reduce tension, they eventually worsen tension because the individual becomes increasingly agitated, unable to decide whether to stop or continue the compulsive act.

Obsessive-compulsive people usually fear that they will harm someone or something. They rely heavily on avoidance and are best understood in terms of their control needs. Individuals who develop obsessive-compulsive symptoms have a great need to control themselves, others, and their environment. Three major psychologic defense mechanisms prominent in obsessive-compulsive disorders are *isolation, undoing,* and *reaction formation.* See Chapter 5 for a discussion of defense mechanisms.

An **obsession** is a recurring thought that cannot be dismissed from consciousness. These thoughts are sometimes trivial or ridiculous, often morbid or fearful, and always distressing and anxiety provoking. An example of a strange but trivial obsession is that of a young adolescent man who could not get the rhyme "Snips and snails and puppydog tails" out of his mind. An example of a much more ominous obsession is that of a woman who could not stop thinking that she must kill her children to prevent a worldwide race war. Other common obsessive thoughts have to do with violence or contamination.

A **compulsion** in contrast, is an uncontrollable, persistent urge to perform certain acts or behaviors to relieve an otherwise unbearable tension. Most compulsive acts are attempts to control or modify obsessions, either because compulsive persons fear the conse-

quences or are afraid that they will not be able to control the primary impulse.

Typical compulsive acts are endless hand washing, checking and rechecking doors to see if they have been locked, and elaborate dressing and undressing rituals. Such defensive compulsive acts are used to contain, neutralize, or ward off the anxiety related to the primary impulse. The young man who could not dismiss the rhyme from his mind developed a compulsion that involved ritualistic washing of his genitals to ward off the anxiety generated by his apparently silly obsession. The woman obsessed with thoughts about killing her children engaged in symbolic rituals of touching religious objects to repel evil influences through magical interventions by the saints. Such compulsive acts as counting and elaborately checking routine duties are frequently associated with the fear of failing or making a mistake, or with the need to be perfect.

Obsessions and compulsions have these features in common:

• An idea or an impulse insistently, persistently, and impellingly intrudes itself into the person's awareness.

• A feeling of anxious dread accompanies the primary manifestation and often leads the person to take countermeasures against the forbidden thought or impulse.

• Both the obsessions and the compulsion are ego-alien—i.e., foreign to one's self-perception.

• No matter how compelling the obsession or compulsion is, the person has enough insight to recognize it as irrational and experience it as a significant source of distress.

• Many of the personality traits associated with obsession and compulsion are highly valued in American culture. Success in many professions and occupations demands cautiousness, deliberateness, and rationality. These traits are usually associated with the tendency toward obsession or compulsion. When these personality traits are carried to an extreme, or when the balance between control and impulse expression leads to paralysis, they become a liability.

Obsessions and compulsions occur together in 75 percent of cases and usually follow a chronic course with waxing and waning of symptoms. In severe cases, extreme preoccupation or compulsive activity disrupts daily life. New knowledge from the fields of pharmacology and brain imaging suggests that severe obsessions and compulsions may be biologically rooted. Several new drugs first formulated as antidepressants relieve them (Rapoport 1989).

Obsessive-compulsive disorder is equally common in men and women. The usual age at onset is in the late teens to mid-twenties, though it has been diagnosed as early as childhood.

Phobic Disorders Like the other anxiety disorders discussed in this chapter, a phobic disorder is a response to experienced anxiety. Unlike people with generalized anxiety disorder, however, whose anxiety is free-floating, people with phobias fear specific places or things. A **phobia** is a persistent and irrational fear of a specific object, activity, or situation that results in a compelling desire to avoid the dreaded object or situation. Nearly all phobic persons panic when in contact with the phobic situation. The fear is recognized by the person as excessive or unreasonable in proportion to the actual danger.

The usual explanation of the development of phobia is that fear arises through a process of displacing an unconscious conflict to an external object symbolically related to the conflict. Thus, in becoming phobic, the individual fears a specific external object rather than an unknown internal source of distress. The phobic person can then control the intensity of the anxiety by avoiding the object with which the anxiety is associated.

A diagnosis of a phobic disorder is generally made when the avoidance behavior becomes so extreme or the problem so pervasive that it interferes with the person's normal functioning at home, work, or school. DSM-III-R divides the phobic disorders into three main types:

1. *Agoraphobia:* Fear of being alone or in public places

2. *Social phobia:* Fear of situations that may be humiliating or embarrassing

3. *Simple phobia:* Fear of specific things, e.g., animals, reptiles, heights, or darkness

Agoraphobia Agoraphobia involves fear of being in public places from which escape might be difficult or in which help might not be available. Often agoraphobic individuals fear leaving the safety of home, worrying that they might develop an incapacitating symptom, such as dizziness, loss of bowel or bladder control, or cardiac distress. Normal activities are increasingly curtailed as the fears dominate the individual's life. Agoraphobic persons often limit travel and need a companion when away from home. Individuals who endure the phobic situation experience intense anxiety. Other common fears associated with agoraphobia include fear of being alone, fear of elevators or enclosed places, fear of falling and of high places or high buildings, and fear of open spaces and public speaking.

Agoraphobia without panic attacks (called agoraphobia without history of panic disorder in DSM-III-R) is considered relatively rare. More usually, agoraphobics have spontaneous panic attacks (see panic disorder with agoraphobia discussed earlier in this chapter).

Most agoraphobics have a history of generalized anxiety or anxiety attacks at the onset of the phobic behavior. Some investigators believe others have had a significant depression preceding the onset of phobia (Cameron 1985, p 5). Onset is usually in the middle to late twenties. Agoraphobia is more frequently diagnosed in women than in men. Separation anxiety in childhood or sudden object loss appear to be predisposing factors. Depression, anxiety, rituals, minor "checking" compulsions, or rumination are frequently associated features.

The prognosis is variable. Some less severely disturbed individuals experience waxing and waning of symptoms and sometimes have periods of remission. The more severely impaired may suffer lifelong disability.

Social Phobia The main characteristic of **social phobia** is a persistent fear and avoidance of situations in which the person may be exposed to scrutiny by others. The person especially fears he or she will act in an embarrassing or humiliating manner. Examples of social phobias are extreme fear of performing or speaking in public, making complaints, or writing or eating in front of others. Others include fear of interacting with the opposite sex, superiors, or aggressive individuals. Usually the individual has only one social phobia.

The incidence of social phobia in the general population is apparently high (Gulledge 1988). Often appearing in late childhood or early adolescence, social phobia usually progresses to a chronic course. Some lessening of symptoms may occur in middle age. The course differs from that of agoraphobia, however, in that waxing and waning of symptoms are not common.

Sex ratio, familial pattern, and predisposing factors are unknown, although some investigators believe that the incidence is more evenly distributed between men and women than in simple phobia or agoraphobia (Tearnan and Telch 1984, p 168). Generalized anxiety, agoraphobia, or simple phobia may coexist with social phobia.

Simple Phobia Sometimes referred to as "specific" phobias, **simple phobias** are more common than any other type of phobic disorder. Simple phobias are isolated fears focused on one situation or object, e.g., a fear of reptiles, darkness, or heights. This category of phobic disorders encompasses all phobias not included in the categories of agoraphobia or social phobia.

Simple phobias generally cause minimal impairment if the phobic object is rarely encountered and easily avoided, e.g., a fear of snakes does not seriously impair an individual living in a high-rise condominium. The phobia can, however, be incapacitating if the phobic situation is frequently encountered and not easily avoided, e.g., a fear of heights or elevators seriously incapacitates the individual living in a high-rise condominium.

Many simple phobias begin in childhood and subsequently disappear. Those that persist into adulthood rarely remit without treatment. Simple phobia is more often diagnosed in females than in males. Complications and predisposing factors are not well understood, and researchers disagree about the contribution of specific occurrences of conditioning of fear in these phobias.

Post-Traumatic Stress Disorder   Although not included in the official psychiatric classification system until quite recently, **post-traumatic stress disorder** has been recognized as a psychologic disorder for many years. Older terms—*shell shock, battle fatigue,* and *war neurosis*—reflect an origin in combat situations. Post-traumatic stress disorder includes traumatic stress reactions to civilian and natural catastrophes as well, e.g., assault or rape, incest, skyjacking, and earthquakes. For a discussion of post-traumatic stress disorder as it relates to the experience of rape or incest, see Chapter 22.

Post-traumatic stress may be defined as the experience of a significant, recognizable stressor or trauma that is followed by recurrent subjective reexperiencing of the trauma. A general numbing of responsiveness followed by cognitive or somatic symptoms of irritability, anxiety, aggressiveness, and depression may follow (Cameron 1985, p 9). The stressor is generally outside the range of usual human experiences, although any environmental stimulus that is perceived as dangerous, whether it produces physical injury or not, can be sufficiently traumatic to precipitate a post-traumatic stress disorder (Scrignar 1984).

The course of post-traumatic stress disorder is variable. Most individuals who have suffered a significant stressor tend to have an acute reaction from which they recover spontaneously. In others, however, the reaction may be delayed or prolonged and eventually become chronic. Delayed onset is defined as symptoms occurring at least six months after the trauma. For example, many Vietnam veterans, upon return from combat, essentially relived their experience through recurrent nightmares. Other sleep disturbances, including insomnia, often occurred. "Psychic numbing"—emotional anesthesia in relation to other people and to previously enjoyed activities—was common. Some veterans reported difficulty in concentrating and remembering. Many veterans felt guilty about having survived when others did not or about actions they took to survive. When veterans were exposed to situations or events that resembled or symbolized the traumatic event, their symptoms often increased, and they felt even greater distress. Reactions such as these continue to disturb some Vietnam veterans even today. The accompanying Assessment box lists common features of post-traumatic stress disorder.

Post-traumatic stress disorder can occur in people of any age, even children. Associated symptoms of depression and anxiety are common, as well as increased irritability, sometimes leading to unpredictable explosions of hostility with little or no provocation. A significant complicating problem is the use of alcohol or other substances to maintain control and soothe emotions.

Somatoform Disorders

The essential features of somatoform disorders are physical symptoms suggesting physical disorders for which there is no positive evidence of organic or physiologic causes. Somatoform disorders are sometimes confused with physical disorders.

Somatoform disorders may also be confused with **factitious disorders.** Factitious means not genuine or natural. DSM-III-R includes in this category disorders in which clients consciously produce physical or psychologic symptoms. For example, a client may take anticoagulants to produce blood in the urine or dislocate a shoulder on purpose for no other reason than to assume a dependent role. The distinction between factitious and somatoform disorders is based on the determination that in factitious disorders the physical symptoms present are under voluntary control. In somatoform disorders, the physical symptoms are *not under voluntary control.* Both conditions must be thoughtfully assessed for the possible presence of a true, primary physical disorder.

 ASSESSMENT

Common Features of Post-Traumatic Stress

Aggressive behavior	Intrusive memories
Avoidance behavior	Memory impairment
Constricted affect	Nightmares
Depression	Panic attacks
Detachment	Phobic responses
Guilty rumination	Poor concentration
Hyperalertness	Repetitive dreams
Impulsiveness	Startle reactions
Insomnia	

Somatoform disorders include the following major clinical pictures described next and summarized in the box below.

Somatization Disorder The diagnosis of **somatization disorder** applies to clients who have sought medical attention for recurrent and multiple somatic complaints of several years' duration and seemingly without physiologic causes. This problem usually begins before the age of 30, has a chronic course, and is often accompanied by anxiety and depressed mood. Clients believe they have been sickly for a good part of their lives and report lengthy lists of symptoms, including blindness, paralysis, convulsions, nausea and other gastrointestinal difficulties, and painful menstruation, among others.

Characteristics of Somatoform Disorders (DSM-III-R)

Somatization Disorder
Many physical complaints or belief of having been sickly for several years before age 30; no organic or physiologic reason.

Conversion Disorder
Loss or alteration in physical function due to psychologic factors; symptom is not consciously produced and is a culturally sanctioned response; not explainable by known physical disorder.

Somatoform Pain Disorder
Preoccupation of at least six months' duration with pain for which there is no organic or physiologic reason; if there is related reason, the complaint is grossly excessive.

Hypochondriasis
Preoccupation with having serious illness despite lack of pathology; duration of at least six months.

Body Dysmorphic Disorder
Preoccupation with an imagined defect in physical appearance out of proportion to actual physical abnormality.

Undifferentiated Somatoform Disorder
Multiple physical complaints with no physiologic basis; if physiologic basis exists, impairments or complaints are grossly excessive; duration in excess of six months.

Conversion Disorder In **conversion disorder**, clients report loss or alteration of physical function that suggests a physical disorder but in fact is related to the expression of a psychologic conflict. Two mechanisms are thought to explain what a person "gets" from having a conversion disorder. The first, **primary gain**, helps the person to keep the psychologic need or conflict out of awareness. For example, a woman may become "blind" to avoid acknowledging a traumatic event she has seen. In this instance, the symptom is a partial solution to the underlying conflict (not having to acknowledge witnessing the traumatic event because she has suddenly been struck blind). The second mechanism, **secondary gain**, helps the person to avoid a distressing, uncomfortable, or repugnant activity while, at the same time, receiving support from others. For example, a soldier with a paralyzed arm could hardly be expected to fire a gun and is also likely to receive sympathy for his paralyzed condition.

The problem usually begins in adolescence or early adulthood, although a conversion disorder may appear at any time during the life cycle. Regardless of the time of its first appearance, a conversion disorder can seriously impede normal life activities.

Somatoform Pain Disorder In **somatoform pain disorder**, clients experience pain in the absence of physiologic findings and the presence of possible psychologic factors. Some of the clinical syndromes in which idiopathic pain may be the predominant complaint are conversion disorders, workers' compensation injuries, and masochistic personality styles. In conversion disorders, pain symbolizes punishment for having an unacceptable wish, perhaps sexual or aggressive, in response to a frustrating life situation. In workers' compensation cases, the client may unconsciously use pain, and the monetary compensation received for the suffering, to strike back against employers or others by whom the client feels unfairly treated. Some individuals seem to need to suffer to achieve any sort of gratification without guilt. They seem to assume they are otherwise unworthy of any pleasure. Often they conduct their entire lives according to a self-destructive pattern of expecting punishment and eliciting it from the environment.

Hypochondriasis Clients with **hypochondriasis** are preoccupied with the fear or belief that they have a serious disease, which on physical evaluation is not present. The unrealistic fear or belief persists for a period of at least six months despite medical reassurance. This fear impairs the social or occupational functioning of the client.

Body Dysmorphic Disorder Clients with **body dysmorphic disorder** are preoccupied with some imagined defect in physical appearance. The preoccupation is out of proportion to any actual abnormality. The belief is overvalued but not of delusional proportion.

Undifferentiated Somatoform Disorder Clients have multiple physical complaints lasting at least six months, and extensive evaluation reveals no organic problem. When there is related organic disease, the complaints or impairments are grossly excessive.

Dissociative Disorders

Dissociative disorders have, as their common base, the defense mechanism of dissociation, in which the client strips an idea, object, or situation of its emotional significance and affective content. Dissociative responses are somewhat uncommon and often bizarre defensive reactions to stress. Dissociative disorders are complex and are usually difficult to distinguish from one another. They share one common characteristic. In any dissociative disorder, a cluster of recent, related mental events is beyond the client's power of recall but can return spontaneously to conscious awareness. **Depersonalization disorder** is included because the client loses the feeling of personal reality, an important component of identity. The most common dissociative disorders are described here and summarized in the accompanying box. None is attributable to an organic mental disorder.

Multiple Personality Disorder Clients with **multiple personality disorder** are dominated by two or more distinct personalities, each of which determines the nature of its behavior and attitudes while it is uppermost in consciousness. The transition from one personality to another is often sudden and dramatic. There are many popular stories about people with multiple personalities. Two of the best known are *Sybil* and *The Three Faces of Eve.* However, these portrayals are popularizations of a disorder that is not always so colorful. The belief that one has been taken over or possessed by another person or spirit may occur as the experience of the alternate personality's influence.

Psychogenic Fugue A person with **psychogenic fugue** wanders, usually far from home and for days at a time. During this period, clients completely forget their past life and associations, but, unlike people with amnesia, are unaware of having forgotten anything. When they return to their former consciousness, they do not remember the period of fugue. Fugue clients are generally reclusive and quiet, and as a consequence their behavior rarely attracts attention. They may assume a completely new and apparently well-integrated identity during the fugue.

Psychogenic Amnesia People with **psychogenic amnesia** suddenly become aware that they have a total

---

Characteristics of Dissociative Disorders (DSM-III-R)

Multiple Personality Disorder
Adoption of two or more distinct personalities. Each personality at some time takes full control of the individual's behavior.

Psychogenic Fugue
Sudden flight from the usual environment or place of conflict and the assumption of a new identity.

Psychogenic Amnesia
A single episode of memory loss of important personal information due to psychologic reasons.

Depersonalization Disorder
One or more episodes of feelings of unreality concerning the environment, the self, or both sufficient to produce significant impairment of social or occupational functioning.

Dissociative Disorder (not otherwise specified)
Experience of dissociative symptoms that do not meet criteria for a specific disorder.

---

loss of memory for events that occurred during a period that may range from a few hours to a whole lifetime. In *localized amnesia,* the most common form, a person forgets only specific and related past times, usually surrounding a disturbing event. *Selective amnesia* for some, but not all, of the events is less common. Least common are *generalized amnesia,* which encompasses the person's entire life, and *continuous amnesia,* in which the person cannot recall events up to a specific time, including the present.

Depersonalization Disorder The essential feature here is one or more episodes of alteration in the perception or experience of the self so that the usual sense of personal reality is temporarily lost or changed with subsequent social or occupational impairment. All the associated feelings are ego-dystonic.

Dissociative Disorder, Not Otherwise Specified (NOS) This is a residual category to be used for disorders in which the predominant feature is a dissociative reaction that does not meet the criteria for any other specific dissociative disorder. An example is a child who enters a trancelike state following abuse or trauma or a person who enters a dissociated state following a period of brainwashing or thought reform.

The Nursing Process and Anxiety Disorders

Chapter 5 covers concepts of anxiety, stress, and coping that are relevant to the care of clients with anxiety disorders; it also covers the general anxiety continuum and the need to identify the level of anxiety. The subject of this section is the nurse's role with clients whose anxiety is severe enough to be classified as an anxiety disorder.

Assessing

Clients with anxiety disorders have impaired psychosocial and physiologic function. The feeling disturbances and physical and intellectual changes that take place as a result of extreme or chronic anxiety affect the client's work, school, and social functioning and frequently impair or threaten previously meaningful interpersonal relationships. These signs and symptoms are listed in the accompanying Assessment box.

For the nurse adopting the humanistic interactionist and psychobiologic philosophy espoused in this text, the goal is to restore the client's function within the family system and to restore biologic and intrapersonal health. Data gathered from both the client and family members are therefore essential to the assessment process.

The occurrence of acute anxiety and its related symptoms is common to a number of other physical conditions and acute medical emergencies. Therefore, a careful evaluation should always be conducted. A history and physical examination should rule out such conditions as hyperthyroidism and other endocrine problems, Ménière's syndrome, brain disorders, caffeine intoxication, mitral valve prolapse, and some medical emergencies (e.g., myocardial infarction).

Differentiation from other psychiatric diagnoses is difficult when anxiety and depression are mixed. The question "Which predominates?" can puzzle many practitioners and demands continued careful evaluation. Anxiety is part of many other clinical syndromes (e.g., schizophrenia and major affective disorders), and

ASSESSMENT

Common Features of Anxiety

Physiologic	Emotional	Cognitive
Increased heart rate	Irritability	Forgetfulness
Elevated blood pressure	Angry outbursts	Preoccupation
Tightness of chest	Feelings of worthlessness	Rumination
Difficulty in breathing	Depression	Mathematical and grammatical errors
Sweaty palms	Suspiciousness	
Trembling, tics, or twitching	Jealousy	Errors in judging distance
Tightness of neck or back muscles	Restlessness	Blocking
	Helplessness	Diminished fantasy life
Headache	Withdrawal	Lack of concentration
Urinary frequency	Diminished initiative	Lack of attention to details
Diarrhea	Tendency to cry	Past rather than present or future orientation
Nausea and/or vomiting	Sobbing without tears	
Sleep disturbance	Reduced personal involvement with others	Lack of awareness of external stimuli
Anorexia		
Sneezing	Tendency to blame others	Reduced creativity
Constant state of fatigue	Excessive criticism of self and others	Diminished productivity
Accident proneness		Reduced interest
Susceptibility to minor illness	Self-deprecation	
Slumped posture	Lack of interest	

the medical diagnosis may be made on the basis of the dominant, most debilitating symptom.

In the assessment phase, the nurse determines not only whether the client is anxious (and, if so, how anxious) but also what the source of the anxiety might be. Knowing the source helps the nurse plan and implement effective care. These two steps can be useful:

1. Help the client to recognize and name the experience as anxiety: "You're trembling. How are you feeling?" Some clients are immediately able to connect their behavior with feeling anxious. For clients who cannot, it is helpful to make the connection: "Often people tremble because they're feeling anxious (or nervous, uncomfortable, or worried). I was wondering if you could be feeling anxious (or nervous, uncomfortable, or worried) right now."

2. Help clients to discuss the experience more fully by moving into the cognitive dimension. It is premature to ask clients why they feel anxious. Encouraging clients to discuss what they are thinking about is more likely to bring their concerns out into the open. Then determine the source of the anxiety and gather data relevant to appropriate nursing diagnoses.

Panicked or extremely anxious clients are an exception; in this case do not use this general strategy. For these clients, suspend formal data gathering in favor of immediate, direct action to reduce anxiety (see "Planning and Implementing Interventions").

Subjective Data Clients with anxiety disorders may report a variety of physical and emotional symptoms. It is important to encourage clients to describe symptoms in their own words and to explain how the symptoms affect their daily activities. Clients with anxiety disorders may report emotional distress, cognitive and perceptual changes, somatic discomforts, or role impairments.

Emotional Distress Clients with anxiety disorders may reveal a number of distressing emotional feelings.

"I have a sense of impending doom—as if something terrible is going to happen."

"I feel helpless; vulnerable for no reason at all!"

"I just can't seem to enjoy life—everything bothers me."

Anger, guilt, feelings of worthlessness, and anguish frequently accompany anxiety. When the anxiety is acute or extreme, as in panic disorder or in post-traumatic stress disorder, the client feels in immediate danger and may seek protection and reassurance from others. If the anxiety is too severe, however, clients may become immobilized and unable to report their terrifying feelings at all, or they may refuse assistance and attempt to flee.

Sometimes clients with anxiety disorders may deny the existence of anxious feelings. They try to protect themselves by dissociating these feelings. The nurse needs to recognize clients' anxiety despite their denials. In such instances, assessment requires an especially careful observation of objective data.

Cognitive and Perceptual Changes Clients frequently have difficulty concentrating and making decisions. Some clients report feeling as if they are "going in circles," unable to think through a problem to make a confident decision. They may worry about their effectiveness at work and fear losing their job as a result of these attention and judgment problems.

In the clinical situation, clients may ask the nurse to make decisions for them or to give directions. At the same time, however, they may express difficulty following through with suggestions, finding many loopholes or possible problems with the plan of action. Other clients become forgetful or misinterpret what they hear.

In extreme anxiety, as in a panic attack, the client is unable to assess a situation accurately and realistically. Such a client needs immediate attention from and orientation by the nurse. The client may later report having had a frightening feeling of personality disintegration.

Somatic Discomfort Clients with anxiety disorders may complain of nausea, indigestion, headache, tightness in the neck or back, lack of appetite, a constant feeling of fatigue, or other psychophysiologic conditions. They may relate these somatic disturbances to having "bad nerves," or they may be unaware of any psychologic component of their discomfort.

The client with an obsessive-compulsive disorder who engages in repetitive activity, e.g., compulsive hand washing or hair pulling, may report special health problems (tissue breakdown or hair loss) as a result.

Clients with post-traumatic stress disorder may report fitful sleep, terrifying nightmares, and a fear of returning to sleep.

Role Impairment Clients may be aware of the impact that the emotional, cognitive/perceptual, and somatic changes have on their social, family, and work roles. They report worry about losing their job, being abandoned by loved ones, or being unable to continue caring for their families.

A young mother despairs that she is unable to take her daughter out to the playground because her phobias prevent her leaving the house.

A middle-aged accountant, obsessed about tallying his firm's financial data, is unable to put his job aside for the weekend and misses his son's football game. He experiences anger, guilt, and self-recrimination as a result.

Objective Data In addition to noting general signs and symptoms of anxiety as discussed in Chapter 5, the nurse notes other specific physical, emotional, and intellectual changes.

Physical Findings Clients with acute or extreme anxiety—e.g., clients with post-traumatic stress disorder or panic disorder, and clients with phobic disorder who cannot avoid the phobic situation—may experience a panic reaction and show extreme discomfort and the desire to flee. The nurse may observe acute physical changes, e.g., difficulty breathing, sweating, trembling, or vomiting, during these incidents. The nurse may note that the client is unable to verbalize or that verbalizations are confused and incoherent. During a panic episode, clients may be so frightened that they may refuse help at the moment and may require firm reassurance and protection until the episode wanes.

The client with an anxiety disorder may develop long-term physiologic effects, e.g., susceptibility to viral infections or development of ulcers, hypertension, or asthma. Alcohol or other substance abuse may develop into a serious complicating problem when clients try to alleviate anxiety through chemical means.

Other physical findings may be the effects of ritualistic or compulsive activity, e.g., skin lesions in a client who obsessively picks at the skin.

Emotional Changes Family and friends of a client with post-traumatic stress disorder may report personality changes in the client, e.g., increased irritability, suspiciousness, angry outbursts, and a tendency to blame others and to withdraw from them emotionally. The nurse may experience such reactions during the assessment interview. The nurse needs to persist in taking a careful history to trace the source of the emotional changes caused by the traumatic event.

Individuals with phobic and obsessive-compulsive disorders show a lack of emotional distress as long as the phobic object or situation is avoided or eclipsed by activity. The nurse may note little spontaneity or active involvement by the client during assessment.

Cognitive Deficits Unrealistic or distorted perception of a real situation is common in anxiety states. During a panic attack, the client may distort or exaggerate details. The client may complain to the nurse about some seemingly insignificant detail. Clients may lose their ability to take in other pertinent data, and thus make errors in judgment.

In the interview, clients with an anxiety disorder are forgetful and unable to concentrate or pay attention to details. Errors in calculation and grammar are common.

Impact on Role Function The symptoms of anxiety disorder affect social, work, and family relationships. It is important to understand the possible effects of anxiety symptoms on interpersonal relationships. Obsessive-compulsive acts, for instance, may become so pervasive that they take the place of relating to other people. In other cases, the client uses obsessions and compulsions to negotiate interaction and social roles. It is not unusual for people to establish a reciprocal pattern of interaction based on obsessions.

Nurses who plan intervention strategies for obsessive-compulsives and other individuals with an anxiety disorder should first assess the impact on the family system of intervening in one member's coping style.

Client or family member reports that the client is having trouble at work are additional evidence of role impairment. The client may be in jeopardy of losing a job due to poor performance. The individual with post-traumatic stress disorder, for example, may have been fired for absences, drug or alcohol abuse, or for outbursts of temper.

Many clients with a panic disorder report that fear of having a panic attack prevents them from seeking employment or from traveling to job interviews. For these individuals, as for many with severe phobic fears, normal activity may be greatly restricted.

Diagnosing

The following sections discuss the implications of nursing diagnoses for the client and the nurse.

Anxiety/Fear/Hopelessness Apprehension, tension, and fright are emotional experiences common to clients with anxiety disorders. Anger and rage may accompany excessive anxiety. A client with post-traumatic stress disorder, for example, may "fly off the handle" without apparent warning or provocation, reacting to an inner stimulus.

Feelings of distress, anguish, fear, hopelessness, and guilt may also accompany anxiety disorders. The focus of emotional expression may be impaired, i.e., clients may worry excessively, ruminating about what might go wrong in the future. They may express anxiety through worry about their physical well-being; somatic preoccupation or hypochondriasis may develop. The potential for substance abuse is high, and suicidal potential is increased. Sexual drive or behavior may be inhibited as well.

Ineffective Individual Coping Excessive anxiety can cause alterations in conduct and impulse control. Some clients, for instance those with post-traumatic stress disorder or panic disorder, manifest unpredictable behaviors in an attempt to cope with the overwhelming fears. Individuals with an obsessive-compulsive disorder are unable to alter behavior, even though they may recognize it as harmful or unnecessary.

Clients with anxiety may turn to abusing drugs. In turn, drug abuse results in disordered conduct and impaired impulse control.

Altered Role Performance Anxiety disorders impair performance in the family, at school, and at work. Anxious clients may become less efficient and accurate at work or school because of distractibility or other perceptual and cognitive difficulties. Clients may withdraw emotionally from formerly important and meaningful relationships, or they may become overly dependent on help from those around them. They may isolate themselves and avoid previously enjoyed activities and recreation. Excessive need for reassurance, decreased productivity, reduced creativity, impaired hygiene, and impaired home maintenance are all possible outcomes for the client with anxiety disorder.

A particularly debilitating consequence of phobic reaction is the incredible restriction it may impose. People who have several phobias concurrently, as is often the case, may become walled off and isolated from many normal activities. A housewife who is afraid of crowds and vehicles becomes gradually less able to carry out her responsibilities of grocery shopping, car pooling, and so forth. The multimillionaire Howard Hughes died a wasted recluse because he had grown so afraid of germs that he refused to leave his hotel room or wear clothing. Such people often consciously recognize the irrationality of their fears but cannot help experiencing them intensely.

Impaired Verbal Communication Clients with anxiety disorders often have difficulty communicating. They may speak too quickly or too loudly and may overelaborate or talk about too many subjects at once. The client is easily distracted and may have trouble understanding explanations or retaining information. A client with severe anxiety may be incoherent, making verbal communication impossible. Written communication may also be impaired.

Risk for Trauma Impairments in motor behavior are often related to hyperactivity and restlessness and place the client at risk for accidental injury. Wringing of the hands, poor coordination, and the appearance of a startle reaction are motor behaviors associated with anxiety disorders. The client with an obsessive-compulsive disorder may perform bizarre repetitive acts, e.g., repeatedly washing the hands or counting, checking, and rechecking activity.

Altered Thought Processes and Sensory/Perceptual Alterations Anxiety disorders can affect perception and thinking. Anxiety reduces the client's ability to solve problems. Judgment, concentration, abstract thinking, and attention are impaired. The client is indecisive but at the same time may make decisions impulsively to relieve tension. In panic, the client may become disoriented, misinterpret reality, and distort the meaning of situations or events.

Loss of self-esteem and a lowered self-concept often result as the client loses previous skills and capacities.

Altered Tissue Perfusion/Diarrhea/Functional Incontinence Alterations in circulation and elimination often occur as a result of stimulation of the autonomic nervous system. The client may experience increased blood pressure, rapid heart rate, dizziness, and palpitations as well as dry mouth, cold or clammy hands, sweating, shortness of breath, and a bad taste in the mouth. Diarrhea, enuresis, and slowed digestion may occur.

In the client experiencing extreme anxiety or panic, these symptoms are intensified, and the client may faint or vomit. A medical emergency may arise if the client has an additional major health problem such as cardiac illness.

Sleep Pattern Disturbance Insomnia is a frequent response to anxiety. Nearly all clients with anxiety disorders complain of trouble sleeping. Sleep may be further disturbed by nightmares or night terrors.

Planning and Implementing Interventions

The planning and implementation phases of the nursing process with anxious persons depend on a careful and accurate assessment of the level of anxiety and the determination of appropriate nursing diagnoses. It is important for planning and implementation to take place as soon as possible. Anxiety not only escalates but is also communicated interpersonally. The client's family and friends, other clients, and staff may be caught up in the tension as well.

Most mental health professionals believe that clients who cope with the stress of anxiety disorders can grow and change with therapeutic intervention. Nursing interventions for clients with anxiety disorders should be geared toward resolving the problems identified in the previous phases of the nursing process.

Reducing Anxiety To deal with clients who are anxious, nurses must understand the operational definition of anxiety. This is the classic definition by Manaser and Werner (1964, p 127):

• Expectations or needs are present.

• Expectations or needs are not met.

• Unexpected discomfort (anxiety) is felt.

• Anxiety is controlled and power is restored through some automatic behavior (e.g., anger, withdrawal, somatization) that has been effective in restoring control in the past.

• The relief behavior is rationalized or justified rather than explained or understood.

Because anxiety is such an uncomfortable feeling, we learn early in life to reduce it or diminish its effect as soon as possible. Although individuals use a variety of behaviors, the most common automatic responses to anxiety are anger, withdrawal, and somatization. Automatic responses are limiting, rigid, and inflexible. Because they are automatic, these responses prevent a creative response to the threat and inhibit learning.

Intervening with Panicked Clients   Clients who are extremely anxious or in panic require more immediate, direct, and structured intervention. During an acute panic attack, perception and personality are disrupted to such a degree that the client cannot solve problems or discuss the source of anxiety. The first priority is to reduce the anxiety to more tolerable levels. The interventions in the Intervention box below help the nurse control the client's panic. The goal is to reduce the client's immediate anxiety to more moderate and manageable levels, since learning cannot occur if the client is experiencing panic. The family of the distressed individual needs counseling about how to respond therapeutically in such events because they are often involved in or present during a panic episode.

Intervening in Cases of Less Severe Anxiety A nurse can frequently detect subtle indications of mounting anxiety and intervene to present a severe attack. Some clients are adept at covering up their anxiety, but they usually transmit something to the sensitive observer. Often the nurse's own feelings of increased tension are a useful cue that the source of anxiety is in the client. Anxiety may make people excessively demanding. The nurse's response to the demands must take into account the consequences for the course of the client's anxiety. In some cases it may be reassuring to set limits and deny the request. In other cases, such a response may place further stress on the client.

The nurses must know how to treat clients who suffer from prolonged anxiety. Here the intervention strategies are intended to help clients use their anxiety to learn about themselves and their coping strategies. This requires that the client endure the anxiety while searching out its causes. The client must then develop more effective and satisfying coping strategies to replace the old ones. To help clients learn to cope more effectively with anxiety, the nurse must first detect the anxiety and then make thoughtful observations and responses that facilitate learning. Hildegard Peplau's five-step plan of action, which includes the interventions shown in the accompanying Intervention box, is now considered a classic model for nursing intervention with the anxious client.

The nurse who is working through this step-by-step intervention approach must avoid getting bogged down in clients' justifications of their usual ways of coping. Often clients try to give plausible explanations for their ineffective anger, withdrawal, or somatization (automatic responses to anxiety; see Chapter 5). However, they do not explain the relief in terms of the factors that caused the anxiety. The relief afforded by

INTERVENTION

Guidelines for Working with the Panicked Client

Strategy	Rationale
Stay with the client	Being left alone may further increase the anxiety
Maintain a calm, serene manner	Knowing that the nurse is calm and in control may be calming to the client
Use short, simple sentences	Because the client's perceptual field is disrupted, the client will experience difficulty in focusing
Use a firm and authoritative voice	Conveys the nurse's ability to provide external controls
Move the client to a quieter, smaller, and less stimulating environment	Prevents further disruption of the perceptual field by sensory stimuli
Focus the client's diffuse energy on a repetitive or physically tiring task	Repetitive tasks or physical exercise can help to drain off excess energy
Administer antianxiety medications if ordered	Antianxiety medications may help reduce anxiety

INTERVENTION

Guidelines for Working with the Anxious Client

Step of Plan	*Nursing Intervention*
1. Observe client for increased psychomotor activity, anger or withdrawal, excessive demands, and tearfulness.	Verbalizations intended to help client recognize and name his experience as anxiety. "Are you feeling uncomfortable?" "Are you anxious or nervous now?" When client says "Yes," he is ready for step 2.
2. Connect feeling of anxiety with relief behavior. Client acknowledges, describes, and names feelings of nervousness or anxiety.	Ask client what he does to feel more comfortable when he feels anxious. When client understands that when he feels anxious he gets angry, withdraws, or somatizes, he is ready for step 3.
3. Investigate situation that immediately preceded feeling of anxiety.	Encourage client to recall and describe what he was experiencing immediately before he got anxious (including thoughts, actions, and other feelings).

4. Help client observe, describe, and analyze connections between what led to his anxiety and what happened after he felt anxious. Only through seeing all parts of this experience can client understand why he became anxious.

5. Formulate causes of anxiety. Help client state causes of the anxiety. Then help him observe and recall similar instances in his experiences of anxiety. Through such extensive discussions, client will eventually be able to recognize and perhaps alter his pattern of handling anxiety.

SOURCE: Peplau H: Interpersonal techniques: The crux of nursing. Copyright © 1962, The American Journal of Nursing Company. Adapted with permission from the American Journal of Nursing, *June, Vol. 62 No. 6.*

the usual coping patterns does not last long because the needs or expectations that originally caused the symptoms still exist. They may even become more intense. Clients can begin to alter disturbed coping patterns only when they understand what their unmet needs are, what they did instead of fulfilling these needs, and what they felt then.

At this point, clients have two alternatives. They can reduce or change their hopes and expectations or they can try new tactics or resources to get their needs met. The nurse should discuss these options with the client and negotiate a contract to work on one or both goals. Realizing either option often involves problem solving. Nurse and client must find ways to alter structural features of the client's environment to reduce or meet the need.

Simple physical activities often help to reduce anxiety to more tolerable levels. Encourage adaptive coping mechanisms that work. Here are a few:

- Soak in a warm bath.
- Listen to soothing music.
- Take a walk or exercise.
- Have a massage or back rub.
- Drink a warm beverage.
- Engage in whatever activity is relaxing.
- Take slow, deep breaths to counteract the effects of hyperventilation, breathing in harmony with the nurse for support.

Nurses use a variety of psychotherapeutic techniques and skills in intervening with clients who experience states of anxiety. Progressive relaxation, meditation, "thought-stopping" techniques, autogenic training, and imagery may help the individual learn new ways to reduce the disturbing affect (see Chapter 27). Other methods of helping clients reduce anxiety include helping them to reality test, because the person's sense of danger is often out of proportion to actual danger. Development of goal-oriented contracts may help to reduce a client's sense of inner chaos by providing structure and direction.

Teaching Clients about Their Medications Education in the use of medications is an essential role of the nurse. Clients should be aware of the major drugs used to manage acute anxiety and their limitations and possible side effects. Anxiety that is secondary to major medical illness or acute trauma (e.g., the death of a child) requires a different dosage than that prescribed for the treatment of primary anxiety.

Short-term use of higher dosage antidepressants has been found to help control panic attacks. The benzodiazepine group of drugs has proved effective and relatively safe in controlling situational anxiety for periods of four to eight weeks. Antianxiety agents such as meprobamate (Equanil), diazepam (Valium), and chlordiazepoxide (Librium) or adrenergic blocking agents such as propranolol (Inderal) may be used (Cole 1988).

The last decade has seen significant progress in pharmacologic treatments for agoraphobia with associated panic attacks. Pharmacologic agents—most notably the tricyclic antidepressants (TCAs), e.g., imipramine (Tofranil); the monoamine oxidase inhibitors (MAOIs), e.g., phenelzine (Nardil); and the second-generation benzodiazepines (BZs), e.g., alprazolam (Xanax)—have been found to reduce or eliminate panic episodes associated with agoraphobia.

Although the antipanic drugs are primarily antidepressants, the existing evidence suggests that panic disorders and agoraphobia are responding to these drugs not because the disorders are types of depression. Instead, the therapeutic effect is thought to be the result of the side effects on the vagal system. Phobic states not associated with panic episodes do not respond well to antianxiety or antidepressant medication.

Antianxiety medication should be used cautiously and sparingly. Certain antianxiety medications (diazepam, for one) are among the most overprescribed and abused drugs in the United States and Canada. Valium overreliance is a serious medical problem that has prompted the formation of a self-help group, Valium Anonymous, to help addicted persons to get off the drug. The elderly are particularly sensitive to the effects of central nervous system depression associated with diazepam.

Although medications may alleviate the symptoms of anxiety, they do nothing to help clients understand its source or manage their own lives in more comfortable ways. At best, these drugs should be used for the short-term treatment of anxiety—meaning days or even weeks, but not months or years.

Promoting Effective Coping

Clients with Obsessive-Compulsive Disorders Clients with obsessive-compulsive disorders avoid anxiety by engaging in compulsive acts and rigid thinking. Nurses working in all practice areas will sooner or later encounter an obsessive-compulsive client whose problem is severe enough to require hospitalization.

Clients use compulsive rituals to control anxiety. Therefore, carefully consider and time any intervention so as not to worsen the client's anxiety. For example, clients with washing compulsions may completely remove the skin from their hands, and nurses have successfully intervened by suggesting surgical gloves. However, it is not usually fruitful, and may be harmful, to interfere prematurely with a ritual unless it threatens the client's or another person's life or health. Generally, the client needs plenty of time to complete the ritual. These clients often have a strong tendency toward negativism, which may cause them to become more firmly entrenched in their defenses if modifications are introduced prematurely or hurriedly. Attempt to develop an affirming, dependable relationship with clients before suggesting that they change their behavior patterns, gradually introducing a substitute behavior. Balance the value of intervening in behavior that protects clients from mental anguish against the need to prevent physical deterioration caused by the behavior.

Clients with Post-Traumatic Stress Disorder Clients with post-traumatic stress disorder frequently experience behavior or conduct disturbances as a result of the intense anxiety triggered by reexperiencing the trauma. Alcohol or other mood-altering drugs, when used to relieve anxiety, may contribute to destructive and impulsive acts. In the acute stage, crisis counseling is essential. Because of the chronic course of the illness and the many psychosocial problems associated with it, a comprehensive treatment approach is needed. Frequently clients experience disordered family relationships, physical disability, social and recreational disruptions, and impaired ability to work or attend school. They may experience symptoms and attitudes of demoralization that further hamper their functioning.

The goal of therapy in treating the client with post-traumatic stress disorder is to desensitize them to the memories of the traumatic events so that the ego, or coping functions, can gain mastery over the anxiety. The following interventions or techniques may be used singly or, more frequently, in combination.

- Education/explanation: Explaining the dynamics of the disability and giving a rationale for the treatment help engage the client's ego in treatment.

- Relaxation training: Typical training programs may include muscle relaxation and imagery. The emphasis is on providing new "tools" or skills that the person may use when faced with memories of the traumatic event (see Chapter 27). Teaching clients about these self-management approaches encourages self-care and provides the clients with tools to use at

RESEARCH NOTE

Citation

Hyman R, Feldman H, Harris R, Levin R, Malloy G: The effects of relaxation training on clinical symptoms: A meta-analysis. Nurs Res 1989;38(4):216–220.

Study Problem/Purpose

This study examined the effects of relaxation training on a variety of clinical symptoms commonly associated with anxiety and tension. The purposes of this study were to determine (a) the overall effects of this training (biofeedback, meditation, and varieties of relaxation exercises) in relieving clinical symptoms, (b) the relative effectiveness of the techniques, (c) the relative sensitivity of outcome measures, and (d) the possible effect on findings of other variables in study design or in characteristics of the subjects.

Methods

In this study relaxation training was defined as a nonpharmacologic, nonmechanically assisted technique to facilitate a relaxed state. Meta-analysis was used to synthesize findings of forty-eight experimental studies of nonmechanically assisted relaxation techniques to control a variety of clinical symptoms. Criteria for inclusion were (a) publication after 1970 and (b) calculation of the size of effect of the training. Three types of comparisons of effect were included: experimental versus control, experimental versus placebo, and pretest versus posttest.

Findings

Relaxation techniques do affect some clinical symptoms. Effect sizes for three types of comparisons ranged from .43 to .66, indicating that treatment of any type included in the analysis moved the client from the 50th to the 67th percentile of an untreated group at minimum and from the 50th to the 75th percentile at maximum. All treatments included in the analysis, except Benson's relaxation technique, demonstrated evidence of effectiveness, particularly for nonsurgical samples with chronic problems such as headache, insomnia, and hypertension.

Implications

The results suggest that future research be designed to test specifically whether the efficacy of specific relaxation techniques varies according to the symptom to be treated, the nature of the problem (acute versus chronic), and the setting (surgical versus nonsurgical).

---

home, at school, and on the job as well as in the health care setting.

• Hypnosis or narcoanalyses (the injection of barbiturates or other drugs to induce partial anesthesia): Some therapists use these techniques to bring to consciousness repressed and suppressed material so that it can be integrated into the ego structure, where it will have a less powerful influence. Self-hypnosis is discussed in Chapter 27.

• Cognitive skill therapies: These include techniques such as "thought stopping" (see Chapter 27), thought substitution, and providing the client with positive reinforcing statements. Cognitive restructuring of events giving new, less noxious interpretations may be used.

• Abreaction/systematic desensitization: The client may derive a therapeutic effect through emotional release or **abreaction** after recalling the painful repressed experience. Systematic desensitization in which the dreaded object, thought, or situation is introduced to the client in gradual amounts may be used as well. Systemic desensitization is discussed later in this chapter.

• Family conferences: Efforts are frequently needed to engage the family in working to resolve the many psychosocial effects caused by the trauma. If successful, the family may provide a crucial supportive function.

• Group treatment: The benefits of group membership have been clearly demonstrated in recent years. Vietnam Veterans, Alcoholics Anonymous, Mothers against Drunk Drivers, and Women against Violence against Women are just a few of the growing number of self-help groups organizing to assist and support victims of trauma and violence.

• Exercise and nutrition: Maintaining a healthy physical state as an adjunct to other therapies strengthens the body's adaptive efforts following trauma.

• Individual therapy: Individual psychotherapy can provide important ego supportive and/or cathartic benefits.

Recent advances in psychopharmacology have led to the use of medication as an adjunct to psychologic treatment of post-traumatic stress disorders. As is true for the other anxiety disorders, however, the nurse should be aware of the heightened potential for drug abuse among clients who suffer disorders of acute distress. The desire for immediate, total relief is powerful and may foster drug dependence and abuse.

BZs, TCAs, MAOIs, lithium, beta-blockers, alpha-adrenergic antagonists, and neuroleptics have all been reported to relieve symptoms of post-traumatic stress disorder, either partially or totally (Elledgrie and

Bridges 1985). During the initial stage (four to eight weeks), the use of benzodiazepines may be helpful in the treatment of the anxiety, insomnia, and nightmares. Longer-term use, however, may lead to habituation and dependence and is a serious limitation to the use (Schuckit 1985). Most recently, preliminary investigations are being conducted using the beta-adrenergic blocker propranolol (Inderal) and the anticonvulsant clonazepam (Clonopin) in an effort to avoid the side-effects of the benzodiazepines.

When depression is a major factor, one of the cyclic antidepressants or an MAOI may be used. Sleeplessness, another common feature, is best treated with a behavioral approach first (e.g., relaxation techniques, imagery, muscle relaxation, and exclusion of daytime naps). Sedatives are discouraged except for very brief use. The nurse's goal is to help the client reestablish the ability to sleep naturally and cope with stress without the use of drugs.

Promoting Effective Role Performance in Clients with Phobia Clients with phobic disorders attempt to avoid anxiety by binding it to a specific object or situation. Many people manage to lead successful productive lives by binding their anxiety up in this way. For others, though, the phobia severely limits their activities, and their performance at work, home, or school may be greatly compromised. It is essential to recognize that forcing clients to come into contact with the feared object or the basic source of their anxiety can create in them an intense, disorganizing flood of panic.

Most clinicians agree that clients with phobic coping patterns are highly resistant to most insight-oriented therapies. These therapies require clients to confront and at least temporarily experience some of their originating anxiety. It is not surprising that they are ineffective with phobic clients, since the phobic's style is basically one of *avoidance*. In recent years, however, some symptomatic improvements have been made using techniques derived from behaviorist learning theory. The most commonly used interventions are desensitization and reciprocal inhibition.

In *systematic desensitization*, the client is exposed, in order, to a series of anxiety-provoking situations that the client has graded in a hierarchy from the least to the most frightening. Through techniques of progressive relaxation, the person becomes desensitized to each stimulus in the scale and then moves up to the next most frightening stimulus. Eventually the stimulus that originally induced the most anxiety no longer elicits the same painful response. For example, a man who is irrationally afraid of ordinary earthworms might first talk about earthworms until the topic no longer evokes the same anxiety. Then he might be shown pictures of earthworms until he masters that level of closeness—and so on, increasing

contact until he can actually hold a live earthworm in his hand.

In *reciprocal inhibition,* the anxiety-provoking stimulus is paired with another stimulus that is associated with an opposite feeling strong enough to suppress the anxiety. Through the use of antianxiety medications, hypnosis, meditation, yoga, or biofeedback training, clients are taught how to induce in themselves both psychologic and physical calm. Once they have mastered these techniques, they are taught to use them when faced with the anxiety-provoking hierarchy of stimuli.

Two other behavior-based interventions may also be used. In *cognitive restructuring* or *"relabeling,"* the client is encouraged to relabel a frightening situation, object, or activity. Closely linked to learning theory, this intervention is based on the belief that anxiety stems from erroneous interpretations of situations. In *exposure* or *"flooding,"* the client is repeatedly brought in prolonged contact with those situations that usually evoke distress until discomfort in their presence subsides.

Using behavioral conditioning techniques to rid the client of a phobia merely eliminates the symptom without removing the original stressor or conflict. If clients give up a phobic reaction without learning a more effective coping strategy, they can usually expect some alternative and equally troublesome disturbed pattern to emerge.

Promoting Effective Communication Nursing interventions that reduce anxiety (see the boxes on pages 330 and 331) are important general measures that promote more effective communication and motor behavior. Many times, simply offering the opportunity to acknowledge and discuss feelings of anxiety helps the client to regain control. Having followed the two steps outlined in the section on assessment, the nurse may find the client's anxiety has already abated somewhat. At this point, clients are more likely to share their concerns because the nurse has already taken the first steps in demonstrating genuine interest and concern in the client's experiences.

After encouraging the client to express feelings, the nurse must, of course, listen. Clients may express fear, anger, sadness, disappointment, or alienation, and it may be difficult to hear about the client's pain. Some nurses feel helpless in the face of their client's catharsis and think they should be able to provide ready answers. Instead, ready answers are more likely to interfere with and thwart the client's communication. Genuine, concerned listening without judgments is an effective intervention in itself.

Explanations should be simple, clear, and concise. Be careful not to overload severely anxious people with more information than they can handle. If anxiety has contributed to knowledge deficit, reduce anxiety before trying to teach about health or provide information. If the client's perceptual field (see Chapter 5) is narrow or disrupted, the client will be unable to assimilate information.

Clients with an obsessive-compulsive disorder require patience and an unhurried attitude, especially in regard to details and ruminations. It is frustrating to try to communicate with people who cope by developing an obsessive-compulsive reaction. If the nurse uses the customary techniques of paraphrasing and reflecting, these clients will say the nurse did not get the details right. They will then go on to correct, qualify, and clarify. Curiously, this pedantic striving for accuracy produces greater vagueness and confusion. It is as if parallel conversations are going on. Clients hear only themselves repeating and correcting insignificant details and completely lose the overall meaning of the message. Developing patience in listening and skill in providing well-timed, simple direction is crucial to working effectively with clients with an obsessive-compulsive disorder.

Promoting Safety Lack of coordination or tremors make anxious clients prone to accidents. Counsel clients not to perform potentially dangerous activities, e.g., driving a car, when anxiety is high. Advise them to move more slowly or to go over instructions carefully when they undertake new tasks or use tools.

Promoting Optimum Tissue Perfusion and Elimination Like communication, circulation and elimination improve when anxiety is reduced. Pay attention to proper nutrition and adequate activity, because clients with anxiety frequently overlook their self-care and health needs. Walking, participating in sports, or developing new hobbies and interests promote physiologic functions and need to be part of a comprehensive nursing treatment plan.

Promoting Effective Sensory Perception and Thought Processes To function more effectively and independently, the client needs to know about normal anxiety and about anxiety disorders. Providing accurate information at the right time and in an appropriate manner is an essential nursing function. Other strategies to promote effective perception and cognition include the following:

• Use adjuncts to verbal communication, e.g., visual aids or role playing, to stimulate memory and retention of information.

• Practice problem-solving vignettes to improve judgment and insight.

• Identify misperceptions that clients hold as a result of a narrowed perceptual field. Begin with comments such as, "I wonder if you've considered this possibility?" or "Perhaps if we tried this tack?"

• Help clients reality test, i.e., help clients explore their opinions in the light of validated experience rather than emotional needs that block accurate perception.

Promoting Sleep Nonpharmacologic nursing measures to promote sleep should be used before medications. These may include any of a variety of relaxation methods. A currently popular method is the use of audio tapes. Like imagery, they provide a relaxing atmosphere—listening to the sounds of a beach or of birds in a wooded forest is soothing and sleep-promoting to some individuals.

Suggest that the client read a boring book in bed, drink warm liquids, or take a warm tub bath before retiring. (See page 655, Visualization for the Bath, and the Psychobiology box on page 647.) The client with post-traumatic stress disorder may fear going to sleep because of nightmares. Having another member of the family nearby and aware of the client's fear may be reassuring.

Evaluating/Outcome Criteria

Anxiety Clients will show no evidence of acute or intense anxiety and be able to perform activities of daily living independently when appropriate. Clients will verbalize feeling less anxious, and they will have fewer somatic complaints. They will state they feel more comfortable.

Clients will have fewer symptoms of physiologic distress, e.g., racing pulse, diaphoresis, or hyperventilation. Clients will be without signs of increased psychomotor activity. They will no longer complain of tearfulness, feelings of rage, or impatience. When appropriate, they will more readily engage in interactions with others. Phobic clients will tolerate the presence of the feared object, activity, or situation without experiencing panic or the need to flee.

Individual and Family Coping The obsessive-compulsive client will limit or cease performing compulsive rituals; for example, a client with a hand-washing compulsion will wash the hands no more than four times a day.

Clients will demonstrate the ability to continue with necessary activities even though some anxiety is present. They will be less likely to panic or flee. Family members will report that the client is "more like himself/herself" and appears less agitated, driven, or explosive in conduct.

Role Performance The client will attend work or school on a regular basis. Family members will report that relationships at home have improved and that the client is once again taking responsibility for family activities.

Text continued on p. 340

CASE STUDY

A Client with Panic Disorder with Agoraphobia

Identifying Information

Mrs R is 43 years old, married, Irish Catholic, and mother of four daughters in their late teens or early twenties. Until very recently she had been employed as a secretary at a local pediatrician's office. She has a high school education and recently attempted attending community college, hoping to fulfill a lifelong dream of getting a college degree. She was referred to the psychiatric outpatient clinic for follow-up counseling by the emergency department of the local general hospital where she had been rushed in acute distress the prior evening with symptoms of a panic attack.

Client's Definition of Present Problem, Precipitating Stressors, Coping Strategies, Goals for Care

At the time of the panic attack, Mrs R believed she was having a heart attack and feared she was dying. She reported racing heartbeat, sweating, and feeling faint. She could not identify any events, thoughts, or feelings that precipitated the incident; it seemed to her to occur "out of the blue." She wanted relief from her fears of a medical emergency and felt unable to cope with the severity of the symptoms of the attack: "I tried to talk myself out of it; to tell myself it would go away, but it only got worse."

History of Present Problem

Mrs R reported she had had similar attacks over the years and that she had always been reassured of her medical and cardiac health, but when these attacks occurred, she "feared the worst" and "lost all perspective." The attacks could last from two minutes to two hours. Her daily routine had become quite restricted as she now sought to have one of her daughters or her husband with her when she went out of the home due to fear of an attack. She sometimes could make it to school on her own but only with great effort, forcing herself to go. She did not feel comfortable when alone in her home and could not go to sleep if the other family members were not home. As an aside, she wondered what she would do when all the girls were off in college and she had no "sidekick." She felt ashamed and angry about her growing disability and often tried to cover up her fears to friends and family.

On interviewing the family, the nurse was able to gather information about a number of significant recent life events preceding the panic episode:

- Recent major surgery. A hysterectomy occurred four weeks earlier.
- Loss of her employment due to her hospitalization. She was abruptly terminated from her position at a new job due to too many absences.
- Recent discovery that her oldest daughter was taking birth control pills.
- The upcoming anniversary date of her father's sudden death from a heart attack.

Psychiatric History

Mrs R had never been hospitalized before for a psychiatric condition, although she had been to the emergency room on three prior occasions with symptoms of panic attack. She had seen a therapist years ago when the attacks first occurred, "about the time I left home to marry." She did not follow up with the therapist, however, saying she felt ashamed ("I've always been a strong and effective person!"), that the episodes were not so severe then, and that she found relief from panic attacks after she had the children.

CASE STUDY (continued)

Family History

Both Mrs R's parents died within the past six years. She was especially close to her father and the second anniversary of his death was approaching. Mrs R's mother was considered a "homebody"; she rarely left the house and took part in social activities only if they occurred at the family home. Mrs R suddenly wondered if her mother had "these fears" too. She did not feel close to her mother in her adolescence, and there were many conflicts over her growing independence. She remembered feeling hurt that her father would not stand up to her mother and "protect me" when she felt her mother was in the wrong or especially harsh. Mrs R had four older sisters and one older brother. They were "always around," and she realized only after she married "how important that was" to her feelings of security.

Social History

Mrs R had always been considered a "doer" and an achiever, "someone people came to for help with problems, not the other way around!" She liked her new position as secretary for a pediatrician's office but felt angry at being terminated from the position due to her many absences. In addition to her absences due to her gynecologic problems she acknowledged that her fears she would have a panic attack at work were interfering with her attendance as well.

She reported she had begun to curtail social and recreational activities, preferring to stay at home where she was most comfortable. She noticed she was "living through the kids" rather than participating actively in golf and church activities as she had previously done with her husband.

She described her relationship to her husband as emotionally warm and supportive. Although she sometimes resented his being away from her, she recognized this as part of her "problem" with being alone.

Her primary relationships had been with her husband and children. She talked of facing the "empty nest" as her daughters, one by one, left for work or college. She "was shocked" to discover that her oldest daughter was using birth control pills but had "gotten over it," concluding that she was being old-fashioned and judgmental "like my mother."

Significant Health History

With the exception of chronic gynecologic problems leading to the recent hysterectomy, Mrs R reported a history of good health. She had no allergies or other chronic illnesses. Her only other hospitalizations were to have her children. The recent hospitalization had been more physically taxing than she expected, and the fact that she was not allowed to return to work after her recovery came as a blow: "Going back to work would have been good for me. I felt discarded."

Current Mental Status

Mrs R presented as an attractive, carefully groomed woman looking her stated age. She sat erect in the office chair, appearing somewhat tense. She answered questions cooperatively, but at times with some hesitation and as if expectant of criticism or judgment from the interviewer. She would say, for example, "Well how would *you* feel?" in response to an inquiry about her emotional reaction to a significant event.

Sensorium

She was oriented to time, place, and person. She exhibited a good fund of knowledge, appropriate for her education and experience. Her memory was intact and recall good. She had no difficulty with calculations. Her judgment was unimpaired. During times of panic, however, sensory and perceptive awareness was greatly impaired.

CASE STUDY (continued)

Feelings

Affect appeared normal, with occasional evidence of anger in the form of irritability and light sarcasm. Mood was within normal limits.

Voice and Speech

Speech was normal in flow and volume. It appeared pressured at times when she attempted to correct an impression she believed the interviewer held.

Motor Behavior

Posture was at times rigid, but she relaxed somewhat as she became more comfortable with the interview.

Thought Content

There were no delusions, ideas of reference, or hallucinations. Obsessive worry about the occurrence of panic episodes and of her safety were present. Embarrassment and shame over her symptoms were apparent. Suicidal or homicidal thoughts were denied.

Thought Processes

Associations and abstractions were appropriate, and there was no evidence of thought process disorder or difficulty in concentration, except during acute panic, at which times concentration was impaired and thought processes were disorganized.

Defenses

Some guardedness toward the interviewer was noted. Rationalization, overintellectualization, and avoidance were other coping and defense mechanisms used.

Insight

Insight into the meaning of the current situation was minimal.

Other Significant Subjective or Objective Clinical Data

Mrs R was considering the use of a trial of antipanic medication, despite "hating the idea" of medication.

Diagnostic Impression

Nursing Diagnoses

Altered role performance
Sensory/perceptual alterations
Altered thought processes
Anxiety
Fear
Ineffective individual coping
Altered health maintenance
Social isolation

DSM-III-R Multiaxial Diagnosis

Axis I: 300.21   Panic disorder with agoraphobia
Axis II: None
Axis III: Gynecologic disorder, under treatment
Axis IV: Psychosocial stressors; recent hysterectomy, acute event; loss of employment, acute event; recent knowledge of daughter's use of birth control, acute event; upcoming anniversary of father's sudden death, acute event
             Severity: 3-moderate
Axis V: Current GAF: 42
             Highest GAF past year: 76

NURSING CARE PLAN

A Client with Panic Disorder with Agoraphobia

Client Care Goals	Nursing Planning/ Intervention	Evaluation
Nursing Diagnosis: *Altered role performance*		
The client will expand activities of daily living.	See interventions for Anxiety and Fear, below.	Client no longer has altered lifestyle. Client conducts normal activities at home, work, or school.
Nursing Diagnosis: *Sensory/perceptual alterations*		
The client will gain mastery over incidents of panic.	See interventions for Anxiety and Fear below.	Client reports feeling able to manage incidents of anxiety. Client demonstrates use of relaxation techniques.
Nursing Diagnosis: *Altered thought processes*		
The client will be able to concentrate better.	Teach client self-relaxation therapy to reduce early signs of anxiety and symptoms.	Client reports that she can concentrate better.
Nursing Diagnosis: *Anxiety/Fear*		
The client will experience less discomfort, including dyspnea, tachycardia, sweating, fear, and anxiety. The client will gain mastery over incidents of panic.	During a panic attack: • Maintain calm manner. • Stay physically with the client. • Acknowledge that he or she will not die. • Use short, simple sentences and firm, authoritative voice. • Consider calling the client's attention to some physically tiring or repetitive task in order to focus energy away from fears. • Consider use of antianxiety medication as an adjunct to psychologic measures.	The client has lessened symptoms of dyspnea, tachycardia, sweating, fear, or anxiety.
The client will not fear that she is dying.	Consider use of specific psychologic treatment approaches: desensitization, hypnosis, "flooding," and imagery therapy to help client master the fear of dying or of having a medical emergency. Encourage verbalization of fears. Validate that fear of dying is a subjective experience.	Client reports no fear of dying.

▶

NURSING CARE PLAN (continued)

Client Care Goals	Nursing Planning/ Intervention	Evaluation
	Recommend dynamic, insight-oriented psychotherapy if unconscious conflicts appear to be motivating force behind mood and affect changes.	Client no longer complains of feeling fearful or anxious.
	Educate client on the proper use of medication, if prescribed.	Client verbalizes an understanding of medications and uses them correctly.

Nursing Diagnosis: *Ineffective individual coping*

The client will develop effective coping strategies.	Assist client in identifying and using own resources and social supports to broaden activities.	Client reports and demonstrates use of effective coping strategies, e.g., use of relaxation techniques. Client no longer uses excessive avoidance. Client uses social supports and has broadened her activities.
	Teach client relaxation techniques.	

Nursing Diagnosis: *Altered health maintenance*

The client will not abuse substances.	Educate client on the proper use of medication, if prescribed.	The client uses medication in correct and safe manner.

Nursing Diagnosis: *Social isolation*

The client will be able to travel away from home.	Teach client relaxation techniques and imagery.	Client travels away from home whenever she desires.

Clients will report engaging in recreational or social activity and independently performing self-care. They will express feeling more comfortable about their performance at home, work, or school. The phobic client will perform daily activities with less restriction or interference from any feared object, activity, or situation.

Communication and Safety Clients will state satisfaction with their communication; they feel heard and understood. They will report being able to perform usual small motor tasks, such as writing, in a competent manner. There will be open lines of communication between client and nurse and client and family. Clients will report no tremors and will not have accidents due to poor motor coordination.

Tissue Perfusion and Elimination Clients will report feeling energetic. Somatic complaints will decrease, and clients will report engaging in daily physical activity. Vital signs will be normal, and weight will be stable.

Thought Processes and Perception Clients will recall information taught by the nurse. They will begin to make decisions about their health care and ask questions about the anxiety process.

Clients will describe what led to anxiety and what happened after they felt anxious. They will state the cause of anxiety and recall similar instances. They will verbalize techniques to reduce anxiety.

The client will correctly verbalize the use, side effects, and limitations of medications used. Clients will verbalize increased awareness of their environment.

Sleep Clients will sleep through the night without medication or with appropriately prescribed medication. They will have fewer nightmares or wake less frequently throughout the night.

The Nursing Process and Somatoform Disorders

Assessing

Assessment of the client with a somatoform disorder is complex because of the many psychobiologic factors involved.

Subjective Data The client with a somatoform disorder reports physical symptoms for which there is no positive evidence of organic or physiologic cause. Clients with hypochondriacal illness, for example, may return many times to the outpatient clinic or emergency room, demanding to be reexamined or retested. They feel sure that they are suffering from some major illness that has been undetected. They are not reassured by the lack of physical findings and may go from doctor to doctor hoping to find someone who will validate their fears.

In conversion disorder, the individual has loss of function or an alteration in function. They may be unable to walk, for instance, complaining, "I woke up this morning with no feeling in my legs; for some reason they won't move." Examination reveals normal sensitivity, however, and no reason for the apparent loss of function. Interestingly, however, the client with conversion disorder seems unconcerned about the presenting problem despite its apparent severity. An inappropriate lack of concern about their disabilities—**la belle indifférence**—is characteristic of these clients.

Clients with somatization disorder or hypochondriacal disorder, in contrast, are overly dramatic and emotional in telling about their symptoms and pain. They report the history in vivid detail and colorful language but often pay more attention to how the symptoms have affected relationships in their lives than in giving careful description of the nature, character, location, onset, and duration of the symptoms.

Clients with body dysmorphic disorder may request unnecessary operations, for example, demanding cosmetic surgery for an imagined or greatly magnified defect in appearance.

Careful interviewing by the nurse frequently uncovers a stressful life situation with which the client is not coping, suggesting that the preoccupation with somatic disorder is a way of avoiding underlying conflict. Helping the client to identify and talk about this is a crucial beginning to psychotherapeutic intervention.

Objective Data Physical examination reveals no evidence for the physical symptoms of the client. Laboratory findings likewise do not substantiate organic or physiologic disorder. Despite this, the client may have undergone many exploratory procedures without relief or diagnosis.

Family members often report the client is moody, self-centered, or demanding. They feel alienated from the client and are frustrated with the client's chronic preoccupation with physical symptoms. In a hospital setting, these clients often create scenes that bring them the attention they need without regard for the needs of either fellow clients or staff. Nurses frequently find it difficult to be kind, understanding, and nonjudgmental with these clients. Nurses who cannot cope with their own reactions to these clients cannot work with them effectively. It may help to remember that these clients do not intentionally produce their symptoms, neither do they appreciate the effects of their behavior on other people. Nurses who appreciate the whole story can sometimes feel more empathy for a client's coping style.

Diagnosing

The following sections discuss implications of nursing diagnoses for the client and the nurse.

Impaired Communication   Clients with somatoform disorders have an impaired ability to communicate their needs. Though they may be highly verbal, careful listening reveals many gaps, oversimplifications, overdramatizations, and overgeneralizations in their communications. These disorders are considered nonverbal substitutes for the expression of underlying conflict that they feel unable to master.

The nurse considers the nonverbal communication function of the symptom itself. Symptoms of blindness, deafness, pain, numbness, itching, swelling, vomiting, paralysis, and so forth may be communicating something as general as "take care of me," "pay attention to me," or "I want out of these responsibilities." Specific symptoms may have more exact or symbolic meanings. The "blind" person may be saying, "I don't want to see something, because not having to see it allows me to escape my feelings about it." The client about to be married may suddenly develop acute pain in the genital area as a way of saying "I'm afraid of becoming sexually involved."

Altered Role Performance and Altered Family Processes The manipulative and dependent traits of the client with a somatoform disorder lead to impairment in social, work, and family relationships and to diminished performance in these roles. Friends and relatives eventually tire of their demands and become less available for support. Clients become emotionally isolated because their self-absorption makes them unable to respond appropriately to the needs of others.

Work performance suffers from frequent absences due to imagined illness. Preoccupation with their health uses up creative energy they could otherwise direct toward their work.

Ineffective Individual Coping   Clients with a somatoform disorder experience anxiety, anger, and feelings of helplessness. They may feel these emotions acutely and demonstrate these feelings excessively, as in somatization disorder and hypochondriacal disorder. Paradoxically, they may show an uncanny lack of feeling where more would be expected, as in the blithe reaction to loss of physical function in conversion disorder.

The emotional life of the client becomes increasingly constricted. The focus of emotional experience becomes somatic concerns, and clients no longer experience meaningful emotional connections with other persons, activities, and events. Range of expression of emotion may be limited to making demands, manipulation, and symbolic manifestation of anxiety.

Altered Thought Processes and Sensory/Perceptual Alterations   These clients show selective inattention, i.e., they filter out stimuli as a response to anxiety. Because they must keep ideas and events out of awareness, their judgment is often impaired. In a further effort to prove their ideas, they distort reality and tend to ramble. It is evident to the nurse that their conclusions are not logical. They may distort memory or show selective memory as well.

Clients with somatoform disorder have a body image disturbance; they sense that they are weak or vulnerable physically. They perceive sensory data incorrectly. For example, they may perceive abdominal discomfort as cancer rather than common indigestion.

Planning and Implementing Interventions

Effective intervention involves the following:

• Recognizing and understanding the life problem or adjustment the client is facing

• Recognizing and understanding the client's self-perception as helpless to cope

• Helping the client learn more effective ways of adapting

These steps may be accomplished by insight-oriented or supportive psychotherapy, behavior modification, hypnosis, or any of several other psychologic, as well as some physical, therapies. None can claim superior effectiveness, and new approaches and techniques are indicated when traditional ones prove inadequate.

It is important to recognize that many clients with somatoform disorders are highly resistant to change. Progress may be slow and recovery partial.

Promoting Effective Communication   After assessing the meaning behind the client's communication patterns, plan intervention strategies that enhance the client's functional verbal communication and self-esteem to the point where the client feels ready to face problems.

It is usually necessary to help these clients tone down their characteristic extravagances and to express respectful skepticism regarding their oversimplifications and overdramatizations. A communication and feelings group gives clients the opportunity to receive feedback about the effect of their behavior on others.

Promoting Improved Role Performance and Family Processes   Working with the family as well as with the client is especially important for clients with somatoform disorders. Educate the family and the client about the disorder, stressing the importance of avoiding unnecessary surgery or medical procedures. Support self-sufficiency, encourage independent functioning, and reduce the possibility of secondary gain by not focusing on physical symptoms. Assume a matter-of-fact, supportive attitude, with the optimistic expectation that the client will return to functioning in work, family, and social roles.

Promoting Effective Individual Coping   The goal of counseling clients with somatoform disorders is to help them express their conflicts verbally rather than acting them out in symptomatic behaviors. The aim of long-term, or insight therapy, is to promote effective emotional expression by exploring the sources of anxiety. Supportive therapy seeks to improve self-esteem, perhaps through such measures as expanding clients' interest in their environment.

In general, try to avoid reinforcing the client's symptoms. A well-known psychiatric axiom that applies to clients in this general category is "ignore the symptoms but never the client." To concentrate on the physical symptom by trying to get a "paralyzed" client to walk or a "blind" client to see again is to give the symptom more importance than it merits, thus increasing the secondary gain associated with it. Ultimately this merely makes it harder for the client to relinquish the symptom.

Promoting Improved Perception and Thought Processes   Help clients improve their capacities of perception and thinking by supporting general measures to reduce anxiety and improve communication of needs. In addition, maintain a calm, unhurried attitude toward the client, listen carefully, and maintain an objective and undistorted view of reality. Avoid a premature challenge to the client's symptoms and complaints.

As clients gradually relinquish their defenses, propose other ways of understanding the condition, e.g., suggesting a psychologic explanation for a physical complaint.

Evaluating/Outcome Criteria

Communication Clients will more regularly express feelings and conflicts verbally. They will have fewer physical complaints and fewer somatic symptoms. Conversation with the client will "flow," with fewer monologues by the client and more natural dialogue between client and nurse.

Role Performance and Family Processes   Clients will attend work regularly without frequent absences due to illness or interference due to worry about physical health. They will be more interested in outside activities and may begin to engage in socialization and recreation. Family and friends will report being more satisfied with their relationship with the client and will be more willing to interact with the client socially.

Individual Coping Clients will be less demanding, manipulative, and attention-seeking in interaction with others. They will appear less anxious and will talk of subjects other than their current physical status. They will appear less helpless and more able to participate in and make responsible decisions about their health care. For example, they may carry out a plan of treatment without voicing innumerable objections or worries.

They will appear more interested and involved in the activities and attitudes of others and more aware of the impact of their own behavior.

Perception and Thought Processes The client will distort and misinterpret reality less frequently. Judgment, insight, and memory will improve as a result of reduced defensiveness in perception and cognition. Clients may report feeling more positive about their bodies. They will be more assertive in physical activities because they no longer tend to feel so vulnerable.

The Nursing Process and Dissociative Disorders

Assessing

The major areas to focus on during assessment are identity, memory, and consciousness.

Subjective Data Clients with dissociative disorders often report sudden loss of memory of events. Clients may report, for example, that they cannot recall certain important personal events or information. They may not recall aspects of their own identity, e.g., how old they are and where they reside.

Sometimes amnesia is only partial, and clients remain conscious of what happened, although they report that they feel no control over it. In cases of complete or nearly complete amnesia, the "lost" memories can be recovered under certain therapeutic circumstances, or they may return spontaneously.

Clients who have sustained loss of their own reality may have adopted an entirely new identity.

If motor behavior is affected in dissociative disorder, clients or their families may report episodes during which clients physically traveled away from home. Clients with depersonalization disorder may report fears that they are going crazy and have great secondary anxiety. In clients with multiple personality disorder, the original personality typically is not aware of the existence of the secondary ones, although the secondary personalities may be aware of the original personality as well as of each other and may report this awareness to the nurse. It is common to find a history of childhood incest or physical or sexual abuse in clients with multiple personality disorder.

Objective Data The nurse conducts a careful assessment of the client's physical condition because of the possibility of organic causes, e.g., brain tumor, of the dissociative disorder. Many of the behaviors of clients with dissociative disorders resemble behaviors associated with organic conditions, including postconcussional amnesia and temporal lobe epilepsy. The Assessment boxes on page 344 summarize the major differentiating points.

The nurse's observations of the character, duration, frequency, and context of the dissociative disorder are crucial firsthand data. Physical examinations are not continued as part of the long-term intervention program, however, because they reinforce the symptoms and provide secondary gain. Therefore the completeness and accuracy of the initial physical assessment are of the utmost importance.

A psychosocial assessment is conducted to discover the fundamental source of the anxiety as early as possible. Although many episodes of dissociation appear to occur spontaneously, there may be a history of a specific, shocking emotional trauma or a situation charged with painful emotions and psychologic conflict. Family or friends may provide clues to the client's conflict and should be included in the psychosocial data gathering.

Diagnosing

The following sections discuss implications of nursing diagnoses for the client and the nurse.

ASSESSMENT

Differentiation of Postconcussional Amnesia and Psychogenic Amnesia

Properties of Postconcussional Amnesia

History of a head injury.

Retrograde amnesia does not extend beyond a week into the past.

Amnesia disappears slowly and memory for events that occurred during the amnesic period is not completely restored.

Properties of Psychogenic Amnesia

No history of head injury.

Retrograde amnesia extends indefinitely into the past.

Client can recover suddenly with total restoration of memory.

ASSESSMENT

Differentiation of Temporal Lobe Epilepsy and Dissociative Trances

Properties of Temporal Lobe Epilepsy

Presence of positive electroencephalographic evidence of temporal lobe dysfunction

Usually does not occur in conjunction with other patterns

Properties of Dissociative Trances

No such evidence

Often occurs with other behavior (stigmata, sleepwalking).

Sensory/Perceptual Alterations and Altered Thought Processes   Clients with dissociative disorder may experience sudden memory loss, disorientation, loss of personal identity, and alteration in state of consciousness. Clients with psychogenic amnesia have partial or total inability to recall or identify past experiences. In clients with depersonalization disorder, feelings of unreality and estrangement can be severe and painful. These can affect clients' perception of the physical and psychologic self and of the world around them. Parts of the body or the entire body may seem foreign. Dizziness, anxiety, and distortion of time and space are common.

Altered Role Performance   Unexplained disappearances, absences from work, unreliability, and unpredictability are common manifestations of dissociative disorders. Of course, the social or occupational functioning of the client is adversely affected.

Symptoms of depersonalization lead to limited or superficial involvement with others and to withdrawal or disengagement in past work or social pursuits. As expected, relationships become highly complicated and disorganized when a client has multiple personalities.

Ineffective Individual Coping   In addition to amnesia, a fugue state may occur in clients with dissociative disorders. In this state, clients defend against perceived danger by active flight. They may wander away from home. Days, weeks, or sometimes even years later they may suddenly find themselves in a strange place, not knowing how they got there and with complete amnesia for the period of the fugue. Fugue clients may adopt a new identity and life pattern.

Planning and Implementing Interventions

In choosing intervention strategies for clients with dissociative disorders, the treatment team must decide whether to alleviate the troublesome symptom or reintegrate the anxiety-producing conflict. Some teams emphasize the disruptions in day-to-day functioning occasioned by dissociative disorders. These include unexplained disappearances, absences from work, unreliability, and unpredictability. The dread associated with them justifies intervention strategies designed to change the disruptive behavior pattern. Others believe that new problems are created by removing the so-called symptoms without considering how they help the client control internal anxiety and maintain some balance in external social life.

Keep in mind that although clients may complain about the difficulties associated with their symptoms, the symptoms often form the basis of relationships with other significant people in their lives. These clients' roles in social groups are likewise built around their coping styles. Anyone who alters these coping styles must offer clients more effective and satisfying ways to handle anxiety and get support in their social network. Such a learning task usually requires long-term psychotherapy. However, behavior-modification strategies can alleviate symptoms.

Promoting Improved Sensory Perception and Thought Processes

Strategies for identifying the source of anxiety that underlies the perceptive and cognitive impairments in clients with dissociative disorders include those for recovering unconscious content, such as free association or dream description. At times more active strategies are used. These may include projective psychometric tests (Rorschach, Thematic Apperception Test) and hypnosis, with or without intravenous administration of sodium thiopental (Pentothal). These techniques are usually employed by psychoanalysts or clinical psychologists rather than nurses.

Supportive insight therapy may be used with the goal of surfacing and integrating traumatic experiences and learning new ways of coping with future anxiety. This is especially relevant for those clients in whom the dissociative phenomena arise primarily against a background of intrapsychic or subjective conflict.

Promoting Effective Role Performance and Family Processes

Including family members in a therapeutic family counseling relationship helps them learn new ways of dealing with the client. As stated earlier, considerable secondary gain is often associated with dissociative behavior: The client can use the illness to escape responsibility and get special treatment. Families may need support in learning to avoid reinforcing dissociative behavior by acting as the source of secondary gain.

Environmental manipulation may be an indicated intervention. For example, it may be necessary to assist the client in problem solving with the goal of minimizing other stressful aspects of the environment. In learning to confront and become desensitized to the underlying conflict, the client will experience some anxiety and discomfort. This anxiety must be kept within manageable limits. Therefore, more obvious and alterable sources of stress and anxiety should be minimized.

Promoting Effective Individual and Family Coping

The nurse may use such measures as psychotherapy (if prepared as a clinical specialist), environmental manipulation, and behavior modification to help the client with a dissociative disorder cope more effectively with impairments of conduct and impulse, e.g., unpredictable and bizarre behavior. Treatment may prove to be long term, and progress may be slow. The establishment of a supportive therapeutic alliance between the client and the nurse and the family and the nurse is crucial. The nurse helps the family and client understand the periodic occurrence of symptoms and guides the family in supporting improved behaviors.

Evaluating/Outcome Criteria

Sensory Perception and Thought Processes

Clients will no longer experience sudden memory loss, disorientation, loss of identity, or alteration in state of consciousness, or they will experience it less frequently. They will correctly recall and identify past experiences.

Role Performance and Family Processes

Clients will experience increased satisfaction with family and work relationships. Involvement with others will occur more often and will be more fulfilling. They will be more successful at work or school. They will attend work or school regularly, without unexplained absences due to dissociative episodes.

Individual Coping

Clients will no longer exhibit bizarre or unpredictable behaviors, or they will experience them less frequently. For example, incidents of being missing from home without explanation will occur less frequently or not at all.

CHAPTER HIGHLIGHTS

• The theoretic frameworks of major importance in the study of anxiety disorders, somatoform disorders, and dissociative disorders include the psychologic, behavioral, and biologic.

• Anxiety disorders, somatoform disorders, and dissociative disorders may be considered disturbed coping patterns and are characterized by loss of freedom to make choices, presence of conflict, repetition despite ineffectiveness, feelings of distress or pain, and the potential for secondary gain.

• Clients with anxiety disorders experience anxiety either as the predominant disturbance or during attempts to master the symptoms.

• Clients with anxiety disorders experience anxiety both as a subjective emotion and as a variety of physical symptoms resulting from muscular tension and autonomic nervous system activity.

• Somatoform disorders are characterized by physical symptoms for which there is no positive evidence of an organic or physiologic basis.

• Dissociative disorders encompass a large group of uncommon and sometimes bizarre conditions in which there is sudden, temporary change in consciousness, identity, or motor behavior so that some part of these functions is lost.

• Nursing assessment to determine the extent of disability in anxiety disorders, somatoform disorders, or dissociative disorders includes, but is not limited to, assessment of subjective emotional experience, presence of physiologic symptoms, altered coping, altered role performance, and altered sensory perception and thought processes.

• Nursing diagnoses for clients with these disorders concern defensive coping and ineffective individual and family coping, e.g., feelings of distress, fear, anger, or anxiety; altered sleep, elimination, and circulation; inappropriate use of or abuse of medication; impaired communication; lack of knowledge about the disorder and its treatment; and distorted perception of the environment.

• Nursing interventions for clients with anxiety disorders, somatoform disorders, and dissociative disorders and their families are integrative and may include the range of psychotherapeutic interventions including providing psychotherapy, increasing social supports, reducing environmental stress, advocating the use of stress-reduction strategies, and administering psychopharmacologic treatment.

• Nursing evaluation for clients with anxiety disorders, somatoform disorders, or dissociative disorders should include assessment of physical and psychologic symptoms, the client's reports of feelings, the client's ability to understand and practice anxiety-reducing skills, demonstration of increase in cognitive capacities, and freedom from restriction in life-style.

REFERENCES

American Psychiatric Association: *Diagnostic and Statistical Manual of Mental Disorders*, ed 3, revised. APA, 1987.

Anderson DJ, Noyes R, Crowe RR: A comparison of panic disorder and generalized anxiety disorder. *Am J Psychiatry* 1984;141:572.

Auden, WH: *The Age of Anxiety*. Random House, 1947.

Beck A, Emery G: *Anxiety Disorders and Phobias: A Cognitive Perspective*. Basic Books, 1985.

Braun BG: *The Treatment of Multiple Personality Disorder*. American Psychiatric Press, 1986.

Breier A et al: Agoraphobia with panic attacks. *Arch Gen Psychiatry* 1986;43(11):1029–1036.

Breuer J, Freud S: *Studies in Hysteria*. Avon Books, 1966.

Cameron OG: The differential diagnosis of anxiety. *Psychiatr Clin North Am* 1985;8(1):3–23.

Cole J: The drug treatment of anxiety and depression. *Med Clin North Am* 1988;74(4):815–830.

Elledgrie E, Bridges M: Posttraumatic stress disorder. Symposium on Anxiety Disorders. *Psychiatr Clin North Am* 1985;8(1):89–103.

Forchuk C, Brown B: Establishing a nurse-client relationship. *J Psychosoc Nurs* 1989;27(2):30–36.

Freud S: *The Problem of Anxiety*. Norton, 1936.

Gulledge A, Calabrese J: Diagnosis of anxiety and depression. *Med Clin North Am* 1988;74(4):753–763.

Hickey J, Baer P: Psychological approaches to assessment and treatment of anxiety and depression. *Med Clin North Am* 1988;74(4):911–927.

Hyman R, Feldman H, et al: The effects of relaxation training on clinical symptoms: A meta-analysis. *Nurs Res* 1989;38(4):216–220.

Insel T, Akiskal H: Obsessive-compulsive disorder with psychotic features: A phenomenological analysis. *Am J Psychiatry* 1986;143(12):1527–1533.

Kamerow D: Anxiety and depression in the medical setting. *Med Clin North Am* 1988;74(4):745–751.

Laage T: Recognizing the drug-resistant patient in anxiety and depression. *Med Clin North Am* 1988;74(4):897–909.

Laraia MP, Stuart GW, Best CL: Behavioral treatment of panic-related disorders: A review. *Arch Psychiatr Nurs* 1989;3:125–133.

Manaser JC, Werner AM: *Instruments for the Study of Nurse-Patient Interaction*. Macmillan, 1964.

Marks IM: Behavioral psychotherapy for anxiety disorders. *Psychiatr Clin North Am* 1985;8(1):25–35.

Nemiah JC: Anxiety states (anxiety neurosis), in Kaplan HI, Sadock BJ: *Comprehensive Textbook of Psychiatry/IV*, ed 4. Williams & Wilkins, 1985a, pp 883–894.

Nemiah JC: Obsessive-compulsive disorder (obsessive-compulsive neurosis), in Kaplan HI, Sadock BJ: *Comprehensive Textbook of Psychiatry/IV*, ed 4. Williams & Wilkins, 1985b, pp 904–917.

Nemiah JC: Somatoform disorders, in Kaplan HI, Sadock BJ: *Comprehensive Textbook of Psychiatry/IV*, ed 4. Williams & Wilkins, 1985c, pp 924–942.

Olson M: The out-of-body experience and other states of consciousness. *Arch Psychiatr Nurs* 1987;1(3):201–207.

Rank O: *The Trauma of Birth*. Robert Brunner, 1952.

Rapoport J: The biology of obsessions and compulsions. *Sci Am* 1989;March:83–89.

Rapoport J: *The Boy Who Couldn't Stop Washing*. E. P. Dutton, 1989.

Rogers B, Nickolaus J: Vietnam nurses. *J Psychosoc Nurs* 1987;25(4):11–15.

Schaffer D: Recognizing multiple personality patients. *Am J Psychotherapy* 1986;40(4):500–510.

Schuckit M: Anxiety treatment progress. *The Psychiatric Times* 1985;June:3.

Schwartz G et al: Anxiety disorders and psychiatric referral in the general medical emergency room. *Gen Hosp Psychiatry* 1987;9(2)87–93.

Scrignar CB: *Post-Traumatic Stress Disorder: Diagnosis, Treatment, and Legal issues*. Praeger Publishers, 1984.

Spitzer RL, Williams JBW: Diagnostic issues in the DSM-III classification of the anxiety disorders, in Grinspoon L (ed): *Psychiatric Update*. American Psychiatric Press, 1984, pp 23–26.

Stinnett J: The functional somatic symptom. *Psychiatr Clin North Am* 1987;10(1):19–33.

Stoudemire A, Sandhu J: Psychogenic/idiopathic pain syndromes. *Gen Hosp Psychiatry* 1987;9(2):79–85.

Sullivan HS: *The Interpersonal Theory of Psychiatry*. Norton, 1953.

Tearnan B, Telch M: Phobic disorders, in Adams H, Sutker P (eds): *Comprehensive Handbook of Psychopathology*. Plenum Press, 1984, Chapter 7.

Teicher M: Biology of anxiety. *Med Clin North Am* 1988;74(4):791–813.

Whitley G: Anxiety: Defining the diagnosis. *J Psychosoc Nurs* 1989;27(10):7–12.

Nutrition Box References

Berkow R (ed): *Merck Manual of Diagnosis and Therapy* ed 15. Rahway, N.J.: Merck and Co, 1987, p. 1086.

Betteridge DJ: Reactive hypoglycemia. *Br Med J* 1987; 295:286.

Chalew S et al.: Diagnosis of reactive hypoglycemia: Pitfalls in the use of the oral glucose tolerance test. *South Med J* 1986;79:285–287.

Foster D, Rubenstein A: Hypoglycemia, insulinoma, and other hormone-secreting tumors of the pancreas, in Wyngaarden J, Smith L (eds): *Cecil Textbook of Medicine,* ed 17. Philadelphia: Saunders, 1985, p. 1801.

Palardy J et al.: Blood glucose measurements during symptomatic episodes in patients with suspected postprandial hypoglycemia. *N Engl J Med* 1989;321(21):1421–1425.

Applying the Nursing Process for Clients with Sexual Disorders

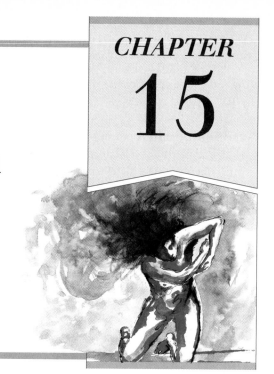

LEARNING OBJECTIVES

- Apply theories of sexuality when providing nursing care with clients to promote, maintain, or regain sexual health

- Describe etiologies of various gender and sexual disorders

- Identify potential side effects of selected drugs that may affect sexual function

- Assess clients' sexual health status

- Elicit a detailed sexual history in which clients express specific sexual concerns

- Formulate nursing diagnoses for clients expressing sexual concerns or having sexual health problems

- Identify principles common to most treatment plans for gender and sexual disorders

- Apply a nursing model for intervening with clients to promote sexual health

- Describe the nurse's role in providing interventions for clients who are experiencing gender or sexual concerns

- Evaluate nursing interventions to promote sexual health with the purpose of making referrals, when needed, to a qualified sex counselor or therapist

Karen Lee Fontaine

CROSS REFERENCES

Other topics relevant to this content are: HIV and high-risk sexual behaviors, Chapter 25; Incest, and rape and rape counseling, Chapter 22.

ALL HUMANS ARE SEXUAL beings. Regardless of gender, age, race, socioeconomic status, religious beliefs, physical and mental health, or other demographic factors, human beings express their sexuality in a variety of ways throughout their lives.

Human sexuality is difficult to define. "Maleness, femaleness, sensuality, sense of self, ego, perception of self in relationship to the world and others, the quality or state of being sexual, the condition of having sexual activity or intercourse, the expression of receiving and expressing sexual interest are all connotative of human sexuality" (Monat 1982, p 1). Sexuality is an individually expressed and highly personal phenomenon whose meaning evolves from objective and subjective experiences. Physiologic, psychosocial, and cultural factors influence a person's sexuality and lead to the wide range of attitudes and behaviors seen in humans. There are no normal, universal sexual behaviors. Satisfying or "normal" sexual expression can best be described as whatever behaviors give pleasure and satisfaction to those involved without threat of coercion or threat of injury to others.

Sexual health is an individual and constantly changing phenomenon falling within the wide range of normal healthy expressions of human sexual thoughts, feelings, needs, and desires. The World Health Organization (WHO) defines sexual health as the "integration of the somatic, emotional, intellectual, and social aspects of sexual being, in ways that are positively enriching and that enhance personality, communication and love" (WHO 1975). An individual's degree of sexual health is best determined by that individual, sometimes with the assistance of a qualified professional. It is helpful for some to view sexual health on the wellness-illness continuum, which allows for changing biopsychosociocultural factors and varied sexual attitudes, values, and needs.

Nursing and Sexual Health Care

Sexual health care is a relatively new area of involvement for psychiatric nurses. Until recently, sexuality has not been viewed as falling within the scope of treatment. Currently, sexuality is increasingly recognized as an important component of a holistic approach to humans and their overall health status. Sexual health care is a legitimate and appropriate nursing concern. The close and often extended relationships that psychiatric nurses have with clients and families foster the rapport necessary to discuss this private area of clients' health status.

Nursing roles in the area of human sexuality are evolving gradually. Psychiatric nurses involved in nursing activities related to human sexual functioning need the following:

- Concrete and comprehensive knowledge about sexual function and dysfunction

- Skill in communication techniques

- Acceptance of, and comfort with, their own sexual values and expressions

- Willingness to explore and separate personal values and attitudes from those of clients

- Proficiency in using the nursing process to assess, diagnose, intervene, and evaluate care to promote optimal sexual health

Historically, human sexuality has been shrouded in myth and controversy. This history has hindered both the delivering and receiving of services that promote sexual health and well-being. Although scientific knowledge has expanded immensely in the past decade, modern North Americans continue to view sex and sexuality with discomfort. Our confusion is complicated by our traditional religious and social values. Nurses may hold some of these negative attitudes and biases. Psychiatric nurses must confront these negative, inappropriate, or stereotypic ideas and opinions before they can meet professional standards of care in helping clients attain optimal sexual health.

Basic to nursing is the notion that the nurse's personal beliefs should not influence the quality of care given a client. It is easier for nurses to live up to this standard if they engage in values clarification before providing sexual health care. Giving nonjudgmental nursing care does not mean that the nurse has to agree with others' beliefs and values about sexuality. However, self-awareness can help psychiatric nurses respect their clients' sexual rights and needs.

Historical and Theoretic Foundations

Human sexual behavior has been studied from various theoretic perspectives. The most significant of these include the (a) historical, (b) psychologic, (c) behavioral, (d) sociocultural, and (e) biologic approaches.

Historical Foundation

One takes a historical approach by examining past sexual behaviors and identifying patterns and influences that have led to present behaviors. Throughout history, people have struggled with sexual ethics, that is, the determination of "good" and "bad" sexual behavior. The sexual ethics of a culture reflect the culture's assumptions about the purpose of sex. In Western society, sexual practices have been strongly influenced by the Judeo-Christian tradition, which historically considered procreation to be the primary purpose of sex. As a result, even modern Western societies are fairly sexually intolerant and are harshly critical of those whose gender identity or sexual behavior is not in the mainstream.

In recent years, new issues have led people to challenge traditional Western values about sexuality. The worldwide concern about overpopulation has forced many people to reexamine the notion that procreation is the purpose of sexual behavior. The development of effective and safe contraceptive methods has given people conscious control of reproduction. The individual rights movement has been extended to the sexually oppressed, who no longer tolerate discrimination and are demanding the same freedoms as others. Thus, society is being forced to become more flexible, adapt to new sexual values, and develop a more humane morality. Because ethical choices are always subjective and based on feelings, beliefs, and moral traditions, many people continue to struggle with conflicting cultural, religious, and personal values.

Psychologic Foundation

Intrapersonal theorists view gender disorders, paraphilias, and sexual dysfunctions as problems occurring within the individual. Some view these as expressions of arrested psychosexual development, some seek an explanation in sexual guilt, and others see the issue as being one of self-punishment. Performance anxiety, negative self-concept, and negative body image are all seen as contributing to sexual problems. Problems to be solved during the treatment process include fears of intimacy, losing control, pain, pregnancy, and sexually transmitted diseases.

Behavioral Approach

Behaviorists believe that gender disorders arise from social learning; that is, that the child was rewarded in some way for adopting behaviors of the other sex. They believe paraphilias are learned responses; the person is conditioned to respond erotically to nonsexual objects or particular sexual acts. In the area of sexual dysfunctions, contributing factors include poor communication skills, lack of sexual experience with oneself or a partner, concern with sexual performance, and ineffective stimulation. The dysfunctions, too, are seen as learned responses.

Sociocultural Foundation

People who grew up with rigid family and religious taboos about sex often experience guilt and anxiety about their adult sexual roles and behaviors. People with little tolerance for cross-gender behavior view transsexuals and transvestites as deviants within the culture. The sexual acts of paraphiliacs conflict with the traditional value of sex for procreation, and they, too, are made to feel like outcasts. Sociocultural theories regarding sexual dysfunctions center on disturbed relationships between partners, negative early learning, and past or present traumatic events.

Biologic Foundation

Those who take a biologic approach are concerned with physiologic aspects of gender identity and sexual behavior. Some believe there is a neurologic basis for gender differences and look to fetal exposure to sex hormones and adult levels of sex hormones as an explanation of gender disorders. They explore sexual dysfunctions to discover factors (e.g., organic disease, injury, medications, pain, or depression) that interfere with the physiologic reflexes during the sexual response cycle.

A review of the various theoretic perspectives shows that human sexuality has been historically characterized by judgments and controversy. This history has hindered both the delivering and receiving of services promoting sexual health and well-being. It is important for health care professionals to remember that *all* individuals are deviant from some physical, social, behavioral, or emotional norm. Some are left-handed, some stutter, some are disabled, some are loners, and some are filled with fears. To achieve the highest level of professional practice, nurses must look beyond the characteristics and respond to the human person.

It is only in the past 25 years that human sexuality has been scientifically studied from a multidisciplinary approach. With the advent of this knowledge came the beginnings of planned interventions for individuals suffering from a variety of sexual problems or disorders. Nursing has been an active participant in the evolution of treatment approaches and programs to provide sexual health care.

Gender Identity Disorders

Gender identity is an individual's personal or private sense of identity as female or male. Gender identity develops from an interaction of biology, identity imposed by others, and self-identity. A newborn is assigned a gender (other's identity) according to the appearance of the external genitals (biology); by 3 years of age, the child says "I am a girl" or "I am a boy" (self-identity). Gender identity can be viewed as a continuum. At one end of the continuum are those persons whose gender identity is congruent with their anatomic sex. In the middle are transvestites, who have both a male and female gender identity. At the other end of the continuum are transsexuals, whose gender identity conflicts with their anatomic sex.

The term **gender roles** refers to learning and performing socially accepted sex behaviors, i.e., taking on a feminine or masculine role. In American culture, roles are more strictly enforced for males than for females, and males are socially punished for female behavior. In many Western countries, however, there is a growing appreciation of **androgyny**, or flexibility in gender roles. Proponents of androgyny view most characteristics and behaviors as human qualities that should not be limited to a specific gender. In an increasingly complex world, adults who can behave flexibly fare better than those who adopt rigid stereotypic gender roles.

Theories of Gender Development

Biologic Imperative   How do gender identity and gender roles develop? One contemporary theory asserts that anatomy is destiny: Because women and men are biologically different, they have innately different characteristics and styles of interacting. In this view, a biologic mechanism directs the fetus to have a female identity with feminine behavior or a male identity with masculine behavior.

Cognitive Switch   Another theory is that children are born neutral, but that one of the central developmental tasks of childhood is to label oneself as female or male. According to this theory, a cognitive switch occurs at age 3 or 4, after which gender identity is irreversible.

Social Learning and Labeling   The third theory, espoused in this text, focuses on social learning. It holds that gender identity and roles are continuously constructed and maintained throughout the life span. The stability of one's gender identity depends not only on biologic differences but also on everyday situations that continuously provide expectations, demands, and feedback. These shape one's conception of self, and people learn role behavior through realizing the consequences of their own behavior and observing the consequences of the behavior of others.

Transsexualism

DSM-III-R identifies **transsexualism** as a gender identity disorder in which a person has consistently strong feelings of being trapped in a body of the wrong sex.

For transsexuals, anatomy is not consistent with gender identity. Most transsexuals report that they have had these feelings since earliest childhood, and their families report that transsexuals insisted since childhood that they were of the other sex. Psychologic gender identity is stronger than anatomy, and most transsexuals develop an aversion to their genitals. Often they hide their problem from family and friends for many years because they fear being considered "crazy." As self-understanding and acceptance increase, many transsexuals live part time or full time as members of the other sex. Cross-dressing (dressing in clothing usually identified with the opposite sex) not only makes their outward appearance consistent with their inner identity and gender roles but also increases their comfort with themselves. Sexually, they are attracted to persons of the same anatomic sex but consider themselves heterosexual because of their gender identity.

At this time there is no clear understanding of the etiology of transsexualism. The biologic theory is based on animal studies, since experimental research cannot be conducted with humans. When exposed prenatally to increased male hormones, the animal exhibits increased male behavior. Decreasing the levels of male hormones prenatally increases female behavior in animals. In humans, the male gonads develop and begin secreting androgen between the eighth and twelfth week of gestation. Differentiation of the hypothalamus to a male pattern, which occurs in the fourth to fifth month of gestation, requires high androgen levels. Thus, one explanation of transsexualism is that prenatal androgen levels were sufficient for the development of male anatomy but insufficient for differentiation in the brain. In transsexuals who are anatomically female, the androgenic influences may have been high at the critical time of hypothalamic development, although not at the time of genital formation.

Psychosocial theories focus on the transsexual's relationship with the parent of the other sex and the processes of identification and introjection. Many believe that gender identity is a learned response and that transsexuals either learn the opposite of what they are taught or are encouraged to adopt the behavior of the opposite sex. It is not yet possible to understand the respective roles of the effect of prenatal androgen on brain tissues on the one hand and the role of social learning on the other in the development of gender disorders (Money 1986).

Gender Identity Disorders of Childhood, Adolescence, and Adulthood

Gender identity disorders occur in children who feel persistent and intense distress about their biologic gender. They state an intense desire to be of the other sex. A girl may insist that she is a boy, has a penis, and will not grow breasts or menstruate. These girls demand to wear boys' underwear and clothing and wish to urinate in a standing position. Similarly, a boy may demand to wear girls' underwear and clothing, express intense dislike of his penis, and voice the desire to grow breasts. This classification by the DSM-III-R refers only to children who have not reached puberty and who express these symptoms persistently (DSM-III-R 1987).

Gender identity disorder may also occur for the first time in adolescence or adulthood. In addition to feeling persistent discomfort and a sense of inappropriateness about one's assigned sex, the person engages in cross-dressing. Cross-dressing behavior ranges from the occasional wearing of a single item of clothing to dressing entirely as a member of the other sex.

The nonfetish transvestite is typically a married heterosexual male who cross-dresses to express the feminine side of his personality. Most transvestites exhibit stereotypic masculine identity and behavior in their public and professional lives. Cross-dressing is a conscious choice and usually occurs at home or in a setting where discovery is unlikely. It is not unusual for nonfetish transvestites to have a female name to go with the female personality and wardrobe. This type of transvestism occurs more frequently in cultures where males are expected to be strong, independent, and unemotional protectors. In a climate of rigid gender roles, it is understandable that some men can express their gentleness and dependency only by creating a separate world and female persona (Peo 1988).

Often these individuals do not tell their spouses about the cross-dressing before their marriage. Some are embarrassed and do not know how to bring the topic into the open. Others view the need to cross-dress as a problem and hope that it will disappear after the marriage. The majority of wives eventually find

RESEARCH NOTE

Citation
Brown GR, Collier L: Transvestites' women revisited: A nonpatient sample. Arch Sexual Behav 1989;18(1):73–83.

Study Problem/Purpose
This study focused on seven adult female partners of transvestites, a group that has rarely been studied. None of these women were in treatment for issues relating to their partners' cross-dressing. The study was done to understand more clearly the women who choose long-term committed relationships with men who cross-dress.

Methods
The sample was recruited from social organization established for cross-dressers. Only women who had been in a committed, exclusive relationship with the transvestite male for a minimum of one year were included. Two women knew of the cross-dressing prior to commitment; three were told within three weeks of the marriage; and two were told after years into the relationship. The group was seen by a female/male team once a month for two-hour sessions over a six-month period. The women were asked to rate their acceptance of transvestism on a scale of A to F, where A represents total acceptance and F represents sadistic rejection.

Findings
Four of seven partners listed transvestism as the biggest problem in their relationships, and five seriously considered leaving their mates at some time in the relationship as a direct consequence of their cross-dressing. On the A to F grading system, two women were A partners; two, B partners; two, C partners; and one, an E partner. The most difficult task for these women was coping with their mate's narcissism, as evidenced by such behavior as primping and spending hours before a mirror.

Implications
Previous studies (of patient populations) described women in a relationship with transvestites as either malicious male-haters, succorers, or symbiotes, all of whom were characterized as moral masochists. An important difference in this study was the finding that, with time, all the women came to view their mates' transvestism as an integral part of their personality and coped with it as an involuntary handicapping condition. Although this study drew on a nonpatient population, the bias was that the women all participated in public cross-dressing at the monthly meetings. Therefore, it is possible that the findings are not representative of women married to transvestites who do not participate in social organizations supportive of cross-dressing.

out. For some women, the discovery raises doubts about their own sexuality and self-worth, and they may decide to terminate the relationship. Other women are not threatened by the cross-dressing but fear it will become public knowledge.

Sexual Disorders

Paraphilias

DSM-III-R classifies **paraphilias** as a group of psychosexual disorders characterized by unconventional sexual behaviors. The person, usually a male, has learned to associate sexual arousal with some environmental stimulus, which triggers the unusual behavior. Paraphilias are not by definition pathologic. Many people engage in mild forms of the noncoercive behaviors and consider them simply love play. The behavior becomes pathologic when it is severe, insistent, coercive, and harmful to the self or others.

Paraphilias can be divided into the noncoercive and coercive types. The coercive paraphilias are described in the legal code, and the sexual behavior is considered a criminal act (Dalley 1988). See the accompanying box for groupings and definitions.

Paraphilias have a strong obsessive-compulsive component. Affected individuals are often preoccupied with and feel compelled to engage in their particular sexual behaviors. One of the distinguishing characteristics is the person's inability to control or stop the behavior.

Humans respond to a wealth of sexual stimuli. Some people are aroused by the strident beat of rock music, while others are aroused by romantic music. Some people prefer making love in a brightly lit room; others, by candlelight; still others, in the dark. Everyone associates sexual arousal with an individual set of stimuli. An association or stimulus that is not typical for the culture is called a **fetish**. A fetish is the sexualization of a body part, such as feet or hair, or an inanimate object, such as shoes, leather, or rubber. Early associations of a particular object or body part with sexual arousal condition the person to respond sexually to that stimulus. Once the initial association is made, repeated viewing or use (fantasized or actual) of the part or object during sexual activity (usually masturbation) reinforces its arousing nature. For instance, a boy may get an erection after trying on his mother's panties. The erection is pleasurable. The next time the boy masturbates, he remembers the panties and puts them on or fantasizes about them. With repeated experiences, seeing the panties or putting them on becomes a sexual stimulus. As with all people, fetishists' responses are highly individual. Fetishism is not considered a problem as long as it is not harmful

---

Characteristics of Paraphilias

Noncoercive

Fetishism Sexual arousal elicited by inanimate objects (shoes, leather, rubber) or specific body parts (feet, hair).

Autoerotic Asphyxia Constriction of the neck to enhance a masturbation experience; often leads to accidental death.

Sexual Masochism Erotic interest in receiving psychologic or physical pain, real or fantasized.

Sexual Sadism Erotic interest in inflicting psychologic or physical pain, real or fantasized.

Transvestic Fetishism Sexual arousal elicited by cross-dressing (most often a heterosexual male dressing in female clothes).

Coercive

Exhibitionism Intentional exposure of the genitals to a stranger or unsuspecting person; may be accompanied by arousal and masturbation either during or after the exposure.

Voyeurism Secret observation of an unsuspecting person (usually a woman) engaged in a private act, e.g., undressing or having sex. The voyeur often masturbates during or after the viewing.

Frotteurism Intense sexual arousal elicited by rubbing the genitals against a nonconsenting person.

Obscene Phone Callers Calling a nonconsenting person and making sexual noises, using profanity, attempting to seduce, or describing sexual activity. The caller often masturbates during or after the call.

Pedophilia Sexual interest in a child. Behavior ranges from exposure, voyeurism, and explicit talk to touching, oral sex, and intercourse.

---

and occurs in the context of consenting adult partners (Sargent 1988).

In contrast with nonfetish transvestites, men who become sexually aroused by dressing in women's clothing are considered **transvestic fetishists**. They are typically heterosexual males and may wear female underclothes or may cross-dress completely. Like other fetishists, they have often undergone conditioning, and female clothing is an intense sexual stimulus. Many report great emotional stress if they try to resist the urge to cross-dress. Like other fetishes, cross-dressing is not a problem among consenting adult partners (Peo 1988).

Sexual **sadism** and **masochism** (S/M) is highly stigmatized in North American culture, and few people admit to being sexually aroused by receiving or inflicting emotional or physical pain. As much as 10 percent of the population may participate in some form of S/M activity, and all groups—heterosexual, bisexual, gay, and lesbians—are represented. Physical behaviors include intense stimulation (scratching, biting, use of ice), discipline (slapping, spanking, whipping), bondage (holding down, tying down), or sensory deprivation (use of blindfolds, hoods, ear plugs). Psychologic behaviors include humiliation or degradation, such as verbally berating others or requiring them to do menial acts. S/M behavior varies in intensity and in its significance in the lives of couples. Some couples engage in the behavior only during sex. Some integrate the roles throughout the relationship, but not at all times. Other couples attempt to live out the dominant/submissive roles continuously. Thus, S/M may be only a part of foreplay or it may be a significant component of life-style. The majority of sado-masochists do not engage in S/M behavior unless the partner is willing. Most typically, both participants agree to safety "rules," and seldom is the behavior dangerous. Sado-masochists do not see the behavior as a problem and therefore do not wish to change (Moser 1988).

A noncoercive but often fatal paraphilia is **autoerotic asphyxia.** At the present time, it is not categorized as a paraphilia in DSM-III-R, but, like paraphilias, it is a compulsive and unconventional sexual behavior. This paraphilia, called head-rushing or scarfing, typically begins in adolescence and is primarily a male affliction. The person fashions a tourniquet-like device that constricts the neck, decreasing the blood and oxygen supply to the brain. The person masturbates and, at the point of orgasm, releases the bonds to enhance the sensation or sexual high. Tragically, this practice causes many deaths. The vagal nerve complex in the carotid artery is stimulated by pressure around the neck, slowing the heart rate and decreasing oxygen flow to the brain even further. The person becomes unconscious, slumps forward, and accidentally hangs himself. Many believe the cause of death is suicide, but family and friends cannot understand the reason for the suicide, since these young men are not mentally ill or even troubled. It is often helpful to the family to explain that the death was a tragic accident.

Coercive paraphiliacs become sexually aroused by including nonconsenting persons in their sexual acts. **Exhibitionists** and **voyeurs,** who are almost exclusively men, have powerful urges to display their genitals to strangers or peep at unsuspecting women involved in intimate behaviors. **Frotteurs** rub up against others, for instance, in a crowded train or elevator, to achieve sexual arousal. The frotteur does not attempt to engage in sex with the victim and has no desire to form a relationship. Many describe the urge to peep, expose themselves, or rub themselves against others as something that just "happens" to them and thus have difficulty assuming responsibility for their behavior (Dwyer 1988).

Most women and many men have been victims of the **obscene phone caller.** Most typically the caller does not know the victim and becomes aroused when the victim reacts with upset, disgust, or shock. Some obscene callers breathe heavily, some make sexual noises, and some utter profanities. The caller may tell the victim that he is masturbating or may suggest they get together for sexual activity. Some pretend to have legitimate reasons for talking about sex (for instance, they may pose as researchers conducting a survey) and continue until the victim is offended. The caller is sexually aroused by the combination of proximity (intimate conversation) and anonymity (Matek 1988).

A **pedophile** is an adult who is sexually aroused by and engages in sexual activity with children. All sexual relationships between adults and children are viewed as criminal in the United States. The courts consider these acts as nonconsensual because minors are presumed to have insufficient knowledge of the consequences of their acts to give meaningful consent. Pedophiliac activity can include exposure, voyeurism, explicit sex talk, touching, oral sex, intercourse, and anal sex. The child usually knows the pedophile, who may be a family member, neighbor, or friend. See Chapter 22 for an in-depth discussion of the dynamics and consequences of sexual abuse of children.

Sexual Addiction

Frequency of sexual activity can be viewed on a continuum, with most people falling in the middle range. Some people have sex frequently in a way that enhances their lives; others have sex infrequently and report contentment and satisfaction. A sexual pattern that falls at either extreme of the continuum, however, can signal problems. At the low extreme are individuals who have great difficulty in choosing to be sexual; such people may have a sexual dysfunction. At the high extreme are people who have lost their ability to choose or control their sexual behavior; these are the sexual addicts. **Sexual addiction** is a disorder in which the central focus of life is sex. People with this addiction spend 50 percent or more of all waking hours dealing with sex, from fantasy to acting-out behavior. Acting-out behavior is often victimless, for instance, having affairs; overindulging in masturbation, fetishism, pornography use, or commercial telephone sex; or visiting prostitutes. Victimizing behaviors (those with a nonconsenting partner) are less frequent and include obscene phone calls, frotteurism, voyeurism, exhibitionism, child sexual abuse, and rape. The incidence of sexual addiction is difficult to determine because of secrecy and shame, but 3 to 6 percent of the population may be affected. Of individuals in treatment, 75 to 80 percent are males (Earle and Crow 1989).

It is unethical to label as sexual addicts people who do not conform to conventional moral codes. Sexual addiction is not simply the frequent enjoyment of sexual behaviors. Many people engage in those behaviors without becoming sexual addicts. Rather, sexual addiction is a progressive disease in which sex is used to numb pain. The payoff is the same as in any other addiction, i.e., an intensely pleasurable high, a short-lived release from pain, and an escape from the problems of daily life. The consequences are also the same in that the addict's life eventually becomes unmanageable.

The components of sexual addiction have the hallmarks of obsessive-compulsive behavior. The first component is *preoccupation*. The person spends hours thinking or obsessing about sex. Preoccupation, in itself, gives a sexual high and is so time-consuming that the person cannot fulfill work, school, or family responsibilities. The second component is *ritualization*. The individual engages in specific behaviors done just the "right" way and in the same sequence each time. Ritual behaviors include wearing certain clothing, taking certain steps to get ready, driving certain routes, or looking for partners only in a certain area. The ritual seems to control anxiety; once addicts begin a ritual, they cannot stop until the cycle is completed. The third component is *compulsivity*. The individual cannot control sexual behavior, and this behavior becomes the most important aspect of life. Some demonstrate sexually compulsive behavior in a regular pattern; others resist for a time and then have a binge cycle. The fourth component is *shame and despair*. At the end of the cycle, the person experiences guilt and shame at the loss of control. The pain of despair creates the need to begin the cycle all over again, because the addict seeks to relieve pain by getting high. Like other addicts, these individuals want to stop their behavior, promise to stop, try to stop, and are unable to stop without treatment (Carnes 1989, Earle and Crow 1989).

Until their lives become totally unmanageable, sexual addicts may successfully live a double life. They work very hard to appear normal, moral, and responsible individuals. Many of them grew up in homes where they were emotionally, physically, or sexually abused. Most of them suffer from low self-esteem and believe themselves to be unlovable. They have a desperate need for love and they equate sex with proof of love. They are so fearful of rejection that they establish only superficial relationships, thus avoiding intimacy and potential abandonment. Often, there is a codependent in the family who is essentially addicted to the addict. The codependent enables the addict by

denying the disease or obsessively trying to reform the addict. Codependents also suffer from low self-esteem, inability to express feelings, fear of abandonment, and resistance to change (Carnes 1989, Earle and Crow 1989). See Chapter 24 for a discussion of codependency.

Sexual Dysfunctions

DSM-III-R classifies problems or difficulties with sexual expression, referred to as sexual dysfunctions, according to the phase of the sexual response cycle that is affected. Not mentioned are dissatisfaction problems, which account for a significant group of individuals seeking sex therapy. Sexual dysfunctions are generally acquired at some point in a relationship but may be lifelong. They may be generalized to all sexual interactions and settings, or they may be situational, i.e., occurring in a specific setting or with specific types of sexual activity.

It is often difficult to sort out the multiple factors contributing to an individual's or couple's sexual problems. Generally a number of past and current factors are implicated. Negative events or situations in the past include lack of sex education, internalization of the teaching that sex is dirty or sinful, parental punishment for normal exploration of one's genitals, or severe trauma, such as rape or child sexual abuse. Current events or situations contributing to sexual dysfunctions include negative feelings, such as guilt, anxiety, or anger, which interfere with the ability to experience pleasure and joy. Fear of failure in sexual performance often becomes a vicious cycle; that is, fear of failure creates actual failure, which in turn produces more fear. *Spectatoring* is the detached appraisal of sexual performance or the body during a sexual act: "Am I going to lose my erection?" "Am I going to have an orgasm this time?" "My stomach is too fat." "When did his thighs get that fat?"

Lack of intimacy and feeling like a sex object inhibit the feeling of communion and connection that is an important part of love making. Fear of intimacy prevents some individuals from truly entering into a trusting and loving relationship. Another factor in dysfunction is the expectation that one's partner read one's mind about one's sexual needs. Lack of sex education and failure to communicate may result in one or both partners not knowing how to please the other. Also, sexual dysfunction may be symptomatic of relationship conflict. Until relationship issues are resolved, sex therapy is largely inappropriate. Even when couples are functioning well in all of these areas, physical changes brought on by illness, injury, or surgery may inhibit full sexual expression. Sexual fulfillment is the result of the positive interaction of psychologic, spiritual, sociologic, and physical factors, and dysfunctions are the result of a negative interaction. See Table 15–1 for an overview of past and current factors.

Disorders of Sexual Desire

Inhibited Sexual Desire   For most people, sexual desire varies from day to day as well as over the years. Some people, however, report a persistently low interest or a total lack of interest in sexual activity; these clients suffer from **inhibited sexual desire disorder.** If both individuals in a relationship are similarly uninterested in sex, there really is no problem. More typically, there is a disparity of sexual needs, and the person with the greater desire becomes dissatisfied with the sexual relationship and often initiates the seeking of help. The key issue in the relationship is not frequency but rather the dovetailing of partners' needs.

Physiologic factors associated with lack of desire are fatigue, illness, pain, use of medications, and substance abuse. Intrapersonal factors may contribute to this dysfunction. Since vulnerability and intimacy are inherent in most sexual relationships, fear of these may lead to avoidance of sex. Others fear that if they allow themselves to experience sexual desire and pleasure, they will lose all control and continually act out sexually. People who believe they must act on all sexual thoughts or desires may prefer to deny all desires than to try to fulfill them.

Relationship problems may be the source of inhibited sexual desire. Conflict and anger with one's partner are not conducive to positive sexual interaction. Some no longer feel physically attracted to one another or feel more attracted to someone else. Unless the partners experiment, sex may in time become boring. If there is a power imbalance in the relationship, the less powerful partner may lose interest in sex as a passive-aggressive way to achieve covert control. Typically, clients have little insight into the association between their lack of sexual desire and their negative feelings and relationship problems.

Sexual Aversion Disorder   **Sexual aversion disorder** is a severe distaste for sexual activity or the thought of sexual activity, which then leads to a phobic avoidance of sex. It occurs in both women and men. Intense emotional dread of an impending sexual interaction also can trigger the physiologic symptoms of anxiety, e.g., sweating, increased heart rate, or extreme muscle tension. The client then stops the sexual interaction or prevents it from even beginning. The most common cause of sexual aversion disorder is childhood sexual abuse or adult rape. This severe trauma can lead to a phobic response to sexual activity (Briere, 1989).

Increased Sexual Interest   Symptomatic of the manic phase of bipolar disorder is an increased interest in sex and sexual activity. The mood elevation is accompanied by a corresponding rise in sexual activity, variety of activity, and, often, number of sexual partners. This behavior occurs despite contrary values and is out of the client's control. The end of the manic episode signals a return to the person's usual level of sexual interest and activity. Since memory is not impaired, the person may feel embarrassment and shame about the uncontrolled sexual behavior during the manic episode.

Some adult survivors of childhood sexual abuse may go through periods of high sexual activity. This is often a desperate attempt to obtain the nurturance, love, care, and power they were denied in childhood.

TABLE 15–1   Factors Contributing to Sexual Dysfunctions

Type	Past Factors	Current Factors
Psychologic	Taught sex is dirty Child sexual abuse	Performance anxiety Spectatoring Fear of failure Guilt Negative thoughts
Spiritual	Taught sex is sinful Child sexual abuse	Not feeling connected to partner Lack of intimacy Fear of intimacy
Sociologic	Punished as child for normal sex play Lack of sex education	Failure to communicate Relationship conflict
Physical	Trauma—abuse, rape	Illness/injuries Organic disorders Medications Substance abuse Failure to engage in effective sexual behavior

CASE STUDY

A Client with Low Desire and Inhibited Orgasm

Identifying Information

Maria is a 46-year-old married woman who has come with her 48-year-old husband, John, to the local mental health outpatient clinic. Neither of them have received mental health services prior to this time.

Client's Definition of Present Problem, Precipitating Stressors Coping Strategies, Goals for Care

Both Maria and John agree that there is a disparity of sexual needs. Maria is satisfied to have sex once a month, and John wants to have sex several times a week. Maria has never been orgasmic with John but does admit to achieving orgasms during masturbation, a fact she has never been able to tell John. Maria states that she would probably like to have sex more often if she would enjoy it. Her fear is that she will not become orgasmic. John thinks that entering therapy is the first big step, and he is hopeful that their sexual relationship will improve.

History of Present Problem

They both describe their sex life at the beginning of their marriage as fine for the first several years, although Maria states that she was never orgasmic during that time. They never talked about their sex life. Some years ago, after reading a "sex book," Maria experimented with masturbation for the first time and began to experience orgasms. She was never able to share this information with John because she felt guilty about touching herself when she was alone. They are verbally and physically affectionate with one another, but, they say, not as much as they used to be. Very seldom do they express their anger to one another, and they manage most relationship conflicts by avoiding the issue.

Psychiatric History

No prior psychiatric history.

Family History

Both Maria and John are second-generation Americans of Eastern European descent. Both describe their parents as very modest and noncommunicative about any sexual issues. No sex education was given in the family. Maria and John have been married 25 years and have two children, a daughter, 19, and a son, 14. John has a good position in sales, and Maria is employed as a bookkeeper.

Sexual History

They both agree that John initiates sexual activity, primarily nonverbally. Sex typically occurs in the bedroom, after midnight, when they are both tired. Maria determines the length of foreplay, which usually lasts five to ten minutes. The only position they use is man-on-top, but both agree they would like to try other positions. John has minimal verbal communication during sex, and Maria says she is too shy to say anything while they are making love. They both have difficulty talking about their sex life with one another. Maria states she is somewhat uncomfortable when John touches her body, except for her genitals and breasts. She is comfortable touching John's genitals but not touching her own genitals in front of him. She likes to receive oral sex but is uncomfortable giving it because she is afraid John will ejaculate in her mouth. Their mutual goals in therapy are to have sex more often, to feel freer to experiment, to discuss sex openly, and to have Maria experience pleasure and orgasms.

Significant Health History

John has no current or past medical problems. Maria had a hysterectomy five years ago for endometriosis and is on hormone replacement therapy.

Current Mental Status

They are both quiet-spoken but articulate individuals. Eye contact is appropriate, mood is stable and appropriate, thought processes are logical, and there are no obvious symptoms of stress. Although they were both uncomfortable discussing sex, it became easier during the two-hour history-taking time.

▶

CASE STUDY (continued)

Diagnostic Impression

Nursing Diagnoses

Knowledge deficit related to lack of sex education and lack of communication with one another.

Altered sexuality patterns related to disparity of needs.

Ineffective individual coping related to masturbatory guilt (Maria)

Sexual dysfunction related to situational nonorgasmic response (Maria)

DSM-III-R Multiaxial Diagnosis

Axis I: 302.71   Hypoactive sexual desire disorder
          302.73   Inhibited female orgasm
Axis II: None
Axis III: Surgical menopause
Axis IV: Avoidance of conflict; ineffective communication patterns
          Severity: 3-mild
Axis V: Current GAF: 81
          Highest GAF in previous year: 81

NURSING CARE PLAN

Client Care Goals	Nursing Planning/ Intervention	Evaluation
Nursing Diagnosis: *Knowledge deficit related to lack of sex education and lack of communication*		
Both will state understanding of sexual anatomy and physiology.	Give reading assignments. Discuss with both their own responses.	Verbalize an increase in knowledge.
They will openly communicate with each other about sex.	Give homework assignment of listing all the sexual words they know. Have them decide on acceptable words.	Come in with list of words; starred items indicated acceptable words.
	Discuss how they can verbally seduce one another.	Agree on verbal signals to indicate sexual interest.
	Encourage them to talk about what they like while they are making love.	Report an increase in verbal sharing that was sexually stimulating for both.
Nursing Diagnosis: *Altered sexuality patterns related to disparity of needs*		
Both will state expectations about frequency of sexual activity.	Analyze the way unspoken expectations lead to disappointments and hurt feelings.	State they shared expectations prior to sexual interactions.
They will agree on average frequency for sex.	Discuss meaning of and methods to compromise.	Agree to do home play exercises 3 times a week.
	Discuss alternative behaviors such as masturbation.	John acknowledges he is comfortable with masturbation when Maria is not interested in sex.

▶

NURSING CARE PLAN (continued)

Client Care Goals	Nursing Planning/ Intervention	Evaluation
Nursing Diagnosis: *Ineffective individual coping related to masturbatory guilt*		
Maria will verbalize less guilt.	Discuss source of guilt.	Identifies family values/beliefs.
	Assign readings on the normalcy of masturbation throughout the life cycle.	
	Assign Maria and John the task of sharing with each other their feelings about masturbation.	
	Encourage them to decide if this is acceptable to try when they are together.	Maria states she enjoys masturbation now and is able to touch herself with John present.
Nursing Diagnosis: *Sexual dysfunction related to situational nonorgasmic response*		
Maria will report achieving orgasms when sexually active with John.	Encourage Maria to demonstrate to John how she achieves orgasms with masturbation.	Maria stimulates self while John watches.
	Encourage John to try these techniques with verbal and nonverbal direction from Maria.	John stimulates Maria; within 3 weeks she begins to achieve orgasm with manual and oral stimulation.
	Suggest they might wish to incorporate the use of a vibrator.	State they are considering buying a vibrator.

Having been sexualized at an inappropriately early age, some have learned to survive in a hostile environment by using their sexual availability to make contact with or control others.

Arousal Disorders   Sexual arousal refers to the physiologic responses and subjective sense of excitement experienced during sexual activity. Lack of lubrication and failure to attain or maintain an erection are the major disorders of the arousal phase. In **female sexual arousal disorder,** the lack of vaginal lubrication causes discomfort during sexual intercourse. The diagnosis of **male sexual arousal disorder** is usually made when the man has erection problems during 25 percent or more of sexual interactions. Some men cannot attain a full erection, and others lose their erections prior to orgasm. The pejorative term commonly applied to this condition, *impotence,* implies that the man is feeble, inadequate, and incompetent. The accurate term is *erectile inhibition,* which is

objectively descriptive and not judgmental. Arousal disorder may also be diagnosed even when lubrication and erection are adequate if individuals report a persistent or recurring lack of subjective sexual excitement or pleasure.

Both male and female arousal phases can be inhibited by physiologic factors interfering with the vasocongestion necessary for lubrication or erection to occur. Lack of vasocongestion may result from disruption of the genital blood supply, from interference with the innervation of the genitals, or, in women, from insufficient estrogen levels. Researchers estimate that 30 to 45 percent of erectile problems are predominantly organic, although the emotional reaction to the disorder must not be underestimated (Rosen and Beck 1988).

Psychologic factors may also be the primary cause of arousal disorders. They include all the previously mentioned factors, such as fear of failure, anxiety, anger, spectatoring, poor communication, and relationship conflict. Insufficient vaginal lubrication is less likely than erectile inhibition to create severe distress for couples, since using saliva or a water-based lubricant such as KY Jelly corrects the immediate problem. Erectile problems are often very threatening because the man often feels his whole sense of masculinity is at stake. Men tend to be dominated by a genital focus more than women are. Thus, any difficulty in getting the penis to "perform" results in feelings of humiliation and despair.

Orgasm Disorders

Inhibited Female Orgasm   The pejorative term commonly applied in the past to women not experiencing orgasm, *frigid*, implies that the woman is totally incapable of responding sexually. The more accurate and objective term is **inhibited female orgasm,** which simply means that the sexual response stops before orgasm occurs. *Preorgasmic* women have never experienced an orgasm; *secondarily nonorgasmic* women have had orgasms in the past but are not currently experiencing them; and *situationally nonorgasmic* women have orgasms in some situations but not in others. Studies indicate that 10 percent of women are preorgasmic, and another 20 percent report irregular orgasms (Rosen and Beck 1988). Compounding the orgasmic difficulty is the associated anxiety. In the preoccupation with orgasm, the real goal of being sexual—mutual pleasuring and intimacy—is lost, and the interchange becomes one of anxiety, frustration, and anger.

Physiologic factors related to inhibited female orgasms include fatigue, illness, neurologic or vascular damage, and drugs interfering with sexual response. In the physically well woman, lack of information or negative attitudes about female sexual response often contribute to orgasm disorder. Women who were taught that masturbation is sinful may not have explored their own bodies. If so, they cannot teach a partner where, how, and when to touch.

Rapid Ejaculation   Rapid ejaculation is one of the most common sexual dysfunctions among men. There are many definitions, with descriptions ranging from ejaculating before being touched, ejaculating before penetration, ejaculating with one internal thrust, to ejaculating within a minute or two of penetration. A more helpful description is the absence of voluntary control of ejaculation. The problem is best self-defined: a man is concerned about his ejaculatory control or the couple agrees ejaculation is too rapid for mutual satisfaction.

There is very little information about the mechanisms causing rapid ejaculation. Possible influences include the man's inability to perceive his arousal level accurately, a lowered sensory threshold due to infrequent sexual activity, early conditioning as a result of hurried masturbation or hurried sexual intercourse, or extreme anxiety during the sexual interaction, resulting in ejaculation triggered by sympathetic nervous system activity.

Inhibited Male Orgasm   The opposite problem is **inhibited male orgasm.** The man with this disorder can maintain an erection for long periods (e.g., an hour or more) but has extreme difficulty ejaculating. In heterosexual intercourse, the difficulty may be limited to ejaculation in the vagina. Some men ejaculate after self-stimulation or manual or oral stimulation by the partner, whereas others have great difficulty ejaculating with any type of stimulation. This disorder is much less common than rapid ejaculation.

Organic causes inhibiting orgasm include spinal cord injuries, multiple sclerosis, Parkinson's disease, and use of certain medications. Psychogenic factors include fear of pregnancy, performance pressure, fear of losing control, and anxiety and guilt about engaging in sexual activity. As with other dysfunctions, the difficulty can adversely affect the sexual relationship and both partner's ability to enjoy sexual interaction.

Sexual Pain Disorders

Vaginismus   Vaginismus is an involuntary spasm of the outer one-third of the vaginal muscles making penetration of the vagina painful and sometimes impossible. The woman often experiences desire, excitement, and orgasm with stimulation of the external sexual organs. Attempts at intercourse, however, elicit the involuntary spasm. She may have similar difficulty undergoing pelvic exams and inserting tampons or a diaphragm.

The partner often becomes fearful and anxious about hurting her or may become resentful and believe she is having the spasms on purpose. The partner may then develop secondary dysfunctions as a result of these negative feelings and interpretations of rejection.

Causes of vaginismus are thought to be psychophysiologic. The vaginismic response may develop initially as a protection against real or anticipated pain. It is often associated with sexual trauma, such as child sexual abuse or adult rape. Emotional conflict, such as extreme fear of pregnancy or intense guilt about engaging in sexual activity, may be additional contributing factors.

Dyspareunia   Both women and men can experience **dyspareunia,** or pain during or immediately after intercourse. It is associated with many physiologic causes, especially those inhibiting lubrication. Thus, skin irritations, vaginal infections, estrogen deficiencies, and use of medications that dry vaginal secretions can cause women to experience discomfort with intercourse. Pelvic disorders, such as infections, small lesions, endometriosis, scar tissue, or tumors, can result in painful intercourse. Engaging in painful intercourse can lead to vaginismus, because the body reflexively becomes guarded and tense. Similarly, in males, infection or inflammation of the glans penis or other genitourinary organs can cause pain with coitus. Also, some contraceptive foams, creams, or sponges can irritate either the vagina or penis, causing pain. For both women and men, fear and anxiety in anticipation of pain can undermine the person's ability to feel pleasurable sexual responses and may lead to an avoidance of sexual activity.

Problems with Satisfaction

Some people experience sexual desire, arousal, and orgasm and yet feel dissatisfied with their sexual relationships. These sexual problems are more related to the emotional tone of the relationship than the physiologic response. Since the giving and receiving of pleasure in a mutually intimate relationship are the primary goals of sex for most people, dissatisfaction problems may be more disturbing than other types of sexual dysfunctions.

At times, satisfaction problems may be *situational*. For example, one partner may choose an inconvenient time, or a partner may feel anxious and therefore cannot experience much pleasure or joy. Some people describe their problems as related to *lack of extragenital satisfaction*. These people describe how much they miss and continue to need all the touching and caressing of their earlier love-making experiences. Unfortunately, people who have been relating sexually for a long time often become genitally focused and neglect the rest of the body. One or both partners may feel touch starved, long for more extragenital loving, and become dissatisfied with sex.

Often satisfaction problems are related to *relationship difficulties*. The inability to communicate effectively in other areas of relationship frequently results in sexual frustration. Partners who are angry at one another and make love without resolving the conflict may feel unhappy about the relationship in spite of having experienced arousal and orgasm. Couples who define their relationships in terms of rigid, unequal power and gender roles may have difficulty negotiating and compromising about sexual issues. Not infrequently, the person with the least amount of power feels helpless and dissatisfied with the sexual interchanges.

Lack of intimacy or a feeling of connectedness is understandably related to satisfaction problems. If one has sex with a stranger, the body may function well but there is often a sense of something missing after the sexual experience. Making love to one person while feeling more attracted to or in love with another person can result in feelings of emptiness or disconnection. Even couples in a committed relationship may complain of lack of intimacy. Dissatisfaction issues include lack of romance, love, tenderness, and nurturance. Fulfillment of sexuality, then, depends on the ability to relate with a partner in an intimate and mutually pleasing manner that is compatible with values and chosen life-style (Ogden 1988, Tiefer 1988).

Sexual Dysfunctions: Gays and Lesbians

Gay men and lesbians may have the same sexual dysfunctions seen in the heterosexual population. However, living in a culture that has fairly strict gender role expectations and is highly homophobic, gays and lesbians experience additional pressures, which may contribute to sexual dysfunctions.

Men, whether gay or straight, may accept stereotypic male gender roles that can lead to ambivalence about intimacy and dependency. Since society teaches that men should be unemotional, competitive, and in control, two men in an intimate relationship are likely to experience conflict if both try to be "macho men." The success of the relationship often depends on the partners' ability to negotiate and compromise on issues of power, control, dependency, tenderness, and nurturance. Some gay men find it difficult to develop a positive sexual self-concept in a culture that does not positively model or reinforce a homosexual identity. Gays who internalize society's negative attitudes about homosexuality have low self-esteem and may have sexual problems as a result. It is not uncommon for gay men to interpret sexual problems in relationships as a sign that the relationship is over as opposed to seeing the dysfunction as a problem to be solved (Coleman and Reece 1988).

Not surprisingly, the reality of HIV infection and AIDS has increased the incidence of sexual dysfunctions in the gay community. Anxiety about past exposure and/or fear of future exposure to HIV is not conducive to pleasurable and joyful sexual relations. Adapting sexual behavior to safer sex practices may be a source of temporary dysfunction for some gay men. Not to be overlooked is the role of grief for gay men. A normal aspect of grief for all humans is a period of decreased sexual desire. With lovers and friends dying from AIDs, gay men begin to see the grief process as never ending and some men wonder if they will ever again be able to experience sexual desire. (See Chapter 25 on HIV/AIDS.)

The most common sexual problem for lesbians in a committed relationship is one of low desire or low frequency of sexual activity. It is highly unusual for lesbian couples to have difficulty with arousal, orgasm, or satisfaction. The pattern of low desire is typically secondary, that is, it develops at a later point in an ongoing relationship. When sexual activity does occur, both partners feel a general sense of satisfaction.

There are several differences between lesbian couples and heterosexual couples experiencing low sexual desire. Unlike heterosexual couples, lesbian couples do not typically withdraw from sex because of a lack of intimacy, a power imbalance, or rigid gender roles in the relationship. A lesbian couple is more likely to report that the nonsexual areas of their relationship are pleasing and agreeable and that there is minimal conflict or arguments about sex. This decreasing sex drive may be related to the socialization of women as passive recipients rather than assertive initiators. Both lesbian and heterosexual women have been taught many sex-negative attitudes, experience more conflict about sex than men do, and may fail to develop their full potential as sexual beings. When two women in an intimate relationship each wait for the other to initiate sex, the result may be low frequency of activity. Thus, many lesbian couples must often make a conscious effort to make love regularly (Coleman and Reece, 1988, Loulan 1988, Nichols 1988).

The Nursing Process and Clients with Gender and Sexual Disorders

Assessing

The psychiatric nurse finds numerous opportunities to apply the nursing process to promote sexual health. Assessment of sexual status is part of a thorough and comprehensive assessment of a client's general health.

Subjective Data   The sexual history provides subjective assessment data needed for formulating nursing diagnoses. Nurses elicit sexual information much as they elicit a general nursing history. However, pay special attention to planning a setting where privacy and uninterrupted time are available. Such a setting helps clients feel comfortable discussing these private aspects of their lives. It is helpful to begin the interview by explaining why you are asking about sexuality, for example: "Sexuality is a part of people's lives. People often have questions about sexual activity when they have changes in their health. I'd like to take this time to talk with you about your sex life."

Move from general to specific questions. This gradual focus on specific sexual behavior promotes trust and rapport. Initially, questions can relate sexuality to health status. Open-ended questions encourage clients to expand on their sexual experiences and concerns. Reassure clients that it is normal to have sexual concerns and questions, for instance: "It is common for many people to feel concerned about. . . . Do you have any questions?" Restate clients' responses to encourage them to expand on feelings. The accompanying Assessment box lists an inventory of questions that the psychiatric nurse can ask as a part of a general nursing history. Questions to ask if the client does identify a sexual problem, or

ASSESSMENT

Sexual History: The ABCs

Affective Assessment

To whom do you feel most intimate and connected?

Describe the type of love and affection in this relationship.

In what way do you experience anxiety about sex?

In what way do you experience guilt about sex?

How depressed are you feeling?

In what way does anger interfere with your sexual functioning?

Do you dislike or feel an aversion to any parts of your body?

Behavioral Assessment

Describe your level of satisfaction with the frequency of your sexual activity.

Describe the positive aspects of your own sexual functioning.

Describe the negative aspects of your own sexual functioning.

What concerns do you have about your future sexual functioning?

What are your partner's concerns about current or future sexual functioning?

Cognitive Assessment

When you were growing up, how did you learn about sex?

How has your religion influenced your sexual values and behaviors?

What "shoulds/should nots," "musts/must nots" do you believe about your sexual behavior/relationships?

How rigidly were gender roles enforced in your family of origin?

How are gender roles enacted in your present relationship/family?

Describe the negative thoughts you have about sex.

Does the use of fantasy increase or decrease your sexual desire?

Sensation Assessment

Describe any physical discomfort you feel during sexual activity.

To what degree do you experience pleasure during sexual activity?

clients often take medications that can affect sexual desire or sexual behavior (see the Assessment box below).

Objective Data   Objective data include the nonverbal behaviors observed by the nurse, laboratory data, test results, medical diagnoses, physical examination results, and other documented sources, such as the chart.

Objective data may also include results of physiologic assessment of sexual function. The nocturnal penile tumescence (NPT) procedure provides a direct measure of erectile capacity. The device measures penile engorgement that occurs during sleep. NPT measurement is considered the best available method to determine if a man's erectile difficulties are physiologic. If so, there is minimal penile engorgement during sleep. Men whose erection difficulties appear to be psychologic in origin have normal engorgement during sleep. Although the NPT procedure is an important source of objective data, its results are not always reliable. Research findings report 28 to 42 percent error in accuracy (Field 1990).

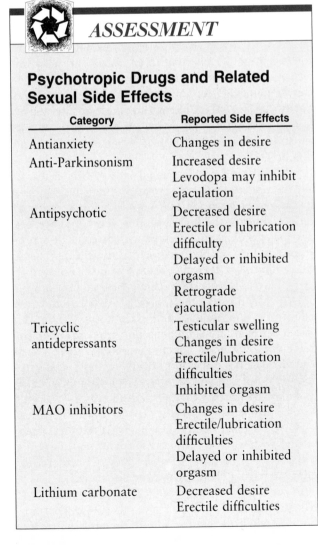

ASSESSMENT

Psychotropic Drugs and Related Sexual Side Effects

Category	Reported Side Effects
Antianxiety	Changes in desire
Anti-Parkinsonism	Increased desire
	Levodopa may inhibit ejaculation
Antipsychotic	Decreased desire
	Erectile or lubrication difficulty
	Delayed or inhibited orgasm
	Retrograde ejaculation
	Testicular swelling
Tricyclic antidepressants	Changes in desire
	Erectile/lubrication difficulties
	Inhibited orgasm
MAO inhibitors	Changes in desire
	Erectile/lubrication difficulties
	Delayed or inhibited orgasm
Lithium carbonate	Decreased desire
	Erectile difficulties

Physiologic assessment of female sexual function is accomplished by use of vaginal plethysmographs or probes. These devices are inserted into the vagina and measure vasocongestion of the vaginal wall tissue.

Several sophisticated and expensive laboratory tests are designed to assess sexual function. For instance, testosterone and estrogen blood levels may be measured. However, laboratory data must be interpreted with caution since test results are not always reliable indicators of clients' actual sexual behavior. Thus clients' self-reports of sexual performance, feelings, and values (the subjective data) are of prime importance in assessment. The nurse evaluates and interprets the data to formulate actual and potential nursing diagnoses.

Diagnosing

The following sections discuss the most likely nursing diagnoses and their implications for clients and nurses.

Anxiety and Fear   Anxiety and fear inhibit the physiologic sexual response as well as the ability to experience pleasure and joy. People who grow up with the teaching that sex is dirty and sinful often experience anxiety in an adult sexual relationship or are so fearful that they develop a phobic avoidance of sex. Adults who have been emotionally, physically, or sexually abused as children often fear intimacy and find they cannot have a trusting relationship with another person. Even individuals with a positive sex history may at some time feel anxious about their sexual performance and develop a secondary fear of failure as a sexual partner.

Spiritual Distress   Lack of fulfillment in a sexual relationship may be related to a temporary feeling of distance from one's partner or an ongoing lack of intimacy in the relationship. Factors relating to lack of intimacy are relationship conflict, multiple fears, adult sexual abuse, or childhood sexual abuse.

Ineffective Family Coping: Compromised   It is difficult to experience sexual fulfillment when the relationship is in trouble in nonsexual spheres. The difficulty may be as straightforward as poor communication or as complex as conflict, anger, and unequal power. When one of the partners is a transvestite, the other partner must come to terms with the behavior if a healthy relationship is to be maintained. To be part of a family with a transsexual means finding ways to reintegrate the person as a member of the other sex, or reject the transsexual and distance the family from this particular member.

Personal Identity Disturbance   In cultures with rigid gender roles, transsexuals and transvestites suffer a great deal of pain as they struggle with their gender identity. Transsexuals completely reject their anatomic sex, and transvestites alternate between their male and their female personas.

Altered Role Performance Sexual addicts often cannot maintain work, family, and social roles. The addiction is so time-consuming that the addict cannot devote time or energy to work or relationships.

Altered Sexuality Patterns Some people cannot achieve sexual arousal and orgasm without the stimulation of an unusual object or situation. These individuals are considered to have one of the paraphilias, which may be coercive or noncoercive. Most often they are preoccupied with and feel compelled to engage in their particular sexual behaviors.

High Risk for Violence: Self-Directed or Directed at Others Autoerotic asphyxia is a noncoercive but often fatal paraphilia. These paraphiliacs are not suicidal and have no intention of harming themselves but often accidentally kill themselves during sexual activity. Coercive paraphilias are considered violence against others because the victim is nonconsenting and offended or hurt by the paraphiliac's sexual behavior.

Pain A nursing diagnosis of pain applies to women who experience vaginismus. The origin may be past sexual trauma or current emotional conflict. The pain of dyspareunia may occur in both women and men and is typically related to organic factors.

Knowledge Deficit People who grow up with no or very limited sex education may have difficulties in their adult sexual functioning. For people who don't know what to expect or how to touch themselves or their partners, sexual interactions can be frustrating rather than pleasurable. Lack of knowledge can contribute to ineffective sexual techniques and sexual dysfunctions.

Sexual Dysfunction Many of the above nursing diagnoses may be contributing factors to the development of sexual dysfunctions. In addition, illness, injury, surgery, medications, or substance abuse may contribute to sexual dysfunction. Problems with satisfaction may be described under either of these diagnoses: Sexual dysfunction or Spiritual distress.

Planning and Implementing Interventions

Nurses play several roles in promoting sexual health. The Mims-Swensen Sexual Health Model (1980) identifies four levels at which nurses can intervene, consistent with their comfort and knowledge.

The *life experience level* of intervention describes a minimal level of effective practice. Interventions are based solely on nurses' own personal experiences. Interventions may be appropriate for clients who share similar life experiences. However, clients holding different values or demonstrating different behaviors may perceive interventions based on the nurses' life experiences as irrelevant.

The *basic level* of intervention to promote sexual health is grounded in nurses' self-awareness combined with a nonjudgmental respect for others' sexual beliefs, practices, and concerns. Nurses at this level have some knowledge about human sexual function. The knowledgeable and nonjudgmental nurse can intervene as a facilitator for clients needing to talk about their sexuality.

The nurse practicing an *intermediate level* of intervention synthesizes knowledge, self-awareness, communication skills, and the use of the nursing process. Nurses are validators of normal sexual behavior and accept the range of sexual expression in our society. Teaching about sexual response is another intervention to resolve client concerns. Teaching is often directed at helping clients understand their stage of sexual development. For instance, teenagers and young adults frequently require accurate information regarding anatomy and physiology, sexual desire, and contraception. Counseling interventions are also implemented in the intermediate level. Counseling is not merely giving advice. The nurse counselor helps clients clarify their sexual problems and decide on alternatives to resolve the problems. Some specific sexual counseling strategies are listed in the accompanying Intervention box.

The Mims-Swensen Sexual Health Model identifies the *advanced level* as requiring that nurses have specialized preparation and knowledge of sexual and gender disorders. Nurses at this level practice sex therapy, develop and present formal education programs, and do sex research. Most nurses refer clients who require sex therapy. Nurses who do function in the sex therapist role should meet the qualifications for practice identified by the American Association of Sex Educators, Counselors, and Therapists (AASECT), which differentiate sex counseling from sex therapy. *Sex counseling* helps clients incorporate their sexual knowledge into satisfying life-styles and socially responsible behavior. *Sex therapy* is a highly specialized, in-depth treatment to help clients resolve serious sexual problems, especially some sexual disorders (AASECT 1979). AASECT publishes a national directory of professionals certified to provide sex education, counseling, or therapy. This directory is a resource for nurses referring clients who need sex therapy.

Reducing Anxiety and Fear Accurate identification of feelings is the first step in the problem-solving

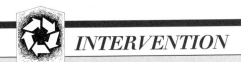

INTERVENTION

Guidelines for Working with the Client with Sexual Difficulties

Male Erectile Disorder
Reestablish a climate of comfort and acceptance for sexual interaction.

Encourage client to masturbate and enjoy touch and body stimulation in general.

Rapid Ejaculation
The man or woman is instructed to stimulate the erect penis until the premonitory sensations of impending orgasm are felt. Then penile stimulation is abruptly stopped. This process is repeated to lower the threshold of excitability and make the client more tolerant of the stimuli. Sometimes the woman uses the squeeze technique: At the point of orgasm, she squeezes the head of the penis with thumb and first two fingers for 3 to 4 seconds. This stops the urge to ejaculate.

The couple is also instructed in ways to reduce friction in the vagina by limiting the frequency of thrusts or the movement within the vagina.

Inhibited Female Orgasm
Intercourse is avoided. Nongenital caressing exercises begin, with man and woman alternating as the initiator of a session of caressing, thus sharing responsibility for sexual interaction.

Next, genital stimulation is added to provide positive sexual experiences without intercourse. When intercourse is attempted, the woman is instructed to assume the superior position and insert the man's penis into her vagina. When setbacks occur, the couple is advised to rely on sexual techniques that do not involve intercourse. The woman is to place her hand lightly on her partner's to indicate her preference for contact. The emphasis is not on achieving orgasm but on learning erotic preferences.

The couple is instructed to use the side-by-side position, which enables both partners to move freely with emphasis on slow, exploratory thrusting. The goal is to develop an ability to enjoy pelvic play with the penis inside the vagina.

Vaginismus
The initial step is physical demonstration of her involuntary vaginal spasm to the woman by inserting an examining finger into her vagina. Then Hegar dilators in graduated sizes are inserted by the man into the woman's vagina. At first she manually controls his insertion of the smallest dilator. Later he can insert larger dilators following her verbal instructions. After larger dilators are successfully inserted, she is instructed to retain the dilator for several hours each night. Most involuntary spasms can be relieved in three to five days with the daily use of dilators.

In addition to physical relief from spastic constriction, therapy is directed toward alleviating the fear that led to the onset of symptoms.

Sexual Acting Out
After identifying increased levels of anxiety, openly discuss the meanings of behaviors. Give feedback about inappropriate behavior, and discuss appropriate ways to meet sexual needs. Reassure clients you are not rejecting them, but the behavior.

---

process, and clients may need help in labeling the feelings they are experiencing. Following this step, help clients identify one anxiety-producing situation within their sexual interactions. At this stage, it is productive to focus diffuse anxiety on a manageable single situation or event. The nurse and client analyze the situation or event to discover negative anticipatory thoughts that may be the source of the anxiety. Together, review how the client has handled anxiety in the past and evaluate the range and effectiveness of this past coping behavior. It may be appropriate to help the client redefine the sensations of anxiety as sensations of sexual excitement, which is more likely to result in positive expectations. Together, explore alternative coping behaviors, and have clients evaluate their effectiveness after implementing them.

Many adult survivors of childhood sexual abuse are periodically overwhelmed by anxiety, fear, and panic. (See Chapter 14 for management of panic states.) Refer adult survivors to support groups as well as individual therapy with a therapist who specializes in this field.

Decreasing Spiritual Distress   Because the origin of spiritual distress is the lack of intimacy or connection within a sexual relationship, the goal of nursing intervention is to help clients achieve and maintain a level of intimacy each partner finds comfortable. In the context of therapy, couples discuss their individual needs for closeness and identify barriers to intimacy. They are instructed to make three or four thirty-minute "dates" each week, during which they share warmth and intimacy. They spend some of the time discussing specific sexual issues; during other "dates," the couple explore intimate, nonsexual topics, such as hopes and expectations for the future. Couples should give these dates top priority, because a common way of avoiding intimacy is by not setting time aside for each other.

Promoting More Effective Family Coping
Good communication is an important part of a sexually fulfilling relationship. Apart from setting specific times to share feelings and beliefs, some couples need training in more effective communication skills. If they give ambiguous signals to indicate sexual interest, they need to learn how to state their interest clearly. Some people expect their partners to "read their minds" about sexual needs and desires; if so, they need encouragement to assert their needs tactfully. Teach couples to avoid "you" language, which evokes a defensive response and results in arguments, and to use "I" language, which expresses personal thoughts, feelings, and needs. The following are some examples of accusatory "you" statements and accountable "I" statements:

"You" language

"You only have sex on your mind. You're a pervert."

"You keep grabbing at me like I'm always ready to go to bed with you."

"You never pay attention to what turns me on. Are you dumb or hard of hearing?"

"I" language

"I'm concerned because we seem to have different expectations of how often we would like to make love."

"I miss all the hugging and caressing we used to do even when we couldn't make love afterward."

"I feel frustrated and hurt when it seems like I'm repeating myself. Maybe I'm not communicating my needs very clearly."

If the relationship is in significant trouble, refer the couple for relationship or sex therapy.

If cross-dressing is a newly divulged secret, offer education and support. If the relationship is to continue, both partners need to agree on where and how cross-dressing will take place. Some couples compromise; for instance, a husband may agree never to cross-dress in front of his wife, and she may agree to give him privacy. Some agree to limit cross-dressing to the home; others are comfortable going out in public with the partner cross-dressed. Some transvestites join a transvestite club where they can express their female personality in a safe social situation. The long-term success of the relationship depends on the couple's ability to negotiate these issues.

Promoting Comfort with Personal Identity
Many adult transsexuals seek hormonal therapy or sex-change surgery to make their bodies congruent with their gender identity. Surgical intervention has been a source of controversy and at this time appears to be decreasing in frequency. This trend may be associated with the cost and practical difficulties of the complex procedures involved, or it may reflect a cultural denial of the reality of the problem. The success rate of hormonal or surgical reassignment appears to be correlated with the degree of gender dysphoria prior to treatment as well as the overall emotional stability of the individual.

Refer transsexuals to therapists who specialize in this area or to gender dysphoria clinics. Because gender identity is stable and nonchangeable, the goal of treatment with transsexuals is to help them live and function in society in the cross-gender role. They need a great deal of support and assistance as they establish themselves in their new role. If the present job is not gender-role stereotyped, they may be able to remain in the same or similar position. Others may need retraining programs to find acceptable employment. A multidisciplinary approach is most effective in helping transsexuals adjust to their situation. Family and friends need support and counseling to reintegrate this person into their lives as a person of the other sex (Satterfield 1988).

Promoting Effective Role Performance Like other addicts, sexual addicts often do not seek help until they literally cannot manage their lives. A sexual addict may lose job, home, and relationships before admitting the consequences of the addiction. When that occurs, sexual addicts may become severely depressed and even suicidal. Refer sexual addicts to self-help groups and specialized professional therapy. Recovery is a long-term process facilitated by individual, group, couple, family, and family-of-origin therapy. The cornerstone of recovery is a twelve-step program modeled on the Alcoholics Anonymous program. Partners and codependents are also referred to appropriate self-help groups. A variety of groups, such as Sexaholics Anonymous, Sex Addicts Anonymous, Sex and Love Addicts Anonymous, S-Anon, and Co-Dependents of Sexual Addicts, have been formed throughout the country.

Promoting Noncoercive Sexuality Patterns
Once paraphilias are a programmed part of arousal, they are very difficult to deprogram. The response to

certain sexual or erotic stimuli tends to persist through life. A noncoercive, nonharmful paraphilia practiced with an adult consenting partner requires no nursing intervention other than client and partner education and possible couple negotiation about the behavior.

Decreasing Violence against the Self and Others   The most important nursing intervention regarding autoerotic asphyxia is community education. Warnings about autoerotic asphyxia should be routinely included in adolescent sex-education programs. Teenagers who practice it must be encouraged to seek immediate professional help. Parents should be taught to look for physical signs of trauma to the neck, such as bruising, abrasions, pressure marks, or rope burns. Ropes, knotted sheets, knotted T-shirts, or the like hidden in the bedroom may be warning signs.

Individuals who practice coercive paraphilias typically end up in the court system. The court may or may not mandate therapy. Therapy for sex offenders is a specialized area that should not be undertaken lightly. Behavior-modification techniques, group therapy, and hypnosis are used but are often not successful. In severe cases, male sex offenders are treated with the antiandrogen drug medroxyprogesterone acetate (Provera or Depo-Provera), which induces a reversible chemical castration. The drug reduces the male sex drive, erections, and ejaculation and decreases the obsessional focus on sex.

Decreasing Pain   Whenever pain is associated with intercourse a thorough physical examination is necessary to find and treat the organic cause of the pain. During vaginal exams, careful attention must be paid to tiny tears in the vaginal wall, which are often overlooked. Even very small tears can cause great pain during intercourse. Vaginismus is treated with education, dilators, and supportive psychotherapy. See the Intervention box on page 365.

Increasing Knowledge   Lack of sex information and education is not unusual among people with sexual dysfunctions. Nurses can intervene by teaching clients sexual anatomy and the sexual response cycle. Encourage couples to talk with one another about their individual responses. Some people may be very uncomfortable with sexual language and need help in learning sexual vocabulary and identifying which words are acceptable for intimate use. Part of the learning and desensitization process is having them repeat the words aloud to one another until they feel comfortable using them.

Managing Sexual Dysfunctions: Sex Therapy
There are many approaches to the treatment of sexual dysfunctions. Masters and Johnson (1970) originated the use of a two-person team (a female and male

cotherapy model) to treat couples on a short-term basis. The focus of treatment is the couple's relationship, with emphasis on their communication. The therapists discuss fears of performance and anxiety about sexual response with the couple and assign behavioral exercises to overcome these concerns. Education about the physiology of sexual response and the natural processes of sexual function is also emphasized.

Since the introduction of the two-person team, many other modes of sex therapy have developed, including individual, couple, and group treatment with one or two sex therapists. The duration of treatment programs also varies. Treatment programs may be for heterosexual or homosexual individuals or couples. The effectiveness of these programs depends on the client's needs and the therapists' skill.

Sex therapy programs have these components in common:

- *Information and education about sexual functions.* The therapist gives clients specific information about their particular needs. The therapist may assign books to read or discuss the information.

- *Experiential/sensory awareness.* The therapist helps clients recognize feelings of anxiety, anger, and pleasure by tuning into bodily cues. Clients focus on and describe feelings both in therapy sessions and at home. If they believe their genitals are ugly and unclean, the therapist assigns desensitization exercises at home to explore and become familiar with their own bodies. Some clients need fantasy training if nonsexual thoughts interfere with sexual arousal.

- *Insight.* The therapist attempts to learn and understand what is causing and perpetuating the sexual problem. The goal is for clients to assume responsibility for their own behavior and recognize that change is possible.

- *Cognitive restructuring.* Clients identify and re-evaluate their fears about sexual interaction. The therapist encourages them to identify and eliminate negative self-statements and irrational expectations.

- *Behavioral interventions.* Focus is on changing nonsexual behavior that contributes to sexual problems. The therapist may assign assertiveness training, communication training, stress-reduction exercises, and problem-solving techniques. Behavioral interventions include assigned pleasuring sessions to discover what is arousing and pleasing to the self and partner. See the Intervention box on page 365.

Evaluating/Outcome Criteria

Anxiety and Fear   Clients will be able to use the problem-solving process as one tool in decreasing anxiety and fear. They will implement effective coping measures and verbalize a decrease in anxiety. Adult survivors of childhood sexual abuse will participate in support groups and engage in psychotherapy to manage the fears and trauma of the past.

Spiritual Distress   Couples will report an acceptable and meaningful level of intimacy in their relationships. They will continue to set aside time for one another and engage in meaningful intimate time.

Family Coping   Couples will increase the use of "I" language and decrease the use of blaming "you" language. They will express their sexual desires, needs, and preferences directly. If the relationship is in significant trouble, they will report a willingness to seek therapy. If one partner is a transvestite, the couple will negotiate the cross-dressing behavior, and both individuals will report satisfaction with their relationship.

Gender Identity   Clients will report increasing comfort and satisfaction in their new gender role, which will be congruent with gender identity. They will be able to function socially and economically as a person of that gender. Family and friends will be supportive and accepting of these clients.

Role Performance   Clients will participate actively in self-help groups as well as professional therapy. They will be able to manage their addiction in such a way that they can maintain intimate relationships and be financially responsible. Family members will participate actively in the appropriate self-help groups.

Noncoercive Sexuality Patterns   Clients and partners will verbalize an understanding that noncoercive paraphilias are lifelong patterns. Couples will be able to negotiate the behavior in a way that is satisfying to both individuals.

Violence   Community and family education programs will be established about the danger of autoerotic asphyxia. Victims of this disorder will be identified and referred for immediate treatment. Clients with this disorder will remain safe. Coercive paraphiliacs will curb their behavior, or society will set strict limits to protect potential victims.

Pain   Individuals will report less pain or no pain during intercourse. Clients suffering from vaginismus will report success in using conscious control to relax vaginal muscles, allowing for pain-free intercourse.

Knowledge   Clients will describe sexual anatomy and the phases of the sexual response cycle. Couples will report an increase in communication about individual responses and preferences using a selected sexual vocabulary.

Sexual Dysfunctions   Clients will report a satisfying and fulfilling sex life. They will experience minimal difficulty with desire, arousal, or orgasm. They will be able to identify and label feelings and acknowledge responsibility for their own behavior. They will implement a chosen variety of sexual techniques.

CHAPTER HIGHLIGHTS

• Nurses must be able to accept and respect the client's sexual beliefs, attitudes, and behaviors as equal in value to, although possibly different from, their own personal beliefs, attitudes, and behaviors.

• Gender disorders have multiple causes. Biologic, environmental, cultural, and learning influences determine the severity and intensity of the disorders.

• Noncoercive paraphilias typically are not harmful, are practiced between consenting adults, and do not require nursing intervention.

• Adolescents must be educated about the dangers of autoerotic asphyxia.

• Coercive paraphilias are described in the legal code and are considered criminal acts.

• Sexual addiction is a progressive condition in which sex is used to numb pain.

• Sexual dysfunctions have psychophysiologic causes. Classification is according to the phase of the sexual response primarily affected as well as difficulties with satisfaction.

• Nurses are appropriate promoters of sexual health by virtue of self-awareness, communication skills, theoretic knowledge, use of the nursing process, and the unique characteristics of the nurse-client relationship.

• Nurses are responsible and accountable for the delivery of care that promotes sexual health, including accurate assessment, diagnosis, education, counseling, and referral.

• Nurses should take a sexual history to assess general sexual health and, if indicated, gather detailed information about specific sexual problems.

• To gauge the effectiveness of nursing interventions for sexual problems, the nurse can evaluate how well the client has understood education and what changes the client reports or the nurse observes.

• Nurses may function in the specialized and expanded roles of sex therapist, researcher, and formal educator after advanced preparation that includes in-depth education and supervised experiences.

REFERENCES

American Association of Sex Educators, Counselors, and Therapists. 435 N Michigan Ave., Suite 1717, Chicago, IL 60611-4067. (312) 644-0828.

American Psychiatric Association: *Diagnostic and Statistical Manual of Mental Disorder,* ed 3, revised. APA, 1987.

Briere J: *Therapy for Adults Molested as Children.* Springer, 1989.

Carnes R: *Contrary to Love: Helping the Sexual Addict.* CompCare Publishers, 1989.

Coleman E, Reece R: Treating low sexual desire among gay men, in Leiblum S, Rosen R (eds): *Sexual Desire Disorders.* Guilford Press, 1988, pp 413–445.

Dalley DM: Understanding and helping the sexually unusual, Dalley DM (ed): *The Sexually Unusual: Guide to Understanding and Helping.* Haworth Press, 1988, pp 3–13.

Dwyer M: Exhibitionism/voyeurism, in Dalley DM (ed): *The Sexually Unusual: Guide to Understanding and Helping.* Haworth Press, 1988, pp 101–112.

Earle R, Crow G: *Lonely All the Time: Recognizing, Understanding and Overcoming Sex Addiction.* Pocket Books, 1989.

Field ML: Psychosomatic sexual dysfunction, in Fogel CI, Lauver D (eds): *Sexual Health Promotion.* Saunders, 1990, pp 553–568.

Fogel CI, Lauver D: *Sexual Health Promotion.* Saunders, 1990.

Gordon S, Snyder CW: *Personal Issues in Human Sexuality.* Allyn and Bacon,1989.

Loulan J: Research on the sex practices of 1566 lesbians and the clinical applications, in Cole E, Rothblum ED (eds): *Women and Sex Therapy.* Haworth Press, 1988, pp 221–234.

Masters W, Johnson V: *Human Sexual Inadequacy.* Little, Brown, 1970.

Matek O: Obscene phone callers, in Dalley DM (ed): *The Sexually Unusual: Guide to Understanding and Helping.* Haworth Press, 1988, pp 113–130.

Mims FH, Swensen M: *Sexuality: A Nursing Perspective.* McGraw-Hill. 1980.

Monat KK: *Sexuality and the Mentally Retarded.* College Hill Press, 1982.

Money J: *Venuses Penuses.* Prometheus Books, 1986.

Moser C: Sadomasochism, in Dalley DM (ed): *The Sexually Unusual: Guide to Understanding and Helping.* Haworth Press, 1988, pp 43–56.

Nichols M: Low sexual desire in lesbian couples, in Leiblum S, Rosen R (eds): *Sexual Desire Disorders.* Guilford Press, 1988, pp 387–411.

Ogden G: Women and sexual ecstasy: How can therapists help?, in Cole E, Rothblum ED (eds): *Women and Sex Therapy.* Haworth Press, 1988, pp 43–56.

Peo RE: Transvestism, in Dalley DM (ed): *The Sexually Unusual: Guide to Understanding and Helping.* Haworth Press, 1988, pp 57–75.

Rosen RC, Beck JG: *Patterns of Sexual Arousal.* Guilford Press, 1988.

Sargent TO: Fetishism, in Dalley DM (ed): *The Sexually Unusual: Guide to Understanding and Helping.* Haworth Press, 1988, pp 27–42.

Satterfield SB: Transsexualism, in Dalley DM (ed): *The Sexually Unusual: Guide to Understanding and Helping.* Haworth Press, 1988, pp 77–87.

Tiefer L: A feminist critique of the sexual dysfunction nomenclature, in Cole E, Rothblum ED (eds): *Women and Sex Therapy.* Haworth Press, 1988, pp 5–21.

World Health Organization: Education and treatment in human sexuality. *The Training of Health Professionals.* World Health Organization Technical Report Series, no. 572. WHO. 1975.

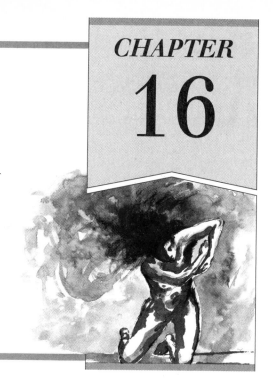

CHAPTER

16

Applying the Nursing Process for Clients with Personality Disorders

LEARNING OBJECTIVES

- Differentiate personality traits and styles from personality disorders

- Compare and contrast characteristics of various personality disorders

- Correlate DSM-III-R with the nursing process in providing care for clients with personality disorders

- Apply the nursing process in a variety of clinical settings with clients identified as having personality disorders

- Distinguish developmental characteristics of the major personality disorders

- Relate theoretical concepts, which are supported by research, to the nursing assessment, diagnoses, planning, implementation, and evaluation of clients who have personality disorders

- Apply the nursing process in caring for clients who manifest angry and/or manipulative behavior

- Discuss positive and negative effects of the nurse's emotional responses to clients who have personality disorders

Judy Banks Campbell
Noreen King Poole

CROSS REFERENCES

Other topics relevant to this content are: Chronicity, Chapter 17; Communication techniques, Chapter 8; Nursing process, Chapter 3; Psychiatric theories, Chapter 4.

Many people demonstrate persistent behavioral patterns that do not significantly interfere with their lives but may charm, annoy, or frustrate others. Such behavioral patterns may be called **personality traits** or styles, and they often define the uniqueness of the individual.

Frank consistently compliments his female coworkers. They, in turn, prepare his lunches, lend him money, and make excuses for his sloppy work performance.

Alice interrupts a supervisory meeting to borrow a stapler. She is surprised when her behavior is criticized.

Whenever Keith is asked a personal question, he responds, "Why do you want to know?"

Jill contributes to daily team conferences only when her input is solicited. She prefaces her comments with, "You probably won't think this is important, but. . . ."

Lance offers detailed descriptions of his personal life to anyone who will listen. Quickly bored with his monologues, his listeners do not return for "seconds."

These lifelong patterns are exhibited in a variety of social and personal experiences, and generally anxiety is absent (Eaton et al. 1976). These relatively stable patterns, however, may become rigid and maladaptive, causing significant personal distress, and impair social functioning. When this happens, these personality traits or styles are called **personality disorders.** Since people with personality disorders experience problems in living rather than clinical symptoms, they may not seek professional help unless there is extreme external stress (DSM-III-R 1987).

The psychiatric nurse encounters people with personality disorders in a variety of settings, including the workplace, counseling centers, general hospitals, and forensic facilities. As Widiger and Frances (1985) point out, the essential features of personality disorders are (a) chronicity, (b) pervasiveness, and (c) maladaptation. All three features must be present to make a psychiatric diagnosis. However, the psychiatric nurse must be aware that personality disorders are extreme exaggerations of personality traits or styles. (A *trait* is a peculiar or unusual mannerism, whereas a *style* is a characteristic way of coping with the environment.) Although the DSM-III-R delineates diagnostic criteria for personality disorders in the Axis II category, human beings rarely manifest clusters of behaviors that have distinct boundaries. Furthermore, persons with personality disorders may or may not view their life-styles as abnormal or intrusive.

If we assume a common developmental course for the emergence of a person's personality, different levels of adjustment may occur. Consequently, one individual may view peculiarities as "natural" or "eccentric" (**ego syntonic**) and seek no change, while a second person may feel tension and conflict as the behaviors become increasingly rigid and lead to difficulties in a variety of social activities (**ego dystonic**). The person may begin to view a characteristic once valued as unique as a weakness. This changed perspective leads to dissatisfaction and disequilibrium, which motivate the person to seek therapy. Our society contributes to such lack of insight by discouraging direct confrontation and feedback about self-defeating behaviors, thus delaying intervention.

Personality disorders may coexist with extreme psychopathology, considered under DSM-III-R Axis I groupings. In addition, under stress, the individual with a personality disorder may progressively deteriorate even to the point of psychosis.

Common Features of Personality Disorders

Three major clusters of personality disorders guide psychiatric nurses in diagnostic, treatment, and research issues (see the accompanying box). These clusters are (a) eccentric, (b) dramatic-erratic, and (c) anxious-fearful. The **eccentric** category includes paranoid, schizoid, and schizotypal personality disorders. The histrionic, narcissistic, antisocial, and borderline personality disorders are included in the **dramatic-erratic group.** The final cluster groups avoidant, dependent, compulsive, and passive-aggressive personality disorders in the category **anxious-fearful.** These clusters establish criteria for distinct disorders accord-

Clusters of Personality Disorders (DSM-III-R)

Eccentric	Dramatic-Erratic	Anxious-Fearful
Paranoid	Borderline	Avoidant
Schizoid	Histrionic	Dependent
Schizotypal	Narcissistic	Obsessive compulsive
	Antisocial	Passive-Aggressive

SOURCE: *Adapted from American Psychiatric Association:* Diagnostic and Statistical Manual of Mental Disorders, *ed 3, revised. APA, 1987, p 337.*

ing to the presence or absence of symptoms that do not characterize major thought, perceptual, or mood disorders. Because individuals often have personality characteristics that overlap DSM-III-R Axis II categories, mental health professionals are encouraged to use multiple Axis II diagnoses when necessary. As the psychiatric nurse becomes familiar with the psychodynamics and behaviors of people with personality disorders, the following common features emerge:

• Restricted or exaggerated development of a particular pattern or trait

• Restricted or exaggerated moral development

• Restricted or exaggerated problem-solving skills

• Seriously impaired ability to develop meaningful interpersonal relationships and communications

• Difficulty in adjusting to social or occupational relationships

• Defensive coping strategies against real or perceived threats to the sense of self

• Lifelong pattern of responding that is consistent in most situations and that becomes accentuated under stress

• Self-stabilizing and self-perpetuating level of functioning despite distorted coping strategies

• Exaggerated or restricted affective responses to the environment, e.g., overly sensitive, unemotional, "cold"

• Conflict with others, either in the immediate family or in society

• Lack of awareness that others view the life-style as different or unusual

Historical and Theoretic Foundations

Our styles of perceiving, thinking, and responding shape our ability to adapt and defend our sense of self (Shapiro 1965). As the individual experiences life, adaptive-defensive operations solidify, ultimately crystallizing into an automatic response style. When the response style is based on misperceived or distorted object relations, a personality disorder may emerge. Given these premises, the psychiatric nurse using a biopsychosocial model views clients with personality disorders as people whose communication and behavior are greatly influenced by past experiences, a need to maintain self-direction and control, and a unique style of interpreting their world.

Martha, a 49-year-old secretary, is a perfectionist and shows exaggerated loyalty to her company. Most of her energies are directed toward work and being indispensable to her employer. She consistently takes work home at night and weekends, even postponing her vacation to complete elaborate, detailed reports. Martha's relationships with coworkers focus on work only; she is unable to socialize with coworkers without experiencing extreme anxiety. Consequently, others view her as rigid, isolated, cold, and tense. They try to avoid relating to her. During a performance evaluation, when her employer pointed out her defensive peer relationships, Martha became irritable and pressured, stating, "I was not hired to socialize. Those people who complain should be doing their work and earning the paychecks they receive."

Martha's definition of any situation is based on her narrow view of the world and her purpose in it. When confronted with her behavior, she does not attend to personal issues but rather focuses on the technical details of the situation. Martha justifies her position by falling back on the rules and regulations that reinforce her own moral convictions. Even with her distorted strategies, Martha is able to achieve stable functioning. As a result, people interacting with Martha generally choose not to confront the frustrating behaviors. Instead, they accept her "peculiarities" as a tradeoff for her work performance. The likelihood that Martha will change her response style is minimal unless she experiences deep dissatisfaction and begins to examine her own personality traits.

In summary, a person's style of functioning is shaped by the following:

• Original biopsychosocial characteristics

• Object relations

• Reinforcement of behavioral responses

Table 16–1 illustrates the preceding developmental concepts and their interaction. It is only when we acknowledge the individual's response style and definition of a situation that we can identify the subjective meaning of a thought, feeling, or behavior for that person.

Little systematic research has been conducted on the causes or treatment of personality disorders (Widiger and Frances 1985). Furthermore, debate continues about the developmental course of personality disorders. Some theorists argue that their course of development is different from that of anxiety-related and psychotic forms of maladaptation. Other theorists see personality disorders as belonging in a developmental continuum that includes personality disorders, anxiety-related disorders, and psychoses. The accompanying box describes the characteristics of the personality disorders discussed in DSM-III-R.

TABLE 16–1 Factors Influencing Style of Functioning

Factor	Definition	Example
Original biopsychosocial characteristics	Unique endowment of qualities, e.g., physical form, mental ability, and social group	An 8-year-old Korean child is adopted by white American parents. The child experiences rejection from his classmates because of his physical characteristics. Consequently, he begins to avoid situations, and he scrutinizes others' behavior for hidden motives.
Object relations	Interaction between the individual and objects in the environment, e.g., people, material things, symbols	An upwardly mobile professional couple demand perfection and conformity from their 7-year-old daughter. They discourage fantasy and creativity. The daughter procrastinates and follows directions half-heartedly in coping with her parents' demands.
Reinforcement of behavioral responses	A reward or punishment that strengthens or weakens a person's responses	A highly anxious mother gives in to her child's demands when the child has a temper tantrum; she fails to respond positively to the child's "good" behaviors. The child rarely makes polite requests, but interrupts, screams, and shouts for attention.

Interaction of Factors
The medicine man of the Hopi Indians sometimes uses meditation to diagnose illnesses. He may even use a crystal ball as his focal point during meditation. At other times the Hopi medicine man chews roots of jimsonweed (datura) to go into a trance as he meditates. The Hopis believe that the ensuing hallucinations are visions of the evil that caused the sickness. After the meditation, he prescribes an appropriate herbal treatment, e.g., fever is "cured" by a plant that smells like lightning. Indeed, the Hopi phrase for fever is "lightning sickness" (Spector 1985).

In 1980, DSM-III grouped the personality disorders into three clusters (see the box on page 374). In presenting the nursing care plans for clients with personality disorders, we shall follow this organization. In addition, DSM-III-R designates a residual category of personality disorders to include people who meet some of the criteria for more than one personality disorder but who do not manifest sufficient responses in any one category to be assigned an Axis II diagnosis.

Eccentric Personality Disorders

The **paranoid, schizotypal,** and **schizoid** personalities are identified as "odd or eccentric" in the DSM-III-R (1987, p 337). The major features of these disorders are social detachment and consequent impairment in social and occupational functioning. These disorders have been observed in family members of schizophrenic persons (Kendler et al. 1984). A 1989 study by Coryell and Zimmerman (1989) did not support the findings of Kendler et al. Rather, only the relatives of mood-incongruent depressed subjects demonstrated a risk for personality disorders higher than that of relatives of subjects with no history of psychiatric illness. People with eccentric personality disorders have been identified as having more cognitive style impairments than people with the disorders in the other DSM-III clusters (Torgensen 1984, Widiger and

Frances 1985). The eccentric disorders are the most peculiar and reflect the most maladaptive defensive styles.

The Nursing Process and Paranoid Personality Disorders

Assessing

Suspiciousness and Mistrust Suspiciousness and mistrust reflect an attitude of doubt toward the trustworthiness of objects or people. The suspicious person is usually preoccupied with being maneuvered, tricked, or framed. Suspiciousness is also a way of thinking and includes such manifestations as expectations of trickery or harm, guardedness, secretiveness, jealousy, doubt of others' loyalty, and overconcern with hidden motives and special meanings. For example, the suspicious person may perceive a birthday gift as a trick to create an obligation.

Rigidity Paranoid people are inflexible in their perception of the world. They are preoccupied with their expectations of others and relentlessly try to confirm these expectations, often through argumentation. They closely examine rational arguments and contrary information, but with prejudice. The paranoid person justifies a position by excessive rationalization, rejecting any evidence refuting the original notion. It is not

Characteristics of Personality Disorders (DSM-III-R)

Eccentric Styles

Paranoid   Is pervasively and unjustifiably suspicious and mistrustful, as evidenced by jealousy, envy, and guardedness. Is hypersensitive and usually feels mistreated and misjudged. Restricts feelings, as evidenced by lack of humor, absence of sentimental or tender feelings, and pride in being cold and unemotional.

Schizoid   Is emotionally cold and aloof. Shows indifference to the praise or criticism of others. Has no desire for social involvement and a tendency to be reserved and reclusive.

Schizotypal   Manifests various oddities of thought, perceptions, speech, and behavior, such as ideas of reference, bizarre fantasies, and preoccupations. Is suspicious and hypersensitive to real or imagined criticism. Isolates self from society.

Dramatic-Erratic Styles

Histrionic   Is overly dramatic and reactive, and responds intensely. Engages in attention seeking, self-dramatization, and irrational outbursts of emotion. Is perceived by others as shallow, self-indulgent, vain, demanding, dependent, and inconsiderate. Is prone to manipulative threats and gestures.

Narcissistic   Has grandiose sense of self-importance. Is preoccupied with fantasies of unlimited success, power, beauty, brilliance, etc. Needs attention and admiration. Is indifferent or reacts to criticism with rage, feelings of inferiority, or humiliation. In relations with others, expects special favors. Takes advantage of others; shifts between overidealizing others to disregarding them. Lacks ability for empathy.

Borderline   Is impulsive and unpredictable in areas of life that are self-damaging. Has unstable but intense interpersonal relationships involving manipulation of others. Displays temper inappropriately. Has unstable moods (including rage); is uncertain about identity, and intolerant of being alone. May inflict physical damage on self. Has chronic feelings of boredom and emptiness.

Antisocial   Engages in behavior that causes conflict with society, e.g., theft, vandalism, fighting, delinquency, truancy. Is unable to sustain consistent work or to function as a responsible parent or spouse. Cannot maintain enduring attachment to sexual partner. Lacks respect or loyalty; is irritable and aggressive. Manipulates others for personal gain, does not plan ahead, lacks guilt, does not learn from past experiences, blames others.

Anxious-Fearful

Avoidant   Is hypersensitive to rejection and interprets innocuous events as ridicule. Is unwilling to become involved with others unless given a guarantee of acceptance. Withdraws socially in interpersonal and work roles. Desires affection and acceptance. Has low self-esteem and is overly dismayed by personal shortcomings.

Dependent   Passively allows others to assume responsibility for major areas of life. Subordinates own needs to those on whom client depends to avoid possibility of having to rely on self. Lacks self-confidence.

Obsessive-compulsive   Is overconscientious, overmeticulous, and perfectionistic. Is excessively concerned with conformity. Adheres rigidly to strict standards. Is prone to self-doubt, unhappiness, and worry. Has limited ability to express warm and tender emotions; is preoccupied with trivial details, rules, schedules, and lists.

Passive-aggressive   Resists demands for adequate functioning through indirect methods, e.g., procrastination, dawdling, stubbornness, intentional inefficiency, and forgetfulness.

unusual for a paranoid person to suspect people with opposing ideas. The paranoid person goes to great lengths to prove a point, making mountains out of molehills. A need to be in control and have power is another characteristic, as is a preoccupation with the rank and status of oneself and others.

Hypervigilance The **hypervigilant** individual is a keen, penetrating observer, far more attentive and acute than the ordinary person (Shapiro 1965, p 58). Constant sensitivity to nuances in social relations, interpretation of both open and hidden attitudes of others, and scrutiny are modes of operation.

Following a bomb threat that occurred one year ago, a unit clerk opens and inspects every package brought into the ICU by staff and visitors, anticipating that someone will bring weapons into the unit.

Distortions of Reality Although paranoid people may perceive facts accurately, they invest them with a special significance. In this way, they create a private reality. They have a special interest in hidden motives, underlying purposes, special meanings, and the like. They do not necessarily disagree with the average observer about the existence of any given fact, only about its meaning and significance. Therefore, even severely paranoid people can recognize various essential facts well enough to achieve a limited adjustment to the normal social world. At the same time, however, they continue to interpret substantial portions of this world autistically. They often have difficulty distinguishing real from imagined offenses. The individual's distorted attitudes antagonize others and may lead to real discrimination.

Ellen is a paranoid woman who is quick to detect signs of anger, jealousy, and rejection in the actions of her coworkers. She magnifies these negative aspects and overlooks such positive behaviors as humor, support, and empathy. Eventually, Ellen's coworkers begin to snicker when she makes public statements, and they gossip about her.

Projection Paranoid people attribute to external figures their own intolerable motivations, drives, or feelings. Some psychiatric theorists believe that paranoid people use projection to attribute to others the evil intentions that they themselves feel. In this way, the idea that one may be harmed really reflects the individual's own wish to harm others.

Nancy's idea that her boyfriend is seeing another woman may reflect her wish to terminate their relationship.

Restricted Affect Lack of emotional expressiveness and spontaneity characterizes paranoid people. They often appear cold, humorless, and devoid of tender, sensitive feelings. They pride themselves on remaining objective and rational and frequently use intellectualization and rationalization to avoid affective experiences. Some paranoid people may appear friendly, but in fact, this friendliness is a "script" that helps them adapt to social situations or achieve their goals.

The Process of Exclusion Because of the paranoid person's antagonism, suspiciousness, and restricted object relations, tension develops between the person and significant others. The persistent strain on relationships causes others to define the paranoid person as more than simply "different." Instead, they see the individual as unreliable or untrustworthy, and others begin to interact according to their perceptions. These behaviors reinforce the suspicions and beliefs of the paranoid person. The effects of this process include the following:

• Blocked communication, which increases the process of exclusion

• Emergence of a crisis, which formally excludes the paranoid person

• Reinforcement of the paranoid person's beliefs, interpretations, or ideas of reference

Because paranoid persons are generally intelligent, persuasive, and creative in justifying their beliefs, these clients may adapt in one of two ways. They may join quasipolitical groups, esoteric religions, or quasiscientific organizations that reinforce their interpretations of reality. Or they may join organizations that challenge societal norms and trends in an effort to direct and thus control hostile feelings. See the Intervention box on page 376 for an example of a paranoid person's behavior and recommended nursing interventions.

Diagnosing

After gathering objective and subjective data about the paranoid client's behavior, the nurse categorizes the information into problem areas designated as nursing diagnostic categories. It is critical to involve the client in all steps of the treatment planning process to enhance participation and promote planned changes. DSM-III-R psychiatric diagnoses and current NANDA nursing diagnoses for the paranoid client are shown in the nursing care plan on the following pages. The general nursing diagnostic groupings that follow for this client focus on psychosocial needs only. The psychiatric nurse develops individualized care plans to address the unique needs of each client assessed.

Defensive Coping The client demonstrates impairment of adaptive behaviors in meeting life's demands. The paranoid personality may exhibit these forms of ineffective coping, among others:

• Suspiciousness

• Limited affect

• Reluctance to confide in others

• Carrying grudges

• Pessimistic regard for others

Altered Thought Processes The paranoid client experiences impaired cognitive functioning without

INTERVENTION

Guidelines for Working with the Paranoid Client

Jim, a 39-year-old engineer, suspects that his employer is withholding significant data from him pertaining to an important job assignment. Jim began to question others about the reliability and integrity of his boss. Jim went to the plant one Sunday morning without authorization. A security guard found him going through the filing cabinets of his employer, who confronted him the following day and sent him to the employee assistance program nurse. During the interview, Jim states, "I knew he [the employer] was dishonest from the start. He never could give me a straight answer. As soon as I was almost on him, he sets me up to lose face and maybe my job."

Nursing Responses

- Remain calm, nonthreatening, and nonjudgmental in all interactions.
- Give clear information regarding confidentiality and job-related consequences of counseling sessions.
- Assist client to identify and verbalize feelings.
- Respond to suspicious ideas by focusing on feelings, e.g., "It must be distressing . . ."; "You see him as vindictive . . ."
- Do not interpret client's beliefs or argue with him about them.
- Include client in formulating the treatment contract.
- Focus on ideas that are reality based.
- Inform client of the emotional cues he gives to others, e.g., suspiciousness, intimidation, or contempt. Encourage him to validate your perceptions.

loss of reality contact. Behaviors often observed include the following:

- Preoccupation with theories of conspiracies
- Hypervigilance and hypersensitivity
- Misinterpretation of benign remarks as threats
- Egocentricity

- Perseveration
- Impaired problem solving

Impaired Social Interaction   The predominant interactional dysfunctions of the paranoid personality are distortions and overuse of defense mechanisms related to high levels of fear and anxiety. Interactional impairments include the following:

- Failure to interpret messages accurately
- Stereotyping others
- Judgmental attitudes toward others
- Failure to listen actively
- Arrogance
- Aggressiveness
- Overuse of defense mechanisms of denial, rationalization, projection, and intellectualization

Planning and Implementing Interventions

Nursing interventions with the paranoid client center around mutual decision making. The goal of all interventions is to diminish the client's pervasive suspiciousness, distortions of thought, communication problems, and resulting impairment of role performance. See the detailed nursing care plan for the paranoid client.

Evaluating/Outcome Criteria

Defensive Coping   It is unlikely that the paranoid client will give up coping responses developed over a lifetime. Consistently used interventions, however, should reduce anxiety and allow the client to identify at least one significant person as trustworthy. At the least, the client should be able to relax sufficiently in the presence of the nurse to explore how personal coping modes have created problems in living and to identify ways to avoid future conflicts with others.

Altered Thought Processes   Consistency and structure help direct the client's thoughts to here-and-now reality. The nurse can use role modeling to reach this goal, i.e., the nurse tests reality appropriately to encourage the client to do the same. When clients begin to voice doubts about their interpretations or to identify alternative interpretations, the nurse is in a position to reinforce their achievements. Many paranoid clients simply learn not to discuss their illogical or irrational beliefs with others.

NURSING CARE PLAN

A Client with a Paranoid Personality Disorder

Client Care Goals	Nursing Planning/ Interventions	Evaluation
Nursing Diagnoses: *Defensive coping (Related factors: exclusion, restricted and controlled affect, guardedness, reclusiveness, and secretiveness) and Social isolation*		
The client will exhibit less suspicious behavior and establish effective and satisfying relationships with staff and significant others.	Respect the client's privacy and preferences as much as is reasonable. Give feedback to client based on observed nonverbal cues of responsiveness, e.g., eye movement, posturing, voice tones. Point out inconsistent behaviors such as affect/verbalization. Provide a daily schedule of activities and inform client of changes as needed. Help client identify adaptive diversionary activities, e.g., leisure, recreation, in one-on-one sessions and groups. Encourage an evaluation of how client behaviors led to the current crisis. Gradually introduce client to group situations. Use role-playing techniques to help client identify feelings, thoughts, and responses brought on by stressful situations.	Attends and spontaneously participates in short one-on-one sessions and activity groups (less than 1 hour). Initiates one-on-one sessions with assigned member. Approaches other clients and staff without encouragement. Identifies personal behaviors that precipitated hospitalization. Demonstrates a variety of moods appropriate to situation encountered. Attends to individual and group tasks without attaching unusual meanings to them. Identifies support systems outside the therapeutic relationship.
Nursing Diagnosis: *Altered thought processes (Related factors: suspiciousness, rigidity, distortions of reality, projection, and hypersensitivity)*		
The client will develop a sense of reality that is validated by others.	Say firmly and kindly that you do not share the client's interpretations of an event but do acknowledge the client's feelings. Follow through on commitments made to client (e.g., contracts). Assign the same staff member to work with the client to establish consistency and trust. Give positive reinforcement for successes in a matter-of-fact manner.	Focuses on ideas that are reality based. Accepts positive feedback without questioning motives or hidden meanings. Accepts responsibility for own feelings and thoughts without attributing them to others, e.g., makes "I" statements. Remains in a group activity for the duration of the activity.

▶

NURSING CARE PLAN (continued)

Client Care Goals	Nursing Planning/ Interventions	Evaluation
	Respond honestly to the client at all times.	Realistically applies the problem-solving process, including making plans for after discharge.
	Refocus conversation to reality-based topics and set limits on the duration and frequency of suspicious concerns during one-on-one sessions and groups.	
	Do not argue with illogical assertions but simply point out that you do not share the same beliefs.	

Nursing Diagnosis: *Impaired verbal communication (Related factors: argumentativeness, critical comments about others, arrogance, aggressiveness, and defensiveness)*

The client will express thoughts and feelings verbally in a nonaggressive manner.	Use an objective, matter-of-fact approach with client.	Expresses feelings without intellectualizing.
	Use concrete, specific words rather than global abstractions.	Consensually validates perceptions of events with a staff member or significant others.
	Give feedback concerning behavior.	
	Identify feelings presented by client during interactions. For example, "I notice some reluctance on your part to tell me about that"; or "From the way you are looking at me, I wonder if you think I'll break my promise."	Makes assertive, nonjudgmental statements to staff and other clients.
		Responds to feedback without rationalizing, projecting, or intellectualizing.
	Direct client to clarify the person or object when pronouns are used.	
	Keep verbal and nonverbal messages clear and consistent.	
	Conduct brief one-on-one sessions daily (avoid prolonged sessions).	
	Encourage client to express feelings through creative modes (e.g., drawing, writing) and to discuss the same.	
	Involve in communication skills groups, e.g., assertiveness training, current events.	

Impaired Social Interaction   The client should learn to make global statements concrete and to clarify verbal expressions. The client may learn to defuse anxiety-producing situations by making "I" statements rather than responding aggressively and judgmentally. Creative modes of expressing feelings are perceived as an acceptable, nonthreatening outlet. Behavior in groups should reflect the client's increasing ability to accept varying opinions without attaching personal significance to them.

The Nursing Process and Schizoid-Schizotypal Personality Disorders

Assessing

Defining Characteristics of Schizoid and Schizotypal Personalities   Persons with schizoid and schizotypal personality disorders generally have a detached and aloof social style. The schizotypal personality, however, has more cognitive impairments than the schizoid personality does. There is a range of adjustment in clients with these personality disorders. Some are fairly well-adjusted individuals who are loners; others live out their lives in protective environments, e.g., group homes, mental hospitals, and prisons. When conducting nursing assessments, the nurse needs to rule out the possibility of a crisis response or chemical dependency.

Lifelong Patterns of Social Isolation   These individuals show a preference for solitary interests and occupations. They have a history of being loners and are indifferent to feedback and insensitive to others.

Blunted Affective Response   The person may appear cool, aloof, humorless, "in a fog," bored, and perhaps even mentally retarded although the IQ would negate this assumption (Cameron and Rychlak 1985).

Detachment from the Environment   The individual appears absent-minded, daydreams, is vague about goals and indecisive, and lacks social skills.

The schizotypal personality demonstrates eccentricities in communication and behavior not seen in the schizoid personality. Examples include (a) such oddities of thought as magical thinking and ideas of reference; (b) altered perceptions, e.g., illusions, depersonalization, and derealization; and (c) speech alterations, e.g., circumstantiality (giving detailed, factual but nonessential information), digression, and metaphorical speech patterns.

Some researchers have found that schizoid and schizotypal personality disorders are significantly more common among relatives of schizophrenic clients. At this time, however, there is no substantial evidence that these personality disorders are early indicators of a future schizophrenic process (Kendler et al. 1984, Torgensen 1984).

Rhoda is a 40-year-old female seen in the emergency room of a large metropolitan hospital. She was brought in after experiencing a hypoglycemic episode at the factory where she has been employed for 15 years as a night maintenance worker. Rhoda's appearance is unkempt and eccentric. She is wearing three layers of clothing and mismatched shoes. Rhoda reports living in a one-room apartment five minutes walk from her place of employment. During the nursing admission interview, Rhoda reports no family or significant others who are available to assist her. Rhoda makes frequent inappropriate grimaces and mutters to herself about getting "back home." She avoids eye contact and direct answers to the nurse's questions. She states, "I don't need any help. I have my own remedies that work just fine. Leave me alone." Following stabilization of her condition, Rhoda is released because she insists she must return to work.

Diagnosing

Persons in the schizoid-schizotypal personality categories are not a danger to themselves or others, a criterion used to authorize long-term hospitalization. They are found among homeless or marginal individuals with limited resources, although some have the financial reserves to lead more adaptive life-styles. They often come to the attention of health professionals as a result of cluttered, negligent life-styles that are considered asocial, unaesthetic, and unhygienic. Assessment of these clients may be hampered by their preference for independence, in spite of the negative consequences such "freedom" may have. If the psychiatric nurse is able to sustain a relationship with these clients, the following NANDA nursing diagnoses are often the basis for guiding nursing care.

Impaired Social Interaction   These clients have a narrow range of coping skills and tend to resist acquiring new skills if they must give up their independence as a result. The following problems signal ineffective coping:

- Social isolation
- Inadequate social skills
- Lack of ongoing support systems

Impaired Communication: Verbal   Schizoid-schizotypal clients have minimal verbal and nonverbal interactions with others. Typical behaviors may include but are not restricted to the following:

- Aloofness
- Restricted affect
- Indifference or excessive social anxiety

Self-Care Deficits: Bathing/Hygiene and Dressing/Grooming These deficits are characteristically seen, particularly in those clients who live on the streets. All aspects of activities of daily living may be involved, including the following:

- Inadequate hygiene
- Bizarre grooming
- Presence of vermin
- Failure to seek health care or adhere to prescribed regimens

Self-Care Deficit: Feeding Feeding self-care deficits may be the result of lack of knowledge, inadequate living arrangements, or lack of interest and motivation. These deficits often lead to physical problems that precipitate visits to emergency rooms and neighborhood clinics. The nurse may be identifying the following problems in this category:

- Obesity
- Anorexia
- Malnutrition
- Dehydration

Impaired Home Maintenance Management Impaired home maintenance is often detected when neighbors report that the person is living in an unhealthy or unsafe environment. This diagnosis includes all aspects of one's ability to make the environment healthful and safe. Problem areas include the following:

- Inadequate housing or lack of housing
- Inadequate sanitation facilities
- Rodent- or vermin-infested living quarters
- Inability to manage finances
- Insufficient income or lack of income

Planning and Implementing Interventions

See the accompanying nursing care plan for the client with a schizoid or schizotypal personality disorder. The goal of nursing interventions is to provide an uncomplicated, supportive environment that is safe and nonthreatening to the client. It is hoped that this approach will prevent deterioration and will enhance the client's level of adaptation and functioning. Because the schizoid and schizotypal personalities have extreme difficulty with emotional commitments, the nurse must be watchful of stressful conditions that could precipitate a psychotic episode.

Evaluating/Outcome Criteria

Although health care providers often address the needs of schizoid-schizotypal persons, it is difficult to persuade them to cooperate with and adhere to structured treatment plans after they are discharged from in-patient settings or halfway houses or crisis intervention programs. In structured settings, these clients perform on the fringe of the group, needing encouragement and reinforcement to become involved in self-care, meal planning, and leisure activities as might be found in a drop-in center providing a variety of services which the client self-selects.

Ineffective Individual Coping These clients may not achieve dramatic behavioral and personality changes. If, however, the client is able to maintain a therapeutic alliance with the psychiatric nurse as an outpatient in individual or group settings, the goal of increasing the client's level of attachment may be met.

Impaired Communication: Verbal If the client remains linked with the support system, increasing levels of interaction should occur. Any appropriate verbal or nonverbal response by the client may indicate motivation and progress toward meeting the goal of effective communication. To encourage the client to use more direct and meaningful speech patterns, focus on low-stress topics during interaction (e.g., weather, travel, current events, games, cards) and use clear, concise speech.

Self-Care Deficits: Bathing/Hygiene and Dressing/Grooming Some of these clients carry all their belongings with them and frequently bathe in bus terminal restrooms. For this reason, it may be difficult to teach and monitor adequate self-care activities. If the client is not homeless, help the client develop weekly schedules for self-care activities.

Self-Care Deficit: Feeding Linking these clients with meals-on-wheels or congregate dining facilities following discharge from in-patient settings not only promotes adequate nutrition but also encourages increased social interactions. Because many of their physical problems are the result of poor nutrition, use a variety of resources to teach nutritional concepts, e.g., pictures, activity groups, cooking classes, and outings to grocery stores.

Impaired Home Maintenance Management Because the schizoid or schizotypal client values independence highly, take into account the client's preferences and former life-style when planning interventions. If the client has a history of transience, provide a list of community resources and discuss other

NURSING CARE PLAN

A Client with a Schizoid-Schizotypal Disorder

Client Care Goals	Nursing Planning/ Interventions	Evaluation

Nursing Diagnosis: *Ineffective individual coping (Related factors: social isolation, inadequate social skills, lack of support system)*

The client will increase level of attachment to available social support systems.	Provide client with schedule of daily activities (in-patient and day treatment programs).	Participates in ongoing support systems offered by community mental health clinic.
	Approach client for one-to-one sessions on a daily basis.	Initiates at least one interaction with a staff member daily.
	Assign same staff members to client to develop rapport and trust.	
	Encourage client to attend and participate in group activities, beginning with those that involve limited interaction and progressing to those of a more verbal nature.	
	Enlist client's cooperation in identifying needs and participating in treatment plan, including goal setting and planning.	

Nursing Diagnosis: *Impaired verbal communication (Related factors: detachment, aloofness, and lack of spontaneity)*

The client will increase effective interactions with others.	Link with case management system at community mental health clinic.	Selects one activity for the group three times weekly.
	Involve in nonthreatening verbal group activities, e.g., current events, social skills groups, leisure skills.	Remains out of room at least six hours daily.
	Focus on low-stress topics to encourage normal speech.	Speaks for ten minutes without introducing circumstantial material.

Nursing Diagnosis: *Self-care deficits: Bathing/hygiene and Dressing/grooming*

The client will maintain adequate hygiene and grooming.	Set up bathing/grooming schedule for client and assist client with tasks, daily.	Bathes and changes clothing at least three times weekly.
		Prepares dirty laundry for washing.

►

NURSING CARE PLAN (continued)

Client Care Goals	Nursing Planning/ Interventions	Evaluation
Nursing Diagnosis: *Self-care deficit: Feeding (Related factors: malnutrition, deficit in normal weight, and vitamin deficiencies)*		
The client will maintain adequate nutrition, hydration, and elimination.	Monitor and record client's intake daily.	Eats three balanced meals daily.
	Refer for dietary consult and implement recommendations.	Participates in a complete physical exam within 48 hours of hospitalization.
	Schedule and assist with physical exam.	Gains 2–3 lbs weekly while hospitalized.
	Administer dietary supplements, as ordered.	Takes vitamin supplements as ordered.
	Discuss with client the minimum requirements for an adequate diet and ways to obtain these necessary foods.	Reports any problems of elimination to nursing staff.
	Monitor bowel patterns daily.	
Nursing Diagnosis: *Impaired home maintenance management (Related factors: inadequate housing, inability to manage finances, lack of sanitation)*		
The client will be physically safe postdischarge.	Refer to social services for assessment and health rehabilitation services link-up.	Accepts social service plan to locate adequate housing, food, and medical care.
	Provide client with list of emergency services, e.g., crisis hotline, Salvation Army, shelters for homeless.	Accepts referral to human services for evaluation and support.

options to prevent life-management crises. Guardianship by government agencies may be necessary and desirable for clients who are incompetent to care for themselves.

Dramatic-Erratic Personality Disorders

DSM-III-R identifies the **borderline, histrionic, narcissistic,** and **antisocial** personality disorders as "dramatic, emotional, erratic" dysfunctions. Individuals with these disorders are often in conflict with society because of their impulsive behavior. Impulsive people view the world as a discontinuous, fragmented conglomerate of opportunities, frustrations, and affective experiences. They live in the present. They lack the ability to examine hunches and to formulate long-range

plans. They act decisively without critical evaluation of consequences. The focus of their intellectual and emotional goals is to achieve immediate gain and satisfaction. This lack of impulse control and inability to delay gratification often result in both verbal and nonverbal outbursts of anger, which may be self- or other-directed. Indeed, clients with dramatic-erratic personality disorders may experience rapid escalation of anxiety when their own angry impulses are not controlled by others. The accompanying Intervention box illustrates some common angry behaviors and offers guidelines for nursing interventions.

Most researchers agree that psychologic fixations in the genital stage of development account for many of the behaviors noted in this cluster of disorders (Cameron and Rychlak 1985). Specifically, parental deprivation; inadequate, excessive, or inconsistent discipline; and failure of the child to develop inte-

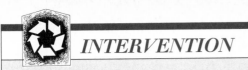

Guidelines for Working with the Angry Client

Defining Characteristics	Nursing Interventions

Nonverbal

Glaring, piercing stares

Tight facial muscles

Facial flushing

Distended neck veins

Hyperalertness

Knitted brows

Tense body posture

Arms crossed over chest or placed on hips

Finger pointing

Fist clenching, waving, or pounding

Slamming, throwing, or punching inanimate objects

Irritability

Overreaction; temper outbursts

Intimidation

Physical assault/injury to animals or persons

Homicide/suicide ideation, plan, or gesture

Verbal

Derogatory statements and sarcasm

Malicious gossiping

Angry voice tone

Pressured speech

Shouting, screaming, cursing

Overly critical, impatient

Threatening

Scapegoating

Negativity

Statements such as, "You make me mad. I could kill you."

Overuse of defense mechanisms of denial, rationalization, projection, and displacement

---

Use a calm, unhurried approach

Do not touch indiscriminately

Respect personal space

Use active listening skills

Remain aware of personal feelings

Use statements to provide feedback and to identify sources of anger, e.g., "I notice your fists are clenched . . . what's happening?"

Set verbal limits on behavior

Use adult-adult rather than parent-child communications

Offer time-out periods/one-to-one sessions in a quiet area

Assure client that the staff will not allow the client to hurt self or others

Observe for escalation of anger (increased activity, verbal and nonverbal acting out)

Institute precautions against suicide, homicide, assault, or escape, as indicated

Document patterns of acting out, including trigger situations

Discuss alternate means of releasing tension and physical energy

Provide physical outlets to reduce tension, e.g., exercise, punching bags, gardening, clay, music, art (avoid competitive or contact sports)

Use humor to reduce tension and avoid a power struggle

Offer medication if appropriate

Be prepared to use seclusion and restraints

Recognize client's potential to act on threats

Initially ignore derogatory statements

Protect other clients from verbal/physical abuse

Clearly communicate and enforce unit regulations concerning acting-out behavior

Postpone discussion of anger and consequences of acting out until client is in control

Role model appropriate assertions of angry feelings, e.g., "I dislike it when . . ."

State desire to assist client to maintain/regain control

Hold client responsible for behavior; remind client that he or she can make choices

Do not argue or criticize

Give feedback regarding client's ability to maintain control in similar situations

Do not threaten punitive action

Involve in treatment planning

Use contracts for behavioral control, including seeking out staff people when feelings emerge

Teach assertive skills, relaxation, imagery, thought stopping, thought control, etc.

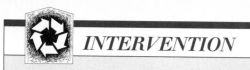

Guidelines for Working with the Manipulative Client

Defining Characteristics	*Nursing Interventions*

Nonverbal

Smiling to excess

Touching inappropriately

Crying, whining in public

Appearing confused and helpless

Drawing attention to self (e.g., falling, dramatic displays of somatic problems, etc.)

Gift giving

Tardiness

Selective forgetting

Refusal to participate in activities

Seductive dressing, eye movements, body language

Decreased frustration tolerance

Self/other destructive acting out

Verbal

Compliments, flattery

Sarcasm

Threats

Demanding behavior

Induction of guilt, e.g., "I thought we had a relationship of trust.'

Excessive criticism of others

Wheeling and dealing

Bargaining for special privileges

Being overly solicitous of others

Requesting exemption from rules, e.g., "Couldn't I have my medication just one hour earlier?"

Mimicking therapeutic responses used by staff, e.g., "I have a feeling you're angry with me."

Confronting staff in the presence of other clients

Lying

Reporting great "insights" early in the relationship

Telling the nurse what he or she "wants" to hear

Using information about others to exploit them

Excessive involvement in the problems of others

Aggressive questioning about personal matters

Rationalizing, projecting, and minimizing blame for behavior

Self-pity

Role reversal

Assign one staff member as primary resource person

Provide for staff conferences on a regular basis

Allow sufficient time to develop a relationship

Use group and peer supervision for staff

Provide for consistency in limit setting

Make limits realistic with enforceable consequences

Give reasons for limits and consequences

Identify personal feelings, e.g., anger, frustration, discomfort, rescuer needs, in response to client's behavior

Model respect, honesty, openness, and assertiveness

Avoid power struggles and focus on need for self-control

Seek times to interact with client when he or she is not acting out

Confront client each time manipulation occurs

Describe impact of client's manipulation in an unemotional way, e.g., "I feel angry when you scream at me in front of all the staff members."

Explore the meaning and effects of the client's manipulations

Discuss with the client alternative ways of dealing with people or situations

Do not express nonverbal amusement (e.g., eye rolling, smiling) when the client manipulates others

Avoid accepting gifts

Explore meaning of gift giving with client

Enlist client's participation in treatment plan

Encourage control over routine ADL decisions

Encourage participation in group activities in both member and leader roles

Assist client to write a self-assessment identifying both assets and liabilities

Remove limits from treatment plan when client adheres to objectives consistently

Evaluate effectiveness of limit setting

Jointly develop contracts for behavioral change

If client refuses to comply with contracts or treatment recommendations, avoid negotiating; enlist staff team to resolve issues

Offer support to other clients who may be targets of manipulations

Involve both client and significant others in identifying and managing manipulative behavior

Teach stress-reduction techniques (e.g., guided imagery, relaxation, thought-stopping)

Involve in assertiveness training and problem-solving

Practice role rehearsal skills

ASSESSMENT

Common Features of the Dramatic-Erratic Personality

- Labile affective responses
- Intense episodes of anger/rage
- Self-centeredness/egocentricity
- Unstable personal relationships
- Superficiality, exploitiveness, and manipulativeness
- Lack of empathy for others
- Inability to postpone gratification
- Boredom or need for constant attention
- Poor judgment
- Failure to learn by experience
- Failure to assume responsibility for behavior
- Poorly integrated sexual identity
- Ability to test reality and absence of major thought or affective disorders

grated cognitive, affective, and behavioral modes in early life may lead to these disorders. Clients have generalized feelings of low self-esteem, need to control people and situations, and are unable to delay gratification. In response, dramatic-erratic clients tend to interact by negatively manipulating others. Although manipulation is a standard response in the repertoire of people with these personality disorders, its occurrence escalates with increased stress. The accompanying Intervention box illustrates some manipulative behaviors and offers guidelines for nursing interventions.

Common features of the dramatic-erratic cluster of personality disorders are summarized in the accompanying Assessment box. Due to its instability and the potential for transient psychotic symptoms, the borderline personality disorder is discussed first.

The Nursing Process and Borderline Personality Disorders

Assessing

Defining Characteristics of the Borderline Personality Although the person with a borderline personality disorder is unstable in a variety of areas, e.g., relationships, mood, and self-image, no single feature

is invariably present. Of the eight criteria in DSM-III-R, at least five must be observed to diagnose this disorder. Some theorists characterize borderline personality disorders as occupying a place on a continuum between neurotic and psychotic disorders. A great deal of research data are being compiled to identify causative factors (Cameron and Rychlak 1985). To date, the data lend support to Mahler's concepts of **separation-individuation** (Mahler et al. 1975) as the psychodynamic basis of this disorder. Benner and Joscelyne (1984) also suggest that the borderline personality is the foundation for the multiple personality disorder.

Among those researchers seeking a biologic basis for the borderline personality, Loranger and Tulis (1985) report that, compared to nonborderline clients, borderline clients have a significantly higher family history of alcoholism. These authors speculate that a biologic or genetic component may account for their findings. Also lending support to the biologic theorists, Andrulonis et al. (1980), in an intensive study of clients with borderline syndromes, report organic involvement, including histories of minimal brain dysfunction and episodic dyscontrol syndromes among their subjects.

Surprisingly, little research has been conducted in the area of family interactional patterns that may predispose to the borderline personality disorder. Feldman and Guttman (1984) recommend further research in this area based upon findings that indicate that **biparental failure,** rather than failures during the separation-individuation process with the primary caregiver, may lead to the development of symptoms. Biparental failure is evident in those homes where the male parent fails to offset the child's troubled relationship with the mother by providing positive experiences for the child. For example, the male parent fails to become involved in day-to-day parenting, generally lacks interest in the child, gives little approval, is passive, or affectively neglects the child.

The following subjective and objective nursing assessment criteria for persons with borderline personality disorders have been adapted from the DSM-III-R diagnostic criteria. Because the majority of individuals with borderline personality disorders are encountered in the workplace or socially, it is important to recognize and intervene appropriately to prevent crises (Wester 1989). The accompanying Nursing Awareness box describes some of the behavioral characteristics of these individuals, along with useful interventions.

Instability or Unpredictability The individual with a borderline personality disorder has fluctuating responses in a variety of situations that are subjectively interpreted and often distorted. This individual often makes such comments as, "I did it. I don't know why I did. I just did." Impulsiveness is manifested in spending habits, sexuality, substance use, eating habits, shoplifting, and frequent job changes.

NURSING SELF-AWARENESS

Recognizing and Working with Borderline Personalities

Patty, a 25-year-old RN has been working on your acute medical-surgical unit for 8 months. During this time she has had several run-ins with the nurse manager and other staff members. After two months of employment, it was obvious that Patty was intent on developing a "special" relationship with the nurse manager. Patty would stay after shift changes to talk with her and frequently asked the nurse manager to go out for drinks after work. When the nurse manager did not respond to these overtures or grant Patty's special requests (vacation, shift changes, time off for personal reasons), Patty became angry and spoke of her supervisor in a disparaging way to the other nurses on the unit. Patty told one coworker, "She [the nurse manager] made me so mad I almost got mugged after I got drunk the night she refused to go out with me." Patty confessed that she had anonymously phoned the nurse manager three times after midnight, hanging up each time, just to "harass her and let her know she isn't as great as she thinks she is."

At the time of her six-month evaluation with the nurse manager, Patty denied that she had abused sick leave even though she had called in sick 10 days and failed to report for duty twice. Patty steadfastly insisted that she did comply with hospital policy even though she had failed to complete CPR and Infection Control inservices, failed to have her PPD test done, and had gone directly to the hospital administrator with a complaint about the nurse manager. Patty had also refused to care for a client diagnosed with AIDS. She tried to justify her behavior by saying that no one had ever explained these policies to her. After Patty was placed on probationary status she became overtly hostile toward the nurse manager and attempted to turn her co-workers against this supervisor. Much of Patty's days were spent gossiping about the unfairness of

her situation and blaming the nurse manager for her own escalating use of alcohol, which Patty said she needed to "calm myself." When Patty's maneuvers failed to elicit a sympathetic response from either her coworkers or the nurse manager, she threatened to sue the supervisor for "harassment and interference with employment stability."

Behavioral Characteristics

- High potential, but low achievement levels
- Excessive interest in the personal lives of those in authority
- Idealistic, oversolicitous responses to supervisory personnel
- Demands for special considerations or privileges
- Inconsistent work performance
- Mood swings, argumentativeness, and manipulativeness with others
- Hostile acting out, including sick calls, dishonesty, noncompliance with policies, and broken promises
- Impulsive behavior, temper tantrums, splitting of work staff and friends
- Substance abuse
- Chronic expressions of boredom
- Malicious gossip; anonymous phone calls and letters of complaint
- Sexual overtures toward physicians, administrators, supervisors, clients, and other nurses
- Verbal attacks on superiors, threats of litigation, failure to follow chain of command

Never underestimate the potential for crisis that these borderline personalities may create. People in supervisory positions should use a consultant to maintain objectivity when identifying and developing strategies to deal with these employees.

▶

Unstable Interpersonal Relationships The person's failure to resolve the separation-individuation process described by Mahler et al. (1975) is reflected in the individual's attitudes toward self and others. Normal autism and symbiosis must occur before the separation-individuation process, referred to as "psychologic birth," can begin. The inability to unify the

"good and bad" objects into one whole is demonstrated by the inability to integrate the self as both "good and bad" or to separate or individuate from the maternal object (see Table 16–2 on page 388).

The sense of self originates with the earliest mother-child interactions. If the mother is not sensitive and attuned to the child's need, she fails to confirm the

NURSING SELF-AWARENESS (continued)

Intervention Strategies

- Establish clear guidelines for workplace behavior; set firm, consistent limits on behavior.
- Give equal treatment in group situations.
- Avoid showing favoritism, emotional involvement, or permissiveness.
- Make work assignments appropriate to level of education, experience, and ability.
- Encourage adult-level communication.
- Be alert for substance use and/or sexual acting out on duty.
- Do not "diagnose"; document problem behavior.

- Avoid behavioral interpretations; document facts only.
- Maintain confidentiality of records.
- Maintain communication with hospital administrators or human resource personnel regarding "problem" employees.
- Carefully screen all applicants for employment to identify borderline characteristics that may result in disruptive activities in the workplace.

SOURCE: Wester CM: Managing the borderline personality. Nurs Management 1989;20(2):49–51.

---

child's emerging sense of reality. Consequently, the child distorts reality and develops an unreal "as-if" personality that shifts to meet the demands of cues in the outer world (Brainerd 1978, Mahler et al. 1975). The implications for the child's later relationships include such behaviors as:

- Manipulation of others
- Pitting individuals against one another
- Intense attachment
- Explosive separations
- Sudden shifts in attitude toward others perceived as good or bad
- Clinging, demanding
- Controlling, exploitive behavior
- Sadism or masochism in close relationships
- Relationships motivated by a need to avoid being alone rather than the need to be with others
- Lack of empathy
- Diminished capacity to evaluate others realistically
- Transient, brief, close relationships

Intense Anger   Borderline individuals, unable to tolerate their own "bad" self-image, project it onto others and rage against those negative attributes. As a consequence of childhood disappointments and frustrations related to insensitive and inadequate parenting, the borderline client seethes with intense, unexpressed rage. The person may direct this rage at anyone who demonstrates the negative attributes that the borderline client sees in the self. However, anger is greatest toward those people who remind the client of nurturing/frustrating parents. Schwarz and Halaris (1984) suggest that this may explain why it is so difficult to maintain these clients in therapy. Borderline clients tend to instigate problems as they become involved in therapeutic relationships. The anger may manifest itself in accusations, frequent displays of temper, inability to control anger (acting out), irritability, sarcasm, argumentativeness, devaluing others, and overreaction to minor irritants. (See the Intervention box on page 383 to review manifestations of anger and nursing guidelines.)

Identity Diffusion   Erikson (1964) coined the term **identity diffusion** to describe the failure to integrate various childhood identifications into a harmonious adult psychosocial identity. The borderline person displays behaviors that show confusion about values and goals in life. Deutsch (1965) describes these individuals as "as-if" people, who assume roles and characteristics of others in a chameleonlike fashion. They persuasively imitate or "play act" others' behaviors. Indeed, they may become "copies" of the people with whom they associate. These clients cannot genuinely experience feelings and emotions; the core personality of the borderline client is hollow. They do not assume responsibility for their actions but project blame and credit onto others.

Problems of identity diffusion are also apparent in the areas of sexual intimacy and gender identity. Sexual intimacy is disturbed as a result of the person's fears of being engulfed and destroyed or abandoned by another. An approach-avoidance conflict emerges as a

TABLE 16–2　Separation-Individuation Subphases

Age	Subphase	Task Versus Failure	Expected Behaviors
5 months	Differentiation	Separation ("hatching") versus increased autistic behavior such as: rocking, bland affect, autoerotic stimulation, and intense stranger anxiety	Is increasingly alert Makes tactile exploration of mother Uses transitional objects to replace mother Compares mother visually with other humans Shows stranger anxiety Begins to separate from maternal object
9 months 10–18 months	Practicing (early) Practicing (late)	Separation ("expansion") versus withdrawal, apathy, and desperate crying	Crawls away while holding on Is capable of upright locomotion Keeps mother "in sight" Is exuberant Continues to use transitional object for comfort Retains memory when person or object is out of sight (object performance)
15–18 months	Rapprochement 1. Beginning 2. Crisis	Establishing optimal distance to maintain psychologic equilibrium versus inability to integrate positive and negative aspects about self and others: "splitting"	Clamors for mother's attention Shadows mother/darts away Shares objects with mother Plays imitation games Has reactions to strangers Has temper tantrums Is shy with strangers Shows ambivalence (clings/pushes) Is indecisive Perceives caretakers as "good" and "bad" Is able to make requests
21 months	3. Resolution		Has wider emotional range Develops verbal language Learns simple rules Expresses wishes and fantasies through symbolic play Begins to establish gender identity Fears loss of live object and/or approval
36 months	Consolidation 1. Individuality 2. Object constancy	Achieving self-boundaries, unifying good/bad aspects of self and others, developing a permanent sense of significant others (object constancy) versus ongoing ambivalence, impulsiveness, intense affective extremes, manipulation	Tolerates separation from mother for longer periods Engages in fantasy play; role playing Shows increased interest in adults other than mother Develops a sense of time Attains gender identity Plays purposefully Communicates verbally Tests reality Can delay gratification

SOURCE: *From* The Psychological Birth of the Human Infant: Symbiosis and Individuation, *MS Mahler, F Pine, A Bergman. Copyright © 1975 by Margaret S. Mahler. Reprinted by permission of Basic Books, Inc., Publishers.*

consequence of the mother having thwarted independence and rewarded dependent behavior during the rapprochement subphase. As a result, the borderline client develops two major fears: the fear of abandonment, which leads to clinging behavior, and fear of engulfment, which leads to distancing from others. The client desperately wants intimate relationships but is terrified of losing the self. These fears are reminiscent of the early choice between mother's love and autonomy, which is the core of the borderline conflict. This conflict is managed by using the primitive dissociation defense, also called *splitting*, which is discussed later in this chapter. Gender identity disturbance may be manifested by the selection of rejecting or abusive partners, the preference for homosexual relationships while maintaining a heterosexual life-style, bizarre fantasies, and transsexualism (Akhtar 1984). False accusations of sexual involvement and sexual acting out with one's therapist are additional examples of identity diffusion problems (Gutheil 1989).

Another area of identity diffusion is temporal discontinuity, which is manifested by a searching for one's origins or keeping detailed chronologic journals. Borderline individuals seem unable to integrate past, present, and future into a continuum. They may frantically plan for the future while reminiscing about past events. These behaviors often lead to difficulty in choosing long-term goals, making career choices, and reassessing personal values.

Affective Instability The failure to resolve object permanence issues is also related to the inability of the borderline person to maintain a consistent, satisfying, affective state. Characteristic of this individual are intense fluctuations of mood, normally of short duration (a few hours to a few days); intense, discrete episodes of depression with accompanying suicidal ideation and gestures; and hypomanic or elated episodes.

Feelings of Emptiness and Aloneness Individuals with borderline personalities report hollow, empty feelings, lack of peaceful solitude, a sense of being disconnected, and **anhedonia** (absence of pleasure in performing ordinarily pleasurable acts). The person may attempt to combat these feelings by compulsive eating, drinking, drug abuse, sexual encounters, and self-mutilation. It is believed that excessive anxiety associated with unresolved separation-individuation issues underlies these behaviors (Perlmutter 1982).

Self-Damaging Acts Impulsiveness, together with identity disturbances, often leads to self-destructive behaviors. Borderline persons are often depressed, but they may make self-destructive gestures to affirm their reality and relieve tension rather than to express a wish to die. Variations in the severity of suicide attempts may be related to age, history of self-directed violence, the presence of an eating disorder, and

psychotic features (Shearer et al. 1988). Additional self-damaging behaviors include self-mutilation (cigarette burns, cutting, taking drug overdoses), recurrent accidents, and physical fights.

Overuse of Primitive Defenses According to Lego (1984, p 419), borderline persons consistently use the following defenses:

• Primitive dissociation (also called **splitting**): The borderline client keeps the opposing affective states of love and hate separate, fearing that the bad aspects (hate) will poison the good aspects (love).

Sharon, a borderline nursing student, loves her instructor during clinical instruction when she receives individual attention but detests the same instructor in the role of distant lecturer.

• Projective identification: The client projects personal feelings onto another, thereby justifying expressions of anger and self-protection.

Paul, a borderline client, accuses a second client, whom he dislikes, of disliking him. Paul refuses to attend any activities at which the other client is present.

• Primitive idealization: Dependent on someone, the client assigns unrealistic powers to that individual.

Francisco tells his nurse, "You are the perfect nurse; I always know nothing bad can happen when you're around."

• Omnipotence: **Omnipotence** is signaled by fantasies of greatness or exaggerated importance.

In response to a question about a suicidal gesture, Brenda states, "Don't worry. I knew I wouldn't die."

• Devaluation: The client criticizes another to defend against a sense of inadequacy.

Phyllis repeatedly criticizes those nursing staff members who do not have master's degrees as being "nontherapeutic."

• Denial: **Denial** is the keeping of disturbing thoughts and feelings out of conscious awareness.

Sue, a nursing student, was expelled from school for academic and clinical incompetence. When the new term began, she attempted to register for the next nursing class. Sue acted dumbfounded when told she could not register.

Distortions of Reality When identity diffusion reaches panic proportions, the borderline individual may experience the following:

• *Depersonalization:* A feeling of strangeness or unreality about one's self.

• *Derealization:* A feeling of disconnectedness from the environment.

Steve has multiple cigarette burns but reports no pain or discomfort and smiles when the lesions are being cleaned and dressed.

Diagnosing

Because of the nature of the borderline personality, the aim of therapy is generally to resolve the immediate crisis and then develop a long-term therapeutic alliance. The long-standing history of affective instability, impulsiveness, and intense, immature relationships leads to persistent maladaptive behavior. The following NANDA nursing diagnoses are integral parts of any nursing care plan for these clients.

Personal Identity Disturbance   Persons diagnosed with borderline personality disorders experience feelings of self-devaluation because of failure to negotiate the rapprochement subphase of separation-individuation. Personal identity disturbances may be identified from the following problems:

• Chameleonlike behavior

• Superficial interactions

• Intense but disruptive relationships

• Play-acting roles

• Mood swings

Ineffective Individual Coping   These clients tend to overuse primitive defenses to the extent that learning adaptive coping skills is highly impaired. These behaviors are frequently observed:

• Splitting, projection, and regression

• Devaluation or idealization of others

• Potential for chemical dependency

• Persistent sense of boredom and loneliness

• Inadequate responses to life stresses and expectations

High Risk for Violence: Self-Directed or Directed at Others   Because of the borderline client's mood swings, limited problem-solving strategies, and self-concept disturbances, the following problems may be observed:

• Intense and often contagious rage

• Impulsiveness

• Self-mutilation or suicidal gestures

• Hostile, threatening verbalizations

• Property destruction

RESEARCH NOTE

Citation
Gallop R et al.: How nursing staff respond to the label "borderline personality disorder." Hosp Community Psychiatry 1989;40:818–819.

Study Problem/Purpose
These researchers attempted to measure the influence of diagnostic labels "schizophrenia" and "borderline personality disorder" on the expressed empathy of psychiatric nursing staff.

Methods
Using the Staff-Patient Interaction Response Scale (SPIRS), the authors surveyed 124 registered nurses from five short-term acute psychiatric settings. The SPIRS instrument assesses the subject's expressed empathy according to written responses to a set of hypothetical client and stimulus statements. The SPIRS instrument possesses both test-retest reliability and validity of $p < .001$.

Findings
A significant proportion of nurses ($p < .001$) gave responses that were belittling or contradictory and displayed a low level of empathy for hypothetical clients with borderline personality disorders. Chi-square analysis showed that subjects in the youngest age group were more empathic and less belittling than subjects in other age groups.

Implications
Findings should not be generalized because the subjects were measured by self-report rather than by an observational instrument. However, differences in attitude may be reflected in actual nurse behaviors. If these findings reflect actual nurse behaviors, clients labeled as having borderline personality disorders may receive a qualitatively lower level of care than clients who are perceived by nurses as being "ill," e.g., schizophrenic clients.

Planning and Implementing Interventions

See the accompanying nursing care plan for the client with a borderline personality disorder. When providing care, be alert to the often intense feelings that the borderline client may precipitate. These feelings (e.g., anger, guilt, overgiving, rescuing, rigidity) may cloud

NURSING CARE PLAN

A Client with a Borderline Personality

Client Care Goals	Nursing Planning/ Interventions	Evaluation

Nursing Diagnosis: *Personal identity disturbance related to history of physical or sexual abuse*

Client Care Goals	Nursing Planning/ Interventions	Evaluation
The client will identify and resolve the immediate crisis and initiate the development of a secure sense of self.	Develop a consistent treatment plan involving all staff.	Behaves and dresses appropriately in social situations.
	Encourage staff to discuss feelings directed toward client in staff meetings.	Develops a realistic view of self by identifying strengths and weaknesses.
	Encourage client to discuss personal body image.	Explores how beliefs and perceptions of situations influence responses and roles played.
	Assist client to deal with loss of body image associated with history of abuse.	Establishes goals that can be reached in a specified time period.
	Help client to examine belief systems and identify how perceptions and beliefs influence responses.	Identifies consequences of behaviors.
	Encourage client to write an autobiography and give feedback.	Evaluates personal progress.
	Encourage client to set daily objectives and assist in meeting goals.	Sustains a situation-appropriate mood, i.e., absence of mood swings.
	Give positive reinforcement for achievement of goals.	Discusses modes of sexual expression and ways of achieving satisfaction.
	Have client evaluate personal progress weekly.	
	Point out to client when affective responses are inappropriate or incongruent to situations.	
	Help client identify rewards of both appropriate and inappropriate responses.	
	Encourage participation in a variety of group situations.	
	Assist to accept disappointments by altering thoughts with such statements as, "It would be nice if . . ." rather than magnifying losses.	
	Confront client with various ways in which he or she denies pleasure.	
	Discuss with client ways to change feelings and behavior.	

▶

Client Care Goals	Nursing Planning/ Interventions	Evaluation

Nursing Diagnosis: *Ineffective individual coping (Related factors: destructive behavior toward self and others; use of defenses such as splitting, projecting, and regression; verbal manipulation)*

Client Care Goals	Nursing Planning/ Interventions	Evaluation
The client will demonstrate moderate and stable means of expressing feelings and relating to others.	Assign nonjudgmental staff to work with client; maintain consistency.	Develops a therapeutic relationship with at least one staff member.
	Schedule frequent staff meetings; establish behavioral expectations.	Verbally acknowledges both positive and negative characteristics about self and others.
	Schedule family meetings if possible.	Explores responses to other's behavior and relates these responses to feelings about oneself.
	Inform client of acceptable behavior and unit rules.	
	Enforce limits when client attempts to manipulate.	Describes feelings rather than somatizing them.
	Delegate to one staff member the final authority and responsibility for the treatment plan.	Identifies situations in which manipulation is employed and verbalizes the consequences.
	Use problem-solving techniques to help the client make changes.	Identifies and uses modes of responding that are assertive and responsible.
	Point out when the client is experiencing both positive and negative responses toward the same person.	Engages in constructive and satisfying activities during free time.
	Challenge client's idealizations of staff.	Sustains a meaningful relationship without using primitive defenses such as projection and splitting.
	Point out discrepancies in client's behavior.	Explores past use of chemicals as a means of coping.
	Tell client you do not feel the way he or she imagines that you do.	Takes times to process a problem, using problem-solving skills rather than acting impulsively.
	Draw a parallel between how you respond to the client's behavior and how others are likely to respond.	Sustains a long-term therapeutic relationship.
	Remain neutral to client's comments, being neither flattered nor offended.	
	Do not seek client's approval.	
	Explore feelings and experiences rather than making interpretations.	
	Use group techniques to teach responsibility for self.	

Client Care Goals	Nursing Planning/ Interventions	Evaluation
	Use role play to demonstrate adaptive communications.	
	Teach client to recognize needs requiring immediate attention and those that may be delayed.	
	Avoid rescuing or rejecting client; rather, deal with the manipulative behavior.	
	Have client record daily experiences, feelings, and responses in a journal; use the journal to enhance the nurse-client relationship.	
	Use a "transitional object" (e.g., appointment card, postcard) when out of town or out of touch with the client.	

Nursing Diagnosis: *High risk for violence: Self-directed or directed at others (Related factors: inability to verbalize frustration and anger, history of impulsive self-mutilating acts, hostile and threatening verbalizations)*

Client Care Goals	Nursing Planning/ Interventions	Evaluation
The client will eliminate destructive acting-out behavior, e.g., suicidal/homicidal threats and gestures.	Assess history of previous self-mutilation.	Verbalizes feelings of anger and frustration when they occur.
	Observe behavior and document every shift.	Requests time-out periods, physical activities, and p.r.n. medications when anger cannot be defused by verbalizing.
	Utilize suicide precautions as necessary.	
	Tell client that staff will not permit injury to self or others.	Identifies precipitating factors, e.g., rejection, separation, loss, disappointment.
	Contract with client to notify staff members when suicidal/self-mutilating thoughts occur.	Seeks out staff member with whom to discuss anger or releases anger in constructive activity.
	Help client identify alternatives to self-destructive behavior.	
	Explore self-destructive fantasies.	Identifies alternatives to self-mutilating behavior.
	Help client identify situations in which self-destructive ideas occur.	Uses "I" statements when dealing with anger and frustration.
	Explore hostile relationships in the past.	
	When client verbalizes anger during one-on-one sessions, point out that the anger is not caused by the current situation but by perceptions of things in the past.	

▶

Client Care Goals	Nursing Planning/ Interventions	Evaluation
	Modulate amounts of warmth shown to the client.	
	Help clients explore ways to express anger constructively.	
	Encourage verbal expression of anger and give positive reinforcement for same.	
	Explore with client how to direct the energy of anger toward positive ends, motivation for change, problem solving.	
	Deal with client's transference phenomena, which are expressions of anger and hatred.	
	Utilize treatment contracts between client and team with mutually agreed upon goals.	
	Give consistent feedback for goal achievement or lack thereof.	

judgment and lead to nursing decisions that the client may interpret as abandonment, distancing, engulfment, or lack of empathy. Staff members who work with these clients should be skillful in nurturing the "adult" side of the client while simultaneously protecting and empathizing with the vulnerable "child" within (Johnson and Silver 1988).

Inez presents herself as a pathetic victim of involuntary hospitalization. As a result, the staff becomes guilt-ridden and prematurely grants an out-of-hospital pass. Inez, in turn, acts out her sense of abandonment by making a serious suicide attempt.

Responding to seductive, angry, or solicitous behavior in either a negative or rescuing manner may reinforce the inappropriate responses of the client. An ideal therapeutic relationship is one in which the nurse: (a) maintains a matter-of-fact but caring approach, (b) establishes and maintains consistent, firm limits, (c) makes regular appointments, and (d) mobilizes the healthy aspects of the client's personality.

As with all clients with personality disorders, use clinical supervision, staff counseling sessions, and team meetings to identify the client's underlying dynamic issues and to work toward decreasing distortions in communications between the client and others.

Wendy is a 27-year-old dental hygienist who comes from a blue-collar family and gives a history of physical and sexual abuse as a child. Her biologic parents were divorced when she was a young child; two younger brothers are addicted to opiates and have had many legal problems related to drug use. Wendy's chemical use was sporadic and primarily recreational until completion of college. At an early age, she married a laborer to escape her home situation. She became pregnant twice but aborted both times. Wendy was divorced a few years later. Prior to her divorce, she lived with her second husband, a chef of Hispanic origin who sought a traditional male-dominated home life. This relationship was marked by verbal and physical abuse, withholding of financial support, sexual indiscretions, and alcohol and cocaine use. Wendy became pregnant three times during this six-year marriage, aborting each fetus prior to five months' gestation.

Wendy presents as a slim, well-groomed, and well-developed young woman with generously applied makeup. She is consistently cheerful on initial contact; she minimizes problems with her husband and is involved in many outside activities. Although she has maintained residence in the community and has worked for many years in the same dental office, she has no close friends, claiming that her husband forbids socializing. Her primary outlet is physical activity. She jogs, bicycles, plays tennis and racquetball, and does daily aerobic exercises. She seeks out sports that involve contact with the opposite sex and always wears designer sports attire when not working.

Throughout the two-year dental hygiene program, Wendy was identified as being very intelligent but manipulative. Instructors documented patterns of tardiness, absenteeism, illness, and accidents in every course. When instructors confronted her behaviors, Wendy gave elaborate rationalizations, which often appeared implausible. However, Wendy was able to meet all course requirements and completed the program as scheduled.

Three weeks prior to taking state board examinations, Wendy cut both wrists, lacerating the tendons and requiring immobilization. She had left her husband, and her new boyfriend had evicted her from his home. She denied any intent to kill herself but stated, "I couldn't help it. I was so confused and desperate." She was able to write the examinations but demonstrated indifference to her injuries by such expressions as, "Oh, I hurt myself." Classmates reported feeling surprised and shocked by both the behavior and her response to it.

After receiving her license, Wendy got a job with a large health maintenance organization. During this time, her supervisor confronted her several times for wearing seductive clothing and makeup. She became very friendly with male clients and saw some of them socially outside the office.

Wendy established residence with a female friend on a house-sharing basis but consistently had difficulty meeting her financial obligations for home maintenance. This placed increased strain on their relationship. Wendy's chemical addiction became apparent to her employer within six months following her licensure. Her rapid mood swings, irritability, and absenteeism led to a confrontation and subsequent admission to a substance-treatment facility. Wendy denied chemical dependency during the first week, displaying intense mood swings and angry outbursts at the staff. When she threatened suicide if not released from the program, she was committed to a psychiatric program.

Within twenty-four hours of admission, Wendy became very calm and identified herself as a "hygienist" to other clients. She participated in all program activities but assumed a therapist role. She lacked insight into her behavior, intellectually accepted "alcohol" as her problem, and requested to be reassigned to the substance-treatment facility. As it was determined that she was no longer actively suicidal, the transfer was made.

When she was transferred to the substance unit, she talked incessantly about the poor standard of care on the psychiatric unit. She focused on staff deficiencies and praised the performance of the substance-treatment staff. She was confronted almost daily about her seductive attire and decision to socialize only with male clients. She attempted to pit one staff member against another and, indeed, had some success. A social worker cried because she felt helpless when Wendy was transferred from the psychiatric unit, while an alcohol counselor raged about Wendy's manipulation of him.

Wendy's treatment program consisted of daily groups and one-to-one sessions, including occupational, recreational, and music therapies, and psychotherapies. Because of her anxiety and depressive components of her disorder, her physician ordered 2 mg of thiothixine (Navane) twice daily. She continued to receive thiothixene until her discharge.

Wendy remained in the treatment facility for five weeks. At the time of discharge, she demonstrated increased consistency of mood, the ability to verbally identify consequences of her behavior, and some capacity for discussing the anger she felt in daily situations. She would not consider long-range goals, especially those pertaining to employment or living arrangements. During her last week on the unit, she called her Alcoholics Anonymous sponsor, who invited Wendy to live with her until Wendy could reestablish herself. A one-year follow-up showed Wendy working as an office manager and public relations coordinator for a busy dental clinic in a large metropolitan area. She was still actively working in her recovery program.

Evaluating/Outcome Criteria

Although borderline clients often appear relatively healthy, the nurse may find it difficult to maintain a therapeutic alliance with them because of their intense and contagious affects, impulsiveness, and the intense feelings they trigger in others. The quality of object relationships, especially that between the therapist and the client, is crucial to the outcome of therapy.

Personal Identity Disturbance   Successful integration of fragmented aspects of the borderline client's personality ("healing the split") depends upon the client's ability to remain in a sustained therapeutic relationship (Platt-Koch 1983). Among clients who do remain in therapy, those who demonstrate likeability, warmth, reliability, interest in people, talents, and social as well as occupational skills have the most favorable treatment prognosis (Woollcott 1985).

Ineffective Individual Coping   The use of primitive defenses may be replaced by more adequate problem-solving skills over time. Encourage the client who has innate cognitive psychomotor talents to sublimate feelings of intense rage into productive outlets (e.g., art, music, dance). Receiving positive reinforcements for these achievements may enhance the development of effective coping strategies.

High Risk for Violence: Self-Directed or Directed at Others   According to Woollcott (1985), those clients who are most infantile and regressed (as opposed to those who have more narcissistic features) tend to achieve greater affective stability. Confront the client's anger during one-to-one sessions by comparing the client's responses to those of others. This strategy may cause the client to think before acting.

The borderline person has established patterns of responding to others in any situation. This pattern may sabotage the client's objectives. Furthermore, these clients usually terminate therapy when the acute crisis has ended. The following are among the factors that influence the likelihood of successful change:

- The severity of the client's emotional deprivation

- The rigidity of the client's personality structure

- The client's ego strengths

- The client's motivation to change

- The nurse's skill and commitment

- Social support systems in the client's family or milieu that favor the desired change

The Nursing Process and Histrionic Personality Disorders

Assessing

Defining Characteristics of the Histrionic Personality Persons with histrionic personalities show a lifelong tendency for dramatic, egocentric, attention-seeking response patterns. Their seeming lack of sincerity and of emotional commitment contributes to disturbances in interpersonal relationships. These people appear to be continually "on stage" and acting a role. Their extensive use of coping patterns based on repression, denial, and dissociation leads them to deal with problems as though they do not exist. Because more females than males are being diagnosed with this condition, the diagnosis of histrionic personality disorder may reflect the bias of the clinician (Ford and Widiger 1989).

Dramatic, Exhibitionistic, and Egocentric Responses Responses are characterized by exaggerated emotional expression; craving for attention, activity, and excitement; overreaction to minor stressors; irrational emotional outbursts; and temper tantrums.

Difficulty Sustaining Interpersonal Relationships Histrionic clients constantly need love, reassurance, and validation of existence because of their feelings of dependency and helplessness. For this reason, histrionic persons have problems with significant relationships. These individuals are likely to manipulate others to hold on to a love object while being highly inconsiderate and lacking empathy.

Sexual Expression The histrionic person is generally provocative and seductive and uses sexual expression to manipulate and control others in relationships. The client is often unaware of this flamboyance and how others perceive it. Individuals are often competitive with those of the same sex and seductive with the opposite sex. This personality disorder is

more frequent in women than men. In males, it may be associated with a homosexual arousal pattern.

Dysphoric Moods Dysphoria is a sense of disquiet or restlessness. Histrionic persons may experience depression when their demands for attention and affection are not met. They may act out in a suicidal fashion. Often, these individuals behave frivolously, acting silly and making nuisances of themselves.

Cognitive Dimensions Histrionic personalities are much more interested in creative or imaginative pursuits than in analytic or academic achievements. They tend to be impressionable and highly suggestible and tend to look to authority figures for magical solutions to problems.

Health Patterns Regression and the development of somatic and/or dissociative disorders are frequent among histrionic people. These disabling symptoms may serve the purpose of calling attention to the person. They generally occur when an audience is present or when an unpleasant situation is anticipated. Substance use, depression, seizurelike activity, blackouts, falling, dizziness, or reactive psychoses may lead to hospitalization.

Linda, a 33-year-old woman who is twice divorced, was observed at the outpatient clinic responding flirtatiously to male staff members. She was neatly groomed but dressed in a low-cut peasant blouse, a tight miniskirt, and bright red knee-high boots. When called by the female therapist for her appointment, Linda screamed that she had waited too long, complaining loudly about patients' rights to rapid treatment. She quickly captured the attention of others in the waiting room. Then Linda feigned dizziness and "fell" as she arose from her chair. During the ensuing session, Linda complained that several men had made passes at her on the bus. When the therapist pointed out that her manner of dress was a probable factor, Linda accused her of being jealous. Linda terminated the interview at that point and left the office, slamming the door behind her and stating, "My problems are physical, and no one cares whether I live or die. You'll be sorry for treating me this way!"

Diagnosing

Although histrionic clients may look and act as though they have few problems, major dysfunctions are present. Nursing diagnoses may include the following:

High Risk for Injury The dramatic, impulsive responses of histrionic clients may lead to injuries or suicidal gestures. Problems often include the following:

- Increased potential for accidents, e.g., falls and automobile accidents

- Self-inflicted injuries/suicide attempts

- Misdiagnosis of physical illness

Ineffective Individual Coping   Ineffective coping is manifested by behavior resulting from high anxiety levels, limited judgment, and need for attention and reassurance. These behaviors are often observed:

- Seductiveness (e.g., in dress, makeup, mannerisms, conversational tone and content)

- Substance use

- Manipulation of others, lack of consideration

- Emotional lability

- Low frustration tolerance

- Irresponsibility, vanity, silliness, frivolity

- Lack of insight

- Overuse of denial

Planning and Implementing Interventions

Nursing care for the histrionic client closely resembles that for borderline persons. Since many health professionals view these clients as feigning illness, it is imperative to carry out a thorough physical assessment. In addition, the potential for self-injury is a risk. Suicidal assessment should be a component of daily interviews when the client is in crisis. Treatment plans need to emphasize that staff should avoid paying attention to the sexual provocations of these clients. Positive reinforcement for appropriate behavior should be stressed.

Evaluating/Outcome Criteria

Even when intervention strategies are implemented consistently, histrionic clients tend to manifest more denial than clients with other disorders in the dramatic-erratic clusters. The treatment plan should emphasize the nurse's need to remain objective.

High Risk for Injury   When acting-out behavior is eliminated, the potential for self-destructive acts should be decreased. The client, however, may develop a conversion or dissociative reaction that impedes optimal functioning and forces others to pay attention to his or her needs.

Ineffective Individual Coping   It is not unusual for histrionic clients to exaggerate all aspects of living and loving. If the client can learn to be less conspicuous and to express emotions appropriately, then many seductive, attention-seeking behaviors will diminish. There is always the possibility that when the client's needs for affection and attention are thwarted, vulnerability to depression may increase.

The Nursing Process and Narcissistic Personality Disorders

Assessing

Defining Characteristics of the Narcissistic Personality   Persons with narcissistic personalities have difficulty regulating self-esteem and self-expression (Masterson 1981). Jacobson (1979, p 431) advises that the term *narcissism* should apply to clients whose self-esteem is too low, as well as inappropriately high. Characteristics most frequently observed include a sense of entitlement, interpersonal manipulations, lack of empathy, and indifference toward others.

Grandiosity   Grandiosity is evidence by expressions of exaggerated self-importance, self-absorption, and egocentricity. This inflated self-concept may be a compensation for feelings of diminished self-worth. Isolating a child from the feedback of others and the parents' failing to mirror the child's behavior may contribute to this disorder. *Mirroring* or "mirror images" reflect what the parents think of and how they treat the child. When coming in contact with people outside the home, the child may discover a discrepancy between the way others treat him or her and the mirror images developed at home. Excessive boasting may result from this inconsistency in self-concept.

Preoccupations   The narcissistic person is generally preoccupied and fantasizes about power, success, idealized love, morals, and intelligence. These behaviors may be the result of overidealization of the child by the parents.

Exhibitionism   Exhibitionistic behavior is evidenced by the constant seeking of support and admiration from others. Because of their limited interests, these clients perseverate about themselves to the point of boring others.

Vacillation of Affective Response   In spite of the narcissistic individual's extensive use of rationalization for failures, there is an underlying sense of rage, shame, and diminished self-esteem. The perceptive nurse may observe cool indifference, emptiness, humiliation, uncontrolled anger, or desire for revenge.

Dysfunctional Interpersonal Relationships   Persons who have narcissistic personalities feel entitled to special favors and attention. Further, they refuse to assume mutual responsibilities in relationships. They tend to exploit others and disregard their rights. Kernberg (1975) emphasizes that chronic, intense envy and defenses against envy lead to idealization or devaluation of others. Responses to others may include lack of empathy, mistrust, lack of intimacy, accusations of incompetence, or demands for unattainable perfection.

Socialization   In addition to having problems forming and sustaining interpersonal relationships, the narcissistic person may experience occupational divergences. Kohut (1971) describes work inhibitions as peculiar to this group. In contrast, Cameron and Rychlak (1985, p 460) note that these individuals often assume active leadership roles, putting their power needs to work and attacking the established working order. One may may also consider the effect of the culture on the development of socialization skills. The post–World War II philosophy of "looking out for number one" may well have contributed to the rise of identification of narcissistic disorders and their inclusion as a diagnostic category in DSM-III (Widiger and Frances 1985).

Sexual Expression　Perverse sexual fantasies, promiscuity, or homosexuality may be associated with this disorder. There may be confusion regarding sex-role behavior as a result of learned defenses against libidinal and ego needs conflicts (Wilson and Prabucki 1983, p 1237).

Alicia is a 40-year-old teacher who seeks professional counseling after dropping out of a graduate program. She presents as a slender, well-groomed individual. Alicia makes it clear upon initial contact that she has a wide circle of friends. Indeed, she devotes the first thirty minutes of the session to recounting sexual encounters and venting anger that concern about AIDS is limiting her sexual partners. She states she had a live-in relationship with one partner for 15 years but that recently this partner became discontented with her need to "party." Consequently the two are not "communicating." Alicia defends her desire to seek out a variety of sexual partners by focusing on her personal needs and the "lack of consideration" of her significant other.

When questioned about dropping out of graduate school, Alicia rationalizes her failure by blaming it on a "hostile major professor" and further proclaiming, "I know more than he does." She describes herself as the "leader" in her group of six graduate students and interprets this to mean that they have great respect for her.

She tells the therapists that she attempted to call two friends following her withdrawal from school. She dramatically and self-righteously expresses anger and disappointment that they were not available to her. (One was vacationing out of state and the other was hospitalized for major surgery.) When the therapist inquires how her friend was doing following surgery, Alicia responded, "How should I know? That's not my problem. She never bothered to call me back."

Alicia requests that the therapist set up Saturday morning appointments (no office hours were normally scheduled on this day), because she became very tired in the afternoons and always took a nap. When the therapist refuses to meet this request, she becomes angry and shouts, "You're just like all the rest of them. No one considers my needs! I'll see to it that your supervisor hears about this and I'll let all my friends know how incompetent you are as a therapist."

Diagnosing

Like people with histrionic and borderline personality disorders, narcissistic people have problems associated with disturbed self-concept and coping abilities. The following dysfunctional behavior may be observed:

Personal Identity Disturbance

- Self-centeredness
- Exaggerated sense of importance and intelligence
- Setting unrealistic goals
- Indifference to the feelings of others
- Interpersonal exploitiveness

Ineffective Individual Coping

- Excessive use of denial of shortcomings, rationalization of errors, and projection of blame
- Inconsistent and intense emotional responses to interpersonal relationships
- Occupational dysfunctions
- Preoccupation with or fantasies of power
- Exhibitionism

Planning and Implementing Interventions

The objectives for care of narcissistic clients are to help clients accept feedback without defensiveness and rationalization, to increase their capacity to tolerate frustration and disappointment, and to help them appreciate the rights and needs of others. Interventions are geared toward using the therapeutic alliance to work through feelings of abandonment, rejection, shame, and self-doubt, thereby heightening self-esteem. Heterogeneous group therapies have been successful with some narcissistic clients (Wong 1980). However, the client often terminates both individual and group work prematurely.

Evaluating/Outcome Criteria

The goal is for the narcissistic individual to learn how to empathize with others by recognizing that it is not necessary to be right all the time—i.e., that imperfections in self and others exist. Although some clients develop positive roles through the use of creativity and humor, most substitute hypochondriacal behavior and a sense of emptiness and lowered self-esteem for previous behaviors and feelings.

The Nursing Process and Antisocial Personality Disorders

Assessing

Defining Characteristics of the Antisocial Personality The antisocial personality was one of the earliest to be identified. It has been labeled *psychopathy, sociopathy,* and *moral insanity.* Without question, it is the most researched and validated of these disorders (Widiger and Frances 1985, p 623). Yet, there have been no great strides in our understanding of the syndrome or the successful treatment of these individuals (Reid 1985). One reason is that most antisocial persons do not seek medical help but often come to the attention of authorities because of criminal activity. Such criminal behavior creates anger toward the person committing it, which precludes medical research support. It is difficult to identify the antisocial personality disorder as an illness when the behaviors are seemingly intentional, antagonistic, and self-serving.

Some clinicians are concerned about the term *antisocial* because it connotes criminality. In fact, the behaviors may be adaptive in people with certain life-styles, e.g., in the transient pieceworker, in people holding high-risk jobs, and even in the chronically mentally ill (Cameron and Rychlak 1985, Reid 1985, Travin and Protter 1982). The nurse must remember that manipulation, which is a hallmark of the antisocial client's behavior, may be a normal, nondestructive mode of meeting one's needs. however, when used to control others, manipulation interferes with interpersonal relationships. In antisocial clients, the drive to manipulate others is paramount, because these clients feel a need to be "number one" at all times.

These are the essential features of the antisocial personality, according to the DSM-III-R:

• A history of continuous and chronic antisocial behavior that violates the rights of others

• A pattern of antisocial behavior that begins before the age of 15 and persists into adult life

• A failure to sustain adequate role performance over a period of several years

The antisocial behavior is not due to severe mental retardation, schizophrenia, or manic episodes.

It is estimated that 3 percent of American men and 1 percent of American women have antisocial personalities, although many researchers predict that the latter figure will increase as female life-styles become more like those of the male population (Reid 1985, Rowe 1984). These statistics may reflect clinician

diagnostic bias in assigning this label predominantly to men (Ford and Widiger 1989). There may also be a relationship between conduct and attention deficit disorders during the prepubertal years and the later development of antisocial personality syndrome. Although Schlesinger (1980) differentiates the psychopath, antisocial personality, and sociopath according to types and motives of criminal activities, all syndromes are classified as antisocial personality disorders in this chapter.

The study of developmental considerations has been hampered by the fact that the majority of investigators have used prisoners as research subjects. Although many criminals are sociopaths, not all sociopaths are found in prisons.

Physiologic Factors Researchers, in an effort to identify biologic markers, have found that antisocial persons have a history of hyperactivity in childhood, a high rate of nonspecific electroencephalographic (EEG) abnormalities, and autonomic nervous system dysfunction manifested by high arousal states. The dysfunctional arousal of the autonomic nervous system may help to explain the early risk-taking behaviors (Cloninger 1978). In 1978, Rowe reported that brain trauma was a plausible precursor to this disorder. More recently, depletion of serotonin and 5-HIAA (the metabolite of serotonin) has been associated with some forms of primitive aggression in mammals. Likewise, impulsive physical violence in humans (including violent suicide) has been negatively correlated with levels of 5-HIAA in cerebrospinal fluid. These data are consistent with the finding that antisocial behavior frequently peaks in late adolescence and young adulthood, when 5-HIAA levels are usually lowest (Reid 1985, p 832).

Cognitive Factors Cognitive development is impaired to the extent that the individual is dominated by interests that are immediate and personally relevant (Shapiro 1965). This would account for the cunning abilities of the antisocial person to capitalize on others' vulnerabilities and quickly achieve personal goals. Gorenstein (1982, p 377) reports that although antisocial persons are able to acquire new ideas, they tend to act in ways that have been previously reinforced. This researcher believes that impaired *cognitive flexibility* characterizes the thinking processes of these persons. Perhaps the long-term planning deficiencies seen in this group are partially explained by this data.

Cognitive theorists, using measures of skill acquisition, hypothesize that developmental arrest of the antisocial personality occurs between the ages of 7–11. During this time, the normal child lacks the ability to reverse roles and seeks retribution for transgressions, showing little empathy or guilt. Around the age of 13, the normal child develops reciprocity with others and is able to abstract and be an empathic partner in a relationship. The antisocial person, however, remains narcissistic and intolerant of the rights of others.

Psychodynamic Factors Psychodynamic theorists propose that antisocial individuals use primitive, global defenses, such as projection and splitting, to distance themselves from others. Antisocial persons stabilize their identities by using these defenses and filling life with action and stimulation to blot out affect and anxiety. Hence, the nurse may observe a "caricature of love" (Cleckley 1964) as the antisocial person playacts relationships (Reid 1985).

Social Factors Social considerations in the development of antisocial personality disorder include the following:

- Failure of early identification experiences

- Excessive, harsh, inconsistent, or overpermissive discipline

- Lower socioeconomic level

- Lack of nurturing

- History of broken homes

- Alcoholic or antisocial parents

- Numerous parent surrogates

- Parental and or community rejection (self-fulfilling prophecy)

- Positive reinforcement of acting out or antisocial behavior during early childhood

Reid (1985) also identifies subtle encouragement of a child's antisocial behavior to bolster pathologic family stability, a finding that is consistent with family systems theory.

It is most likely that the antisocial personality disorder has multiple causes. The nurse is cautioned not to make hasty judgments regarding the issue of criminality versus illness. If one views psychopathy as an internal defect, the antisocial person does not feel satisfaction with this disruptive life-style. Nonetheless, it is wise to consider the adaptive nature of this disorder, as well as its encouragement in an increasingly pleasure-seeking Western culture. The public anger aroused by antisocial persons and their behavior is likely due to fear and a sense of powerlessness to stop or prevent their actions (Figure 16–1). The following example illustrates the typical behavior of an antisocial person who has become disruptive without overt criminality.

Jack is a handsome, charming man of 38 who was the vice-president of a prominent general construction company. Jack is the second of three boys. Both his parents were alcoholics, and his father had spent many years

putting together unsuccessful business deals. Jack was encouraged and applauded by his father, even as a child, whenever he outsmarted someone else, particularly those in authority, such as teachers and police. Jack's first legal involvement occurred at the age of 14, when he stole a neighbor's car and went joyriding. His charm and persuasiveness, as well as his neighbor's perception that Jack was a neglected child, kept the neighbor from pressing charges. Jack continued to be involved in antisocial activities, financing his college education by stealing and selling exams and dealing drugs on campus.

Jack initially sought consultation due to marital problems arising from his repeated acts of infidelity and lying. His third wife was contemplating a divorce after finding a two-carat diamond engagement ring in his briefcase. He heatedly denied the ring was for someone else. He did not give it to his wife, however, stating, "You spoiled the surprise." The few people who know him well in social and work relationships view Jack as unreliable, unethical, unpredictable, and insincere. They call him a "pathological liar." Three months prior to this visit, Jack had been caught embezzling over $300,000 from the construction company. His response to the discovery was, "Somehow there's been a big misunderstanding on the part of the accountants." He was able to charm the company owner out of pressing charges against him. Jack paid back only a part of the embezzled funds, citing high entertainment and travel expenses on company business for his need for the money.

When news of the embezzlement reached the community, Jack denied the story and stated, "He [the owner]

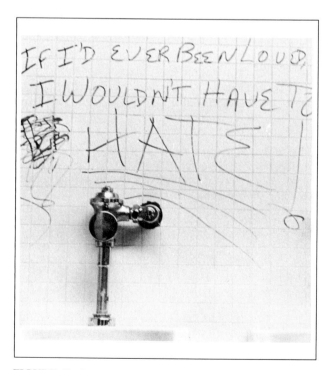

FIGURE 16–1 People with antisocial personality disorders are storm centers in their social relations and sometimes thrive on the trouble they create. Underlying their behavior and attitudes may be feelings they seldom express.

is jealous of my intelligence and was looking for a way to get rid of me." After leaving this company, Jack formed his own business. He again engaged in illegal and unethical business practices. He spent large sums skydiving, flying to Switzerland to ski, and having cosmetic surgery. He became preoccupied with both his own and his wife's appearance. He demanded that she have cosmetic surgery, dye her hair, and wear tinted contact lenses to alter the color of her eyes. Jack had several hair transplants and exercised excessively. As the marriage began to deteriorate, Jack began to use cocaine and drink alcohol daily. On one occasion, while intoxicated, he beat his wife severely because "she was losing her sex appeal." He told the therapist during the first interview, "Any problems we have are due to my wife's behavior; I'm here only to please her."

Jack canceled appointments for both his second and third sessions, stating, "My tax accountants have to spend some time with me. The IRS thinks I've cheated them out of some money."

Lifelong patterns of antisocial behavior often emerge during childhood and adolescence. However, this diagnosis is not applied to people younger than 18. DSM-III-R criteria for the antisocial personality disorder are shown in the accompanying box. The following subjective and objective data have been adapted from this source:

- Has impaired superego (conscience) development associated with faulty identification process

- Is relatively free of anxiety; shows free-floating anxiety only when under external stress

- Is unable to defer pleasure; wants immediate gratification

- Cannot feel guilt, although easily verbalizes or playacts a remorseful role

- Lacks interest in morals or values

- Is impulsive without considering the alternatives or consequences

- Is insincere and lies

- Uses people as objects for gratification of needs and discards them when they are no longer useful

- Commits frequent sexual indiscretions

- Lacks responsibility for commitments, including marriage, family, and occupation

- Manipulates situations and people for personal gain without concern for the rights or feelings of others

- Is extroverted; makes good first impressions due to charm and persuasiveness

- Is financially and emotionally dependent on others but fears intimacy

- Has few close friends but many casual relationships

- Changes jobs frequently, has long periods of unemployment, and is belligerent

- Has poor school and work history

- Abuses or is dependent on drugs

- Is intellectually competent; however, does not profit from experience or mistakes

- Is often involved in socially unacceptable or criminal activities, including crimes of violence such as rape

- Has no major disorders of thought, affect, or brain function

Diagnosing

Despite the quantity of assessment data, the primary nursing diagnoses for the antisocial client are **Ineffective individual coping** and **Impaired social interaction**. These problems are often observed:

Ineffective Individual Coping

- Altered participation in society

- Verbal and nonverbal manipulation

- Destructive behavior toward self and others

- Overuse of defense mechanisms of denial, splitting, projection, rationalization, and intellectualization

- Impaired problem-solving abilities

Impaired Social Interaction

- Altered self-esteem evidenced by affective disturbances (grandiosity, depression)

- Lack of responsibility, accountability, or commitment

- Lying

- Distancing relationships

- Nonparticipation in therapy

- Impulsiveness

Planning and Implementing Interventions

Because antisocial people manipulate others so successfully, it is unlikely that the individuals will seek change unless faced with severe external stress. In clinical situations, the nurse's responses to these clients are critical to developing and maintaining a therapeu-

Diagnostic Criteria for 301.70
Antisocial Personality Disorder

A. Current age at least 18.

B. Evidence of Conduct Disorder with onset before age 15, as indicated by a history of *three* or more of the following:

1. Was often truant
2. Ran away from home overnight at least twice while living in parental or parental surrogate home (or once without returning)
3. Often initiated physical fights
4. Used a weapon in more than one fight
5. Forced someone into sexual activity with him or her
6. Was physically cruel to animals
7. Was physically cruel to other people
8. Deliberately destroyed others' property (other than by fire-setting)
9. Deliberately engaged in fire-setting
10. Often lied (rather than to avoid physical or sexual abuse)
11. Has stolen without confrontation of a victim on more than one occasion (including forgery)
12. Has stolen with confrontation of a victim (e.g., mugging, purse-snatching, extortion, armed robbery)

C. A pattern of irresponsible and antisocial behavior since the age of 15, as indicated by at least *four* of the following:

1. Is unable to sustain consistent work behavior, as indicated by any of the following (including similar behavior in academic settings if the person is a student):
   a. Significant unemployment for six months or more within five years when expected to work and work was available
   b. Repeated absences from work explained by illness in self or family
   c. Abandonment of several jobs without realistic plans for others
2. Fails to conform to social norms with respect to lawful behavior, as indicated by repeatedly performing antisocial acts that are grounds for arrest (whether arrested or not), e.g., destroying property, harassing others, stealing, pursuing an illegal occupation
3. Is irritable and aggressive, as indicated by repeated physical fights or assaults (not required by one's job or to defend someone or oneself), including spouse- or child-beating

4. Repeatedly fails to honor financial obligations, as indicated by defaulting on debts or failing to provide child support or support for other dependents on a regular basis
5. Fails to plan ahead, or is impulsive, as indicated by one or both of the following:
   a. Traveling from place to place without a prearranged job or clear goal for the period of travel or clear idea about when the travel will terminate
   b. Lack of a fixed address for a month or more
6. Has no regard for the truth, as indicated by repeated lying, use of aliases, or "conning" others for personal profit or pleasure
7. Is reckless regarding his or her own or others' personal safety, as indicated by driving while intoxicated, or recurrent speeding
8. If a parent or guardian, lacks ability to function as a responsible parent, as indicated by one or more of the following:
   a. Malnutrition of child
   b. Child's illness resulting from lack of minimal hygiene
   c. Failure to obtain medical care for a seriously ill child
   d. Child's dependence on neighbors or nonresident relatives for food or shelter
   e. Failure to arrange for a caretaker for young child when parent is away from home
   f. Repeated squandering, on personal items, of money required for household necessities
9. Has never sustained a totally monogamous relationship for more than one year
10. Lacks remorse (feels justified in having hurt, mistreated, or stolen from another)

D. Occurrence of antisocial behavior not exclusively during the course of Schizophrenia or Manic Episodes.

SOURCE: Reprinted with permission of the American Psychiatric Association: Diagnostic and Statistical Manual of Mental Disorders, *ed 3, revised. APA, 1987, pp 344–346.*

INTERVENTION

Guidelines for Working with the Antisocial Client

- Use a concerned but matter-of-fact approach.
- Set, communicate, and maintain consistent rules and regulations for all clients.
- Do not argue, bargain, or rationalize.
- Confront inappropriate behaviors without anger, punitiveness, or personalization.
- Do not seek approval.
- Set limits on all interactions.
- Be alert for flattery or verbal attacks.
- Do not permit client to dictate therapeutic regimen.
- Using contracts and relaxation techniques, teach client how to delay immediate gratification and impulsiveness.
- Teach client to redirect thrill-seeking impulses into socially acceptable outlets, e.g., race car driving versus speeding.
- Use peer pressure (e.g., groups, buddy systems) to modify manipulative behaviors.
- Use reinforcing techniques to achieve desired behaviors.
- Role model self-discipline.
- Participate in staff meetings and clinical supervision to work through transference and countertransference phenomena.

tic alliance as well as preserving the hospital or prison milieu. The accompanying Intervention box illustrates some guidelines for developing a relationship. It is important to recognize, however, that these clients identify unit power structures and pit staff members against one another. Because these clients tend to be intelligent and charming, staff may fail to identify manipulations or excuse these behaviors. In addition, these clients may often actively resist directives while appearing to be compliant. Short-term therapy is usually ineffective, and long-term hospitalization or incarceration may be indicated.

In general, the nurse must present the "brick wall" against which the client can butt (Dighton 1986) as the antisocial person attempts to manipulate others to achieve personal ends. Because of their charm, facade of superiority, and persuasiveness, antisocial people sometimes manipulate nurses to assume the roles of nurturers and rescuers. Nurses should never give out telephone numbers, assign special privileges, or make themselves available to these clients outside the therapeutic relationship. The clients have lifelong patterns of victimizing others.

Evaluating/Outcome Criteria

Extensive studies indicate that antisocial clients: (a) do not respond to drug therapy, (b) remain in psychodynamic therapies only long enough to decrease their anxiety and ingratiate therapists, and (c) respond to cognitive-behavioral therapies only as long as someone is available to reinforce the desired behaviors. Court-ordered hospitalization tends to be more successful than voluntary treatment because the antisocial individual is generally highly manipulative and may easily disrupt the milieu or leave the facility. Some therapeutic success has been observed with back-to-nature, survival programs in which survival depends on developing skills and relationships with others (Reid 1985). The treatment outcome may improve if the antisocial client is able to form a working relationship with the therapist (Gerstley et al. 1989).

Some antisocial people "burn out" in later life (over age 35), giving up extreme forms of antisocial responses. Narcissism continues, but family stability and occupational adaptation are evident in about 25 percent of the population (Cloninger 1978). These people do not become model citizens, but they tend to avoid the criminal and welfare systems.

When evaluating short-term in-patient objectives, the nurse looks for the following client behaviors as evidence that coping abilities and self-concept are within normal boundaries.

Ineffective Individual Coping

- Increased impulse control and ability to delay gratification
- Decreased verbal and nonverbal manipulations
- Adherence to unit rules and regulations
- Acceptance of personal responsibility and accountability for actions

Impaired Social Interaction

- Realistic identification of assets and liabilities
- Identification of personal problem areas
- Absence of aggression directed to self or others
- Assertive communications with others

See the nursing care plan on page 404 for a client with an antisocial personality disorder.

NURSING CARE PLAN

A Client with an Antisocial Personality

Client Care Goals	Nursing Planning/ Interventions	Evaluation

Nursing Diagnosis: *Ineffective individual coping (Related factors: inability to delay gratification, manipulation of others, failure to learn behaviors, and overuse of defensive mechanisms, including denial, projection, rationalization, intellectualization, splitting)*

Client Care Goals	Nursing Planning/ Interventions	Evaluation
The client will assume personal responsibility for behavior and its consequences.	Develop a plan for dealing with manipulative behavior and instruct all staff to use the same approaches.	Verbally identifies manipulative responses.
	Help client to identify patterns and consequences of manipulative behavior by pointing them out when they occur.	Identifies unfulfilled needs that lead to manipulation of others.
	Set firm, consistent limits and expectations of behavior and review these with the client.	Delays immediate gratification when appropriate.
	Discuss with client what he or she hopes to achieve by manipulations.	Develops appropriate outlets for aggressive impulses.
	Listen matter-of-factly when client verbalizes frustration or annoyance, at the limits established.	Verbalizes the consequences of actions.
	Observe for escalating behavior of a violent nature (assault, suicide) and take precautions as necessary.	Develops alternative strategies for dealing with frustration.
	Encourage client to identify consequences of behavior.	Minimizes use of defense mechanisms of denial, projection, splitting, rationalization, and intellectualization.
	Contract with client to express feelings verbally without acting out.	
	Teach client differences between immediate needs and those that can be delayed.	
	Establish privilege system compliance with treatment program activities.	

NURSING CARE PLAN *(continued)*

Client Care Goals	Nursing Planning/ Interventions	Evaluation
	Point out to client defensive behaviors and encourage expression of underlying feelings.	
	Assist client to write behavioral options for dealing with situations of anger, frustration, or desire.	
	Give consistent feedback and positively reinforce appropriate behaviors.	
	Identify personal feelings about client and the behaviors they manifest; use clinical supervision to deal with issues.	
	Use peer pressure to modify manipulative behaviors.	

Nursing Diagnosis: *Self-esteem disturbance (Related factors: impulsivity, lying, failure to meet role expectations, sexual indiscretions, lack of support system)*

The client will exercise honesty and increased impulse control within societal guidelines.	Help client assess strengths and weaknesses via feedback, peer reviews, verbal dialogue in one-to-one sessions and journals, and "homework" tasks of a self-evaluative nature.	Realistically identifies assets and liabilities.
	Give positive reinforcement when client is able to delay gratification.	Uses self-control and appropriate judgment in meeting short-term objectives.
	Help client to problem solve, identifying alternative actions and probable consequences.	Refrains from deceitful communications, e.g., lying, breaking promises, "stretching" the truth, intentional forgetting.
	Confront client with lies and insist on truthfulness in all interactions.	Develops and maintains a support system that encourages adherence to group norms and mutual respect.
	Be firm and courteous when client becomes angry or hostile.	
	Role play situations, demonstrating direct and adaptive responses.	

Common Features of the Anxious-Fearful Personality

Aloof, Ambivalent Social Style

The anxious-fearful person restricts social contact to those individuals typified as safe and nonrejecting. Because they anticipate rejection and criticism from others, their relationships may be either clinging or detached.

Restricted Affect

The affective responses of anxious-fearful persons range from insensitivity to the feelings of others to overconcern and oversensitivity to the evaluation by others. The inability to express underlying feelings is generally based on a fear that others will reject them unless they are perfect. The avoidant and dependent personalities tend to see themselves as inferior to others and subordinate their needs accordingly. In contrast, the compulsive and passive-aggressive personalities view authority as overly restrictive; consequently, they are insensitive to others' needs.

Fear of Success or Failure

Active or passive avoidance of responsibility characterizes all the anxious-fearful personalities. Resistant behavior may be deliberately avoidant, as seen in dependent and avoidant persons. The behavior may be covert, as evidenced by the compulsive person's obsessive attention to details, leading to ineffective overall performance. Passive-aggressive persons set themselves up to fail by dawdling, intentional forgetting, and procrastination.

Fear of Loss of Control

When a person's quest for autonomy is thwarted at an early age, response patterns manifested by rigidity are often noted. The needs to control, to have guarantees of others' love, to avoid relaxation and fun, and to maintain structure and orderliness are seen in anxious-fearful people. These responses seem to provide some reassurance of predictability and control in their lives.

Fear of Embarrassment

Persons with all the personality disorders in the anxious-fearful cluster manifest response patterns indicating low self-esteem and lack of self-confidence. An insignificant act by a waitress or salesperson may be construed as rejecting or overly solicitous.

Difficulty with Decision Making

Related to low self-esteem and fear of criticism is a fear of making an incorrect choice or recommendation. Consequently, anxious-fearful people either tend to focus on details and procrastinate, or they may give responsibility for decision making to others.

Negativity

Anxious-fearful people view the world as potentially disappointing. They exude an air of pessimism, irritability, sulkiness, discontent, and submissiveness that colors all their interactions. They tend to dampen everyone's spirits, thus confirming their perceptions and expectations.

Anxious-Fearful Personality Disorders

Individuals with personality disorders who present primarily as anxious or fearful may be diagnosed as **avoidant, dependent, obsessive-compulsive,** or **passive-aggressive** under the criteria established in the DSM-III-R. Anxious-fearful persons generally experience both social and occupational impairments as a result of their restricted affect, nonassertiveness, problems expressing feelings, unrealistic expectations of others, and impaired decision making and problem solving. These individuals tend to have arrested development during the oral or anal stages of psychosexual development (Cameron and Rychlak 1985). Developmental precursors to these disorders include early anxiety associated with parental attitudes and fears of abandonment and rejection. Overly critical, demanding, and punitive parenting practices coupled with diminished opportunities to express feelings may be contributing factors. Reich's (1989) study indicates the significance of family history in the development of the anxious-fearful personality disorder cluster. The lifestyle of the anxious-fearful person is characterized by intense emotional repression and behaviors that are socially isolating and self-defeating. Because the behaviors of the disorders in the anxious-fearful cluster tend to overlap, common features of these conditions are shown in the accompanying Assessment box.

The Nursing Process and Avoidant Personality Disorders

Assessing

Defining Characteristics of the Avoidant Personality The essential features of the avoidant personality are fear and hypersensitivity to potential rejection and shame. These people withdraw socially although they avidly desire affection and acceptance. They want guarantees that people will uncritically accept them. Their avoidant behavior results in their often visiting public places, e.g., movies, museums, and ballparks, simply to experience the presence of other people because they do not enjoy being alone. When in public places, however, they maintain a safe distance from others. For example, in a movie theater one can be physically close to people without feeling that one's personal space is being invaded. Avoidant people devalue their own achievements. They appear overly serious, humorless, and painfully shy. Speech is often slow, and they do not express feelings. Though content is generally serious.

Mary Jane is a 27-year-old single female who sought counseling due to feelings of loneliness and lack of friends. She describes herself as having grown up on a Midwest farm where she was "pretty much a homebody." In high school she made good grades but did not participate in any extracurricular activities. She studied library science in college and admits to receiving secondhand pleasure from reading about the experiences of others. Historical novels are her favorites. She is currently employed as a reference librarian in a large aerospace company where she has minimal contact with other people. She says she wants to establish both male and female friendships but feels afraid that "people will laugh" at her. Mary Jane joined the company bowling team at the suggestion of a coworker but quit after the first evening because she felt she would "hold them back." Mary Jane rationalized her decision by stating, "I think I would be more comfortable pursuing an intellectual hobby."

Although the schizoid and avoidance personalities have many similar characteristics, the avoidant person's motivation to form a therapeutic relationship differentiates the two. The avoidant person also tends to lead a fairly productive life, particularly regarding occupation and self-care maintenance.

Diagnosing

Social isolation and **Self-esteem disturbance** are the major nursing diagnoses for the avoidant client. The social isolation is self-induced, and the feelings that promote distancing are very painful.

Social Isolation

- Feelings of being "different"
- Lack of significant purpose
- Insecurity in public
- Verbalized fears of rejection

Self-Esteem Disturbances

- Inability to accept positive reinforcement
- Inability to evaluate one's own worth realistically
- Belittling oneself in daily activities
- Condemning oneself for failing to develop adequate social skills

Planning and Implementing Interventions

Intervention strategies are focused on developing a therapeutic alliance with the client. In this relationship, the nurse confronts clients' illogical beliefs about themselves and their perceptions of others. Systematic desensitization techniques are useful in helping the clients form social relationships. Behavioral techniques, e.g., contracting with the client to network with others in support groups and employment activities, may also be useful. Underlying any intervention strategies should be the knowledge that avoidant personalities, because of their intense fear, are prone to episodes of depression, phobias, and periods of intense inner-directed rage. Consequently, be prepared to prevent and deal with intermittent crises as psychodynamic issues are uncovered.

Evaluating/Outcome Criteria

Unless the cycle of timidity and fear in social situations is interrupted, avoidant clients continue to reinforce their apprehension by their own interpersonal restraint. Cognitive-behavioral therapies are often useful in helping these clients look at their own behaviors and the erroneous meanings that they may assign to the comments of others.

The Nursing Process and Dependent Personality Disorders

Assessing

Defining Characteristics of the Dependent Personality The essential features of the dependent personality include lack of self-confidence, inability to

INTERVENTION

Guidelines for Working with the Dependent Personality

- Evaluate the client's ability to perform self-care activities; encourage grooming and personal hygiene.
- Schedule regular sessions as a way to anticipate clients' needs *before* they demand attention through inappropriate responses.
- Help the client identify assets and liabilities, including plans for change; emphasize strengths and potential.
- Encourage the client to take responsibility for own opinions; point out when the client negates own feelings or opinions.
- Encourage the client to verbalize feelings of anxiety related to independent functioning.
- Encourage the client to talk about how needs for affection, control, and responsibility are currently being met.
- Share with the client your observations of his or her manipulative behavior. For example, a client may offer to accompany a physically impaired client to a group activity in order to minimize the amount of time spent in productive therapy.
- Set realistic limits about what can and cannot be done for any client.
- Using group therapy to provide support, emphasize that the client is not alone in experiencing fear of failure or of success.
- Work through feelings of disappointment with the client when new behaviors are not immediately successful.

- Explore with the client the consequences of behaviors; for example, clinging tends to result in avoidance by others.
- Discuss personal responsibilities and make the client aware that he or she has choices.
- Teach the client problem-solving techniques, including goal setting, making alternative responses, and evaluating consequences.
- Provide opportunities for the client to have successful experiences and encourage participation in such activities.
- Help the client develop a realistic time frame in which to achieve independent living activities (e.g., getting a job or apartment).
- Do not do for the client what he or she is capable of doing without help.
- Give positive reinforcement for successful achievements.
- Teach and role model assertive behavior; teach client to develop strategies for confrontations by others.
- Prevent secondary gains from negative statements about self by refocusing interactions.
- State goals for nursing care in terms that the client and staff can understand.
- Involve staff members in conferences and clinical supervision to deal with transference and countertransference issues.

make decisions, and inability to function independently. In sharp contrast to the avoidant person, dependent people cling to others and passively accept their dictates and leadership. Dependent people view themselves as "helpless" or "stupid" and seek out dominant others or objects to lean on for guidance, control, and support as well as for "permission" to behave. The dominant other/object relationship stems from the normal life-sustaining bond between mother and infant. In dependent people, this normal symbiotic relationship has been excessively prolonged, impairing their capacity for thinking, feeling, and responding on their own. They believe they must be taken care of and

consequently rely on others to mirror their feelings to them. Dependent people subordinate their desires and needs to the wishes of others in order to maintain relationships. They often appear friendly, helpful, and indispensable. When the dominant other or object is unavailable, or perceived as unavailable, dependent persons experience intense anxiety. This may lead to feelings of unhappiness, anger, resentment, or depression. It is also noteworthy that significant others may eventually respond to dependent people with anger and resentment because of their continuous clinging and ingratiating behaviors.

The early childhood environment, which is characterized by premature separation from parents, neglect, overprotection, or lack of parental responsiveness, may predispose to dependent personality disorders (Moyer and Snider 1984). Like people with other personality disorders discussed in DSM-III-R, the dependent person may have multiple Axis II diagnoses. The following example illustrates how a dependent client might behave.

Marie is a 40-year-old single parent of two teenage daughters. She has gained seventy pounds since her divorce two years ago. Currently, Marie is sporadically attending a group for displaced homemakers, where she has shared a great deal of information about herself. She states that she is essentially a "homebody" and feels most satisfied when baking, cooking, and sewing for her daughters. Marie describes her secondhand pleasure in their activities, including ballet, gymnastic, and modeling. In fact, Marie becomes visibly saddened when she discusses her daughters' eventual departure for college. When her daughters expressed concern about Marie's weight gain and general health, Marie giggled and said, "Better to be fat and jolly than skinny and mean." Marie has made no attempt to develop new friendships or social outlets since her divorce. She is poorly groomed and haphazardly dressed, in contrast to her impeccably groomed daughters. When confronted by group members about her priority setting and the need to direct some energy toward herself, Marie responded, "My life is devoted to my daughters; their needs are more important than mine, and that's why I agreed to make the thirty costumes for their dance recital next week."

Diagnosing

Nurses frequently avoid or voice dislike for dependent clients because of their cloying, clinging, and demanding behaviors. This avoidance response tends to reinforce these clients' perceptions that other people are unwilling to help and that they are unable to help themselves. As a result, clients increase their clinging responses because they know no other way to behave. This increased clinging only leads to further avoidance by others. The primary nursing diagnoses and problem areas are as follows:

Self-Esteem Disturbance

- Is verbally and nonverbally compliant
- Lacks initiative
- Avoids decision making or changes mind frequently
- Is unable to meet own needs independently
- Is unwilling to make assertive requests of others for fear of rejection
- Belittles personal assets and abilities

Self-Care Deficits: Bathing/Hygiene, Dressing/Grooming, Feeding

- Altered activities of daily living, e.g., grooming, hygiene, and nutrition
- Self-indulgence in food, alcohol, and drugs
- Inattention to medical and dental needs

Planning and Implementing Interventions

The goal of nursing interventions is to help the client achieve independent functioning. Guidelines for nursing interventions are shown in the accompanying Intervention box.

Evaluating/Outcome Criteria

Dependent personalities commonly experience crises when the dominant support system is altered. During crisis episodes, these clients may be open to cognitive-behavioral strategies, but the outlook for major personality restructuring is dim. Instead, dependent people tend to transfer dependency needs to others.

The Nursing Process and Obsessive-Compulsive Personality Disorders

Assessing

Defining Characteristics of the Obsessive-Compulsive Personality   The obsessive-compulsive individual demonstrates anxiety and fearfulness by behavior that shows fear of losing control over situations, objects, or people. The obsessive-compulsive personality strives at all times to keep the world predictable and organized. The major features of this disorder are an excessive dedication to work, productivity, and perfectionism to the exclusion of feelings and pleasure. The obsessive-compulsive individual may be likened to a drill sergeant in the military who is rigid, serious, detail oriented, and stingy with emotions.

A focus on trivial details often leads this person not only to "miss the forest for the trees, but also fail to see the tree while counting its leaves" (Eaton et al. 1976, p 106). Although these people may be highly praised for their organizational skills and work ethic, eventually their rigidity causes them to fear making mistakes. Consequently, they postpone making decisions. They tend to resent authority but rarely express this resentment openly. Instead, they may engage in passive-aggressive behavior, e.g., procrastination and stubbornness. To manage their procrastination, obsessive compulsive people often initiate work on a project far in advance of the due date, as shown in the following example:

Peter set himself a deadline in early fall for ordering his family's Christmas gifts. His family found this deadline something of an annoyance. Yet Peter persisted in his attempts to get commitments from everyone about what they wanted. Often, he would mislay his early purchases by the time Christmas arrived, and he would rush out to do last-minute shopping anyway.

Peter appears to be concerned with his family and interpersonal relationships, but he is really more concerned with meeting the Christmas deadline and checking off his list than in his relatives' enjoyment of their gifts. Although Peter suffers under the pressure of his deadlines, he sets them for himself. He functions as his own overseer, issuing commands, directives, reminders, warnings, and admonitions about what should be done. People like Peter are also keenly aware of society's and other people's expectations, of the threat of possible criticism, of the weight and direction of authority, of rules, regulations, and conventions, and of a great collection of moral or quasimoral principles. These people feel required to fulfill unending duties, responsibilities, and tasks that are, in their view, not chosen, but simply there.

Compulsive people do not view taking work home and working long hours as an imposition, since work organizes their lives and binds their anxiety. Indeed, the compulsive person will make work out of pleasurable activities, as the following example shows:

Jennifer planned her European vacation in meticulous detail. She scheduled exhausting daily tours and activities from 6:30 A.M. until 12:00 P.M. Jennifer planned to visit every attraction available as quickly as possible. So as not to waste time, she wrote her postcards to her family while she rode tour buses. The cards were crammed with information about weather, prices of goods and services, menus, and daily time tables. She wrote nothing about how she felt or what she was experiencing. Upon returning home, she spent two weeks cataloging all her photographs and typing short paragraphs to accompany each photo. She passed her album around at work during lunch hour expecting that her coworkers would read all the captions. She became insulted and irate when several coworkers flipped through the album quickly. Jennifer found it difficult to forgive them for "slighting" her in this way.

When a coworker was planning a trip, Jennifer suggested that he record details of the trip in a diary so that he could compile an album similar to her own. Jennifer was not aware of the resentment, hurt, and irritation her behavior generated in others.

Specific defining characteristics of the obsessive-compulsive personality are listed in the accompanying Assessment box. However, the nurse should always consider how clients will react to the realization that years of denying themselves satisfaction, working hard, saving, and restricting the quality of life have not produced the expected rewards (e.g., career advancement, status, promotions). This realization often leads to the potential for depression, especially during middle life. As the following example shows, the obsessive-compulsive person may even postpone acting on major decisions to avoid the reality of life without work.

Millie, a 61-year-old college professor, seeks counseling one year prior to her planned retirement. She complains of insomnia, weight loss, and pervasive anxiety about "what life will be like without anything to do." Millie is retiring early because she feels that in spite of twenty-five years of loyal service to the university and diligent work,

ASSESSMENT

Common Features of the Obsessive-Compulsive Personality

- Shows excessive dedication to work
- Is sensitive to criticism and rejection
- Is preoccupied with organization, details, procedures, and rules
- Is a perfectionist
- Is indecisive and ambivalent
- Demands conformity to his or her standards
- Resists authority of others
- Excludes pleasure; makes work out of play
- Is moralistic and judgmental about self and others
- Concentrates on minute details and trivia
- Restricts emotional expression
- Is stingy with both emotions and material objects
- Harbors anger and resentment against others
- Shows little empathy
- Expresses anger indirectly
- Is status conscious
- Fears making mistakes
- Has potential for depression

she has been passed over repeatedly for promotion to the position of department chairperson. Millie is an unmarried, slender woman who is meticulously dressed in very conservative clothing.

During the interview, she says that she made most of her own clothing and purchased only items that were on sale. In describing her daily activities, Millie states that she is a "hard worker who always took things home to finish." She voices resentment that neither the department chairperson nor other faculty did likewise. Millie says that she spent more than ten years caring for an elderly mother because "my sister didn't have time for her." Millie devoted a great deal of time to church and university activities. The therapist's impression is that Millie performed these functions out of duty rather than for spontaneous enjoyment or satisfaction. Millie states that she volunteered to be secretary of the local humane society because she knew she could keep the detailed records better than any of the other members.

When questioned about her relationships with other faculty, Millie says that she communicated with them by memos to avoid being misquoted. She further states that she kept copies of all these memos because "They can't keep things straight most of the time." Millie becomes visibly angry when relating a recent experience: She overheard two colleagues ridiculing a memo requesting, six months in advance, that guest lecturers be permitted to use the colleagues' parking spaces. When challenged about the lack of immediacy of her request, Millie states that she has "stopped speaking to them [the faculty] entirely." When the therapist questions Millie about her interests for retirement, Millie says, "I don't really know; I've never had time for frivolous activities." By the end of the session, Millie has become indecisive about whether she should retire, after all.

The obsessive-compulsive personality, according to some theorists, evolves from the need to exert control and autonomy over one's bodily functions and the world during the second stage of psychosexual development. The struggle with parental figures over bowel control and the resultant anxiety and frustration may lead to characteristics of stinginess, pompous bookishness, and touchiness. Consequently, there is a lifelong struggle for independence, which is hampered by equally strong feelings of inadequacy, self-doubt, and ambivalence toward authority figures (Cameron and Rychlak 1985).

Interestingly, excessively conscientious, rigid people often exhibit a contradictory pattern of slovenliness, which is also compulsive. Thus, a compulsive housewife may scrub her kitchen floor daily but allow bags of garbage to accumulate and become infested with maggots.

If one looks to learning and behavioral theories for explanations for the obsessive-compulsive personality, it is clear that society positively reinforces the ritualistic patterns that the person uses to adapt to the world. It is also likely that the parents of the obsessive-

compulsive individual disciplined the child excessively during the early years of development. Whether a compulsive response is adaptive or symptomatic depends on: (a) its effectiveness and (b) the person's ability to modify the response when it is inappropriate.

Diagnosing

Ineffective individual coping is the primary nursing diagnosis with obsessive-compulsive clients. This is evidenced by responses that show restricted cognitive, affective, and motor behavior. "Social isolation" related to resentment, self-doubt, and exclusion of pleasure is the other major nursing diagnosis.

Planning and Implementing Interventions

The goal is to help clients examine and evaluate their life-styles and goals so that they can modify troublesome compulsive traits. The nurse intervenes to help these clients express dissatisfaction with their lives and to encourage realistic planning for future changes. Guidelines for nursing interventions are shown in the Intervention box on page 412.

Evaluating/Outcome Criteria

As always, when evaluating any client with a personality disorder, consider the potential for major psychiatric conditions such as depression and anxiety-related disturbances. Even though people with obsessive-compulsive personalities often seek treatment for subjective distress, the course of treatment may be drawn out and ineffective due to the rigidity of their defensive operations. If the behavior is confronted directly, the client might develop acute psychiatric conditions because of intense anxiety.

The Nursing Process and Passive-Aggressive Personality Disorders

Assessing

Defining Characteristics of the Passive-Aggressive Personality The DSM-III-R (1987) definition of and criteria for identifying the passive-aggressive personality disorder are substantially different from those in the 1980 edition. The Assessment box on page 412 shows the new DSM-III-R criteria for diagnostic purposes. Resistant behaviors often observed are listed in the Assessment box on page 413. Simply stated, passive-aggressive behavior is the indirect expression of anger.

INTERVENTION

Guidelines for Working with the Obsessive Compulsive Personality

- Confront nonconstructive, compulsive responses gently and be alert for anxiety when you confront the client.

- Discuss the importance of these responses with the client.

- Show approval of recreation and enjoyment.

- Do not demand that the client engage in leisure or recreational activities (clients will "work" at them instead of enjoying them).

- Make a contract with the client stating how much time during one-to-one sessions will be used to discuss obsessive thoughts or rituals; gradually decrease the time allotted to these activities.

- Help the client identify feelings of anxiety generated in stressful situations and the usual responses to this anxiety.

- Help the client identify alternative coping methods to deal with stressful situations.

- Help the client identify and differentiate between "shoulds" (behaviors expected by others) and "wants" (desirable activities).

- Explore activities that were or are pleasurable or satisfying.

- Plan activities and interventions around pleasurable memories.

- Encourage physical activity.

- Encourage verbalization of feelings, especially those of anger and resentment.

- Provide examples of appropriate ways to handle emotion through role modeling, skills training, and group activities.

- Discuss with the client how to recognize behavior changes.

- Monitor levels of compulsive behavior after initial baseline assessment.

- Give gentle feedback, identifying weaknesses as well as strengths.

- Provide progressive opportunities to make decisions.

- Encourage the client to evaluate progress in meeting goals.

ASSESSMENT

Common Features of the Passive-Aggressive Personality Disorder

The client who is passive-aggressive passively resists demands requiring adequate social and occupational performance. A diagnosis of passive-aggressive personality disorder may be made if the client consistently demonstrates five or more of the following behaviors:

- Puts off jobs that need to be done and thus misses deadlines (procrastination)

- Deliberately works slowly or does a bad job on those tasks that he or she really doesn't want to do

- Protests, unjustifiably, that others make unreasonable demands

- Claims "forgetfulness" to avoid meeting obligations

- Becomes pouty, sulky, irritable, or argumentative when asked to do something that he or she does not want to do

- Overestimates the value of his or her work, i.e., thinks that he or she is doing a much better job than others think is being done

- Becomes resentful when others offer useful suggestions to enhance his or her productivity

- Obstructs task accomplishment by failing to do his or her share of the work

- Is unreasonably critical or scornful of people in positions of authority

SOURCE: *Adapted from American Psychiatric Association:* Diagnostic and Statistical Manual of Mental Disorders, *ed 3, revised. APA, 1987, pp 358–359.*

All passive-aggressive behaviors are eventually self-defeating. Consider the dynamics presented in the following example:

Antonio is asked to work overtime to cover a very short-staffed unit. If he chooses to accept the assignment willingly and does his best, he receives the approval of his employer. If he flatly refuses the assignment, he avoids the work but possibly risks his job. His third option is to compromise in a mutually satisfactory way with his employer. However, if he chooses to respond in a passive-

ASSESSMENT

Resistant Responses of Passive-Aggressive Personalities

- Is stubborn and complies half-heartedly
- Is inefficient
- Is forgetful
- Procrastinates
- Is negative
- Is pessimistic
- Is sarcastic, makes snide remarks
- Is envious, resents others
- Dawdles
- Is sullen and moody
- Sees self as a victim of circumstances
- Assumes no responsibility for control of situations
- Is subtly antagonistic
- Complains chronically
- Sulks and pouts
- Is critical of advice or direction from others
- Avoids open hostility or expressions of anger
- Sabotages the work of others
- Is chronically late
- Is verbally abusive toward others
- Has repeated educational, vocational, and social failures
- Is crude and rude in social situations, e.g., cracks gum, does needlework, belches, is flatulent, or falls asleep during working meetings
- Deliberately dresses inappropriately for social or occupational activities
- Has frequent somatic complaints or disability claims

dependency needs were not met through nurturing and protective parental behavior. Consequently, the child learned to deal with anger by passively responding to those in authority with seemingly polite and undemanding behavior. This behavior, however, is marked by inefficiency and subtle resistance. Because these passive-aggressive maneuvers (which were unconsciously selected to protect the person from fear of abandonment) are so irritating to others, a self-defeating situation is perpetuated. Significant people continue to withdraw from the passive-aggressive person, who then increases the use of these maladaptive responses (Mahler et al. 1975).

Diagnosing

The major nursing diagnosis for passive-aggressive clients is **Ineffective individual coping.** Problem behaviors are identified in the accompanying Assessment box on resistant behaviors.

Planning and Implementing Interventions

See the nursing care plan on page 414 for clients with a passive-aggressive personality. In addition to implementing the interventions in the care plan, the psychiatric nurse may find it helpful to teach the families of passive-aggressive clients how to interact with and relate to their significant others in order to disrupt ineffective patterns of behaving. In general, the dawdling, resistant behaviors of the passive-aggressive personality are best viewed as ineffective coping strategies. In specific situations, passive-aggressive responses may be adaptive. For example, a prison inmate who openly complies with authority may be at high risk of violence by other inmates. In this situation, slow-downs and careless workmanship would satisfy the authorities without antagonizing the other inmates. Consequently, assess the client's responses within the context in which they occur. The following example shows how one therapist learned to cope with a passive-aggressive client.

Greg, a 22-year-old medical student, visits the university counseling service requesting assistance with time management. During the initial interview, he was soft-spoken, submissive, and polite, but his affect was sullen and pouting. He was evasive when asked for information concerning his daily activity schedule, making such comments as, "Well, sometimes I spend a lot of time thinking about how easy my classmates have it and how hard I have to work." Greg initially contracted to work on a list of problems, and he cooperated with the therapist. However, by the third session he had not only established a pattern of arriving late but also was interrupting role playing and counselor modeling, stating, "The real problem is something else." When the therapist tried to focus him on one

aggressive manner, he will stay, do the work hurriedly and carelessly, and complain frequently about how unfair the employer is. By choosing the passive-aggressive option, he forfeits the advantage of winning approval but still has to do the task.

The example demonstrates the underlying dynamics of the passive-aggressive person. It is believed that early during the person's childhood, the parents were assertive or aggressive toward the child but blocked the child's need to express anger. In addition, the child's

NURSING CARE PLAN

A Client with a Passive-Aggressive Personality

Client Care Goals	Nursing Planning/ Interventions	Evaluation

Nursing Diagnosis: Ineffective individual coping (Related factors: behavioral responses such as belching in public, leaving room early, cracking gum during meetings, habitual lateness, sulking, pouting, moodiness)

Client Care Goals	Nursing Planning/ Interventions	Evaluation
The client will develop assertive strategies for coping with stress.	Establish a relationship based on mutual responsibilities, minimizing authoritarian approaches.	Verbalizes the belief that he or she can control the outcomes of a situation.
	Assess client's perceptions of his or her situation, including underlying assumptions.	Identifies feelings of anxiety in stressful situations.
	Evaluate if client's perceptions of situations are realistic.	Uses appropriate assertive responses in a variety of situations without experiencing undue anxiety.
	Deal initially with minor problems to generate successful experiences.	Verbalizes anticipated outcomes of assertive behavior.
	Give feedback on client's ability to create and control successful experiences.	Identifies and uses coping responses to reduce anxiety that are not passive-aggressive.
	Involve client in setting short- and long-term objectives and stick to the plan of action.	
	Avoid focusing on negative responses, e.g., whining, tantrums, angry outbursts.	
	Point out to client when hostility is being shown in a passive rather than in an open assertive manner.	
	Use active, directive approaches in helping the client identify and express feelings.	
	Discuss ultimate positive and negative consequences of choice.	
	Model assertive responses for the client.	
	Encourage client to try different approaches to problem solving.	
	Use cognitive approaches, e.g., homework assignments, journals, explanation of illogical beliefs.	

NURSING CARE PLAN *(continued)*

Client Care Goals	Nursing Planning/ Interventions	Evaluation
	Involve in assertiveness training groups.	
	Avoid arguing when the client offers excuses for passive-aggressive behavior; focus on the meaning that "giving in" has for client.	
	Teach anxiety-reducing and relaxation techniques.	
	Use humor to defuse argumentativeness and resistant behavior.	
	Use clinical supervision or staff meetings to work through transference and countertransference phenomena.	

problem at a time, Greg would become angry, sulk, and make whining complaints about not being "understood." He repeatedly "forgot" to do his homework assignments, stating, "I would have done it, but. . . ." By the fourth session, the therapist was feeling helpless and demoralized by Greg's habitual partial compliance. It was only after the therapist sought clinical supervision and cut back on the demands she made on Greg that a successful therapeutic alliance was established.

Evaluating/Outcome Criteria

Two factors influence the outcome of therapeutic strategies. The first is the degree of insight the client and family have concerning the passive-aggressive behavior. The second is the attitude of the family system toward assertiveness or open aggression. If insight is lacking and the attitude toward change is negative, then the passive-aggressive person will go through life feeling frustrated and victimized. These individuals will never comprehend the part they play in their own misery.

CHAPTER HIGHLIGHTS

• When personality traits (consistent, enduring response patterns) become inflexible, maladaptive, and cause social or occupational impairments, they may be diagnosed as personality disorders.

• Personality disorders are modes of functioning that include ways of thinking and perceiving, ways of experiencing emotion, and modes of subjective experience that are generally consistent patterns over broad areas of living.

• Personality disorders are characterized by life-style responses that may create problems both for clients and, to some extent, for society.

• Personality disorders are best understood as defensive modes of living rather than as psychiatric illnesses.

• Examples of personality disorders include three major DSM-III-R clusters, as follows: (a) eccentric, (b) dramatic-erratic, and (c) anxious-fearful.

• The eccentric life-style is generally associated with people who are emotionally cold, aloof, guarded, and reclusive and who exhibit various degrees of odd behavior.

• The dramatic-erratic life-style is generally associated with people who are impulsive, demonstrative, emotionally labile, needy, lacking in empathy, and unmindful of the consequences of behavior.

• The anxious-fearful life-style is generally associated with people who are hypersensitive, fearful of losing control, and lacking in spontaneity.

• The interactionist view of personality disorder focuses on those complex processes of perception and interpretation of people and the situations in which we encounter each other.

• Nursing interventions for clients with personality disorders are based on the understanding that defensive operations such as anger and manipulation allow the client to avoid anxiety and maintain an ego syntonic state.

REFERENCES

Agras WS: *Behavior Modification Principles and Clinical Applications.* Little Brown, 1978.

Akhtar S: The syndrome of identity diffusion. *Am J Psychiatry* 1984;141:1381–1385.

American Psychiatric Association: *Diagnostic and Statistical Manual of Mental Disorders,* ed 3. APA, 1980.

American Psychiatric Association: *Diagnostic and Statistical Manual of Mental Disorders,* ed 3, revised. APA, 1987.

Andrulonis PA, et al.: Organic brain dysfunction and the borderline syndrome. *Psychiatr Clin North Am* 1980;4:47–66.

Benner DG, Joscelyne B: Multiple personality as a borderline disorder. *J Nerv Ment Dis* 1984;172:98–104.

Brainerd CJ: *Piaget's Theory of Intelligence.* Prentice-Hall, 1978.

Braverman B, Shook J: Spotting the borderline personality. *Am J Nurs* 1987;2:200–203.

Cameron N, Rychlak JF: *Personality Development and Psychopathology: A Dynamic Approach.* Houghton Mifflin, 1985.

Chitty KK, Maynard CK: Managing manipulation. *J Psychosoc Nurs Ment Health Serv* 1986;24:8–13.

Cleckley H: *The Mask of Sanity.* Mosby, 1964.

Cloninger CR: The antisocial personality. *Hosp Pract* (Aug) 1978;97–106.

Coryell WH, Zimmerman M: Personality disorders in the families of depressed, schizophrenics, and never-ill probands. *Am J Psychiatry* 1989;146:496–502.

Cull A, Chick J, Wolff S: A consensual validation of schizoid personality in childhood and adult life. *Br J Psychiatry* 1984;144:646–648.

Deutsch H: *Neuroses and Character Types.* International Universities Press, 1965.

Dighton S; Tough-minded nursing. *Am J Nurs* 1986;86:48–51.

Eaton Jr MT, Peterson MH, Davis JA: *Psychiatry,* ed 3. Medical Examination Publishing, 1976.

Ellis A: *Humanistic Psychology.* McGraw-Hill, 1973.

Erikson EH: *Childhood and Society.* Norton, 1964.

Feldman RB, Guttman HA: Families of borderline patients: Literal-minded parents, borderline parents, and parental protectiveness. *Am J Psychiatry* 1984;141:1392–1396.

Ford MR, Widiger TA: Sex bias in the diagnosis of histrionic and antisocial personality disorder. *J Consult Clin Psychol* 1989;57:301–305.

Frank H, Paris J: Recollections of family experience in borderline patients. *Arch Gen Psychiatry* 1981;38:1031–1034.

Freeman SK: Inpatient management of a patient with borderline personality disorder: A case study. *Arch Psychiatr Nurs* 1988;2:360–366.

Frosch J: The psychosocial treatment of personality disorders, in Frosch J (ed): *Current Perspectives on Personality Disorders.* American Psychiatric Press, 1983.

Gallop R: The patient is splitting: Everyone knows and nothing changes. *J Psychosoc Nurs Ment Health Serv* 1985;23:6–10.

Gallop R, Lancee W, Garfinkel P: How nursing staff respond to the label "borderline personality disorder." *Hosp Comm Psychiatry* 1989;40:815–819.

Garfinkel T: A reconsideration of psychotherapy of narcissistic personality disorder. *Am J Psychoanal* 1982;42:207–220.

Genetic traits predispose some to criminality. *U.S. News* (Sept) 1985;54.

Gerstley L, McLellan AT, Alterman AI, Woody GE, Luborsky L, Prout M: Ability to form an alliance with the therapist: A possible marker of prognosis for patients with antisocial personality disorder. *Am J Psychiatry* 1989;146:508–512.

Gorenstein E: Frontal lobe functions in psychopaths. *J Abnorm Psychol* 1982;91:368–379.

Gutheil TG: Borderline personality disorder, boundary violations and patient-therapist sex: Medicolegal pitfalls. *Am J Psychiatry* 1989;146:597–602.

Haaken J: Sex differences and narcissistic disorders. *Am J Psychoanal* 1983;43:315–324.

Hickey BA: The borderline experience: Subjective impressions. *J Psychosoc Nurs Ment Health Serv* 1985;23:24–29.

Jacobson G: Personality disorders, in Lazare A (ed): *Outpatient Psychiatry.* Williams and Wilkins, 1979, pp 431–437.

Johnson AG: *Human Arrangements: An Introduction to Sociology.* Harcourt-Brace-Jovanovich, 1986.

Johnson M, Silver S: Conflicts in the inpatient treatment of the borderline patient. *Arch Psychiatr Nurs* 1988;2:312–318.

Kendler KS, Gruenberg AM: Genetic relationship between paranoid personality disorder and the schizophrenic spectrum disorders. *Am J Psychiatry* 1982;139:1185–1186.

Kendler KS, et al.: A family history study of schizophrenia-related personality disorders. *Am J Psychiatry* 1984;141:424–427.

Kernberg O: *Borderline Conditions and Pathological Narcissism.* Aronson, 1975.

Kohut H: *Analysis of the Self.* International Universities Press, 1971.

Kuhlman TL: Gallows humor for a scaffold setting: Managing aggressive patients on a maximum-security forensic unit. *Hosp Comm Psychiatry* 1988;39:1085–1090.

Lego S (ed): *The American Handbook of Psychiatric Nursing.* Lippincott, 1984.

Loomis ME, Horsley JA: *Interpersonal Change: A behavioral Approach to Nursing Practice.* McGraw-Hill, 1974.

Loranger AW, Oldham JM, Tulis EH: Familial transmission of DSM-III borderline personality disorder. *Arch Gen Psychiatry* 1982;39:795–799.

Loranger AW, Tulis EH: Family history of alcoholism in borderline personality disorder. *Arch Gen Psychiatry* 1985;42:153–157.

Mahler MS, Pine F, Bergman A: *The Psychological Birth of the Human Infant: Symbiosis and Individuation*. Basic Books, 1975.

Masterson JF: *The Narcissistic and Borderline Disorder*. Bruner/Mazel, 1981.

McEnany GW, Tescher BE; Contracting for care: One nursing approach to the hospitalized borderline patient. *J Psychosoc Nurs Ment Health Serv* 1985;23:11–18.

Moyer RL, Snider MJ: Interpersonal problems of adults, in Howe J et al. (eds): *The Handbook of Nursing*. Wiley, 1984, Chapter 37.

O'Brien P, Caldwell C, Transeau G: Destroyers: Written treatment contracts can help cure self-destructive behaviors of the borderline patient. *J Psychosoc Nurs Ment Health Serv* 1985;23:19–23.

Perlmutter R: The borderline patient in the emergency department: An approach for evaluation and management. *Psychiatr Q* 1982;54:190–197.

Perry JC, Flannery RB: Passive-aggressive personality disorder: Treatment implications of a clinical typology. *J Nerv Ment Dis* 1982;170:164–173.

Platt-Koch LM: Borderline personality disorder: A therapeutic approach. *Am J Nurs* 1983;83:1666–1671.

Poldrugo F, Forti B: Personality disorders and alcoholism treatment outcome. *Drug Alcohol Depend* 1988;21:171–176.

Reich JH: Familiality of DSM-III dramatic and anxious personality clusters. *J Nerv Ment Dis* 1989;177:96–100.

Reid WH: The antisocial personality: A review. *Hosp Community Psychiatry* 1985;36:831–837.

Rowe CJ: *An Outline of Psychiatry*. Brown, 1984.

Runyon N, Allen C, Ilnicki S: The borderline patient on the med-surg unit. *Am J Nurs* 1988;88:1644–1650.

Schaefer RT, Lamm RP: *Sociology*. McGraw-Hill, 1986.

Schlesinger LB: Distinctions between psychopathic, sociopathic, and anti-social personality disorders. *Psychol Rep* 1980;47:15–21.

Schwarz G, Halaris A: Identifying and managing borderline personality patients. *Am Family Physician* 1984;29:203–208.

Shapiro D: *Neurotic Styles*. Basic Books, 1965.

Shearer SL, Peters CP, Quaytman MS, Wadman BE: Intent and lethality of suicide attempts among female borderline inpatients. *Am J Psychiatry* 1988;145:1424–1427.

Slavney PR, Teitelbaum ML, Chase GA: Referral for medically unexplained somatic complaints: The role of histrionic traits. *Psychosomatics* 1985;26:103–109.

Smoyak SA: Borderline personality disorder (editorial). *J Psychosoc Nurs Ment Health Serv* 1985;23:5.

Spector RE: *Cultural Diversity in Health and Illness*. Appleton-Century-Crofts, 1985.

Standage K, et al.: An investigation of role-taking in histrionic personalities. *Can J Psychiatry* 1984;29:407–411.

Togensen S: Genetic and nosological aspects of the schizotypal and borderline personality disorders. *Arch Gen Psychiatry* 1984;41:546–554.

Travin S, Protter B: Mad or bad? Some clinical considerations in the misdiagnosis of schizophrenia as antisocial personality disorder. *Am J Psychiatry* 1982;139;1335–1338.

Waldinger R: Intensive psychodynamic therapy with borderline patients: An overview. *Am J Psychiatry* 1987;144(3):267–274.

Wester CM: Managing the borderline personality. *Nurs Management* 1989;20:49–51.

Widiger TA, Frances A: Axis II personality disorders: Diagnostic and treatment issues. *Hosp Community Psychiatry* 1985;36:619–627.

Wilson JP, Prabucki K: Psychosocial antecedents of narcissistic personality syndrome. *Psychol Rep* 1983;53:1231–1239.

Wong N: Combined group and individual treatment of borderline and narcissistic patients: Heterogeneous versus homogeneous groups. *Int J Group Psychother* 1980;30:389–494.

Woollcott Jr P: Prognostic indicators in the psychotherapy of borderline patients. *Am J Psychother* 1985;39:17–29.

PART FOUR

Contemporary Clinical Concerns

CONTENTS

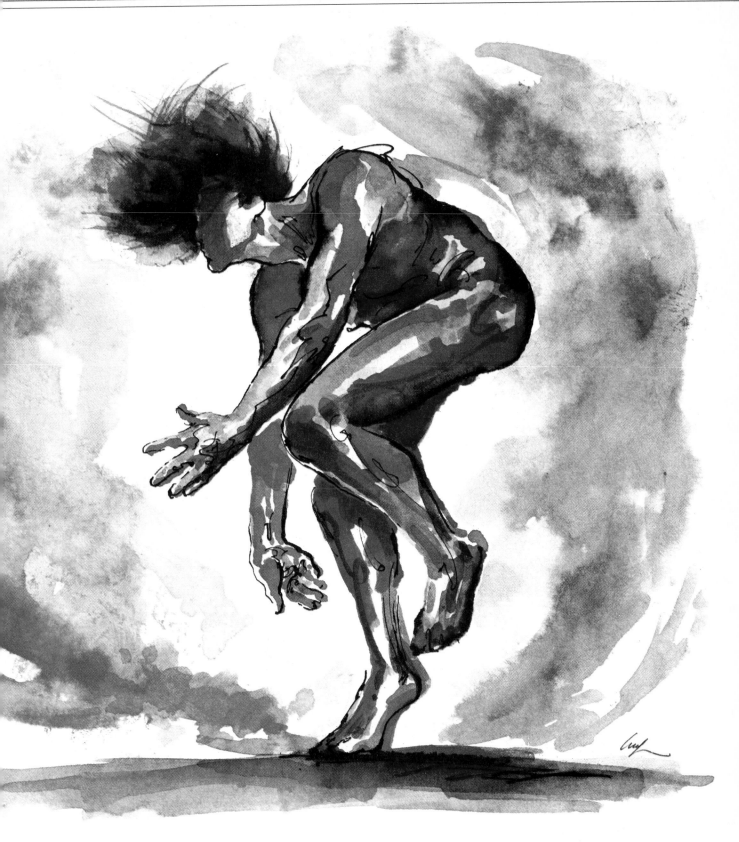

Love, joy, compassion, and grief—the cornerstones of emotion—
are often manifested in the movement of the human body.

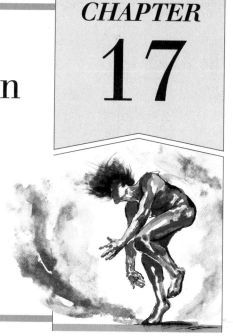

CHAPTER 17

Psychosocial Rehabilitation with the Severely and Persistently Mentally Ill

LEARNING OBJECTIVES

- Define psychiatric chronicity

- Describe the stages of debilitation in chronic illness

- List three or more of the problems of the chronically mentally ill in the community

- Distinguish the components of assisted employment

- Differentiate among the suggested theories for disability in the persistently and severely mentally ill

- Identify factors that burden the families of the chronically mentally ill

- Describe the characteristics of effective support programs in the community

- Suggest ways in which the nurse can support the caregivers of clients

Linda Chafetz

Nan Rich

Candace Furlong

Patricia Underwood

CROSS REFERENCES

Other topics related to this chapter are: Community mental health, Chapter 38; Mood disorders, Chapter 13; Organic mental disorders, Chapter 10; Psychotropic medications, Appendix B; Schizophrenia, Chapter 12; Substance abuse, Chapter 11.

P SYCHIATRIC CHRONICITY REFERS TO persistent functional impairment due to a mental disorder. In contemporary terminology, these clients are referred to as the **severely and persistently mentally ill.** Chronic disorders carry a high potential for impairment. Despite all we know about diagnosis and treatment of specific disorders, psychiatric chronicity remains one of the most puzzling phenomena in psychiatric nursing. We cannot always predict which client will experience a disabling course of illness or what factors influence this course. However, strategies are being identified with which to intervene in the complex needs of the chronically mentally ill, and we need to consider the phenomenon of chronicity as a nursing issue in its own right.

Who are the chronically mentally ill, and what perspectives may help to explain psychiatric chronicity? What effect does chronic illness have on individuals and groups? This chapter addresses these questions and then examines some of the theories being developed to explain these problems. Certainly, the issues of the chronically mentally ill in our communities are urgent ones, because social and economic disadvantage go hand in hand with chronicity. New service models for responding to the needs of the severely and persistently mentally ill—particularly psychosocial rehabilitation, self-care, and case management—are discussed, as well as contemporary issues and special needs areas. The chapter concludes with an investigation of the nursing process in caring for the chronically mentally ill and implications for further investigations and research in this dynamic area of concern.

Defining Chronic Mental Illness

Although the term **chronically mentally ill** is used in this text, it is not without its problems: it is difficult to define, it stigmatizes individuals with connotations of hopelessness and inevitable deterioration, and it obscures the heterogeneity of the population (Goldman and Manderscheid 1987). *Persistently and severely mentally ill* may be an alternative descriptor; however, the term *chronically mentally ill* continues to be widely accepted. It may be useful to investigate what makes an illness "chronic."

A definition developed by Goldman in 1984 may still be one of the most meaningful: a chronic mentally ill person has an illness that has prevented functioning in at least three of the following areas: personal hygiene and self-care, self-direction, interpersonal relationships, social interactions, learning, and recreation. These deficits prevent economic self-sufficiency. Often, prolonged mental health services are required (Goldman 1984). Other definitions take into account diagnosis, duration, and disability; however, it is difficult to give these qualities precise meaning and definition because of frequent disagreement over one or all of the components (Bachrach 1988). See Figure 17–1.

Psychiatric Disorders Linked to Chronicity

Certain psychiatric disorders are linked to chronicity. Schizophrenic disorders account by far for the largest subgroup of the chronically mentally ill and dominate much of the literature on psychiatric chronicity and disability. However, the major mood disorders, as well as anxiety disorders, somatoform disorders, and personality disorders can also lead to chronic disability, as can progressive mental disorders (such as Alzheimer's dementia). Alcohol and other substance abuse may add to the disability, as can mental retardation. All age groups are vulnerable to psychiatric chronicity.

These chronic disorders have common features, including the tendency to affect the personality in a

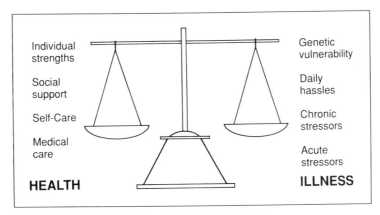

FIGURE 17–1   The balance between health and illness.

pervasive sense. Pervasive impairment implies impairment in multiple areas of function, leading to global difficulties. For example, persecutory delusions produce a fearful affect and bizarre and inappropriate behaviors, frequently including social withdrawal and isolation. Residual symptoms frequently persist between acute episodes of these illnesses. The unpredictable course of these disorders contributes to a fear of relapse in the affected persons between episodes, as well. This may result in an avoidance of environmental stressors, restriction of activities, and a general withdrawal from overstimulation in an attempt to reduce the risk of relapse.

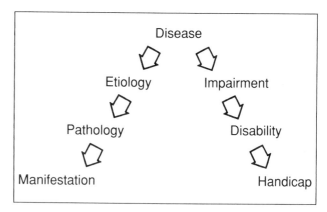

FIGURE 17-2 The WHO parallel sequence for long-term illness.

Stages in Chronic Illness

No matter how inclusive, a disease model rarely accounts for the consequences of illness, particularly of long-term, persistent illness. Understanding this, the World Health Organization (1980) developed and published a classification that proposes a parallel sequence for long-term illness (see Figure 17-2).

The etiology, known or unknown, gives rise to changes in structure or functioning. These pathologic changes are manifested as signs and symptoms. The disease is externalized when either the person or someone else becomes aware that there are abnormalities of structure or function. This awareness is the basis of **impairment,** which is defined as "any loss or abnormality of psychological, physiological or anatomical structure or function" (WHO 1980, p 27). Impairment is disturbance at the organ level.

The impairment may alter the functional performance or behavior of the individual. The alteration usually interferes with everyday living. This alteration is disability. Disability is said to be objectified because it restricts common activities and becomes the focus of the person's attention. **Disability** is defined as "any restriction or lack (resulting from an impairment) of ability to perform an activity in the manner or within the range considered normal for a human being (WHO 1980, p 28). Disability is disturbance at the level of the person.

When the impairment or the disability places the person at a disadvantage with others, handicap occurs. **Handicap** is defined as "a disadvantage for a given individual, resulting from an impairment or a disability, that limits or prevents the fulfillment of a role that is normal (depending on age, sex, social and cultural factors) for the individual" (WHO 1980, p 29). Handicap is disturbance at the level of society. The WHO classification provides a way to understand the consequences of illness and to include the responses of the individual and society in service delivery. Further,

it supports the idea that, in long-term illness, treatment of the disease alone is not enough.

Epidemiologic Considerations

When most of the chronically mentally ill resided in state mental hospitals, census data made it relatively easy to estimate their numbers. Since the transition to community-based care, this has become much more complex. Most of the chronically mentally ill are now dispersed throughout the community, in a myriad of treatment and living situations.

To resolve the problem of counting the chronically mentally ill, Goldman, Gatozzi, and Taube (1981) employed three overlapping criteria:

1. Chronic diagnosis. Information about the prevalence of major mental disorder was used to estimate the size of the population.

2. Duration of hospital treatment. Census data from institutional settings were used to count the mentally ill.

3. Disability. The number of persons receiving disability benefits for psychiatric disorders were counted.

Using these criteria, researchers estimated the chronically mentally ill population at the beginning of the 1980s at between 1.7 and 2.5 million. Data from the 1990 census are not yet available. Clinical conditions and functional limitations of persons in this population not only vary widely at any point in time but also change over time, making any exact accounting extremely difficult.

The 1990 census figures will no doubt be evaluated to expand our awareness of this major public health problem and to guide service delivery. Statistical evaluation of this group will remain a challenge to nurse researchers.

Historical Cycles

Society in all ages has been organized to furnish some type of protection to those perceived as group members against threats to security from natural forces or from other human beings, alien in behavior, customs, or beliefs. See Figure 17–3. The mentally ill, whether regarded as possessed by demons or blessed by the Holy Spirit, have always been considered unpredictable if not inherently dangerous. They have been outcasts or barely tolerated in the community. In short, they have been considered anything but other human beings with problems.

Support systems are now more readily available to provide basic needs, and research is being done to assist in promotion of mental health. Efforts are being made in the fields of maintenance and rehabilitation as well to prognosticate future needs and trends. However, it is still routine to speak of crisis in mental health

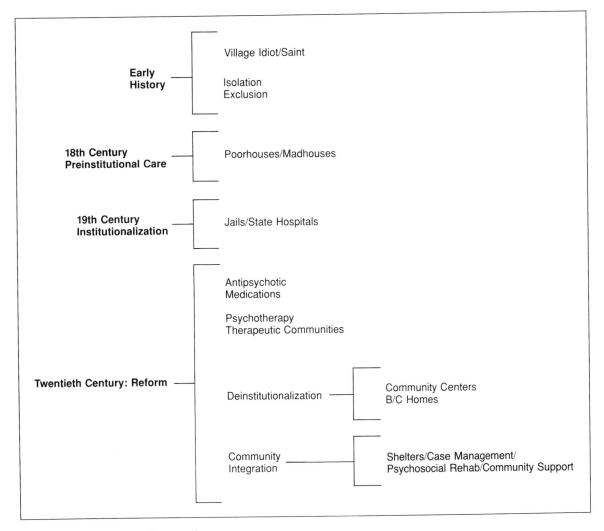

FIGURE 17–3   Historical perspectives.

care and funding and, indeed, it is accurate to say that this system is organized from one crisis to the next (Scott and Black 1986). At least the potential for improving the quality of life for the mentally ill is more than just a vision.

Persistent Problems

Limits of Medication Management

Medication regimens have become the mainstay of treatment programs for the chronically mentally ill. Research on the efficacy of medication, particularly neuroleptic regimens in schizophrenia, demonstrates that these agents reduce rates of relapse and hospital readmission. However, they have not been problem free. Drug regimens demand compliance, tolerance of temporary side effects, and acceptance of the risk of long-term problems such as tardive dyskinesia. Secondary effects of medications can be uncomfortable. They can also be embarrassing, since their effects on motor behavior (e.g., muscular stiffness, a shuffling gait) are visible to others (Estroff 1981).

In addition, psychoactive medications do not cure severe mental illness. Medications do not work with equal success for every individual or solve all the problems of chronic disorder. Many individuals who use psychoactive medications competently continue to experience some symptoms. For example, it is possible to suppress acute symptoms of schizophrenic illness without changing deficits in the area of social skills.

Economic Factors

Community mental health systems in many regions of the United States emphasize the importance of self-support and gainful employment whenever possible. However, surveys of the chronically ill suggest a low rate of competitive employment and indicate that expectations for autonomy may be unrealistic for some clients. A 1982 survey of the chronically mental ill found only one quarter to be employed, while less than half held full or part-time competitive jobs (Tessler et al. 1982). These figures reflect conditions in the job market, as well as individual disability. General unemployment tends to increase competition for jobs that might fit the skills of the mildly disabled.

Programs such as Supplemental Security Income (for the disabled) address the financial needs of some of the chronically mentally ill. Such programs, however, simply provide a small, fixed income and do not address the need for vocational programs and other meaningful activities for clients in the community.

Limits of Outpatient Therapies

As community-based systems develop, they form around a core of outpatient services, and rates of ambulatory service use climb dramatically. Clinics offer some services (such as medications and day treatment) for the severely ill, but they also provide individual, family, and group treatment to the larger population. Individuals with less severe or persistent problems account in part for the 120 percent rise in outpatient visits reported in national statistical data (Chafetz et al. 1983). In fact, some of the chronically mentally ill fail to connect with ambulatory services or to follow through with outpatient treatment.

Today we recognize that traditional outpatient programs (therapeutic services, generally on an appointment basis) may not meet the needs of all the varied population of chronically mentally ill. Although some clients use traditional outpatient care modalities, others require broader support services and do not benefit from psychotherapy. Some of the more successful outpatient services for this group emphasize coordination of comprehensive and continuous services rather than traditional therapies alone (Test and Stein 1978).

The Enduring Need for Acute Care

The chronically mentally ill continue to require access to acute care. Twenty-four-hour emergency and crisis units, in-patient services, and outreach programs were mandated in community mental health statutes to provide for people with problems (e.g., dangerous behavior, suicidal ideation, or grave disability) exceeding the resources of the outpatient sector. Many community health planners hoped to use hospitals as a last resort, treating only the most urgent problems in expensive acute care components of the service system.

Residential Placements

One community response to the presence of the chronically mentally ill has been proliferation of proprietary boarding homes and residential placements. Benefits from the federal Supplemental Security Income program (or other disability or general-assistance programs) often pay only residential costs, leaving very little in the way of extra funds for personal use.

These placements vary in size and quality, making it difficult to generalize about them. Some boarding arrangements encourage autonomy and provide a warm, stable environment for residents. Others, however, fall far below standards that should be applied to living environments for the disabled. Even satisfactory boarding facilities may provide limited opportunities for active treatment and community participation. For this reason, the movement of the chronically mentally ill to proprietary boarding homes is sometimes called *transinstitutionalization*, referring to movement from one custodial setting to another.

Community Exclusion

Boarding homes and other group residences for the mentally ill sometimes cluster in neighborhoods where few opportunities for community participation or integration exist. Movement to marginal urban districts has been called *ghettoization* (Chafetz et al. 1983), since it reflects containment of a disadvantaged group within special areas. It applies to more than boarding homes. For example, many of the chronically mentally ill reside in central city areas where single-room rentals can be found.

Single-room rentals have become a dwindling resource in many cities. Conversion of resident hotels to other uses reduces the overall housing supply and obliges the chronically mentally ill to compete with less stigmatized or disabled groups for limited resources. Loss of low-cost housing has been linked to residential instability (moving from place to place) among the chronically mentally ill and to their merging with the urban homeless (Baxter and Hopper 1982, Chafetz and Goldfinger 1984).

A Theoretic Perspective on Rehabilitation

When we look at psychiatric chronicity today, it is clear that not every individual who is mentally ill faces homelessness or even ostracism. Many clients manage well in existing treatment programs, participate in social and occupational activities, and demonstrate that serious disorder need not be synonymous with isolation or poverty. Their success is inspiring both for the mental health professional and for others who are afflicted with mental illness.

It is, however, equally clear that the chronically mentally ill comprise a population at risk for overwhelming social limitations. Their vulnerability raises many questions for mental health professionals concerning rehabilitation, in the broadest sense, for the heterogeneous groups that fall under the shadow of severe and persistent mental illness. Rehabilitation for them may be learning to paint in old age or holding a satisfying job for the first time. The question of potential for rehabilitation has particular relevance for nursing, because of its foundation in community health and its history of service to the disadvantaged.

What factors increase the risk of isolation and alienation? Do clinical problems beget social difficul-

ties? Can we develop a theoretic perspective on these problems that can guide the nursing process and help us prevent or reverse a loss of social and economic resources? To shape viable models for practice, we must consider intrinsic factors of genetics, the social environment, and the treatment system that make some people extremely vulnerable to poor clinical outcomes, exclusion from community living, isolation, and poverty.

Even though these causes and their consequences are not fully understood, mental health providers need models that give some structure to rehabilitation for this difficult and diverse group of people.

A Biopsychosocial Phenomenon

The concepts of genetic or biologic precipitants, social causation, social selection, and social reaction all play a role in the ongoing debate about "nature versus nurture" in psychiatry. This debate concerns the comparative importance of innate factors (the illness, personal competence) and environmental factors (child-rearing practices, social resources) in the incidence and course of chronic mental illness. There have been many swings of the pendulum in this discussion, with biologic or social theories gaining prominence at different points in history.

During the early deinstitutionalization period, professionals and laypeople widely believed that some of the more unfortunate effects of long-term illness, e.g., withdrawal and loss of initiative and social skills, were caused by the institutional environment. The persistence of some of these problems in community settings has rekindled debate on how they come about and on how much responsibility for chronicity should be borne by the individual and how much by the social and physical surroundings.

Recent advances in biologic psychiatry (Chapter 6) make it impossible to consider psychiatric chronicity a purely social construction. Because biologic processes appear to play a role in both incidence and course of illness, it is difficult to dismiss them with discussions of social adjustment. At the same time, we are gaining knowledge about the effects of environmental variables on functional adaptation, even when biologic factors are clearly operating. Psychiatric chronicity appears to be a complex biopsychosocial phenomenon, determined by multiple factors and amenable to as many interventions.

Stress-Vulnerability

Several investigators have proposed the stress-vulnerability model to explain the interaction of biologic, psychologic, and social factors in the onset and course of illness in the severely and persistently mentally ill.

This model proposes that certain individuals are born with genetic vulnerability for certain mental disorders, activated by environmental stressors, which then continue to influence the course of the disease.

This model provides a way to account for the biologic factors without ignoring the influence of societal and psychologic factors. It also supports the need for interpersonal and environmental as well as biologic interventions.

Since the stress-vulnerability model views the person as having a disease rather than being a diseased person, all behavior need not be viewed as pathologic. This model also allows for the incorporation of primary and secondary symptoms, and support interventions such as psychoeducation. Rather than promoting an exclusive emphasis on pathology, the perspective of this model directs our thinking toward matching persons with environmental resources and increasing their capacity to function at more individually satisfying levels.

Social Resources

The relationship between social resources and chronic psychiatric disorder has preoccupied clinicians and social scientists since the beginnings of psychiatric epidemiology. The reason for this relationship remains a matter of debate. One point of view considers poor treatment outcomes a function of individual factors. From this perspective, severity of illness reduces individual ability to maintain interpersonal and economic assets. The **social selection** hypothesis places locus of causation within the individual and suggests that social disadvantages are the result of illness (Turner and Gartrell 1978).

It is also possible that social characteristics could cause poor clinical outcomes. The poor, the powerless, and the socially isolated are more likely than others to bear the negative consequences of psychiatric labeling. This is the social reaction hypothesis, which places the site of causation in the social environment (Turner and Gartrell 1978). It follows from this line of reasoning that a disenfranchised population living in poverty on the fringes of society would be helped by human contact and support in meeting basic human needs. Provision of adequate shelter, nourishing food, and health care would be of greatest benefit.

Community studies have also attempted to examine the persistent relationships between mental illness (particularly schizophrenia) and socioeconomically deprived environments. Epidemiologic studies dating back to the 1930s demonstrate that rates of mental illness rise in socially disorganized parts of the central city and drop in more affluent or socially integrated areas (Faris and Dunham 1939). More recent reports continue to document the movement of the mentally ill to marginal areas (Baxter and Hopper 1981). A social causation explanation considers urban alienation and poverty as stressors that help produce psychiatric symptoms. However, the same phenomenon has been explained in terms of social selection; that is, sicker and more isolated people "drift down" to pockets of urban poverty.

The **National Alliance for the Mentally Ill (NAMI)** and its state and local chapters have grown tremendously over the past decade. Originally composed of family members organized to support one another, these groups now include politicians and concerned health care workers who influence mental health policy and funding.

The activist efforts of the mentally ill, their families, and people in their support systems may in time increase the flow of needed resources from both public and private funds, thereby improving the lot of mentally ill clients in the community. Many of these persons also need help in utilizing the system and linking with available services to raise their functional level.

The Service System

Social disadvantage and isolation have been tied to the mental health system itself, specifically its complexity and lack of flexibility. The most successful programs for the chronically mentally ill have sometimes selected clients with superior treatment histories and intact social resources (Braun et al. 1981). The system as a whole may respond best to clients who "fit" into programs, people who resemble the ideal client anticipated by the treatment system. Others, less attractive, unaware of how to navigate the seas of red tape, or less able to fit into existing programs, receive less attention.

Segal and Baumohl (1980) use the concept of **social margin** to describe clients who seem to slip through the cracks of the mental health system. This term refers to a decrease in the attributes and assets a person can trade on to obtain services, material, and interpersonal resources. These assets are interpreted as an indication that the individual will be able to use services and remain in treatment. People who appear to be "bad risks," including the transient mentally ill and volatile younger chronic clients, receive little follow-up. This means that those with multiple needs sometimes receive the least support. In this sense, the system actually contributes to its clients' difficulties.

Rehabilitation

Complete social and economic rehabilitation for the persistently mentally ill has been dismissed as a pipe dream by all but the most visionary reformers until fairly recently. Rehabilitation approaches seem to encounter strong resistance among providers trained in a treatment/cure rather than a rehabilitative philoso-

TABLE 17-1   **Elements of Rehabilitation**

Stage	Examples	Interventions
Pathology	Brain tumor or infection	Lab and radiographic tests
Impairment	Positive and negative symptoms of schizophrenia (delusions, anhedonia)	Diagnosis, hospitalization, pharmacotherapy
Disability	Deficient self-care, social skills	Assessment, skills training, social support
Handicap	Unemployment, homelessness	Supported employment, case management

phy. Farkas and Anthony (1989) suggest that, to expedite change, pressure needs to be brought to bear on service deliverers: people (professionals or laypersons), programs (to support these people), and systems (to provide resources on many levels).

Empowerment of this often-isolated and disenfranchised population has been a difficult principle to operationalize in the practical world of mental health today, hindered as it is by overextension of staff and underfunding of programs. But progress is being made. Practitioners are employing physical rehabilitation and psychotherapeutic techniques already widely utilized in helping physically disabled persons. (See Table 17-1.) The emphasis is on the principles of impairment, disability, and handicap discussed earlier (Farkas and Anthony 1989).

The program for rehabilitation follows the nursing process model and has similar tools for assessing function and setting goals. It may contain groups that deal with social skills and vocational skills, as well as traditional support groups for medication management or accessing financial assistance and budget making. One manager usually coordinates the activities of several different clients and periodically evaluates their individual needs and desires, at times giving them emotional support. Success is measured by how good the match is between what the client wants and how well the client is actually functioning.

This approach incorporates a wide repertoire of technologies from medicine, social work, psychology, and physical rehabilitation. The nurse is ideally educated to coordinate such a mix, because the nursing process already incorporates many of the techniques and the language from these various disciplines.

Contemporary Issues and Rehabilitation

Age of the Population

While the U.S. population has tripled since 1900, the group over age 65 has grown eightfold. Although increased morbidity and mortality are associated with chronic mental illness, persons with persistent and severe mental disorders can be found in increasing numbers in the older age groups. It is estimated that 15 percent of elderly psychiatric outpatients are schizophrenic, and this figure does not take into account institutionalized clients. Currently there are approximately two million chronically mentally ill elderly in the United States. This number is growing continually, reflecting the aging of the "baby boom" population (Perse et al. 1986).

The nursing home has become one of the major care providers for the chronically mentally ill elderly. With little consultation from mental health professionals, geriatric staff feel poorly prepared to deal with these clients (Fopma-Loy 1989). Frequently abusive, dependent, wandering, and demanding, the clients may be shifted from one care facility to another (transinstitutionalization), with no consistent supportive services (Richter 1989). Their frequent concomitant medical problems may lead to fragmentation of care, and negative attitudes toward aging may add to the stigma and problems caused by their chronic psychiatric disorder. This aging group of the chronically mentally ill may present the most critical challenges of the future.

The Young Chronically Mentally Ill

The young chronic population is defined on the basis of age (18–44) and chronicity (as indicated by diagnosis and number of admissions in a given time frame). This group is very heterogeneous and difficult to study or categorize. It has been classified according to energy level, functional ability, and demand on available mental health services (Sheets et al. 1982). The young chronic element is seen as a major trend in the definition of the client in the 1990s, and its growing numbers are among the most difficult to engage in rehabilitation programs. Many have not been previously hospitalized and unlike the generation before them, do not exhibit the traits of institutionalization. They may constitute over a third of the functionally impaired population.

These less mature clients seem to have more difficulty adjusting to the demands of society and often turn to alcohol and drug abuse, with resultant cycles of acting-out behaviors and withdrawal in an acute setting, such as jail or the psychiatric hospital. They are generally not amenable to offers of help except on their own terms.

Dual-Diagnosis Clients

Dual-diagnosis clients have concurrent problems: substance abuse and a psychiatric diagnosis. Many of the young chronic population are included in this group. Researchers are studying dual-diagnosis clients to ascertain relationships between diagnosis and substance category, proper treatment modalities, and prognosticators of successful rehabilitation, including return to the community. The complexities of their behavior make it difficult to sort them into categories or to predict their functional levels. Especially interesting are hybrid programs, which integrate both conventional psychotherapy and substance abuse treatment modalities (Minkoff 1989). These parallel programs hold some promise for the dual-diagnosis client, but progress is slow and painstaking, with little guarantee of rehabilitation.

Caregiver Stress

When families assume a caregiving or supervisory function, they take on roles that involve additional stress. Medication supervision may often raise concerns about policing the client. Liaison activities with health and social agencies take time and effort, since they often demand negotiation of services with complex and poorly coordinated systems. These activities can also involve high levels of frustration, since mental health and social welfare systems are designed to communicate with clients as individuals, not their relatives. Families may be rebuffed if they act on behalf of the clients and feel negligent if they leave them to fend for themselves. Acute episodes may raise intense feelings in the family, including fears of betraying the client by calling for outside help, self-doubts about what might have been done to prevent recurrence, and bitter disappointment about the relapse.

Emotional problems seem to burden families as much as practical or economic concerns. The stigma of mental illness, as well as guilt arising from many psychodynamic theories that stress the role of family dynamics in etiology, distance families from sources of support and assistance. In fact, current psychiatric theory counters the notion that family interactions causes a chronic illness, although expressed emotion theory does propose that families can influence the course of illness (Falloon et al. 1984).

Aging parents functioning as caregivers present a unique set of problems. Frequently the responsibility falls on the mother (Ascher-Svanum and Sobel 1989), taking a significant economic, emotional, and physio-logic toll. Lefly (1987) recommends that placement of chronically mentally ill clients with aging parents should not be considered a viable option for community management of the mentally ill, as it increases the stress on an already vulnerable group.

As supportive family members grow older and their energy diminishes, many of the mentally ill who reside with them will lose their homes and support. It is estimated that over the course of the next decade, this loss will affect the majority of clients now with family caretakers (Perlman et al. 1988). The implications for the mental health system, both economically and in sheer numbers of clients needing services, need to be addressed now. Planning agencies must prepare for alternative care, to prevent even greater swelling of the ranks of the homeless mentally ill.

The Forensic Population

It has been noted that prevalence rates of major psychiatric disorders in the jails have increased gradually but continuously over the past twenty years. This increase may be attributable at least in part to deinstitutionalization policies (Jamelka et al. 1989). Society has low tolerance for disordered behavior, and the lack of services for the persistently and severely mentally ill in the mental health system may lead to a funneling of these persons into the criminal justice system.

Unemployment, homelessness, and drug and alcohol abuse contribute to the profile of the chronically mentally ill forensic client (Whitmer 1989). Nearly one-fourth of forensic in-patient services are filled over capacity (Way et al. 1990). Most mentally ill offenders end up in county jails rather than forensic mental hospitals; these persons rarely become connected with local mental health networks and are frequently counted among the homeless, because they have no residence of record (Rossi et al. 1987). Inappropriate arrest and incarceration cannot be judged the treatment of choice for the person who needs psychiatric treatment.

The Homeless

The 1980s saw an increasing awareness of the scope of homelessness. The rise in homelessness is explained in part not only by deinstitutionalization but also by increased joblessness, the loss of low-rent housing due to gentrification of many cities, and the loss of federal housing monies (Mechanic 1987). Although the homeless are a very diverse population that is very difficult to count, estimates are that there are 2–3 million homeless in urban areas, and that 40 to 60 percent of these persons have severe mental disorders (Goldman and Manderscheid 1987).

RESEARCH NOTE

Citation

Grunberg J, Eagle PF: Shelterization: How the homeless adapt to shelter living. Hosp Comm Psychiatry May, 1990;41(5):521–525.

Study Problem/Purpose

Emergency shelters have become the backbone of the service delivery system to the homeless, and crime in such shelters is a way of life. Despite the dangers of shelter living, many residents don't leave but instead adapt according to a process termed "shelterization" by the authors. The purpose of this study was to describe the process of adapting to shelter life.

Methods

The findings in this report are based on a case study of the Fort Washington's Men's Shelter on 168th Street off Broadway in New York City. This shelter is one of the 20 New York City shelters located in converted buildings such as National Guard armories and unused public schools in 1988. This particular shelter houses nightly more than 1000 homeless men, who plan their lives around the various pressures of shelter life, e.g., appointments with social workers, finding the safest time to take a shower, borrowing money, and so on. Although data collection and analysis procedures are not specific in this report, findings were clearly based on fieldwork observation and interviewing strategies.

Findings

Like institutionalization, shelterization is a social process of adapting. It is described by the investigators as a *process of acculturation endemic to shelter living* and is characterized by a decrease in interpersonal responsiveness, a neglect of personal hygiene, increasing passivity, and an increasing dependence on others. The residents show decreasing interest in leaving the shelter, increasing attachment to shelter routines, and rejection of any outside groups to which they may have belonged. In short, they become isolated in the shelter and lose their motivation to reenter mainstream society.

Implications

If the process of shelterization is to be ameliorated, strategies must include the establishment of positive social networks and affiliations between the homeless, social service, and mental health providers. On-site psychosocial rehabilitation programs can be developed to offer a therapeutic alternative to the subculture that exists within the shelter. Programs that promote improved self-esteem, improved social relations and social skills are essential if the disaffiliation-shelterlife-shelter reaffiliation sequence is to be supplanted with optimal functioning for the homeless mentally ill.

There is much debate over the etiology of this portion of the homeless. Do homelessness and its severe stressors lead to increased mental illness, or do impairment and disability lead to a higher risk and vulnerability to homelessness, as some reports (Chafetz and Goldfinger 1984) suggest?

Data obtained on the homeless mentally ill to date indicate that they are a clinically heterogeneous group, with a range of psychiatric problems. They share social isolation, poverty, and the medical illnesses their conditions impose. Lost prescriptions and medications, lost personal belongings, and lack of contacts for social and financial support are all part of the specter of homelessness. Substance abuse and disruptive behaviors are not uncommon reactions to this experience (Lamb and Talbott 1986). The chronically mentally ill homeless are often victimized by other homeless persons and therefore can have great difficulty trusting others.

Some members of this group may prefer the freedom and independence of life on the streets, as well as the personal distance and anonymity it provides (Gullberg 1989). This attitude is perhaps a response to enforced participation in alternative housing programs with mandatory treatment components.

Many of this population have become so entrenched in the social life of the shelters ("shelterized") that they seldom leave these refuges and have little energy to pursue reintegration into society (Grunberg and Eagle 1990). The individual needs and issues of each of the homeless mentally ill are unique to their own situation and past experiences, and solutions cannot be standardized or generalized.

The homeless require subsistence services as well as psychiatric services. Completing long application procedures may mean missing a place in line for a bed or a meal. Certain areas still require an address for the provision of public assistance, leading to a significant and seemingly insurmountable dilemma for the mentally ill homeless person.

Federal, local, and private agencies, such as the Robert Wood Johnson Program for the Chronically Mentally Ill (Krauss 1989), are attempting to find meaningful ways to deliver services to this group. Block grants are being used to fund public health programs delivering primary medical care to clients in shelters and on the streets and to develop outreach programs for psychiatric service provision. The nurse working in mental health centers, crisis services, and shelters must be creative to address the unique needs of this group. Some of these programs may be tenuously funded and depend on year-to-year budget allocations.

A regrettable consequence of homelessness is the image that these persons acquire with providers of services; they appear to be "poor risks," "noncompliers," or "manipulators" (Goldfinger and Chafetz 1984). This image makes working with the homeless even more difficult and reduces the possibility of engaging them in services that might address their needs. To be effective, service providers must begin by accepting the alienation and suspicion of homeless people and by attempting to build trust, beginning with efforts to meet their basic subsistence needs (Goldfinger and Chafetz 1984).

AIDS

Although comprehensive data are not yet available, the incidence of AIDS may become a problem for the mentally ill population. Their minimal ability to function in the mainstream makes them vulnerable to sexual abuse by opportunists. There is also an increasing prevalence of AIDS in the homeless population due to IV drug use (Froner 1988). Still not classified as severely and persistently mentally ill are people who manifest AIDS-related symptoms. Many people with HIV disease have become homeless and suffer from AIDS-related dementia, which is becoming increasingly prevalent in urban psychiatric wards (Baer 1989).

Comprehensive Models

The medical model and the psychosocial model need to be synthesized into a structured treatment modality. Such a synthesis has been attempted in the comprehensive service models, which go beyond psychiatric treatment in a narrow sense. These models offer a range of support services to correct some of the problems of deinstitutionalization and promote quality of life in the community. The "basic and specialized needs of the chronically mentally ill," identified in *Toward a National Plan for the Chronically Mentally Ill* (DHHS 1980), include a continuum of services for

structured or independent settings, including: food, clothing, and household management; financial support and budgeting; recreation; transportation; general medical and mental health services; habilitation and rehabilitation; vocational and social services; and integrative services that bring together and coordinate other areas of care.

Community Programs

There are many movements today to enlist the support of communities of residence, especially important in urban areas (Davies et al. 1989), to help the mentally ill to live fuller, more productive lives on their own terms. These include volunteer friend and fund-raising activities, activist groups such as the Alliance for the Mentally Ill, programs that enhance social and employment skills, and supported and sheltered work environments.

Vocational rehabilitation, which at its inception referred to sheltered employment in a workshop away from the mainstream marketplace, is now becoming a functional reality for those clients willing to make the commitment of time and energy to the systems available. A current program, receiving recognition from the business community because of federal incentives, offers opportunities for supported employment in more public and satisfying situations. For people with psychiatric disabilities, a new model based on personal choice, called choose, get, keep, has been developed (Danley and Anthony 1987). This model (see Table 17-2) delineates three basic competencies that are necessary for employment and offers classes that prepare the client to set goals and choose a job focus. Once clients are placed, they are supported by job coaches, who act as role models, provide feedback, and act as liaisons to employers.

Depot-medication therapy, usually consisting of an injection every two to four weeks, does not require the client to remember to take medications several times a day and is a valuable adjunct to the success of community involvement.

Social skills training has been shown to be the basis for re-entry into the community after the disease process is stabilized and client is ready for discharge. Such training, however, is not always applicable to the novel situations that the client may encounter in the real world outside the hospital (Hogarty et al. 1987) and does not appear to prevent rehospitalization, although it may increase the time spent outside of the hospital.

Social dramatics, including having clients view themselves on videotapes (Whetstone 1986), seems to be a promising area not only for functional-skills training but also for assessing self-concept and increasing self-esteem. Both motor skills and cognitive functions must be addressed in a social skills program

TABLE 17–2 **Phases of Supported Employment**

Choose	*Get*	*Keep*
Identifying interests	Identifying assets	Appropriate behavior
Assessing capabilities	Locating potential employment	Being on time
Matching traits to job	Writing a resume	Responding well to training
Evaluating options	Job applications	Interacting well with others

(Bellack et al. 1989). It is most important to empower even the most psychotic patients (Bechnel and Gurgone 1987) to give them an opportunity for interpersonal communication with staff and to encourage their optimal growth.

Case Management

Being the case manager for mentally ill clients can challenge psychiatric nurses to use all their skills and see beyond individual clients to a larger perspective. The case-management model is fundamental to the community-support program of care developed through the Federal Community Support Program (a demonstration project with federal-state collaboration that began in 1978). This program employs a case manager to coordinate therapeutic and support services.

The case manager assesses the total needs of the chronically ill individual, establishes goals, and obtains the set of services required to meet them. Because service needs can change over time, the goals and referrals for a given client may change as well. Unlike clients receiving conventional treatment, however, these clients remain in contact with the same provider in spite of alterations in their clinical status.

Case managers often find that they are filling many roles for their clients that have not been provided by other clinical resources and that, as a result, their clients may make less frequent use of in-patient treatment (Harris and Bergman 1988). At first they need to build relationships, assess their clients, and connect them with pertinent services. As time passes, these functions evolve into monitoring the client's needs by touching base with them and responding to periodic crises. This population varies in type and extent of service requirements but case management may require a longer time than previously assumed.

The case-management philosophy has generated enthusiasm in many quarters because it seems to respond to the special needs of the psychiatrically disabled. It acknowledges the pervasive nature of their problems and their needs for multiple services. It anticipates an oscillating or unpredictable course of illness and acknowledges the possibility of prolonged dependence. It is likely that many clients will receive case management within community support programs in the future.

Ms L is a 67-year-old widow who comes into the medication clinic for her monthly injection, accompanied by her case manager. Ms L has carried a diagnosis of schizophrenia, paranoid type, for many years. She was able to stay at home with her husband and was maintained well with outpatient care and medications, requiring only brief crisis intervention and two short hospital stays by the time she was 60. She was unable to maintain employment. Her husband participated in a support group at the local clinic.

After her husband died, Ms L had a severe decompensation: she experienced frightening hallucinations and delusions and was threatening her neighbors. Police were called and she was hospitalized. During this time, all her belongings were stolen from her apartment. She was stabilized on depot medications and was referred to a Community Support Program (CSP) for assistance with both housing and rehabilitation. Ms L was assigned a case manager who helped her apply for SSI. The case manager also arranged for a shared apartment, facilitated medication and clinic appointments, visited her weekly, and encouraged regular participation in a social rehabilitation program. Ms L has not required hospitalization in the six years since being enrolled in the CSP. She participates in several small social groups and has been able to take two trips to California to visit her son and his family. Although she stills "hears voices," she is able to monitor her symptoms and advises her son or her case manager when her symptoms increase.

Applying the Nursing Process with the Chronically Mentally Ill

The nursing process for the chronically mentally ill addresses individual problems and environmental supports. To find a conceptual framework that can help us to understand the practice of nursing care for the severely and persistently ill, we can turn to Orem's Self-Care Deficit Theory, as operationalized by Underwood (Underwood in press, Morrison 1985). This framework, combined with an understanding of the stages of chronic illness, helps nurses apply the nursing process. The focus of nursing is the individual's health, well-being, and quality of life (Meleis 1981). The self-care model expands on the individualized focus by assuming that the person's ability for self-care and self-determination affects health, well-being, and quality of life.

While nurses usually encounter individuals who are identified as having illness or disease, the intent of nursing remains assisting the person to maintain, regain, or attain self-care and self-determination in day-to-day living. The goal is to help the individual sustain health, well-being, and quality of life.

The nurse uses the nursing process to organize care and utilizes the complementary contractual nurse-client relationship to develop the mutually negotiated individual plans of care. The components described above, along with a knowledge of the stages of chronic illness, provide a basis for understanding severe and persistent mental illness and the nurse's role in both treatment and rehabilitation.

Chronic mental disorders (disease) produce a wide range of signs and symptoms (impairment). Nurses must have in-depth knowledge of both psychiatric and medical disease processes to assess disease and strengths not only in clients but also their families and others in their environment. Basic medical needs are frequently unmet in this population (Roca et al. 1987), and nurses may be among the most appropriate caregivers to address this area of concern (Mechanic 1986).

Assessing

A concise history of the client's life should include functional level, specific areas of impairment (such as self-care and hygiene, community living, social or family relationships, and control of inappropriate behavior), as well as current psychiatric treatment, including medication compliance. The client's perception of difficult areas and expectations for treatment should also be addressed. The data-collection process should focus on the types of events or experience that the individual finds difficult.

Comprehensive data collection focuses simultaneously on the environment. The nurse looks not only at problems but also at supports that protect the clients. Attention to the environment should occur in any settings where nursing care is delivered: family home, boarding facility, apartment, or hospital. See the accompanying Assessment box for a complete list of assessment data.

Planning and Implementing Interventions

The psychiatric nurse analyzes information about client and environment to identify areas where nursing intervention may buffer environmental stress, increase

ASSESSMENT

Comprehensive Data Assessment

- Physical health
- Self-care/Hygiene
- Medication compliance
- Self-acceptance/Self-esteem
- Vocational history
- Family involvement
- Personal relationships
- Decision-making abilities
- Philosophy: Expectations/hopes
- Recreation/Community involvement
- Management of emotions
  —Self-directed violence
  —Violence toward objects/others
- Substance use: past/present
- Legal problems
- Resource utilization/social services

support, or decrease individual vulnerability. Nursing care plans vary according to the setting where the care is delivered. Psychiatric nurses in hospitals, for example, care for clients experiencing acute exacerbations of illness and needing symptomatic treatment and a safe, structured environment. Rehabilitation planning for them is inappropriate until they are more stable. Nurse clinical specialists in a community setting may have a caseload of outpatients with very different needs, among which rehabilitation planning would figure prominently. In both situations, nursing diagnoses and nursing care plans should reflect a comprehensive, flexible view of the person in a given environment. See the accompanying Nursing Care Plan.

Intervening with Clients   Impairment associated with the chronic mental diseases often results in disability. Rehabilitation efforts generally focus on teaching clients skills to improve daily functioning. Nurses help individuals by promoting self-care in daily living. Medication regimens, psychotherapeutic services, social skills training, and psychosocial rehabilitation, including day treatment and vocational training, emphasize control of the illness process or development of skills to reduce individual behavior deficits.

It should be emphasized that many clients seem to benefit from interventions that address functional

NURSING CARE PLAN

A Client in a Day Treatment Program

Client Care Goals	Nursing Planning/Intervention	Evaluation
Nursing Diagnosis: *Self-care deficit: Bathing/hygiene, Dressing/grooming*		
The client will arrive at center without noticeable body odor, wear clean clothes, and maintain neat appearance for entire day.	Monitor appearance. Give verbal feedback. Supply used clothing if possible.	By the end of one month, client improves in specified areas.
Nursing Diagnosis: *Altered role performance*		
The client will be able to formulate career goals, evaluate assets, and review options for employment.	Participate in skills training. Give encouragement and feedback. Suggest methods of transportation.	After skills training workshop, client role-plays job interview and fills out applications.

problems, such as referrals to socialization groups or vocational rehabilitation programs. These approaches promote development of skills that help clients live in the community. Traditional psychotherapists do not place this emphasis on living skills and assume instead that personal growth will lead to better functional skills. In fact, at least among some persons diagnosed as schizophrenic, intense psychosocial interventions may prove too stressful and may actually increase vulnerability to relapse (Falloon et al. 1984). It appears that, at least for a subgroup of the severely and persistently mentally ill, treatment should focus not on gaining insight but on working toward improvement in maintenance goals, such as improved self-care and social skills.

Impairment and disability may result in handicap. The severely and persistently mentally ill are a stigmatized group that suffers disadvantages in housing, education, and work. Nurses can influence program and policy decisions that could reduce the handicap of mental illness. In the process of promoting self-care and self-determination, nurses work with client advocacy groups, consumer groups, families, and non-kin networks and encourage the formation of self-help groups and use of peer counselors.

The nurse working with the severely and persistently mentally ill applies the nursing process at many levels. The most basic focus is the individual needs of assistance with daily living and impulse control. The nurse must also make an effort to match these needs with environmental supports, such as medical manage-

ment and psychotherapeutic intervention. When the client's acuity level is at a manageable level, the nurse may be able to initiate a process of normalization or integration into a therapeutic community.

Intervening with Systems People with psychiatric disabilities tend to have small social networks, yet clients rely heavily on these networks for practical or instrumental assistance (Falloon et al. 1984). Social networks serve a vital function in helping vulnerable individuals live in the community. Research is being done on how to analyze these systems and encourage their stability in the lives of the mentally ill person (Morin and Seidman 1986). To prevent the erosion of support that often accompanies chronicity, nurses and other mental health professionals have turned their attention to interventions that not only help the individual, but also "support the supporters."

Family therapies once placed the responsibility for the client's illness on the family itself (for example, on communication patterns in the family of a schizophrenic). Increasing awareness of the biologic basis of major mental disorders and growing recognition of the burden that these disorders impose on families have shifted attention to enhancing the client's natural support networks.

While the idea that families engender chronic illness may have been discredited, family factors remain important determinants of success in treatment and rehabilitation. A family's ability to cope with psychiatric chronicity appears to influence the course of schizophrenic illness and possibly other disorders (Falloon et al. 1984). The management of "expressed emotion" in families is currently the subject of rigorous research (see Chapter 12). Expressed emotion is a topic of great concern in the context of rehabilitation because it appears that persons with schizophrenia are more prone to relapse if their families are emotionally overinvolved with them, either verbally critical or excessively positive, sometimes infantilizing the client (de Cangas 1990). It appears that when families modify the type and amount of contact with a chronically ill member, the risk of acute exacerbation may diminish. This psychoeducational approach to care minimizes blame for the illness by educating family members about its biologic basis and offers constructive ways to manage psychiatric chronicity.

Relatives who maintain a disabled member in the household and assume caregiving responsibilities (such as supervising the taking of medication and maintaining a safe environment) may require very practical assistance. Information about homemaking or legal services can be as welcome as information about treatment. Family caregivers often face seemingly insurmountable obstacles when they plan vacations and trips. Respite services (or short-term placements to relieve the family of the burden of care) allow families the help they require to continue in a caregiving role. Such services have been widely recommended as a way to reduce family burden and enhance the quality of life for both the client and the relatives on a long-term basis.

Nurses working with families of the severely and persistently mentally ill need to become attuned to their concerns about the future and their inability to control or predict changes in the client's condition that may affect the household. Families may express ambivalence about caregiving. For example, they may want to promote the client's autonomy yet feel discomfort or guilt about the type of living situation the client is able to maintain independently. Clear information and nonjudgmental attitudes from nurses and other providers can do much to alleviate a family's distress and assure them that there may not be a perfect way to deal with their problems. In addition, self-help groups and advocacy organizations formed· by families of the mentally ill promote sharing and support.

Family may not be the best resource for every individual with chronic psychiatric illness. Family relationships can be fraught with conflict; the familial responsibilities may preclude psychiatric caregiving; or the client may simply prefer an independent living situation. Under these circumstances, the client's network of interpersonal resources must go beyond the family.

Persons residing in proprietary boarding homes and residential hotels benefit from contacts with managers and fellow residents. Despite the problems described in some residential placements, there are conscientious and competent managers who occupy a pivotal position in the individual's support system. Like families, these "support persons" need access to assistance from the mental health system. For example, residential care managers or hotel staff are more willing to retain a difficult or volatile client in their facility if they feel that outreach and emergency services are available. In a similar sense, clients with strong links to health care and social service systems place fewer demands or inappropriate burdens on support systems in residential placements.

The chronically mentally ill sometimes establish support systems that seem idiosyncratic. Clients living in hotels or other urban rentals, for example, may benefit from casual contacts with local merchants, workers in local restaurants, or other neighborhood residents. Clients may feel closer to other recipients of psychiatric services than to the larger community. In a study of the community-based mentally ill, Estroff (1981) noted that "insiders" feel a special rapport or mutual understanding.

It is important for psychiatric nurses to recognize that clients have their own life experiences and preferences, which should be respected. Although the literature indicates that chronic mental illness alters social networks, there is no basis for active intervention to alter the individual's social support system. Overintensive or interventionist approaches may contribute to rather than alleviate environmental stress.

This does not mean that nurses and other mental health professionals should follow a hands-off policy about environmental conditions that appear inadequate or even dangerous (e.g., hazardous or unsanitary living situations). It does mean that the nurse should attempt to assess interpersonal environments from the client's perspective, with an understanding of the client's unique needs and preferences.

Evaluating/Outcome Criteria

The chronically mentally ill contend with an unpredictable and oscillating course of illness. Unlike acute health problems with a clear resolution, chronic psychiatric disorders may change over time, though underlying symptoms persist. These changes can occur in reaction to shifting individual factors (e.g., aging with general changes in health status) and external factors (e.g., living conditions and life events). Mental health nurses working with clients in extended care settings (e.g., community clinics) can monitor changes over time. In this way, nursing evaluation can identify shifting needs and match them with available resources.

A thorough evaluation requires recognition of personal characteristics. No matter what constellation of services the client requires, they must be delivered in a manner that is meaningful to the individual. This meaning is a function of multiple factors such as culture, ethnicity, age, sex, values, and beliefs about health and illness. Diagnostic differences alone suggest a variety of environmental needs. Interpersonal factors, such as dependence or distance, and more material environmental properties, such as crowding or noise, have different meanings for different people. In fact, environmental needs do not remain static for any person, and the mentally disordered, like anyone else, experience dynamic changes related to their own growth and development. If an environment is to be considered supportive, personal characteristics and individual potential for change must be valued.

In the same sense, although psychosocial stressors influence the course of illness, events are more stressful or less so according to individual meanings and values. The client or support persons, for example, can often identify the events that trigger episodes of acute illness. These events may not appear universally stressful, but they have personal significance.

The goal of going beyond the brokerage of resources and services for an individualized response to each person's needs encourages psychiatric nurses to develop rapport and enter a relationship of mutual trust and understanding with the client. Through this interactive approach the nurse can assess each person's unique needs and wishes. The nursing process for the chronically mentally ill, as for other client groups, occurs through a human exchange and shared understanding. As an interactive process, it involves both acceptance of clients' problems and consideration of their potential for change and growth.

Humanistic Care

It is sometimes difficult for nurses to maintain a humanistic perspective on care for the severely ill. Like some client's families, and the mentally ill themselves, nurses may interpret long-term impairment or increased acuity as treatment failure, thereby investing the idea of chronicity with negative meanings. The persistence of the disorder may be seen as a sign of the client's lack of compliance or the system's inability to deliver effective services. In either case, the message is one of disappointment, lowering the client's already compromised self-esteem and exacerbating alienation and loneliness.

Nurses occupy a pivotal position in mental health systems serving the chronically ill population. Because of nursing's traditional concern with such issues as self-care, environmental support, and family-oriented health services, psychiatric nurses can apply their skills to the planning of comprehensive care more easily than mental health professionals prepared for narrower

psychotherapeutic activities. As McCausland (1987) urges: "An opportunity exists for psychiatric nursing to become a corporate actor with influence on health policy. Visionary leaders and nurse researchers should join forces to design and evaluate model treatment and case management programs that would justify transferring some of the two thirds of public mental health dollars currently budgeted to hospitals to true community-based programs for the mentally ill" (p 33).

Possibly the most ambitious effort for a nurse is to start a free-lance agency that promotes a type of mental health care within the community (Worley and Albanese 1989). Such nurses are in effect independent case managers following the prototype of the primary nurses for an in-patient setting. Worley and Albanese believe that "of all the health care disciplines, nurses are probably the most skilled at crossing lay-professional boundaries and marshalling resources where there appear to be none."

Nursing Research and Education

Nursing is now in an important position to provide impetus and leadership in the field of care for the persistently and severely mentally ill. Judith Krauss (1989) identifies the chronically mentally ill as a population that needs what nursing has to offer: "Comprehensive care, continuity of care, community-based care—these words have a far better chance of being actualized through the practice and research of nursing than through the work of any of the other four core disciplines." If nursing is to meet this challenge, educators and researchers must focus intensely on this population (Connolly 1989, Lefley et al. 1989). Becoming more involved with this population during education can give the nurse a sense of the positive value of working with the chronically ill, helping to destigmatize their condition. We need to emphasize the positive aspects and outcomes of current therapies, as outlined in this chapter and others, to generate enthusiasm and to initiate action.

Aggressive energy needs to be directed toward conducting nursing research on relapse-prevention strategies and developing and evaluating nontraditional modalities of care (e.g., training volunteers and community members to work with the client). Alternative delivery systems and approaches, e.g., the use of nurses in shelters and as case managers, need to be outlined and investigated. The implications of the increasing body of psychobiologic information need to be incorporated into nursing interventions, especially as regards cognition and thought processing in the psychotic client. Interventions directed to decreasing impairment lead to less disability. Social and societal interventions by nurses can prevent handicap. Attempts to define and codify the nursing body of knowledge are necessary as both a mechanism of identifying ourselves to the community and a way to regulate reimbursement. Efforts at increasing the monies available through all channels is work that nurses can and should pursue.

The chronically mentally ill are certainly a difficult population with which to work. Long-term problems and impairment may invest the idea of chronicity with negative meanings and cause frustration. However, because of nursing's traditional concern with such issues as self-care, environmental support, and family-oriented health services, psychiatric nurses can apply their skills to the planning of care for this group of clients. Treatment of disease is not enough. Rehabilitation is a key component in the treatment of the severely and persistently mentally ill, and nurses can take a lead in this opportunity for care.

Chapter Highlights

• The persistently and severely mentally ill, also called the chronically mentally ill, have illnesses that prevent functioning in personal hygiene and self-care, self-direction, interpersonal relationships, social interactions, learning, and recreational activities.

• Schizophrenic disorders account for the largest subgroup of the chronically mentally ill.

• Impairment is defined as any loss or abnormality of psychologic, physiologic, or anatomic structure or function. Disability is any restriction of ability to perform human activities resulting from an impairment. Handicap is a disadvantage resulting from an impairment or disability that limits or prevents the fulfillment of normal roles.

• Most of the chronically mentally ill are dispersed throughout the community.

• Traditional outpatient therapy services may not meet the needs of the varied population of chronically mentally ill.

• One community response to the presence of the chronically mentally ill has been the proliferation of boarding homes and residential placements. Loss of low-cost housing has been linked to residential instability and homelessness.

• Recent advances in biologic psychiatry make it impossible to consider psychiatric chronicity a purely social construction. Instead, it appears to be a complex biopsychosocial phenomenon.

• Empowerment of this often isolated and disenfranchised population has been difficult to operationalize in the practical world or mental health world, but

rehabilitation principles used in helping physically disabled persons are providing important tools.

• The emphasis of psychosocial rehabilitation is on addressing impairment, disability, and handicap through wide-ranging services that include medication management, financial assistance, social skills training, and case management.

• Treatment of the disease is not adequate; nurses can take the lead in providing rehabilitation as well.

REFERENCES

American Psychiatric Association: *Diagnostic and Statistical Manual of Mental Disorders,* ed 3, revised. APA, 1987.

Anthony WA, Cohen MR, Cohen BF: Philosophy, treatment process, and principle of psychiatric rehabilitation approaches. *New Directions for Mental Health Services.* Jossey Bass, 1983.

Anthony WA, Liberman RP: The practice of psychiatric rehabilitation: Historical, conceptual, and research base. *Schizophr Bull* 1986;12(4):542–559.

Ascher-Svanum H, Sobel TS: Caregivers of mentally ill adults: A woman's agenda. *Hosp Community Psychiatry* 1989;40(8):843–845.

Bachrach LL: Defining chronic mental illness: A concept paper. *Hosp Community Psychiatry* 1988;39(4):383–388.

Baer J: Study of 60 patients with AIDS or AIDS-related complex requiring psychiatric hospitalization. *Am J Psychiatry* 1989;146(10):1285–1288.

Baxter E, Hopper K: *Private Lives/Public Spaces: Homeless Adults in the Streets of New York City.* Community Service Society, 1981.

Baxter E, Hopper K: The new mendicancy: Homeless in New York City. *Am J Orthopsychiatry* 1982;52:393–408.

Bechnel A, Gurgone D: Personal growth in chronic psychiatric patients: A new look at an old problem. *Int J Partial Hosp* 1987;4(4):291–301.

Bellack AS, Morrison RL, Mueser KT: Social problem solving in schizophrenia. *Schizophr Bull* 1989;5(1):101–116.

Braun P, Kochansky G, Shapiro R, Greenberg L, Gudeman JE, Johnson S, Shore MF: Overview: Deinstitutionalization of psychiatric patients, a critical review of outcome studies. *Am J Psychiatry* 1981;138:736.

Chafetz L, Barnes LE: Issues in psychiatric caregiving. *Arch Psychiatr Nurs* 1989;3(2):61–68.

Chafetz L, Goldfinger SM: Residential instability in a psychiatric emergency setting. *Psychiatr Q* 1984;56(10):20–34.

Chafetz L, Goldman HH, Taub CA: Deinstitutionalization in the United States. *Int J Mental Health* 1983;11(4):48–63.

Church OM: From custody to community in psychiatric nursing. *Nurs Res* 1987;36(1):48–55.

Connolly PM: The homeless mentally ill: Strategies for improving education. *J Psychosoc Nurs* 1989;27(6):2428.

Danley KS, Anthony WA; The choose-get-keep model: Serving severely psychiatrically disabled people. *Am Rehab* 1987;3:6–11.

Davies MA, Bromet EJ, Schulz SC, Dunn LO, Morgenstern M: Community adjustment of chronic schizophrenic patients in urban and rural settings. *Hosp Community Psychiatry* 1989;8(40):824–831.

de Cangas JPC: Exploring expressed emotion: Does it contribute to chronic mental illness? *J Psychosoc Nurs* 1990;28(2):31–34.

Department of Health and Human Services Steering Committee on the Chronically Mentally Ill: *Toward a National Plan for the Chronically Mentally Ill.* US DHHS, December 1980.

Estroff SE: *Making It Crazy: An Ethnography of Psychiatric Clients in an American Community.* University of California Press, 1981.

Falloon IRH, Boyd JL, McGill CW: *Family Care of Schizophrenia.* Guilford Press, 1984.

Faris REL, Dunham HW; *Mental Disorders in Urban Areas.* University of Chicago Press, 1939.

Farkas MD, Anthony WA: *Psychiatric Rehabilitation Programs: Putting Theory into Practice.* Johns Hopkins University Press, 1989.

Fopma-Loy J: Geropsychiatric Nursing: Focus and setting. *Arch Psychiatr Nurs* 1989;3(4):183–190.

Froner G: Aids and homelessness. *J Psychoactive Drugs* 1988;20(2):197–202.

Goldfinger SM, Chafetz L: Developing a better service delivery system for the homeless mentally ill, in Lamb HR (ed): *The Homeless Mentally Ill: A Task Force Report of the American Psychiatric Association.* APA, 1984.

Goldman HH; Mental illness and family burden: A public health perspective. *Hosp Community Psychiatry* 1984;33:557–560.

Goldman HH, Gatozzi AA, Taube CA: Defining and counting the mentally ill. *Hosp Community Psychiatry* 1981;32(1):21–27.

Goldman HH, Manderscheid RW: Chronic mental disorder in the United States, in Manderscheid RW and Barrett SA (eds): *Mental Health, United States, 1987.* US DHHS, 1987.

Grunberg J, Eagle, PF: Shelterization: How the homeless adapt to shelter living. *Hosp Community Psychiatry* 1990;41(5):521–525.

Gullberg PL: The homeless mentally ill: A psychiatric nurse's role. *J Psychosoc Nurs* 1989;27(6):9–13.

Harris M, Bergman HC: Misconceptions about use of case management services by the chronic mentally ill: A utilization analysis. *Hosp Community Psychiatry* 1988;39(12):1276–1281.

Hogarty GE, Anderson CM, Reiss DJ: Family psychoeducation, social skills training, and medication in schizophrenia: The long and short of it. *Psychopharmacol Bull* 1987;23(1):12–13.

Jamelka R, Trupin E, Chiles J: The mentally ill in prisons: A review. *Hosp Community Psychiatry* 1989;40(5):481–491.

Krauss JB: New conceptions of care, community, and chronic mental illness. *Arch Psychiatr Nurs* 1989;3(5):281–287.

Lamb HR, Talbott JA: The homeless mentally ill: The perspective of the APA. *JAMA* 1986;256(4):498–501.

Lefly H: Aging parents as caregivers of the chronically mentally ill: An emerging social concern. *Hosp Community Psychiatry* 1987;38(10):1063–1070.

Lefly HP, Bernheim KF, Goldman CR: National forum addresses need to enhance training in treating the seriously mentally ill. *Hosp Community Psychiatry* 1989;40(5):460–470.

McCausland M: Deinstitutionalization of the mentally ill: Oversimplification of complex issues. *Adv Nur Sci* 1987;9(3):24–33.

Mechanic D: The challenge of chronic mental illness: A retrospective and prospective review. *Hosp Community Psychiatry* 1986;37(9):891–901.

Mechanic D: Correcting misconceptions in mental health policy: Strategies for improved care of the chronically mentally ill. *Milbank Q* 1987;65(2):203–230.

Meleis AI: The inaugural Helen Nahm lectureship: The new age of nursing scholarliness: Now is the time. San Francisco School of Nursing, University of California, San Francisco, 1981.

Minkoff K: An integrated treatment model for dual diagnosis of psychosis and addiction. *Hosp Community Psychiatry* 1989;40(10):1031–1036.

Morin RC, Seidman E: A social network approach and the revolving door patient. *Schizophr Bull* 1986;12(2):262–273.

Morrison E et al.: The nursing adaptation evaluation (NSGAE): A proposed axis VI of DSM III. *J Psychosoc Nurs Mental Health Serv* 23(8):14–18.

Pepper B, Kirshner MC, Ryglewicz H: The young adult chronic patient: Overview of a population. *Hosp Community Psychiatry* 1981;32:463.

Perlman BB, Kentera A, Melnick G, Wile L: The aging of caretakers of those with chronic mental illness. *N Y State J Med* 1988;7:351–352.

Perse T, Howell T, Jefferson JW: Depression in the chronically mentally ill elderly, in Abramson NS, Quam JK, Wasow M (eds): *The Elderly and Chronically Mentally Ill.* Jossey-Bass, 1986, pp 15–32.

Richter JM: Providing nursing home care for the chronically mentally ill. *J Gerontol Nurs* 1989;15(6):18–23.

Roca RP, Breakey WR, Fischer PJ: Medical care of chronically mentally ill outpatients. *Hosp Community Psychiatry* 1987;38(7):741–744.

Rossi PH, Wright JD, Fisher GA, Willis G: The urban homeless: Estimating composition and size. *Science* 1987;235:1336–1341.

Segal SR, Baumohl J: Engaging the disengaged: Proposals on madness and vagrancy. *Soc Work Health Care* 1980;25:358–365.

Scott WR, Black BL: *The Organization of Mental Health Services: Societal and Community Systems.* Sage Publications, 1986.

Sheets JL, Prevost JA, Reihman J: Young adult chronic patients: Three hypothesized subgroups. *Hosp Community Psychiatry* 1982;33(3):197–203.

Tessler RC et al.: The chronically mentally ill in community support systems. *Hosp Community Psychiatry* 1982;33(3):208–211.

Test LI, Stein MA: Community treatment of the chronic

patient: Research overview. *Schizophr Bull* 1978;4(3): 350–364.

Turner RJ, Gartrell JW: Social factors in psychiatric outcome: Toward the resolution of interpretive controversies. *Am Soc Rev* 1978;43:368–382.

Underwood PR: Orem's self-care model: Clinical application, in Reynolds and Cormack (eds): *Psychiatric Mental Health Nursing: Theory and Practice*. Crom Helm, in press.

Way BB, Dvoskin JA, Steadman HJ, Huguley HC, Banks S: Staffing of forensic inpatient services in the United States. *Hosp Community Psychiatry* 1990;41(2):172–174.

Whetstone WR: Social dramatics: Social skills development for the chronically mentally ill. *J Adv Nurs* 1986; 11:67–74.

Whitmer GE: From hospitals to jails: The fate of California's deinstitutionalized mentally ill. *Am J Orthopsychiatry* 1989;50(1):65–75.

World Health Organization. *International Classification of Impairments, Disabilities, and Handicaps*. WHO, 1980.

Worley NK, Albanese N: Independent living for the chronically mentally ill. *J Psychosoc Nurs* 1989;27(9):18–23.

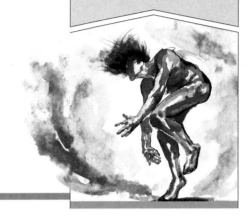

Psychophysiologic Conditions

LEARNING OBJECTIVES

- Explain the multicausational concept of illness

- Define the term *psychophysiologic disorders*

- Relate psychologic and physiologic factors to the syndromes presented in this chapter

- Choose specific nursing interventions to augment the client's medical regimen

Jerry D. Durham

CROSS REFERENCES

Other topics related to the content in this chapter are: Caring for clients in a general hospital setting, Chapter 19; Influence of anxiety and stress on coping, Chapter 5; Psychobiology, Chapter 6; Stress-management techniques, Chapter 27.

Portions of this chapter were contributed to the third edition by Mary-Eve Zangari.

THIS CHAPTER AND THE chapter that follows present material about the intriguing ways in which our bodies and our minds interact to produce a variety of behaviors and symptoms. **Psychophysiologic disorders** (having both physiologic and psychologic components) have an important emotional component in their onset and course. It is important to note, however, that many clinicians no longer use the term *psychophysiologic*. The psychophysiologic disorders appear in DSM-III-R as "Psychological Factors Affecting Physical Condition." The physical condition or syndrome is noted on Axis III of the multiaxial evaluation system. Until 1968, and today in some circles, *psychosomatic disorder* was the official term for such conditions. Bartol and Eakes have found that the term *psychosomatic* has negative connotations for many nurses (see the accompanying Research Note). The new terminology is more consistent with the systems approach to clients who have illnesses with marked organic and emotional components.

See Table 18–1 for examples of physical conditions having a psychologic component. The list of conditions in Table 18–1 is by no means complete. A review of such journals as the *Journal of Psychosomatic Research, Psychosomatic Medicine, Psychosomatics, Psychotherapy,* and *Psychosomatus* reveals the extent to which clinicians and researchers see a mind-body (*psyche-soma*) connection.

The revised DSM-III-R classification reflects the role of psychologic factors that lead up to, worsen, or perpetuate *any* physical illness. Therefore, even disorders not traditionally viewed as psychosomatic or psychophysiologic can be evaluated according to the new model. The revised classification is expected to encourage greater collaboration between mental health professionals and strictly medical professionals in the treatment of ill persons.

The DSM-III-R diagnostic criteria for "Psychological Factors Affecting Physical Condition" are as follows:

1. Psychologically meaningful environmental stimuli related to the initiation or exacerbation of a specific physical condition or disorder (recorded on Axis III).

2. The physical condition involves either demonstrable organic pathology (e.g., rheumatoid arthritis) or a known pathophysiologic process (e.g., migraine headache).

3. The condition does not meet the criteria for somatoform disorder.

Because all illnesses may ultimately be termed psychophysiologic, a holistic theory of illness serves as a basis for understanding all human disorders. By

RESEARCH NOTE

Citation
Bartol G, Eakes G: The connotative meaning of the term "psychosomatic." J Prof Nurs 1988; 4(6):453–457.

Study Problem/Purpose
The purpose of the study was to investigate the connotative meaning nurses attach to the term *psychosomatic*.

Methods
An open-ended questionnaire designed to elicit information regarding the connotative meanings that nurses ascribe to the term *psychosomatic* was administered to sixty nurse subjects. Subjects were asked to describe ideas and feelings that came to mind when they heard this term and to give an example of how *psychosomatic* would be used in their practice. Both qualitative and quantitative data analyses were conducted.

Findings
Only 8 percent of respondents acknowledged a continuous and joint interaction between body and mind in their definition. Only 15 percent of concepts submitted by respondents could be classified as positive. The remainder were negative (30 percent) or neutral (55 percent). Subjects reported feelings about the term *psychosomatic* as infrequently positive (20 percent of responses). The other responses were negative (56 percent) or neutral (24 percent).

Implications
The researchers concluded that the connotative meanings assigned to the term *psychosomatic* by nurses in the study contradict the word's original meaning and are often associated with negative or ambivalent feelings. Nurses need to be aware of the impression such terms create, both in themselves and in their clients.

appreciating the complex, interwoven pattern of emotional and physical elements, the nurse can more fully comprehend the essential unity of the body and the mind.

Clients who come to the attention of health care professionals because of physical complaints frequently have their psychologic needs neglected. Often,

TABLE 18–1 **Examples of Physical Conditions Having Psychologic Components**

System	Condition
Circulatory	Essential hypertension, angina pectoris, tachycardia, arrhythmia, cardiospasm, coronary artery disease, mitral valve prolapse, myocardial infarction, migraine headache
Gastrointestinal	Irritable bowel syndrome, gastric ulcer, duodenal ulcer, pylorospasm, regional enteritis (Crohn's disease), ulcerative colitis, nausea and vomiting, gastritis, chronic diarrhea
Hormonal	Hypoglycemia, diabetes mellitus, hyperthyroidism, hypothyroidism, hyperparathyroidism, hypoparathyroidism, premenstrual syndrome, obesity
Immune	Allergic disorders, cancer, autoimmune disorders (systemic lupus erythematosus, rheumatoid arthritis, Hashimoto's thyroiditis, myasthenia gravis, psoriasis)
Integumentary	Neurodermatitis (atopic dermatitis), pruritus, psoriasis, hyperhidrosis, urticaria, alopecia, acne
Neuromuscular/skeletal	Chronic pain, sacroiliac pain, temporomandibular joint (TMJ) pain, rheumatoid arthritis, Raynaud's disease
Respiratory	Asthma, hyperventilation syndrome

those unmet needs may be contributing to the complaint, may be the primary cause of symptom development, or may be the reason for the client's decision to seek help. Even if the most technologically advanced diagnostic and treatment approaches are applied, ignoring the psychologic components of illness can be as disastrous as ignoring the biologic components. Such psychologic components can undermine medically appropriate treatment.

Therefore, in all illness, a holistic approach is necessary if each facet of the client's overall problem is to be addressed. For each of the disorders, we suggest nonmedical interventions that reduce stress while increasing the client's understanding and control over troublesome symptoms. Promoting healthy life-styles and advocating life-style modifications are important nursing responsibilities regardless of the clinical area in which nurses practice.

Historical and Theoretic Foundations

The relationship between the mind and the body has always been a subject for speculation. Early humans had a holistic approach to disease, making no distinction between physical and mental illness. From Socrates, we have, "As it is not proper to cure the eyes without the head, nor the head without the body, so neither is it proper to cure the body without the soul." And from Hippocrates, "In order to cure the body it is necessary to have a knowledge of the whole of things." Then, during the Middle Ages, medicine became dominated by mysticism and religion. Sin was thought to be the cause of disease. In reaction to this view, and in conjunction with the scientific discoveries of the Renaissance (autopsy and microscopy), the study of the psyche was completely divorced from the study of medicine. In the nineteenth century, the rift was deepened by further scientific advances. It was thought that all disease must be associated with structural cell changes. Hence, the disease and not the client was the focus. Now, in the twentieth century, we have come full circle, and the mind and body are again united. How they are united is still unknown, although many theorists have attempted to explain the nature of the relationship.

The Specificity Model

One theory is the specificity model of Franz Alexander (1950). Alexander believed that prolonged psychologic stress could sometimes lead to a medical condition via activation of the autonomic nervous system. The development of the disorder is mediated by genetic predisposition and vulnerability. According to Alexander, specific types of emotional conflict cause anxiety in the individual. In defending against this anxiety, the individual regresses to an earlier psychologic and physiologic stage of development. For instance, a person may regress into the oral receptive stage, in which there is an unconscious wish to be fed by the mother. This results in gastric hypersecretion. If the person has a vulnerable duodenal mucosa, peptic ulcer may result. Alexander hypothesized seven psychosomatic disorders: essential hypertension, neurodermatitis, bronchial asthma, rheumatoid arthritis, hyperthyroidism, ulcerative colitis, and peptic ulcer. The following case example illustrates how the specificity model is applied.

Linda, a 20-year-old nursing student, has been diagnosed with a small peptic ulcer, treatable with diet and medication. Because she mentioned that she was having difficulties at school, she is also referred to the psychiatry service, where she meets with a psychoanalytically inclined therapist. He asks Linda about her childhood and discovers that she was cared for by her grandmother while both her parents were away at work during the day. Later, Linda had to take care of a younger sister and brother after school and on weekends. The student says she never had a "real childhood" and doesn't ever remember her mother being there when she needed her. According to Alexander's model, the therapist would deduce that Linda has a dependency conflict deriving from her early childhood. Current academic stress causes her to wish for a time when she was protected and nurtured by her mother. These unconscious feelings produce gastric hypersecretion, and eventually a peptic ulcer.

Other investigators made further attempts to relate specific personality characteristics to certain diseases. People with ulcerative colitis were found to be passive, conforming, and dependent. Those with hypertension had counterdependency strivings. Diabetic people were passive, needed affection, and wished to be cared for. Women with dysmenorrhea were infantile and expressed hopelessness and self-denial. Cancer clients were found to be selfless and undemanding (Sachar 1975).

On closer scrutiny, the specificity theory is not very specific after all. Certain emotional states, such as dependency, appear to be common to all disorders. Furthermore, research does not indicate whether dependence is a cause or an effect of the disease process. Another criticism is that some of the relationships described above have been based on faulty physiologic premises. For instance, ulcerative colitis was thought to be caused by an inability to express anger openly. Instead, the client's rage "explodes" in uncontrollable bouts of diarrhea. It was believed that the frequent evacuations caused inflammation of the bowel lining. However, recent research has shown that *before* the persistent diarrhea appears, small ulcerations are already forming in the bowel (Sachar 1975).

The Nonspecific Stress Model

A second theory is the nonspecific stress model of Gustav Mahl (1953). Unlike Alexander, who focused on specific types of emotional conflict, Mahl theorized that the psychosomatic process can be activated by any stressful event, such as an earthquake, or a more subtle intrapsychic event, such as a fear of elevators. Whatever the source of the stress, the physiologic responses are identical for everyone. Selye (1950, 1976) also studied these physiologic responses. Selye's general adaptation syndrome has been widely featured in nursing literature and is the theoretic underpinning of much stress-related nursing research (see Chapter 5). These responses include gastric and cardiovascular hyperfunctioning and hormonal changes, such as increased adrenal steroid secretion. A person who experiences chronic stress may develop a biologic symptom, whose nature is determined by organ susceptibility and early learning experiences involving pathologic responses.

This nonspecific model can be applied to the same case study used to illustrate Alexander's specificity model. Linda, the nursing student, still has a small peptic ulcer, but with this model it is explained differently.

Linda experienced the usual school stresses along with the rest of her classmates. But Linda develops an ulcer because her stomach is particularly vulnerable to stress. She may naturally produce an excess of hydrochloric acid, or her stomach lining may have some congenital defect. Along with organ susceptibility, Linda may have a parent who also had a peptic ulcer. She may have seen a parent react to stress with abdominal disturbances and learned to react in a similar manner.

This viewpoint is consistent with the clinical research data that have been gathered from studying people under stress. However, this theory fails to account for the influence that meaning has in an individual's interpretation of stressful events.

The Individual Response Specificity Model

A third theory is the individual response specificity model formulated by Lacey, Bateman, and Van Lehn (1953). According to this model, individuals tend to show highly characteristic and consistent physiologic responses to a wide range of stimuli. These responses were formed in childhood. This model contradicts the nonspecific model in which everyone is seen as responding in much the same way to stress. Instead, according to the individual response model, there are "cardiac reactors," "gastric reactors," and "hypertensive reactors."

To illustrate this model, we return to Linda and her peptic ulcer.

Linda always has indigestion when she becomes upset. However, Monica, her roommate, never has indigestion. Instead, she frequently has migraine headaches.

This theory is compatible with the previously mentioned theories of organ susceptibility and early learning experiences. Because it encompasses much of the current research data, this theory has become increasingly popular.

The Multicausational Concept of Illness

It is readily apparent that the preceding models do not fully illuminate the relationships between emotions and physical functioning. By taking some other factors

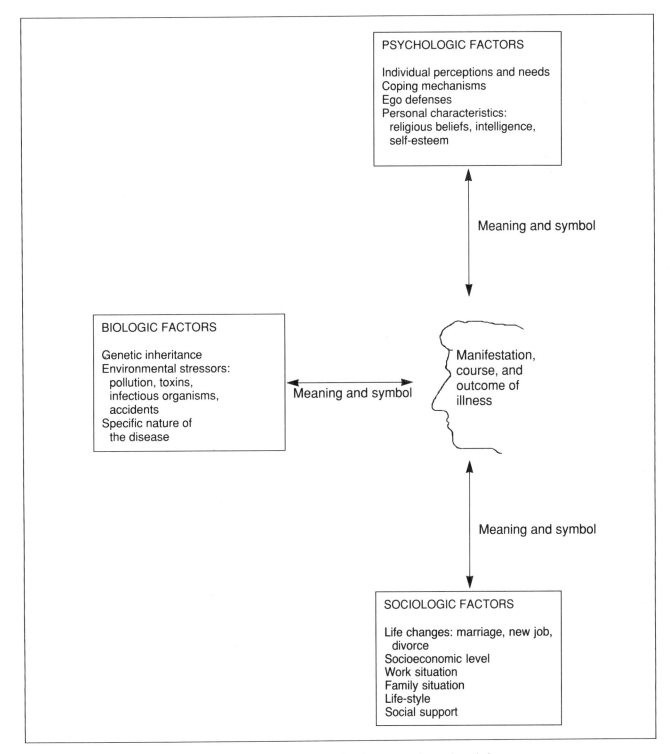

FIGURE 18-1   Multicausational concept of the illness process. The phrase *meaning and symbol* in the figure refers to the fact that the client interprets all experiences in a highly individual manner according to their specific meaning for that client and their broader meaning in the client's culture.

into account, researchers developed a more useful model. Some of these factors are presented in the research by Holmes and Rahe (1967), Mutter and Schleifer (1966), and Rahe and Arthur (1978). These studies show that physical illness is commonly preceded by stressful life changes. Their findings thus indicate that emotions play a role in all disease processes. The studies further suggest that physical disorders, like mental disorders, are related to social class. Furthermore, individuals in similar social situations defined those situations differently and consequently had different reactions to the similar situations.

These findings underscore the following:

• The concept of separation of mind and body is not useful in understanding the total disease process.

• Stress comes in many forms—psychologic, physiologic, and sociologic—and is a causative factor in all illness.

• Stress is perceived differently, depending on the individual and the specific context.

Figure 18–1 on page 443 and the following clinical example illustrate these ideas.

Peter G, 5 years old, was admitted for the fourth time in six months because of an acute asthma attack. While Peter was being treated medically, his parents waited in the family room. Mrs G sat crying and wringing her hands while Mr G paced the floor with a strained expression on his face. A staff nurse was able to talk to them and trace the sequence of events leading up to Peter's admission to the hospital.

It was a Saturday afternoon, and Mr and Mrs G had been arguing about whether to send Peter to kindergarten in the fall. Two points of view had emerged. Mr G was all for it. He wanted Peter to grow up quickly and leave his "babyish ways" behind. Mrs G was against it. Peter was the baby of the family, and Mrs G felt that her husband was always pushing him to do things too advanced for a 5-year-old. Peter had awakened from his nap to hear his parents shouting at each other. The quarrel ended abruptly when Peter started to wheeze, and both parents rushed to his bedside, united in their concern for him.

What factors brought on Peter's asthma attack at that particular time? The biologic factors include Peter's physiologic makeup. His mother had been a child asthmatic. She and Peter are both allergic to chocolate, eggs, feathers, and dust. Peter inherited certain genetic features that make him susceptible to certain environmental stressors, in this case, the specific allergens. Sociologic components of Peter's illness revolve around his family's functioning. Mr and Mrs G have different viewpoints on what Peter's role in the family should be. Their conflicts create a second source

of stress for Peter. A third component is Peter's psychologic state. A 5-year-old boy views the integrity of his family as extremely important, and parental conflicts may threaten his sense of security. Peter had discovered that his parents rallied together when he was ill.

In view of these contributing factors, the treatment plan for Peter should not end when Peter stops wheezing. To reduce the number of such emergencies, caregivers need to devise a long-range treatment plan. This plan should encompass the physiologic, psychologic, and sociologic components of Peter's asthma attacks.

Psychophysiologic Disorders

The following sections review the characteristics of syndromes traditionally considered psychophysiologic disorders. For most of the syndromes, an exact etiology is unknown. Current research focuses on the complicated interrelationships among such factors as stress, personality, environment, and hormones.

Peptic Ulcer

Peptic ulcer has been one of the most thoroughly studied psychophysiologic illnesses. Still, many questions remain unanswered. Peptic ulcer incidence rises in response to stress (e.g., in times of war) and is prevalent among those persons with stressful life-styles (e.g., city dwellers, air traffic controllers, and police officers). It is often associated with "getting ahead" in Western culture. Peptic ulcers seem to run in families. Other related causational factors are nutritional deficiencies, allergies, remote infections, alcohol and caffeine ingestion, and situations prompting prolonged responses of anxiety and resentment. The overall rate of ulcer disease has declined in recent years.

Peptic ulcers of the duodenal type occur about three times more often in men than in women. Most persons with duodenal ulcer secrete excess acid. Among people with the gastric type of ulcer, 50 percent secrete normal or less than normal amounts of acid. This evidence illustrates the mixture of emotional and psychologic factors involved in ulcer formation and in the progression of the illness. The following clinical example illustrates this point.

A 42-year-old trial lawyer, married and the mother of two children, is referred for consultation by her gastroenterologist following her third hospitalization for duodenal ulcer disease. Her ulcer disease was first diagnosed four years ago, but an upper gastrointestinal (GI) series at that time showed evidence both of an active ulcer and of scarring secondary to previously healed ulcers. The gastroenterologist has requested the consultation for help in considering the possibility of surgery, prompted by the seriousness of the bleeding episode that precipitated the client's last admission and by the fact that she seems to "ignore pain." His referral note indicates that he sees no clear connection between the bleeding episodes and her highly stressful occupation.

The client appears exactly on time for her appointment; she is neatly and conservatively dressed. She presents an organized, coherent account of her medical problem and denies any past or immediate family history of significant mental disorder. She appears genuinely worried by her recent hospitalization, frightened by the prospect of surgery, and doubtful that speaking to a psychiatrist will produce any meaningful help. As she points out, "Ulcers are supposed to be related to stress, and that just isn't true with me." She then produces a detailed, written outline of her professional life over the past five years side by side with a chronology of her ulcer attacks. Indeed, there seems to be no temporal relationship between her attacks and several highly taxing court cases in which she has appeared.

During the second evaluation session, the client discusses her background. She is the oldest of four children and the clear favorite of her father, also an attorney. He communicated a strong expectation that she would become a lawyer and that she would succeed in his field. The client sees herself as having fulfilled this expectation admirably and displays a rare smile while describing several of her more dramatic courtroom triumphs. There is no evidence that she experiences these difficult cases as stressful; in fact, she seems to enjoy them.

She married a law-school classmate, who is also quite successful and who works noncompetitively in an unrelated legal field. Their marriage seems sound. As she begins to talk about her two sons, aged 8 and 4, the client becomes noticeably more tense and appears much more concerned and upset than usual while describing minor crises they have experienced with friends or in school. With great surprise, she discovers that the chronology of these crises corresponds clearly to five of her seven ulcer attacks, including all of those that resulted in hospitalization. She admits that despite being upset by her sons' problems, she finds it difficult to share her concerns about parenting with her husband or friends. At the end of the session she comments: "You'd have made a good lawyer. I'm glad I'm not arguing against you." She herself suggests that some further sessions may be in order.*

The classic ulcer personality type is said to be competitive and aggressive, and appears lean and hungry. Psychoanalysts explain these characteristics as defenses against dependency needs. These traits have not been consistently demonstrated by research. Other psychologic constructs have more obvious validity.

Gastric functioning becomes intimately tied to dependency needs in humans through the feeding

process from earliest infancy. The baby's mouth and digestive system are its early means of relating to the external world and its principal sources of gratification and frustration. Through complex learning processes, humans associate feeding and being taken care of and nurtured in a general sense. The mouth, through biting and chewing, also becomes the first mechanism through which the human infant can express anger and disappointment at being frustrated. It is well known that gastric secretion increases when infants and children are emotionally involved in either a positive or a negative sense.

Along with medical, surgical, and nutritional treatments, the care of these clients may include stress-management techniques designed to decrease stress or the response to it. Psychotherapy may be appropriate if a dependency conflict exists and the client wishes to resolve it.

Bowel Disorders

Ulcerative colitis and Crohn's disease are chronic inflammatory disorders of unknown etiology. They are characterized by diarrhea, abdominal pain, anorexia, fever, weight loss, vomiting, urgency to defecate, and incontinence. In severe cases, an ileostomy or colostomy may be necessary.

Clients with ulcerative colitis are said to display a compulsive personality style with the following features: neatness, orderliness, punctuality, indecisiveness, emotional guardedness, humorlessness, conscientiousness, obstinacy, conformity, moral rigidity, and worry.

Contemporary researchers say that the psychologic traits these clients display are similar to those of clients with other chronic illnesses, with dependency being the most common trait. In many cases, onset and flare-ups seem linked to stressful life events, e.g., separations, failures, and disappointments.

Regardless of the source of the client's illness, treatment should focus on present troublesome areas. The plan may include individual psychotherapy, family therapy, and environmental manipulation along with the medical regimen. These persons do best when they are involved in solid and long-term supportive relationships with their nurses and physicians.

Cardiovascular Disorders

The cardiovascular system is a sensitive indicator of emotional arousal, whether fear, anger, or pleasurable excitement. High levels of stress are suspected to have harmful effects on the heart and vascular system, especially if stress is chronic or repeated. Experience, learning, and symbolic meaning, along with their emotional content, can influence the heart rate, heart rhythm, and blood pressure. These cardiovascular

---

*Adapted from Spitzer RL et al.: *DSM-III Casebook*. American Psychiatric Association, 1981, pp 23–24.

changes can in turn create emotions, mostly unpleasant, that affect perception and ideation.

A number of factors have been identified as associated with high risk of heart disease. They include genetic, physiologic, social, and psychologic factors:

- Family history of heart disease

- Diet high in saturated fats, cholesterol

- High level of blood cholesterol, triglycerides, sugar, uric acid

- Hypertension, diabetes, hypothyroidism, renal disease, gout

- Low level of physical activity

- Heavy smoking and eating

- High-pressured life-style (type A personality)

- Suppressed anger and hostility

The highly competitive, driving **type A personality** displays the classic constellation of personality characteristics associated with coronary disease, angina pectoris, and myocardial infarction. Adverse conditions in the client's environment, either social or economic, can also create the stress that leads to cardiac dysfunction.

Essential hypertension, cardiac dysrhythmias, and so-called cardiac neurosis are three syndromes of cardiovascular functioning with major psychologic inputs. The classical hypothesis in hypertension has been that people have conflict between their dependent and aggressive inclinations. This causes chronic repression of all displays of anger or resentment. The repressed emotions are eventually transformed into disorders of blood pressure regulation. Although this specific hypothesis has been difficult to prove, experiments have shown that fear, anger, frustration, and guilt all cause rises in diastolic blood pressure in vulnerable individuals. Likewise, anxiety, hostility, depression, interpersonal conflict, and disruptive life events have all been shown capable of precipitating dysrhythmias, e.g., sinus tachycardia, paroxysmal atrial tachycardia, and both atrial and ventricular ectopic beats.

Cardiac neurosis is a syndrome consisting of cardiac distress, exercise intolerance, easy fatigability, respiratory discomfort, and dizziness. These features are very similar to those found in panic disorder and mitral valve prolapse.

The treatment of cardiac disease must be multifaceted. In addition to medical or surgical treatment, other approaches involve stress management, relaxation training, biofeedback, weight control through diet and exercise, and behavioral interventions to help people give up smoking. More efforts are being geared toward prevention, including programs by industry and corporations to promote healthy life-styles among employees.

Asthma

Asthma is among the most widely studied psychophysiologic illnesses of the respiratory system. Because breathing is essential to life, there has been much speculation about the emotional and symbolic significance that can become attached to the processes of air exchange. Asthma is characterized by labored breathing and wheezing resulting from spasm, secretions, and swelling in the bronchial tree.

There are allergic, immunologic, and emotional inputs to asthmatic attacks. The emotional components may lead directly to alterations in bronchus size. They may also affect the allergic and immunologic systems through hypothalamic nuclei in the central nervous system.

Asthmatic persons may be extremely frightened by asthmatic attacks, particularly in childhood. This may make them feel more helpless and vulnerable. In response, they often adopt a clinging style of relating. The emotional and the physical aspects of the illness seem to interrelate in a complex system of feedback loops. See the case history of Peter G on page 444 for an example.

Each person with asthma must be assessed individually to determine what factors are contributing to the disease process. A treatment plan may include, along with medication, family therapy, relaxation training, behavior modification, and hypnosis. Psychotherapy, if employed, must proceed cautiously so as not to precipitate an asthma attack.

Arthritis

Rheumatoid arthritis (RA) has long been identified as an illness that is strongly influenced by emotional life. Written records over 1500 years old attest to this. Basically, RA is a progressive inflammatory disease, primarily of the joints, of unknown cause. Family prevalence studies indicate a genetic predisposition to the disease. RA is three times more common in women than men.

Psychologic stresses are thought to precipitate attacks and flare-ups. The mechanism of transformation from idea or affect into tissue alteration appears to be hormonal and autonomic nervous system pathways. Specifically, levels of growth hormone, sex hormones, thyroid hormone, and adrenal corticosteroids all change in stages of emotional arousal, and all are involved in the production of connective tissue, especially collagen. The hypothalamus and the limbic system also mediate. Heredity and stress may operate in inverse proportion, according to a study by Rimon

(1969). Rimon found that arthritic clients without genetic predisposition developed the illness under severe stress, and others with a heavy genetic loading developed it despite little evidence of life conflict. In a follow-up study, Rimon and Laakso (1985) found that in those persons who developed RA amidst serious emotional trauma, later flare-ups were also linked to such circumstances.

In another study, Baker (1982) studied the relationship between stressful life events and the onset of RA. Baker suggests that severe emotional stress can bring on RA by decreasing the body's resistance to a virus, which then activates an autoimmune response.

People with RA appear to have difficulties with control, especially of hostility. Most clients appear to be overcontrolled, highly responsible, sensitive to criticism, and self-sacrificing. The diagnosis cannot be based on personality type, however, because there are many exceptions to the rule. Physical findings, deformities, subcutaneous nodules, and blood studies remain the criteria for identification.

A treatment plan for the arthritis client may include pain control, surgery, drugs, vocational counseling, occupational therapy, and interventions to alleviate or prevent depression and to deal with hostility more directly.

Headache

The experience of headache resulting from emotional tension is common. Headaches may be divided into the five following types:

1. Vascular headache of migraine type

2. Muscle contraction headache (tension headache)

3. Combined vascular–muscle contraction headache

4. Delusional, depressive, conversion, or hypochondriacal headaches

5. Structural or disease-related headaches

The mechanism of vascular headache seems to involve the release of various vasoactive substances in the brain, such as serotonin, catecholamines, histamine, bradykinin, and prostaglandins. This release frequently occurs with stress. In genetically susceptible individuals, the substances cause vasodilation and inflammation of the arterial walls. There are generally early warning symptoms of migraine attacks. These range from mood changes and gastrointestinal upset to gross neurologic findings in the visual and contralateral sensorimotor systems. A number of upsets in physiologic functioning can actually be migraine equivalents. These include nausea and vomiting, diarrhea, tachycardia, cyclical edema, vertigo, periodic fever, pain, depression, confusion, and insomnia.

Tension-induced headache results from muscular contraction in the neck, shoulders, face, or scalp. These are steady, persistent headaches with no warning signs and commonly feel like a "band wrapped around the head." Some theorists support the notion that headache sufferers are likely to maintain rigid control over emotions, feel hostility toward others, use introjection as a defense, and be perfectionists.

Structural or disease-related headaches arise from: systemic infections, primary or metastatic tumors, hematomas, abscesses, cranial infections, cranial nerve inflammations, and eye, ear, nose, sinus, or tooth diseases. Interventions are based on the diagnosis and the contributing factors that have been identified. Possible treatments include measures that increase circulation, e.g., massage or heat application; use of medications; alterations in diet, rest, and exercise patterns; psychotherapy; and biofeedback, transcendental meditation, hypnosis, relaxation, and other stress management approaches (Kneisl and Ames 1986).

Endocrine Disorders

A large number of disorders of endocrine functioning are associated with psychologic factors. The endocrine system has particular significance for psychiatry, because there is a close relationship between the emotions and a variety of active chemical substances released in tissues by nerve impulses. In physical medicine, the feedback loop has long been accepted as the model for the functioning of the endocrine organs.

Extensive research on the endocrine feedback system has led to a sophisticated model that includes three kinds of feedback loops. The levels of circulating hormones released by endocrine glands, such as the thyroid or sex glands, are controlled by long feedback loops that send information to the cerebral cortex and limbic system. Short feedback loops of pituitary hormones affect the hypothalamus. Very short loops of releasing hormones from the hypothalamus determine their own production and control. Studies on the relationship of emotions to endocrine function have shown that:

• Various neurotransmitters affect hormone-releasing factors.

• Psychoactive drugs whose action is mediated by neurotransmitters also affect the release of releasing factors.

• Stress stimulates the autonomic nervous system, which can stimulate the adrenal medulla to produce epinephrine or the pancreas to secrete insulin.

• Corticosteroid production of the adrenal cortex increases greatly during acute psychotic episodes of schizophrenic clients.

• Steroid levels also increase in agitated or anxious depressive people.

It seems fair to conclude that the emotional centers of the brain—the cortex and limbic systems—are intimately tied to the endocrine organs, through the axis of the hypothalamus and the anterior pituitary. Their secretions act as communication messengers. It is not surprising, then, to find expressions of emotional arousal through endocrine changes and major effects on emotional states from endocrine diseases. These are both, in fact, common. Endocrine diseases and conditions and their physical and mental symptoms are listed in the accompanying Assessment box.

Adrenal dysfunction characteristically produces prominent mental as well as distinctive physical symptoms. Thyroid disorders commonly are accompanied by cognitive or emotional changes. Stress has been implicated, though inconclusively, in the precipitation of thyrotoxic crises. Stress may influence the course of diabetes, either directly by promoting a flare-up or indirectly by causing the client to neglect a usually rigid medical regimen. So many mental symptoms are associated with hypoglycemia that many clients are classified and treated as "classic neurotics."

It is evident that numerous problems can be caused by endocrine dysfunction. The treatment approach

ASSESSMENT

Common Features of Endocrine Disorders

Disease	Physical Symptoms	Mental Symptoms
Cushing's syndrome (adrenal cortex hyperfunction)	Truncal obesity, moon facies, abdominal striae, hirsutism, amenorrhea, hypertension, osteoporosis, weakness	Impotence, decreased libido, anxiety, increased emotional lability, apathy, insomnia, memory deficits, confusion, disorientation
Addison's disease (adrenal insufficiency)	Weakness, fatigue, anorexia, weight loss, nausea and vomiting, pigmentation of skin, hypotension	Depression, irritability, psychomotor retardation, apathy, memory defect, hallucinations
Hyperthyroidism	Staring, exophthalmos, goiter, moist warm skin, weight loss, increased appetite, weakness, tremor, tachycardia, heat intolerance	Anxiety, tension, irritability, hyperexcitability, emotional lability, depression, psychosis, or delirium
Hypothyroidism	Dull expression, puffy eyelids, swollen tongue, hoarse voice, rough dry skin, cold intolerance	Psychomotor retardation, decreased initiative, slow comprehension, drowsiness, decreased recent memory, delirium, stupor, depression or psychosis
Diabetes mellitus	Polydipsia, polyuria, polyphagia, weight loss, blurred vision, fatigue, impotence, fainting, paresthesia	Stupor, coma, fatigue, impotence
Hypoglycemia	Tremor, light-headedness, sweating, hunger, nausea, pallor, tachycardia, hypertension	Anxiety, fugue, unusual behavior, confusion, apathy, psychomotor agitation or retardation, depression, delusions, hallucinations, convulsions, coma
Premenstrual syndrome	Headache, breast engorgement, lower abdominal bloating, GI complaints, increased sweating, craving for sweets, other appetite changes	Irritability, depression, anxiety, emotional lability, fatigue, crying spells

must be individualized to meet the client's physical and psychologic needs.

An important role for the nurse is primary prevention. Adequately preparing a person for developmental changes by offering accurate information about likely physical and emotional alterations can help prevent severe psychiatric disturbances during these periods. Reliable support and open channels of communication are necessary. New coping strategies can be successful, if their ingenuity, timing, and presentation are appropriate.

Skin Disorders

Allergic illnesses, particularly those involving the skin, have been shown to have psychologic elements in etiology or course. The skin, with its critical sensory functions, mediates between the outside world and internal states. Itching (pruritus), excessive sweating (hidrosis), urticaria, and atopic dermatitis are all common classified as psychophysiologic conditions.

A variety of stressful or emotional states are associated with flare-ups of allergic skin disorders. Attempts have been made to correlate the following specific emotional states or stresses with individual disorders:

• Generalized pruritus: aggression

• Genital and anal pruritus: sexuality (heterosexual and homosexual)

• Hyperhidrosis: anxiety

• Urticaria: anger

• Atopic dermatitis: longing for love

In truth, these feelings and conflicts are seen in normal, disordered, and other psychophysiologic states. Nurses should therefore be cautious about accepting pathogenic mechanisms and explanations.

The location of the lesions has, historically, had symbolic significance. Thus, conflict over an extramarital affair has been associated with dermatitis in the wedding ring area. Head and face locations have been classically associated with conflict over affective display. Affliction of the hands is associated with practical or professional conflicts. A genital distribution is associated with sexual concerns.

Resistance to Psychosocial Intervention

Behavior therapy, biofeedback, hypnotherapy, and psychotherapy have all been used with success with appropriate clients. However, despite the wealth of psychosocial interventions available to persons with psychophysiologic disorders, many clients are resistant to approaches that are not strictly medical. Some reasons for this are:

• These clients are believed to lack insight, since they express conflict through somatic complaints rather than verbalization.

• Conflicts over unresolved dependency and aggressive wishes may make it difficult to relate to these clients interpersonally.

• These clients focus steadfastly on their somatic complaints, apparently indicating that alternative defense mechanisms are unavailable or inadequate.

• They are rarely highly motivated to heighten their self-awareness, which is the goal of many forms of psychotherapy.

• Even when they are somewhat motivated, they may be unable or unwilling to delay gratification and thus are impatient with the slow process of growth usually required in psychotherapeutic work.

For these reasons, traditional psychotherapy is not the most useful intervention. Approaches that enhance medical and surgical intervention and allow the client's primary bond to remain with nonpsychiatric health care providers are more successful. Programs geared toward stress management are very useful because they present stress as part of the human condition and the participants do not feel labeled as having psychiatric problems.

CHAPTER HIGHLIGHTS

• The multicausational concept of illness acknowledges the biologic, psychologic, and sociologic components of the illness/disease process.

• Psychologic factors should always be considered among those factors that lead up to, worsen, or perpetuate any physical illness.

• Ignoring the psychologic components of illness can undermine appropriate treatment.

• Psychophysiologic disorders are those that have an important emotional component in their onset and future course.

• The psychophysiologic disorders in particular illustrate the complicated interactions of mind, body, and environment because they present physical symptoms with a strong psychologic component.

• Syndromes in which physical and psychologic factors interact by means of feedback loops include peptic ulcer; asthma; arthritis; headache; and certain bowel, cardiovascular, endocrine, and skin disorders.

- Promoting healthy life-styles and advocating life-style modifications are important nursing responsibilities.

- Regardless of the clinical area in which they practice, nurses must have a knowledge of stress-management approaches to offer clients a useful plan of care.

- Many clients resist the idea that emotions may play a part in their disorders. Therefore, the plan of care should be thoughtfully managed by a health care professional that the client trusts.

REFERENCES

Alexander F: *Psychosomatic Medicine: Its Principles and Application.* Norton, 1950.

American Psychiatric Association: *Diagnostic and Statistical Manual of Mental Disorders,* ed. 3. APA, 1980.

American Psychiatric Association: *Diagnostic and Statistical Manual of Mental Disorders,* ed 3, revised. APA, 1987.

Baker GHB: Life events before the onset of rheumatoid arthritis. *Psychother Psychosom* 1985;43:38–43.

Bohachick P: Progressive relaxation training in cardiac rehabilitation: Effect on psychologic variables. *Nurs Res* 1984;33:283–287.

Burckhardt CS: The impact of arthritis on quality of life. *Nurs Res* 1985;34:11–16.

Castleberry K: Rules for disease: An interactional model for psychosomatic illness in families. *Issues Ment Health Nurs* 1988;9:363–371.

Cohen S, Evans G, Stokols D, Krantz D: *Behavior, Health, and Environmental Stress.* Plenum Press, 1986.

Conte HR, Karasu TB: Psychotherapy for medically ill patients: Review and critique of controlled studies. *Psychosomatics* 1981;22:285–315.

Engel GE: Clinical application of the biopsychosocial model. *Am J Psychiatry* 1980;137:535–544.

Green SA: *Mind and Body: The Psychology of Physical Illness.* American Psychiatric Press, 1985.

Hart CA: The role of psychiatric consultation liaison nurses in ethical decisions to remove life-sustaining treatments. *Arch Psychiatr Nurs* 1990;4(6):370–378.

Holmes TH, Rahe RH: The social readjustment scale. *J Psychosom Res* 1967;11:213–218.

Janisese M: *Individual Differences, Stress, and Health Psychology.* Springer-Verlag, 1988.

Julkunen J, Hurri H, Kankainen J: Psychological factors in the treatment of chronic low back pain. *Psychother Psychosom* 1988;50:173–181.

Justice B: *Who Gets Sick.* Jeremy P. Tarcher, 1988.

Kneisl CR, Ames SA: *Adult Health Nursing: A Biopsychosocial Approach.* Addison-Wesley, 1986.

Koskenvuo M et al.: Hostility as a risk for mortality and ischemic heart disease in men. *Psychosom Med* 1988;50:330–340.

Krakowski A, Kimball C: *Psychosomatic Medicine.* Plenum Press, 1983.

Lacey JI, Bateman DE, Van Lehn R: Autonomic response specificity. *Psychosom Med* 1953;15:8.

Lesser I: A review of the alexithymia concept. *Psychosom Med* 1981;43:531–543.

Lesser I, Lesser B: Alexithymia: Examining the development of a psychological concept. *Am J Psychiatry* 1983;140:1305–1308.

Mahl GF: Physiological changes during chronic fear. *Ann N Y Acad Sci* 1953;56:240.

Mennies JH et al.: Overview of adult allergy. *Nurs Pract* 1985;16:19–23.

Mutter AZ, Schleifer M: The role of psychological and social factors in the onset of somatic illness in children. *Psychosom Med* 1966;28:333–343.

Orth-Gomer K, Unden A: Type A behavior, social support, and coronary risk: Interaction and significance for mortality in cardiac patients. *Psychosom Med* 1990;52:59–72.

Pollock SE: Human responses to chronic illness: Physiologic and psychosocial adaption. *Nurs Res* 1986;35:90–95.

Ragland D, Prand R: Type A behavior and mortality from coronary heart disease. *N Engl J Med.* 1988;318:65–69.

Rahe R, Arthur R: Life change and illness studies: Past history and future directions. *J Hum Stress* 1978;4:3–15.

Rahe R et al.: Simplified scaling for life change events. *J Hum Stress* 1980;5:22–27.

Rimon R: A psychosomatic approach to rheumatoid arthritis. *Acta Pehumatol Scand* (Suppl) 1969;13:1–154.

Rimon R, Laakso RL: Life stress and rheumatoid arthritis. *Psychother Psychosom* 1985;43:38–43.

Sachar EJ: Current status of psychosomatic medicine, in Strain J, Grossman S (eds): *Psychologic Care of the Medically Ill.* Appleton-Century-Crofts, 1975, pp 54–56.

Schwab JJ: Psychosomatic medicine: Its past and present. *Psychosomatics* 1985;26:583–593.

Selye H: *The Physiology and Pathology of Exposure to Stress.* Acta, 1950.

Selye H: *The Stress of Life.* McGraw-Hill, 1976.

Shaver JA: Biopsychosocial view of health. *Nurs Outlook* 1985;33:186–191.

Spacapan S, Oskany S: *The Social Psychology of Health.* Sage, 1988.

Sparacino J: Blood pressure, stress, and mental health. *Nurs Res* 1982;31:89–94.

Sparacino LL: Psychosocial considerations for the adolescent and young adult with inflammatory bowel disease. *Nurs Clin North Am* 1984;19:41–49.

Spitzer RL et al.: *DSM-III Casebook.* American Psychiatric Association, 1981.

Talbott J, Hales R, Yudofsky S: *Textbook of Psychiatry.* American Psychiatric Press, 1988.

Toner B et al.: Self-schema in irritable bowel syndrome and depression. *Psychosom Med* 1990;52:149–155.

Valdes M, Treserra J, Garcia L, Pablo J, Flores T: Psychogenic pain and psychological variables: A psychometric study. *Psychother Psychosom* 1988;50:15–21.

Psychosocial Nursing in Non-Psychiatric Settings

LEARNING OBJECTIVES

- Discuss the coping tasks of the hospitalized client
- Evaluate the usefulness of the client's coping skills
- Explain the process of helping clients to develop effective coping skills
- Describe the role and functions of the psychiatric nursing consultant

Jerry D. Durham

CROSS REFERENCES

Other topics relevant to this content are: Coping strategies, Chapter 5; Crisis management, Chapter 28; Family dynamics, Chapter 30.

Portions of this chapter were contributed to the third edition by Carol Ren Kneisl and Mary-Eve Zangari.

Nurses working in general hospitals face the challenge of combining what futurist Naisbett has called "high tech and high touch." They not only must keep abreast of the latest technology but also must apply it with an understanding of the emotional and psychologic ramifications for each client.

Nurses have always practiced holistically, paying attention to their clients' families, life-styles, values, and beliefs. In health care in general, the trend is toward the delivery of more humanistic care. Some of the change is in response to public demand for more personalized and effective health care. Another influence is the steady accumulation of research that points to a biopsychosocial model of illness. Among hospitalized persons in general, studies indicate that 30 to 60 percent have significant psychologic problems secondary to their medical illness (Strain 1982).

Chapter 18 presented the theoretic base for a holistic approach to all physically ill persons. Here we apply the nursing process to the psychosocial needs presented by clients in nonpsychiatric settings. This chapter also describes the process of coping with the stresses of hospitalization.

To help nurses deliver care to clients with diverse psychosocial needs, many general hospitals have added master's prepared **consultant-liaison psychiatric nurses** to their staffs. This role has helped nurses to apply psychiatric nursing principles to their work with the general hospital client. Clinical examples in this chapter demonstrate the application of theory to practice.

The Hospital Experience

Hospitalization As a Crisis

Illness and hospitalization can be viewed as crisis situations for clients and their families. This section discusses what the nature of this crisis is, how clients and their families can learn to cope, and how nurses can facilitate the coping process.

Hospitals are ideal places in which to see crisis brewing. The emergency room and the cardiac and intensive care units are designed specifically for clients who are experiencing an unexpected illness or accident. However, general medical and surgical floors, where clients are admitted by schedule or following stabilization of their medical condition, also include clients in states of crisis.

Any hospitalization is extremely stressful. Clients are in a strange environment away from their customary supports of family and friends. They literally fear for their lives. Never knowing from minute to minute what to expect, they are subjected to all sorts of indignities. Often no one informs them of procedures more than a few minutes ahead of time, and even worse, they are the last to know the results of their many tests. In a large teaching hospital, the client has a specialist for everything and consequently may not develop a supportive relationship with any one physician or nurse. These clients lie passively in bed, while the parade of hospital personnel work on their various parts. In 1975, Volicer and Bohannon developed the Hospital Stress Rating Scale, which ranks stressful events commonly experienced by hospitalized persons such as:

- Having strangers sleep in the same room

- Having strange machines around

- Having nurses or doctors talk too fast or use words they can't understand

- Not getting pain medication when they need it

- Thinking they might lose a kidney or some other organ

- Thinking they might have cancer

The scale consists of forty-nine events, a sober reminder of the number of stressors a hospitalized person confronts.

In addition to this lack of customary support systems and the fear of bodily injury, clients suffer a psychologic reaction to hospitalization. They are expected to assume the *sick role* described by Parsons (1951). While occupying this role, they are exempt from responsibility and from their normal social role obligations: they are expected to depend on others, not to be self-directed, and to be compliant. Essentially, clients can be left almost totally without their usual supports, including the coping mechanisms on which they usually rely.

Coping with Illness and Hospitalization

How does someone manage to survive so many obstacles? Several authors have studied the coping processes of the physically ill (Lambert and Lambert 1985, Miller 1983, Moos 1977, Weisman 1978). Moos (1977, p 12) identifies seven coping skills common to clients with a variety of physical problems:

1. Denying or minimizing the seriousness of a crisis

2. Seeking relevant information

3. Requesting reassurance and emotional support

4. Learning specific illness-related procedures

5. Setting concrete, limited goals

6. Rehearsing alternative outcomes

7. Finding a general purpose or pattern of meaning in the course of events

These coping skills are behaviors that can be practiced and learned. They can be used at various times and in no special order of sequence. Sometimes they are labeled "positive," as in the case of the diabetic who learns to inject insulin. However, when a person constantly bombards the staff with questions about treatment, the skill may be labeled "negative." Coping with illness is a *process* that takes place over time. It necessitates the guidance of the hospital staff to help the client develop a workable coping style. The nurse must identify the client's present coping skills, evaluate their effectiveness, and intervene if necessary to help the client develop new methods of coping. This process is called **anticipatory guidance.**

The following questions help the nurse explore clients' coping styles:

• What has bothered you most about this illness?

• How has it been a problem for you?

• What have you done (or are you doing) about the problem?

• Is this helping?

• What has been the most difficult thing you've had to face until now?

• What did you do then?

• Whom do you rely on most, or expect will be most helpful to you?

• In general, how do things usually turn out for you?

The nurse can also evaluate the client's coping style by assessing key areas: Is the client emotionally distressed by anxiety, depression, and hostility? How does the client deal with significant others? Does the client's coping style interfere with *necessary* medical or surgical treatment or with other components of the treatment plan?

There are many approaches available to nurses who want to guide their clients toward optimal coping. Among them are the following:

• Being knowledgeable about the usual responses to a given illness so that the client's behavior can be properly evaluated

• Accepting the client's feelings and behavior as the best response the client can make at the present time

• Educating the client and the client's significant others about the reactions the client and others may have to the illness

• Knowing what the client is likely to be struggling with (i.e., the developmental tasks at the client's age and stage of life)

• Allowing the client the opportunity to try out new ways of being (e.g., talking about feelings with the nurse)

• Listening to clients solve problems out loud and providing feedback without giving direct advice

• Teaching such skills as relaxation and assertiveness

• Giving information (e.g., the relationship between anxiety and pain)

• Providing referrals to other resources (e.g., self-help groups, specialists, or other clients)

• Helping the client to manage the hospital environment, thereby increasing the client's sense of control and competence

• Developing written contracts with clients

• Separating the nurse's own personal responses from those of the client

Clients who develop effective coping styles will be strengthened in many ways. They will feel more capable of dealing with future problems, and, should the current illness prove to be chronic, will have developed the beginning skills to cope with a lifelong source of stress.

In the following sections, the nursing process is applied to selected clinical examples. Many of these examples reflect the input of a consulting psychiatric nurse.

The Nursing Process and the Demanding Client

Ruth was a resident of a home for the permanently disabled. She had been admitted to the hospital for a possible bowel obstruction. She was 65 and had lived most of her life in a wheelchair. Her body was misshapen from cerebral palsy, and she had no use of her legs or left hand. Recently she had developed arthritis in her right hand and could use it only for short periods each day. She had also been born with megacolon and was obsessed with the use of various laxatives. Ruth's appearance belied the fact that she was very intelligent, although humorless, as the staff soon found out.

According to the staff, Ruth was the "worst client they'd ever had." Ruth wanted to direct her own care in meticulous detail. She had to be bathed at a certain time and in a certain sequence, out of bed in time for breakfast and dressed by her own idiosyncratic method. It took two nurses one half hour to make her bed—they declared they needed a ruler to make sure the bedclothes hung precisely even. Medications were a real problem. Ruth had many p.r.n. medicines and constantly experimented with various combinations of laxatives, antispasmodics, and tranquilizers. No matter how one tried to please Ruth, she always found some fault with her nurse for the day, until finally she had been through the entire staff, and they all dreaded seeing her name on their assignment list.

Since Ruth inspired such strong feelings from the staff, the psychiatric clinical nurse specialist was consulted to ensure an objective plan of care.

Assessing

Discussions aimed toward connecting Ruth's behavior with theory to understand the *meaning* of her actions and attitude.

Ruth's demanding attitude was a life-style that had been exaggerated by the current hospitalization. The consultant helped the staff understand Ruth's behavior by looking at the underlying dynamics. Ruth had a distorted **body image** that reached back to her childhood, when she was confined to her bedroom and had to deal with body casts and braces. She had had to rely on others all her life and apparently had never resolved this dependency issue. To counteract her rage at being so helpless, she devised ways to control her environment by making incessant demands on others. In this way she vented her anger toward those with normal bodies. At the same time, she felt as if she had some degree of control over her surroundings. Ruth had behind her a lifetime of maladaption to her handicap, and it was not to be expected that she would change overnight. In fact, the current loss of functioning of her right hand constituted a crisis situation for Ruth. Behind Ruth's demands lay a myriad of feelings: anger, helplessness, frustration, jealousy, fear, and ambivalence.

Diagnosing

Here is a list of some of the nursing diagnoses that apply to Ruth:

- Impaired social interaction

- Chronic low self-esteem

- Ineffective individual coping related to loss of right hand function

- Body image disturbance

- Impaired physical mobility

A possible DSM-III-R diagnosis for Ruth is obsessive-compulsive personality disorder.

Planning and Implementing Interventions

In this situation, the consultant found herself performing a *parallel process*. This means that she was fulfilling parallel needs for both the staff and the client. She would meet with Ruth and allow her to *vent her feelings* of anger and frustration—some of which were justified and some of which were distortions of reality—toward the staff and the world in general. She encouraged Ruth to use her coping mechanism of intellectualization to recognize how she distorted reality because of fear and frustration.

At the same time the clinician *worked with the staff*, allowing them to express their feelings about Ruth. These feelings were also justified. Here, the clinician worked toward helping the staff recognize their anger at the client—a very difficult task for most nurses. Once the anger has been identified, steps can be taken to control it. Otherwise nurse and client engage in a no-win battle over control. The clinician demonstrated that anger was acceptable between nurse and client. She taught the staff how to *set limits* without being punitive or feeling guilty. This is also a difficult task for nurses who often feel they must fulfill everyone's wishes without paying any attention to their own needs.

A demanding person needs to have limits set and to be treated in a consistent and nonconflicted manner. Thus, Ruth's nurse conveyed to her that she wanted to make her as comfortable as possible, but that she couldn't spend a half hour making and remaking the bed until she got it just right. It was OK for the nurse to tell Ruth when she was angry, to be clear about what had provoked the anger, and to demonstrate that this did not mean that she would abandon or punish Ruth. The staff and clinician hoped that Ruth would begin to learn how to handle her own anger.

A client as difficult as Ruth always elicits feelings that nurses usually find unacceptable for themselves. But before we can accept anger from a client, we must learn to accept it in ourselves and learn that it will not overwhelm us. Working with demanding clients involves looking behind the external behavior for the reasons that are always there, although not always obvious.

In summary, these were the key interventions:

- Daily meetings between Ruth and nurse consultant

- Weekly meetings between staff and nurse consultant

- One staff nurse assigned to Ruth to coordinate *all* care

- Limit-setting approach discussed with Ruth and consistently used by all staff

Evaluating/Outcome Criteria

By the end of one week, tension on the unit had visibly decreased. Ruth had fewer outbursts of anger; staff was no longer hostile toward her. Ruth was discharged without further incident.

Applying the Nursing Process with the Client in Pain

Many nurses remember receiving an order to give an injection of sterile water for pain. Feeling guilty about carrying out such an order, we wondered why the client would "pretend" to be in pain. Who'd *want* to get injections, anyway?

The whole issue of pain and the use of medication to alleviate it is laden with myths and value judgments. References are made to psychogenic pain versus "real" pain. In fact, pain is both an objective and a subjective experience. A nurse can observe pain behaviors like wincing, limping, or splinting. And a nurse can listen to a client's reports of feeling pain. How a client manifests pain depends on many factors:

- The client's background
- Previous experiences with pain
- Family's attitude toward the expression of pain
- Immediate environment
- Type of illness
- Emotional state

The nurse's perception of a client's pain depends on the same factors. A nurse who thinks that people should suffer in silence will be intolerant of a client with a low pain threshold. It is important to realize that whether it is labeled psychogenic or physiologic, the client experiences the same pain.

An accompanying factor is the emotional component of pain. Anxiety, depression, guilt, anger, and hostility can all be associated with the experience of pain and can, in fact, become indistinguishable from one another.

In the general hospital, the nurse encounters pain in all its variations, from the post-cardiac-surgery client, to the cancer client with pathologic fractures, to the adolescent who has just had a tonsillectomy. Each client has an individual response to particular stimuli. Therefore, the nurse should evaluate each client's needs individually. Here is a case in point.

Mr S had been a client on the oncology service for eight months. He had come to America from his home in Brazil when he discovered that he had a mandibular tumor. He had heard that the United States had the most advanced methods of chemotherapeutic and surgical treatment of cancer. During his eight months of hospitalization, Mr S had undergone numerous courses of chemotherapy and four operations. Now he was ambulatory and self-sufficient. He had facial scars and a left-sided facial paralysis, but he could communicate clearly. His treatment had come to a standstill, and the doctors were planning discharge. However, Mr S complained of constant severe pain that he reported kept him awake all night and prevented him from thinking about anything else. At this point the psychiatric clinical nurse specialist was asked to see Mr S and help with the discharge planning.

Assessing

The consultant suggested a comprehensive assessment of Mr S's situation. This involved learning about his family background, his present relationship to his family, his plans for the immediate and distant future, and his perception of his illness. It also involved obtaining a detailed account of his pain experience.

Mr S had left all his friends and relatives in Brazil. He was divorced and had a 12-year-old daughter. In Brazil, he had held a university position, but he was not interested in returning either to his job or to his family. His reasons were not very clear, but he kept saying that he wanted to get a doctoral degree and a teaching position in the United States. He had written to several universities to inquire about their programs but had not made any definite plans. Apparently, money was no problem, but Mr S repeatedly returned to the issue of his pain. This pain kept him from making progress—he couldn't rest until he knew whether the pain was from another tumor growing in his jaw. For this reason he felt he had to stay in the hospital for further tests.

Diagnosing

Four key nursing diagnoses in this situation are:

- Ineffective individual coping
- Pain (acute)
- Altered role performance
- Body image disturbance

Mr S's pain behavior was related to his fear of dying, his fear of rejection due to disfigurement, his fear that he had lost his status and role in his own country, and his fear of leaving the hospital. All these issues were considered in his treatment plan.

Planning and Implementing Interventions

A coordinated approach was planned with the primary nurse as the client's primary contact. First, she obtained information about Mr S's medical status and asked the physicians to communicate clearly to Mr S his present condition and his prognosis. He was told that there was no evidence of another tumor, that no further treatment was indicated at this time, and that they were willing to help him make plans for discharge. Next, the nurse carefully evaluated the client's pain behavior. Exactly where was the pain? When was it most severe? What medications helped most? What activities made it worse or better? Together with Mr S, the staff nurses, and the physicians, the consultant implemented a plan whereby Mr S could gradually be weaned from his present analgesics. The client was also taught how to meditate and use distraction and relaxation techniques.

Underlying the entire plan was the relationship formed between Mr S and the primary nurse. It was understood that Mr S had developed a strong dependency on the hospital and indeed believed that he could not survive outside its walls. The nurse aimed to reduce this dependency gradually, guiding Mr S through the process of regaining his autonomy.

In summary, these were key interventions:

- Evaluate pain
- Learn status of tumor
- Wean client from analgesics
- Teach client meditation and relaxation techniques
- Increase client's independence gradually

Evaluating/Outcome Criteria

Within one month, Mr S returned to Brazil to his former position, needing only a nonnarcotic analgesic.

The Nursing Process and the Dependent Client

Some degree of dependency is a normal, necessary, and expected part of the person's new role as client. To be cured, clients allow us to take control of most of their bodily functions. They obediently open their mouths for the thermometer at six in the morning. They cooperate while we record everything they eat, drink, and eliminate. They answer questions in minute detail about their most intimate parts. Dependency and regression are aspects of their new role that allow clients to tolerate hospital life.

American culture values self-reliance and independence. But when we become ill, it becomes socially acceptable to ask for help. In fact, this is exactly what is expected. But sometimes the system backfires, and instead of giving up the sick role after the appropriate convalescent period, the client continues to act helpless. Whether or not clients return to their prior level of functioning depends on many factors. These include the length and severity of the illness, the client's personality, the client's family situation, and the attitude of the nursing staff, as illustrated in the following case.

Mrs C was admitted to a neurology unit amid rumors that she probably had Guillain-Barré syndrome, a rare disease that sometimes ends in total paralysis. The nurses were afraid to leave her bedside, expecting that at any moment she would stop breathing. After the diagnosis had been confirmed, Mrs C was intubated and transferred to the intensive care unit, where she remained for four weeks. When she returned to the neurology unit, the nurses met a severely regressed young woman who needed complete and total nursing care. Mrs C was off the respirator, and she was able to blink her eyelids. Otherwise she could move her limbs only with excruciating pain. Imagine the sensation one feels when one's leg has fallen asleep and one is trying to move it—that was only a fraction of what Mrs C felt.

At first the nurses were awed and sympathetic. Mrs C had survived. Now the staff's goal was to return her to her former role as a wife and mother. After several weeks, however, staff members became disillusioned. It seemed that Mrs C did not always share the staff's grand design for her rehabilitation. She cried that getting out of bed was too painful. She couldn't possibly brush her own teeth. At times Mrs C was too exhausted even to talk and seemed scarcely better than she had been on admission.

Assessing

The consultant liaison psychiatric nurse began to meet with the staff to discuss Mrs C's lack of progress. It was established that the nurses were anxious for her to improve because they wanted to deny the extreme severity of Mrs C's illness. The woman had suffered a catastrophic event, and it reminded the nurses that sickness is often meaningless and uncontrollable. Staff members discussed their need to control her progress. In their heads, they had formulated a time chart on which to record Mrs C's expected progress. It was very difficult to accept that the client didn't meet their expectations, because to them this meant that they were failures as nurses. It is interesting to observe that the nurses' need for control was actually aggravating the client's dependency. Mrs C was to give up her dependency according to the nurses' schedule! This is like demanding that someone "be spontaneous!"

Another factor was the prolonged period of immobility and complete helplessness that Mrs C had experienced. Her regression had been severe, and she needed time to relearn how to function on her own. This was a fearful and bewildering period for Mrs C and her family. For the first time, she contemplated how close she had come to death. Because Mrs C had been mercifully unconscious for much of the time in the ICU, this period was analogous to a rebirth for her. Psychologically and physically she had to learn to live again.

Diagnosing

The following nursing diagnoses apply to the psychologic problems Mrs. C experienced:

• Anxiety related to fear of death

• Powerlessness related to illness and health care environment

• Ineffective individual coping

Planning and Implementing Interventions

Out of weekly nursing care conferences with the nurse consultant, the staff developed a plan that allowed the client to gradually increase her independence. The staff allowed Mrs C to "pace" herself and gave her increased attention for her progress.

In summary, these were key interventions:

• Weekly care conferences with nurse consultant

• Schedule and priorities developed in collaboration with Mrs C

• Use of behavior-modification principles

Evaluating/Outcome Criteria

Because the nurses were insightful and perceptive enough to recognize their part in the situation, and because Mrs C had the desire to regain her former role, this case had a satisfactory ending. When the nurses were able to let go of their own objectives, Mrs C gained the ability to progress at her own rate.

The Nursing Process and the Client's Family

Hospital personnel speak of "the client with breast cancer," as if that phrase defined the target of their treatment. It may be more appropriate and accurate to talk about "the family of the client with breast cancer." This is because family members constitute a system, each part of which affects the functioning of all the other parts. Each family member fills a certain role, and if one member is hospitalized, that role is left vacant. The remaining members must make adjustments to compensate for the missing role.

The illness of a family member constitutes a family crisis. A crisis represents a turning point, the outcome of which can be adaptive or maladaptive, depending on the contributing factors. The nurse consultant is often called on when the nursing staff believe that the client's family is not making a positive contribution to their efforts to treat the client. That is what happened in the following situation.

Mrs W was recovering from a stroke that had left her aphasic and with right-sided weakness. Her treatment included physical therapy, speech therapy, and a weight-reduction, low-salt diet. The client, a widow, had been living alone at the time of her stroke. Her daughter had found her collapsed on the kitchen floor and had brought her to the hospital.

Mrs W's daughter and son visited her every night, bringing her presents of candy, fried chicken, and potato chips. They literally spoon-fed her and were horrified when the nurse suggested that Mrs W show her family how she could feed herself. The nurses were angry, believing that the family was encouraging Mrs W to remain dependent and interfering with her dietary regimen.

Assessing

The staff asked the nurse consultant for suggestions on how to deal with Mrs W's family.

One evening during dinner, the consultant dropped in on Mrs W and her family. She commented to the children that they showed great concern for their mother, and that it must sometimes be a strain to visit the hospital every night when they had families of their own. The son nodded agreement, but the daughter's eyes filled with tears and she asked to talk to the clinician alone. She began to tell her how guilty she felt about her mother's stroke. She had not visited Mrs W for several weeks prior to the stroke, saying she was too busy. When she finally had visited, it was to find Mrs W unconscious. If only she'd been a better daughter! Now the barrage of food and attention became understandable. Mrs W's children needed to assuage their guilt over what they believed to be neglect of their mother. The consultant made it clear that the staff did not view them as neglectful and indeed needed their help in rehabilitating Mrs W.

Diagnosing

The major nursing diagnosis in this instance was **Ineffective family coping.**

Planning and Implementing Interventions

Mrs W's family was included in a care planning session in which family members were designated certain tasks. The primary nurse determined which members were interested in and capable of giving her bed baths and back care and feeding her.

Evaluating/Outcome Criteria

The family became very helpful to both Mrs W and the nursing staff, allowing the client to progress more rapidly. They felt they had been an important part of her recovery and had been allowed to stay close to her during the long hospitalization.

Another situation frequently encountered is that of the angry, demanding family. They complain about the nursing care, ask to talk to the supervisor, and may even ask to see the hospital administrator. This behavior is one way a family can cope with the rage and impotence they feel. It is not acceptable to express anger toward the ill family member, although many spouses *do* experience anger. A wife is angered and frightened by her heavy new responsibilities and by the possibility of her husband's death. She cannot express this anger to her husband. Nor can she direct it toward the doctors, who seem to have the power of life and death. Often she takes her feelings out on the nurse, who is less threatening and more accessible. A husband whose wife is ill is also angry and frightened and feeling particularly left out in caring for his wife. He may overcompensate by keeping a close watch on the care the nurses are giving.

Nurses can provide this kind of family with a safe place to express their anger, fear, and frustration. They can let these families know that their feelings are not unusual and that the nurse doesn't find them selfish or insensitive. The staff can also be helped to understand the meaning of the family's behavior. This often leads to a decrease in hostility and allows everyone to spend more energy on adaptive methods of coping.

The nursing staff are often instrumental in helping the family cope successfully.

Ella visited her mother four times a week. Mrs R was 87 and had suffered a severe stroke three months ago. She had been hospitalized all that time, awaiting placement in a nursing home. Ella was upset that she couldn't take her mother home, but she had a full-time job and realized that she couldn't give her mother the proper care. Mrs R was fully bathed every morning by the nursing staff. Nevertheless, Ella always gave her mother a complete bath on each visit, checking her carefully for any sign of pressure ulcers and finishing off with a cloud of dusting powder. Often one of the nurses would assist Ella with the second bath. The staff did not consider this a comment on their ability to give adequate care. Instead, they recognized the pleasure Ella received in caring for her mother. Mrs R was eventually discharged to a nursing home.

Several months later the staff learned that Ella was a client on the psychiatric unit. Mrs R had died, and Ella had reacted with a psychotic episode. One of the nurses went to visit Ella on the psychiatric ward. Ella immediately recognized her and embraced her warmly. Excitedly, she began to ask the nurse, "Didn't I take good care of my mother? She never had a sore on her body when she was here!" Then she told how the nursing home staff had refused to let her bathe her mother, and how one day she had discovered an ugly pressure ulcer on Mrs R's hip. Shortly thereafter, Mrs R had died.

This example illustrates the powerful bonds that exist between family members. These bonds are strained when one member becomes seriously ill. Nurses can help maintain the integrity of the family unit, thus providing the client with this very crucial element of support.

The Nursing Process and the Client in the Intensive Care Unit

Throughout this chapter we have emphasized the importance of recognizing that the hospitalized client is under stress, and that this stress is both physiologic and psychologic. Because the stress is multifactorial, we have stated that meeting the client's physical needs alone will not restore the client's equilibrium. In an intensive care unit—that is, in any specialized acute care area such as cardiac care or respiratory care—the stress is magnified many times because the client's life is acutely threatened. All efforts are directed toward keeping the client's body functioning, a task that involves using sophisticated machinery and highly trained personnel. It is understandable that amid these valiant efforts, the client's psychologic state may well be overlooked. However, now that the intensive care unit is no longer a novelty, more attention is being paid to making it a more humane place for clients, their families, and the staff.

Clients in these units commonly develop an **ICU psychosis,** or intensive care syndrome. These terms are not exact and may refer to any combination of the following: depression, withdrawal, anxiety, hallucinations, delusions, paranoia, and delirium. A typical case is described below.

Mr W, a 55-year-old man, was admitted with a possible myocardial infarction. After forty-eight hours in the unit, he began to call for the nurses constantly. He would clutch their hands and plead with them to stay at his bedside. He would cry when the technicians came to draw

RESEARCH NOTE

Citation

Scherck KA: Coping with acute myocardial infarction. Unpublished dissertation, Rush University, 1989.

Study Problem/Purpose

This study examined how acute myocardial infarction (AMI) clients cope during the first three days of illness. Using the coping theory of Lazarus and colleagues, this study explicated clients' appraisals and use of various behavioral and cognitive coping strategies.

Methods

This study used a descriptive, exploratory design with a nonrandom sample of thirty acutely ill AMI patients. Data were collected on the fourth or fifth day of hospitalization through open-ended interview and administration of the Jalowiec Coping Scale (JCS). Interview content was analyzed using qualitative methods; JCS-related data were quantitatively examined as recommended by the instrument's author.

Findings

Clients' appraisals were conceptualized as coming to recognize illness, evaluating stakes, appraising the type of stress, considering coping options, experiencing emotions, and appraising and reappraising stress. From these appraisals emerged a unique description of coping with an AMI differing from that proposed by earlier investigators. Most clients reported they had to accept the AMI, although initial symptoms were difficult to recognize. Clients reported twenty-five different coping strategies, including positive thinking, humor, controlling feelings, controlling the situation, and handling things one step at a time. Optimistic, confrontative, and self-reliant strategies contributed most to total coping efforts.

Implications

Nurses should recognize and facilitate AMI clients' varied coping behaviors. Although nurses should be alert to the life-threatening nature of an AMI, clients may not share their perspective of their illness. Clients' appraisals change and may be unpredictable, although many AMI clients can describe their perspective of and their adaptation to their situation.

blood, or when he received injections. Mrs W reported that her husband could not keep track of her visits and was very much afraid that he would be left in the hospital all alone. This behavior lasted twenty-four hours. At that point Mr W was transferred out of the unit onto a general medical floor. His progress thereafter was uneventful, and there was no recurrence of any confused behavior.

Assessing

The stresses on such a client can be divided into three categories: environmental, psychologic, and physiologic. The following list includes some stressors that belong in each category.

1. Environmental stressors

   a. Sensory overload from constant noise, lights, unfamiliar treatments

   b. Sensory deprivation from immobility, restraints, bandages

   c. Lack of familiar orienting cues such as clocks, calendars, windows, meals, radio, television

   d. Close proximity to other clients who are also very ill

   e. Constant attendance by physicians, nurses, and technicians

   f. Lack of personal belongings

2. Psychologic stressors

   a. Fear of mutilation or death

   b. Little or no understanding of medical jargon or procedures

   c. Separation from family and friends

   d. Separation from familiar environment

   e. Depersonalization and physical exposure

   f. Powerlessness

   g. Pain

   h. Inability to release tension in accustomed fashion

3. Physiologic stressors

   a. Metabolic changes

   b. Decreased cardiac output

   c. Neurologic status

   d. Fever

   e. Electrolyte imbalance

   f. Drugs

g. Pain

h. Length of time spent on pump or under anesthesia

i. Sleep deprivation

Diagnosing

Among the relevant nursing diagnoses for clients in the intensive care unit are:

- Fear

- Anxiety

- Ineffective individual coping

- Powerlessness

- Sleep pattern disturbance

- Altered thought processes

- Impaired social interaction

A DSM-III-R diagnosis would be delirium.

Planning and Implementing Interventions

All clients in acute care areas experience some of these stressors. What can be done to reduce the occurrence of an ICU psychosis? Obviously, the stressors themselves should be eliminated, if possible. Many intensive care units are now being remodeled to create a less frightening environment for the client. When structural alterations are not feasible, other innovations can be made, such as adding color and pictures, arranging beds for maximum privacy, and turning lights down at night. In essence, any manipulation of the environment that will reduce stress and increase positive meaningful sensory input is helpful.

Clients and their families should be adequately prepared if circumstances permit. Clients who know what they can expect are much less frightened by the strangeness of the unit. Ideally, clients should meet some of the staff who will be caring for them. A familiar face is a welcome sight to someone who is recovering from anesthesia or waking from a fitful sleep.

Clients should be provided with consistent nursing personnel. This will diminish the process of depersonalization and isolation that always occurs to some degree in an intensive care unit. Family members can be encouraged to visit as the situation permits. An often overlooked feature is a room where family members can spend their many hours of waiting.

One way to reduce client stress in the acute care areas is to attend to the frustrations and needs of the staff. Work in a high-pressure unit affects staff dramatically, causing a high turnover rate and some-

times intrastaff conflict. The nursing staff should identify ways in which they can support one another. This may range from weekly meetings with the psychiatric nursing consultant to regular intrastaff volleyball games. It is crucial that the staff have some means of dealing with the enormous pressures they face. Perhaps this is where the consultant can be most helpful—as a vital link in the chain of support.

In summary, these are the key nursing interventions:

1. Educational preparation of clients

2. Use of orientation devices, e.g., clocks, windows

3. Reduction of environmental stressors

4. Provision of support for family

5. Staff support sessions

Evaluating/Outcome Criteria

Mr W's problems ended upon transfer out of the unit. With appropriate interventions, his "syndrome" could have been prevented or minimized.

The Nursing Process and the Client Manifesting Overt Sexual Behavior

Sexual acting out is psychiatric jargon for overt sexual behavior. For example, male or female clients may make flirtatious comments, attempt to touch or hold a male or female nurse, boast about sexual experiences, or deliberately expose their genitals while bathing or changing.

One sees a wide range of staff reactions toward this kind of behavior. Some nurses react by chastising clients verbally and then shunning them or reporting them to a supervisor or doctor. Other nurses simply ignore it, pretend not to notice it, or do not consider this kind of behavior important enough to comment on. Part of the reason for these varied responses to sexual behavior lies in the differences among clients and the perceptions and values of staff members. A young, attractive man who flirts with the female nurses may be acceptable, while a paunchy middle-aged man who exhibits the same behavior may be labeled a sex maniac or a dirty old man. A young woman client who wears makeup and sexy nightgowns may be criticized, whereas an elderly woman who habitually exposes herself may be virtually ignored.

Another reason for staff members' varied responses is that regressive behavior in the hospital is expected and even encouraged. *Regression* means that the client role includes, among other things, loss of identity, especially one's sexual identity. Clients are dressed in flimsy hospital gowns, they are left lying naked under the sheets on a stretcher, and they are often examined without much attention to discretion or modesty. Because hospitalization encourages sexual regression, a client's acting out may not be seen as anything unusual.

A third factor to consider is the attitude of the individual nurse about his or her own sexuality. These personal values will determine how nurses view the client's behavior and how they will choose to interact with the client who acts out sexually. The following case history illustrates many of these points.

Mr H was a 19-year-old male who had been admitted for a crush injury of the right hand. He was a frequent drug abuser, lived in a slum area, and was unemployed. From the beginning, he was not a popular client. He complained constantly of pain and demanded narcotics by name and dosage. No amount of medication seemed to hold him for very long, and he began threatening to call his friends and have them bring in the drugs he needed. Indeed, some shady-looking visitors were often seen in Mr H's room. This unpleasant situation reached crisis proportions when Mr H hung a pornographic poster in his room. At this point the staff called the psychiatric nursing consultant, and a staff conference was arranged.

Everyone was noticeably unnerved by the situation and needed to verbalize individual reactions to seeing the poster. One nurse had demanded that he take it down immediately. This confrontation had ended in a heated argument between the nurse and the client, and the poster was back on the wall the next day. Another nurse had quickly averted her eyes and pretended not to have noticed it. Thereafter, she avoided entering his room. A third nurse, alone on the night shift, became very frightened when Mr H asked to have his back rubbed. She spent a very uncomfortable eight-hour shift, feeling both afraid and guilty. The consultant accepted and understood all these reactions. However, none of them had proved a useful intervention.

Assessing

The consultant now explored with the group some of the possible dynamics behind Mr H's behavior. Mr H was only 19, an age when one's sexuality is extremely important. But both his injury and the hospitalization were threats to his image of himself as an active sexual male. The clinician discussed several issues. She explained the depersonalization and desexualization of a hospitalized client. Added to this, she pointed out, is the powerlessness and dependence of the client role. Many clients, especially unpopular ones, also experience emotional and touch deprivation. Another important concept in understanding Mr H was the insult to his body image. What was his perception of himself without the use of his right hand? Also, what significance did deformity to his right hand have for him?

Diagnosing

Appropriate nursing diagnoses are:

- Body image disturbance
- Self-esteem disturbance: situational
- Pain

Planning and Implementing Interventions

The staff responded readily to these ideas. They began to see Mr H as someone who was trying to maintain some control and self-esteem in a situation that was very threatening to him. It was decided that the staff would talk to him on a one-to-one basis and state their true reactions to his poster: "Mr H, I feel very uncomfortable being in your room since you hung that poster. I would appreciate it if you'd keep it in a more private place." Mr H soon complied, and overall relationships improved rapidly as other suggestions were made. These included allowing Mr H time to be alone with his girl friend; being more aware of his need for privacy; and giving him more control over his daily activities.

These new policies resulted in more open communication with the client in other areas as well. The nurses explained to Mr H that they wanted to keep him pain-free, but that it was impossible to assess the effects of analgesics when he was suspected of taking drugs on his own.

In summary, these were the key interventions used with Mr H:

- Use of assertive communication by staff nurses
- Meetings with the nurse consultant to plan a nonjudgmental approach
- Increased client control over activities

Evaluating/Outcome Criteria

The medication issue remained a problem, but the nurses felt much less judgmental and were better able to tolerate Mr H's behavior. This interaction with the consultant allowed the staff to explore some of their own values about sexuality. It also showed them how these values affected their ability to give optimal client care.

The case example that follows illustrates some further issues in dealing with the sexual concerns of clients.

Mr M, a 68-year-old man, had been on the unit for four weeks. During this time he had received cancer chemotherapy, and he was now in a state of remission. The psychiatric clinical nurse specialist had not been consulted for this particular client, but while she was spending time on the unit, she noted some unusual behavior. Mr M would pinch the nurses whenever they got near enough. They would respond by making a disapproving face that Mr M couldn't see, or by completely ignoring him. He also made suggestive remarks, which the staff also ignored. On one occasion, Mr M approached the consultant, saying he wanted to kiss her for "good luck." The consultant thought it important to understand the meaning of his behavior. Reading his chart, she learned that he had been impotent for the last six months.

Because the consultant already had a good working relationship with the staff, she approached them with the data she had gathered, instead of waiting for them to consult her. A staff conference was held. At this conference the nurses discussed why they had not taken direct measures to deal with Mr M's behavior. An important point was that the staff consisted mostly of newly graduated female nurses. Several nurses said they thought they were the only ones that Mr M was bothering and felt that they personally had done something to provoke him. Others said they were afraid that the doctors or nursing supervisors would laugh if they voiced their concerns. Another issue was documentation—they were uncertain whether such behavior should be noted in the client's chart. Was this information important? Would it be harmful to the client to document his behavior?

It became clear that the nurses were missing the meaning of Mr M's behavior because they became uncertain and embarrassed when the behavior was overtly sexual. Looking further, they could see the behavior as a defense against the actual impotence Mr M was experiencing. The consultant developed a therapeutic relationship with Mr M, who subsequently ceased his sexual acting out but became depressed instead. He and the consultant began working their way through the natural grieving process he had to undergo in relation to having cancer.

As this example illustrates, it is important for nurses to understand that all client behavior has meaning. It also points again to the all-important task of exploring one's own sexuality to understand the sexual behavior of clients during hospitalization.

The Nursing Process and the Noncompliant Client

The noncompliant client is both poorly understood and poorly tolerated. Many people fall under this label: the man with a recent myocardial infarction who refuses to stay in bed; the new diabetic who won't test his urine; the hypertensive who "forgets" to take her medicine. These clients may verbally state their understanding of the prescribed regimen, but their behavior indicates an underlying problem. Research indicates that at least one-third of clients studied did not follow their prescribed regimen (Young 1986). Noncompliance also causes frustration for the nurse whose task it

is to promote the highest possible level of client learning and functioning.

Mrs Schwartz is a 54-year-old woman who has been diabetic since age 30. She is divorced, has no children, and lives alone in a small apartment. She works as a cashier in a parking lot. Over the years, she has controlled her diabetes with diet and later with insulin. Recently she injured her left foot but did not seek treatment for several weeks until her foot became black and swollen. Now she is hospitalized for a below-the-knee amputation of her left leg. Mrs Schwartz is very aggressive and controlling. Because she has been diabetic for so long, she views herself as an expert and taunts the younger nurses about their ignorance on the subject of diabetic teaching. Mrs Schwartz does not comply with the hospital routine; instead she follows her own regimen of self-care, which is not sound in principle.

Assessing

There is always a reason for noncompliance, although neither the nurse nor the client may initially understand the dynamics involved. Many nurses respond to such clients with anger and impatience, which serves only to increase the distance between client and nurse. It is admittedly very difficult to watch self-destructive behavior that thwarts what we believe to be the correct therapeutic route. The nurse can reach an understanding of the client's behavior only through careful thought and observation.

In general, the factors that contribute to noncompliance can be summarized as follows:

• *Psychologic*—lack of knowledge; clients' attitudes, beliefs, and values; denial of illness and other defense mechanisms; personality type (e.g., rigid, defensive); very low or very high anxiety levels

• *Environmental and social*—lack of support system; other problems that distract from health care; finances, transportation, and housing

• *Characteristics of the regimen*—demands too much change from client; not enough benefit realized; too difficult, complicated; distressing side effects; leads to social isolation and stigma

• *Properties of the provider-client relationship*—faulty communication; client perceives provider as cold, uncaring, authoritative; client feels discounted and treated like an "object"; both parties engage in struggle for control.

The example of Mrs Schwartz illustrates many of the above factors. Her psychologic profile includes long-standing rigidity. She is extremely independent and strong-willed. Presently, she has the added need for control to compensate for the loss of her leg. This client should not be expected to accept a new regimen from an unfamiliar hospital staff. The fact that Mrs Schwartz lives alone and has no family will contribute to her difficulty in learning new behaviors because she will have no one to *reinforce* her new behaviors. Also important is the nature of the regimen itself. If Mrs Schwartz follows the regimen set out for her, will she see results quickly, and will those results be worth the effort of following the plan?

In addition, the nurse must examine the nature of the relationship with the client. Research points out that clients respond negatively to nurses and doctors who are cold, disapproving, rigid, and controlling. Mrs Schwartz could easily engage such a nurse in a battle for control. An added detriment would be a frequent turnover of nurses, none of whom feel responsible for the client, and hence do not form a stable relationship with her.

Diagnosing

Relevant nursing diagnoses are:

- Noncompliance related to diabetic regimen

- Powerlessness

- Body image disturbance

Planning and Implementing Interventions

Mrs Schwartz's noncompliance can be dealt with through contracting. One nurse should be assigned to her for the duration of her hospitalization. This would foster mutual communication, commitment, and understanding. Nurse and client would explore the *client's* goals, which would undoubtedly include prevention of further complications. They could establish the steps to take to meet the goals.

As the steps are discussed, the nurse should acknowledge Mrs Schwartz's self-care activities and ask her to review the basics of a diabetic regimen. Since the client's goal is to reduce complications, she should agree to review this material with the nurse. Mrs Schwartz will probably respond to being treated like an individual, not like another client who "needs diabetic teaching." Ideally, in this atmosphere of mutual respect, the client can relearn some important principles without having to admit the flaws in her own routine.

Evaluating/Outcome Criteria

Even when nurses understand the dynamics leading to noncompliance and take measures to prevent it, clients may not always respond to their efforts. In these circumstances, nurses must deal with their own feelings of frustration. This frustration is resolved only when the nurse accepts that clients are ultimately responsible for their own actions.

The Nursing Process and the Client with Body Image Alteration

Because every illness results in some change in body image, this is an important concept for all nurses in health care settings to consider. The **body image** is the individual's concept of the shape, size, and mass of the body and its parts. This image allows a person to evaluate the space the body occupies and to move about freely in the environment. It is the internalized picture a person has of the physical appearance of the body. Sensations arising inside the body and the attitudes and responses of others influence the individual's body concept. In this way, body image is closely allied with self-concept or self-image. Changes in the body image are threatening. Of necessity, people attempt to maintain the integrity of their own bodies.

The body image extends beyond the physical body. Objects of daily use that are intimately connected with the body surface, such as a cane, dentures, clothes, a tattoo, makeup, and jewelry, are incorporated into the body image. Without these, a person may feel incomplete and anxious. Objects connected with and symbolizing a profession, such as the police officer's gun or the nurse's white uniform, may be even more intensely incorporated into the body image, not only by the wearer but by the public as well.

All these factors form an inner mental diagram called the body image. This diagram is fluid and dynamic—it changes in response to the current sensory and psychic stimuli it receives.

Assessing

Certain consistent elements are important in assessing the significance of the body image and its alteration.

First, body characteristics that people have from birth or acquire early in life seem to have less emotional significance for them than those that arise in adolescence or later. The boy born lacking a limb formulates an image of himself that accounts for the limb's absence. His healthy self-concept naturally excludes that limb from the "me." Children with crossed eyes, protruding teeth, or disfiguring facial birthmarks often similarly incorporate these features into their body images. The school nurse or teacher who recommends correction of such a "defect" is often astounded by the resentment that greets this well-meant suggestion. Attempts to change a characteristic are unwelcome and resisted because they require changing the loved "me."

A second factor to consider in evaluating the significance of alterations in body image is that a defect, handicap, or change in body function that occurs abruptly is far more traumatic than one that develops gradually. For example, crippling arthritis that eventually impairs the use of an extremity is less disturbing than traumatic amputation of an extremity during an auto accident. A person has time to adjust to the effects of arthritis on body function and body image, whereas the person whose extremity has been suddenly amputated is not allowed the healing effects of time. The person suddenly discovers the absence or loss of function of a loved part of self.

Third, the location of a disease or injury greatly affects the emotional response to it. Internal diseases are generally less distressing than external diseases that can be seen by the person and by others. For example, radical head and neck surgery, with its consequent disfigurement, is devastating to the body image and to the psyche, since the face is one of the primary means by which people communicate. Most people focus on the face in interacting with others. When that face becomes less pleasing to the eye, radical changes in body image may also occur.

People generally experience a great threat when the genitals or breasts are involved in change. Breast surgery is of particular significance to many women, because breasts symbolize femininity and sexual attractiveness in Western culture. In men, such surgical procedures as circumcision and inguinal hernia repair pose a far more disturbing threat to the body image than major operations such as gastrectomy or cholecystectomy. Fears about sexuality and virility are reawakened and reinforced when illness or injury threatens genital areas. Those parts of the body are important to people's mental view of themselves as men or women.

Diagnosing

These nursing diagnoses may apply to persons with body image problems:

- Body image disturbance
- Self-esteem disturbance

A DSM-III-R diagnosis would be depersonalization disorder.

Planning and Implementing Interventions

Individuals develop new body images when they *interact* with the new body part. Nurses can begin this process with the client.

Mrs M has returned from the operating room after undergoing an above-the-knee amputation. When she is alert enough, the nurse orients Mrs M and tells her that her stump is now bandaged and the dressing will be changed tomorrow. The nurse encourages Mrs M to look at her leg and touch the dressing. The nurse herself uses touch frequently in changing the stump dressing. She is gentle and caring toward this "new" body part. Mrs M and her family will soon be involved in looking at Mrs M's stump and learning to dress and care for it.

Nurses need to be aware of their own reactions toward clients' altered bodies. Nurses who can accept imperfections in their own bodies accept those of a client more readily.

It is important for nurses who may work with "repulsive" body alterations to learn to *look past* the unpleasantness to the person inside the body. Nurses who can accomplish this find that over time the initially unbearable becomes secondary to the nurse-client relationship that develops.

Mourning a Body Image Alteration or the Loss of a Body Part Loss is the general theme in all body image alterations. To cope with the loss of a loved person, loved object, or loved body part, a person must mourn. Clients may need to be helped to acknowledge the loss in order to move from a stage of shock and disbelief into developing awareness. Health professionals sometimes believe that ignoring or minimizing the loss is helpful to clients and their families. This is not true. Those who fail to acknowledge the loss or minimize it hinder grief work.

Clients need a supportive person to help them move toward the resolution phase of mourning. It may be necessary to create opportunities for discussing the disability, its meaning to the client, the problem of compensating for the loss, and the reaction of persons with whom the client will come in contact. Attitudes of disapproval, repulsion, or rejection toward a person with a physical disfigurement or defect hinder the person's social adaptation. Nurses can help family and friends to overcome such attitudes, if they experience them, by creating similar opportunities for them to discuss their fears and concerns.

Providing Anticipatory Guidance Anticipatory guidance aims to help people cope with a crisis by discussing the details of an impending stressful occurrence and solving problems before the event occurs. Anticipatory guidance is needed not only for clients but also for the significant persons in their lives, both family and friends. Anticipatory guidance lays the foundation for effective grief work. It consists of brief psychotherapeutic intervention to discuss the meaning of the body part to the client and significant others, their beliefs and feelings concerning previous losses, and the beliefs they hold about the body image. A discussion of the phantom phenomenon should be included for all clients who experience the loss of a body part. The **phantom experience** can be defined as the sensation of feeling a part of the body that is no longer there. The phantom limb phenomenon is the most well known. It is far more common than is generally believed. Phantom limb experiences increase markedly if amputation occurs after the client is 4 years of age, and they are almost universal when the client is age 8 or older.

Phantom experiences occur in an attempt to redefine the lost part and to maintain the stability and integrity of the body image. In fact, some theorists view the phantom as an indication of a stable body schema. Too stable a body schema can prove troublesome, however, when the individual recognizes that the phantom is unreal and that others do not share the perception of it. Problems also arise when the phantom is experienced as painful.

Although phantoms are considered universal, **phantom pain** is relatively rare. Phantom limb pain has been hypothesized to have a neurophysiologic basis. In the psychoanalytic view, the painful phantom is thought to be psychopathologic in nature and rooted in the loss of the limb. People experiencing them have described the pain as acute, burning, grinding, tearing, and crushing. The severity of the pain may account for the high incidence of addiction to narcotics and suicidal tendencies among persons with painful phantoms. Therapeutic preparation of a person who is to undergo amputation can help prevent the painful phantom.

The nonpainful phantom eventually disappears, although there are recorded instances in which phantoms have persisted for as long as twenty years. Phantoms of the upper limb are generally stronger and last longer than phantoms of the lower limb. They often begin to disappear through a process known as *telescoping*—i.e., the hand or the foot appears to be shrinking toward the stump. The final parts to disappear are usually the thumb, the index finger, and the big toe.

Explore the client's fears and determine how the client wishes to dispose of the body part to be amputated. Fantasies and superstitious beliefs about amputated parts of the body can increase a client's anxiety and discomfort.

Evaluating/Outcome Criteria

Nursing interventions for a client with altered body image are successful if the client is able to express thoughts and feelings about body changes, to look at and touch a body deformity, to participate in self-care

related to the body part, and to discuss the alterations in life-style (if any) resulting from the body change.

Role of the Psychiatric Nursing Consultant

Almost every general hospital has some kind of mental health professional available to work with clients directly or to support and educate the staff toward handling clients' emotional problems. Here, we discuss the psychiatric nurse in the consulting role.

History of Consultation in the Hospital Setting

Physicians were the first to practice **consultation-liaison psychiatry**— providing psychiatric consultation to clients in the general hospital—based on the concepts of psychophysiologic medicine and preventive psychiatry. Liaison psychiatry originated in the late 1950s. Paralleling this trend, psychiatric nurses also began to act as consultants to their colleagues in medical and surgical settings. At first, the **liaison nurses** remained based on their psychiatric units, providing indirect assistance when it was requested. Later, they began to work directly with clients and their families. Currently, psychiatric nurse clinicians perform both direct and indirect consultative functions. (See the work of Caplan [1970] and Lewis and Levy [1982] for in-depth information on the consulting process.)

Qualifications of the Consultant

The psychiatric nurse consultant should be prepared at the graduate level in psychiatric-mental health nursing. Some graduate programs are specifically geared to liaison nursing and provide clinical experiences in a general hospital setting. Other programs are oriented toward the community mental health center or the psychiatric in-patient unit. In any case, the consultant's education includes classroom and supervised clinical experiences in individual, group, and family therapy, since all these modes are used in practice. Most graduate programs include courses in organizational theory in which the principles of power and influence and planned change are emphasized. Because a hospital is an incredibly complex organization, a successful consultant needs a solid theoretic and experiential base, along with confidence, competence, and concern.

Consultants who have actual staff nursing experience in a nonpsychiatric general hospital setting have an invaluable advantage over the inexperienced clinician. They have firsthand knowledge of the day-to-day problems facing the staff nurse: what is it like having to rotate shifts; having to work weekends; being the only registered nurse in charge of forty clients; dealing with complaints from X-ray, dietary, and operating room departments—and on top of it all, having clients say they would get better service for less money in a hotel down the street. It is definitely true that nursing educators and administrators gain respect by having "paid their dues." Consultants with staff experience start out with two advantages. They are *nurses,* and they share a common background of experience with their consultees.

Guidelines for the Consultation Process

The consulting psychiatric nurse usually works according to the classic consultation process developed by Caplan. The staff nurse who seeks a nurse consultant's help can expect the relationship to be guided by the following precepts:

* Mental health consultation is a process of interaction between two professionals with respect to a client or a program for clients.

* Ideally, the consultant has no administrative responsibility for the consultees' work. The consultant is under no compulsion to alter the consultee's handling of the case.

* The consultee has no obligation to accept the consultant's ideas or suggestions.

* The basic relationship between the two is egalitarian. This allows the consultee to accept or reject what the consultant says and to incorporate any ideas the consultee feels are appropriate to the situation.

* Consultation can take various forms. These include individual and group consultation and work with staff as well as with clients, depending on the particular situation.

* The exact form of the consultation is made explicit in the contract—a verbal or written agreement between consultant and consultees.

* The goals of consultation are to help the consultees improve their handling or understanding of the current work problem and to generalize this learning to future similar situations.

* The consultative process is not therapy, but it can be therapeutic. Increasing a consultee's competence in the work situation gives the consultee an overall sense of accomplishment and self-worth (Caplan 1970, pp 28–30).

CHAPTER HIGHLIGHTS

* Nurses working in general hospitals face the challenge of combining "high tech" and "high touch."

* Illness and hospitalization can be viewed as crisis situations for clients and their families.

* Hospitalized clients can be left almost totally without their usual supports, including the coping mechanisms upon which they usually rely.

* The nurse must identify the client's present coping skills, evaluate their effectiveness, and intervene if necessary to help the client develop new methods of coping.

* Clients who develop effective coping styles will feel more capable of handling future problems and, should the current illness prove to be chronic, will have developed the beginning skills to cope with a lifelong source of stress.

* Working with demanding clients involves looking behind the external behavior for the reasons that are always there, although not always obvious.

* A comprehensive assessment and a coordinated approach are needed for the client in pain.

* Although some degree of dependency is a normal, necessary, and expected part of a person's new role as client, it is essential to help clients regain their former independence and autonomy.

* The illness of a family member constitutes a crisis for a family. The nursing staff are often instrumental in helping the family cope successfully.

* The stress of hospitalization is magnified many times for the client in the intensive care unit because the client's life is actually threatened.

* Nurses must explore their own sexuality to understand the sexual behavior of clients during hospitalization.

* There is always a reason for a client's noncompliance with the treatment regimen; this reason can be understood only through careful thought and observation.

* Clients who undergo a body image change should be provided with anticipatory guidance and the opportunity to prepare for the body image alteration or mourn the loss of a body part.

* In complex client situations, nurses may need input from case conferences and nurse consultants to remain objective and to attend to all aspects of the client's problems.

REFERENCES

American Psychiatric Association: *Diagnostic and Statistical Manual of Mental Disorders,* ed 3, revised. APA, 1987.

Antai-Otong D: Dealing with demanding patients. *Nursing* 1989;19(1):94–95.

Baer CL (ed): Patient compliance: Issues and outcomes. *Top Clin Nurse* 1986;7:entire issue.

Benner P, Wrubel, J: *The Primacy of Caring: Stress and Coping in Health and Illness.* Addison-Wesley, 1989.

Boehm S: Patient contracting. *Annu Rev Nurs Res* 1989; 7:143–153.

Brown L: The experience of care: Patient perspectives. *Top Clin Nurs* 1986;8:56–62.

Buchanan D, Mandell A: The prevalence of phantom limb experience in amputees. *Rehab Psychol* 1986;31(3): 183–188.

Cameron K et al.: Chronic illness and compliance. *J Adv Nurs* 1987;12(6):671–676.

Caplan G: *Theory and Practice of Mental Health Consultation.* Basic Books, 1970.

Christman N et al.: Uncertainty, coping and distress following myocardial infarction. *Res Nurs Health* 1988;11(2): 71–82.

Chyum D: Patient perceptions of stressors in intensive care and coronary care units. *Focus Crit Care* 1989; 16(3):206–211.

Cousins N: *Anatomy of an Illness as Perceived by the Patient: Reflections on Healing and Regeneration.* Norton, 1979.

Dalton J: Nurses' perceptions of their pain assessment skills, pain management practices, and attitudes toward pain. *Oncol Nurs Forum* 1989;16(2):225–231.

Damrosch SP: Perceived loss of body parts in nursing and nursing students. *Health Care Women Int* 1988;9(4): 305–315.

Dracup K: Are critical care units hazardous to health? *Appl Nurs Res* 1988;1(1):14–20.

Dulaney P et al.: Ten years in liaison nursing: Concepts, models, and conventional wisdom. *Issues Ment Health Nurs* 1988;9(4):425–431.

Fife BL: Establishing the mental health clinical specialist role in the medical setting. *Issues Ment Health Nurs* 1986;8:15–23.

Fitzpatrick R et al.: *The Experience of Illness.* Tavistock, 1984.

Groves JE: Taking care of the hateful patient. *N Engl J Med* 1978;298:883–887.

Holm K: Effect of personal pain experience on pain assessment. *Image* 1989;21(2):72–75.

Hussey LC et al.: Compliance, low literacy, and loss of control. *Nurs Clin North Am* 1989;24(3):605–611.

Lambert V, Lambert C: *Psychological Care of the Physically Ill.* Prentice-Hall, 1985.

Leahey M, Wright L: *Families and Life-Threatening Illness.* Springhouse, 1987.

Lewis A, Levy JS: *Psychiatric Liaison Nursing.* Prentice-Hall, 1982.

Loomis M: Levels of contracting. *J Psychosoc Nurs* 1985;23(3):8–14.

McCaffery M: *Pain: Clinical Manual for Nursing.* Mosby, 1989.

Miller JF: *Chronic Illness.* F. A. Davis, 1983.

Miller T: Advances in understanding the impact of stressful life events on health. *Hosp Community Psychiatry* 1988;39(6):617–621.

Miller T, Kraus R: An overview of chronic pain. *Hosp Community Psychiatry* 1990;41(4):433–440.

Mishel M: Uncertainty in illness. *Image* 1988;20(4):225–232.

Montgomery C: How to set limits when a patient demands too much. *Am J Nurs* 1987;87(3):365–366.

Moos R (ed): *Coping with Physical Illness,* vol 2. Plenum, 1984.

Nemeroff CB: Clinical significance of psychoendocrinology in psychiatry. *J Clin Psychiatr* 1989;50(5)(Suppl):13–20.

Norris CM: Body image, in Carlson CE, Blackwell B (eds): *Behavioral Concepts in Nursing Intervention.* Lippincott, 1978.

Parsons T: *The Social System.* The Free Press, 1951.

Pelletier LR, Kane J: Strategies for handling manipulative patients. *Nursing* 1989;19(5):82–83.

Podrasky D: Nurses' reactions to difficult patients. *Image* 1988;20(1):16–21.

Postone N: Phantom limb pain: A review. *Int J Psychiatry Med* 1987;17(1):57–70.

Ribbers G et al: The phantom experience: A critical review. *Int J Rehab Res* 1989;2(2):175–186.

Riegel B, Ehrenreich D: *Psychological Aspects of Critical Care.* Aspen, 1989.

Rutherford D: Consultation: A review and analysis of the literature. *J Prof Nurs* 1988;4(5):339–344.

Sabo K: ICU family support sessions: Family perceived benefits. *Appl Nurs Res* 1989;2(2):82–89.

Scherck KA: *Coping with Acute Myocardial Infarction.* Unpublished dissertation, Rush University, 1989.

Sherman R, Sherman C, Bruno G: Psychological factors influencing chronic phantom pain: An analysis of the literature. *Pain* 1987;28(3):285–295.

Sontag S: *Illness as Metaphor.* Vintage, 1984.

Strain JJ: Needs for psychiatry in the general hospital. *Hosp Community Psychiatry* 1982;33:996–1001.

Taylor AG: Chronic pain: A guide to nursing intervention. *Appl Nurse Res* 1988;1(1):8–13.

Teasdale K: The concept of reassurance in nursing. *J. Adv Nurs* 1989;19(1):94–95.

Volicer BJ, Isenberg MA, Burns, MW: Medical-surgical differences in hospital stress factors. *J Human Stress* 1977; June:3–13.

Weisman AD: Coping with illness, in Hacket TB, Cassem NH (eds): *Handbook of General Hospital Psychiatry.* Mosby, 1978.

White C: The psychiatric clinical nurse specialist as mental health consultant. *Nurs Manage* 1988;19(6):80,82.

Whitley MP: Seduction and the hospitalized person. *J Nurs Ed* 1978;17(6):34–39.

Williams M: Physical environment of the ICU and elderly patients. *Crit Care Nurs* 1989;12(11):52–56.

Wilson V: Identification of stressors related to patients' psychologic responses to the surgical intensive care unit. *Heart Lung* 1987;16(3):267–273.

Yarcheski A: Uncertainty in illness and the future. *West J Nurs Res* 1988;10(4):401–413.

Young SM: Strategies for improving compliance. *Top Clin Nurs* 1986;7:31–39.

Eating Disorders

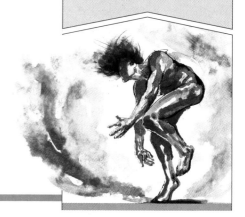

LEARNING OBJECTIVES

Kay K. Chitty

- Define anorexia nervosa, bulimia nervosa, and compulsive overeating
- Describe the historical and theoretic foundations essential to the understanding of eating disorders
- Compare and contrast the characteristic clinical features of eating disorders
- Assess individual and family problems of clients with eating disorders
- Identify nursing diagnoses for clients with eating disorders
- Develop individualized nursing care plans for clients with eating disorders who are treated in in-patient settings
- Describe the nurse's role and appropriate nursing interventions for clients with eating disorders and their families
- Evaluate the effectiveness of nursing interventions with clients with eating disorders and their families

CROSS REFERENCES

Other topics relevant to this content are: Adolescents, Chapter 34; Codependence, Chapter 24; Mood disorders, Chapter 13; Personality disorders, Chapter 16; Psychophysiologic conditions, Chapter 18; Stress, anxiety, and coping, Chapter 5; Visualization, guided imagery, and other stress-management techniques, Chapter 27.

IN THE PAST TWENTY years, the United States has experienced what has been described as an epidemic of eating disorders. The emphasis on slimness in North American culture has made increasing numbers of adolescents and young adults obsessively concerned about eating, weight, and body shape, size, and appearance. In a desperate attempt to achieve perfection, the need for which is often psychologically obscure, some individuals go to extreme lengths to achieve thinness. While they starve themselves, sometimes to death, others apparently reject the cultural norms, overeat, and become obese.

For many, eating symbolizes parental nurturing—the love and care that are the prototype of and basis for all future intimate relationships. For some, however, eating creates anxiety because of its association with unsatisfactory and unpleasant parent-child interactions. Clearly, food and eating have greater individual and cultural meaning and importance than merely an activity undertaken to sustain life.

The three major eating disorders discussed in this chapter—anorexia nervosa, bulimia nervosa, and compulsive overeating—create biologic, psychologic, and social imbalances that interfere with the individual's normal functioning. Changes in biochemistry, metabolic rate, emotional state, family relationships, and social status brought about by eating disorders can create depression, isolation, and sometimes self-destructive behavior.

Because eating is closely bound up with emotions, disorders of eating indicate emotional difficulties that fall within the scope of psychiatric nursing. Most psychiatric nurses begin their work with clients once an eating disorder has been suspected or has been diagnosed. The primary prevention role of the nurse should not be underestimated (Chitty 1991). Although the development of eating disorders is complex, community-wide education by nurses about nutrition and feeding at successive developmental levels from infancy to old age can decrease the incidence of eating disorders in the community. To move from a treatment mode to a prevention mode, psychiatric nurses change the focus of attention from individuals and families as the unit of treatment to the entire community as the unit of treatment.

Anorexia Nervosa

Anorexia nervosa is a potentially life-threatening disorder characterized by extreme weight loss, intense fear of gaining weight, body image disturbances, strenuous exercising, and peculiar food-handling patterns. Hilde Bruch (1978) has called it "the relentless pursuit of thinness." Clients usually undergo a single episode of anorexia nervosa and experience full recovery; unchecked, the course of anorexia nervosa results in a mortality rate between 5 percent and 21 percent, depending on time elapsed since onset (Halmi 1985). It is estimated that 95 percent of anorexia nervosa clients are female, usually between the ages of 12 and the mid-30s (Herzog 1988). The onset of the disorder is sometimes associated with a stressful life event.

Simone is a tall, quiet girl who was considered polite, well liked, and a good student. She was given responsibility beyond her years both at school and home because of her quiet competence and maturity. When she was 15 she entered a beauty contest at a local amusement park as a lark but did not win. She became convinced that she lost because her legs were too large and her abdomen protruded. She decided to diet. To radically control her own intake without arousing the family's suspicions, she began preparing all the family's meals. She did not eat herself, but played with her food during mealtimes.

Simone spent long hours alone in her room studying, dancing, and exercising vigorously. She began weighing herself several times daily, and if the scales showed an unacceptable number, she exercised even more frenziedly.

As she lost weight, Simone disguised her gauntness with loose clothes. One day, when she and her mother were shopping, her mother saw her without her blouse and was dismayed. She insisted that Simone see the family physician, who encouraged her to eat more and prescribed nutritional supplements.

When Simone collapsed at a shopping mall a few weeks later, her parents prevailed on the family doctor to admit her to the psychiatric unit of the community hospital. As an IV was started in the emergency room, Simone asked the nurse, "How many calories are in that bag? It won't make me gain weight, will it?"

Bulimia Nervosa

Bulimia nervosa is a disorder characterized by **binging,** the frequent compulsion to eat large quantities of food in a short period of time. These periods of overeating are usually followed by **purging,** self-induced vomiting and/or use of large doses of laxatives and diuretics. Enemas may also be used to rid the body of all traces of food consumed during a binge. Abraham and Llewellyn-Jones (1985) estimate that 40 percent of anorexia nervosa clients also indulge in binging. There must be a minimum average of two binge-eating episodes per week for at least three months to warrant this DSM-III-R diagnosis. Most bulimics are young females of high school or college age of normal or slightly above average weight. Recent statistics show bulimia is escalating among older women and young men as well. Like anorectics, bulimics are preoccupied with body shape and size.

Beth, a 17-year-old student, came to the mental health center because of binge eating. She complained that although she was very concerned with her weight and very invested in her physical image, she regularly went on gluttonous eating binges for one to two days. These would leave her nauseated, exhausted, and disgusted with herself. Her inability to control the behavior voluntarily was making her depressed.

In the course of her therapy, it became apparent that although Beth consciously wanted to make certain improvements in her academic and social life and her appearance, she had subtle ways of sabotaging any movement in that direction. Binge eating destroyed any attempts she made to control her weight and thus feel positive about her body image.

Movement in a self-interested direction had become attached in Beth's mind to repudiation of her depressed mother, with whom she felt very close. Individual successes, she felt, were antagonistic toward her mother, since they might lead to her own greater independence. Although she wished such independence for herself, she also feared losing her mother's support, which she needed. Thus, she developed ways of undermining her own efforts.

Psychotherapeutic work with Beth involved discovering these meanings, bringing her concerns to the surface for discussion, and attempting to resolve issues of fear of separation and dependency needs. When this material was directly discussed, Beth had less need for indirect expression of conflict, and the binge-eating behavior subsided.

Compulsive Overeating

Obesity can be defined as "excessive storage of energy in the form of fat" (Wurtman and Wurtman 1987). Although obesity has adverse effects on both longevity and health, it also may adversely affect mental health. There is considerable controversy as to whether obesity by itself should be classified as an eating disorder. It is not included under that category in DSM-III-R, and many obese individuals are apparently quite well adjusted. Many others, however, experience anxiety, depression, low self-esteem, and poor body image. These are individuals whose **compulsive overeating** may be an attempt to compensate for the love and nurturing they did not receive as children or to relieve stress. Obesity and compulsive overeating, therefore, are included in this chapter on eating disorders. Compulsive overeating can be diagnosed under the DSM-III-R category, "psychological factors affecting physical condition."

Joan, an obese 45-year-old secretary, is 63 inches tall and weighs 167 pounds. She came to the outpatient department of a private psychiatric hospital because of depression over her weight. She reported her weight problem began about ten years ago when her husband left her on the day of her parents' twenty-fifth wedding anniversary. She and her 10-year-old son moved back in with her parents, and the family had many long discussions concerning what Joan should do. At about the same time, she lost her job. It took Joan nearly six months to find a comparable job, and she suffered severe financial stresses. Again, her parents helped. She felt trapped by, yet dependent on, her parents.

Joan described herself during that period as "tense and angry all the time." Her weight gradually crept up. She tried to diet, but the problems remained and eating seemed to be the only way to dull the pain. "When I'd look at myself in the mirror, I would be so discouraged that I'd eat a whole pan of brownies, just to feel better."

Psychotherapy with Joan involved exploration of the meaning of her obesity and focused on her concerns about her attractiveness to men. Her relationship with her parents, particularly dependence/independence issues, were also explored. Joan, who has been in therapy for only four months now says, "My behavior is destructive; I am using food as an escape from emotional stress and pain. I still wish I were thinner."

Historical Foundations

With few exceptions, for most of recorded history women were considered desirable when they had plump breasts, hips, and thighs. Plumpness was fashionable, demonstrated that the male was a good provider, and symbolized sensuality.

During medieval times, however, saintly women fasted, mortifying the flesh to achieve spiritual enlightenment (Rossi 1988). Food practices were used to express religious ideals. Physical evidence of fasting in women was felt to reveal the inner beauty of saintliness (Rossi 1988), and many women, particularly of the upper classes, fasted.

The Renaissance signaled a return to popularity of the plump, full-figured beauty seen in paintings by Titian, Raphael, and Michelangelo. A very practical societal need was at the basis of this emphasis on robust women; the bubonic plague, which swept Europe in the Middle Ages, wiped out fully half of the population (Gottfried 1983). Repopulating Europe was of great importance. Voluptuous, padded contours were associated with fertility, and both were highly prized in women for the next several centuries.

In the late 1800s another serious epidemic occurred, an outbreak of syphilis so severe that the survival of Western society was in question (Brumberg 1988). The only means of survival in that preantibiotic age was a retreat to the repressive morality that came to characterize Victorian society. Middle- and upper-class women portrayed themselves, both in clothing and conduct, as asexual creatures, thus avoiding being labeled "loose women." A thin, wan appearance was cultivated as the proper Victorian lady's look. Thus, Victorian women protected society from its sexuality through denial of their own (Brumberg 1988).

Denial of sexuality continued throughout the early twentieth century. The flappers of the 1920s achieved their flat-chested prepubertal bodies through breast binding, severe exercise, and starvation diets leading to the first reported epidemic of anorexia and bulimia (Fontaine 1991). Narrow waists, larger busts, and shapely legs became erotic symbols during the Depression and World War II.

The 1940s, 1950s, and 1960s brought dramatic social changes. World War II created the first generation of females to work outside the home. Outside employment caused some women to feel guilty and confused about their roles. The development of birth-control pills in the mid-1960s set the stage for a sexual freedom previously unknown, creating additional role conflicts and insecurities in both sexes. These, and the emerging women's movement, required a rethinking of all female experiences, including mothering.

The voluptuous but tiny-waisted look continued to be popular through the 1950s. In 1966, Twiggy, a very thin model from London, came on the scene, signaling a change in taste. According to Fontaine (1991), the 1970s and 1980s saw only slight modifications of the lean and hipless look. A more muscular and healthy, lean, strong, and graceful ideal and a new emphasis on physical fitness characterize the late 1980s and early 1990s. There are both positive and negative impacts of physical fitness on women, notes Fontaine. Improved physical and mental health is counterbalanced by a demand to control and master the body.

Richard Morton, a physician, published the first report of anorexia nervosa in 1689. He described a young woman with a condition he termed "nervous atrophy," which he attributed to her "sadness and anxious cares" (Halmi 1985). In 1873, an English physician, Sir William Gull, coined the term "anorexia nervosa" in his paper discussing the case of "Miss A." Infrequent reports were published in the next century, and it was not uncommon for physicians to practice for an entire lifetime without seeing a single case of anorexia. Modern psychiatric understanding of anorexia nervosa did not begin until 1961, when Bruch (1978) published a paper based on her observations of twelve anorectic women. The professional literature concerning anorexia has proliferated in the last thirty years as the incidence of the disorder has increased.

Descriptions of bulimic symptoms first appeared in the literature in 1873, although bulimic disorders were not recognized as a syndrome until more recently. Until the 1940s, bulimic symptoms were discussed only in association with anorexia, diabetes mellitus, and obesity. The case of "Ellen West," published in 1944, was the first well-documented account of bulimia nervosa (Garfinkel and Garner 1982). Not until 1979 was there published a systematic investigation of bulimia as a distinct eating disorder. In that report, Russell (1979) described a group of women who had long histories of difficulty in regulating food consumption.

This brief review shows the influences of historical events and the link between women's eating and sexuality. Throughout history, the female form has been an object of pleasure for men. This emphasis has, to this day, powerfully affected each woman's relationship with her body. Viewed in historical context, eating disorders can be interpreted as an understandable, although extreme, response to disturbances in that relationship. The rapid and sweeping societal changes of the last fifty years have created the right climate for the proliferation of eating disorders in Western society.

Theoretic Foundations

Although many clinical studies have been published, the literature on eating disorders shows no theoretic consensus on etiology and treatment. Psychoanalytic theory, cultural theory, family systems theory, behavioral theory, feminist theory, and physiologic theory all contribute to an understanding of the development and dynamics of eating disorders.

Psychoanalytic Theory

Since Freud first identified it as such, food ingestion has been regarded as a critical aspect in the psychologic growth and development of infants, children, and adults. It is widely recognized that the infant at the breast already is beginning to internalize certain primitive knowledge about life through the quality of the feeding experience.

Psychoanalytic theory considers eating disorders symptoms of unconscious conflicts that the individual resolves by gaining insight into the nature and meaning of the conflicts. Little attention is given to the biologic or cultural domains. Aspects of psychoanalytic theory related to eating disorders include the concept of regression to prepubertal phases of development and repudiation of developing sexuality. In psychoanalytic thinking, compulsive overeating represents overcompensation for unmet oral needs during infancy; obesity is also thought to represent a defense against intimacy with the opposite sex.

The basic treatment modality in the psychoanalytic model is long-term individual psychotherapy, sometimes accompanied by group therapy. The goal of both therapies is the development of insight and subsequent "working through" of underlying issues to resolve the unconscious conflicts manifested in the eating disorder.

Cultural Theory

Culture profoundly affects food choices, attitudes toward food, food rituals, preferences, and taboos. Eating behaviors are learned in the family and reflect the ethnic background of the family group. Culture also affects perceptions of beauty, which include cultural norms regarding body size and shape.

The cultural approach to eating disorders assumes that Western society's current emphasis on thinness plays a pivotal role in the development of eating disorders. People in Western cultures are preoccupied with the importance of creating a body that "fits" contemporary norms of size and shape exemplified by fashion models, dancers, and Hollywood stars. Gourmet cooking, "designer foods," and the sensual pleasures of preparing and consuming foods are emphasized simultaneously, creating confusion and conflict. Bruch (1978) reports that the cultural emphasis on sexual freedom is also a problem, particularly to the female adolescent most likely to be affected by eating disorders.

Family Systems Theory

Hilde Bruch (1978) was a pioneer in the application of family systems theory in her work with individuals with anorexia nervosa. Others have incorporated systems theory into work with other eating disorders as well. According to Bruch, the eating disorder itself expresses unconscious intrapersonal and interpersonal conflicts of the client and the family. The symptom stabilizes the family by allowing them to focus on the client, thus ignoring their own unresolved conflicts.

Bruch described the anorectic family as consisting of parents with overly rigid expectations of an overly compliant child. The child's conflict is between enslavement to parental expectations and the drive for independence and autonomy. Anorectic adolescents sometimes see controlling their own body size as the only way to assert control in their lives.

Treatment in the family systems model focuses on defining the family conflicts for which the eating disorder compensates. Through both individual and family therapy, indirectly expressed conflicts are resolved. Healthier and more direct means of expressing family conflicts are learned. An interesting aspect of Bruch's therapeutic orientation is her insistence on the client's "physiological restoration." She refuses to work with families until the psychologic effects of starvation have been ameliorated through weight gain.

The family systems approach to compulsive overeating includes a working theory that ambivalence of a parent or parents toward a child sets the stage for the child's obesity. Conflict between parents and subsequent scapegoating of a child also are seen as contributing factors.

Behavioral Theory

The behavioral model views eating disorders as learned behaviors. It focuses on changing cognitive and behavioral responses to physiologic, psychologic, and social stimuli. Insight into the nature of the maladaptive behavior, i.e., the eating disorder, is integrated with new and healthier responses to emotional stimuli. Because food cannot be entirely avoided, education about the psychology of compulsive behavior and the physiologic effects of starvation and purging behaviors is usually incorporated into the therapeutic process. Cognitive approaches include correction of perceptual disturbances and elimination of irrational thoughts and beliefs such as, "Eating any food is too much," "Eating makes me feel better when I'm anxious or insecure," and "I have always been fat and I will always be fat."

Both individual and group therapy are useful in the behavioral treatment of eating disorders. Group support over the long term is helpful in reinforcing and solidifying new behaviors as they are adopted.

Feminist Theory

In her feminist model of the etiology and treatment of eating disorders, Orbach (1978) emphasizes female issues and resulting conflicts that contribute to abnormal eating patterns. The issues include those surrounding nurturance, sexuality, individuality and boundaries, and societal limitations on the power of women. Orbach asserts that women select abnormal eating patterns as a means of coping with these conflicts when healthier and more direct means of coping are not available. Overeating is thought to reflect a need to fill oneself "up and out" to attain the stereotypic, all-giving, nurturing role that women have been encouraged to assume. Anorexia, by contrast, can be interpreted as a rejection of that stereotype.

For Orbach, the goals of therapy include differentiating between the desire to eat and the physiologic need for food, understanding the meaning of food and eating to the individual, and developing an understanding of the meaning of "being fat" and "being thin." Psychologic, cognitive, and cultural insights are goals of therapy, which may combine individual sessions with either therapy or self-help groups, or both.

Physiologic Theory

The biologic forces that shape the behavior of individuals with eating disorders have received relatively little attention. Because the neurochemical control of eating is the result of complex interactions between neurotransmitters and the brain (see Chapter 6 for a discussion of neurotransmitters), it has been much simpler to explain eating disorders as based on cultural, family, and intrapsychic phenomena. These explanations are incomplete without further examination of the biologic factors influencing disordered eating behaviors.

Some research has focused on the hypothalamic sites that control feeding and has led to speculation about the exact nature of physiologic bases of eating disorders. A neurochemical model has been proposed for anorexia nervosa (Morley et al. 1986), but it is clearly not useful for bulimia nervosa. Heredity is thought to be a factor in obesity, but environmental factors may be equally or more important (Wurtman and Wurtman 1987).

We cannot overlook the fact that both extreme weight loss and excessive weight gain can be caused by physical conditions. Certain conditions must be ruled out before an eating disorder diagnosis can be made. Such wasting conditions as advanced cancer, tuberculosis, acquired immune deficiency syndrome (AIDS), hyperthyroidism, pyloric obstruction, and drug abuse must be considered when weight loss is a feature. Rapid weight gain can result from brain tumor or endocrine disorders. A good history and physical examination usually provide enough information to eliminate the possibility of a physical basis for sudden weight loss or gain.

Currently there is renewed research interest in possible physiologic bases of eating disorders. Further investigation will undoubtedly reveal new knowledge about the biology of these disorders. For now, an understanding of the relationship of physical-biologic processes to eating disorders is just emerging.

Biopsychosocial Factors

Biologic factors, sociocultural pressures to over- or undereat, and intrapsychic or interpersonal fears and conflicts cannot—and should not—be dealt with separately. The interaction of these factors creates a cyclical pattern. For example, clients suffering from severe obesity may experience shame and helplessness as they attempt to cope with fears of rejection and loss of love. These feelings can lead to compensatory overeating behaviors, which in turn may create interpersonal conflict with family members. The client may withdraw from others, thus reinforcing the feelings of rejection and increasing social disability. Only by understanding the interrelated factors leading to eating disorders can psychiatric nurses take a holistic approach to the care of affected individuals and their families.

Why do some individuals develop eating disorders while others do not? Despite research efforts, no satisfactory answer has been found.

Biologic Factors

Caloric Intake/Metabolic Requirements Even in today's calorie-conscious society, the quality of care a mother gives to her infant is measured, at least in part, by the infant's "healthy" appearance. A chubby baby is seen as a healthy baby who outwardly embodies the nurturing and love of the mother. Some mothers encourage food intake exceeding the infant's metabolic requirements. The resulting fat cells, once in existence, remain throughout life.

During childhood, activity level is high. Children learn to consume an abundance of food, often snack foods rich in refined carbohydrates and fat, on a daily basis. They are also encouraged to eat larger portions at meals as they grow.

Over time, obesity results from the imbalance between caloric intake and energy expenditure. During adolescence, both boys and girls experience growth spurts that require additional energy. Because boys continue to increase in muscle mass well beyond puberty, they need additional calories. By the age of 16, girls' energy requirements have fallen off considerably. If they continue to eat as they did during childhood and early adolescence, they are bound to gain weight at a time when they are most concerned about their appearance and attractiveness to the opposite sex.

Neurochemical Abnormalities/Genetic Factors Anorectic and bulimic clients have various neurochemical abnormalities. Whether these changes are a result of the starvation state or a cause of it has not been determined, but nearly all the abnormalities disappear with weight restoration (Herzog 1988).

Studies of bulimia suggest possible central neurochemical abnormalities of the serotonergic and noradrenergic systems. Serotonin studies in animals have linked *satiation,* the sensation of being full after a meal, to serotonin levels. Bulimics appear to have low levels of serotonin, which may predispose them to bingeing behavior. Studies of twins support the hypothesis that genetic factors predispose to eating disorders, even when environmental factors are different (Holland et al. 1984).

Psychologic Factors

Some studies have suggested that people with eating disorders are more neurotic and obsessive than normal eaters. The idea that people eat to compensate for the emptiness of their lives has been hypothesized as a causative factor in obesity. Anorectics are thought to fear sexual maturity; the anorexia is seen as a rejection of the feminine form and a desperate attempt to regain the contours and dimensions of a prepubertal child. Study results are so mixed, however, that clear-cut personality traits predisposing to these disorders are difficult to validate.

Although personality traits are difficult to identify, it is possible to identify common feelings and experiences. Between 25 percent and 50 percent of people with eating disorders are thought to have major depressive disturbances. Controversy surrounds the chicken-or-egg relationship between depression and eating disorders. Research continues into the relationship between mood and eating behaviors.

It is commonly recognized that people with eating disorders almost universally have distorted attitudes about food, eating, and the size of their bodies. Early developmental failure is common, as is family dysfunction. Anorectics in particular are excessively concerned about achieving perfection and avoiding self-indulgence. They equate weight gain with being "bad" or "out of control."

Common feelings reported by anorectic, bulimic, and obese individuals include a sense of ineffectiveness and preoccupation with food and eating. Most have interioceptive disturbances, such as not feeling satiated even after a large meal.

Sociocultural Factors

The incidence of anorexia nervosa in the United States has doubled over the past 25 years. Reports on the frequency of bulimia nervosa vary. Between 4 percent and 10 percent of the female high school and college students in one study were bulimic. A survey of medical students revealed that 12 percent of the female students reported lifelong history of bulimia (Herzog 1988). Estimates of obesity range as high as 80 million North Americans, depending on criteria used (Stunkard 1980).

In the past, most anorectics were from middle-class or upper-middle-class families. Recent studies show greater representation of all classes. Obesity, by contrast, is clearly related to social class, with a higher incidence among socioeconomically disadvantaged groups than others.

Women are at greater risk than men for developing eating disorders, partly because of the cultural bias that bigness is OK for men and not for women. In television and magazine ads, women portrayed as successful, attractive, healthy, and popular are invariably slim. Becoming slim is a major pursuit in this country. The diet and exercise industry, earning $5 billion per year, is based on the desire to achieve that cultural norm. Some populations at higher risk for the development of weight-loss eating disorders are dancers, long-distance runners, flight attendants, high school and college wrestlers, and fashion models. Housewives, mothers of young children, professional cooks, and people who prepare family meals are at high risk for obesity.

A 1980 study of *Playboy* magazine centerfolds and Miss America contestants from 1960 to 1980 revealed that the bust and hip measurements of these idealized women showed a steady downward trend, as did their weights (Garner et al. 1982). Their waists became larger and their body shapes more tubular, a departure from the traditional "hourglass" shape. While the rest of the population was growing heavier, women who wished to be perceived as desirable were receiving strong messages to be thinner than ever. Society has thus created the potential for tremendous secondary gains for anorectic behaviors.

Coexisting with the emphasis on thinness is a renewed interest in preparing and consuming food. Gourmet food stores and kitchen supply firms have burgeoned in response to the emphasis on cooking and entertaining at home. In women's magazines, photographs of beautifully prepared foods are shown side by side with the latest diet information and tips on effortless weight loss. Women thus receive the conflicting messages "Food is love," "Eat what you are given," and "Stay slim so that you will be attractive to men." It is hardly surprising that these conflicting messages confuse the young who, because they are just beginning to develop their own sexual identities, are at high risk for the development of eating disorders.

The Nursing Process and Anorexia Nervosa

Assessing

The nurse assessing clients with anorexia nervosa must take into consideration the multiple biopsychosocial factors involved in this complex disorder. Although anorexia nervosa and bulimia nervosa are discussed separately in this chapter, the two disorders often coexist. Indications for hospitalization include deteriorating physical condition, increasing parental discord leading to either scapegoating of the client or unhealthy coalition between client and one parent, or a request by the client for hospitalization. In-patient treatment within the therapeutic milieu in conjunction with behavior therapy generally yields positive results. See the accompanying box for DSM-III-R criteria.

DSM-III-R Diagnostic Criteria for Two Eating Disorders

Anorexia Nervosa

A. Refusal to maintain body weight over a minimal normal weight for age and height, e.g., weight loss leading to maintenance of body weight 15 percent below that expected; or failure to make expected weight gain during period of growth, leading to body weight 15 percent below that expected.

B. Intense fear of gaining weight or becoming fat, even though underweight.

C. Disturbance in the way in which one's body weight, size, or shape is experienced, e.g., the person claims to "feel fat" even when emaciated, believes that one area of the body is "too fat" even when obviously underweight.

D. In females, absence of at least three consecutive menstrual cycles when otherwise expected to occur (primary or secondary amenorrhea).

Bulimia Nervosa

A. Recurrent episodes of binge eating (rapid consumption of a large amount of food in a discrete period of time).

B. A feeling of lack of control over eating behavior during the eating binges.

C. The person regularly engages in either self-induced vomiting, use of laxatives or diuretics, strict dieting or fasting, or vigorous exercise in order to prevent weight gain.

D. A minimum average of two binge eating episodes a week for at least three months.

E. Persistent overconcern with body shape and weight.

SOURCE: *American Psychiatric Association:* Diagnostic and Statistical Manual of Mental Disorders, *ed 3, revised. APA, 1987, pp 67–69.*

Subjective Data Clients with anorexia nervosa perceive themselves as overweight, no matter how thin they may be. However emaciated their bodies, they can always find some body part they believe is fat.

They are preoccupied with thoughts of food and simultaneously obsessed with rigidly controlling their own intake. They often collect cookbooks, cook prodigious amounts of food, and insist others eat while not taking a morsel for themselves. They are fearful of even the slightest weight gain and view with suspicion anyone who encourages them to eat.

Another preoccupation is with exercise; it is not uncommon for anorectics to engage in extremely lengthy sessions of calisthenics, or to run, bike, or walk to excess, even when in an emaciated condition. They push themselves to greater and greater levels of endurance and deprive themselves of sleep as a measure of self-control.

Anorectics frequently deny that they have a weight problem. They insist that they have never felt better and simply wish to be left alone about food. They report feeling strong, powerful, and good as a result of self-denial. They therefore resist treatment, although they may admit to feeling isolated and lonely and may even describe themselves as exhausted with the effort it takes to achieve the perfection they seek. They tend to have difficulty accepting nurturing behavior from others and therefore have difficulty forming therapeutic alliances (Deering 1987). They report a loss of interest in sex but do not perceive this as a problem.

Objective Data Anorectic clients are most often well-educated teenage females from middle- and upper-middle-class families (Herzog 1988). There is evidence of extreme and/or rapid weight loss of at least 15 percent of original body weight. In women, amenorrhea is a cardinal sign. The client has extensive knowledge of the nutritional and caloric value of foods.

The anorectic client appears emaciated, with a sunken-eyed, skeletonlike look. In very young clients, growth failure may be present. Lanugo growth (babylike, fine hair) on the face, extremities, and trunk may occur. Other physical symptoms include bradycardia, hypotension, arrhythmias, delayed gastric motility, and a hypothyroidlike state manifested by dry skin, listlessness, and dry, falling hair. Peripheral edema may be a feature in advanced starvation.

Laboratory tests may reveal leukopenia, mild anemia, low serum potassium, and elevated blood urea nitrogen (BUN). High serum calcium levels indicate osteoporosis is occurring, and renal calculi may result.

Diagnosing

The major NANDA diagnoses for clients with eating disorders are given in the Nursing Diagnosis box on page 476. The following sections discuss the implications of several priority nursing diagnoses for the anorectic client and the nurse.

Altered Nutrition: Less Than Body Requirements By the time anorectic clients are hospitalized, their physical condition is often so deteriorated due to self-imposed starvation that it becomes the priority for nursing care. Life-threatening malnourish-

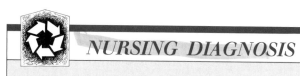

NURSING DIAGNOSIS

Common NANDA Diagnoses for Clients with Eating Disorders

Activity intolerance

Anxiety

Body image disturbance

Body temperature, Altered: High Risk

Constipation

Coping, Ineffective family: Compromised

Coping, Ineffective individual

Diarrhea

Diversional activity deficit

Family processes, Altered

Fatigue

Fear

Fluid volume deficit: High risk

Growth and development, Altered

Hopelessness

Infection: High risk

Knowledge deficit

Nutrition, Altered: Less than body requirements

Nutrition, Altered: More than body requirements

Oral mucous membrane, Altered

Role performance, Altered

Self-care deficit: Feeding

Self-esteem disturbance

Self-esteem, Low: Chronic

Sexuality patterns, Altered

Skin integrity, Impaired

Sleep pattern disturbance

Social interaction, Impaired

Social isolation

Tissue perfusion, Altered: Peripheral

Violence, High risk: Self-directed

food for others, is due to suppression and sublimation of the client's own hunger. Overexercising creates even more extreme nutritional deficits. In those anorectic clients who also purge by vomiting or using laxatives, nutritional status is further endangered.

Clients in a state of starvation experience hormonal, metabolic, and emotional changes. Some of those changes are manifested in amenorrhea or delay of onset of menses, ketosis, severe vitamin deficiencies, depressed immune response, lethargy, weakness, and irritability (Miner 1988), conditions that vitally affect nurse-client relationships.

Ineffective Individual Coping Clients experiencing anorexia nervosa demonstrate impairment of adaptive behaviors, such as self-care in activities of daily living (ADL). They have difficulty meeting daily demands, and role performance may be affected. Their preoccupation with the pursuit of thinness deprives them of the energy necessary for adaptive behavior and distracts them from interest in role fulfillment. The quest for thinness is the entire focus of these clients' lives.

In addition, developmental issues such as the desire for independence and the longing for dependence combine with traditionally adolescent resentment of authority to influence the quality and character of the nurse-client relationship. Family overprotectiveness and unwillingness to allow the client to separate contribute to self-doubt and inability to accept responsibility for self.

Body Image Disturbance Clients with anorexia nervosa are unable to make realistic appraisals of their own body size, although they can accurately evaluate the size of others. They drastically underestimate their own bodily needs, even in the face of overwhelming evidence of malnutrition. Profound disturbances in accurate perception of size and intense client denial indicate a poor prognosis. The client's body image disturbance is often the source of conflict in family and therapeutic relationships.

Self-Esteem Disturbance Anorectic clients' lack of confidence in themselves and feelings of inferiority are main factors in the disorder. Their self-deprivation and self-denial make them feel powerful and superior to others who cannot muster such profound self-control. The quest for perfection is never-ending, but they can never achieve a level of thinness that is satisfying; there are always a few more pounds to shed. They often present the picture of "model clients," in contrast to seemingly more disturbed clients in the in-patient setting. As a result, novice nurses may have difficulty assessing the severity of their illnesses accurately.

ment is seen in 5 percent to 20 percent of these clients. Death may occur from malnutrition, infection, or cardiac abnormalities related to electrolyte imbalances. Intravenous therapy, tube feedings, and hyperalimentation are required in cases of medical emergency.

The client's preoccupation with food, evidenced by reading recipes, discussing food, and preparing

The low self-esteem of anorectic clients stems from unrealistic expectations by self and others, complicated by unmet dependency needs. The clinical picture is further complicated because cultural norms of thinness reinforce maladaptive behavior. The nurse-client relationship is affected by the extreme difficulty these clients have in accepting positive feedback and by their nonparticipation in self-care and therapeutic activities. Their preoccupation with their appearance and with others' perceptions of them may be irritating to other clients. The nurse-client relationship is also affected by these clients' needs to control, which often lead to manipulative behaviors. (See the accompanying Nursing Self-Awareness box for possible reactions of nurses working with clients with eating disorders.) Self-aware nurses recognize their own emotional reactions to clients and view clients' self-absorption and manipulativeness as symptoms of the disorder.

Planning and Implementing Interventions

When a client's behavior meets the criteria for a diagnosis of anorexia nervosa, effective nursing intervention is directed toward ensuring that the client will not die and helping the client learn more effective ways of coping with the demands of life. A variety of approaches, including behavioral, insight-oriented, and cognitive therapies may be useful; pharmacologic therapy may be used as an adjunctive measure. Nurses must recognize that many, if not most, anorectic clients are extremely resistant to change. Progress may be slow, and recovery may be defined as lessening of symptoms.

Promoting Improved Nutrition To establish adequate eating patterns and fluid and electrolyte balance, assume a calm, matter-of-fact attitude and positive expectation of the client. Meeting minimal nutritional goals is non-negotiable.

Nursing interventions may include tube feedings or intravenous therapy, which are administered in a nonjudgmental manner. Weighing the client daily, recording intake and output, observing the client during meals, and observing bathroom behavior may be necessary if the nurse suspects the client is discarding food or inducing vomiting. Avoid discussing food, recipes, restaurants, and eating with the client because these conversations reinforce maladaptive behaviors. Providing a pleasant mealtime environment and adopting realistic expectations of how much the client will eat are critically important aspects of nursing care. Clients find frequent, small meals more acceptable than three large meals. Setting a time limit of about one-half hour is a good way to forestall mealtime "marathons"—protracted meals during which the client eats little.

The nurse collaborates with the hospital dietitian to determine appropriate weight gain expectations. Acknowledge and recognize the efforts of clients who

---

NURSING SELF-AWARENESS

Nurses' Potential Reactions to Working with Clients with Eating Disorders

- The nurse feels exhausted and defeated by the structured demands of the client's care plan.
- The nurse feels resentment at client's attempts to manipulate and attempts at "staff splitting."
- The nurse identifies with the client due to personal body image concerns.
- The nurse feels overprotective of the client and allows a coalition between self and client to form.
- The nurse feels annoyance and anger toward the client and is unnecessarily rough during physical care.

- The nurse has difficulty recognizing that the client's symptoms are as serious as those of the hallucinating or delusional client.
- The nurse fails to monitor the client's mealtime and after-meal behaviors, allowing the client to continue maladaptive patterns of coping.
- The nurse allows the client to reenact power struggles from home, e.g., about food, weight, and exercising.
- The nurse believes that the client is deliberately engaging in maladaptive coping behaviors to upset the staff and family.
- The nurse feels repelled by the client's eating habits or the appearance of the client's body.
- The nurse feels hopeless and is affected by the client's despondency.

meet weight gain goals but avoid praise or flattery. Education about adequate eating patterns is a necessary part of discharge planning.

Consistency and coordination among hospital personnel are essential to avoid manipulation by clients. Interdisciplinary planning conferences and adherence to written care plans promote effective care. Behavior-modification programs, which base privileges on weight gain, may be useful if nurses focus on emotional issues and not just on eating behaviors. The nurse and client may engage in a contract for weight gain, such as the one in Figure 20–1. Usually a target weight is chosen by the treatment team.

Discharge planning can include referral to self-help groups such the American Anorexia/Bulimia Association, Anorexia Nervosa and Related Eating Disorders, and Anorexia Nervosa and Associated Disorders.

Promoting Effective Individual Coping

The best way to promote individual coping is by involving clients in their own treatment planning while they are hospitalized. Self-determination fosters adaptive coping mechanisms in clients' day-to-day hospital experiences; this process carries over to daily life outside the hospital setting and helps clients meet its demands.

Although trust is difficult to establish with anorectic clients, it is the basis for all therapeutic relationships. Being honest, available, and matter-of-fact helps establish trust and encourages clients to express their feelings. If they must, allow clients to assume a dependent patient role at first, but as trust is developed and physical condition improves, encourage clients to take more responsibility for themselves. Participating in the planning of care gives clients opportunities to practice making decisions. Letting clients have input into their treatment plans also fosters compliance. Provide flexibility in activities of daily living, type and timing of exercise, and choice of occupational and recreational therapy activities. This autonomy increases clients' sense of responsibility for themselves.

Giving clients the opportunity to practice problem solving can lead to power struggles if the nurse disagrees with clients' choices. Demonstrate positive belief in clients' abilities to regain healthy functioning and a willingness to tolerate "mistakes." The team must set firm and clear limits, however, to provide the secure environment clients need to learn more effective coping behaviors. Also help clients identify ways to feel in control by other than anorectic and manipulative behaviors.

Clients need to explore their extreme fears of gaining weight before they can relinquish maladaptive behaviors. It is helpful to explore clients' feelings about their families, their roles in the families, and their autonomy within the family system. This process

often helps to heal the hurt inner child. Bradshaw (1990) believes that a child whose development is arrested by having to repress feelings, especially feelings of anger and hurt, grows to be an adult with an angry, hurt child inside. Psychotherapeutic strategies directed toward healing the hurt inner child can help clients with various types of eating disorders to begin to understand their unmet needs, a necessary step in the path toward recovery (Kneisl 1991). Because this type of therapeutic work is insight-oriented, the nurse needs exceptional clinical skill and advanced preparation.

Promoting Improved Perception of Body Image

To help clients regain an accurate perception of their body size and nutritional needs, first encourage clients to express feelings about body size. Reframe clients' misperceptions by using language that emphasizes health, strength, and evaluation. For example, if the client says "My thighs are huge," reply "Your thighs are becoming stronger now that you're gaining weight. Healthy muscles are rounded and firm, like yours." With practice, clients can replace negative thinking with positive self-talk. Teach and reinforce this skill, and help the client practice it. For example, ask clients to make three positive statements (positive affirmations) about their bodies each day.

For clients who are unable or unwilling to discuss their feelings about body size, Miller (1991) recommends asking them to draw themselves as they are now and as they desire to be. These drawings not only focus the discussion of body size and nutritional needs but also help the nurse understand how clients view their bodies. Because clients with bulimia nervosa and compulsive overeating also have distorted body images, this activity can be incorporated into their plans of care as well.

When clients share feelings honestly, show improvement in accurate perception of body image, or demonstrate healthier eating behaviors, reinforce their efforts through verbal recognition. It is also useful to examine with clients the ways in which the fashion and advertising industries support unrealistic cultural norms of excessive thinness that are incompatible with healthy functioning.

Promoting Improved Self-Esteem

Help clients reexamine negative feelings about themselves and identify their positive attributes. Encourage clients to record in a diary thoughts that are difficult to share directly. Essential elements are nonjudgmental acceptance of negative feelings and positive reinforcement of honest expression of all feelings. Encouragement is particularly important when clients experiment with independently made decisions, even when outcomes are not entirely positive. The client needs to interpret

Client's Name: _____ Weight: _____

Date of Birth: _____ Age: _____ Height: _____

Goal Weight Range: _____

You will be weighed daily in the morning after voiding, wearing only a johnny coat and no jewelry. Nothing is to be consumed prior to being weighed.

No exercising, jogging, etc. is to be done.

Ensure or Ensure Plus is given as a medication. It must be taken within 15 minutes while sitting at the nurses' station. No conversation, reading, knitting, other activity while drinking Ensure.

Must drink _____ cans of Ensure per day if weight gain is 1/4 pound or more over your last highest weight.
Ensure will be dispensed at: _____   _____   _____   _____   _____   _____

Must drink _____ cans of Ensure per day if weight gain is less than 1/4 pound over your last highest weight.
Ensure will be dispensed at: _____   _____   _____   _____   _____   _____

Weights to be attained for status change/privileges:

    Independent Status: _____ pounds
    Monitor Status: _____ pounds for _____ consecutive days
    Buddy Status: _____ pounds
    Passes: _____ pounds for _____ consecutive days

Ensure can be made optional, at the discretion of your primary clinician, once you reach Buddy Status weight.

To use Buddy Status or take passes, a weight gain of 1/4 pound above your last highest weight must be attained on that day.

Participation in dance therapy and walks: at Monitor Status weight and/or with staff permission.

Participation in gym: at Buddy Status weight and/or with staff permission.

Additional comments/issues:

Signature of Client _____
Signature of Primary Clinician _____

Date: _____

FIGURE 20–1   Client contract for weight gain   SOURCE: Courtesy Patricia Worthy, Head Nurse, and the nursing staff of the Adolescent and Young Adult Treatment Unit, Yale-New Haven Hospital, New Haven, Connecticut

each experience as worthwhile. Stress the feeling of control gained through independent decision making.

Together, client and nurse explore the client's attempt to achieve perfection by controlling weight. The idea is for the client to realize that perfection is an unrealistic goal. The nurse is a role model of the person who accepts imperfection yet retains self-esteem. One way to model strong self-esteem is to admit errors willingly. Also model appropriate expressions of anger and teach clients the destructive effects of unexpressed anger.

Evaluating/Outcome Criteria

Identifying the desired outcomes of nursing interventions is an essential part of the nursing process that rarely receives the attention it deserves. The following sections give sample outcome criteria for nursing interventions with clients with anorexia nervosa.

Nutrition Clients will regain and maintain at least 90 percent of normal weight for height and age. Clients will follow eating patterns that demonstrate they recognize the importance of adequate nutrition. They will regain and maintain normal elimination patterns, vital signs, fluid and electrolyte balance, and muscle tone. Female clients will have normal menstrual cycles.

Individual Coping Clients will participate actively in treatment planning and discharge planning using problem-solving skills. They will demonstrate interest and competence in self-care activities such as hygiene, sleep, activity, rest, diversional activities, and nutrition. They will accurately identify both maladaptive coping behaviors and adaptive coping behaviors that can be integrated into daily routines. Clients will express less anxiety about weight gain and will verbalize other means of feeling in control of their lives.

Body Image Clients will accurately assess their own body size and nutritional needs. They will use criteria such as strength and health, rather than appearance alone, to evaluate body size. They will verbalize less preoccupation with body size. They will easily verbalize positive statements about their own bodies.

Self-Esteem Clients will verbalize their own positive attributes. They will demonstrate less preoccupation with their own appearance and will focus increasingly on others. They will accept compliments and positive feedback and show greater interest in activities around them. They will verbalize that perfection is an unrealistic life goal. Clients will express anger appropriately without experiencing incapacitating guilt. They will demonstrate interpersonal relationships substantially free of manipulation.

The Nursing Process and Bulimia Nervosa

Assessing

Although they are described separately, the boundary between anorexia and bulimia is blurred. Many bulimics were formerly anorectic, while others may become anorectic in the future. As many as half of all anorectics are estimated to binge and purge at some time during their illnesses. During the assessment phase of the nursing process, nurses must keep in mind that these two conditions, although distinctly different, often coexist. See the box on page 475 for DSM-III-R criteria.

Subjective Data Clients with bulimia nervosa have feelings of low self-esteem, worthlessness, inadequacy, and guilt. They experience shame and embarrassment over their secret binges (eating several quarts of ice cream, buckets of popcorn, or eight or more candy bars is not unusual) and subsequent purging activities. This shame may be manifested in self-deprecating remarks. Clients report feeling out of control, but at the same time they feel an excessive need to control. Unlike anorectics, clients with bulimia nervosa recognize that their eating behaviors are abnormal and bizarre.

Anxiety and unsatisfactory interpersonal relationships are a feature of this disorder. Anxiety is intensified when others see the bulimic as successful and in control, and they often appear so to others. They are impulsive and cannot delay gratification. Preoccupation with food, weight, and diets is a prominent feature. Bulimic clients may report feeling weak and lethargic.

Objective Data Like anorectic clients, bulimic clients tend to be young females. Bulimia first manifests itself later than anorexia, typically during late adolescence or young adulthood. Clients are likely to be white, middle-class females with a history of weight-control problems. They are usually of normal or slightly above average weight. Appearance does not provide diagnostic clues, hence the term *normal-weight bulimics*. Weight tends to fluctuate but does not get dangerously low unless anorexia occurs concurrently (Herzog 1988).

Clients with bulimia nervosa are more outgoing than anorectics and they tend to be more comfortable with sexual relationships. They sometimes manifest impulsive behaviors such as substance abuse, shoplifting, and self-inflicted injury (Herzog 1988). On the unit, they may steal others' food and hoard food in their rooms.

Physical signs of bulimia nervosa include hoarseness and esophagitis, dental enamel erosion, enlarged parotid glands, abrasions or calluses on knuckles from inducing vomiting, and amenorrhea in about 40 percent of cases (Herzog 1988). The client may also have symptoms of fluid volume deficit: concentrated urine, decreased urine output, hypotension, elevated temperature, poor skin turgor, and weakness.

Laboratory tests may reveal electrolyte abnormalities, particularly low serum potassium. Potentially fatal cardiac arrythmias may result. Overuse of syrup of ipecac, an emetic agent, can create cumulative systemic toxicity affecting the gastrointestinal, neuromuscular, and cardiovascular systems, potentially leading to death from cardiotoxicity (Parks and Fischer 1987).

Diagnosing

The major NANDA diagnoses for clients with eating disorders are listed in the Nursing Diagnosis box on page 476. The following sections discuss the implications of several diagnoses pertinent to the bulimic client and the nurse.

Anxiety Clients with bulimia nervosa experience anxiety—vague, uneasy feelings of moderate to intense severity and unknown cause. (The symptoms of anxiety are discussed in Chapter 5.) A rise in the client's anxiety level is usually a forerunner of binge/purge behaviors and may lead to hoarding food in preparation for a binge.

Fluid Volume Deficit Depletion of body fluids in clients with bulimia nervosa is usually due to self-induced vomiting and excessive use of laxatives and diuretics, combined with decreased fluid intake. Extreme dehydration may lead to changes in mental status such as lethargy and confusion.

Ineffective Individual Coping Binge and purge behaviors are ineffective ways to cope with the stresses of life. Other impulse control problems, such as alcohol abuse, drug abuse, and shoplifting, are equally ineffective ways to reduce stress. The bulimia nervosa client is often dealing with adolescent issues such as independence/dependence, identity, and self-determination. Ineffective coping is manifested in the bulimic client's preoccupation with body size, poor self-esteem, distorted body image, and excessive overeating followed by purging.

Ineffective Family Coping The families of clients with bulimia nervosa perceive themselves as unable to deal effectively with the client's eating disorder. They, too, may have distorted perceptions of the problem. Parents may have difficulty allowing the client to grow up and may be overprotective; at the same time, they may have overly high expectations of the client. The

bulimic client's behavior may become the family's focus, preventing the fulfillment of essential family roles. If disruption is extreme, the family may not be able to interact effectively with the larger community. Usual problem-solving methods are only partially adequate to deal with the stress of having a bulimic family member.

Planning and Implementing Interventions

In addition to the interventions discussed below, tricyclic antidepressants have been found to be effective in the medical treatment of bulimia nervosa (Pope and Hudson 1989).

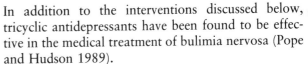

Promoting Effective Coping with Anxiety The goal of nursing interventions with anxious bulimic clients is to help them recognize events that create anxiety and to avoid binging and purging in response to anxiety. Initially, being available to the anxious client is useful. Project a calm, reassuring attitude and provide a quiet, nonstimulating environment. After trust is established, help the client identify anxiety-producing situations. Clients experience anxiety as occurring "out of the blue" and are often unaware that it is related to emotional issues and situations. Help clients identify previously used coping behaviors to determine if they might be useful in current situations. How did the client handle anxiety before starting to binge and purge? Help bulimic clients identify feelings that precede binging and purging episodes and explore healthier ways of dealing with those feelings.

Teach clients to recognize anxiety early, before it is severe, and to manage increasing anxiety. Energy-consuming activities, such as walking, running, and exercising, are useful but must be used very judiciously if the client's prehospital behaviors included overexercising. Clients can benefit from being taught progressive relaxation techniques and meditation. Administer antianxiety medications as ordered, but use caution because of the tendency to habituation.

Client contracts are useful with bulimic clients. The contract is jointly developed by the client and the nurse and renegotiated at periodic intervals, depending on the client's goals, severity of symptoms, and compliance with the contract. Such a contract might include agreements about binging, vomiting, or hoarding food, such as these:

> I will sit at the nurses' station for one half hour following my meals.
>
> I will not vomit after my meals.
>
> I will not hoard food.
>
> I will not take laxatives or diuretics.

I will not bring any such substances onto the unit.

I will tell the nursing staff if I feel like binging.

I will stay away from the kitchen if I feel like binging.

Client _____

Nurse _____

Date _____

Using a contract encourages clients to assume responsibility for themselves.

Promoting Improved Fluid Volume The importance of accurate intake and output records cannot be overstated. Daily consumption of 2000 to 3000 mL of liquid promotes rehydration. Accurate daily weights are needed. Always weigh the client at the same time of day (immediately upon arising is preferred) and on the same scale. Assess and document the condition of the skin and oral mucous membranes daily, and monitor laboratory values, reporting significant alterations to the physician. Observe clients for at least one hour after meals to prevent purging. To promote comfort in the dehydrated client, give frequent mouth care.

Promoting Effective Individual Coping Clients with bulimia nervosa can learn adaptive coping mechanisms to replace the out-of-control, binge-purge cycle. During hospitalization, once trust is developed, help the client plan and practice strategies for dealing effectively with intense feelings and the demands of daily living. It is important for clients to identify situations and patterns of events that precede episodes of binging and purging. Clients learn to identify, name, and express feelings that they formerly perceived only as "bad." Once this is accomplished, client and nurse explore alternative ways to express those feelings.

Help clients identify times when they are at risk for binging and lack impulse control, for instance, times when they are bored, frustrated, angry, lonely, or feeling unloved. Teach clients ways to nurture themselves during these times other than binging and purging. Suggest taking a warm bath, calling or visiting an old friend, or a hobby not involving food.

Clients with bulimia nervosa often perceive feelings of guilt and underlying resentment as overwhelming. They need to learn effective ways of expressing these feelings and assertive techniques (see Chapter 2) to diminish guilty interactions in the future. Role playing with the nurse is a good way to practice assertiveness.

Involve the client in discharge planning. Topics covered in discharge planning include the productive use of time, identification of diversional activities not related to food, and participation in support groups.

Promoting Effective Family Coping Certain family dynamics reinforce maladaptive eating behaviors; therefore, families must also develop effective coping mechanisms to support the client's healthier coping behaviors. Assess the family's feelings and perceptions of the client's bulimia, listening carefully for what is most stressful and threatening to family members. Correct misperceptions about the disorder. Encourage family members to explore together their usual coping strategies and determine if any previously used strategies can be useful in the present situation.

Help the family identify their strengths and weaknesses. Encourage family members to share their thoughts and feelings, including feelings of guilt, blame, and resentment, with one another and with the client. Teaching families to make "I statements," thereby acknowledging feelings, is useful.

If the client's disorder impairs family functioning, help the family reorganize roles to reduce stress and ensure that members' needs continue to be met during the client's recovery. Help the family understand that two normal developmental needs of adolescents and young adults are to develop autonomy and to establish identities outside the family. Make appropriate referrals to community resources, such as Anorexia Nervosa and Associated Disorders, Inc.

Home visits for an evening or weekend can help both the client and the family learn to use their new coping behaviors. Planning before visits and evaluating the success of visits afterward are essential parts of nurse-client and nurse-family interventions.

Evaluating/Outcome Criteria

Anxiety Clients will verbally identify situations and events that evoke anxiety. They will identify ways of structuring the environment to prevent feeling out of control. Clients will eliminate binge/purge behaviors and demonstrate the use of anxiety-reduction strategies unrelated to eating. They will verbalize acceptance of normal body weight without intense anxiety.

Fluid Volume Dryness of oral mucosa and skin will not be evident. Skin turgor will be normal. Clients' vital signs and results of laboratory studies will be within normal limits. Clients will verbalize understanding of the relationship between dehydration and self-induced vomiting, laxative abuse, and diuretic abuse. Clients will verbalize understanding of the physiologic and psychologic consequences of dehydration.

Individual Coping Clients will accurately assess maladaptive coping behaviors. They will demonstrate healthier ways to deal with stress and intense feelings. They will identify times of risk and verbalize alternative self-nurturing behaviors. They will demonstrate assertive communication techniques. Clients will demonstrate self-control in eating behaviors. They will verbalize increased self-confidence in the ability to handle demands of day-to-day life. They will follow through with recommended self-help or support groups and therapy following discharge.

Family Coping Families will verbalize accurate perceptions of their situation. They will verbalize their feelings about having a family member with an eating disorder. They will identify useful strategies for coping with the impact of bulimia nervosa on the family. They will use "I statements" during communication with one another, the client, and the nurse. They will verbalize an understanding of the developmental needs of adolescents and young adults. The family will reorganize family roles as necessary. They will identify community resources available to them and will follow through on referrals.

The Nursing Process and Compulsive Overeating

Assessing

The assessment of compulsive overeating is not as straightforward as it might seem. Many obese individuals are apparently content and well adjusted. The nurse cannot assume that all obese people are emotionally distressed. The following discussion pertains to those clients who suffer psychologically from their excessive weight and who seek treatment for the resulting psychologic pain.

Subjective Data Being overweight in a culture that equates attractiveness with thinness can cause depression, anxiety, low self-esteem, anger, and isolation. These psychologic stresses in turn create the desire to eat, and a pathologic cycle begins. Most obese individuals report a lifelong inability to maintain normal weight. They tend to use food as a substitute for other forms of gratification, such as companionship, attention from others, and emotional nurturing. They may also eat when happy or to reward themselves.

When obesity has its onset in childhood, the child may have a permanently distorted body image (Stunkard 1980). These individuals view themselves as fat, even following weight loss. The resulting negative feelings impair social functioning and may lead to withdrawal and isolation. Isolation intensifies the obsessive preoccupation with food.

Attitudes toward food and eating are strongly influenced by cultural and ethnic background. These attitudes are firmly established by adulthood and are difficult to change. Family traditions and beliefs about food are influential. Parents' use of food to punish or reward a child or to deal with negative feelings teaches children to do the same. They learn that they need not deal with feelings directly as long as they can eat. Obesity is thought to be related to ambivalence in the parent-child relationship (Orbach 1986). In homes where there is marital conflict, children may become scapegoats, and they may seek protection by becoming obese (Orbach 1986). In some families, children are punished unless they eat everything they are served. This teaches them to disregard satiety messages and contributes to overeating in later life. Because the tendency toward obesity may be genetic, a family history is useful (Wurtman and Wurtman 1987).

Be sure to obtain a medication history. A number of medications, including birth-control pills, some antipsychotics, the cortisones, some antidepressants, and antacids, may contribute to weight gain. Some postmenopausal women attribute increased appetite to hormone replacement therapy.

Objective Data In our culture, obesity is generally defined as body weight exceeding by 20 percent recommended weights on standard height and weight tables. Although obesity is more common among women of all ages, many men are obese. Obesity is most prevalent in individuals between 20 and 50 years of age.

Obese people tend to be inactive, which further widens the gap between calorie intake and expenditure of energy. Obesity-related disorders include hypertension, shortness of breath, and palpitations upon exertion.

Diagnosing

The major NANDA diagnoses for clients with eating disorders are given in the Nursing Diagnosis box on page 476. The following sections discuss the implications of several major diagnoses for obese clients and the nurse.

Knowledge Deficit Clients suffering from obesity, despite their preoccupation with food and eating, often lack sufficient information about nutrition to make healthy decisions about diet. This knowledge deficit may be related to lack of interest, anxiety, denial of the need for information, or other factors.

Evidence of nutritional knowledge deficit includes a history of noncompliance with dietary regimens, statements indicating lack of knowledge, misconceptions about the hospital diet plan, and requests for information.

RESEARCH NOTE

Citation
Allan JD: Knowing what to weigh: Women's self-care activities related to weight. Adv Nurs Sci 1988;11(1):47–60.

Study Problem/Purpose
The purpose of this study was to determine how women interpret and use the health-related information that obesity is detrimental to health. An additional purpose was to learn about women's self-care activities in weight management.

Methods
Thirty-seven working-class and middle-class white women were selected to obtain a broad community-based sample. The sample subjects were between 18 and 55 years of age, white, living in the study geographic area, United States-born, not pregnant, normal to moderately obese, and without major health conditions (except obesity) involving dietary treatment. Data were collected over a seven-month period through the use of a semistructured interview and anthropometric measures of height, weight, and skinfold thickness.

Findings
Most informants reported they had developed their own norms of what to weigh and had identified three levels: ideal, acceptable, and overweight weights. The ideal weights were acknowledged as probably unrealistic and unattainable. The acceptable weight was based on experiences with dieting and appearance, and was felt to be realistic and attainable. The overweight weight served as a signal to action,

because the individual had reached the outer limits of what she felt she should weigh. The poundage range of these three weight classes changed over time with age and childbirth. Normal-weight women had narrower weight ranges than obese women.

Informants used three major means of determining whether or not they were within their own weight norms—appearance, both naked and clothed (51 percent), physical feelings, such as energy level and bodily comfort (46 percent), and weight charts, which none of the informants really agreed with but consulted anyhow (43 percent). Professional contacts were not used in developing weight-management activities. Informants depended instead on television and magazines, weight charts, and peers, or coworkers. Few had discussed weight during medical visits.

Implications
These data suggest that nurses and their clients may be depending on different explanatory models of weight norms, which can interfere with communication, collaboration, and self-care practices. Nurses should ask clients what their weight norms are and how these were developed, as well as their major concerns about weight. Nurses and other health professionals need to reexamine their traditional emphasis on the connection between weight control and health, since most women in this study were motivated more by appearance than health concerns in controlling their weights. Since the sample size was small, caution must be exercised in the generalization of these findings. More studies are needed in this important area of self-care.

Altered Nutrition: More Than Body Requirements The obese client consumes more calories than required while expending few calories in exercise and activity. A sedentary life-style and occupation are common. Unhealthy eating patterns, such as night eating and binging, complicate the picture.

Recognize that the client's negative self-concept reinforces the desire for nurturance, i.e., food, and that all negative feelings may be identified as hunger. These clients often ignore internal cues to hunger and eat in response to external cues, such as the time of day or stressful situations.

Obese clients are vulnerable to a variety of weight-loss fads such as appetite suppressants, fad

diets, and expensive "get-thin-quick" programs at diet centers. The failure of these efforts leads to guilt and a sense of hopelessness about ever losing weight. Depression and loss of faith in self are common in obese clients.

Hopelessness Clients who compulsively overeat frequently feel hopeless about their repeated failure to lose weight or to control their eating behavior. The inability to feel positive about the present life situation is manifested in a despondent and passive approach to living. Any effort seems too extreme; every task is too great. "What's the use?" is a question characteristically posed by the hopeless client.

Hopelessness debilitates because clients cannot mobilize energy on their own behalf; nor do they believe that anyone else can help. Hopelessness is characterized by apathy and lack of involvement in activities that profoundly affect the nurse-client relationship. Clients may lose interest in self-care activities; oversleeping, decreased affect, and decreased response to stimuli are associated features. The speech of hopeless clients is filled with despondency. They may verbalize loss of faith in a higher power or God.

Social Isolation   Obese clients are sometimes rejected by others or choose to withdraw from social interaction because of self-consciousness and fear of rejection. Regardless of the cause, the resulting alienation and loneliness increase depression and preoccupation with food. Obese clients want to participate in social situations, but negative past experiences have conditioned them to expect rejection and possible ridicule.

Planning and Implementing Interventions

Promoting Knowledge of Nutrition   Providing basic nutritional education is the goal of interventions with clients who have a knowledge deficit in this area. First determine what knowledge or misconceptions the client has and begin teaching at that level. If the client's information base is minimal, begin by showing pictures of the basic food groups. Provide lists of foods in each group and encourage the client to select favorite foods in each group. Discuss the body's need for proteins, carbohydrates, fats, vitamins, and minerals. Help the client plan a day's menus, keeping the client's food preferences in mind. Teach the client to analyze labels on prepared foods to determine foods with high nutrient value and reasonable caloric content. Supplement educational sessions with written materials the client can keep for later reference. Opportunities for teaching clients about nutrition can be used as a trust-building strategy.

Promoting Improved Nutrition   In planning interventions to help obese clients improve their nutritional status, collaborative goal setting is essential. The client must set a personal goal of controlling eating behaviors and establish a realistic weight-loss goal. Help the client explore measures for changing eating habits. For instance, clients can keep a food diary to monitor the types and amounts of foods they eat. Slowing the rate of eating by chewing more thoroughly, placing implements on the plate between bites, conversing with table companions, and avoiding eating alone are helpful. Establishing a program of gradually increasing physical activity helps to narrow the gap between caloric intake and energy expenditures.

The food diary also helps clients identify the link between feelings and eating behaviors. Encourage clients to voice their feelings, maintaining a calm and accepting attitude as they do. Help clients develop new, non-food-related coping strategies for dealing with troublesome feelings.

Cognitive restructuring techniques, such as correcting clients' irrational beliefs, are helpful. Help the client practice replacing negative self-talk with positive self-talk.

Give positive reinforcement and recognition when clients achieve any small weight loss. On the other hand, small "slips" should be viewed as such and not allowed to assume major importance or to impede steady progress. Teach the client how to select balanced, nutritionally sound meals when dining outside the home.

Provide information about community resources for exercise, such as YMCA and YWCA. As part of discharge planning, make referrals to support groups and self-help groups, such as Overeaters Anonymous, Weight Watchers, and the National Association to Aid Fat Americans.

Promoting Hopefulness   Personal hygiene and good grooming promote a sense of well-being. Spending time with obese clients at mealtimes, engaging them in conversation, can slow the eating process and demonstrate that change is possible. Assume an unhurried and caring attitude.

Unresponsive, apathetic clients become more responsive when exercise becomes part of their daily routine (Parent and Whall 1984). Encourage daily exercise or activity for obese clients.

Also encourage clients to express both positive and negative feelings as a step toward accepting their feelings as valid. Adopt an empathic, nonjudgmental attitude and, over time, help clients move from expressing feelings to exploring ways of coping other than by eating.

Attaining an intellectual understanding of one's condition promotes hope and a sense of control. Teach clients about obesity and its psychologic impact, and involve them in decision making regarding their care.

Visualization and guided imagery (see Chapter 27) are useful with hopeless clients. Encourage them to focus on happy experiences from the past and to envision themselves as they wish to be—healthy, energetic, and filled with vitality. Reinforce any expression of hopefulness, no matter how tentative.

Promoting Social Interaction   For the socially isolated obese client, the goal of nursing interventions is to increase time voluntarily spent in group settings. The first step is to offer companionship; just sitting quietly with the client while making no demands for interaction signifies the nurse's acceptance. Frequent, brief contacts indicate interest and foster the development of a therapeutic nurse-client relationship. Next, engage the socially isolated client in a noncompetitive one-to-one activity, such as working on a jigsaw puzzle. After the client feels comfortable during one-to-one activities, offer to accompany the client to a group activity. Help the client plan ahead, making sure the client realizes that leaving is OK if anxiety becomes too high. Positively reinforce any amount of time in groups, however brief.

As the client becomes more comfortable in groups, withdraw gradually, but remain available. Role playing social skills helps clients increase their repertoires of socially acceptable behaviors. Teach assertive techniques, because passivity and aggressiveness both invite rejection by others.

Evaluating/Outcome Criteria

Nutritional Knowledge   Clients will demonstrate nutritional knowledge by identifying the correct food group for each food in a sample daily menu. They will recognize missing food groups and identify overrepresented groups. Clients will accurately assess the nutritional value of prepared foods, using label information. They will demonstrate the ability to select a nutritious, low-calorie, balanced daily menu for themselves.

Nutritional Status   Clients will verbalize feelings that trigger overeating. They will verbalize feelings of increased self-control and greater self-esteem. Clients will progress steadily toward their personal weight-loss goals. They will demonstrate slower eating behaviors and avoid eating alone. They will describe how to order food in a restaurant yet adhere to their meal plans. They will participate in regular, structured exercise programs as well as self-help/support groups following discharge.

Hopefulness   Clients will voluntarily assume responsibility for hygiene and grooming. They will demonstrate commitment to a program of daily exercise. Clients will verbalize both positive and negative feelings and recognize life events over which they have no control. Clients will verbalize intellectual understanding of compulsive overeating and techniques for its control.

Social Interaction   Clients will demonstrate willingness to socialize with others. They will voluntarily attend client group activities. Clients will approach individuals appropriately for one-to-one interactions. They will report minimal anxiety during social interactions.

CHAPTER HIGHLIGHTS

• Major theoretic frameworks of importance in the understanding of eating disorders are psychoanalytic, behavioral, sociocultural, feminist, and biologic.

• Eating disorders can be considered maladaptive coping patterns characterized by obsession with food and compulsive overeating or undereating behaviors.

• Clients with anorexia nervosa and bulimia nervosa are predominantly young females from middle-class backgrounds.

• Obese clients are of both sexes; obesity is related to social class, being more common among the disadvantaged.

• Clients with anorexia nervosa experience fears of weight gain and markedly restrict their daily caloric intakes, denying hunger.

• Clients with bulimia nervosa are preoccupied with body size and shape. They experience hunger and respond to intense feelings with binging-purging behaviors.

• Clients who overeat compulsively may use food as a substitute for psychologic nurturance, which they desire.

• Nursing assessment of clients with eating disorders includes, but is not limited to, assessment of subjective emotional experiences, physiologic alterations, alterations in impulse control, impairment in family function, and impairment of social function.

• Nursing diagnoses for clients with eating disorders include altered nutrition, ineffective individual and family coping, body image disturbances, self-esteem disturbances, anxiety, fluid volume deficit, knowledge deficit, hopelessness, and social isolation.

• Nursing interventions for clients with eating disorders and their families include a wide range of psychotherapeutic, behavioral, insight-oriented, cognitive, pharmacologic, environmental, family-oriented, and stress-reduction approaches.

• Nursing evaluation criteria for clients with eating disorders include reduction in physical and psychologic symptoms, increased cognitive understanding of the disorder, ability to use stress-reducing skills, accurate perception of body size, decreased preoccupation with food and eating, increased interest in others, and improved social skills.

REFERENCES

Abraham S, Llewellyn-Jones D: *Eating Disorders: The Facts.* Oxford University Press, 1985.

Akridge K: Anorexia nervosa. *J Obstet Gynecol Neonatal Nurs* 1989;18(1):25–30.

Allan JD: Knowing what to weigh: Women's self-care activities related to weight. *Adv Nurs Sci* 1988;11(1):47–60.

American Psychiatric Association: *Diagnostic and Statistical Manual of Mental Disorders,* ed 3, revised. APA, 1987.

Boskind-White M, White WC: *Bulimarexia: The Binge/Purge Cycle.* W. W. Norton, 1983.

Bradshaw J: *Home Coming: Reclaiming and Championing Your Inner Child.* Bantam, 1990.

Bruch H: *The Golden Cage: The Enigma of Anorexia Nervosa.* Harvard University Press, 1978.

Brumberg JJ: *Fasting Girls: The Emergence of Anorexia Nervosa as a Modern Disease.* Harvard University Press, 1988.

Carter JA, Duncan PA: The practice of self-induced vomiting among high school females. *J Sch Health* 1985;54(11):450–452.

Chitty KK: The primary prevention role of the nurse in eating disorders. *Nurs Clin North Am* 1991; in press.

Deering CG: Developing a therapeutic alliance with the anorexia nervosa client. *J Psychosoc Nurs* 1987;25(3):11–17.

Deering CG, Niziolek C: Eating disorders: Promoting continuity of care. *J Psychosoc Nurs* 1988;26(11):6–15.

Dippel NM, Becknal BK: Bulimia. *J Psychosoc Nurs* 1987;25(9):13–17.

Edmands MS: Overcoming eating disorders. *J Psychosoc Nurs* 1986;24(8):19–25.

Fontaine KC: The conspiracy of culture: Women's issues in body size. *Nurs Clin North Am* 1991; in press.

Forisha B, Grothaus K, Luscombe R: Dinner conversation: Meal therapy to differentiate eating behavior from process. *J Psychosoc Nurs* 1990;28(11):12–16.

Garfinkel PE, Garner DM: *Anorexia Nervosa: A Multidimensional Perspective.* Brunner/Mazel, 1982.

Garner DM, Garfinkel PE (eds): *Handbook of Psychotherapy for Anorexia Nervosa and Bulimia.* Guilford Press, 1985.

Garner DM, Garfinkel PE, Bemis KM: A multidimensional psychotherapy for anorexia nervosa. *Int J Eat Disord* 1982;2(1):3–46.

Geary MC: A review of treatment models for eating disorders: Toward a holistic nursing model. *Holistic Nurs Pract* 1988;3(1):39–45.

Gottfried RS: *The Black Death.* Macmillan, 1983.

Halmi KA: Anorexia nervosa, in Kaplan HI, Freedman AM, Sadoch BJ (eds): *Comprehensive Textbook of Psychiatry/IV.* Williams and Wilkins, 1985.

Herzog D: Eating disorders, in Nicholi AM (ed): *The New Harvard Guide to Psychiatry.* Belknap Press, 1988.

Holland AJ, Hall A, Murray R, Russell GFM, Crisp AH: Anorexia nervosa: A study of 34 twin pairs and one set of triplets. *Br J Psychiatry* 1984;145:414–419.

Jacobson J: Speculations on the role of transitional objects in eating disorders. *Arch Psychiatr Nurs* 1988;2(4):110–114.

Kallen DJ, Sussman MB (eds): *Obesity and the Family.* Haworth Press, 1984.

Kneisl CR: Healing the neglected, wounded inner child of the past. *Nurs Clin North Am* 1991; in press.

Kopeski LM: Diabetes and bulimia: A deadly duo. *Am J Nurs* 1989;89(4):483–485.

Leininger MM: Transcultural eating patterns and nutrition. *Holistic Nurs Pract* 1988;3(1):16–25.

Maceyko SJ, Nagelberg DB: The assessment of bulimia in high school students. *J Sch Health* 1985;55(4):135–137.

McBride AB: Fat: A women's issue in search of a holistic approach to treatment. *Holistic Nurs Pract* 1988;3(1):9–15.

Miles MW: Bulimia nervosa and gender identity: Symbols of a culture. *Holistic Nurs Pract* 1988;3(1):56–66.

Miller KD: Body image therapy. *Nurs Clin North Am* 1991; in press.

Miner CD: The physiology of eating and starvation. *Holistic Nurs Pract* 1988;3(1):67–74.

Morley JE, Levine AS, Willenburg ML: Stress-induced feeding disorders, in Carruba MV, Blundell JE (eds): *Pharmacology of Eating Disorders: Theoretical and Clinical Developments.* Raven, 1986.

Muscari ME: Effective nursing strategies for adolescents with anorexia nervosa and bulimia nervosa. *Pediatr Nurs* 1988;14(6):475–482.

Oehler JM, Burns MJ: Anorexia, bulimia, and sexuality: Case study of an adolescent inpatient group. *Arch Psychiatr Nurs* 1987;1(3):163–171.

Orbach S: *Fat Is a Feminist Issue.* Medallion Books, 1978.

Orbach S: *Hunger Strike: The Anorectic's Struggle as a Metaphor for Our Age.* W. W. Norton, 1986.

Parent C, Whall A: Are physical activity, self-esteem, and depression related? *J Gerontol Nurs* 1984;10(3):8.

Parks BR, Fischer RG: Misuse of syrup of ipecac. *Pediatr Nurs* 1987;13(4):261.

Pope HG, Hudson JI: Pharmacologic treatment of bulimia nervosa: Research findings and practical suggestions. *Psychiatr Ann* 1989;19:9–17.

Potts NL: Eating disorders: The secret pattern of binge/purge. *Am J Nurs* 1984;84(1):32–35.

Reed G, Sech EP: Bulimia. *J Psychosoc Nurs* 1985;23(5):16–22.

Reighley JW: *Nursing Care Planning Guides for Mental Health.* Williams and Wilkins, 1988.

Rosenfield S: Family influence on eating behavior and attitudes in eating disorders: A review of the literature. *Holistic Nurs Pract* 1988;3(1):46–55.

Rossi LR: Feminine beauty: The impact of culture and nutritional trends on emerging images. *Holistic Nurs Pract* 1988;3(1):1–8.

Russell GFM: Bulimia nervosa: An ominous variant of anorexia nervosa. *Psychol Med* 1979;9:429–448.

Sanger E, Cassino T: Eating disorders: Avoiding the power struggle. *Am J Nurs* 1984;84(1):31–33.

Santopinto M: The relentless drive to be ever thinner: A study using the phenomenological method. *Nurs Sci Quart* 1989;2(1):29–36.

Schultz JM, Dark SL: *Manual of Psychiatric Nursing Care Plans,* ed 2. Little, Brown, 1986.

Staples NR, Schwartz M: Anorexia nervosa support group: Providing transitional support. *J Psychosoc Nurs* 1990;28(2):6–10.

Stuart GW, Laraia MT, Ballenger JC, Lydiard RB: Early family experiences of women with bulimia and depression. *Arch Psychiatr Nurs* 1990;4(1):43–52.

Stunkard AJ (ed): *Obesity*. Saunders, 1980.

Twiss JJ: The plight of a female adolescent—Anorexia or bulimia: An overview. *Issues Compr Pediatr Nurs* 1986;9(5):289–298.

White JH: Feminism, eating, and mental health. *Adv Nurs Sci* 1991;13(3):68–80.

Wurtman RJ, Wurtman JJ (eds): *Human Obesity*. New York Academy of Sciences, 1987.

Violence and Victims in the Psychiatric Setting

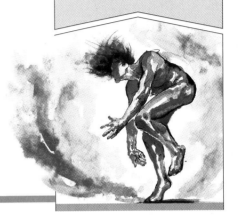

LEARNING OBJECTIVES

- Define three theoretic frameworks useful in understanding violence
- Identify and describe strategies for managing violent behavior
- Define in-patient psychiatric violence
- Assess a client's potential for violent behavior
- Plan nursing interventions for clients assessed as violent
- Explain staff responses to violent assault
- Recognize the factors that increase staff vulnerability to violent assault

Anastasia Fisher

CROSS REFERENCES

Other topics relevant to this content are: Ethics, Chapter 7; Legal issues, Chapter 37; Milieu therapy, Chapter 31; Rape and abuse, Chapter 22; Suicide, Chapter 23.

THERE ARE RELATIVELY LITTLE data on institutional violence or systematic description of the frequency, types, or consequences of assaults on nursing personnel (Ryan and Poster 1989). The three reasons generally offered for this deficiency are (1) a lack of nursing research in the area, (2) the tendency to deny the frequency and severity of resulting injuries, and (3) the tendency to hold nurses accountable for the assaults (Levy and Hartocollis 1976).

The information that does exist tells us not only that institutional violence occurs frequently, but also that psychiatric nurses are the most frequent victims of psychiatric client assault (Fottrell 1981, Lanza 1983). A study of formal incident reports determined that almost five times as many assaults occurred as were reported (Lion et al. 1981). The reasons postulated by the authors for the underreporting of assaults were: staff expectations of assault, the effort required to complete the report, and the admission of a performance failure. The authors also speculated that staff feared legal investigation of the event.

A survey of university-affiliated psychiatrists working within various settings reported that 42 percent have been assaulted by their clients during their careers (Madden et al. 1976). Another study noted that 24 percent of therapists—including psychiatrists, psychologists, and social workers—were assaulted during a year by one or more clients (Whitman et al. 1976). Conservative estimates suggest that clinicians can expect 7 percent to 10 percent of in-patients to be assaultive just prior to or shortly after admission to a psychiatric unit (Craig 1982), and that one in four therapists may be assaulted at some time during their careers (Whitman et al. 1976). Whatever the precise dimensions of psychiatric violence, mental health professionals have the responsibility for its prediction, prevention, and management.

For the purpose of this chapter, **psychiatric client violence** is defined as behavior by a psychiatric in-patient that threatens or actually harms or injures persons or destroys property (APA 1974). Although there are no simple approaches to the topic of violence, several frameworks can be used to stimulate our thinking about in-patient psychiatric violence.

Theoretic Foundations

Descriptive frameworks are ways to organize our thoughts, observations, and intuitive notions into coherent patterns. They do not explain the causes of violence on a case-by-case basis or tell us what to do about it. Because of the complexity of individuals,

situations, and interactional components to violence no one framework is sufficient. It is necessary to approach psychiatric violence from a variety of perspectives. The frameworks useful in understanding psychiatric violence are the importation theory, situationism, and an interaction model.

Importation

The "importation" theory reflects the position that the client brings or imports certain values, attitudes, and behavior patterns conducive to violence into the treatment setting (Armstrong 1978). Most of the literature on violence represents this position, identifying such client characteristics as social and cultural factors, psychiatric diagnosis and personality traits, and demographic characteristics. The social and cultural conditions often associated with violent behavior include:

- Low socioeconomic status

- A history of childhood abuse

- Life experiences from a subculture condoning or expecting the use of violence to resolve conflicts

- A history of violent behavior

Research findings on the role of psychiatric diagnosis in the production of violent behavior are conflicting and unclear. Violent behavior has been observed across the entire spectrum of diagnoses, but violent clients are more likely to have a diagnosis of schizophrenia, personality disorders, psychotic organic brain syndrome, or mental retardation (Lion et al. 1981, Tardiff and Sweillam 1980, 1982). Most current thinking suggests that the degree of psychopathology, or severity of the illness, is the more significant contributor to violent behavior, not the specific diagnostic classification. A central psychodynamic theme repeatedly described in the literature is that violent clients perceive themselves to be hopeless and powerless (APA 1974; Lion et al. 1981). Violent clients are also three to four times more likely than nonviolent clients to have attempted suicide at least once (Tardiff 1983).

Age and sex are the demographic characteristics typically included in research on psychiatric client violence. Young males tend to be overrepresented in the samples. Whether this reflects a subculture that

---

The author of this chapter prefers the use of "patient" instead of "client" in institutional work. "Client" is retained for the text's overall consistency.

condones violence or the frustration of a deprived status is not clear.

Of all the characteristics noted, the only one found to be predictive of future violence is a history of violent behavior. This generalization requires some modification since a past episode of violent behavior in the community appears to be the best predictor of future violence in the community and a past event of violent behavior in the hospital setting is a good indicator of a future event in the same setting (Steadman 1981).

If one were to use the importation theory to construct a profile of a client most likely to exhibit violent behavior, it might look like the following. He would be a young male (under 44 years of age) from a subculture or minority group that condones the use of violence to resolve conflicts (APA 1974, Tardiff and Sweillam 1982). He would be poor, have little formal education, and possess few employment skills and poor verbal communication skills (APA 1974, Tardiff and Sweillam 1980). He would come from a home in which there was violence or parental deprivation. His parents would have had problems with alcoholism, and he would have experienced abuse as a child. He would have engaged in some expression of violent behavior in the recent past. His psychiatric diagnosis would be anything from psychiatric conditions such as schizophrenia or organic brain syndrome to a severe personality disorder. He would exhibit severe psychopathology and impairment in function. He would see himself as helpless and powerless. He would have a history of at least one previous suicide attempt.

In-Patient Management Strategies The in-patient management strategies suggested by the importation theory include verbal techniques, medications, behavioral techniques, seclusion, and restraint. Typically these strategies are targeted to individuals who are currently violent or are perceived to be imminently dangerous. However, such strategies are also common in the long-term management of violent behavior.

The overall goal of these strategies, whether considered individually or used in combination, is to strengthen clients' ability to control themselves. Implementation of these management strategies must be considered within the context of the principle of least restrictiveness. This principle requires that staff demonstrate attempts to use less restrictive measures of control before resorting to more restrictive interventions. For example, staff must document their efforts to intervene with a client using verbal strategies before they intervene physically.

Verbal Technique Forming a verbal alliance with the potentially violent client is often the first step to containing the violent behavior. Two common errors occur during the initial efforts to intervene with the potentially violent or violent client (Nigrosh 1983):

1. Confusion between control and confrontation

2. Overemphasis on supportive concern characterized by statements such as, "I know how you feel and I'm here to help"

It is important to convey control in the situation by using clear, calm statements, and a confident physical stance rather than through remarks or cues that can be interpreted as challenging the client. A confrontive, aggressive, or threatening manner or a tendency to overidentify with the client's experience can make the staff member a target of violence.

Several strategies are suggested as guidelines to assist in establishing quick rapport and alliance with the potentially violent client. Clinical judgment and the situation must dictate the appropriateness of their use. Some violent behavior occurs impulsively and without warning. Most episodes, however, involve an escalation of behavior and are therefore more amenable to verbal intervention. An example of verbal intervention useful in working with some potentially violent clients is summarized in the Intervention box on page 492. The overall goals of these verbal techniques and positional strategies are to establish a relationship that minimizes the client's projection on the helper, and to protect the client's already damaged self-esteem as much as possible, thereby decreasing the potential for violent behavior.

Sometimes verbal techniques are insufficient to contain the situation, particularly when the violent behavior occurs impulsively. In these instances, additional interventions—including medications, behavioral techniques, and seclusion and restraint—can be used with or instead of the verbal strategies just presented.

Medication Although daily use of neuroleptic medication is the most widely used treatment for the control of violent behavior in institutional settings, it is important to recognize that pharmacologic agents alone are not the answer to violence (Lion 1983). Whether these medications are being prescribed in response to the degree of psychotic symptomatology or in response to the violent behavior remains an issue for future research.

Choice of neuroleptic medication is often a function of the clinician's preference and the client's medication history. Among those medications routinely used are haloperidol (Haldol), chlorpromazine (Thorazine), thioridazine (Mellaril), and thiothixene (Navane). Long-acting injectable fluphenazine (Prolixin) and haloperidol are used with clients discharged to the community to be followed as out-patients, as well as with clients who have histories of noncompliance. Dosages vary for each medication. Younger clients with previously documented histories of violent behavior tend to receive higher doses of neuroleptic

INTERVENTION

Verbal Techniques and Positional Strategies for Potentially Violent Clients

Technique	*Goal of Intervention*
1. Approach the client from the side, symbolically facing what the client faces. Do not stand face to face with the potentially violent person.	1. Focusing the interaction away from the client-staff dyad can decrease the tendency of the violent person to project and externalize the attack.
2. Avoid direct eye contact.	2. Avoid becoming a target of the client's violent expression.
3. Center the verbal content on the figures or issues of concern to the client. For example, if the client states, "The nurse said I'm too sick to leave the hospital," a response such as, "That's a real drag," will likely be more effective than "I can see how you must be upset by that." The latter statement draws attention back to the client and staff member (Nigrosh 1983).	3. Deflect attention away from the staff member as a potential target for the violent behavior.
4. Express affect similar to the client's. For example, when responding to the client's anger at not being allowed to leave, state, "That really is crummy."	4. Avoid sounding too clinical. Identify and verbalize some part of the client's feelings toward the object(s) or person(s) of concern to the client (Nigrosh 1983).

medications. Refer to Chapter 32 for a thorough analysis of antipsychotic medications, frequent side effects, and treatment of their symptoms. See also Appendix B.

Behavioral Techniques   Various behavioral strategies established around the principle of progressive isolation are often attempted before initiation of seclusion and restraint. The therapeutic intent of this technique is to reduce disruptive stimulation and provide the client with a contained, well-defined space for reassurance, protection, and defense. Depending on unit construction, the client can be encouraged to seek quiet refuge at the back of the unit or in a private room. Isolation can progress from the back of the unit,

to the client's room, to open seclusion or a quiet room as indicated. These strategies are typically used in conjunction with the medications previously mentioned and to avoid the more aggressive and restrictive procedures of seclusion and restraint.

When efforts to contain the client's behavior using verbal techniques separately or in combination with administration of medications and behavioral techniques do not prevent the violent behavior, or if an assault occurs without warning, staff must intervene to restrain the client physically and protect the milieu.

Seclusion and Restraint   Seclusion and restraint are techniques used to contain violent clients who do not respond to less restrictive verbal, chemical, or behavioral interventions. Using seclusion or restraint as punishment, divorced from the treatment interests of the client, cannot be justified and represents a serious mismatch between the needs of the client and those of the treatment setting (Soloff 1983).

Facilities using seclusion and restraint as a means of controlling violent behavior generally require staff attendance at assault training programs. These programs teach hospital policies and procedures for dealing with assaultive clients, including legal and clinical documentation requirements, as well as appropriate physical contact skills for use with violent psychiatric in-patients. While all courses in contact skills must emphasize the concept of team building, variations do exist. Some courses emphasize situation-specific skills, such as standard therapeutic holds and "release from hair pull," while others provide practice for more general strategies such as evasive techniques and deflection and neutralization of blows (Nigrosh 1983). The most comprehensive programs provide analysis and opportunities to role play interview situations, as well as other noncontact techniques, in addition to specific contact skills training. Evidence in the literature indicates an association between participation in staff training programs and not being assaulted. In other words, nursing personnel who participate in staff training workshops are less likely to be assaulted than staff who do not participate (Infantino and Musingo 1985).

Whichever type of program is offered, it is desirable to provide monthly on-unit reviews for each shift. These reviews, emphasizing the team orientation, provide opportunities for practice, role modeling, and evaluation of performance. In addition, it is important to integrate these physical contact skills into a larger training program that places the physical interventions into proper clinical perspective.

The decision to use medication, seclusion, or restraint to control violent behavior depends on an understanding of the individual client. For example, the use of repetitive neuroleptic medication to control violent behavior in an organically impaired client is not as desirable as using restraint or seclusion as the first intervention option. On the other hand, involuntary medication may be preferred to the use of seclusion and restraint in the case of a schizophrenic client whose violent behavior is a response to paranoid delusions.

Techniques of Seclusion and Restraint Psychiatric nurses have a major responsibility in the decision to seclude and restrain as well as in caring for the client while in seclusion and restraints. Once the decision has been made to seclude and restrain a potentially violent client, a "leader" is chosen from among the available staff. The leader is responsible for designating roles to be played by the remaining staff and for directing the steps in the seclusion-restraint procedure. Choice of the leader is important and can be based on numerous factors, including familiarity with the client. It is important to remember that the goal in the procedure is to gain maximum cooperation from the client and minimize violence. For example, one would not choose a large male staff member to confront a psychotic client in homosexual panic (Tardiff 1984a).

After a leader is chosen a sufficient number of personnel must be gathered. This support staff should convey confidence and calm reflecting a detached, professional approach to a familiar procedure. The staff should avoid intimidating language and physical stances as these behaviors may provoke the client's potential for violence. It is often sufficient to have the support staff gather around the leader the first time the client is approached. This **show of force** may be interaction enough and the client may comply without further escalation. It is important for the client to perceive that sufficient strength is available to control his or her behavior. From the staff's perspective, the show of force provides confidence with minimal physical risk to staff, client, and the remaining milieu (Tardiff 1984a).

One staff member is assigned responsibility for managing the unit environment and other clients. This person is responsible for supporting and calming the other clients, who may become anxious during the procedure. In addition, the area near the seclusion room must be cleared of clients or physical obstructions to minimize the potential of injury.

Once the unit environment is safe, the team approaches the potentially violent client. The leader offers a clear, brief statement of the purpose and rationale for seclusion or restraint. For example, the client is told that his or her behavior is out of control and that time in seclusion is required to help him or her regain control. The other team members position themselves around the client for easy access to the client's limbs. The leader then asks the client to walk into the seclusion room accompanied by staff. At this point, further discussion or negotiation should be avoided as it frequently aggravates the situation. The behavioral options given to the client must be kept simple, clear, and minimal. Time allowed for client cooperation must be brief, measured in seconds rather than minutes, to avoid an escalation of the behavior into an uncontrolled episode of violence (Tardiff 1984a).

If the client does not begin to walk toward the seclusion room, on cue from the leader, the team members positioned around the client move in to restrain the client physically. Using practiced techniques the team brings the client to the ground and restrains each limb at the joint.

Once the client is safely controlled to the ground, additional staff may be needed to transport the client to the seclusion room where mechanical restraints can be applied. These clients can be carried in the recumbent position with arms pinned to sides, legs held at the knees, and head controlled. Other clients may be walked into the seclusion room with staff maintaining adequate control over both arms.

In the seclusion room the client is routinely positioned on the bed on his or her back. Street clothes are removed and the client is placed in a hospital gown. Belts, shoes, jewelry, and glasses are usually removed to avoid self-injury. In situations of high risk, elastic bras, shoe laces, and the like may also be removed. If the client is to be restrained, one limb at a time is secured in the restraint with staff announcing as each limb is secured and pressure released. The client's head should be secured until all staff members have withdrawn their holds to reduce the chance of staff being bitten. Medications are frequently injected at this time. Once the client is safely restrained and medicated, the leader reassures the client that he or she will be carefully monitored and the staff will assess his or her capacity for control. Then the team can exit one at a time, with the final member moving backward out of the seclusion room door, which is then quickly locked.

The final step in the seclusion or restraint process is a rehash of the procedures and techniques used. During the rehash staff must be allowed to express their emotional reactions to the episode. The client community should also be given an opportunity in community meetings or other forums to ventilate their feelings and verbalize their concerns about the restraint and seclusion procedure. Clear therapeutic rationales for the use of seclusion or restraint should be openly discussed with the client community (Tardiff 1984a).

Care of the Client in Seclusion and Restraint Once a client requires seclusion or restraint, observations of the client's behavior are usually made every 15 minutes by nursing staff. These checks include a description of the client's behavior (e.g., yelling or sleeping), as well as routine care activities, including meals, circulation checks, and toileting needs. When the client is quiet, these checks should be conducted by nursing staff entering the seclusion room and participating in a verbal exchange with the client. The nurse should document content of these dialogues, paying particular attention to a reduction in the client's symptoms, responsiveness to limits, capacity to discuss options, and increased capacity to tolerate frustration. Documentation of these behavioral checks and routine physical care activities are required and can be accompanied in a checklist format. A sample of a nursing care checklist is presented in Figure 21–1.

Release from Seclusion and Restraint Clients may be released from seclusion and restraint when the goals of the intervention have been accomplished, that is, when the client's behavior is under control and no longer poses a danger to self, others, or the milieu. The decision to release from seclusion or wean from restraint and seclusion is based on an assessment of data gathered while the client is in seclusion. The ability of the client to control his or her behavior has been observed many times during the course of seclusion or restraint and is the basis for the decision to release. Each time nursing staff enter the seclusion room for the purpose of feeding, bathing, or toileting the client, responsiveness to verbal direction can be assessed. If a client has been secluded and not restrained, the first entries into the seclusion room should always be preceded by specific behavior requests. For example, the nurse should ask the client to sit on the bed before entering. The capacity of the client to follow simple directive statements is a first step in gathering assessment data for making a decision to release (Tardiff 1984a).

The release process follows a behavioral course that can be outlined in the nursing care plan. The initial step may be opening the seclusion room door for brief periods of time and monitoring the client's tolerance. With the door open, the client is expected to remain in the room and converse with staff across the open door. Deviation from the stated expectations of staff leads to a relocking of the door and a requirement to begin the process again. Once the client has demonstrated cooperation with medications, meals, hygiene care, and interaction with staff from an open seclusion setting, staff can consider a return to the client's room and the milieu. See the Nursing Care Plan on page 496.

The client in restraints should be released from restraints gradually. There are many different types of restraints, from cloth camisoles and posey vests to locked leather restraints. Locked leather restraints are frequently used in acute psychiatric facilities. These restraints are secured to the frame of a bed that is often bolted to the floor of the seclusion room. A restraint is applied to each limb of the client and locked. With this type of restraint it is possible to vary the placement based on an assessment of the client's need for external control. It is common when assessing the client's

capacity for control to move gradually from a condition of four-point restraints (two ankle, two wrist), to three-point restraints (two ankle, one wrist), to two-point restraints (opposite ankle and wrist). This strategy allows the staff a margin of safety while providing the client gradual release. Once released from restraints, clients require the same assessment as indicated above for individuals in seclusion (McCoy and Garritson 1983, Soloff 1983, Tardiff 1984b).

Limitations of Importation Theory Although the in-patient management strategies of verbal techniques, medication, behavioral techniques, seclusion, and restraint are among the most frequently used, the importation theory on which they are based has limited value. Knowing the numerous individual characteristics that are the basis of the importation theory has not helped in predicting psychiatric client violence. In spite of its popularity, the importation theory is limited because the characteristics identified are not descriptive of all clients who are violent, and not all clients fitting this profile exhibit violent behavior. The two frameworks discussed next address dimensions excluded by the importation theory and define the problem of violence in terms of the environment or the interactional process as integrated components contributing to violence.

Situationism

Situationism proposes that violence is a response to the unique, coercive, and regimented hospital environment in which the client feels devalued and dehumanized (Armstrong 1978). Research conducted in this area suggests the environmental elements that contribute to the violence process on in-patient psychiatric units are space and location, time of day, unit construction, staffing patterns, activity levels, and population composition.

Space and Location Space and location factors include territoriality, privacy, overcrowding, and place of the incident (Depp 1983, Dietz and Rada 1983, Kinzel 1970). The concept of territoriality involves defense of physical objects or the space a client has identified or "staked out" as personal space. For example, often a client "claims" a special chair on the unit, and a new client comes along and sits in it. The resulting conflicts over special territory also raise the issue of privacy.

Overcrowding Overcrowding is also related to the issue of privacy. Evidence suggests that assaultive clients have unusual and consistent difficulty tolerating people near them or touching them (Depp 1983, Kinzel 1970).

Date _____   Time in _____

Renew R/S order at _____

Seclusion only _____

Type of restraint _____

Client I.D.

Level of search:
  I. Clothing and belongings _____
  II. In hospital gown _____
  III. Body search _____

Time every 15 minutes	Check circulation q 15 min.	Fluids offered every hour	Exercise/limb massage q hour	Hygiene needs assessed q 2⁰	Need for elimination assessed q 2⁰	Observations (include client behavior, sleep, etc.):	Staff Initials

CRITERIA FOR RELEASE MET

Time	Accepts limits	Tolerates frustration	Contracts	Other	Staff initials

Initials	Staff signatures/title	Initials	Staff signatures/title

FIGURE 21−1 Nursing care check-list for clients in seclusion or restraint.

NURSING CARE PLAN

A Client in Seclusion

Client Care Goals	Nursing Planning/ Intervention	Evaluation
Nursing Diagnosis: *High risk for violence: Self-directed or directed at others*		
Client will gradually gain control of impulses during episode of seclusion.	Provide clear and firm limits to supplement the client's lack of internal controls.	Client verbalizes one option to hitting others, e.g., talking, requesting meds, requesting a "quiet place," before release from seclusion room.
	Assess client's ability to respond to limits:	
	Instruct client to sit on bed before staff enters seclusion room.	
	Evaluate client's cooperation taking oral meds.	
	Graduate from locked to open seclusion room during the next 2 hours if client can tolerate.	
	Teach client alternative ways to deal with assaultiveness.	
	Use medications as ordered for increasing control.	
	Restrain if client demonstrates violent behavior toward others.	
Nursing Diagnosis: *Activity intolerance*		
Client will be able to tolerate environmental stimuli.	Provide a low stimulus environment of seclusion room.	Client tolerates open seclusion door, staff contact, following instructions.
	Graduate from locked to open seclusion during next 2 hours if client can tolerate.	
Nursing Diagnosis: *Self-care deficit: Feeding*		
Client will maintain an adequate intake of food and fluid.	Offer client food and fluids at meal time.	Client accepts food and fluids at least every 2 hours and actual intake is documented.
	Offer supplemental fluids every 2 hours while client is in seclusion.	
	Physically assist client with eating and drinking if necessary.	
	Document client's actual intake of food and fluids.	

NURSING CARE PLAN (continued)

A Client in Seclusion

Client Care Goals	Nursing Planning/ Intervention	Evaluation
Nursing Diagnosis: *Self-care deficit: Toileting*		
Client's need for toilet facilities will be met.	Offer client opportunity to use bathroom facilities every 2 hours or as requested.	Client is offered facilities at least every 2 hours.
	Physically assist client in meeting toileting needs if necessary.	
	Document client's use of facilities.	
Nursing Diagnosis: *Self-care deficit: Bathing/hygiene*		
Client will have hygiene needs met during seclusion.	Offer client opportunity to wash face and hands.	At time of release from seclusion, client indicates opportunities were given to brush teeth, change gown, and so on.
	Offer client dental hygiene after meals, at bedtime, or on request.	
	Provide clients with clean gown and linens if needed or requested.	

Place on the Unit Observation of the location or place on the unit where assaults take place can be instructive. For instance, one study of assaults on a forensic service revealed that most assaults occurred in the dining room during mealtime (Dietz and Rada 1983). In another study, the highest number of incidents occurred in the corridors or in clients' rooms, with fewer assaults occurring in the dining room (Quinsey and Varney 1977). The difference in results appeared to be related to institutional policy. In the first example, all clients except those in seclusion were required to go to the dining room for meals, while in the second instance access to the dining room was obtained only after the client had demonstrated the ability to handle that social environment.

Specific management strategies suggested by these data include options such as structural enlargement of communal ward areas, or diversion of some clients to alternative areas at times of highest use (Dietz and Rada 1983). The frequency of dining room incidents might be reduced by staggering mealtimes, seating fewer clients at a table, or increasing selectivity over which clients go to the dining room. On units where assaults are highest in client rooms, consideration

might be given to issues of negotiating ward census, structural changes providing a higher proportion of single rooms, and flexibility in moving clients to decrease density or establish a better match of room-mates.

Time of Day The example of incidents in the dining room indicates that the time of day may be closely linked to the location of violent incidents. Although the times of assaults vary across research studies, assaults appear to occur with greatest frequency at the times and places with the highest level of interaction among clients (Dietz and Rada 1983).

Architectural Design Another reported precondition for violence is architectural designs that create blind spots and opportunities for nonobservation. Research suggests, however, that rather than a lack of staff monitoring contributing to violence, fights between clients occur around scarce items that require sharing, often creating an atmosphere of competition (Depp 1983). Placement of the radio, telephone, piano, or washer and dryer in out-of-the way places (to decrease noise on the unit) often contributes to incidents. Mirrors have been used effectively to cope with particular architectural design problems in psychiatric units. But how a unit and staff choose to handle scarce items is far more complex and is related not only to institutional policy and unit philosophy but also to individual clinical judgment. Many units monitor these items, either through using signup procedures or by locking them up and distributing them at the discretion of the staff or a member of the client government. The significant issue is developing an awareness that location of these items often creates areas where violence occurs. Sometimes the simple installation of one additional client telephone or a minor structural alteration on a unit can significantly reduce the number of incidents.

Staffing Patterns   The relationship between staffing patterns and violence is not well understood. The notion of optimal staffing, often cited as a prerequisite for attainment of treatment objectives, is ambiguous and appears more complex than "more staff equals less violence." Whether a given hospital milieu has sufficient staff to manage potentially violent clients depends on the amount of care required by the total client population at that period of time. Most units are prepared to deal with a certain amount of acting-out, disorganized, agitated, or violent behaviors, but beyond that they may become overwhelmed.

Although a number of researchers have attempted to clarify the relationship between staffing patterns and violence, they report conflicting results. Some have found increased numbers of assaults on days with higher staffing levels (Depp 1983, Kalogerakis 1971). The researchers attributed this finding to the idea of activity level (see the next section) or the potential for physical coercion that occurs with an increased presence of staff authority. Other researchers exploring the problem of understaffing and its relationship to psychiatric violence have found that the presence of one or two staff members is associated with a significant decrease in violent episodes (Rogers et al. 1980). In this case it is not clear whether staff passively provide an audience that inhibits violent behavior or whether staff actively model more acceptable role behaviors (Cobb 1984). In addition to confusion over optimum numbers of staff, there is controversy over the relationship between client violence and nursing staff gender. It has been suggested that female staff are less likely to provoke violence than male staff (Levy and Hartocollis 1976).

Because of the difficulty comparing across studies due to differences in unit and staffing compositions, the relationship between staffing and violence remains unclear. It is likely that the staffing question will not be answered by studying such survey characteristics as number or gender of staff, but by pursuing an understanding of the quality, content, and variations in staff to client interactions.

Activity Level   Activity level refers to the requirement that clients participate in therapeutic activities. As mentioned previously, peak times for violent incidents tend to be mealtimes and periods of concentrated treatment programming. In both situations there is a high concentration of clients, and performance and participation are demanded. Ways of handling the problems suggested by activity level include scheduling, coordinating, and withdrawing. Scheduling staff breaks and mealtimes during client meals can create a situation of temporary understaffing on the unit. Whether this contributes to staff anxiety that is communicated to clients is not clear, but staggering mealtimes for clients and staff is a simple alternative and may prevent violent behavior. Coordinating client activities with the nursing staff schedule, although a tedious process, is an important consideration.

Staff who are expected to cajole or coerce clients into participation often create a situation in which the client feels trapped, and striking out becomes the only defense. Sometimes the most valuable intervention with any client—but particularly with one who is agitated, angry, and frightened—is temporary withdrawal. This allows the client quiet time free from the anxiety of interpersonal demands. Making frequent, short, individualized contact with the client is more reassuring and does more to de-escalate a situation than forcing the client to attend a community meeting or other activity where the client's behavior is likely to be the focal point of the community's discussion. Individualizing the milieu activities of clients may be as important to advancing their treatment and preventing violence as the proper medication regimen.

Client Population Composition   The last element evolving from the situationism framework is client population composition, which involves the risks and benefits of segregating violent clients or establishing special units for them. This raises clinical as well as ethical issues. On the one hand, designating one unit for "assaultive clients," while creating a homogeneous treatment unit, may actually create an assaultive unit. On the other hand, admitting violent clients to all units contributes to an increased risk from assault for more vulnerable clients. Although the latter is by far the most popular and pragmatic approach, danger of serious injury to other clients by ward violence is a factor of growing concern in many hospitals (Depp 1983).

It has been suggested that much of the violent and disruptive behavior within settings reflects the success with which the institutional environment conveys the message that clients are expected to act violently (Dietz and Rada 1983). This is particularly true in forensic services, but every treatment unit contributes to these messages, either implicitly or explicitly. Physical characteristics, such as the posted notice "High Assault Risk" on the front door of the unit or the storage of leather restraints in plain view, alert clients as well as staff to potential problems.

While it is important to attend to issues such as space and location, time of day, and unit construction, their contribution to psychiatric violence is not well understood. However, the situationism framework provides an additional perspective from which to understand violence and generate assessment data. These data can then be used to plan individual interventions that take into account the environmental component in violent behavior. The major limitation of the situationism framework is that it fails to account for the vast majority of clients in these settings who do not engage in violent behavior. Like the importation framework, this perspective fails to address the complexity of psychiatric violence. The framework discussed next emphasizes client-staff interaction as a contributing element in psychiatric violence.

Interaction

Emphasizing the interactional process as the trigger or cue for violent assault, this framework concentrates on client and staff interaction. The specific interactional processes identified as cues to violence between staff and clients tend to cluster around three elements: (1) provocations, (2) expectations, and (3) conflicts. While the emphasis here is on client-staff violence, and these elements have been noted typically in relation to this specific interactional pattern, they may also be important in understanding client-client violence.

Provocation Several studies suggest that provocative styles of interaction contribute to violence (Hatti et al. 1982, Madden et al. 1976, Ruben et al. 1980, Straker et al. 1977). In each of these studies the therapist interviewed thought he or she had done something to trigger the violence. These provocations to violence were described as frustrating clients by not granting requests regarding hospitalization or medications and making clients do something they were unwilling to do, such as attend group activities.

Individual therapist's behaviors that increase the likelihood of assault are irritability, a tendency to speak up when angry, and a tendency to fight when confronted with physically threatening situations (Ruben et al. 1980). Although nurses may not know what part they play in the violent encounter, repetitive incidents of assault or threats of assault on the same

nursing staff member may provide clues. A tendency in staff toward a controlling, rigidly authoritarian, and intolerant stance toward clients increases vulnerability to assault (Soloff 1983). These attitudes are often communicated unwittingly through tone of voice, physical demeanor, or choice of language. Abusive language or actual assault on clients may provoke a violent defense from clients. These provocations and abusive interactions increase nurses' vulnerability to violent assault. Strategies for providing supervision and staff support are discussed in the next section. At this point, it is important to suggest that some nurses may not be able to work successfully with certain types of clients at certain times.

Nurses working with the violent need to monitor themselves and each other with regard to the following:

- Their ability to use anger constructively and not to take clients' anger personally

- Their capacity for clear verbal communication

- Their capacity for self-analysis

- Their capacity to listen

- Their capacity both to establish and maintain empathic linkages with clients and to disengage

- Their capacity to understand their fears and anxieties about violence

- Their belief that violent psychiatric clients are treatable

Nurses with long-standing difficulties in these areas and the previously mentioned controlling interpersonal style may be more successful in other clinical settings.

In addition to the behavior styles and provocations that increase vulnerability to violence, two major staff expectations have been associated with psychiatric violence:

1. Expectations that clients will act violently

2. Expectations that clients are hopeless and cannot be treated

Expectations Within the hospital setting, persistent expectations and fears of assault may set up a self-fulfilling prophecy (Levy and Hartocollis 1976, Straker et al. 1977, Whitman et al. 1976). Seeing the danger of being assaulted as part of the work hazard in psychiatric nursing (Duvall 1984) and expecting to be assaulted at work are related but separate experiences. A greater need for staff vigilance in recognizing that they work with assaultive individuals is necessary, but this does not require that assaultive behavior be expected or acceptable. The client may interpret such

RESEARCH NOTE

Citation

Poster EC, Ryan JA: Nurses' attitudes toward physical assaults by patients. Arch Psychiatr Nurs 1989;3(6):315–322.

Study Problem/Purpose

This study examined nurses' attitudes toward physical assault by clients.

Methods

This descriptive study was conducted in seven psychiatric units (two child, two adolescent, two adult, one geropsychiatric, and two neurology). All nursing staff (*n*=258) were requested to volunteer for the study. Questionnaires were returned by 184 staff members. The questionnaire, called Attitudes Toward Patient Physical Assault, was developed by the authors and consisted of thirty-one items related to client assault. The items concerned four major attitude areas: client responsibility for behavior, staff competence and performance, legal/ethical issues, and safety concerns. Participants were asked to respond on a five-point Likert scale as to their degree of agreement.

Findings

It was determined that there was consistency in attitude across the demographic factors of age, gender, educational preparation, and history of a previous assault. Data also indicated that staff competency, performance, and personality traits did not correlate with being assaulted by clients. In addition the findings reinforced nurses' concern with their own safety, and the authors suggest various ways to increase the nurses' safety while at work.

Implications

Studies describing issues related to physical assault increase our knowledge and ability to care for assaultive psychiatric clients. The present study is significant for its exploration of the nurses' attitudes toward assaultive clients, a previously neglected area of inquiry.

attitudes to mean that violence is not serious (Madden 1983).

Staff hopelessness about clients has also been associated with psychiatric violence. As noted previously, the major presenting psychodynamic theme describing violence-prone individuals is their self-perception as hopeless and powerless. It is believed that communications by staff supporting these perceptions provides another interpersonal cue to violence (Depp 1983).

Conflicts It has long been suggested that conflicts between staff can become the basis for acting-out behavior in clients (Stanton and Schwartz 1954). As a result of philosophic splits or competitive rivalries among staff, clients can be scapegoated into behaving violently to release ward tension (Straker et al. 1977).

In conjunction with provocations, expectations, and staff conflicts, it is important to consider the concept of timing; knowing when to engage in interaction is as crucial as knowing how to engage. Single episodes of provocation, assault expectations, or staff conflicts may have no adverse effects, but repeated interactions involving these dynamics may culminate in violence.

In-Patient Management Strategies Management strategies specific to the interaction framework focus on the client-staff dyad, rather than the individual client or the environment. Among the strategies are clinical supervision, staff development, and staff meetings. These techniques are discussed in the next section.

This final management approach is based on integration of the frameworks of importation, situationism, and interaction. This integrated approach to managing in-patient psychiatric violence recognizes violence as a response to the complex social processes between actors. Using this integrated approach to understand psychiatric in-patient violence has implications for assessment, planning, intervening, and evaluating the nursing care delivered to these clients.

Figure 21–2 is a comprehensive violence assessment tool addressing clinical, situational, and interactional factors that helps the nurse collect and organize data. This tool seeks information relevant to each of the frameworks presented. Information from the assessment tool can be used to plan meaningful, individualized integrated interventions to decrease the incidence of violent behavior.

These interventions can be coordinated around the factors that contribute most significantly to increasing the individual's potential to violent behavior. Clients and their families are important sources of information. Interview questions about the violent client's history should be open and direct, much as though one were questioning a suicidal individual. The nurse should ask, "How much have you thought about violence?" "What have you done about it?" "What

I.   Clinical history

    A.   Diagnosis at discharge
        Axis I: _____
        _____

        Axis II: _____
        _____

    B.   Age: _____
    C.   Sex: ___ M ___ F
    D.   Admitting status
        ___ 72-HR hold   ___ Vol.
        ___ 14-DAY cert.   ___ Other
        ___ Temp conservatorship
    E.   Previous experience in seclusion/restraint
        ___ Yes   ___ No
        Reaction to seclusion/restraint
        _____
        _____
        _____

F.   Age at onset: _____
G.   Psychotropic medications:
    ___ Taking prior to admission
    ___ Not taking prior to admission

    Medications:
    _____
    _____
    _____
    _____

    Previous criminal history
    ___ Yes   ___ No
    _____
    _____

I.   Use of ETOH/street drugs
    ___ Yes   ___ No
    _____
    _____
    _____

II.   Violence history

    A.   Previous institutional violence   ___ Yes   ___ No

        Type of institution: _____ Date(s): _____ _____
        Number of incidents: _____ _____ _____
        Type of violence:

Against person	___ Yes	___ No	Date _____
Family	___ Yes	___ No	Date _____
Stranger	___ Yes	___ No	Date _____
Inmate/client	___ Yes	___ No	Date _____
RN/LPT/MD	___ Yes	___ No	Date _____
Other	___ Yes	___ No	Date _____
			Who _____
Weapon used	___ Yes	___ No	Date _____
Against property	___ Yes	___ No	Date _____
Type	_____		
Verbal threat (only)	___ Yes	___ No	Date _____

        Situational factors: Time of day   _____
                                     Location   _____
        Engaged in therapeutic activity   ___ Yes   ___ No
                         Type of activity   _____
               Other factors _____
                            _____
                            _____

        Interactional factors: Engaged in interaction with victim ___ Yes ___ No
                          Type of interaction _____
                                        _____
                        With whom: _____
                        Content of conversation, request:
                        _____
                        _____

FIGURE 21–2   Violence assessment tool.

Response to violence: Medications ___ Yes ___ No

Type and dose: _____

_____

_____

Seclusion only ___ Yes ___ No
Seclusion/restraint ___ Yes ___ No
Milieu management ___ Yes ___ No
Combination ___ Yes ___ No
(list) _____

_____

_____

Client's response to intervention(s): _____

_____

B. Community violence
Previous violence: ___ Yes ___ No
Number of incidents: _____ Date(s): _____ _____

_____ _____

_____ _____

Type of violence: Against person ___ Yes ___ No Date _____
Family ___ Yes ___ No Date _____
Stranger ___ Yes ___ No Date _____
Inmate/patient ___ Yes ___ No Date _____
RN/LPT/MD ___ Yes ___ No Date _____
Other ___ Yes ___ No Date _____
Who _____

Weapon used ___ Yes ___ No Date _____
Against property ___ Yes ___ No Date _____
Type _____
Verbal threat (only) ___ Yes ___ No Date _____
Situational factors: ETOH ___ Yes ___ No Amount _____
Street drugs ___ Yes ___ No
Type _____

_____

_____

Time of day _____ Activity _____

_____

Location _____ _____
Other factors _____

_____

Interactional factors: Engaged in interaction with victim ___ Yes ___ No
Type of interaction: _____

_____

_____

Others present: _____

_____

Content of conversation, request, argument, or dispute: _____

_____

FIGURE 21–2 Violence assessment tool (continued).

weapons are available to you, and what preparations have you made?" "How close have you come to being violent, and what is the most violent thing you have done?" (Monahan 1981).

The nurse can use this assessment tool to gather data throughout the hospitalization or during multiple hospitalizations, adding data with each admission. Nurses should not become discouraged if the data prove difficult to obtain. At this time, few practitioners use such a comprehensive framework when thinking about violence.

Integrated Management Approach

Clustering around three considerations—the client, the unit, and the staff—the integrated strategies capitalize on contributions from the importation, situationism, and interaction frameworks. These strategies emphasize negotiation, collaboration, and sensitivity to the multiple meanings each actor brings to the situation. Although the strengths and limitations of this approach to management have yet to be discovered, the strategies emphasized are compatible with the theoretic frameworks presented.

Client-Focused Strategies   The five client-focused strategies discussed below represent an extension to the strategies mentioned in the previous discussion of the importation framework.

History Taking   It is important to begin by taking comprehensive violence histories on admission. In taking the history nurses should think of each acute violent episode as an event in a life history and establish a longitudinal picture of violence in and out of the hospital. The goal of the history is to find patterns or trends in the violent behaviors to understand the conditions under which an individual is likely to act violently. (See Figure 21–2.)

Planning   After obtaining a comprehensive history and assessment data, planning treatment and setting goals with the client are the next steps. Nurses can begin to address and minimize the coercive regimentation of the hospital environment by developing a sensitivity to the individual's habits, strengths, and perceived needs. A treatment plan reflecting awareness of the client's capacity and tolerance for participation in therapeutic activities, as well as specific "cues" to violent behavior, is the goal.

Role of Catharsis in Treatment   When planning the client's treatment, be cautious in using catharsis as a way of handling the violent feelings of an individual. Encouraging clients to hit punching bags and pillows may actually increase emotions and lead to violent acts. Consult with the therapist involved in the client's treatment before recommending or initiating this technique. Teaching the client how to talk about violence and develop options to the violent behavior is a more useful intervention.

Rehash Violent Episodes   If a violent act occurs on the unit, use a rehash format for client witnesses to the violence, as well as with the individual client(s) involved if possible. A rehash is a small, spontaneous group led by staff that discusses what happened, the outcome, and the feelings of the community members about the incident (see the section "Seclusion and Restraint"). The goal is to decrease anxiety, increase understanding about violence and its management, and reduce the potential for others in the client group to behave violently.

Reintegration   If a client assaults another client or a member of the staff, it is important to reintegrate that client with the assaulted individual. If the client has been secluded after the incident, reintegration can begin after the client has regained control but before release from the seclusion room. Too often no effort is made to establish a therapeutic understanding of the events of the assault. Failure to reintegrate the individuals involved in the violent act can result in lingering anxieties for them and the larger milieu.

Unit-Focused Strategies   The six strategies presented here provide nurses with additional management strategies and are consistent with the situationism framework.

Unit Philosophy   Nurses can help develop a unit philosophy of prevention of violent behavior. No one professional discipline can assume responsibility for the prevention of violent behavior. It is important to articulate a unit philosophy that identifies shared responsibility among all disciplines for the maintenance of acceptable client behaviors.

Unit Policies   Nurses can also help establish and regularly evaluate unit policies regarding the management of violent incidents. The policies should include client consequences for violent behavior and a careful delineation of areas of responsibility among the disciplines in the management of violence in the milieu.

Team Approach   Staff members should develop a unit attitude of collaboration and negotiation and a team approach to prevention and violence management. Developing a consensus about the unit's position on violent behavior and its consequences decreases arguments and anxieties among staff and clients.

Record Keeping   Comprehensive unit record keeping of violent incidents is important. In addition to the formal unusual occurrence reports with their administrative orientation, it is useful to collect clinical documentation on incidents, which provides a basis for structured clinical audits. Contents of the clinical documentation include identification of the who, what, where, when, and how of a violent act. These notations are behavioral rather than interpretive and serve multiple purposes, including:

- Increasing understanding of violence by looking for patterns among episodes

- Teaching and clinical supervision

- Establishing and revising policy

- Conducting research

Clear Authority While no one person or discipline can prevent and manage violent behavior alone, there must be a clearly identifiable authority who makes decisions about violent incidents. Nurses who have responsibility for milieu management must have authority for decisions regarding violence management. This authority must be clearly articulated and supported by unit leaders and departmental administrators.

Review Committee A unit-based committee should be established for periodic review of incidents, policies, and mechanisms for handling client and staff issues about violent incidents. All the disciplines on the unit should be represented, with nursing as chair.

Staff-Focused Strategies The following staff strategies are suggested as the last element in the integrated management model. These staff strategies are compatible with and complementary to the client and unit strategies outlined.

Supervision The department should provide ongoing clinical supervision with an expert in management of in-patient violence.

In-Service Education Continuous in-service training on violence helps staff:

- Understand ways in which they increase their vulnerability to assault

- Develop provocation profiles of staff members to increase sensitivity and awareness among the staff

- Role play conversations with violent clients

- Practice teamwork for physical restraint procedures

- Promote a safe, nonblaming environment for staff to discuss their experiences of working with violent clients

- Develop sensitivity to the effects their own experiences of violence have in their daily work

These discussions are not a license to act in abusive or punishing ways toward clients or other staff members.

Research Nursing staff should encourage and participate in nursing research in the area of psychiatric violence and establish contact with doctoral programs in nursing, inviting interested researchers to discuss their studies and providing them access to the unit.

Rehash Nurses can encourage and ritualize the use of rehash after each incident to understand, not blame, those involved in the episode. These sessions can focus on identifying precipitants to the violence, reinforcing the client's own control, and working together as a team. The overall goal of the rehash sessions is improved competence and confidence for staff.

Support for Victims Staff victims of violence need a safe, supportive environment. When nursing staff are assaulted on the unit, establishing a "buddy system" with another nursing staff person may decrease the isolation and denial of the incident (Dawson et al. 1988, Lanza 1983, 1984). In addition, providing emotional support for the staff may decrease the potential for retaliation.

Evaluating Effectiveness of Strategies There are many elements to consider in evaluating the effectiveness of strategies for violence management. As suggested by the three theoretic frameworks, individual characteristics of the actors, conditions in the social environment, and the interactional styles of both clients and staff contribute to violent behavior. In spite of these theoretic understandings of violent behavior and efforts to implement management strategies that decrease the likelihood of its occurrence, we are not yet able to predict with certainty when someone will act in a violent manner. The fact is that violence occurs in our health care settings and that psychiatric nurses are victims of assault from psychiatric in-patients.

Victimatology

The study of victims of violent assault, whether from psychiatric in-patients or other sources, is called **victimatology**. This section focuses on the psychiatric nurse as the target of violence from psychiatric in-patients. Literature on client-nurse violence is almost nonexistent (Lanza 1983). Although much more research must be conducted on client-nurse violence, the limited information available reveals three general issues:

1. Staff reactions to the assault

2. Impact on the institutional setting

3. Services required by the victims

Staff Reactions

Lanza (1983) reports two interesting and contradictory findings:

1. Reactions of staff members who have been assaulted can last much longer than the time they are away from work.

2. Staff members often report having no reaction to the assault.

Research findings suggest that client-nurse assaults result in acute or immediate responses as well as long-term sequelae for the staff member (Lanza 1983, Ryan and Poster 1989). In addition, denial of any reaction may be the most frequent immediate response to the assault, possibly due to fear of being overwhelmed by the event if it were acknowledged.

Among the emotional reactions reported by staff who were assaulted are anger, anxiety, irritability, depression, shock, disbelief, apathy, self-blame, fear of returning to work and of other clients, disturbed sleep patterns, and other somatic symptoms, as well as a change in relationships with their coworkers and feelings of professional incompetence (Engel and Marsh 1986, Lanza 1983). In one study of psychiatric nurses, physical violence in the workplace was most frequently cited by the respondents as the reason for leaving the psychiatric nursing profession (Melick 1982). Whether these responses are typical of members from other disciplines or across different work settings is a subject for further research. It is apparent, even from the scarce information available, that for many nursing personnel, being assaulted on the job has serious personal and professional ramifications.

Institutional Implications

Violence in the context of the work environment has an impact on the setting. Although it is difficult to draw clear distinctions between the consequences for the individuals and the impact on the institution, there are several identifiable implications for the work setting. When either physical or emotional injuries occur, staff often lose time from work. The need to hire a temporary worker strains the budget. Morale is often lower among the remaining staff, who frequently share guilt and a sense of responsibility for the incident. Other staff members can feel afraid and vulnerable after an incident, and their effectiveness decreases as a result.

Often an incident of violence leads to an overemphasis on control among staff. This attitude of control takes precedence over treatment and sound clinical judgment. These measures and efforts to overcontrol can actually increase the staff's vulnerability to future assaults.

The staff may also limit their interactions with certain clients who they perceive as likely to be violent. This withdrawal and avoidance, coupled with staff anxiety, can also increase their vulnerability to assaults.

Institutional Services

Staff victims of psychiatric assault require a variety of services as well as emotional support from their unit leaders and coworkers. The employee health service or an employee assistance program can provide these services. Among these are opportunities for medical attention, trauma-crisis counseling, legal advice, and information regarding insurance, workers' compensation, and rights to health and safety in the workplace (Engel and Marsh 1986). Because of the number of incidents occurring in health care settings, many institutions have developed a policy and procedure for filing assault charges against a client. While this remains controversial, and nursing personnel report ambivalent feelings about using this option, it is being used more frequently and is considered a major institutional support for staff (Hoge and Gutheil 1987, Phelan et al. 1985, Sales et al. 1983).

Much of our understanding of staff victims of psychiatric violence is speculative. Recognizing that staff assaults occur and assuming a multidimensional response approach are important first steps. As research studies increase our knowledge about the phenomena of staff victims, their needs and the impact on the institutional setting, more specific interventions will evolve.

CHAPTER HIGHLIGHTS

• Violence is a complex human behavior with individual, environmental, and interactional components.

• In-patient psychiatric violence represents a specific type of violent behavior.

• A theoretic understanding of violence helps staff design management strategies.

• Nurses are frequent targets of in-patient psychiatric violence.

• Comprehensive assessment and treatment planning can decrease the likelihood of violent behavior among psychiatric in-patients.

• Nurses frequently deny the impact and significance of a violent assault by psychiatric clients.

• Psychiatric nurses are in a key position to contribute a unique perspective on psychiatric violence.

• Not all violence is committed by psychiatric clients and not all psychiatric clients are violent.

REFERENCES

American Psychiatric Association: *Clinical Aspects of the Violent Individual.* Task Force Report No. 8. U.S. Government Printing Office, 1974.

Armstrong B: Conference report: Handling the violent patient in the hospital. *Hosp Community Psychiatry* 1978;140:301–304.

Cobb BA: *A Descriptive Correlational Study Exploring the Relationship between Adult Psychiatric Patient Role Strain and Violence in an Inpatient Setting,* thesis. University of California, San Francisco, California, 1984.

Craig TJ: An epidemiologic study of problems associated with violence among psychiatric inpatients. *Am J Psychiatry* 1982;139:1262–1266.

Dawson J, Johnston M, Kehiayan N: Responses to patient assault: A peer support program for nurses. *J Psychosoc Nurs* 1988;26(2):8–15.

Depp FC: Assaults in a public mental hospital, in Lion JR, Reid WH (eds): *Assaults within Psychiatric Facilities.* Grune and Stratton, 1983, chap 2.

Dietz PE, Rada RT: Interpersonal violence in forensic facilities, in Lion JR, Reid WH (eds): *Assaults within Psychiatric Facilities.* Grune and Stratton, 1983, chap 3.

Duvall J: Violence is hazard for psych nurses. *American Nurse,* 1984; June:4.

Engel F, Marsh S: Helping the employee victim of violence in hospitals. *Hosp Community Psychiatry* 1986;37: 159–162.

Fottrell E: Violent behavior by psychiatric patients. *Br J Hosp Med* 1981; Jan:28–34.

Hatti S, Dubin WR, Weiss KJ: A study of circumstances surrounding patient assault on psychiatrists. *Hosp Community Psychiatry* 1982;33:660–661.

Hoge SK, Gutheil TG: The prosecution of psychiatric patients for assaults on staff: A preliminary empirical study. *Hosp Community Psychiatry* 1987;38:44–49.

Infantino JA, Musingo S-Y: Assaults and injuries among staff with and without training in aggressive control techniques. *Hosp Community Psychiatry* 1985;36: 1312–1314.

Kalogerakis MG: The assaultive psychiatric patient. *Psychiatr Q* 1971;45:372–381.

Kinzel AF: Body-buffer zones in violent prisoners. *Am J Psychiatry* 1970;127:99–104.

Lanza ML: A follow-up study of nurses' reactions to physical assault. *Hosp Community Psychiatry* 1984;35: 492–494.

Lanza ML: The reactions of nursing staff to physical assault by a patient. *Hosp Community Psychiatry* 1983;34: 44–47.

Levy P, Hartocollis P: Nursing aids and patient violence. *Am J Psychiatry* 1976;133:429–431.

Lion JR: Special aspects of psychopharmacology, in Lion JR, Reid WH (eds): *Assaults within Psychiatric Facilities.* Grune and Stratton, 1983, chap 19.

Lion JR, Snyder W, Merrill GL: Underreporting of assaults on staff in a state hospital. *Hosp Community Psychiatry* 1981;32:497–498.

Madden DJ: Recognition and prevention of violence in psychiatric facilities, in Lion JR, Reid WH (eds): *Assaults within Psychiatric Facilities.* Grune and Stratton, 1983.

Madden DJ, Lion JR, Penna MW: Assaults on psychiatrists by patients. *Am J Psychiatry* 1976;133:422–425.

Maier G et al.: A model for understanding and managing cycles of aggression among psychiatric inpatients. *Hosp Community Psychiatry* 1987;38:5:520–524.

McCoy SM, Garritson SH: Seclusion: The process of intervening. *J Psychosoc Nurs Ment Health Serv* 1983;21:8–15.

Melick ME: *Factors Associated with Psychiatric Nurse Turnover: A Report on an Exit Survey and Some Recommendations.* Funded by Grant No. 5T23MH-15378-04. Manpower programs for a changing mental health system, National Institute of Mental Health, January 1982.

Monahan J: *Predicting Violent Behavior: An Assessment of Clinical Techniques.* Sage Publications, 1981.

Nigrosh BJ: Physical contact skills in specialized training for the prevention and management of violence, in Lion JR, Reid WH (eds): *Assaults within Psychiatric Facilities.* Grune and Stratton, 1983.

Phelan LA, Mills MJ, Ryan J: Prosecuting psychiatric patients for assaults. *Hosp Community Psychiatry* 1985;36:581–582.

Poster EC, Ryan JA: Nurses' attitudes toward physical assaults by patients. *Arch Psychiatr Nurs* 1989; 3(6):315–322.

Quinsey VC, Varney GW: Characteristics of assaults and assaulters in a maximum security hospital unit. *Crimes and Justice* 1977;5:212–220.

Rabkin JG: Criminal behavior of discharged mental patients: A critical appraisal of the research. *Psychol Bull* 1979;85:1–27.

Rogers R, Ciula B, Cavanaugh JL: Aggressive and socially disruptive behavior among maximum security psychiatric patients. *Psychol Rep* 1980;46:291–294.

Ruben I, Wolkon G, Yamamoto J: Physical attacks on psychiatric residents by patients. *J Nerv Ment Dis* 1980;168:243–245.

Ryan JA, Poster EC: The assaulted nurse: Short-term and long-term responses. *Arch Psychiatr Nurs* 1989; 3(6):323–331.

Sales BD, Overcast TD, Merrikin KJ: Worker's compensation protection for assaults and batteries on mental health professionals, in Lion JR, Reid WH (eds): *Assaults within Psychiatric Facilities.* Grune and Stratton, 1983.

Soloff PH: Seclusion and restraint, in Lion JR, Reid WH (eds): *Assaults within Psychiatric Facilities.* Grune and Stratton, 1983.

Stanton AH, Schwartz MS: *The Mental Hospital.* Basic Books, 1954.

Steadman HJ: Special problems: The prediction of violence among the mentally ill, in Hays JR, Roberts TK, Soloway KF (eds): *Violence and the Violent Individual.* Spectrum, 1981.

Straker M et al.: Assaultive behaviors in an institutional setting. *Psychiatr J Univ Ottawa* 1977;II:185–190.

Tardiff K: The use of medication for assaultive patients. *Hosp Community Psychiatry* 1981;33:307–308.

Tardiff K: A survey of assault by chronic patients in a state hospital system, in Lion JR, Reid WH (eds): *Assaults within Psychiatric Facilities*. Grune and Stratton, 1983.

Tardiff K: *The Psychiatric Use of Seclusion and Restraint*. American Psychiatry Press, 1984a.

Tardiff K: Violence: The psychiatric patient, in Turner JT (ed): *Violence in the Medical Care Setting*. Aspen, 1984b.

Tardiff K, Sweillam A: Assaultive behavior among chronic psychiatric inpatients. *Am J Psychiatry* 1982;139: 212–215.

Tardiff K, Sweillam A: Assault, suicide and mental illness. *Arch Gen Psychiatry* 1980;37:164–169.

Whitman RN, Armao B, Dent OB: Assault on the therapist. *Am J Psychiatry* 1976;133:426–429.

Rape and Intrafamily Abuse and Violence

LEARNING OBJECTIVES

- Discuss the incidence of rape and intrafamily physical and sexual abuse

- Discuss theories related to the dynamics of rape, intrafamily physical abuse, and intrafamily sexual abuse

- Identify the behavioral, affective, cognitive, physiologic, and sociocultural characteristics related to rape-trauma syndrome, intrafamily physical abuse, and intrafamily sexual abuse

- Repudiate myths about rape and intrafamily violence with facts about rape and intrafamily violence

- Assess a client and family behaviorally, affectively, cognitively, physiologically, and socioculturally

- Formulate appropriate nursing diagnoses for rape victims, victims of intrafamily physical or sexual abuse, and their families

- Plan and implement interventions for victims of rape or intrafamily physical or sexual abuse and their families

- Evaluate the effectiveness of nursing interventions for these clients and their families

Karen Lee Fontaine

CROSS REFERENCES

Other topics relevant to this content are: Anxiety disorders, Chapter 14; Elder abuse, Chapter 35; Family dynamics and family therapy, Chapter 30; Multiple personality, Chapter 16; Post-traumatic stress disorder, Chapter 14; Sexual disorders, Chapter 15; Substance abuse, Chapter 11.

VIOLENCE THAT IS DEMONSTRATED as rape or occurs as physical or sexual abuse within the family is a national health problem that confronts not only psychiatric nurses but also nurses in many different clinical settings. Victims are seen in the community, in pediatric units, in intensive care units, in medical-surgical units, in maternal care settings, in ambulatory care facilities, in geriatric units, and in psychiatric settings.

Nurses need to assess and provide appropriate intervention for the emotional consequences, as well as the physical trauma, of rape. Nurses may be called on to give legal evidence in the prosecution of a rapist. Within the community, nurses can establish, or refer victims to, support groups. They can also become active in increasing public awareness of rape through formal and informal teaching activities. Because of their unique position, nurses can be active in the prevention of rape and treatment of its victims.

Nurses also need to be involved in the prevention, detection, and treatment of intrafamily violence. Developing a knowledge base and being able to identify factors that contribute to intrafamily violence help nurses assume a preventive role. Part of this role is providing public education and becoming active in changes in public policy. This knowledge, along with increased awareness of the extent of the problem, helps nurses arrive at earlier, more accurate detection of intrafamily violence. Nurses also need to comply with state laws on the reporting of violence and referral for treatment. Some nurses with advanced education in family therapy are part of the therapy teams that intervene with violent families.

Rape

Rape is a crime of violence second only to homicide in its violation of a person. The issue is not one of sexuality but one of force, domination, and humiliation. In this text, **rape** refers to any forced sex act. The key factor is lack of adult consent. Legal definitions vary from state to state. In many states, rape is defined as forced sexual intercourse against a female who is not married to the perpetrator. Other states have broadened the definition to include other sex acts. The legal climate in regard to marital rape is beginning to change. In many states a husband cannot be charged with rape if he sexually assaults his wife. But other states have recognized that rape can be committed within a marriage and that the husband can be prosecuted.

From the perspective of the victim, rape occurs very suddenly. There is often no warning of the attack, which most frequently occurs between 6:00 P.M. and midnight. However, the majority of rapes are not sudden and impulsive; indeed, 60 to 75 percent of all rapes are well planned.

The perpetrators often use guns or knives and may tie the victim or use verbal intimidation, such as a threat of death. Some victims attempt to offer physical resistance, and some succeed. Others may reason or plead with the perpetrator. However, fear of death and the suddenness of the event make many victims unable either to flee or to fight.

Victims of Rape

There is no typical rape victim although, of reported rapes, 93 percent of the victims are female, and 90 percent of the perpetrators are male. One can be a victim of rape at any age, from childhood through old age. The average age of female children who are raped is 7.9 years, and in 80 percent of the cases, the perpetrator is someone the child knows. The rapist may attack strangers, acquaintances, friends, or family members. With increased awareness of the possibility of rape, women are becoming more sensitive to preventive measures. Since this means being suspicious of men in potential rape environments, all women and men are, in one sense, victims of rape. Women have become fearful for their safety, and men, in general, are the recipients of this fear and suspicion. Thus, everyone is affected, at least indirectly, by the crime of rape.

Male victims of rape are just beginning to come to the attention of the general public. Like females, males can be raped at any age. The myth of male rape has been that it occurs only where heterosexual contact is not possible, such as in prisons or in isolated living conditions. As more male rape victims report the crime, however, this myth has been exploded. Male rape is not a homosexual attack. Again the issue is one of violence and domination rather than one of sexuality. Some rapists, who define themselves as heterosexual, will rape both males and females; at times, they rape whoever is available.

In the past, men have been afraid to report rape for fear of being ridiculed or not believed. As was true for females in the past, society has a tendency to blame the male victim by saying such things as, "He must have thought you were trying to pick him up," "You must have made him angry," or "You could have resisted if you had really wanted to." Male rape victims undergo the same emotional trauma that female victims do, and

Portions of this chapter appeared in another form in Cook JS, Fontaine KL: *Essentials of Mental Health Nursing*, ed 2. Addison-Wesley, 1991.

they need the same protection, interventions, and understanding accorded to female victims (Seeley 1985).

Incidence of Rape

It is difficult to determine the incidence of rape, since it is the most underreported crime. Because of shame and fear of being blamed, victims have been hesitant to report and testify. It is projected that one woman in six will experience an attempted rape sometime in her lifetime, and one woman in eight will be forced to submit. Between the ages of 16 and 19, females are at the highest risk for being raped. Nonwhite victims are more likely to be raped at an earlier age, with the highest risk being between 12 and 19 years of age. The highest risk for white victims is between the ages of 20 and 34. Most often, the rapist is of the same race as the victim (Erickson 1989).

It was not until 1974 that the first case of **marital rape** was prosecuted in the United States. Before then, the law viewed married women as the property of their husbands. Even today, some women are beaten and raped by their husbands, often in full view of their children. Not infrequently, marital rape is accompanied by extreme violence. Current estimates are that 8 million women in the United States are at risk for marital rape, which may be the most underreported type of rape. Among battered women, 35 to 50 percent are also raped. The time of greatest danger is when the woman leaves or threatens to leave her partner. He perceives her leaving as a challenge to his dominance and control, and he often responds by using sex to humiliate and dominate (McLeer 1988, Pagelow 1988).

Also often unreported is **acquaintance rape,** or **date rape,** which is growing in incidence. Of all women raped on college campuses, 50 percent are raped by acquaintances. Women very rarely report rapes when they know their attackers and especially if they were in a dating relationship. Failure to report such rapes in part reflects the cultural value that under certain circumstances it is acceptable for a man to coerce or force a woman to have sex. The victim is often blamed, by herself and others, for being naive or provocative. Another cultural value, slow to die, is that a woman who accepts a date and allows the man to pay for all the expenses somehow "owes" him sexual access. To combat this problem, many universities have established antirape seminars and counseling services for both women and men (Shotland 1989).

Rape-Trauma Syndrome

Burgess and Holmstrom (1979) first described **rape-trauma syndrome** as a two-phase syndrome of *disorganization* (the acute phase) and *reorganization.* An intermediate phase, *outward adjustment,* was proposed by others (Golan 1978). These phases and the rape victim's accompanying responses are described in Table 22–1. The characteristics of rape victims in each of these phases are discussed next.

Behavioral Characteristics Many victims of rape do not report the crime, sometimes because of guilt or embarrassment about what has occurred. Other victims are fearful of how their families or the police will react to the information. Some perpetrators threaten victims by saying they will return to rape them again if the police are notified. Because many of the crimes are committed by acquaintances, friends, dates, or husbands, victims fear they will not be believed. This has been termed the *silent reaction.* It dooms the victim to experiencing the rape-trauma syndrome without the help of support systems.

Some rape victims respond immediately with agitated and nonpurposeful behavior. They are brought to the emergency room emotionally distraught and unable to respond to questions about what has occurred. So great is their level of anxiety and fear that they may be unable to follow simple directions.

Other rape victims may return home and shower or bathe before notifying the police or going to the emergency room. In the past, this behavior has been viewed with suspicion of a false charge of rape. It is now recognized that people who have been violated by

---

TABLE 22–1 **Phases of the Rape-Trauma Syndrome**

Phase	Response
Acute phase	Fear, shock, disbelief, desire for revenge, anger, denial, anxiety, guilt, embarrassment, humiliation, helplessness, dependency; victim may seek help or may remain silent.
Outward adjustment phase	Victim appears outwardly composed, denying and repressing feelings; for example, she returns to work, buys a weapon, adds security measures to her residence, and denies need for counseling.
Reorganizational phase	Victim experiences sexual dysfunction, phobias, sleep disorders, anxiety, and a strong urge to talk about or resolve feelings; victim may seek counseling or may remain silent.

SOURCE: *Niehaus MA: Rape, in Griffith-Kenney J:* Contemporary Women's Health. *Addison-Wesley, 1986, p 226.*

rape experience extreme feelings of helplessness. Often, this cleaning-up behavior is an attempt to regain control of the self and return to the normality that was so suddenly disrupted.

The majority of victims appear in good control of their feelings and behavior immediately after the rape. This appearance of outward calmness usually indicates a state of numbness, disbelief, and emotional shock: "This whole thing doesn't seem real," "I must be dreaming. This couldn't have happened," or, "I just can't believe this has happened to me."

Doreen, a graduate student at the local university, was brought to the hospital by the police who found her running down the street half clothed. In the hospital she was able to tell the staff that she had been raped by her date, Mike, another graduate student. She exhibited outward calmness but kept repeating "This cannot have happened to me. My friends introduced us and he seemed so nice." She could not decide whom to call to take her back to the dorm or what to tell her friends about what had happened.

Nurses need to recognize that underneath the facade of control and calmness is a person in acute distress. The nurse should support the victims' need to control until they are able to manage the reality of their situation. Nurses who assume that the calmness indicates no distress will miss the victims' needs for emotional support and intervention.

Rape may have long-term effects on behavior. Some rape victims are prone to crying spells that they may or may not be able to explain. Some may have difficulty maintaining or forming interpersonal relationships, especially with people who remind them of the perpetrator. Many victims develop problems at work or school. Some report nightmares and have difficulty sleeping. Others develop secondary phobic reactions to people, objects, or situations that remind them of the rape (Resick 1983). A woman who is a victim of marital rape suffers additional problems. Often she must continue to interact with her rapist because she is dependent on him. She may be forced to pretend, to herself and to other family members and friends, that the rape never occurred. Until it becomes more socially acceptable and legally feasible to report marital rape, many of these victims will suffer in silence.

Affective Characteristics Victims of rape suffer immediate and long-lasting emotional trauma. After a period of shock and disbelief, many experience episodes of anxiety and depression. Anxiety is a response to a threat or assault on one's integrity, and depression may be a response to loss. Rape victims have been threatened, both physically and emotionally. They

have experienced a loss of autonomy, control, safety, and self-esteem. Thus, anxiety and depressive reactions in response to rape are not unusual (Hartman and Burgess 1988).

Many victims feel ashamed and embarrassed about the rape, because sexual behavior is normally an intimate, private act. They often feel unclean or contaminated. These feelings are unique to victims of rape as opposed to victims of other crimes. Many women are humiliated by having to disclose the details of the rape to police officers and in a courtroom, particularly since women have been socialized not to talk about sexual behavior in public. Victims who do not report rape generally say it was too private or personal for them to talk about it with strangers.

Rape victims feel physically and emotionally violated. The loss of control over their bodies and their autonomy leads to feelings of helplessness and vulnerability. They may feel alienated from friends and family, particularly if there is not a strong supportive network. Feeling angry is a healthy response to the violation that has occurred, but the victim needs to discharge the energy of anger appropriately so that she does not later become consumed with fantasies of revenge.

Cognitive Characteristics During the actual rape, some victims use the defense mechanisms of depersonalization or dissociation to cope with the attack. By perceiving the attack as "not really happening to me" the victims protect their sense of integrity. Other victims rely on denial to block out the traumatic experience. The victim may continue to use these defense mechanisms through the initial stages of treatment, and the nurse should support their use until the person is able to face the reality of the attack (Resick 1983).

Victims often enter the emergency room in a state of confusion. They may have great difficulty concentrating and appear unsure of exactly what has occurred. This confusion and uncertainty are not evidence that a rape did not occur, but indications of emotional shock. Moreover, the victim's problem-solving and decision-making abilities are greatly reduced during the immediate aftermath of the rape as the result of anxiety and fear.

Some victims are unable to discuss the attack at all. Some may not even be able to report the rape until the next day when they feel better prepared to cope with the event and the subsequent procedures. Other victims are very concerned about which family members and friends they should tell. They may be uncertain about how significant others will react to the information that a rape has occurred. They also may not know how to tell others about the experience and may depend on the nurse for guidance and support.

Some victims blame themselves for the rape during the initial stages. This self-blame is reflected in statements such as, "If only I had taken a different way home," "I should have been able to escape because he didn't have a gun," or "I should have fought harder than I did." Marital rape victims may also blame themselves: "If I were a better wife, he wouldn't have raped me," or "If I tried harder to please him sexually, he wouldn't have to force me."

Some victims develop obsessional thoughts about the rape, which may be severe enough to interfere with daily functioning. Some, though not obsessed, experience periodic flashbacks of the event. Others are preoccupied with thoughts of future danger, and violent dreams are common.

Rape may profoundly affect one's beliefs about the environment. Victims assaulted at home generally lose the sense of home as a safe place. Some victims, especially those who know the rapist, fear retaliation by the perpetrator for reporting the crime. Other victims, particularly young women and girls, may generalize their fear to all men or all strange men. Women who have been raped by their husbands often state that they have lost their ability to trust the husband or any other man.

Physiologic Characteristics Rape usually results in a number of physical injuries. Generally, the vagina or rectum is sore and swollen. There may be tearing of the vaginal or rectal wall from forceful insertion of the penis or a foreign object. The throat may be traumatized by forced oral sex. The victim may also be beaten, stabbed, or shot. Profuse bleeding and injuries to vital organs may be critical problems.

Female victims of child-bearing years may become pregnant as a result of the rape. Victims of all ages and both genders may contract a sexually transmitted disease from the perpetrator. This could be transmitted to mucous membranes in the vagina, mouth, or throat.

In addition to the immediate physical trauma, there may be serious, long-term physiologic effects. Victims may experience insomnia or anorexia a long time after the event. Some victims complain of fatigue or generalized aches and pains, and may experience gynecologic problems. They may also experience the long-term effects of a beating, stabbing, or shooting. Victims are also at risk for developing a psychophysiologic disorder in response to a chronically high level of anxiety and fear.

Future sexual functioning may be adversely affected. The likelihood of developing a sexual dysfunction depends on the quality of sexual experience and relationships before the attack, the behavior used to cope with the attack, and the quality of future relationships. Women victims of marital rape often have more difficulty adjusting sexually in a subsequent relationship. Nearly all adult rape victims need to withdraw from sexual activity for a time. For some, the period of celibacy is necessary to reestablish control and autonomy. Others may choose abstinence because they feel unclean or contaminated. Both the victim and the sexual partner need to understand that the need for closeness and nondemanding physical contact continues. Giving comfort through touch decreases the partner's feelings of rejection and the victim's feelings of self-blame or uncleanness.

Sociocultural Characteristics Families experience many of the same thoughts and feelings as the rape victim. They may talk about guilt, doubts, fears, hatred toward the perpetrator, and feelings of helplessness. They need to be educated about the nature and trauma of the rape and the immediate and long-term potential reactions of the victim. They need support and direction in helping the victim so that they do not overprotect the victim or minimize the impact of the rape.

Many cultural myths surround the crime of rape. Examples of these myths and the facts that nurses can use to dispel them are presented in the accompanying Client/Family Teaching box. In the past twenty years, great strides have been made to abolish these myths from the legal system and to treat rape as the crime of violence it is.

Changing the personal belief system of the general public has been a slower process. Many people continue to believe the myth that the victim rather than the perpetrator is to blame. In one study, 50 percent of both women and men accepted the myths without question. The greatest predictors of acceptance of the myths were rigid gender role stereotyping and the acceptance of interpersonal violence by the participants (Burt 1980). Thus, people who are more flexible in gender roles and abhor violence are more likely to support the victim and blame the perpetrator.

Theoretic Perspectives

Intrapersonal Theories Rape is a crime of violence generated by issues of power and anger rather than by sexual drive. According to the intrapersonal view, rapists are emotionally immature persons who feel powerless and unsure of themselves. They are incapable of managing the normal stresses of everyday life. The causes of rape are multidetermined, but the dynamics of the act are that perpetrators abuse their own and others' sexuality to discharge anger and frustration. From this perspective, there are three types of rape: the anger rape, the power rape, and the sadistic rape.

The **anger rape** is distinguished by physical violence and cruelty to the victim. The rapist believes he is the victim of an unjust society and takes revenge on others by raping. He uses extreme force and vicious-

CLIENT/FAMILY TEACHING

Rape Myths versus Rape Facts

Myth: Sexual assault is caused by uncontrollable sex drives.

Fact

Sexual assault is an act of physical and emotional violence, not of sexual gratification. Men assault to dominate, humiliate, control, degrade, terrify, and violate. Studies show that power and anger are the primary motivating factors.

Myth: Women provoke sexual assault, and sex appeal is of prime importance in selecting targets.

Fact

Women who have been sexually assaulted range in age from infants to the elderly. Appearance and attractiveness are not relevant. A man assaults someone who is accessible and appears vulnerable.

Myth: Women are usually sexually assaulted by strangers.

Fact

Studies show that the majority of those sexually assaulted are acquainted with their assailants.

Myth: Most sexual assaults are interracial.

Fact

As a national average, more than 90 percent of all sexual assaults occur between people of the same race, although attacks by men of color against white women are given more publicity.

There is evidence of racial bias in our legal system: Although men of color are estimated to constitute a small proportion of sexual assailants, they are 48 percent of those convicted and 80 percent of those jailed for assault.

Myth: Sexual assault is unplanned and spontaneous.

Fact

Studies show that a majority of sexual assaults are planned in advance.

Myth: Women make false reports of sexual assault.

Fact

Statistics show that 2 percent of reports of alleged rape are unfounded; this is the same proportion as for all other crimes.

Myth: Men do not have to be concerned about sexual assault because it affects women.

Fact

Men, both straight and gay, suffered 10 percent of the sexual assaults treated last year at the San Francisco Sexual Trauma Services. In addition, men have wives, friends, mothers, and daughters who may someday need help coping with the aftereffects of sexual assault. Last, rape will not cease until men stop raping.

SOURCE: *Adapted from* Resources Against Sexual Assault. *Rape Prevention Education Program, University of California, San Francisco, 1987, pp 5–6.*

---

ness to debase the victim. The ability to injure, traumatize, and shame the victim provides an outlet for his rage and temporary relief from his turmoil. Rapes occur episodically as the rage builds up and he strikes out at others to relieve his pain.

In the **power rape,** the intent of the rapist is not to injure the victim but to command and master another person sexually. The rapist has an insecure self-image and feelings of incompetence and inadequacy. The rape is the vehicle for expressing power, potency, and might. Seeing the victim as a conquest, the rapist temporarily feels omnipotent.

The **sadistic rape** also involves brutality. The use of bondage and torture is not an expression of anger but necessary for the rapist's sexual excitement. The

assault is eroticized and is sexually stimulating. To achieve sexual gratification, he needs an unwilling sexual partner who will resist his advances. Rape becomes a source of excitement in his life (Pagelow 1988).

Interpersonal Theories Some rapists are unable to develop intimate and strong relationships with other men and women. The relationships they do have are unequal and characterized by a lack of mutuality and an inability to share. With this model for relationships, the rapist sees no need for consent to sexual activity, particularly within a marital relationship. The husband may view the rape as merely a disagreement over sexual activity. Unless he is extremely brutal, the wife may not regard the forced sex as an assault and rape either. Both of them may view sexual relationships as exploitive rather than a process of mutual sharing. If the wife has said she does not want to engage in sex and the husband uses force, her control and autonomy have been violated. When sex occurs without consent, it is, in fact rape. What appears to be a conflict over sex in the marriage is actually a conflict over power and the right to consent to or refuse a given activity (Pagelow 1988).

Sociocultural Theories   The acceptance of interpersonal violence in a culture contributes to a higher incidence of rape within that culture. Society's approval of the use of intimidation, coercion, and force to achieve one's goals promotes violence. It becomes an issue of power and strength rather than a consideration of individuals' rights.

Rigid gender role expectations and stereotypes may be correlated with the incidence of rape. The belief that women are inferior to men gives tacit approval to coercion and force. These stereotypes support the false beliefs that at times women deserve to be raped, that they may want or need to be raped, and that it does not cause them much physical or emotional damage.

More than half of sexually abused women are the victims of marital rape or date rape. Some theorists propose that the reason for this type of rape are sociocultural and can be traced to societal attitudes toward females. These stereotypes are perpetuated when, in cases of marital or date rape, the woman's actions, rather than the man's, are questioned. It is believed that elimination of stereotypes and sexism will decrease men's use of rape as a way to demon-

strate power and control (Resick 1983). Russell (1975, p 16) describes it this way:

Rape is the ultimate sexist act. It is an act of physical and psychic oppression. Eradicating rape requires getting rid of the power discrepancy between men and women, because abuse of power flows from unequal power.

Steps that men can take to prevent rape are presented in the Client/Family Teaching box below.

Ageism, which defines the older person as weak and incompetent, is a correlate to the crime of rape. Older people, especially those who are socially isolated or live alone, are seen as easy victims. Some older people, believing the myth that only young women are raped, do not protect themselves as well as they could. Especially vulnerable are older people who have established patterns of daily activities that can be readily observed. If they depend on walking or public transportation, they can be more easily accosted, particularly if their vision and hearing are impaired. Moreover, they may have neither the physical strength to resist a rape nor the ability to outrun the rapist.

Prevention and Resistance

Awareness, trusting intuitive feelings, and assertive behavior are the key to preventing rape. Although awareness can be taught, it may be difficult for women to rely on their intuition or be assertive because they do not want to appear suspicious or unfriendly. However, politeness and friendliness may signal to the rapist that one is an "easy mark" and unlikely to resist. Rape prevention strategies in various environmental settings are presented in the Client/Family Teaching box on the opposite page.

 CLIENT/FAMILY TEACHING

Steps Men Can Take to Prevent Rape

- Tell other men that you do not think rape jokes are funny.
- Set time aside to talk with the women in your life about working toward equal relationships.
- Confront men who are harassing women on the street or at a party.
- Point out sexist comments and behavior to your friends and coworkers.
- Be aware of situations that increase a woman's vulnerability. How would you respond if you witnessed an intoxicated woman at a party being escorted by two or three men to a bedroom?

- If a woman says no to your sexual advances, respect that no at face value. Do not accept the myth that no means yes.
- In a dating or intimate relationship communicate clearly how you feel and what you want. Do not assume that your date or partner feels the same way. Respect the other person's feelings and needs.
- Learn new skills to help you express your anger in constructive, rather than destructive, ways.

SOURCE: *Adapted from* Resources Against Sexual Assault. *Rape Prevention Education Program, University of California, San Francisco, 1987, p 4.*

CLIENT/FAMILY TEACHING

Rape Prevention Strategies

At Home

In an apartment or house:

- Good locks on doors and windows make it difficult for assailants and burglars to get in. If you have a deadbolt, use it. For information on window locks and other home security measures consult the crime prevention unit of your local police department.

- When you're home alone, pull the shades or curtains after dark. If you let someone in and have second thoughts, be assertive: (1) tell him to leave; (2) leave if you can; (3) call a friend or neighbor and ask her or him to come over; (4) pretend you're not alone; mention a family member or a friend who is sleeping or about to return.

- Make sure hallways, entrances, garages, and grounds are well lighted. (Timers or photosensitive devices may be installed to conserve electricity.) Leave porch light on all night. When away from home at night or if you expect to return after dark, leave an interior light on in a room or two with shades drawn, and leave a radio on.

- Install a peephole in your door.

- When someone is at your door, never open it without first asking who's there. Repair and sales people, police and survey takers carry identification; ask to see it and then call the company to verify before letting the person in. If someone wants to use your phone, make the call for him, while he waits outside.

- Leave spare house keys with a friend, not under the doormat, in planter boxes, and so on.

- Get to know your neighbors so you can get help if necessary and are familiar with who's coming and going in the neighborhood.

- List last name and two initials only on mailbox and door and in phone book. Consider not listing your address in the phone book.

- Avoid giving out information about yourself or making appointments with strangers over the phone.

- Have a preconceived escape plan.

In residence halls and student housing:

- Living groups are only as safe as the residents make them. *Take your share of responsibility.* Always keep outside doors locked. Ask strangers to wait outside while you get their friends. Lock your room when you leave—even if only for a few minutes. Look out for one another.

In Public Places

On the street:

- *Be alert.* Look around you; be aware of who else is on the street; make it difficult for anyone to take you by surprise.

- Wait a few minutes so that you can walk or bike with others. If you have a choice, don't walk alone.

- Stay on populated, well-lighted streets when you can.

- If possible, avoid dark or concealed areas— consider open areas—walk in the street if it appears to be safer.

- If you think someone is following you:
  - Turn around and check so you're not caught off guard.
  - Cross the street, change direction.
  - Walk or run toward people, traffic.
  - Consider confronting the man with a loud, firm voice, "Don't follow me!"
  - Do anything necessary to enter an occupied building; throw something through a window if necessary.

- If a car follows you or stops, do not approach the car. Change directions, walk or run toward other people, stores, or a house.

In the car:

- Park in well-lighted areas at night; pay for parking. Check the street before leaving the car.

- Walk to your car with key ready.

- Check the back seat before you get in to make sure no one is hiding there.

- While driving, keep doors locked so no one can jump in at a red light.

- Keep enough gas in your tank for emergencies.

- If you're followed by another car, drive to a

CLIENT/FAMILY TEACHING (continued)

police or fire station, or hospital emergency entrance or any open business or gas station. DON'T go home or to a friend's home. If necessary, call attention to yourself by honking the horn or speeding.

- If your car breaks down, lift hood, put on flashers, and wait inside with the doors locked. Ask people who stop to call the Highway Patrol (or AAA if you are a member).
- Don't stop for a stranded motorist; call the Highway Patrol, local police, or sheriff's department, who can help him.

Elevators:

- Trust your intuition; if you feel uncomfortable you don't have to get on or off.
- Stand near the controls. If necessary, you can press all the buttons or use the telephone.

Jogging:

- Be aware.
- Try to avoid jogging alone, even in daylight.
- Stay on well-lighted paths in open areas.
- Vary your route.
- Be suspicious of people you pass many times.

Hitchhiking:

Hitchhiking increases your vulnerability to sexual assault. However, if you do risk it:

- Consider taking rides only from women.
- Ask first where a driver is going before you

volunteer your destination; never go with someone who offers to take you wherever you want to go.

- If there is more than one man in a car, do not accept a ride.
- Always jot down the license number of the car.
- While entering the car, check to be sure there is an inside handle to the door on the passenger side.
- Mention that someone is waiting for you and will be anxious if you are late.

Using public transportation:

- If possible, wait for buses at well-lighted stops.
- *Be alert* so you can't be grabbed from behind.
- If possible, join other people at a nearby stop.
- If anyone bothers you on the bus:
  - In a loud, firm voice say "Leave me alone!"
  - Let other riders and the bus driver know what's happening.
  - If the bus is radio dispatched, ask the driver to call the police.
  - Don't get off in an isolated area.
- Notice who else gets off at your stop. If someone is following you, practice the tips for street safety.

SOURCE: *Adapted from* Resources Against Sexual Assault. *Rape Prevention Education Program, University of California, San Francisco, 1987, pp 13–17.*

There is no one easy answer to the question of how one should behave if attacked. According to the Rape Prevention Education Program at the University of California, research indicates that while an immediate aggressive response increases one's possibility of escape when rape is threatened, it can sometimes slightly aggravate the situation (*Resources Against Sexual Assault,* 1987). Suggestions for resisting attack are discussed in the Client/Family Teaching box on the opposite page.

The Nursing Process and the Rape Victim

Before rape victims are assessed or treated, they need to be informed of their rights, which include the right to have:

- A rape crisis advocate accompany them to the hospital
- Their personal physician notified
- Privacy during the assessment and treatment process
- Family, friends, or an advocate present during the questioning and examination
- Confidentiality maintained by all staff
- Gentle and sensitive treatment
- Detailed explanations and consent for all tests and procedures
- Referrals for follow-up treatment and counseling

The nurse functions as an advocate for rape victims in supporting these rights.

CLIENT/FAMILY TEACHING

Suggestions for Resisting Attack

- Evaluate the situation for possible ways of escape. If one method doesn't work, try another, and another; often women have had to try several before one worked.

- Resist only as long as you feel it is safe to do so. If resistance proves to be too dangerous, stop. It may be less dangerous, however, to risk minor injury in order to escape than to remain in an assault situation.

Women have deterred assailants in a variety of ways. Talking and thinking about what you might do if attacked increase your chances for successfully defending yourself. We provide the following brief list to stimulate your thinking.

Verbal

- Deep, guttural yell that is simply a startling sound, not any word.

- Yell directions, e.g., "Call the police, this man is after me!"

- Yell "fire" rather than "help" or "rape." Though our intent is not to hide sexual assault from the community, yelling "fire" is more apt to bring a response, because people are concerned with protecting their own property. If *you* ever hear a yell of "help" or "rape," take it seriously and respond.

- Do something unpredictable.

- Assertive verbal confrontation, e.g., "Leave me alone!" "Stop bothering me!"

- Make noise, e.g., throw a heavy object through your window if someone attempts to enter your home.

Physical

- Escape, or put something between you and him.

- Run

- Fight (see information on self-defense).

- Use available objects as weapons.

- Use tear gas. In the State of California you must take a class to obtain a license to carry tear gas legally. We recommend taking a class that informs you of the drawbacks of tear gas as well as the situations in which it is effective. Using tear gas is one of several options and cannot be relied on to work in every situation. It works best when used in conjunction with physical self-defense techniques.

Only the person being attacked can decide whether resistance or submission is the safer thing to do. If you do submit, it doesn't mean you asked for it, enjoyed it, or wanted it. Rather, you chose the best survival technique available to you at the time.

Self-Defense Classes

As previously mentioned, an immediate aggressive response is more likely to result in rape avoidance than in further violence. We urge women to take classes in street-fighting techniques that can be learned in a relatively short period of time. The benefits of learning self-defense include increased options for self-protection, self-confidence, and verbal and nonverbal assertiveness skills. If you decide to resist physically, know how to do it effectively. The Rape Prevention Education Program recommends classes that combine street-fighting techniques with sexual assault prevention information.

SOURCE: *Adapted from* Resources Against Sexual Assault. *Rape Prevention Education Program, University of California, San Francisco, 1987, pp 19–21.*

Assessing

First assess the rape victim physically from head to toe for any serious or critical injuries resulting from the assault. With the victim's permission, a vaginal examination is performed to determine the need for treatment and to obtain documentation for legal proceedings. Again with permission, photographs of the injuries may be taken for legal documentation (Foley 1984). The physical assessment process must be carefully documented in writing to assist with possible prosecution of the perpetrator. Guidelines to assist with physical assessment are given in the Assessment box on page 518.

Next, assess the victim's mental status. Behavioral, affective, and cognitive responses to the traumatic event need to be gathered. A sociocultural assessment

ASSESSMENT

Physical Assessment of the Rape Victim

Complete a head-to-toe physical assessment with particular attention to the following:

Head

Evidence of trauma

Facial bruises

Facial fractures

Eyes: swollen, bruised, hemorrhages

Skin

Bruises

Genital trauma

Rectal trauma

Musculoskeletal

Fractures of the ribs

Fractures of arms/legs

Dislocated joints

Impaired mobility

Abdomen

Bruises or wounds

Evidence of internal injuries

Other

Have physical injuries such as scratches, bruises, and cuts been recorded and photographed?

Have fingernail scrapings been taken and preserved?

Has blood typing been done?

Have smears for sexually transmitted diseases been taken of the mouth, throat, vagina, and rectum?

Have combings of the pubic hair been made and preserved?

Has genital trauma been recorded and photographed?

Has rectal trauma been recorded and photographed?

Have semen specimens been preserved?

When was the client's last menstrual period?

Has the clothing been inspected for rips, blood, and stains?

Has the clothing been preserved?

---

provides additional data for planning appropriate interventions. Guidelines for assessing the rape victim's mental status are given in the Assessment box on the opposite page.

Victims who present a controlled style may be able to respond to assessment questions, but those in a state of emotional shock and disbelief may find it difficult to engage actively in the assessment process. The method by which the nurse completes the assessment obviously depends on the person's response to the trauma.

Diagnosing

The central NANDA diagnosis for clients who have been raped is rape-trauma syndrome. This is a general category for clients experiencing the phases described in Table 22–1, earlier. Several other nursing diagnoses may also be appropriate, depending on the client's needs and the results of both physical and mental status assessment.

There is no corresponding DSM-III-R diagnosis. Rape is, however, mentioned specifically as the type of trauma that may result in post-traumatic stress disor-

der. Rape victims may also experience one of the anxiety disorders or sexual dysfunctions discussed in DSM-III-R.

Planning and Implementing Interventions

Acute Phase   The health care team quickly establishes physical and mental status priorities. Attention is then given to long-range physical, emotional, social, and legal concerns of the victim.

It is advantageous to assign the client a primary nurse in the emergency room. The client needs a warm, accepting, understanding, and respectful relationship with the nurse. If police officers are involved, the nurse acts as an advocate in helping the client decide when to talk with the police about the rape. The nurse also needs to provide breaks in the questioning if the client appears overwhelmed and distressed by the interview. See the Nursing Care Plan on page 520.

Outward Adjustment Phase   In their roles as school or industry nurses, mental health counselors,

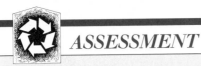

ASSESSMENT

Nursing History Tool for Assessment of the Rape Victim

Behavioral Assessment

Is the client able to respond verbally to questions?

Is the client able to follow simple directions?

Has the client bathed, douched, changed clothes, or done any self-treatment before coming to the hospital?

Affective Assessment

Which of the following emotions is the client experiencing? Describe with objective and subjective data.

Disbelief

Shame

Embarrassment

Humiliation

Hopelessness

Vulnerability

Anxiety

Fear

Guilt

Anger

Depression

Alienation from others

Cognitive Assessment

Evidence of defense mechanisms.

Is the client confused?

Has the client been informed of her rights?

Describe the client's attention span.

Is the client able to describe what occurred?

Is the client able to make decisions?

Who has the client informed about the rape? Family? Friends? Police?

Does the client need assistance in telling others?

Is the client blaming self for the attack?

Is the client experiencing flashbacks to the attack?

What does this event represent to the client?

Sociocultural Assessment

Who and where are the available support systems for the client? Family? Friends? Advocate? Clergyperson?

Is the client in need of temporary shelter?

Does the client know about available counseling?

---

citizens, or community members, nurses may have contact with rape victims and their families in the outward adjustment phase. Encouraging, but not forcing, rape victims and their families to obtain mental health counseling may help them cope with their feelings during this time.

Reorganization Phase   During the reorganization phase, many victims have a strong urge to discuss their feelings and experiences. Rape counseling may be especially helpful during this phase.

Foley and Davies (1983) have identified three phases of rape counseling;

1. *Self-exploration* revolves around establishing a relationship with the client and helping the client verbalize thoughts and feelings.

2. *Self-understanding* focuses on working to identify the source of the feelings and exploring the behaviors the client can undertake to resolve feelings.

3. *Action* involves making specific, often step-by-step, plans for action and testing out alternatives. A major emphasis in this phase is resuming control over one's life.

Some clients find family therapy or social networking activities, such as women's groups or self-defense classes, helpful. These may be an adjunct to, or a substitute for, rape counseling.

Evaluating/Outcome Criteria

The long-term goal of intervention with rape victims is to have them return to their level of functioning before the rape, or a higher level. These three outcomes must occur for rape clients to resolve the crisis adaptively:

1. Verbalization of accurate cognitive perceptions of the rape

NURSING CARE PLAN

A Victim of Rape During the Acute Phase

Client Care Goals	Nursing Planning Intervention	Evaluation
Nursing Diagnosis: *Rape trauma syndrome*		
The client will return to prerape level of functioning within six weeks.	Give client time to respond to simple questions.	
	If client is unable to express feelings, acknowledge the difficulty (e.g., "I understand that it is difficult for you to describe your feelings right now. That's okay. You may be able to talk about them later.").	
	Communicate your knowledge and understanding of usual emotional responses to rape (e.g., "People usually experience a number of feelings such as anxiety, fear, embarrassment, guilt, or anger.").	Client identifies and expresses feelings about the rape.
	Encourage client to talk about the rape.	Client talks about the rape.
	Identify distortions related to self-blame or guilt.	Client identifies self as a victim.
	Identify specific coping behavior client used during the rape (e.g., screaming, fighting, talking, blacking out).	Client identifies adaptive behavior.
	Encourage client to discuss the personal meaning of the rape.	Client verbalizes anticipated problems.
	Help client identify and arrange immediate concerns in order of importance.	Client identifies most important concerns.
	Assist client to use the problem-solving process in developing solutions to concerns.	Client develops short-term plan for concerns.
	Support client's making own decisions and acting in own behalf.	Client makes necessary decisions.
	Assist client to identify who to tell and how to tell about the rape.	Client uses significant others for support.
	Discuss beliefs about postcoital contraception and abortion if appropriate.	Client verbalizes understanding of available choices.

▶

NURSING CARE PLAN (continued)

A Victim of Rape During the Acute Phase

Client Care Goals	Nursing Planning Intervention	Evaluation
	Discuss need for follow-up medical evaluation and treatment for sexually transmitted diseases.	Client verbalizes importance of medical care.
	Provide anticipatory guidance about common physical, emotional, and social reactions to rape.	Client acknowledges understanding of potential reactions.
	Provide written list of referrals to community resources.	Client verbalizes need for short-term counseling.
	Make follow-up phone contact within two to four days.	Client implements immediate plans.

2. Emotional equilibrium

3. Adaptive coping behaviors

Crisis intervention ends when the nurse determines that the client has met the outcome criteria. Some clients need or desire long-term counseling to adjust to the trauma of rape.

Intrafamily Violence— Physical Abuse

In the 1970s, family violence gained public attention as a social problem of great magnitude. Before that time, the beating of children, wives, and the elderly was often justified as necessary discipline. Those who wanted to intervene had no legal basis on which to do so. More recent public awareness of family violence has been due mainly to the efforts of feminist organizations.

Intrafamily physical abuse, violence within the family, occurs in all strata of society. The myth is that physical abuse occurs only among the poor and undereducated, but in reality physical abuse also occurs among white-collar workers and professionals. In the past, intrafamily abuse among the wealthy or prominent people was kept hidden from the general public. With an increase in national concern, however, more publicity is being given to cases of intrafamily physical abuse at all levels of society. The United States has a higher incidence of violence than other Western countries. In 1985 the U.S. Surgeon General, C.

Everett Koop, declared interpersonal violence, including intrafamily abuse, a priority public health problem (Bersani and Chen 1988).

The popular image of the North American nuclear family is of a happy, cohesive, and harmonious unit. This ideal public image is often in conflict with the underlying reality of abuse and violence. In fact, the family home may be the most dangerous place to live since violence is more likely to occur within the family than between strangers. Children are beaten by their parents, brothers and sisters beat one another, spouses beat each other, and even elderly parents are beaten by family members. Beatings often escalate into more severe violence, with 20 to 40 percent of all murders occurring within the family unit (Bullock et al. 1989, McLeer 1988).

Incidence of Physical Abuse

Child Abuse   Each year approximately 4 percent of children between the ages of 3 and 17—about two million children—are physically abused (Humphreys and Campbell 1989). As the general public has become more aware of the problem, more cases are being reported, but these are probably only a small percentage of the total. We do not know if the incidence is increasing, because we have no historical data. Laws mandating the reporting of child abuse were not passed in all 50 states until 1968 (Straus et al. 1980).

The sex of the child does not appear to be significant in the incidence of abuse. Of abused children under the age of 3, as many as 25 percent die as a result. Some studies say the most dangerous age for abuse is 3 months to 3 years. Of abused children less than 6 years old, 64 percent suffer major physical injuries. In this age group, girls are abused as often as boys. In contrast, some studies say the incidence of abuse increases during adolescence, and that boys are more likely to become victims. Perhaps because older children are better able to defend themselves or escape, the rate of serious injury drops to 16 percent after the age of 11. By the time the abuse is discovered and reported, most acts of violence have been going on for one to three years (Starr 1988).

In past studies, mothers have been described as more physically abusive of their children than fathers. The proposed reasons were that mothers typically spend more time with their children than fathers do and are more likely to feel that society judges their competence as parents by the behavior of their children. Thus, mothers were thought to use more physical force to make their children obey. More recent studies indicate that men and women abuse younger children equally. However, adolescent children are more likely to be abused by the father (Bolton and Bolton 1987).

Sibling Abuse The most common and unrecognized form of family violence occurs between siblings. Many people assume it is natural and even appropriate for children to use physical force with one another: "It's a good chance for him to learn how to defend himself," "She had a right to hit him. He was teasing her," or "Kids will be kids." These attitudes teach children that physical force is an appropriate method of resolving conflicts. Sibling violence is highest in the early years and decreases with age. In all age groups, girls are less violent toward their siblings than are boys.

Spouse Abuse Spouse abuse has come to national attention more recently than child abuse. The woman's movement in the 1970s brought the issue into the public domain. In 1976 efforts were begun to establish resources for battered wives. There has been a continuing focus on providing counseling and shelters and passing new laws to protect the abused spouse.

No one knows how many adults are abused by their spouses or live-in partners. The estimates range from 11 to 50 percent of the population. It is believed that as many as 80 percent of the cases are unreported because the victims are ashamed, feel responsible, or fear reprisal in the form of increased violence (Bullock et al. 1989). One of six couples in the United States will commit at least one act of violence against each other in any given year.

Violence is not confined to marriage relationships. It is estimated 30 percent of couples dating or living together have been involved in violence. Half of battered women receive beatings several times a year.

Of the remainder, many are beaten as often as once a week. The intensity and frequency of attacks tend to escalate over time. Compared to nonabused women, battered women are five times more likely to attempt suicide, fifteen times more likely to abuse alcohol, and nine times more likely to abuse drugs (Sachs 1988, Stark and Flitcraft 1988, Tilden and Shepherd 1987).

Among couples filing for divorce, most abuse cases involve violence by husbands. Among cases of violence by both partners, it is unknown what proportion of women are acting in self-defense. Women are more vulnerable to violence because of their disadvantage in size and strength and their social and economic dependence on men.

Elder Abuse The abuse of the elderly by family members is just beginning to receive national attention. Elder abuse may take the form of physical neglect. Victims may suffer from dehydration, malnutrition, and oversedation. Families may deprive them of necessary articles, such as glasses, hearing aids, or walkers. Some elderly people are psychologically abused by verbal assaults, threats, humiliation, or harassment. Abuse may include failure to provide appropriate medical treatment, isolation, unreasonable confinement, lack of privacy, an unsafe environment, and involuntary servitude. Some are financially exploited by relatives who steal from them or misuse their property or funds. Others are beaten and even raped by family members.

The rate of elder abuse is unknown because many older people are ashamed to admit that their children have abused them and often fear retaliation if they seek help. At present, between 4 and 11 percent of older persons are being abused. The majority of the victims are between the ages of 59 and 90, with most experiencing two or more forms of abuse. Older women are more likely to be abused and account for 75 percent of the reported cases. Two-thirds of the abusers are over the age of 40, and half of them are either sons or daughters of the victims. Abuse by a spouse accounts for 12 percent of the cases among the elderly; the remainder are cases of abuse by other relatives, such as grandchildren, siblings, nieces, and nephews. As the proportion of elderly increases in this country, it is likely that abuse of the elderly will become a greater problem (Hudson 1986, Quinn and Tomita 1986).

Homosexual Abuse Although the issues of homosexual battering by heterosexuals (street violence) has received open attention in the gay community, physical abuse occurring in lesbian or gay relationships continues to be minimized or denied. Particularly among lesbian couples, battering contradicts the belief that women are nonviolent and peaceful. The following myths have contributed to the silence: only "bar dykes" engage in violence; only couples who have stereotyped male/female roles are violent; and feminist lesbians are not involved in violence toward one another. The fact is that battering occurs in some lesbian families regardless of class, race, age, and life-style.

The reasons for abuse are the same in lesbian or gay contexts and heterosexual contexts: to demonstrate, achieve, and maintain power and control over one's partner. In addition to engaging in physical, sexual, or emotional abuse, the violent partner may use homophobic control, which is the threat of publicizing the victim's sexual orientation to family, friends, neighbors, or employers. Lesbian and gay communities are currently making an attempt to bring this problem out in the open (Hart 1986, Strach and Jervey 1986, Walker 1986).

Emotional Abuse Although the focus of violence in this chapter is on physical abuse, emotional abuse is often equally damaging. Words can hit as hard as a fist, and the damage to self-esteem can last a lifetime. Emotional abuse involves one person shaming, embarrassing, ridiculing, or insulting a loved one. It may include the destruction of personal property or the killing of pets in an effort to frighten or control the victim. Statements such as these are devastating to the victim's self-esteem: "You can't do anything right." "You're ugly and stupid—no one else would want you." "I wish you had never been born."

Characteristics of Intrafamily Violence

Behavioral Characteristics   Acts of violence within the family range from light slaps, to severe beatings, to homicide. The hitting or spanking of children is condoned and even considered necessary and good for the child, and 84 to 94 percent of all parents use this form of discipline at some time in the life of a child. Many parents, however, do not realize that spanking conveys these underlying messages to the child (Straus et al. 1980):

- If you are small and weak, you deserve to be hit.

- People who love you hit you.

- It is appropriate to hit people you love.

- Violence is appropriate if the end result is good.

- Violence is an appropriate method of resolving conflict.

Parental violence can become extreme and often occurs periodically or regularly. Many times, it ends in the death of the infant or child.

A mother was convicted of beating to death her HIV-infected, heroin-addicted, infant twin sons. The four-month-old, five-pound infants died of skull fractures induced by severe beatings (*Chicago Sun-Times,* June 10, 1988).

The boyfriend of the mother of a 2-year-old boy was charged with the boy's murder. While caring for the child, the boyfriend bit him on the face, abdomen, and buttocks. The child bled to death from deep bite wounds into the abdominal cavity (O'Connor 1985.)

The father of a 17-year-old young man was convicted of solicitation to commit murder. There was evidence of previous physical abuse, with the son testifying that he had been beaten with a broomstick and a hose, and at one point his father had held a cocked, loaded gun to his head. Previously, the father told the son: "I can't wait until you die. When you die, I'll put your name on my trucks to show my appreciation" (Rossi 1985).

Acts of violence between adult family members fall along the same continuum, with women committing fewer violent acts than men. Women do more hitting, kicking, and throwing of objects when involved in violent conflict with men. Acts of violence by men against women are more dangerous and result in more severe injuries. Men are likely to push, shove, slap, beat up, and even use knives or guns against their wives or girlfriends (Straus et al. 1980). In one study (Giles-Sims 1983) of abused women, it was found that 50 percent of the abusing men had threatened their partners with a knife or gun, and 25 percent had actually assaulted their partners with a knife or gun. Verbal abuse always accompanies battering.

There is real danger that women may be killed by a violent male family member. A study of 538 women murdered in 1981 found that 29 percent were killed by their current husbands or boyfriends. If the data had included former husbands or boyfriends, the percentage would have been higher. In one study of domestic killings, there was a history of wife abuse in 71.9 percent of the murders. Women are more likely to kill their husbands or boyfriends as an act of self-defense when battering has been a continual problem in the home (Campbell 1984a).

A pattern of behavior usually develops in violent families. The first incident may be precipitated by frustration or stress. If a pattern of violence is to be avoided, the victim must immediately refuse to accept the violence. Outside help may be necessary to put a stop to the behavior. If the victim submits to the violence, physical force, without the stimulus of frustration or stress, becomes a way of relating to one another, and the pattern becomes difficult to change. Intrafamily violence is typically cyclic. Conflict escalates into a violent episode. After the episode, the perpetrator, feeling regret and shame, begs for the victim's forgiveness. The victim stays in the system because the perpetrator promises to reform and perhaps because of material rewards for remaining. During the next episode of conflict, the cycle begins again, and violence becomes a stable pattern of family behavior (Giles-Sims 1983, O'Leary 1988).

Michael, age 45, is a very successful physician. During recent divorce proceedings, he has confessed to beating his wife, Maria, periodically. At times, he would yank her around by the hair or hold her out of a second-story window and threaten to let her fall. During each of Maria's three pregnancies, Michael would beat her, particularly in her abdomen, saying he wished he could kill both her and the unborn child. This periodic abuse has continued throughout the 20-year marriage but was kept a family secret until the divorce proceedings.

Perpetrators lack impulse control, and their behavior is immature and self-serving. These behaviors indicate pathologic jealousy in a husband: keeping his wife under surveillance, calling home repeatedly during the day, locking her in the house and disconnecting the phone while he's away, and prohibiting social life with other women. An abusive man may publicly humiliate his wife and alienate her friends, increasing her isolation and thus making it more difficult for her to leave the relationship. Unpredictable behavior is typical of the perpetrator. At times he may be kind and generous to his wife and is able to present this "good" side when he needs to, such as in the presence of the police (Okum 1986).

Abused children often try to please the abusing parent and may become overly compliant to all adults. They may avoid peers and withdraw from outside contact. It is not unusual for the victim to act out with aggressive behavior during adolescence.

Many adult victims of abuse attempt to cope by becoming compliant. They try to placate the abuser, hoping that conflict will not escalate into physical abuse. However, the more submissive the victim, the more severe and frequent the abuse. If victims are dependent on the security of the home, they often accept the abuse rather than risk disrupting the family. Some victims, immobilized by fear, are unable to leave the abuser. Others attempt to leave but are tracked down and forced back into the home by the abuser. Both fear and inability to escape contribute to further compliant behavior in the victim.

Affective Characteristics Physically abusive people are often described as extremely jealous and possessive. They view other family members in terms of property and ownership. Within a culture that historically condones violence as a method of protecting property rights, these people believe violence is an acceptable method of maintaining the family unit. Extreme jealousy can escalate to hostility toward the victim and even the entire world as the abuser feels forced to defend his or her rights of ownership.

Some abusers have strong dependency needs and fear the loss of intimate relationships. They may beat a child because of the competition for the love and attention of their spouse. Some men are so dependent and fearful of loss that they respond with violence when their wives attempt to become more independent.

Closely related to the dependency needs of abusers is the feeling of inadequacy. Abusers use violence in an attempt to prove to themselves and others that they are superior and in control. The use of physical force temporarily decreases their fears of inadequacy and compensates for the lack of other internal resources. People who feel inadequate in relationships may use violence to create emotional distance and thereby avoid the fears of closeness and intimacy (Bolton and Bolton 1987).

Victims may be immobilized by a variety of affective responses to the abuse. In one study, it was found that 25 percent of the victims felt guilty, 50 percent felt helpless, and 75 percent experienced feelings of depression (Resick 1983). The feelings of guilt and self-blame may be expressed in statements such as, "If I were a better wife, he wouldn't beat me," or "If I hadn't talked back to my mother, she wouldn't have hit me." Victims who feel responsible for the abuser's behavior may also experience guilt if they are unable to change the pattern of violence within the family. Many victims feel helpless to prevent the violence and fear greater injury or death if they attempt to defend themselves. Guilt can contribute to distorted thinking and depression, which further keep the victim from leaving or seeking help for the family system.

Fear helps to keep a woman in an abusive relationship. Not infrequently, the man threatens to kill her if she tries to leave, and the woman lives in fear of physical reprisal. Fearing loneliness, the woman may believe that being in a bad relationship is better than being alone. Multiple potential or real losses contribute to an immobilizing grief reaction. Losses include self-esteem, a caring relationship, trust, safety, and financial security. To leave the relationship does not ensure the end of abuse. The abuser is often most dangerous when threatened with separation or after it. As many as 26 percent of the incidents occur after separation or divorce (Okum 1986, Tilden and Shepherd 1987).

Fear also contributes to a lesbian's failure to leave an abusive relationship. Since many couples have friends in common, the victim may fear shaming her partner. She may also fear friends will either deny the problem or take the abuser's side. Homophobia contributes to the victim's fear of seeking help. She may fear ridicule or hostility from police officers if she calls for help. A lesbian may fear seeking help from her family because the disclosure of abuse might reinforce negative stereotypes and increase her family's homophobia (Hammond 1986).

Cognitive Characteristics   Many abusive people set perfectionistic standards for themselves and members of their families. They convey a sense of rigidity and have an obsession with discipline and control. This inflexibility decreases their ability to find alternative solutions to conflict. Some abusers are self-righteous, believing it is their right to use physical force to get others to comply with their wishes. Many abusers don't understand the effect of their behavior on the victims and may even blame their abusive behavior on the victims. Often they deny or minimize the problem and refuse to accept responsibility for their behavior. Low self-esteem contributes to feelings of impotence and they seek power to counteract this negative self-evaluation.

Many parents who abuse their children suffered emotional deprivation when they themselves were children. As a result, they may have unrealistic expectations of their own children. Anger may turn to violence when the children are unable to fulfill the unrealistic emotional needs of the parent.

Other parents may have minimal information about children's growth and development and unrealistic expectations of what the child is capable of performing. Child abuse may ensue—for example, when the child is not toilet trained by the age of 9 months, an unrealistic expectation.

Adult children of elderly parents may also have minimal understanding of the developmental changes of aging. Not infrequently, the adult children view the changes of aging as deliberate and under the control of the parent. Abusers of the elderly use the defense mechanisms of minimization, denial, and projection of blame (Bolton and Bolton 1987, Broome and Daniels 1987).

Victims of abuse often develop low self-esteem. People who are beaten begin to believe that the violence is evidence of personal worthlessness. The verbal abuse accompanying the beating further lowers self-esteem, and the victim comes to believe the derogatory remarks. This distorted thinking process contributes to guilt and toleration of the violence.

Some victims believe they are helpless to change the pattern of domination or to leave the relationship. Some victims rationalize that the abuser was not responsible for the abuse, but that the behavior was due to stress or alcohol. Victims of abuse often exhibit the Stockholm syndrome, or hostage response. This includes a feeling of personal responsibility, a sense of unworthiness, and an affinity with and sympathy for the perpetrator. The belief in reform is a common characteristic among victims. When the abuser promises never to strike again, the victim is seduced by the hope of reform and the belief that perhaps this was the last incident of violence. Wives who believe that women are responsible for keeping the family together may stay in an abusive relationship in an attempt to do so. This responsibility may also be a factor for the woman who submits to abuse for fear that the children will become victims if she does not submit (Bolton and Bolton 1987, Valenti 1986).

Physiologic Characteristics   Victims of physical abuse may suffer a variety of injuries. In general, small children may be retarded in the areas of growth and development. In victims of all ages, any combination of the following may be observed (Mittleman et al. 1987):

• Bald patches where hair has been pulled out, or subdural hematomas from blows to the head

• Bruised or swollen eyes, hemorrhages into the eyes, or petechiae around the eyes from attempted strangulation

• Bruises, burns, or scars of past injuries on the skin, genitals, and rectal areas

• Fractures, or evidence of previous fractures, particularly of the face, arms, and ribs

• Dislocated joints, especially in the shoulder, when the victim is grabbed or pulled by the arm

• Intra-abdominal injuries, especially in pregnant women

• Paresthesias or numbness from old injuries and hyperactive reflexes due to neurologic damage

Sociocultural Characteristics   The abuser's family of origin is an important factor in understanding intrafamily violence. It is common for each generation to perpetuate violence unless circumstances alter the family dynamics.

Much of adult behavior is determined by childhood experiences in the family. Parents model marital interactions and parent-child interactions for their children. When the children grow up and form their own nuclear families, they unconsciously attempt to recreate the same interactions in the new family system. They repeat negative patterns, despite the pain, because they represent security. Also, the new generation has not learned other problem-solving skills. Thus, the experience of violence in the family of origin teaches that the use of physical force is appropriate. Violence is integrated into the family dynamics in such a way that violence and love are fused, or violence is perceived as morally right when used to achieve good results. Children may cope with exposure to abuse by identifying with either the aggressor or the victim. Not infrequently, these children grow up to become another abuser or another adult victim. There is evidence that some adult abusers were emotionally neglected or abandoned as children. Because their early security and dependency needs were not met, these adults cannot meet their own children's needs for affection and trust (Bennett 987, Valenti 1986).

Traditional gender roles foster violence in the family. Violent families are more likely to enact sex-role stereotyping and to have a hierarchical family structure. Some men get caught up in compulsive masculinity and feel a need to be tough, strong, aggressive, and unemotional. These husbands see an egalitarian marital relationship as evidence of a lack of masculinity. To support their superior position, they tend to marry women who are younger, less educated, and less economically productive. In addition, they may view women as childlike and needing to be overprotected.

When the wife or the children threaten the man's position of dominance or leadership, violence is more likely. Men whose sense of masculinity is not tied to the need for superiority and who can adapt to egalitarian relationships are less likely to use violence against their wives and children (Bersani and Chen 1988, Goodrich 1988).

The violent family is often socially isolated. In some families, the isolation precedes the violence. With few network support systems, the isolated family is less able to manage life stresses and may resort to violence to cope with frustration. In other families, social isolation is a response to the violence. Family members, ashamed of the violence and fearing public humiliation, withdraw from interactions with others.

Violent families may have experienced significant life stressors before the onset of physical abuse. This stress hampers the family's ability to adapt to change. The draining of emotional, physical, or financial resources may cause violence to erupt in the family system.

It is difficult for many women to leave an abusive relationship. Women have been socialized to be self-sacrificing for the good of others. They feel responsible for keeping the family together at almost any cost. Cultural beliefs about loyalty and duty reinforce the role of victim. Women who do leave an abusive relationship attempt an average of three to five separations before finally ending the relationship. Many women are financially dependent on their abusive partners. If they have outside employment, they are unlikely to earn as much as their male counterparts. If there are children, the woman may desperately need child support, and many fathers do not honor this obligation and default on the payments. The burdens of child care have traditionally been assigned to the mother. Lack of affordable and adequate child care facilities is a major problem for the single mother seeking employment. Also, single parents may experience some social disapproval because

of the separation or divorce. The cultural belief continues to be that two parents are always better for the children than one parent (Burden and Gottlieb 1987, Gilligan 1982).

The criminal justice system has not significantly decreased the amount of intrafamily violence in North America. Police officers and lawyers have minimal or no training in crisis or family violence intervention. There may be long delays in obtaining court orders or peace bonds to protect the victims. Court cases are often rescheduled, causing long delays in legal relief. The victims need advocates in the court so that they are not revictimized by the trauma of the judicial system (Giles-Sims 1983, Straus and Hotaling 1980). Male and female defendants often receive unequal treatment in the courts. Walker (1984, p 135) points out this difference in cases involving family violence: "Women who kill their husbands are more likely to be charged with first-degree murder, while men who kill their wives are more likely to receive a manslaughter charge." Changes must be made within the criminal justice system to allow all victims legal relief from family violence.

Theoretic Perspectives

The violent family is easy to describe but difficult to explain. There is no single cause of family violence. Violent behavior takes many forms and has many origins. Aggressive behavior involves the internal and external systems of both the abuser and the victim. This multidimensional approach to understanding family violence includes biologic, intrapersonal, social learning, sociologic, and system theories.

Biologic Theories The *instinctivist theory* suggests that people possess a natural fighting instinct that preserves the species. The animal kingdom is cited as proof that it is natural to protect territory and prey on smaller or weaker victims. Many authorities refute this theory stating that it confuses hunting for food with indiscriminate violence. In animals, competitive struggles for territory or mating privileges are not marked by the cruelty that characterizes human violence. In addition, most animal groups work to keep fighting incidents at a minimum.

The *neurophysiologic theory* proposes that the limbic system and the neurotransmitters are implicated in violent behavior. It is thought that an increase in norepinephrine, dopamine, and serotonin increases irritability and may result in various types of aggression. Stimulation of the lateral and medial hypothalamus in animals produces attack behavior, whereas stimulation of the dorsal hypothalamus prompts escape behavior. It is also thought that the septal area of the limbic system normally has an inhibiting influence, since lesions that destroy the septal region cause ferocious and vicious behavior in animals. Research is also continuing into the increased tendency toward aggression in women experiencing severe premenstrual syndrome (PMS). Theories center around the decrease in progesterone or dopamine hyperfunction occurring before menstruation (Keye 1988).

Substance abuse, especially of alcohol, is often implicated in violent behavior. In some people, alcohol may decrease the normal inhibitions against violence and thereby increase its probability. Alcohol decreases verbal ability, increases fear of attack from others, and decreases recognition of inappropriate behavior. These factors may contribute to a violent outburst. This, however, is not a direct cause because many alcoholics are not violent to their loved ones (Humphreys and Campbell 1989).

Intrapersonal Theories The intrapersonal theories suggest that violence has its roots in the individual personalities of the abusers. Aggression is seen as a basic drive within the personality, and violence is the result of an inability to control the impulsive expression of anger and hostility. People who feel helpless or inadequate may use physical force in an attempt to defend themselves and increase their low self-esteem.

Intrapersonal theories of child abuse describe rejection of the child and failure of bonding between parent and child. Parents may also project their own negative characteristics on to the child and then abuse the child for the perceived problems. Parents' own early rejections or childhood identifications with an abusive parent contribute to the cycle of family violence.

Other explanations involve personality traits or disorders. Abusers are often obsessive-compulsive, jealous, suspicious, paranoid, or sadistic. Violent behavior may be used to enforce absolute discipline, protect one's "property," or protect one's self from being attacked. Some abusers are described as having an aggressive-impulsive personality style. These individuals have a lifelong history of physical fighting. Successful outcomes of childhood fights reinforce the aggressive behavior and increase the likelihood of child, spouse, and elder abuse (Campbell 1984d, McLeer 1988, O'Leary 1988).

Social Learning Theory The social learning theory proposes that violence is a learned behavior rather than an instinctive one. It is believed that stimulation of the neurophysiologic mechanisms for violence are under cognitive control. Both the abuser and the victim learn their roles during childhood. Children learn about violence by observing it, being a victim, or behaving violently themselves. If the use of violence is rewarded by a gain in power, the behavior is reinforced. If there is immediate negative reinforcement within the family, violent behavior decreases (Hum-

phreys and Campbell 1989, Walker 1984). In addition to family models, media models of violence influence children. Westerns, cartoons, police shows, and adventure movies all demonstrate that "good" people use force to achieve "good" ends. Much of the violence in the media is not even rationalized by the use of force for "good" ends but rather is just endless, senseless cruelty. With these family and media examples, children develop values of tolerance and acceptance of violence.

Sociologic Theory The social environment can place additional stress on the family unit. Violence tends to occur in multiproblem families that have experienced a prolonged series of significant stressors, such as illnesses, accidents, economic crises, and the entrance of new persons, such as babies, or aged parents. Factors such as underemployment, unemployment, and poverty contribute to feelings of anger and deprivation. When financial, physical, or emotional resources are limited and strained, there is a greater probability that conflict will end in violence.

Identifiable factors contribute to the abuse of elders within the family. With the trend to smaller family size, there are fewer family members to share in the care of older parents, and with the longer life expectancy, the number of years of caring for a dependent parent have increased. As people live longer, they often develop many medical problems, and the cost of medical care can be a financial burden.

Middle-aged adults often look forward to freedom from the demands and responsibilities of child care. Before they can experience this freedom, an aged parent may move into the family system, and the adult children may find themselves limited socially and economically. The feeling of being caught between their children's needs and their parent's needs, with no time for themselves, may contribute to the abuse of elderly parents. Some daughters and sons have difficulty redefining the relationship with their parents. It is difficult for them to see the parent as dependent, rather than all powerful and resourceful. They may feel angry that aged parents are no longer a source of support.

When older parents move into the homes of their adult daughters and sons, the level of intrafamily stress may rise. The physical environment may become crowded with few places, or opportunities for privacy. Power struggles often ensue with strong differing opinions on how the household should be managed. The subsequent increase in stress and frustration may be a contributing factor in the abuse of the elderly (Phillips 1986).

Family Systems Theory System theorists believe violence does not occur in isolation but results from the interrelationships between people, events, and behavior. Understanding the interrelationships is not the same as saying each family member is equally responsible for the violence. Systems theory describes the process of intrafamily violence in the following way (Giles-Sims 1983):

- The taboo against violence is broken.

- A rise in expectations of further violence occurs.

- The family system denies that violent behavior is deviant.

- The abused person does not label himself or herself as a victim.

- Violent behavior is reinforced when it produces the desired results.

The abused child may be the scapegoat in a dysfunctional family system. One particular child may be labeled as the deviant member of the family. In this situation, marital conflict is displaced onto the scapegoated child, who becomes the target of hostility and violent attacks.

In the enmeshed family system, boundaries may be diffused, increasing stress and conflict. Family member roles may be constantly shifting. If the parents are unable to meet each other's needs for support and affection, they may turn to the child for this type of adult love. Each parent then begins to view the child as his or her special support system, and the parents begin to compete for the child's attention. When the child is unable to meet all the emotional needs of the parents, frustration builds and often ends in violent behavior. This type of family system may become disorganized and chaotic when the parents are unable to provide consistent leadership functions.

A closed family system is characterized by rigidity, inflexibility, and highly repetitive patterns of behavior. Input from larger social systems, such as friends or community resources, is discouraged and avoided. Solutions to problems must be found within the family system, whose resources are eventually depleted. The closed family system is rigid in its authoritarianism; it needs children who conform and comply with the family rules. When children begin to question the rules or challenge the power structure of the family, violence may be used to reinforce the authoritarian structure (Okum 1986).

Feminist Theory Feminist theories describe the sexist structure of the family and society as an important factor in intrafamily violence. The patriarchial organization gives men dictatorial authority over women and children. Women are viewed as childlike, passive, unreasonable, and overly emotional individuals who need to be dominated and controlled. The sexist economic system helps to entrap women, who must choose between poverty and battering. It is difficult for women to find advocates and solutions in the legal, religious, mental health, and medical systems, which are male-dominated (Humphreys and Campbell 1989, Okum 1986).

The Nursing Process and Intrafamily Physical Abuse

Assessing

Battered women enter the health care system for a variety of conditions associated with abuse. Failure of nurses to be alert to signs of abuse contributes to inappropriate diagnoses and interventions. Some battered women may not offer the information or minimize the impact. However, it is the nurse's responsibility to assess for and not deny the reality of violence. In one study (Stark and Flitcraft 1988) 75 percent of abused women volunteered the information that they had been battered, but only 5 percent of the assigned professionals acknowledged this information. Another study (Rose and Saunders 1986) of 86 physicians and 145 nurses identified the gender of the professional as the most significant factor in the recognition of abuse. Female nurses and physicians were less likely than males to believe the beatings were justified and that the victims were responsible for preventing the abuse.

The most important outcome of nursing assessment is the identification of domestic violence. Following this, a team assessment takes place. The victim's medical condition and emotional state must be assessed. The severity and potential fatality of the situation must be considered, as well as the needs of dependent children and the legal ramifications.

Nurses in all clinical settings must routinely assess clients for evidence of violent attacks. Because of the extent of the problem of intrafamily violence, one or two introductory questions should be asked of every client. In assessing a child, the nurse may ask, "Moms and dads try to help their children learn how to behave well. What happens to you when you do something wrong?" In assessing an adult, the nurse may ask, "One source of stress in all our lives is family disagreements. Could you describe how disagreements affect you?" If the responses to these questions indicate violence, conduct a detailed assessment, based on the nursing history tool and the guidelines for physical assessment in the Assessment boxes on pages 529 and 530. Obviously, the assessment must be adapted to the client's age, gender, and family situation.

Because of the increased incidence of violence toward pregnant women, nurses in these clinical settings must routinely look for evidence of violence through history taking and physical assessment. There are more incidents of beating during pregnancy than of either diabetes or placenta previa; indeed, one out of every fifty pregnant women is physically abused.

Nursing History Tool for Assessing Victims of Family Violence

Behavioral Assessment

Tell me about how people communicate within your family.

What types of things cause conflict within your family?

How is conflict managed or resolved?

Who in your family loses control of themselves when angry?

Have you received verbal threats of harm?

Have you ever been threatened with a knife or gun?

In which ways have you been at the receiving end of a family member's violent outbursts? Slapped? Hit? Punched? Thrown? Shoved? Kicked? Burned? Beaten up?

Is there a history of need for emergency medical treatment?

In what ways have you attempted to stop the violence?

Have you attempted to leave the situation in the past?

What occurred when you attempted to leave?

Describe the use of alcohol in the family.

Describe the use of drugs in the family.

Affective Assessment

Who do you think is responsible for the use of physical force within the family?

In what way is this person(s) responsible?

How much guilt are you experiencing at this time?

Tell me about your fears. Lack of security? Financial problems? Child care problems? Living apart from spouse? Further physical injury?

What kinds of factors contribute to your feeling of helplessness to leave or stop the abuse?

How hopeless do you feel about your situation?

How would you describe your level of depression?

Cognitive Assessment

Describe your strengths and abilities as a person.

If you were describing yourself to a stranger what would you say?

What are your beliefs about keeping your family together?

Tell me about your reasons for remaining in this situation. Promises of reform? Material rewards?

Do you believe/hope the violence will not recur?

What are your expectations of how children should behave?

What rights do parents have with their children?

What rights do spouses have with each other?

What are the rules about physical force within your family?

Sociocultural Assessment

How did your parents relate to each other?

Who enforced discipline when you were a child?

What type of discipline was used when you were a child?

What was/is your relationship like with your mother?

What was/is your relationship like with your father?

How did you get along with your siblings?

In your present family, who is the head of the household?

How are decisions made in your family?

How are household jobs assigned in the family?

Describe the recent and current stresses on the family. Unemployment? Financial problems? Illness? New family members? Deaths or separations? Child rearing problems? Change in job status? Increase in conflict? Change in residence?

Who can you turn to for support in times of stress?

Describe your social life.

What types of contact have you had with the legal system? Phoned police? Peace bonds? Obtained a lawyer? Court cases? Protective services?

ASSESSMENT

Physical Assessment of the Victim of Family Violence

Complete a head-to-toe physical assessment, paying particular attention to the following:

Head

Evidence of trauma

Evidence of hematoma

Bald patches on scalp

Facial bruises

Facial fractures

Eyes: swollen, bruised, hemorrhages

Skin

Swelling or tenderness

Bruises

Burns

Presence of scars from burns or injuries

Genital trauma

Rectal trauma

Musculoskeletal

Fractures of the ribs

Fractures of arms/legs

Dislocated joints

Impaired mobility

Abdomen

Bruises or wounds

Evidence of internal injuries

Neurologic

Reflexes

Paresthesias

Numbness

Pain

Nonpregnant women are usually beaten about the face and chest, but many pregnant women receive blows to the abdomen and often suffer injuries to the breasts and genitals. This behavior may represent prenatal child abuse, since violence during pregnancy is associated with subsequent child abuse. It may also represent attempts to abort the fetus. It is estimated 30 to 56 percent of women beaten during pregnancy experience at least one miscarriage. Pregnant adolescents still living at home may be physically abused by

their parents. Unfortunately, medical personnel often overlook this abuse even when the victim appears in the emergency department with bruises, cuts, broken bones, and abdominal injuries (Bullock et al. 1989, Hillard 1988, Okum 1986).

Ensure privacy during the assessment interview. It may be difficult for the client to admit to the reality of family violence until a trusting nurse-client relationship evolves. Many clients are afraid that the nurse will respond judgmentally, blaming the victim for being abused and remaining in the situation or demonstrating malice toward the abuser. Assure the client of genuine desire to help the entire family system (Sengstock and Barrett 1984).

Diagnosing

These nursing diagnoses are appropriate for the family in which physical abuse occurs:

- Altered family processes
- Altered parenting
- High risk for violence: Directed at others
- Ineffective family coping: Disabling
- Ineffective individual coping
- Powerlessness
- Self-esteem disturbance

Obviously, other nursing diagnoses might apply, depending on the individual family's needs.

Planning and Implementing Interventions

The majority of people involved in intrafamily violence are disturbed by this behavior and would like it to end. Even though they want help in stopping the abuse, they may not know how to seek the assistance they need. It is extremely important to be nonjudgmental in interactions with all family members. The abusers feel condemned by society at large and may therefore be distrustful of the motives of the nursing staff. Initially, the victims may be unwilling to trust the nursing staff because of family shame and fears of being accused for remaining in the violent situation. Approach victims in a nonsexist manner; in other words, do not blame the victim or look for pathologic elements in the victim's behavior. It is vital not to impose personal values on the family by offering quick and easy solutions to intrafamily violence.

Treatment of violent families requires a multidisciplinary approach and a broad range of interventions. Nurses, social workers, physicians, family therapists, vocational trainers, police, protective services personnel, and lawyers need to coordinate their skills to

RESEARCH NOTE

Citation

Campbell JC: A Test of Two Explanatory Models of Women's Responses to Battering. Nurs Res 1989;38(1):18–24.

Study Problem/Purpose

This study had two primary purposes. The first was to compare the responses of battered women to responses of nonbattered women who were having serious problems in their intimate relationships. The second purpose was to determine if the models of learned grief and helplessness were explanatory of these responses.

Methods

The sample consisted of 97 battered women and 96 nonbattered women having relationship difficulties. Only 23 percent of the battered women were shelter residents. Thirty-six percent were from minority ethnic groups, 60 percent were under the age of 35, 35 percent were married, and 71 percent were either employed or in school full time.

Several standardized measurement instruments, as well as an in-depth interview, were used. The tools were: Tennessee Self-Concept Scale (TSCS), Beck Depression Inventory (BDI), Denyes Self-Care Agency Instrument (DSCAI), SCL-90 Modification, Blame Operationalization, and Conflict Tactics Scale (CTS).

Findings

The nonbattered women were significantly older, less poor, less likely to belong to a minority ethnic group, and in a relationship of a longer duration. Battered women were more likely to suffer from organic symptoms of stress and grief. Battered women more actively utilized the problem-solving process in attempting to find solutions to their relationship problems.

Implications

The data suggest very similar responses to relationship problems by both battered and nonbattered women. Both were below established norms of self-concept. Battered women were more likely to suffer from a more serious level of depression than their nonbattered counterparts. This finding supports the theory that being a victim of violence is an important component of suicide by women. In assessing women, nurses must be alert to symptoms of grief and stress, which may be the only cue to ongoing abuse. The ability of battered women to use the problem-solving process was in contrast to the learned helplessness model. It was when battered women finally recognized that the violence was not going to change that they decided to take direct action to remove themselves from the situation.

---

intervene effectively. The family is the most open and accepting of professional intervention during periods of crisis. When identified during a crisis, the violent family should be immediately referred for multidisciplinary treatment. They will be most open to developing new patterns of behavior in the four to six weeks following the crisis. If no interventions are made during that time, they are likely to return to the familiar patterns of interaction, including the use of physical force (Campbell 1984c).

Nurses need to be knowledgeable about the laws regarding the reporting of physical abuse. In all fifty states, nurses are required by law to report suspected incidents of child abuse, and in every state there is a penalty—civil, criminal, or both—for failure to report child abuse. Child protective services and the courts make decisions in the best interests of the child. The child may remain with the parents under court supervision, the child may be removed from the home, or if abuse is severe, parental rights may be terminated.

State laws vary for reporting abuse of adults and the elderly. Adult protective services provide health, housing, and social services. Currently the resources are inadequate to meet the needs of abused adults. Domestic violence is now considered to be a violent crime; for this reason the victim has the right to be protected and the perpetrator is often arrested and prosecuted (Bolton and Bolton 1987). To maintain trust, tell the family that a report is being made to protective services. To keep the family adequately informed of the process, nurses need to know the procedures that follow a report of abuse. Many families are fearful that the only function of protective services is to remove family members from the home; in fact, protective services can be very supportive to the family by offering counseling and other social services.

Nurses in all clinical settings are able to intervene with violent families at the basic level shown in the Nursing Care Plan on page 532. The referral process is a vital component of nursing care since the family will

Text continues on p. 535

NURSING CARE PLAN

A Victim of Family Violence

Client Care Goals	Nursing Planning Intervention	Evaluation
Nursing Diagnosis: *Ineffective family coping: Disabling related to inability to manage conflict without violence.*		
Family will resolve conflict without the use of violence.	Teach communication skills to family. • Blocks that occur • Active listening with feedback • Clear and direct communication • Communication that does not attack personhood of family members	Communication is more direct and clear. Family members actively listen to one another.
	Discuss how violence is learned and transmitted from generation to generation.	Family members verbalize need for violence to be stopped now if it is not to be perpetuated.
	Discuss how disagreement in a family is inevitable.	Family identifies the normality of conflict.
	Explore with family the democratic process.	Family verbalizes understanding of democratic process.
	Using a minor, nonemotional family problem, have family solve the problem in a democratic manner.	Family uses democratic process.
	Discuss nonviolent ways of expressing anger.	Family identifies alternative modes of expressing anger.
	Have family identify times and places that each member can have privacy and time alone.	Family establishes private times for family members.
Nursing Diagnosis: *Ineffective individual coping related to being a victim of violence*		
Client will manage feelings and physical disorders related to violence.	Listen carefully to client's difficulties, and treat client with respect.	
	Give verbal recognition of client's hesitancy to trust staff.	Client identifies fears of trusting staff.
	Assist client in identifying feelings related to being the recipient of violent behavior.	Client decreases use of denial, identifies feelings.
	Assist client in identifying ambivalent feelings (e.g., love/hate, hopelessness/hopefulness, or terror/security).	Client verbalizes understanding of ambivalent feelings.
	Help client use anger to implement change.	Client uses anger appropriately.

▶

A Victim of Family Violence

Client Care Goals	Nursing Planning Intervention	Evaluation
	Discuss her right and ability to make own choices.	Client identifies self as chooser.
	Do not make decisions for client.	Client formulates own decisions.
	Discuss how stress is related to psychophysiologic disorders.	Client verbalizes understanding of physical illness and stress.
	Refer to physician for diagnosis and medical intervention of psychophysiologic disorders.	Client follows up on medical care.
	Prepare client for any referrals that are made.	Client follows through on referrals.

Nursing Diagnosis: *Family coping, potential for growth related to desire to stop family violence*

Family will maintain the family unit without the use of violence.	Assist family in seeing that the use of violence is a family problem, that is, that all members are involved in maintaining the violent behavior, but are not equally responsible for the violence.	Family identifies each member's role in maintaining the dysfunction.
	Assist family in problem solving alternative behaviors for each family member.	Family identifies possible changes in behavior.
	Help family redefine intrafamily relationships as ones in which physical force is unacceptable.	Family defines family as a nonviolent place of refuge.
	Assist family to see relationship between developmental crises and coping with physical force.	Family verbalizes understanding of future crises.
	Encourage family to formulate alternatives for coping with elderly parent in the home. • Investigate day-care centers. • Investigate extended care centers. • Enlist help from other family members. • Investigate short-term care so family can take vacation.	Family develops plans to provide relief.
	Refer for family therapy.	Family follows through on referral.

Nursing Diagnosis: *Altered parenting role related to physical abuse of children*

Parents will not abuse their children in the future.	Express concern for all family members including parents.	Parents verbally recognize nurse is nonjudgmental.

▶

A Victim of Family Violence

Client Care Goals	Nursing Planning Intervention	Evaluation
	Give recognition for positive parenting skills.	Parents identify areas of strengths in parenting.
	Give recognition that use of violence is a desperate attempt to cope with children.	Parents identify need to cope more effectively.
	Discuss with parents how they were punished as children.	Parents discuss childhood experiences.
	Teach parents about normal growth and development of their children.	Parents verbalize knowledge of growth and development.
	Discuss problems they experience with raising children.	Parents identify problems.
	Help parents identify parenting tools other than physical force that are age appropriate for their children.	Parents identify alternative skills.
	Help parents identify ways to spend time together without children.	Parents plan times together as a couple.
	Refer to community resources (e.g., crisis hot lines, Parents Anonymous, family therapy, or group therapy).	Parents follow through on referrals.

Nursing Diagnosis: *Powerlessness related to feelings of being dependent on abuser*

Client Care Goals	Nursing Planning Intervention	Evaluation
Client will not feel forced to remain in an abusive, dependent relationship.	Help client identify past dependency relationships.	Client identifies lifelong process of dependency.
	Have client formulate a list of ways she is dependent on abuser (e.g., emotional and economic areas of dependency).	Client formulates list.
	Help client identify intrapersonal and interpersonal strengths.	Client identifies strengths.
	Help client identify aspects of her life under her control.	Client identifies situations of control.
	Provide assertiveness training.	Client behaves more assertively with abuser.
	Caution use of assertiveness if partner still battering.	Client decides on appropriateness of assertive behavior.
	Refer to community resources for financial aid, legal aid, or job training.	Client follows through on referrals.

need multidisciplinary interventions to halt the use of physical force.

Nurses should strive to eliminate homophobia in clinical settings. This mean that a battered woman's sexual preference should not be used against her in a way that blames the victim for the violence. Battered lesbians have the same needs for support, safety, and positive regard as do heterosexual women.

Evaluating/Outcome Criteria

Nurses in acute care settings may not have the opportunity for long-term evaluation of the family system. Sengstock and Barrett (1984) state that short-term evaluations center on the following:

• The identification of intrafamily abuse

• The family's ability to recognize that a problem exists

• The family's willingness to accept assistance and to follow through with referrals

• The removal of the victim from a volatile situation

Nurses in long-term care settings or in the community have the opportunity to evaluate the effectiveness of the multidisciplinary treatment plan over an extended period. Sharing in the process of family growth and healthy adaptation in the ceasing of violence can be a tremendous source of professional satisfaction.

All nurses can evaluate their professional obligations and practice in counteracting those aspects of the society that foster violence. Violence is a mental health problem of national importance, and nurses should be leaders in preventing violence in future generations. Campbell (1984c) suggests these as questions to guide evaluation of nursing practice:

• What action have I taken to decrease violence in the media?

• Have I been an advocate for gun control?

• Have I volunteered to teach parenting classes at the grade school and high school level?

• Have I confronted the use of physical punishment in the school system?

• How have I supported programs to assist the elderly?

Intrafamily Violence— Sexual Abuse

Sexually abused children and adult survivors of incest are crying out for help. A few cry out loudly in protest, but the majority cry inwardly in silence. It is estimated that as many as one in four girls and one in ten boys are abused sexually before the age of 18. More recent studies give evidence that the actual rate may be one in two girls and one in five boys (Wolfe et al. 1988, Wyatt et al. 1988). Intrafamily sexual abuse occurs in all racial, religious, economic, and cultural subgroups. The perpetrators are not monsters; they love their children, may be steady workers, provide for the family, and are often seen as good family men.* Among forms of child abuse, sexual abuse is the most denied, concealed, and distressing.

Intrafamily sexual abuse is defined as inappropriate sexual behavior, instigated by an adult family member or surrogate family member, whose purpose is sexual arousal of the adult or the child. Behaviors range from exhibitionism, peeping, and explicit sexual talk to touching, caressing, masturbation, and intercourse (Trepper and Barrett 1986a). The term is often used interchangeably with *incest*.

Incest is defined as the occurrence of sexual relations between blood relatives. A broader definition includes sex between two persons related to one another by some form of kinship tie. Social taboos against incest have psychologic as well as sociologic roots. Although accurate figures of the incidence of incest are difficult to obtain because of the shame associated with it, most authorities believe that contemporary social, cultural, physiologic, and psychologic variables have all contributed to a breakdown in the incest taboo. For example, incestuous behavior has been associated with alcoholism, overcrowding, and rural isolation. Major mental disorders and intellectual deficiencies are also associated with cases of incest.

Intrafamily sexual abuse creates different problems for the family system from sexual abuse by neighbors, friends, or strangers. Within the family system, all the participants—that is victim, perpetrator, and conspirator—must continue to interact and function as a unit. There is no way of avoiding one another or dealing directly with the anger and rage aroused. Strangers must use physical force or threats of physical violence to rape another person, but most typically, physical force is not used in intrafamily sexual abuse. Rather, the adult uses psychologic coercion to ensure the silence and compliance of the child (Waterman and Luck 1986): "You must not tell anyone what we are doing, or they will take me away, and you won't have a father anymore," or "You are very special to me, and we don't want anyone else to know how special or they might feel bad," or "You know I'll buy you lots of toys and gifts as long as you don't tell anyone about our secret."

---

*This text uses the male adult–female child configuration, unless otherwise noted, since this is the most frequently reported type of intrafamily sexual abuse.

Incest is considered violence because it causes psychologic and physical injury to the victim. Because of age and level of development, children are unable to consent to sexual activity with an adult. The sexual activity is forced and thus constitutes violence against the child. Additionally, incest is a form of violence because the adult uses the child to meet his needs without regard for the needs and safety of the child.

Incidence of Sexual Abuse

It is difficult to estimate accurately the incidence of intrafamily sexual abuse. Because of increased public awareness, there has been an increase in the reporting of cases. It is believed that the actual rate has not increased but that the secrecy around current and past occurrences is decreasing. Despite more public acknowledgment, a tremendous number of cases of sexual abuse go unreported: estimates range from 100,000 to 500,000 children each year. About 75 to 80 percent of the abusers belong to affinity systems, that is, family, relatives, friends, and neighbors. Male perpetrators account for 92 to 98 percent of the cases; grandfathers and uncles are frequently reported. Not uncommon is successive victimization of children in the family; 30 percent of perpetrators have sexually abused other relatives as well. Unclear at this time is the rate of abuse in young boys. Gender role norms and homophobia are factors in the underreporting of sexually abused boys: The abuse involves the breaking of two taboos, incest and homosexuality. In the past, it was thought that intrafamily sexual abuse began when the child was around 10 or 12 years old. Current research has shown that many victims are under the age of 5, and some are as young as 3 to 6 months. The average age for sexual molestation is 4 years, and the average age for intercourse with a family member is 9 years (Courtois 1988, Urbanic 1987, Wolfe et al. 1988).

Characteristics of Intrafamily Sexual Abuse

It is difficult to predict which of the following characteristics a given child or family will exhibit in the face of intrafamily sexual abuse. Some exhibit most of the characteristics, others exhibit some, and still others exhibit none. These characteristics should be taken as cues for further investigation since they may also be signs and symptoms of other emotional problems in children and families.

Childhood sexual abuse may be a hidden feature of adult mental disorders. In one study of women being treated in an in-patient setting, 72 percent reported a history of sexual abuse, with 59 percent of these incidents occurring before the age of 16. Com-pared to the nonabused clients, they had more severe symptoms and were more suicidal. The link may be managing not only the severe trauma of sexual abuse but also the secrecy and denial affecting all subsequent relationships. Secondary disorders include depression, anxiety, eating disorders, substance abuse, somatization disorders, personality disorders, dissociative disorders and post-traumatic stress disorder. This victim-to-client process is an area of current research (Bryer 1987, Courtois 1988).

Although it is known that many victims suffer long-term problems such as anxiety disorders, sexual dysfunctions, sleep disorders, and multiple personality, there are also instances where there appear to be no lasting negative consequences. In studies of women who were not in therapy and who had been victims as children, 25 percent reported that the abuse had a great effect on their lives, 25 percent reported some effect, 25 percent reported little effect, and 25 percent reported no long-term effects. The severity of long-term effects seemed to be correlated with the presence of violence, the duration of the abuse, and the type of sexual activity. Most harmful was sexual abuse by fathers/stepfathers. Less harmful was abuse by brothers or other relatives outside the nuclear family. Again, nurses must find the balance between the extremes of denial of effects and excessive victimization of the individual and family (Herman 1988, Trepper and Traicoff 1983).

Behavioral Characteristics   Not uncommonly, adult perpetrators believe in extreme parental restrictiveness and domination. The use of threats or violence is unusual. More typically, the adult coerces the child and misrepresents the relationship and the activity. Sexual abuse may begin under the guise of affection or education and is often presented as something fun or a game. Perpetrators are typically viewed as having poor impulse control.

Children who are victims of intrafamily sexual abuse may exhibit regressive behavior. This may take any form of regression, but the most common is bedwetting. Sleep disturbances are common in children, particularly among those who have been molested during their sleep. Some return to a clinging form of attachment to one or both parents. Children may become extremely affectionate, both within the family and with others outside the family. Other children isolate themselves at school and in the neighborhood and limit the majority of their interpersonal interactions to family members. They may become overly compliant in hopes that the abuse will stop.

Victimized children may act out sexually with other children or adults. This must be distinguished from the normal childhood behavior of mimicking sexual behavior observed between parents or in the media. Sexual acting out behavior is seen in child victims who initiate genital or oral sex with other children or adults.

Adolescent victims of intrafamily sexual abuse may run away from home to escape an intolerable situation. Some of the victims turn to prostitution, since they have learned in the family that sexual behavior is a way to receive affection, love, and attention. Other victims attempt or commit suicide if they experience the hopelessness of being trapped in a pathologic family system (Courtois 1988, Herman 1988, Wolfe et al. 1988).

Long-term behavioral effects in adult survivors include indiscriminate sexual activity or sexual dysfunctions, such as inhibited sexual desire, orgasmic difficulties, or compulsive sexual behavior. They may also experience sleeping problems, chemical abuse, social isolation, depression, and suicide (Wolfe et al. 1988).

Affective Characteristics Under the facade of dominance, perpetrators often feel weak, afraid, and inadequate. They inappropriately view the relationship with the child as a safe and less threatening source of nurturance and caring than adult relationships. Additionally, perpetrators are unable to distinguish between nonsexual and sexual affection for children (Bolton and Bolton 1987).

Victims of incest may experience many fears. They fear that if they tell another adult, they will not be believed or that they themselves will be blamed, and the nonmolesting parent will side with the molesting parent. They may have fantasies of being thrown out of the family if the molesting behavior becomes known to other family members. Some victims fear loss of parental love. They may fear the family will be separated, especially if this threat was made by the abusing parent. Some fear that if they resist the sexual advances or tell the secret, they will be physically abused, even if the parent has never before used or threatened physical abuse.

The affective responses to sexual abuse are often confusing to the child. Opposing feelings may occur simultaneously, which creates ambivalence within the child. Developmentally, the child may not have the skills to manage the conflict that arises from ambivalent feelings. Victims often experience physical pleasure in the sexual interactions. In addition, they may enjoy being the "special" child in the family and exerting power over the molesting parent and the other siblings. At the same time, they may feel responsible for the sexual behavior and guilty that they have not been able to stop the abuse. Further, because they are emotionally and physically dependent on the abusing parent, they may feel helpless and powerless. The ambivalence leads to a pervasive sense of confusion and self-blame.

Extremely prevalent is the feeing of powerlessness—the victim feels that what she says and does makes no difference. The associated rage typically does not emerge until adolescence. When the suppressed rage comes to the surface, the victim may direct it inwardly in self-defeating and self-destructive ways.

Adult survivors most frequently describe long-term effects of fear of sex and distrust and fear of men. They may suffer from chronic anxiety attacks or demonstrate the affective characteristics of borderline personality disorder. Anger may be the only emotion they experience and express, and all other feelings may be severely constricted.

Cognitive Characteristics Perpetrators believe their needs are most important in the family system. When confronted with their behavior, some deny the abuse and accuse the child of lying. Others may acknowledge the abuse but minimize the impact: "Better for her to learn about sex from her father than from some horny teenager" or "She really didn't mind. In fact, we have a very close relationship." Others use the defense mechanism of projection and blame the child for the abuse: "She is a very provocative child and she seduced me" or "If she hadn't enjoyed it so much I would not have continued" (Bolton and Bolton 1987).

Victim denial of intrafamily sexuality may take several forms. Some victims deny that the abuse ever occurred. Others, acknowledging that sexual activity occurred, minimize the impact and say it was not important: "It's not so bad. It only happens once a month," or "It's all right because it stopped when I was 11 years old." Still others acknowledge the sexual activity and the negative consequences but deny the parent's responsibility and assume they are to blame for their parent's behavior: "It's my fault, I seduced my grandfather," or "If I had not been running around in my swimming suit it would not have happened" (Barrett et al. 1986). Denial may be used to protect the family system as well as the individual victim. The fear that the family may be separated by the removal of the parent or the removal of the child to a foster home may be so overwhelming that the secret is kept in the family.

Not uncommonly, dissociation is the victims' major defense mechanism. They separate the mind from the body so as not to feel and not to be present during the sexual activity: "I put myself in the wall, where he couldn't reach all of me" or "When he would come into my room I would close my eyes and go to my favorite place. Only my body stayed on the bed. The rest of me was not there." When sexual abuse is severe and sadistic, the victim may develop the dissociative disorder of multiple personality.

Children molested during the night may experience nightmares as a result. They may begin to dream they are being molested. They may become unable to distinguish the reality from the dream and begin to believe that the abuse did not happen but was simply a dream.

Quite frequently, adult survivors have total amnesia for episodes of incest. This is a defense mechanism in response to repeated abuse during childhood. A significant life event, such as getting married or having a child, or psychotherapy may trigger recall of the events.

Self-blame and self-hatred contribute to low self-esteem in adult survivors. Male victims may have a diminished sense of masculinity because they were unable to protect themselves. Victimization contributes to an external locus of control, which may continue into adulthood and carry over to other situations.

It may be difficult for adult survivors to develop an adequate self-esteem. They may continue to feel responsible for the incest, worthless, and different from other people. They may believe they are good only as sexual objects to be used and abused by others. Not uncommonly, they experience either amnesia for the events or flashbacks, nightmares, and other symptoms of post-traumatic stress disorder (Courtois 1988).

Sarah, age 19, describes her relationship with her father when she was 12 years old in this way: "I don't remember how it started, but my father conned me into soaping up his stomach, testicles, and erect penis when he was in the bathtub. This took place at his apartment when my brothers and I went there for the weekend. I didn't particularly enjoy it, but my father encouraged it. I got completely turned off by it when he offered to do me. One time, while I was sleeping on the bed, I woke up from a violent shaking of the bed. I was dressed in a shirt and shorts. I realized my father was rubbing his penis between my thighs and feeling on my vagina. I didn't let him know I was awake, and I turned slightly, hoping he would stop. I never wore that tee shirt or shorts again. I've never told anyone. Even my father doesn't know that I know. I think my experiences have had a deep effect on my relationships. Every time I get close to a man, I become afraid. I think what I'm most afraid of is being used. My childhood experiences seem to bother me the most when my friends talk about their childhood with their fathers and how they were 'Daddy's little girl.' Feelings of rage, anger, and total disgust burn deep inside me."

Physiologic Characteristics The obvious physical signs of sexual abuse in a child are irritated or swollen genitals or rectal tissue, or both, or the presence of a sexually transmitted disease. About 12 to 24 percent of female victims become pregnant. In an effort to protect the family from conflict and distress, girls may try to conceal the pregnancy (Krueger 1988, Zolanuk et al. 1987). Chronic vaginal or urinary tract infections, with no known medical cause, may be indicators that

the child is being sexually abused. Some children may have sexually transmitted diseases of the mouth and throat. Because oral sex is frequent in these interactions, the child's throat may be irritated. The child may also exhibit a hyperactive gag reflex and, at times, unexplained vomiting. Younger children may complain of tummy aches with the discomfort located near the diaphragm. The penis is seen as so huge that when penetration is attempted or completed, the child imagines that it reaches the chest area.

Some children attempt, consciously or unconsciously, to abuse their bodies to prevent or halt the sexual abuse. They may gain weight in hopes that the abuser will no longer find them desirable. Anorexia may also be a response to intrafamily sexual abuse. If an older child is being abused, a younger sister may become anorexic so as not to mature and experience the same abuse. This lack of care for the body may continue into adult life as an unconscious attempt to keep distance and avoid intimate relationships (Herman 1988, Wolfe et al. 1988).

Sociocultural Characteristics A number of sociocultural characteristics may contribute to intrafamily sexual abuse. Rigid or compulsive gender roles increase the vulnerability of the children within the family. It is difficult for a child to protest any type of abusive treatment in a highly structured, authoritarian family system. Rigid gender roles place women and children in a submissive and obedient position. In a culture that has traditionally supported male supremacy and viewed women and children as the property of males, it is not surprising that sexual abuse has been, and even continues to be, tolerated (Trepper and Barrett 1986b, Waterman 1986).

There is a widespread belief that the mother always knows when her husband is sexually involved with one or more of the children. In reality, mothers are rarely aware of intrafamily sexual abuse and with disclosure often react in a concerned and protective manner (Trepper and Traicoff 1983). Some women deny any evidence of the abuse because they feel inadequate to cope with the family problems. Others use denial because they fear their husbands' retaliation against them if the accusation of incest is brought into the open. Denial may be a defense mechanism used by women who fear financial, social, and emotional problems if their husbands are removed from the family (Barrett et al. 1986). When cues to intrafamily sexual abuse are discovered, some women begin to question their own thinking processes. Believing their husbands are incapable of this behavior, they believe something must be wrong with themselves.

Cherenia has recently become somewhat suspicious that her husband, Joe, may be sexually abusing their daughter. In response to her fears, she says the following things to herself: "You must really have a dirty mind, Cherenia. How could you possibly think those things about Joe? He's a very good husband. He works hard and loves all of us. He goes to church every week, and everyone knows what a good family man he is. How could you even consider that he might be doing something so awful? You must be really sick, Cherenia."

Chronic stress in the family system may contribute to intrafamily sexual abuse. Families that are socially isolated and have few support systems are more vulnerable to the effects of acute and chronic stress. When internal and external resources are depleted, the family dynamics may become pathologic. In some incestuous families, alcohol abuse may be a factor. Alcohol abuse does not cause incest but rather intoxication decreases inhibitions and is often used as an excuse for irresponsible behavior (Trepper and Barrett 1986b).

Survivors are at greater risk for revictimization as adults, and many end up in relationships with physically abusive partners. Some develop only superficial relationships because they have difficulty trusting others. Some adult survivors continue to function as caretaker of their family of origin and are unable to set limits on demands. Others may cut off all contact with their family of origin or interact only with certain family members (Courtois 1988).

Theoretic Perspectives

There is no single cause of intrafamily sexual abuse. In fact, the abuse is not a primary diagnosis but a symptom of dysfunction in the individual, family, and societal systems. The nurse must consider all these systems to understand the dynamics of a particular family (Trepper and Barrett 1986b). Individual and family systems theories of incest are presented in this section. (See the section on physical abuse for the sociologic theories of causation.)

Intrapersonal Theories   There are many descriptions of the perpetrators and victims of intrafamily sexual abuse. Many of these descriptions are contradictory, and there is no agreement on a personality pattern peculiar to all perpetrators or victims (Barrett et al. 1986). Many people experience these same factors of vulnerability without participating in intrafamily sexual abuse. These theories are guidelines for assessment, not absolute proof of sexual abuse.

The intrapersonal theories view the adult perpetrator as the "sick" or pathologic family member. These people may be insecure and have low self-esteem. They may be fearful of interacting with adults and more secure in interpersonal interactions with children. This fear of failure may contribute to a sexual dysfunction in adult relationships. Lack of sexual dysfunction in the sexual relationship with the child provides positive reinforcement to continue the behavior. Some perpetrators were emotionally deprived as children and thus have a great need for constant, unconditional love, which is more easily obtained from children than from adults. If they were sexually abused themselves as children, they may have learned to associate all feelings of love with sexual behavior (Trepper and Barrett 1986b).

Some perpetrators are described as lacking impulse control and the inability to experience feelings of guilt. Others have been described as rigid and overcontrolled. They may be dominant and aggressive. Lack of parenting skills or the loss of the mother from the family may result in role confusion among the family members. The father may turn to the daughter for companionship when he feels deprived of it in adult relationships (Trepper and Barrett 1986a, Waterman 1986).

The mothers of victims may be emotionally and financially dependent on the marital relationship. Denial may be the major mechanism that allows them to remain in the marriage. They may have been victims of sexual abuse during their own childhoods, and in consequence they may have an adult dysfunction such as female sexual arousal disorder. The mother's lack of parenting skills may contribute to the daughter's assuming responsibility for the younger children in the family. In addition to fulfilling the role of parent, the daughter may be expected to fulfill the role of sexual partner (Barrett et al. 1986).

Daughters who are victims may feel emotionally deprived and need unconditional love and attention. If their self-esteem is low, the "special" attention from their fathers may help them feel attractive, desired, and needed. The daughter may exhibit seductive and provocative behavior, a learned response to the father's inappropriate sexual behavior, not the cause of the incest (Trepper and Barrett 1986a).

Family Systems Theory   In the family systems perspective, intrafamily sexual abuse arises from and is maintained by the interactions of all family members. Rather than looking at *why* the behavior occurs, as the intrapersonal theorists do, family systems theorists look at *how* the behavior occurs.

Family Structure   The structure of the family is organized around hierarchical membership according to age, roles, and distribution of power. Typically, the adults, who are older, assume the parental roles and are the most influential members of the family system. The structure of incestuous families, however, is often quite different. An adult may move downward in the structure, or a child may move upward in the structure in terms of roles and influence. If the father moves downward, he assumes a childlike role and is cared for and nurtured by his wife, as are the children in the family. In this position, the father assumes little parental responsibility. He may then turn to the daughter, as a peer, for sexual and emotional gratification. In other family systems, the daughter may move upward and replace the mother in the hierarchical structure. Usually the mother does not move downward in the structure but rather moves out of the structure by distancing herself emotionally or physically from the family. As the daughter assumes the parental roles and responsibilities, the father may turn to her for fulfillment of emotional and sexual needs (Barrett et al. 1986, Trepper and Barrett 1986b).

Family Cohesion Family cohesion is the degree of emotional bonding in a family. At one end of the continuum of cohesion is the family system that is disengaged, that is, the family members are isolated and alienated from one another. At the other end of the continuum is the enmeshed family system in which the members are immersed in and absorbed by one another. The most adaptive family systems function between these two extremes.

Intrafamily sexual abuse usually occurs in an enmeshed family. The need to be overinvolved in one another's lives is accompanied by intense fears of abandonment and family disintegration. In an attempt to maintain closeness, the family closes itself off from external input and support. If the parent's marital dyad does not provide adequate emotional and sexual fulfillment, the father turns to the daughter for these needs rather than searching outside the family system for a different partner (Barrett et al. 1986, Zolanuk et al. 1987).

Family Adaptability Family system adaptability to change is also described along a continuum. At one extreme is the rigid family system and, at the other end, the chaotic family system. Incestuous families tend to fall on either end of the continuum. Rigid family systems have strict rules and stereotyped gender role expectations with minimal emotional interaction. Children are given no power and authority, even over their own bodies. They are not allowed to question or protest inappropriate sexual behavior within the family. In contrast, chaotic family systems have either no rules or constantly changing roles. The parents are unable to assume parental roles or leadership positions. Within the chaotic system, there may be no assigned roles or no rules regarding appropriate sexual behavior, which may contribute to the incidence of intrafamily sexual abuse (Trepper and Barrett 1986b).

Family Communication Communication patterns within the family system may contribute to the occurrence of intrafamily sexual abuse. Within some families, messages between two persons are communicated through a third family member. This indirect communication perpetuates secrecy and avoidance of conflict (Barrett et al. 1986, Trepper 1989). Intrafamily sexual abuse is dependent on keeping the secret within the family. In family systems that avoid conflict, accusations of sexual abuse are not tolerated. Peace must be kept at all costs, even the cost of abuse.

The Nursing Process and Intrafamily Sexual Abuse

Assessing

Nurses must acknowledge the reality of intrafamily sexual abuse. Nurses who deny the existence of the problem miss the individual and family cues and fail to complete a more detailed assessment. Nurses knowledgeable about the incidence and characteristics of the problem at all levels of society are alert for cues that suggest the need for an in-depth nursing assessment. A note of caution must be added, however. Some families have been torn apart by rumors and false accusations. Nurses need to assess carefully and maintain a balance between denying incest and assuming it exists.

When assessing children, remember that some will exhibit most of the characteristics presented, others will exhibit only some, and still others will exhibit none. These same behavioral, affective, and cognitive characteristics may be signs and symptoms of other emotional problems in children. Also, assess family dynamics before making an assumption of intrafamily sexual abuse. Routine questions on nursing histories, such as that in the accompanying Assessment box, may provide an opportunity for survivors of incest to share their pain and obtain treatment as adults. Do not wait for clients to broach the topic, because shame and confusion may inhibit the adult survivor. By avoiding the topic, nurses contribute to the problem by supporting the client's denial of reality. Now that intrafamily sexual abuse has been identified as a major health problem, nurses in every clinical setting must be alert to cues from both individuals and families. Guidelines for physical assessment are in the Assessment box on page 542.

Diagnosing

These are common nursing diagnoses for families in which sexual abuse exists:

- Ineffective family coping: Disabling

- Ineffective individual coping

- Altered family processes

- Altered parenting

Additional nursing diagnoses will be determined by the individual needs of family members and by the family system as a whole.

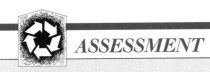

ASSESSMENT

Nursing History Tool for Assessment of Individuals and Families for Intrafamily Sexual Abuse

Behavioral Assessment

Individual child

Have there been any signs of regressive behavior in the child?

Is the child having sleeping problems?

Is the child exhibiting clinging behavior to the parents or others?

Does the child have friendships with other children?

Has there been any sexual acting out on the part of the child?

Has the child ever run away or threatened to run away?

Has the child ever attempted suicide?

Perpetrator

Describe how discipline is handled in the family.

Do you see yourself as the dominant person in the family?

At what age do you believe parents should give up control of their children?

How many adult friends do you have?

Describe your relationship with these friends?

Describe your relationships with your spouse.

What kinds of sexual difficulties are you and your spouse experiencing?

When you were young, who was the closest family member with whom you had any sexual activity?

Family system

Describe who has responsibility (mother, father, both parents, or children) in the following areas of home management:

Caring for the younger children?

Cooking?

Cleaning?

Paying bills?

Shopping?

Outside home maintenance?

Budget planning?

Decisions about leisure time?

Supervising children's homework?

Taking children to activities?

Putting children to bed?

Who are the best communicators in the family?

Who talks to whom the most?

Who is unable to talk to whom very much?

How are secrets kept from one another within the family?

How are secrets prevented from leaking outside the family?

Affective Assessment

Individual child

How helpless do you feel about changing any of the family's problems?

In what way are you responsible for family problems?

Do you get enough love within the family?

Are you more loved than the other children in the family?

Tell me about the fears you may have if any family secrets are told?

Fears of not being believed?

Fears of being blamed for the problems?

Fears that your parents will not love you?

Fears that you will be moved to a foster home?

Fears that your parents will be taken away?

Fears of physical abuse?

Perpetrator

Who loves you most within the family?

Who is able to give you unconditional support and affection?

How do you see yourself responsible for family problems?

How does fear of failure affect your life?

Family system

Describe the emotional relationships among family members.

▶

ASSESSMENT *(continued)*

Does everybody know each family member's business?

How is privacy protected within the family?

Do you have any fears of the family unit disintegrating?

What will happen if the family is separated?

Cognitive Assessment

Individual child

Tell me about your nightmares.

How would you describe the family's problems?

What effect do these problems have on you?

What effect do these problems have on the rest of the family?

Who do you believe is responsible for these problems?

Perpetrator

Describe what kind of a person you are.

What are your personal strengths?

What are your personal limitations?

Describe how you handle new situations.

Do you enjoy changing situations?

Family system

Who sets the family rules?

Tell me about the most important family rules.

How do rules get changed within the family?

What are the expectations of the males in the family?

What are the expectations of the females in the family?

Sociocultural Assessment

What significant events have occurred for your family in the past year?

What support systems do you have outside the family?

How often do you visit with friends?

Who are the problem drinkers in the family?

How is the issue of drugs managed within the family?

ASSESSMENT

Physical Assessment of the Sexual Abuse Victim

Complete a head-to-toe physical assessment with emphasis on the following:

Weight and nutritional status

Throat irritation

Gag reflex

Episodes of vomiting

Abdominal pain near diaphragm

Smears of the mouth, throat, vagina, and rectum for sexually transmitted diseases

Genital irritation or trauma

Rectal irritation or trauma

Chronic vaginal infections

Chronic urinary tract infections

Pregnancy

Planning and Implementing Interventions

The long-term goals of intervention are to act in the best interests of the child; support the nonabused children, who may be very frightened; and prevent trauma from the legal process. Resolution of anger, hostility, shame, and fear may be a goal in healing the family and decreasing the stigma of incest. See the accompanying Nursing Care Plan.

It is important to identify, reinforce, and support individual and family system strengths. Because family therapy is critical to the healthy resolution of intrafamily sexual abuse, referral to therapists who specialize in treating incestuous families is a priority in nursing intervention.

Intrafamily sexual abuse is an emotionally laden health problem. Nurses need to identify their personal values and determine if these will interfere with the ability to care for all members of the family system. Beliefs about maintaining or splitting up of the family unit will influence nursing care. Many nurses feel anger and hostility, both toward the perpetrator and the parent who was not able to prevent or stop the abuse. If the nurse is a survivor of childhood sexual abuse,

NURSING CARE PLAN

A Victim of Sexual Abuse

Client Care Goals	Nursing Planning Intervention	Evaluation
Nursing Diagnosis: *Ineffective family coping: Disabling related to enmeshed family system that is either rigid or chaotic in which a child is being sexually abused*		
Family will no longer engage in inappropriate sexual behavior.	Help family identify how some members cross generational boundaries by discussing roles and role reversals.	Parents function in parental roles and children function in age-appropriate roles.
	Discuss ways that parents can maintain generational boundaries.	Family makes decisions on ways to change roles.
	Discourage secrecy within the family.	Family communicates openly.
Family will move to a moderate position between the extremes of rigid and chaotic.	Discuss ways family can increase flexibility of roles and rules.	Family demonstrates flexibility of rules and roles.
Nursing Diagnosis: *Altered parenting related to being a perpetrator of sexual abuse*		
Client will develop adaptive coping skills.	Discuss client's family of origin in regard to sexual abuse and parenting styles.	Client discusses childhood as it relates to present problem.
	Help client discuss feelings around being discovered as an abuser.	Client shares feelings.
	Help client problem solve to find alternative coping behavior.	Client identifies specific changes in behavior.
Nursing Diagnosis: *Ineffective individual coping related to being a victim of intrafamily sexual abuse.*		
Client will develop adaptive coping skills.	Use play and art therapy with children under the age of 5.	Client participates in therapy.
	Help older children to identify and discuss feelings about the abuse.	Client shares feelings.
	Group therapy may be utilized with preteens and teens.	Client participates in group therapy.
	Help client learn methods to avoid future abuse such as telling others about advances, saying "No," and refusing to be left alone with the abuser.	Client lists methods of coping in the future.

▶

NURSING CARE PLAN (*continued*)

A Victim of Sexual Abuse

Client Care Goals	Nursing Planning Intervention	Evaluation
Nursing Diagnosis: *Post-trauma response related to being an adult survivor of incest*		
Client will resolve associated anger, anxiety, fears, and ineffective coping.	Ask client about relationship with parents.	Client discusses incest when ready.
	Discuss feelings of guilt. Repeat often that children are never responsible for the incest but rather the adult perpetrator is totally responsible.	Client verbalizes a decrease in guilt.
	Discuss feelings of anger toward the perpetrator and anger toward the nonabusing parent for not protecting client.	Client verbalizes anger appropriately.
	Connect feelings of low self-esteem to feelings of guilt and anger.	Client acknowledges lack of responsibility for the past.
	Help client move to an internal locus of control by identifying areas of life over which client has control.	Client identifies situations of control.
	Assess for sexual dysfunctions; refer to sex therapy or adult survivors groups if this is a serious problem.	Client follows through on referrals.
Nursing Diagnosis: *Spiritual distress related to being an adult survivor and asking questions such as "Why did this happen to me?" and "How could a loving God allow this to happen?"*		
Client will verbalize decreasing spiritual distress.	Provide empathy rather than a theologic discussion of God.	Client acknowledges the unfair and tragic aspect of incest.
	Pay attention to religious concerns and refer to appropriate religious counselor.	Client verbalizes faith as a source of comfort and support.
	Discuss how suffering might be managed.	Client discusses plan on how to manage suffering.

personal issues and feelings may interfere with effective nursing care. Some nurses may need to disqualify themselves from caring for incestuous families because of their personal values and feelings.

Evaluating/Outcome Criteria

Evaluation of the incestuous family and adult survivors of sexual abuse is similar to that of the violent family. In addition, these questions are used to guide the evaluation of the treatment plan:

• What are the implications for the family if (a) the family stays intact, (b) the abuser is removed, (c) the child is removed, or (d) the child and the abuser are both removed?

• Have the family members learned to communicate directly?

• Has the family structure become more flexible in terms of gender roles?

• Have the parents demonstrated more effective parenting skills?

• Is the family less socially isolated?

• Is the family able to use support systems?

CHAPTER HIGHLIGHTS

• Rape is a crime of violence perpetrated against victims of all ages.

• Date rape/marital rape often goes unreported. Victims may feel responsible or fear other's disbelief.

• Behavioral characteristics of rape victims include agitation, outward calmness, crying, nightmares, sleeping problems, or phobias.

• Affective characteristics of rape victims include shock, anxiety, fear, depression, shame, embarrassment, helplessness, and vulnerability.

• Cognitive characteristics of rape victims include disbelief, depersonalization, dissociation, denial, confusion, self-blame, obsessions, and fears for future safety.

• Causative theories relating to rape involve revenge, dominance, eroticized assault, inadequate interpersonal relationships, rigid gender role expectations, and agism.

• Nurses must function as client advocates for rape victims to prevent additional victimization.

• The family home is a place of danger for many women, children, and elderly people.

• Behavioral characteristics related to intrafamily violence include hitting, kicking, shoving, beating, and use of weapons. The pattern of violence tends to escalate in frequency and severity.

• Affective characteristics related to intrafamily violence include jealousy, hostility, dependency, inadequacy, guilt, helplessness, depression, and multiple fears.

• Cognitive characteristics related to intrafamily violence include self-righteousness, low self-esteem, unrealistic expectations, rationalization, and hope for reform.

• There is a higher risk for intrafamily violence under conditions of rigid gender roles, social isolation, high stress, and highly dependent family members.

• Causative theories relating to intrafamily violence include substance abuse, projection, impulsiveness, learned behavior, poverty, enmeshed family systems, and sexist structure of the family.

• Intrafamily sexual abuse occurs in all racial, religious, economic, and sociocultural subgroups.

• As many as 50 percent of girls and 20 percent of boys may be sexually abused before the age of 18.

• Behavioral cues to victims of sexual abuse include regression, sleep disturbances, isolation, extreme affection, sexual acting out, running away, or suicide.

• Affective cues to victims of sexual abuse include fears, ambivalence, guilt, helplessness, powerlessness, distrust and self-hatred.

• Cognitive cues to victims of sexual abuse include denial, self-blame, low self-esteem, and external locus of control.

• Causative factors related to intrafamily sexual abuse include rigid gender roles, chronic stress, low self-esteem, fear of adult relationships, impulsivity, altered family structure, and low adaptability to change.

• It is vitally important that nurses acknowledge the reality of intrafamily sexual abuse and be alert to cues demanding an in-depth nursing assessment.

REFERENCES

Barret MJ, Sykes C, Byrnes W: A systematic model for the treatment of intrafamily child sexual abuse, in Trepper TS, Barrett MJ (eds): *Treating Incest: A Multiple Systems Perspective.* Hayworth Press, 1986.

Bennett G: Group therapy for men who batter women. *Holistic Nurs Pract* 1987;1(2):33–42.

Bersani CA, Chen HT: Sociological perspectives in family violence, in Vanhasselt VB et al. (eds): *Handbook of Family Violence.* Plenum Press, 1988, pp 57–86.

Bolton FG, Bolton SR: *Working with Violent Families*. Sage, 1987.

Broome ME, Daniels D: Child abuse: A multidimensional phenomenon. *Holistic Nurs Pract* 1987;1(2):13–24.

Bryer JB et al.: Childhood sexual and physical abuse as factors in adult psychiatric illness. *Am J Psychiatry* 1987;144(11):1426–1430.

Bullock L et al.: The prevalence and characteristics of battered women in a primary care setting. *Nurs Pract* 1989;14(6):47–54.

Burden DS, Gottlieb N: *The Woman Client*. Tavistock, 1987.

Burgess AW, Holmstrom LL: *Rape: Crisis and Recovery*. Prentice-Hall, 1979.

Burt MKR: Cultural myths and supports for rape. *J Pers Soc Psychol* 1980;38:217–230.

Campbell J: Abuse of female partners, in Campbell J, Humphreys J (eds): *Nursing Care of Victims of Family Violence*. Reston, 1984a, pp 74–108.

Campbell J: Nursing care of abused women, in Campbell J, Humphreys J (eds): *Nursing Care of Victims of Family Violence*. Reston, 1984b, pp 246–280.

Campbell J: Nursing care of families using violence, in Campbell J, Humphreys J (eds): *Nursing Care of Victims of Family Violence*. Reston, 1984c, pp 216–245.

Campbell J: Theories of violence, in Campbell J, Humphreys J (eds): *Nursing Care of Victims of Family Violence*. Reston, 1984d, pp 13–52.

Campbell JC, Sheridan DJ: Emergency nursing interventions with battered women. *J Emerg Nur* 1989;15(1):12–17.

Courtois C. *Healing the Incest Wound*. Norton, 1988.

Davis LV: Battered women: The transformation of a social problem. *Soc Work* 1987;32(4):306–311.

De Nitto D et al.: After rape: Who should examine rape survivors? . . . Nurse rape examiners? *Am J Nurs* 1986;86(5):538–542.

Elvik SL: Child sexual abuse: The role of the NP. *Nurs Pract* 1986;11:15–22.

Erickson CA: Rape and the family, in Figley CR (ed): *Treating Stress in Families*. Brunner/Mazel, 1989, pp 257–289.

Foley TS: The client who has been raped, in Lego S (ed): *The American Handbook of Psychiatric Nursing*. Lippincott, 1984, pp 475–491.

Foley TS, Davies MA: *Rape: Nursing Care of Victims*. Mosby, 1983.

Freunk K et al.: Males disposed to commit rape. *Arch Sex Behav* 1986;15(2):23–27.

Giles-Sims J: *Wife Battering: A Systems Theory Approach*. Guilford, 1983.

Gilligan C: *In a Different Voice*. Harvard University Press, 1982.

Golan N: *Treatment in Crisis Situations*. Free Press, 1978.

Goodrich TJ et al.: *Feminist Family Therapy*. Norton, 1988.

Hafen B, Frandsen K: *Psychological Emergencies and Crisis Intervention*. Morton, 1985.

Hammond N: Lesbian victims and the reluctance to identify abuse, in Lobel K (ed): *Naming the Violence: Speaking Out about Lesbian Battering*. Seal Press, 1986, pp 190–197.

Hart B: Lesbian battering: An examination, in Lobel K (ed): *Naming the Violence: Speaking Out about Lesbian Battering*. Seal Press, 1986, pp 173–189.

Hartman CR, Burgess AW: Rape trauma and treatment of the victim, in Ochberg FM (ed): *Post-Traumatic Therapy and Victims of Violence*. Brunner/Mazel, 1988, pp 152–174.

Herman JL: Father-daughter incest, in Ochberg FM (ed): *Post-Traumatic Therapy and Victims of Violence*. Brunner/Mazel, 1988, pp 175–195.

Hillard PJA: Physical abuse and pregnancy. *Med Aspects Human Sex* 1988;22(10):30–41.

Hudson MF: Elder mistreatment: Current research, in Pillemer KA, Wolf RS (eds): *Elder Abuse*. Auburn House, 1986, pp 125–166.

Humphreys J, Campbell JC: Abusive behavior in families, in Gilliss CL et al. (eds): *Toward a Science of Family Nursing*. Addison-Wesley, 1989, pp 394–417.

Keye WR: *The Premenstrual Syndrome*. Saunders, 1988.

Krueger MM: Pregnancy as a result of rape. *J Sex Ed Theory* 1988;14(1):23–27.

Limandri BJ: The therapeutic relationship with abused women. *J Psychosoc Nurs* 1987;25(2):9–16.

Lowery M: Adult survivors of childhood incest. *J Psychosoc Nurs* 1987;25(1):27–31.

McLeer SU: Psychoanalytic perspectives on family violence, in Vanhasselt VB et al. (eds): *Handbook of Family Violence*. Plenum Press, 1988, pp 11–30.

Mittleman RE, Mittleman HS, Wetli CV: What child abuse really looks like. *Am J Nurs* 1987;87(9):1185–1188.

O'Connor PJ: Sitter charged with biting boy to death. *Chicago Sun-Times*, February 24, 1985.

Okum L: *Women Abuse:* State University of New York, 1986.

O'Leary KD: Physical aggression between spouses, in Vanhasselt VB et al. (eds): *Handbook of Family Violence*. Plenum Press, 1988, pp 31–55.

Pagelow MD: Marital rape, in Vanhasselt VB et al. (eds): *Handbook of Family Violence*. Plenum Press, 1988, pp 87–118.

Phillips LR: Theoretical explanations of elder abuse, in Pillemer KA, Wolf RS (eds): *Elder Abuse*. Auburn House, 1986, pp 167–196.

Quinn MJ, Tomita SK: *Elder Abuse and Neglect*. Springer, 1986.

Resick PA: Sex-role stereotypes and violence against women, in Franks V, Rothblum E (eds): *The Stereotyping of Women*. Springer, 1983, pp 230–256.

Resources Against Sexual Assault. Rape Prevention Education Program, University of California, San Francisco, 1987.

Rose K, Saunders DG: Nurses' and physicians' attitudes about women abuse. *Health Care Women Int* 1986;7(6):427–438.

Rossi R: Dad convicted of plot to kill son, 17. *Chicago Sun-Times*, February 7, 1985.

Russell DE: *The Politics of Rape: The Victim's Perspective*. Stein and Day, 1975.

Sachs A: Swinging-and-ducking-singles. *Time*. September 5, 1988.

Seeley D: Encountering rape: Not for women only. *Chicago Tribune*, February 7, 1985.

Sengstock MC, Barrett S: Domestic abuse of the elderly in Campbell J, Humphreys J (eds): *Nursing Care of Victims of Family Violence*. Reston, 1984, pp 145–188.

Shotland RL: A model of the causes of date rape in developing and close relationships, in Hendrick C (ed): *Close Relationships*. Sage, 1989, pp 247–270.

Stark E, Flitcraft A: Personal power and institutional victimization, in Ochberg FM (ed): *Post-Traumatic Therapy and Victims of Violence*. Brunner/Mazel, 1988, pp 115–151.

Starr RH: Physical abuse of children, in Vanhasselt VB et al. (eds): *Handbook of Family Violence*. Plenum Press, 1988, pp 119–155.

Strach A, Jervey N: Lesbian abuse: The process, in Lobel K (ed): *Naming the Violence: Speaking Out about Lesbian Battering*. Seal Press, 1986, pp 88–94.

Straus MA, Gelles RJ, Steinmetz SK: *Behind Closed Doors: Violence in the American Family*. Anchor Press/Doubleday, 1980.

Straus MA, Hotaling GT: *The Social Causes of Husband-Wife Violence*. University of Minnesota Press, 1980.

Tilden VP, Shepherd P: Battered women: The shadow side of families. *Holistic Nurs Pract* 1987;1(2):25–32.

Trepper TS: Intrafamily child sexual abuse, in Figley CR (ed): *Treating Stress in Families*. Brunner/Mazel, 1989, pp 185–208.

Trepper TS, Barrett MJ: Introduction to a multiple systems approach for the assessment and treatment of intrafamily child sexual abuse, in Trepper TS, Barrett MJ (eds): *Treating Incest: A Multiple Systems Perspective*. Hayworth Press, 1986a, pp 5–12.

Trepper TS, Barrett MJ: Vulnerability to incest: A framework for assessment, in Trepper TS, Barrett MJ (eds): *Treating Incest: A Multiple Perspective*. Hayworth Press, 1986b, pp 13–25.

Trepper TS, Traicoff ME: Treatment of intrafamily sexuality: Issues in therapy and research. *J Sex Educ Ther* 1983;9:14–18.

Urbanic JC: Incest trauma. *J Psychosoc Nurs*. 1987;25(7):33–35.

Valenti C: Working with the physically abused woman, in Kjervik DK, Martinson IM (eds): *Women in Health and Illness*. Saunders, 1986, pp 127–133.

Walker L: Battered women's shelters and work with battered lesbians, in Lobel K (ed): *Naming the Violence: Speaking Out about Lesbian Battering*. Seal Press, 1986, 73–79.

Walker LE: Violence against women: Implications for mental health policy, in Walker LE (ed): *Women and Mental Health Policy*. Sage Publications, 1984, pp 121–156.

Waterman J: Family dynamics of incest with young children, in McFarlane K, Waterman J (eds): *Sexual Abuse of Young Children*. Guilford Press, 1986, pp 204–219.

Waterman J, Luck R: Scope of the problem, in McFarlane K, Waterman J (eds): *Sexual Abuse of Young Children*. Guilford Press, 1986, pp 3–12.

Wolfe DA, Wolfe VV, Best CL: Child victims of sexual abuse, in Vanhasselt VB et al. (eds): *Handbook of Family Violence*. Plenum Press, 1988, pp 157–185.

Wyatt GE, Peters SD, Guthrie D: Kinsey revisited. *Arch Sex Behav* 1988;17(3):201–239.

Zolanuk JM, Harris CC, Wisian NL: Adolescent pregnancy and incest: The nurse's role as counselor. *J Obstet Gynecol Neonatal Nurs* 1987;16(2):99–103.

Suicide and Self-Destructive Behavior

LEARNING OBJECTIVES

- Describe the historical and theoretic foundations pertinent to understanding suicide and self-destructive behaviors

- Identify social, demographic, and clinical variables that influence suicidal or self-destructive behavior

- Explain the process of a lethality assessment

- Develop a plan for nursing intervention with suicidal clients

- Apply the nursing process with clients who experience suicidal ideation

- Suggest strategies for intervention with survivors of suicide

- Discuss potential staff responses to suicide and clients with suicidal ideation

- Differentiate conceptually among suicidal behavior, indirect self-destructive behavior, and self-destructive behavior

Carol Ren Kneisl
Elizabeth A. Riley

CROSS REFERENCES

Other topics relevant to this content are: Anxiety and panic, Chapter 14; Crisis intervention, Chapter 28; Ethics, Chapter 7; Legal issues, Chapter 37; Mood disorders, Chapter 13; Personality disorders, Chapter 16; Psychoactive substance abuse disorders, Chapter 11; Rape and intra-family abuse and violence, Chapter 22; Stress, anxiety, and coping, Chapter 5; Stress-management techniques, Chapter 27; Violence and victimatology in the psychiatric setting, Chapter 21.

SUICIDE IS A MAJOR public health problem in many countries. In the United States, suicide is the eighth leading cause of death across all age groups, the third leading cause of death among adolescents and young adults, and the leading cause of preventable death in the elderly (age 60 and over). The suicide rate among males 15–24 increased 50 percent from 1970–1980. The rate of suicide for all age groups and both sexes in the U.S.A. is 11.9 per 100,000 and this has remained fairly constant since the 1960s (U.S. Bureau of the Census 1989).

Suicide as a response to overwhelming life crises cuts across all cultures, ages, religions, classes and can affect every kind of person. It is conservatively estimated that 300,000 people will attempt suicide each year. However, these statistics are at best estimates of suicide and suicide attempts. No one knows for sure how many deaths that are labeled as accidents are truly suicides. Officials may be pressured not to cite a death as suicide, perhaps because of religious or insurance reasons. Some coroners will not rule a death as a suicide unless a suicide note is present. Many doctors, families, and hospitals remain reluctant to label a youth or adolescent accident as a suicide.

Nurses frequently find themselves face to face with suicidal or self-destructive people, and yet few clients elicit such intense feelings of anxiety and helplessness in nurses. The clients below have all considered suicide in the preceding two hours.

Kelly, age 17, is a petite brunette cheerleader. She comes to the school nurse stating that she just found out that she has been rejected from the college of her choice.

Frank is 68 years old. His wife died last year and his children live two states away. He comes to the family nurse practitioner stating he just "feels sick."

Natalie is a 36-year-old divorced mother of two. She comes into the outpatient clinic stating she has taken thirty-two Valium, 10 mg tablets.

Tom is 24 years old. He is in the emergency room of the hospital and is comatose. He was found that way in his apartment by the landlord. There were bottles and pills all around him.

Suicide or suicidal ideation can be a component of any client's situation in any health care or community setting. Thus, all nurses must be competent in assessing and analyzing suicide and self-destructive behaviors, and planning, implementing, and evaluating effective interventions while they manage their own feelings, attitudes, and beliefs toward what may seem to be their clients' unreasonable or irrational behavior.

Historical and Theoretic Foundations

Historical Perspectives

Suicide and ambivalence about suicide have been a part of history since the beginning of civilization. Suicide is considered appropriate at times and against the law at other times. Some early societies even forced members to commit suicide during rituals. During some eras, suicide was viewed as an appropriate alternative to military defeat, rape, or being taken hostage. Although suicide was mentioned in the Old Testament, it was not until the sixth century that suicide was viewed as "sinful" and the church refused certain religious rites or privileges—such as burial in sanctified ground or a religious cemetery—to people who committed suicide (Schneidman 1985).

In the fifteenth century, the bodies of people who committed suicide were often dragged through the streets, and their personal property was seized by the church or state. In countries such as India and Japan, suicide was expected of the widows and slaves of husbands or masters who died. In those cases, suicide was an expression of duty and fidelity.

Modern culture and laws reflect the ambivalence that has surrounded this issue. We abhor youth or adolescent suicide and may believe that the person who opts for death over life is weak. At the same time, we hold public forums to discuss euthanasia or rational suicide and believe that suicide may be appropriate when the quality of life deteriorates. American law is generally lenient in regard to suicide, yet suicide is considered a felony in some states (Curran 1987).

Theoretic Foundations

Although a multitude of theories about suicide and self-destructive behavior have been postulated, none of these theoretic models has been effective or precise in identifying or predicting who is at risk. Some of the more common theoretic models for understanding suicide are discussed below.

Psychodynamic Theories   Psychodynamic theories focus on the role of aggression and the inner world of the suicidal person. Freud (1964) conceptualized the act of suicide as a conflict between the instinct for life and the instinct for death. Suicide occurs when the wish for death predominates. Menninger (1938) postulated that the individual turns aggression intended for others inward against the self. This may not only be

CLIENT/FAMILY TEACHING

Suicide Myths versus Suicide Facts

Myth: A suicide threat is just a bid for attention and should not be taken seriously.

Fact: All suicidal behavior should be taken seriously; a bid for attention may be a cry for help.

Myth: It is harmful for a person to talk about suicidal thoughts. The person's attention should be diverted when this occurs.

Fact: Of prime importance in planning nursing care is an accurate assessment of the lethality of the person's suicide plan.

Myth: Only psychotic persons commit suicide.

Fact: The majority of successful suicides are committed by persons who are not psychotic.

Myth: People who talk about suicide won't do it.

Fact: Most people do talk about their suicide intention before making a suicide attempt.

Myth: A nice home, good job, or an intact family prevents suicide.

Fact: Persons of all emotional, social, and economic backgrounds may commit suicide.

Myth: A failed suicide attempt should be treated as manipulative behavior.

Fact: Failed attempts are more likely to be evidence of a person's ambivalence toward suicide.

Myth: People who commit suicide are always depressed.

Fact: People who commit suicide are not always depressed, although depression is common. Also, people can be psychotic, agitated, organically impaired, or have personality disorders.

Myth: Once suicidal, always suicidal.

Fact: Often a suicide attempt is made during a particularly stressful time in one's life. If managed properly, people can go on with their lives without recurrent thoughts of suicide.

Myth: The tendency to commit suicide is passed along in families.

Fact: Suicide does not run in families. It has no genetic quality.

Myth: There is no connection between alcohol/drug use and suicide.

Fact: Alcoholism and suicide often are closely connected: a person who commits suicide may be an alcoholic or may become depressed, impulsive, and suicidal after using alcohol.

Myth: Suicidal people rarely seek medical help.

Fact: In retrospective studies of suicides, 50 to 60 percent of those people had sought help within six months preceding the suicide.

---

the reason for suicide but also a way of understanding self-destructive behaviors such as self-mutilation, smoking, eating disorders and more indirect self-destructive behaviors such as self-neglect, excessive gambling, and compulsive overeating (Adam 1985).

Sociologic Theories Sociologic theories of suicide propose that the social and cultural contexts in which the individual lives influence the expression of suicidality (Adam 1985). Many of the sociologic concepts of suicide follow the initial work of Durkheim (1951), who described four types of suicide:

1. *Egoistic suicide.* An individual's ties to the community are too loose or tenuous, and the individual is not invested in maintaining his or her relationship with the community. This person does not benefit from the usual social constraint on behavior. Individuals who have no close relationships are more likely to kill themselves.

2. *Anomic suicide.* An individual experiences the aloneness or estrangement that occurs when there is a precipitous deterioration in one's relationship with society (e.g., loss of a job or a close friend).

3. *Fatalistic suicide.* An individual is excessively regulated, or there are no personal freedoms or no hope of these, e.g., suicide of slaves.

4. *Altruistic suicide.* Rules or customs demand suicide under certain situations, or self-inflicted death is honorable.

Perhaps the most significant contribution that sociologists have added is the understanding that suicide is not only an expression of intrapsychic conflict. Sociologists have been instrumental in reviewing the additional interpersonal, societal, and community components that we now know are critical to the understanding of suicide.

Biopsychosocial Factors   Suicide and self-destructive behavior are not well understood by the public or by the scientific community. (See the accompanying Client/Family Teaching box for a list of suicide myths and realities.) Suicide is a complex phenomenon. There is no single explanation for this complicated process. There are as many reasons for suicide attempts as there is variation in the profiles of people who do commit suicide.

The psychoanalytic and sociologic theories of suicide are limited in that they do not give a comprehensive overview of all the factors, influences, or conditions that may have an impact on an individual who is considering suicide. Suicidologists (those who study suicide and suicide prevention) have focused on studying all the biopsychosocial factors associated with suicide. They tell us that although there are many reasons why people commit suicide, there are also some commonalities among people who commit suicide. The following factors have been identified as having great significance to individuals who are suicidal. The following factors are useful to consider when working with suicidal people (Aguilera and Messick 1990, Schneidman 1985):

- The meaning and motivation of suicide

- The cognitive style of the suicidal person

- Ambivalence and its relationship to suicide prevention

- Communication and its relationship to self-destructive behavior

- The importance of the significant other

Direct and Indirect Self-Destructive Behavior

Self-destructive behavior is action by which people emotionally, socially, and physically damage or end their lives (Hoff 1989). Typical self-destructive behaviors include, but are not limited to, biting one's nails, pulling one's hair, scratching or cutting one's wrist, smoking cigarettes, driving recklessly, drinking alcohol, or using drugs. In general, these behaviors range from relatively innocuous acts, such as overeating and gambling, at one end of the continuum, to more lethal ones, such as driving recklessly in a blinding snowstorm, at the other.

A completed suicide is the most violent self-destructive behavior. In addition to completed suicide, there are four varying levels of self-destructive behavior:

- **Chronic self-destructive behavior:** Behavior that harms the self may be chronic or habitual and generally poses a low level of lethality to the individual. These may include such behaviors as smoking, gambling, substance use, and self-mutilation.

- **Suicidal threat:** A threat that is more serious than a casual statement of suicidal intent and that is accompanied by other behavior changes. These may include mood swings, temper outbursts, a decline in school or work performance, characterologic changes, sudden or gradual withdrawal from friends, or other significant changes in attitude.

- **Suicidal gesture:** A more serious warning signal than a threat that may be followed by a suicidal act that is carefully planned to attract attention without seriously injuring the subject. A superficial scratch across the wrist, if its goes unheeded, may be followed by a more dramatic display.

- **Suicidal attempt:** A strong and desperate call for help. It is often the final call, for unlike the suicidal gesture, it involves a definite risk. The outcome frequently depends on the circumstances and is not under the person's control. For example, someone who takes a heavy overdose of sleeping pills may or may not be discovered in time.

People who are self-destructive may manifest several of the four behaviors listed here. For example, people who are chronically self-destructive may also make suicide attempts or complete suicides. This section focuses on chronic self-destructive behavior that is not highly lethal or imminently suicidal. Suicide, suicide attempts, and suicide threats are discussed in greater detail later in this chapter.

According to Valente (1983), people who are chronically self-destructive share these common family characteristics:

- Prior family history or tendencies

- Early trauma

- Rigid, disorganized, or dysfunctional family system

- Disturbed parent-child relationship
- Unresolved loss
- History of abuse

Van der Kolk (1988) posits the possibility that the self-destructive behavior of self-mutilation is related to early childhood abuse or neglect and trauma. It may have a physiologic component. In human beings, elevations of plasma endorphins have been reported following stress, surgery, gambling, and marathon running. Another study (Coid et al. 1983) indicates the possibility that metenkephalins are elevated in some who habitually mutilate themselves. No single theory or scientific study explains why some people are self-destructive.

Self-destructive persons under stress perceive themselves as having very limited options. They tend to select self-destructive behaviors because: (a) these behaviors make the most sense to them, and (b) these behaviors relieve them, at least temporarily, of their acute discomfort.

Indirect self-destructive behavior may injure one's health and hasten one's own sometimes premature death. The goal of the behavior distinguishes direct from indirect self-destruction. When the primary conscious goal of the behavior is self-injury, then the term *direct self-destructive behavior* is accurate. Suicide is its most extreme form. In *indirect self-destructive behavior,* self-injury is an undesired effect rather than the primary conscious goal.

The exact reason for indirect self-destructive behavior is unknown, although there is much speculation about it. Several interpretations are possible. For example, indirect self-destructive behavior may help people deny mental pain or cope with it, thus avoiding helpless depression. Indirect self-destructive behavior may also result from impulsivity in persons who are unable or unwilling to consider the long-term results of their behavior. Another possibility is that indirect self-destructive behavior is a coping mechanism that enhances flagging self-esteem by denying helplessness. A self-punishing act tends to relieve unconscious guilt. Taking risks and overcoming them increase self-esteem.

People in crisis often resort to indirect self-destructive behavior in attempts to cope. They may get into fights, drink heavily, overeat, overwork, become preoccupied, and neglect their own health. When asked why they do what they do, clients often report that they have been experiencing or trying to avoid mounting anxiety, racing thoughts, depersonalization, inner rage, or a high level of distress. To work effectively with this group, the nurse must:

- Find out what the self-destructive behavior means at this time to this client

- Perform a lethality assessment (discussed later in this chapter)
- Consider the possibility of a neurophysiologic component that may respond to medication, and evaluate the client for this
- Help the client cope with dysphoria and loneliness
- Help the self-destructive person by enlarging their repertoire of adaptive coping behavior available
- Focus on interventions that diminish self-hatred, instill hope, build support, and stabilize the client's life-style (Farazza et al. 1989)

Meaning of and Motivation for Suicide

Suicide is never a random act. Whether committed impulsively or after painstaking consideration, the act has both a message and a purpose. In general, the purpose or reason for suicide is to escape; to get away from or end an intolerable situation, crisis, difficulty, or relationship, such as the following:

- Escaping a terminal (especially a painful) illness

Helen has advanced lung cancer that has metastasized to her bones. The slightest exertion causes spontaneous fractures, and she is in constant pain. She has been asking friends, family, and health care workers to help her escape her illness by ending her life.

- Avoiding being a burden to others

Joan is a widow. She fell three times last year and is now in a nursing home. She decided upon suicide so that she would no longer be a burden to her family. Joan has not eaten in seven days.

- Resolving an untenable family situation

Matt, age 7, attempted to run into the path of a car. He had heard his mother say many times, "If it weren't for you, your Daddy and I would never have broken up." Matt believed that if he were dead, his parents would reunite, thus solving what he believes to be an untenable family situation.

- To avoid punishment or exposure of socially or personally unacceptable behavior

John, 34, was a successful businessman. Last night, he was charged with drunken driving and vehicular homicide. Horrified that his unacceptable behavior would be exposed, he committed suicide after learning that his picture and the story would be in the morning newspaper.

The Cognitive Style of the Suicidal Client

Suicidologists have speculated about the cognitive style (method of thought processing) of the client who commits or attempts suicide. Although there is no single suicidal logic, some cognitive styles predispose to suicidal behavior. These are generally destructive ways of thinking.

Dichotomous thinking (the belief that there is only an either/or choice) is commonly seen in the suicidal person. The person falls into an imminently suicidal state when death seems the only escape. The thought processing of the suicidal client is generally constricted. People who are suicidal have great difficulty (if they can do it at all) in considering alternatives to their current dilemma. This may account for clients who agree to a request even if they have no intention of following through. Constriction in thought generally results in the dichotomous ideation that there are only two choices: a magical solution or death. The first nursing task is to maintain the client's safety and provide time and opportunity for discussion of alternatives. Then the nurse can intervene by helping the client explore other options.

Ambivalence

People who are considering suicide are divided within themselves. They have two conflicting desires at the same time: to live and to die. To understand the thinking of someone who is acutely suicidal, the nurse must understand the concept of ambivalence.

Ambivalence accounts for the fact that a suicidal person often takes lethal or near-lethal action but leaves open the possibility for rescue. This ambivalence allows for the possibility of intervention with the suicidal client (Aguilera and Messick 1990). A nurse may avert suicide by recognizing a cry for help (discussed later in this chapter) and intervening appropriately. However, failure to intervene and provide life choices increases the person's desperation. When this happens, death becomes the more focused choice.

Communication

Many people who are self-destructive have lifelong difficulties communicating their needs to others (Hoff 1989). Some people cannot express their needs or feelings to others, or, when they do, they do not obtain the results they hope for. For them, suicide becomes a clear and direct, if violent, form of communication.

Suicidal thoughts and plans can almost always be traced back to feelings of hopelessness and helplessness, often as the result of separation from or loss of a significant person, place, or thing. People usually resort to suicide only when they believe there is no other way to express the depths of their despair. Clients feel driven to suicide because they believe they have exhausted their coping abilities or that they cannot influence the behavior of others.

The message inherent in suicide is often aimed at a specific person, usually the significant other. The significant other's ability to recognize this message is the key to understanding and resolving the suicidal person's unmet need. Interrupting a suicide plan or suicidal thoughts requires hearing, understanding, and responding appropriately to messages of pain, loneliness, or hopelessness.

Intended Effect of Suicidal Behavior on Significant Others

Suicide is often thought to be an act, thought, or behavior that exists solely within one person. However, suicidologists tell us that suicide is more accurately described as a dyadic event between two unhappy people (Schneidman 1985), motivated by real or perceived rejection, abandonment, guilt, revenge, or pity. Suicide can be better understood if viewed in the context of the relationship between two people: the suicidal person and the significant other. Broadly defined, the significant other can be a spouse, child, boss, landlord, friend, nurse, or other health care worker.

Suicidal people almost always communicate their intent to the significant others before the fact or attempt. Schneidman (1985) found a clear communication of intent in 80 percent of cases studied. Suicidologists have learned from such studies that another way to understand suicidal behavior is to look at the intended effect on significant others. A suicide attempt, gesture, or verbalization can arouse feelings of sympathy, anger, hostility, anxiety, or desire for connectedness on the part of a significant other, thus altering the current relationship to meet the need of the suicidal person.

The Nursing Process and Self-Destructive Behavior

This section discusses the nursing process for suicide and self-destructive behavior in general. Specific guidelines for assessing and intervening with special populations, such as children, adolescents, the elderly, psychiatric clients, and substance abusers, are discussed in the next section.

Assessing

Social Variables   Low suicide rates are noted among the following:

• Developing communities and groups in which hope and optimism are high

• Cultures that are warm and nurturing, such as the Irish, Italians, and Norwegians

• Communities in which there is strong disapproval of suicide as an act, such as in Italy, Spain, and Ireland, where the Catholic Church is highly influential

High suicide rates are associated with the following:

- Societies in which social unrest, internal governmental problems, or pessimistic outlooks for the future predominate

- Subcultures that are uncaring and cold and lack concern for people in trouble, such as skid rows and disorganized inner-city areas

- Societies, such as the United States, Japan, Russia, and Germany, that value independence and individual performance

- Social roles, occupations, and professions in which people exhibit high concern and nurturance toward others (e.g., physicians and police)

- Both ends of the socioeconomic scale

Demographic Variables   Suicide rates are higher among the following:

- Single people (two times the rate of married people)

- Divorced, separated, or widowed people (four to five times the risk of married people)

- People who are confused about their sexual orientation

- People who have experienced a recent loss: divorce, loss of a job, loss of prestige, or loss of social status or who are facing the threat of criminal exposure

- Caucasians, Eskimos, and Native Americans

- Protestants or those who profess no religious affiliation

Clinical Variables   Suicide rates are higher among the following:

- People who have attempted suicide before

- People who have experienced the loss of an important person at some time in the past or the loss of both parents early in life, or the loss of or threat of loss of their spouse, job, money, or social position

- People who are depressed or recovering from depression or a psychotic episode

- People with physical illness, particularly when the illness involves an alteration of body image or life-style

- People who abuse alcohol or drugs, especially among people who use two or more substances

- People who are recovering from a thought disorder combined with depressed mood and/or suicidal ideation (especially people experiencing command

hallucinations that tell them to kill or harm themselves or to join someone in the afterlife)

Clues or Cries for Help   People bent on suicide almost always give either verbal or nonverbal clues of their intent. Suicidologists and crisis workers who work with suicidal people believe that people bent on self-destruction actually make a powerful attempt to communicate to others their hurt and desperation. They are crying out for help.

Seventy-five percent of persons who commit suicide signal their need for help by making contact with the health care system three to six months before the suicide because of various physical complaints (Roberts and McFarland 1986). But, when questioned, many express feelings of depression and thoughts of suicide. The nurse should be alert to patterns that may at first seem coincidental.

A 21-year-old man was referred to a therapist by his physician. Although he described chronic "aches and pains" and "not feeling well," a physical exam revealed no physical problems. He did talk about how life was just not worth living, and he had a recent history of driving recklessly. After further discussion, he said that he had recently broken up with his girlfriend and admitted that his reckless driving had a suicidal intent.

The cry for help may be indirect or subtle. A person may say: "I just can't take it anymore," "There's no reason to go on," "Sometimes I think I'd be better off dead," "I won't be seeing you anymore," "Take care of my dog and cat," "Too bad I won't get to see my little brother grow up," "Will you be sorry when I'm gone?" Sometimes their behavior provides the clue. They may:

- Give away prized possessions

- Make out or change a will

- Take out or add to an insurance policy

- Cancel all social engagements

- Be despondent or behave in unusual ways

- Be unable to sleep

- Feel hopeless

- Have trouble concentrating at school or on the job

- Suddenly lose interest in friends, organizations, and activities

- Have a sudden, unexplained recovery from a depression

- Plan their funeral

- Cry for no apparent reason

An assessment for suicide should *always* be done whenever the nurse suspects suicidal thought or intent.

Because a Korean nursing student had failed the same major clinical course twice, she was asked to leave the BSN program. She desperately fought to be allowed to continue even though the faculty had deemed her unsafe in the clinical area. The faculty could not understand her refusal to accept failure until they considered her cultural and family background, which sees failure as dishonorable. They decided to have the student speak with the psychiatric nursing instructor who assessed the student's emotional state and found that she had no intentions of self-harm.

Nurses and others who may have contact with potentially suicidal people must be alert to both clear and veiled communications about suicide. Once clues have been identified, the next step is to undertake an accurate lethality assessment.

Lethality Assessment A lethality assessment is an attempt to predict the likelihood of suicide. Certain signs (see the Assessment box on page 556) help predict suicide risk. An accurate lethality assessment is essential in formulating a plan for helping a suicidal person. It also gives the nurse cues about the client's possible need for hospitalization. Carrying out a lethality assessment requires direct communication between client and nurse concerning the client's intent. Part of assessment is a consideration of the lethality of the proposed suicide method. Table 23–1 on page 557 compares the lethality of suicide methods.

Assessment of suicide risk is not easily accomplished. One barrier is the nurse's fear of asking the appropriate questions. It is not possible to "cause" a person's suicide by assessing feelings and thoughts. Suicide is not a spontaneous behavior, and inquiring about suicidal thoughts may alleviate the anxiety of someone considering suicide rather than "give them the idea." Begin with "How bad are things for you?", "How down do you get?", "Are you worried about yourself?", "Do you ever think of harming yourself when you're down?" Then proceed with questioning the client gently, but directly.

Do not use euphemisms. Some sample phrases might be: Do you have any thoughts of harming yourself? Have you ever thought of taking your own life? Have you ever been so sad that you wanted to end it all, maybe by dying?

The client who asks the nurse to promise not to tell anyone about a suicide plan poses a serious assessment problem. A nurse should never promise to keep clinical information a secret and should explain to the client that information is shared with the treatment team. The nurse will probably need to discuss the issue of confidentiality further and to explore the dynamics of the nurse-client relationship.

Many institutions and crisis centers use protocols for assessing suicide risk and have published these forms in the literature. However, research efforts to *predict* suicide by testing, use of scales, or clinical judgments have not been successful.

A comprehensive assessment, including a lethality assessment, helps nurses decide which interventions are indicated for the client. Correct assessment of level of lethality can prevent unnecessary hospitalizations. Hospitalizations in and of themselves can create a crisis. At times, mental health staff hospitalize a client because of their own fears and anxiety about possible suicide. However, admission should be considered and encouraged when the suicide plan is highly lethal and there are inadequate supports to maintain the client in the community. This assessment tool helps the clinicians to develop and review the clinical rationale for the resulting treatment plan. The Assessment box on page 557 presents a lethality assessment scale.

Diagnosing

These are core nursing diagnoses that apply to most suicidal persons:

- High-risk for violence: Self-directed
- Hopelessness
- Ineffective individual coping
- Low self-esteem

Several other nursing diagnoses (e.g., anxiety, impaired verbal communication, and spiritual distress) may be appropriate, depending on the situation.

Planning and Implementing Interventions

Do people have the right to commit suicide, and can or should nurses intervene when people try to kill themselves? Nurses should know that, ethical concerns aside, they may be prosecuted under state laws, making it a crime to aid or abet a suicide, under any circumstance, even when a terminally ill person decides to end his or her life. Questions about a client's right to suicide and society's right to control suicide have not been answered. The nursing interventions discussed below are based on the traditional belief that mental health professionals should do everything possible to prevent suicide. Engaging in the process of ethical reflectiveness suggested in Chapter 7 will help nurses in their search for a personal position.

General Guidelines for Any Setting The essential task of the nurse is to work with the client to stop

Signs That Help Predict Suicide Risk: Comparing People Who Complete or Attempt Suicide with the General Population

Signs	Suicide	Suicide Attempt	General Population
Suicide plan*	Specific, with available, high lethal method; does not include rescue	Less lethal method, including plan for rescue; risk increases if lethality of method increases	None, or vague ideas only
History of suicide attempts*	65% have history of high lethal attempts; if rescued, it was probably accidental	Previous attempts are usually low lethal; rescue plan included; risk increases if there is a change from many low lethal attempts to a high lethal one	None or low lethal with definite rescue plan
Resources* • psychologic • social	Very limited or nonexistent; or person *perceives* self with no resources	Moderate, or in psychologic and/or social turmoil	Either intact or able to restore them through nonsuicidal means
Communication*	Feels cut off from resources and unable to communicate effectively	Ambiguously attached to resources; may use self-injury as a method of communicating with significant others when other methods fail	Able to communicate directly and nondestructively for need fulfillment
Recent loss	Increases risk	May increase risk	Is widespread but is resolved nonsuicidally through grief work, etc.
Physical illness	Increases risk	May increase risk	Is common but responded to through effective crisis management (natural and/or formal)
Drinking and other drug abuse	Increases risk	May increase risk	Is widespread but does not lead to suicide of itself
Isolation	Increases risk	May increase risk	Many well-adjusted people live alone; they handle physical isolation through satisfactory social contacts
Unexplained change in behavior	A possible clue to suicidal intent, especially in teenagers	A cry for help and possible clue to suicidal ideas	Does not apply in absence of other predictive signs
Depression	65% have a history of depression	A large percentage are depressed	A large percentage are depressed
Social factors or problems	May be present	Often are present	Widespread but do not of themselves lead to suicide
Mental illness	May be present	May be present	May be present
Age, sex, race, marital status	These are statistical predictors that are most useful for identifying whether an individual belongs to a high risk group, not for clinical assessment of individuals		

*If all four of these signs exist in a particular person, the risk for suicide is very high regardless of all other factors. If other signs also apply, the risk is further increased.

SOURCE: *Hoff LA:* People in Crisis, *ed 3. Addison-Wesley, 1990, pp 207–208.*

TABLE 23–1   **Lethality of Suicide Methods**

Less Lethal Methods	Highly Lethal Methods
Wrist cutting	Gun
House gas	Jumping
Nonprescription drugs (excluding aspirin and acetaminophen [Tylenol])	Hanging
	Drowning
Tranquilizers, e.g., diazepam (Valium), flurazepam (Dalmane)	Carbon monoxide poisoning
	Barbiturates and prescribed sleeping pills
	Aspirin and acetaminophen (Tylenol) (high doses)
	Car crash
	Exposure to extreme cold
	Antidepressants, e.g., amitriptyline (Elavil)

ASSESSMENT

Lethality Assessment Scale

Key to Scale	Danger to Self	Typical Indicators
1	No predictable risk of immediate suicide	Has no notion of suicide or history of attempts, has satisfactory social support network, and is in close contact with significant others
2	Low risk of immediate suicide	Person has considered suicide with low lethal method; no history of attempts or recent serious loss; has satisfactory support network; no alcohol problems; basically wants to live
3	Moderate risk of immediate suicide	Has considered suicide with high lethal method but no specific plan or threats; or, has plan with low lethal method, history of low lethal attempts, with tumultuous family history and reliance on Valium or other drugs for stress relief; is weighing the odds between life and death
4	High risk of immediate suicide	Has current high lethal plan, obtainable means, history of previous attempts, has a close friend but is unable to communicate with him or her; has a drinking problem; is depressed and wants to die
5	Very high risk of immediate suicide	Has current high lethal plan with available means, history of high lethal suicide attempts, is cut off from resources; is depressed and uses alcohol to excess, and is threatened with a serious loss, such as unemployment or divorce or failure in school

SOURCE: Hoff LA: People in Crisis, *ed 3. Addison-Wesley, 1989, p 209.*

the constricted processing of suicidal thinking long enough to allow the client and the family to consider alternatives to suicide. The nature of the nursing interventions are in large part determined by the setting in which the nurse encounters the suicidal client. The following list of interventions and suggestions offers general guidelines that are applicable in most settings:

• Take any threat seriously. Evaluate the threat before dismissing it.

• Talk about suicide openly and directly. Asking about it will not put the notion in the client's head.

• Implement suicidal precaution status that includes checking on the client at least every 15 minutes or requiring the client to remain in public spaces.

Text continues on p. 563

CASE STUDY

A Suicidal Client

Identifying Information

Mr G is a 67-year-old white male who is widowed. He is the father of two children, now both in their early 40s. He has been unemployed for the last three years. Prior to this, he was an architect for a major construction company. He has a master's degree in engineering and has authored texts on his particular area of expertise. He was transferred to this psychiatric unit after a seven-day stay at the intensive care unit of a nearby hospital.

Mr G was hospitalized after a suicide attempt when he shot himself. He has a superficial wound to the chest.

Client's Definition of Present Problem, Precipitating Stressors, Coping Strategies, Goals for Care

At the time of transfer to this hospital, Mr G states he has "no psychiatric problem, and don't know why I am coming to the psychiatric unit." Mr G states that he "just had a problem" and tried to work it out in the only logical way.

Mr G believes there may be a way for others to help him, but it has never "occurred to me to ask." He does not acknowledge any precipitants to current problems but states he had finally had it when "the car wouldn't start."

History of Present Problem

Mr G relates the details of his present problem in a matter-of-fact manner. He says that for the last three to four years things have been going downhill. His wife died three years ago after having breast cancer for a year. She died slowly and needed much physical care in the last few months. After that time, Mr G experienced great difficulty going out or meeting other people. He became more reclusive, began drinking every day for most of the day, and had difficulties at his job. Approximately one year ago, he lost his job at the construction company. He had held a high-ranking position, but after appearing intoxicated at work several times, he "retired early." For the last four months, the client has done little but drink alcohol for most of the day every day. His "nest egg" has been slowly dwindling. When he realized he was running out of money, he began to plan his death. Prior to the attempt, he wrote a will and destroyed all his private papers and personal communications. He then took his shotgun and went to a heavily wooded area to shoot himself. Apparently, the gun misfired, and he suffered a flesh wound to the chest area. Mr G lost a great deal of blood and passed out. Unexpectedly, there were others in the area who found Mr G and notified the police. Mr G was subsequently treated in the ICU for the chest wound and alcohol detoxification.

An interview with the family yielded the following information: The client had ongoing difficulties with alcohol prior to his wife's illness. His daughter and son both indicated interest in having him be more a part of their lives, but felt he was uninterested in doing so. Interpersonal relationships with the extended family have always been strained and uncomfortable.

Psychiatric History

Mr G has never been hospitalized for any psychiatric condition. In the past, on at least three occasions, he was referred for alcohol detox or rehabilitation. Mr G never attended any of those programs.

CASE STUDY (continued)

Family History

Mr G was raised in an affluent but emotionally cold family. Although his parents had both died many years ago, the client still talked of the anxiety and fears he felt as a young boy. He related being "excessively worried if I didn't know the right answer" to his parents' questions. He was sent away to boarding school from first grade through high school. He relates having a brother who was a better student and more athletic than he. This brother did not go away to boarding school as Mr G had to. At age 21, he met and married his first and only girlfriend. They subsequently had two children, a son now aged 42 and a daughter aged 40. He states his wife kept things together for the family since he traveled a great deal in his position. Since her death three years ago he has had "little contact" with his children and believes that "they don't care" about him.

Social History

Mr G has always been an active man who enjoyed intellectual stimulation. He remains a recognized expert in his field. He traveled a great deal in his position and now says that he has probably missed the most significant parts of his children's growth and development. He describes his marriage as "a good one." He says he depended heavily on his wife to maintain the family. He states, "We had our problems, but we worked them out." When discussing his wife and their marriage, Mr G becomes teary and quickly changes the subject. Since the death of his wife, Mr G has had little contact with his son and daughter. He has had difficulty dealing with leisure activities and uses alcohol to fill up his time.

He has not pursued his hobbies, which were flying his own plane and being a member of the Flying High Club, for the last two years.

He now relates that he has a few acquaintances, but no real friends. He has not maintained a relationship with his brother for many years.

In looking at his life over the past three years, he states "I'm just a broken-down machine." He believes he has outlived his usefulness.

Significant Health History

The client, subsequent to the suicide attempt, has a superficial chest wound. He apparently just missed shooting himself in the heart. The client was kept in the intensive care unit for seven days for observation. During his stay in the intensive care unit, he was also detoxed from alcohol. During this time, he did not evidence seizures but was irritable and shaky and had an elevation in vital signs for four days. In addition, the client is a four-pack-a-day smoker and has emphysema and a history of hypertension. He denies any additional medical problems, and the physical exam revealed no additional concerns.

Current Mental Status

Mr G presents as a casually groomed male who looks younger than his stated age. He participated in the interview process in an informed and matter-of-fact fashion.

Sensorium

Mr G was oriented to person, place, and time. He exhibited an above average fund of knowledge and at times tended to use multisyllabic words to either gain distance from or impress the interviewer. He appears hyperalert to any nuance or change in the environment. Judgment is seen as impaired because client does not see himself as having any problems.

CASE STUDY (continued)

Feelings

Mr G denied having any feelings about his current life situation. His affect was limited to either sarcasm or laughter when questioned about the past. He denied anger at self or others. Mood appeared to be superficially within normal limits, but there is evidence of guardedness and depression. One gets fleeting glimpses of sadness from the client, but he cannot tolerate these feelings for longer than a few seconds.

Voice and Speech

Speech was normal in flow and volume. When challenged by the interviewer he began to use polysyllabic words. He also would intersperse German, Italian, and French into the conversation when he appeared increasingly stressed.

Motor Behavior

Posture during interview was relaxed and comfortable. There were no overt signs of restlessness or agitation. No atypical movements were noted. Client denies past use of medications that might result in abnormal involuntary movements.

Thought Processes

Client's thoughts were coherent and logical but did tend to drift. He appeared preoccupied at times.

Thought Content

There are no signs of any delusions, illusions, or hallucinations. Client, at this time, denies suicidal ideation or plan, but cannot relate why things have changed from a week ago. Client's plan prior to admission should be considered highly lethal as he had a calculated plan with violent means to accomplish it. He was discovered by accident, not by design.

Defenses

The most obvious coping methods are intellectualization, denial, and rationalization. It is clear that this client has used these defenses for most of his life.

Insight

There is no evidence that this client has any insight into his current situation. He denies current intent for suicide despite his recent elaborate plan to end his life.

Other Significant Subjective or Objective Clinical Data

Client's chest wound is judged to be healing properly, and client has some residual pain. He is currently able to change his own dressing, and thus this will not be the major focus of treatment on the psychiatric unit. His vital signs are within normal limits. Prior to his transfer here, he was treated for alcohol withdrawal and initially showed signs of irritability and anxiety. No other overt signs were noted. Mr G denies that his use of alcohol is a problem.

Diagnostic Impression Nursing Diagnoses (NANDA)

High risk for violence: Self-directed
Self-esteem disturbance
Ineffective individual coping
Dysfunctional grieving
Altered role performance

DSM-III-R Multiaxial Diagnosis

Axis I: 296.23   Major depression, severe, without psychotic features
           305.00   Alcohol dependence
Axis II: Narcissistic personality traits
Axis III: Status post chest wound; emphysema, hypertension
Axis IV: Psychosocial stressors; loss of wife, loss of job; no family connection; Severity-5
Axis V: Current GAF = 10; Highest GAF past year = 30.

▶

NURSING CARE PLAN

A Suicidal Client

Client Care Goals	Nursing Planning/ Interventions	Evaluation
Nursing Diagnosis: *Ineffective individual coping related to alcohol dependence*		
Client will verbalize acceptance of alcohol as an ongoing life problem.	Utilize 2 × weekly psycho-therapy groups to allow client time to review problems of the past and investigate the presence of alcoholism in these areas; provide health teaching on the interaction of alcohol dependence and depression.	Client verbalizes acceptance of his alcoholism.
Client will verbalize knowledge of the disease process and use self-help groups to aid in recovery.		Client verbalizes knowledge of disease process.
Client will attend AA groups.		Client attends two AA meetings per week.
	Help client explore the use of alcohol as a learned coping mechanism in his family.	Client requests a sponsor.
	Encourage client to verbalize feelings about loss of control over alcohol use.	
	Staff familiar with 12-step models should discuss the process with client and encourage active participation into the program.	
Nursing Diagnosis: *Dysfunctional grieving related to death of wife*		
Client will verbalize need to begin grief work.	Establish a working relationship with client.	Client discusses losses and begins to work on grief process.
Client will verbalize and experience feelings about loss of wife.	Utilize individual sessions twice weekly to allow for ventilation and exploration of feelings about loss of wife.	Client verbalizes stages of grief work.
	Educate client about grief process and potential effects of not resolving grief.	Client verbalizes plan to obtain follow-up mental health services.
	Discuss grief groups with client.	Client attends grief group.
	Encourage client to attend grief groups in community.	
Nursing Diagnosis: *Altered role performance related to unemployment*		
Client will develop alternatives to his current unemployed status and follow through on finding employment or other pursuits in his field.	Discuss with client his loss of prior positions.	Attends session with vocational counselor.
	Encourage client to review the factors leading to his termination.	Verbalizes insight into reason for losing last position.

▶

NURSING CARE PLAN (continued)

Client Care Goals	Nursing Planning/ Intervention	Evaluation
	Support client while he realistically examines the problems so that he avoids blaming or self-deprecating behaviors.	Discusses possible methods to avoid recurrence of this problem in the future.
	Encourage client to attend meeting with vocational counselor.	
	Encourage client to follow up on recommendations of vocational counselor, e.g., discuss how he would have his resume prepared.	
	Encourage client to prepare a plan for obtaining employment.	

Nursing Diagnosis: *High risk for violence: Self-directed*

Client will be free of self-inflicted injury.	Assess the client as to his level of suicidal ideation. Evaluate for feelings, ideations, plans, and future orientation. Evaluate client's potential for self-harm at least every shift. Implement suicide precautions as indicated. Check on client at irregular intervals.	Client complies with suicide precaution.
Client will decrease suicidal ideation.		Client verbalizes decreased desire for self-harm.
Client will verbalize alternatives to suicidal behavior.		Client discusses two alternatives to suicide.
Client will resolve his ambivalence about suicidal behavior.	Encourage discussion of alternatives to suicide.	Client participates in forming no-suicide contract with primary nurse.
	Encourage client to verbalize ambivalence about suicidal ideation and plan. Consider the use of a no-suicide contract, if indicated.	

Nursing Diagnosis: *Ineffective individual coping*

Client will develop additional coping strategies.	Encourage client to discuss current and past coping methods.	Client reports having used three additional coping strategies.
	Encourage him to investigate alternate methods of effectively coping, e.g., communicating with others, asking for help when he needs it, developing leisure and recreational skills.	
	Help client to try out new coping styles with staff support.	

NURSING CARE PLAN (continued)

Client Care Goals	Nursing Planning/ Intervention	Evaluation
	Give positive feedback about his attempts at new behaviors. Help client identify how not having coping skills has led to his current problems.	

Nursing Diagnosis: Self-esteem disturbance related to perceived feelings of loss of control

Client Care Goals	Nursing Planning/ Intervention	Evaluation
Client will verbalize the full range of feelings associated with current losses: of his vocational status, of his physical well-being, and of his wife. Client will verbalize increased self-esteem. Client will gain skills in resolving losses.	Use therapeutic sessions twice weekly to encourage verbalization of his losses. Encourage client (as much as feasible) to assume responsibility for his own treatment, e.g., setting discharge date, deciding what groups to attend, selecting an outpatient therapist. Encourage client to review his part in these losses, if appropriate. Encourage client to decide what areas can be changed and which need acceptance. Discuss past vocational success and support a future focus about jobs or other vocational pursuits that will enhance self-esteem. Utilize milieu activities to enhance self-esteem, e.g., participating in client government, participating in groups.	Client verbalizes connections between significant losses and his low self-esteem.

• Expect that the client will be experiencing shame, and work to assist the client toward self-acceptance.

• Remove the client from immediate danger by confiscating pills or other harmful objects in the client's possession, or by moving the client to a physically safe environment.

• Relieve the client's obvious immediate distress. Does the client need a bath, clean clothing, food, sleep?

• Find out what, in the client's view, the most pressing need is. This may be to see a friend or family member, or to arrange for someone to pick up the children after school.

• Assume a nonjudgmental, caring attitude that does not engender self-pity in the client.

• Ask why the client chose to attempt suicide at this particular moment. The answer will shed light on the meaning suicide has for the client and may provide information that can lead to other helpful interventions.

• Provide for the client's safety through close observation and careful monitoring (see the section on safety).

• Review the safety of the environment (see the section on milieu factors).

INTERVENTION

Do's and Don't's of No Self-Harm/No-Suicide Contracts

No self-harm/no-suicide contracts are effective in many situations, and they work well with certain groups of clients. They can be used in hospital or outpatient settings as a means of providing additional support to people who are likely to harm themselves. It is imperative to establish a trusting relationship with the person prior to making a contract.

Do's

• Do fully assess a client to decide if a contract will be a helpful aid to treatment.

• Do establish a relationship with the client prior to initialing the contract.

• Do use the contract as a way of connecting with and staying connected with the client.

• Do specify in the contract the intervals for re-evaluation. In outpatient work the interval may be one week; the inpatient interval may range from every shift to every one to three days.

• Do have both nurse and client sign the contract and date it.

• Do have the client write out the contract if at all possible. Be creative if a client is unable or unwilling to write it out; the contract could be audiotaped, or client and nurse might each write half.

• Do include possible alternatives in the contract such as "If I'm feeling like hurting myself I'll call _____, or I'll ask for _____."

Don't's

• Don't use a no-suicide contract before performing a full nursing assessment.

• Don't place more trust in a contract or emphasis on it than in clinical judgment. The contract is a helpful therapeutic tool but does not replace good clinical judgment. Clients who are acutely suicidal may agree to the contract even though they have no intention of adhering to it.

Sample No Self-Harm/No-Suicide Contract

I, Cathy Smith, will not harm myself in any way. If I feel I am going to lose control, I will tell the staff (call the crisis unit, call my therapist, etc.)

I will not bring nor will I ask others to bring harmful articles or substances on the unit.

This contract lasts until 1/10/92 and is renewable at that time.

Signed

Cathy Smith   1/3/92

Nancy Jones, RN   1/3/92

• Search the client's room, especially if suicidal ideation or a suicide attempt occurs after admission.

• Decide (usually along with other members of a team) if a no-harm, no-suicide contract will be used (see the accompanying Intervention box).

• House the client in areas that are accessible for easy observation.

• Select a room that is near the nurses' station. A two-person room is best.

• Be careful not to encourage staff behaviors that give clients or staff members a false sense of security. In one instance, staff members took a client's shoes and reduced safety checks on the client thinking that, without shoes, he would not run away from the unit.

He ran from the unit barefoot and suffered lacerations on both feet.

• Organize a plan of care with the client. Discuss all important problems, prioritize them, and list several approaches to each problem. Write down this plan, noting who is responsible for which actions.

• Do not make unrealistic promises such as, "Don't worry, I won't let you kill yourself." Remain honest, but hopeful. Making unrealistic promises diminishes the nurse's credibility with the client.

• Encourage the client to continue daily activities and self-care as much as possible. Assign tasks for the client that are distracting, but not taxing.

• Decide with the client which family members and friends are to be contacted and by whom.

• Be prepared to deal with family members who may be confused, angry, or uninterested. Strive to remain neutral and do not make assumptions about the family's behavior.

• Evaluate the client's need for medication.

• Evaluate the plan developed in collaboration with the client and arrange for appropriate follow-up.

• Monitor your personal feelings about the client and decide how they may be influencing your clinical work.

• Work with other team members to evaluate the issues fully. The nurse doesn't always have all the pieces of the puzzle.

• Do a body examination. One woman had cut herself severely prior to coming to the hospital, but this injury was not discovered until the physical examination was performed.

• Recognize that people can and have hanged or strangled themselves with shoelaces, brassiere straps, pantyhose, robe belts, craft materials, and so on. Remain alert: Razor blades have been found in pages of books; matches are relatively easy to hide; pills have been hidden in plastic wrap in a cake box and stuffed animals; light bulbs can be broken and used to cut oneself, as can wire from spiral notebooks. Clients can also drown in a bathtub, go through a plate-glass window, set themselves on fire, or drink bleach from the cleaning person's cart.

In the emergency department, the main goal of treatment is to save the person's life. Although the ER staff may be excellent at technical interventions, the staff may voice or feel contempt for the client who is a "repeater," especially if the attempt is not a serious one. The client needs a professional, nonpunitive approach and a smooth transition to other caretakers or agencies. Leaving the person alone or with access to harmful objects is obviously a hazard to be avoided in a busy emergency department.

Safety: Observing and Monitoring Client Behavior   Maintain the client's safety in the least restrictive manner possible. The length of time on restrictive status is of concern to both the client and the staff. Remember that restrictions meet the safety needs of the client, but they do not constitute treatment. On an in-patient unit, times of highest risk for suicide are evenings, nights, and weekends. Two factors account for this. During these periods, clients' time is less structured, and fewer staff members are available.

Most psychiatric in-patient units have developed a system for observing clients or a set of protocols or guidelines for observing and monitoring client behavior. Systems of observation may have three to six

levels. Restrictions often require a physician order but can be implemented on an emergency basis by privileged clinical staff. These protocols are often labeled to reflect the rationale for their use and are known by such names as *suicide precautions, special awareness, observation, constant observation,* and *constant awareness.* See the Intervention boxes below and on page 566 for sample protocols.

It is of critical importance that all staff members be familiar with the system that is used and know the rationale for its use. The responsibility for maintaining and observing clients on these protocols remains with the registered nurse.

Restrictive status should be reserved for the safety management of suicidal clients. Restrictions can con-

INTERVENTION

Basic Suicide Precautions: Sample Protocol

• The client is to remain in the room with the door open unless accompanied by staff or a family member. The client may use the bathroom alone.

• Check the client's whereabouts and safety every 15 minutes. Have a check-off sheet on client's door to document safety checks.

• Stay with the client while all medications are taken.

• Search the client's belongings for potentially harmful objects. Make the search in the client's presence, and ask for the client's assistance while doing so.

• Check articles brought in by visitors.

• Allow the client to have regular food tray, but check whether the glass or any utensils are missing when collecting the tray.

• Allow visitors and telephone calls unless the client wishes otherwise.

• Check that visitors do not leave potentially dangerous objects in the client's room.

• The plan may be started without a physician's order, but a psychiatric consultation must be arranged as soon as possible.

• Maintain the protocol until it is canceled by a psychiatrist.

• Inform the client of reasons for and details of precautionary measures. This explanation must be made by nurses and physician and documented in the chart.

INTERVENTION

Maximum Suicide Precautions: Sample Protocol

The following is a protocol for maximum suicide precaution. These measures can be instituted without a physician's order under emergency conditions. However, a psychiatric consultation must be obtained as soon as possible.

- Provide one-to-one nursing supervision. The nurse must be in the room with the client at *all* times. When the client uses the bathroom, the bathroom door must remain open. Stay within arm's reach of the client at all times. Staff should sit next to the client's bed at night.

- Use no restraints on general hospital floors.

- Do not allow the client to leave the unit for tests or procedures.

- Allow visitors and telephone calls unless the client wishes otherwise. The nurse maintains one-to-one supervision during visits.

- Look through the client's belongings in the client's presence and remove any potentially harmful objects, e.g., pills, matches, belts, razors, tweezers, and mirrors or other glass objects.

- If suicide precautions are initiated after the client has been on the unit for any length of time, make a complete search of the room.

- Check that visitors do not leave potentially harmful objects in the client's room.

- Serve the client's meals in an isolation meal tray that contains no glass or metal silverware.

- Prior to instituting these measures, explain to the client what you will be doing and why. A physician must also explain this to the client. Document this explanation in the chart.

- Do not discontinue these measures without an order from a psychiatrist.

found therapeutic management, and their use simply to restrict the free movement of clients diminishes their effectiveness. In general, privileges and other components of unit restriction are better dealt with by other measures such as privilege systems. If staff are in doubt as to the appropriate safety status, the client should remain on a more restrictive status until the team decides what measures are appropriate. If there is doubt or concern about moving a client to a different status, it is best to retain the more restrictive status until the direction of treatment is clarified.

As the team begins to move clients off special status, it is important for all team members to keep communicating openly about the client. As the client begins to improve, the risk of suicide increases temporarily (especially if the client has increased energy and ability finally to act on the suicidal ideation). The following times are critical and call for careful evaluation:

- When the decision is made to *move the client off the suicide precaution status*. Clients, especially those who have come to be dependent upon the around-the-clock safety, comfort, and nurturance provided by a staff member, may experience discontinuance of suicide precaution status as a loss. Gradual removal from suicide precaution status and careful monitoring of its impact on the client is indicated for these clients.

- When the decision is made to *increase access to "sharps"* (dangerous objects). This increased access may make it possible for a client to act on a suicidal impulse. Assess the client carefully before granting this access.

- During the *second or third week of antidepressive drug therapy*. At this time, clients have increased energy but their depression has not been resolved.

- When the decision is made to *grant a pass*. Decisions to grant pass privileges should be evaluated carefully. Where is the client going and with whom? What time frame is being considered and why? The nurse must perform a careful assessment both before and after the client goes on a pass. Additional searches may be needed at these times.

- *Prior to discharge* and while formulating the *discharge plan*. It is crucial to evaluate the "holding environment" in the community. The client should be referred to resources in the community, and a follow-up appointment should be scheduled at the time of discharge. Family and significant others should participate in discharge planning. It is generally not a good idea to discharge a client (especially one who lacks immediate family supports and must rely on agencies or clinics for support) on a Friday, over a long weekend, or when the mental health care provider will be on vacation or otherwise unavailable.

Once a client has been recognized as a suicide risk and a safety plan has been implemented, the therapeutic work of addressing the depression, psychosis, and precipitating factors needs to begin. As the client begins to show signs of clinical improvement, there are critical intervals at which the treatment focus shifts from safety to investigation and treatment of the depression or precipitant of the suicidal ideation.

The following signs usually indicate clinical improvement. They often signal the need to review and possibly change treatment plans, to grant privileges, or to plan discharges:

• Verbalizing a range of options other than suicide

• Making long-term plans or discussing future events

• Verbalizing hope

• Responding to antidepressant and/or antipsychotic medications

• Wanting to reconnect or moving toward reconnecting with family or significant others

• Showing more energy

• Sleeping better

• Feeling less hopeless

• Demonstrating a wider range of affective responses to situations that occur on the unit

Restrictions should be changed gradually, rather than all at once. A realistic plan is to change one or, at the most, two variables at a time while observing, monitoring, and documenting client responses.

Monitoring Safety in the Milieu   The safety of the milieu should be evaluated periodically. Does it meet the needs of the current client population, and is the level of restrictions consistent with the milieu philosophy? Here are some specific questions to ask:

• Are areas free of glass or sharps?

• Are hazardous objects and areas kept locked?

• Are closet or shower rods of the breakaway type?

• Are craft items safe?

• How many clients are there? What is the client population like now? Do they have character disorders? Serious depression?

• If the milieu is temporarily deemed unsafe, that is, if there are objects (liquor, razors, drugs) on the unit that can harm others, is there a need to do a "health-and-welfare search," examining all areas of the unit for contraband or other potential hazards?

The nurse also needs to educate the family and visitors about safety measures and their rationale. This helps to ensure that family members and other visitors do not bring unsafe objects on the unit. Visitors must understand visit limits and unit policies in relation to passes. The need for searches is also explained. Families and friends who repeatedly violate safety measures require additional attention, and their visiting privileges may have to be restricted.

Documenting Client Behavior and Treatment
Documentation is an essential duty for nurses working with suicidal clients on an in-patient unit. Documentation helps all staff to understand the rationale for changes and to comply with ethical and legal requirements. In general, follow agency rules about documentation. Nurses should also be sure to document the following:

• All team reviews of client status and the names of the team members involved

• Any decision to remove the client from a more restrictive status to a less restrictive one

• The rationale for any changes in the treatment approach, especially changes in the level of restriction

• Statements from clients about self-harm or denial

• Client responses to changes, passes, family, visitors

• All telephone calls or interactions with family members

• All searches done and the reason for them

Evaluating/Outcome Criteria

Suicide, like all crisis situations, calls for ongoing evaluation of the plan made by the nurse and client. Because events often occur rapidly, initial care plans may need to be changed almost daily. In addition to evaluating individual care plans, a staff who deals with suicidal clients needs to evaluate its overall approach and philosophy periodically.

Suicide in Special Populations

Children

Not long ago most people believed that it was impossible for children to be depressed or suicidal. However, the truth is that suicide by children has increased threefold over the last two decades. In 1986, for example, there were 300 suicides among children aged 1–14 (U.S. Bureau of the Census 1989), and the numbers continue to rise despite increasing awareness by parents and professionals. These statistics probably underestimate the scope of the problem, because professionals and families still collude to label suicidal acts as accidents. Depending on age, children may not see death as irreversible, and to that degree suicide may be accidental (Valente 1983).

Some people cannot believe children would want to end their lives. Suicide attempts by children belie the myth of the "happy child" in our culture. One study revealed that, among children or adolescents who come to a general hospital emergency room with indications of suicidal intent or behavior, at least one-half are diagnosed as victims of accidents rather than suicide attempts, and no follow-up is planned (Hawton 1986). The following example illustrates denial and lack of information in parents of a suicidal child.

A 10-year old boy set up a rope over a door to hang himself. His attempt was stopped by his parents. The door, a second entrance to the room, was painted shut, and the subject of suicide was not discussed. His parents failed to recognize the same symptoms in the child two years later. However, at this time, severe behavior problems in school and pressure by school personnel forced the parents to bring in the child for a psychiatric evaluation.

Children commit suicide by simple but lethal methods such as poisoning, shooting themselves with firearms, hanging, or darting into the path of moving cars.

It is unclear what drives a child to commit suicide. Several authors have described characteristic presuicidal symptoms and life circumstances of the suicidal child. The symptoms are known as depressive equivalents; that is, the symptoms may indicate a masked depression. The symptoms of a masked depression are:

- Boredom and restlessness

- Irritability or lethargy

- Difficulty in concentration

- Apparently purposeful misbehavior

- Somatic preoccupation

- Excessive dependence on or isolation from others, notably adults

Orbach (1984) and others reviewed many life and family factors that place a child at risk for suicide. These include depression, psychosis, impulsive traits, substance abuse, failure to complete developmental tasks, lack of family cohesion, overemphasis on achievement, frequent exposure to aggression, lack of religious identification, losses (e.g., peers, relationships), poor school performance, and family factors such as frequent moves, deprivation of love and attention, marital conflict, parental unemployment, parental loss, suicidal behavior in other family members, and poor management of divorce.

Adolescents

Adolescent suicide is a serious concern. This decade has seen a dramatic rise in the rate of adolescent suicide. The rates among 15-to-19-year-olds increased from 8.5 per 100,000 in 1980 to 10.2 per 100,000 in 1986. Among 15-to-24-year-olds, the rate of completed suicides over the past 20 years has doubled (Curran 1987). Suicide is now the third leading cause of death among 15-to-24-year-olds in the United States. Only homicides and accidents account for more deaths.

The rate of attempted suicide is also a major public health issue. Information on attempts is elusive, and some researchers speculate that many "accidents" of adolescents are actually suicide gestures or attempts. The ratio of adolescent suicide attempts to completed suicides is now estimated at 200:1; approximately one million young people annually engage in self-harmful behavior. As with suicide statistics for all age groups, it is likely that suicide rates for this group have been underestimated.

There are no known reasons for the 173 percent increase in adolescent suicide since 1950. Many link it to decreased family stability, greater pressure in childhood, or heightened competition for grades in the schools and jobs in the workplace. Some speculate that our complex and dangerous world (nuclear threats, terrorism, war) contributes to a sense of depression or futility.

Some maintain that the very nature of adolescence greatly contributes to the problem: that adolescent grandiosity and narcissism make the potentially suicidal adolescent believe, for instance, "I cannot die. Someone will find me before this overdose kills me." Others blame the increase in adolescent suicides on the media reporting of suicides. They insist that the sensational and romantic quality of the reporting actually precipitates suicides, particularly suicide clusters. The critics allege that suicide clusters would never have happened in the absence of publicity.

Although there are no studies that allow us to predict with certainty which adolescents will commit suicide, the presence of certain stressors and risk factors can help the nurse identify a potentially suicidal adolescent. Most suicides or suicide attempts are preceded by verbal or action threats, a statement of intent, or a suicidal gesture. However, this is less true of adolescents, unless they have a history of long-standing problems and behavior changes. Adolescent suicides often occur without warning. They are frequently triggered by a seemingly trivial incident, such as a fight with a boyfriend or a quarrel with parents. The suicide is a sudden, impulsive reaction to a stressful situation or a perceived loss, such as a separation, a divorce, a death, a loss in self-esteem (for instance, being cut from a high school team), or a transition or move that symbolizes loss (for instance, going away to college). The loss can also be an imagined one, e.g., "No one likes me," or "I'll never be pretty enough (or good enough)." The need to work through loss is a necessary developmental task of adolescents.

RESEARCH NOTE

Citation

Schneider SG, Farberow NL, Kruks GN: Suicidal behavior in adolescent and young adult gay men. Suicide Life Threat Behav *1989;19(4):381–393.*

Study Problem/Purpose

The purpose of this study was to examine the relationship of homosexuality to suicidal ideation and attempts in self-identified gay youth.

Methods

The subjects consisted of two groups of self-identified gay men between 16 and 24 years of age. One group was drawn from gay and lesbian student organizations from fourteen Los Angeles colleges. A second group was drawn from rap groups conducted by the local gay and lesbian community center. Participation was voluntary. Subjects were judged by their respective group leaders to be representative of all persons attending meetings, and over 90 percent of those present when the questionnaires were distributed participated.

Subjects completed a questionnaire requesting information on suicidal thoughts and feelings, with items specifically focused on fleeting thoughts of suicide, and serious consideration of acting on the suicidal thoughts. Items were ranked on a seven-point scale from "never" to "chronically" over three time periods: (1) before age 14 (2) after age 14 (3) during the last 6 months. Subjects noted a number of suicidal plans and attempts they had made for each time period. Information was also obtained on the age at which each attempt occurred, accompanying thoughts and feelings and treatment received. Demographic data were obtained, and levels of current support were measured. The degree to which each support source accepted or rejected

the subject's sexual orientation was also reviewed. Also reported were the ages when the subjects reached critical stages in the process of "coming out," when they had "come out" to relationships, and what degree of acceptance or rejection they encountered upon "coming out."

Results

The results of the study indicate that family dysfunction, particularly paternal alcoholism and physical abuse, may be a significant characteristic in the backgrounds of those gay male youths most likely to report suicidal ideation in adolescence. Suicidal ideation in gay male youths is often accompanied by perceived (or actual) rejection by important and needed social supports for an emerging homosexual identity. Suicide attempts among gay male youths are mostly intrapersonal acts carried out as these adolescents grapple in basic isolation with difficult aspects of an emerging homosexual identity or with rejection for being homosexual.

Implications

This research supports current theories about populations at risk for suicide i.e., given a lack of situational supports, homosexuality may place the adolescent at higher risk for suicide. Nursing assessments should include questions that elicit information about sexuality, sexual orientation, and presence or absence of situational supports. Nurses need to be aware of these factors and include them when assessing individuals with these characteristics or life-styles. Assessment and interventions should be directed toward developing supportive relationships, devising conflict-resolution strategies, and building self-confidence.

Adolescence is a time of increased internal and external stressors. Adolescents experiencing an abnormal number of life changes appear to be at even higher risk for suicide (Parker 1988). What may be extremely stressful to one adolescent, however, may be a minor matter to another. The nature and severity of the precipitating stress can reveal a great deal about the adolescent's coping abilities. Events and situations that have special significance as potential stressors and the possible meanings they may have for the adolescent are

listed in Table 23–2 on page 570. Rather than assume a meaning, however, the nurse should, before developing a plan of care, explore a stressor with the client to identify the significance of the event.

Which adolescents are most likely to commit suicide? Certain risk factors can help the professional identify the potentially suicidal adolescent. For example, it is possible to recognize individuals who are suffering from depression before it interferes with their ability to function in everyday life and before the

TABLE 23-2 Stressors That Have Special Significance for the Adolescent

Stressor	Possible Meaning
Anniversary date of death of loved one (particularly if death was suicide)	Can rekindle feelings of loss and mourning; may evoke feelings of guilt or anger, if unresolved; may prompt ideas of "rejoining" the loved one
Developmental milestone (e.g., menarche, leaving grammar school and entering high school)	Can represent loss of childhood and decreasing dependency on parental figures; can evoke performance anxiety and fear of failure or embarrassment
Holidays	Can represent unfulfillment and disappointment; can trigger or intensify needs and longings; can be a source of increased family tension and fighting
Loss, real or imagined	Can intensify feelings of low self-esteem and unworthiness; can cause feelings of acute loss and loneliness, resulting in depression and despair
Performance failure (e.g., failed exam, embarrassing school situation)	Can devastate the adolescent, particularly the overachieving adolescent with uncompromising parents; at the other extreme, can be the "last straw" for an adolescent with many failures

depression becomes so oppressive that the adolescent considers suicide. The accompanying Assessment box lists warning signals of the need to explore and assess further.

The nurse assessing the youth or adolescent for suicide or evaluating suicide attempts should consider some additional factors to determine the lethality of the behavior:

• Does the adolescent have a "suicide model" (a family member or close friend who has attempted or completed suicide)?

• What is the motivation for the act, e.g., wanting to die, to get help, to get relief?

• How lethal is the suicide intent? More importantly, how lethal does the adolescent consider the act to be? (If the adolescent took ten aspirin tablets thinking this constituted an overdose, the attempt has high lethality.)

• What is the nature of the precipitating stress?

• What resources are available to the adolescent?

• What is the history of prior problems, and how good are the adolescent's coping skills?

How can the nurse effectively assess depression in individuals who characteristically act out their feelings rather than express them verbally? In fact, largely because of this acting-out behavior, the nurse in a setting frequented by adolescents has numerous opportunities to make such assessments. The nurse not only observes depressed adolescents for certain behavioral cues but also compares their behavior with that of peers who are not depressed. Assessments and interventions by the school or community nurse can be critical in this respect. The accompanying box lists possible behavioral cues indicative of adolescent depression.

The most common precursor of adolescent suicide is certainly depression. Adolescence is a volatile time characterized by rapid mood swings and great intensity of feelings. For this reason, adults may have trouble recognizing depression in adolescents. Moreover, adults tend to idealize adolescence and may refuse to accept the idea of adolescent depression. Adults, including mental health professionals, are likely to view suicide attempts by adolescents as manipulative and hostile acts designed to punish or control significant others. A survey by Curran (1987) concluded that adults may view suicide attempts by adolescents as insincere acts because they are often of low lethality. However, the rising numbers of adolescents who complete suicide indicate the need to view all attempts as serious requests for help. For adolescents—for all clients—it is imperative to assess and answer cries for help.

The Elderly

The elderly are also at high risk for suicide. Suicide is the ninth leading cause of death and the leading cause of preventable death in this age group. It has long been recognized that the risk in the elderly is inordinately high (roughly two to three times that of all age groups). For example, in the United States in 1986

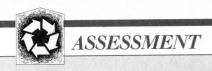

Factors Increasing the Risk for Suicide among Adolescents

- Depression, usually related to the loss of someone or something of great value to the adolescent. Depression is usually marked by the following group of symptoms: feelings of helplessness, hopelessness, worthlessness, loss or deprivation, and guilt or rejection.
- Low self-esteem and lack of basic trust in self and others.
- Family unit problems such as:
  - Psychiatric illness in the family, particularly in one or both parents
  - Chronic depression in the family, particularly in one or both parents
  - Chronic or extensive history of family problems; conflicts in family, especially about discipline
  - Marital discord and unhealthy interactions between parents or among parents and the adolescent. Parents may scapegoat the adolescent, displacing their feelings of dissatisfaction and disappointment and leading the adolescent to accept blame.
  - Situations characterized by long-term neglect, abuse, or unstable home and family life.

- A handicap that makes the adolescent "different" and unworthy (e.g., a learning problem, a chronic illness, or a physical deformity). It is not the handicap that leads to the feelings of unworthiness but the negative messages the adolescent may receive if family and significant others do not provide frequent and consistent positive and accepting emotional experiences.
- Intrapersonal/interpersonal problems such as:
  - School problems
  - Pregnancy
  - Drug use/abuse
  - Worries about sexuality, sexual feelings, or sexual orientation
  - Worries about breaking the law
  - Feelings of anxiety
  - Problems with a romantic relationship
- Presence of a "suicide model": Forty-four percent of adolescents who attempted suicide had a close friend or relative who had either attempted or completed suicide. Twenty-five percent of adolescents who attempted suicide had a parent who attempted suicide.

Behavioral Cues Indicative of Adolescent Depression

Changed mood	Reflects a persistent and pervasive unhappy mood rather than the transient and situation-specific mood typical of adolescence; may project a global anger that interferes with interpersonal relationships.
Low self-esteem	Results in feelings of unworthiness, guilt, and rejection; leads to behaviors that "set up" failure and rejection.
Decreased energy	Marked by extreme fatigue that is incapacitating at times; adolescent may "wake up tired"; leads to concern about possible underlying illness.
Problems with school involvement	Includes both academic performance and social activity; low grades or decline in academic performance can be marker of emotional difficulty; changes in interpersonal relationships, particularly social withdrawal and isolation, are cues for the nurse.
Somatic complaints	Will most likely be reason to see nurse in school or community clinic; symptoms usually fall into three major categories; physical complaints with fatigue, alterations in sleep patterns, and changes in appetite and body weight.

there were 6275 suicides among people 65 and older (U.S. Bureau of Census 1989). The statistics of elderly suicide do not include deaths that are labeled as accidents. They also do not include deaths that are a result of indirect self-destructive behavior, e.g., the client who "forgets" to take his cardiac medication and subsequently dies of "natural causes." Suicidologists speculate that the true suicide rate is at least double the reported rate (Boxwell 1988). Thus, suicide assessment and prevention should be a significant concern for the nurse working with this population in any health care setting.

The lethality index (ratio of suicide attempts to completed suicides) is also high in the elderly. For all age groups, this ratio is between 10:1 to 20:1 (the ratio for adolescents is as high as 200:1). Among the elderly, the ratio of attempts to completed suicides is 4:1. Here are two significant concerns for this age group:

• High lethality of intent in the elderly. There is a notable lack of ambivalence around the decision to suicide.

• High lethality of the methods utilized. In one recent study, older males most commonly shot themselves with guns (Boxwell 1988).

The elderly are also less likely to have the physiologic strength to recuperate after a suicide attempt.

The elderly tend to underutilize mental health services for several reasons. An elderly client may avoid seeking help from mental health professionals because of the ethical, moral, and social stigma associated with suicide and suicide ideation and psychiatric illness. It is estimated that only 1 to 3 percent of calls to suicide prevention centers are from clients over the age of 65. Elderly people who have suicidal ideation or plans may have attempted to get help from primary health care providers (usually medical sources) and may complain of depression or somatic symptoms. Thus, nurses are in an ideal position to identify people at risk and provide services or make appropriate referrals.

These factors place the elderly at increased risk for suicide:

• Serious illness (terminal illness, debilitating illness, or chronic pain)

• Bereavement and loss (loss of spouse, significant friends, family)

• Use of alcohol and mood-altering drugs to cope with stress

• Neuropsychiatric disorders (organic brain disease)

• Changes in socioeconomic status, work status, prestige

• History of prior suicidal behavior or prior requests for help

• Use of medication that may precipitate depression (antidepressants, steroids, phenothiazines, rauwolfia derivatives)

To assess suicide potential in elderly clients, the nurse must be perceptive, listen actively, and pose direct questions. The suicidal elderly individual may give the following cues:

• Verbal cues ("I'm going to end it all." "Life is not worth living." "I won't be around much longer.")

• Behavioral cues (completing a will, making funeral plans, acting out, withdrawing, somatic complaints)

• Situational cues (recent move, loss of a loved one, diagnosis of a terminal illness)

• Atypical cues (cognitive changes similar to organic brain disease, excessive preoccupation with physical symptoms, a resigned attitude—"I'm supposed to feel this way; I'm old.")

Psychiatric Clients

There is a serious risk of suicide among those persons diagnosed with a psychiatric illness. Roy (1985) suggests that the risk of suicide among this group is three to twelve times greater than the risk among the general population and that 10 percent of all persons labeled schizophrenic die by suicide.

Among psychiatric clients in general, these factors are associated with increased suicidal risk:

• Female sex

• Young age

• Diagnosis of depression or schizophrenia

• History of past attempt, living alone, unemployment, and being unmarried and recently admitted to psychiatric care

The suicide rate for schizophrenics may be increasing because of stress from community living and frequent brief hospitalizations. The schizophrenic client most at suicide risk is a young white male who is in remission. He is well educated (several years of college) and has high expectations of himself. He feels hopeless, depressed, inadequate, and unable to cope with the chronicity of his illness. Other factors are previous suicide attempts and current threats or ideation. Suicide occurs most often early during hospitalization or soon after discharge.

The incidence of self-destructive behavior and suicide is also high among characterologically impaired people. Suicidal behavior is an integral part of the clinical presentation of clients with personality disorders, especially clients with a diagnosis of borderline personality disorder or histrionic personality disorder. In their study of suicidal behavior, Raczek et al. (1989) found the following:

• Suicidal behavior appears to be related to character pathology; the higher the number of pathologic personality traits, the higher the suicide risk.

• Borderline personality traits are the most common characterologic traits among clients with suicidal behavior.

• The combination of borderline and avoidant personality traits seems to be the most "lethal."

Substance Abusers

What is information about substance abuse doing in a chapter about suicide and self-destructive behavior? It is estimated that 35 to 40 percent of completed suicides are alcohol related, as many as 50 to 60 percent of all suicide attempts are alcohol related, and the risk of suicide in alcoholics is thirty-two times the risk for suicide in the general population (Estes and Heinemann 1986). Substance abuse is also related to many fatal automobile and boating accidents. It is often difficult to distinguish suicides from accidental overdoses and accidents. When more than one substance is used, (e.g., alcohol and sedatives, alcohol and cocaine) the impact on a person's mood and psychologic stability is even greater, increasing the risk for suicide or self-destructive behavior.

 It is important to remember that drugs react chemically with the brain to produce altered moods, alter thought processes, and increase impulsivity. In general, the abuse of substances tends to:

• Diminish control and inhibition

• Uncover or release impulses or thoughts

• Diminish memory and concentration

• Promote relaxation and feelings of stability (People believe that they are seeing and understanding the situation exactly as it is. In these circumstances, suicide may seem to be the rational course, adopted without the anxiety or ambivalence that might normally accompany suicidal thoughts.)

• Increase depression, especially after the initial response of relaxation

Abrupt cessation or withdrawal from alcohol or other drugs is likely to precipitate suicidal thoughts or impulses. Habitual cocaine use can lead to life-threatening depression. This depression can last months and may require in-patient treatment.

Nurses' Attitudes about Self-Destructive/Suicidal People

Nurses' attitudes toward suicidal clients have many sources. In addition to direct experience with suicidal persons, societal and ethical issues as well as historical antecedents influence nurses' attitudes toward suicide and self-destructive behavior. These controversial issues include rational suicide, euthanasia, abortion rights, right to commit suicide, and responsibility to prevent suicide. Nurses often get caught up in the dilemma of how much responsibility to take for the self-destructive person and for how long.

Hoff (1989) points out that self-destructive people run counter to the socialized sick role that most clients assume in health care settings. They seemingly defeat our best efforts by choosing death over life, or by being self-destructive. Although it is the responsibility of the nurse to promote and maintain life, the nurse cannot battle the client to do so. Rather, the nurse joins clients in examining and understanding how it is that they have gotten to this point.

Nurses working with self-destructive or suicidal clients may feel frustrated and angry. Aggressive responses by nurses (e.g., choosing the largest nasogastric tube for gastric lavage in the emergency room, complaining that self-destructive clients are taking up the time they should be spending on their "real patients") are not unknown. Before working with someone who is suicidal or self-destructive, nurses need to assess personal feelings, experiences, conflicts, and memories that might render them ineffective in performing this task.

Survivors of Suicide

A 27-year-old woman called her former boyfriend and told him to look out of his window so that he could watch her die. He hung up on her. Only minutes later he heard a crash. She had driven her car into a tree in front of his apartment building. The impact killed her instantly.

A 17-year-old high school student killed himself in his home after holding his mother hostage for three hours and forcing her to type his suicide notes. The young man tied his mother to a chair and forced her to type four suicide notes. When she finished, he shot himself in the head.

The act of suicide has long-lasting ramifications for the survivors. Nurses who are working with the families or staff who have worked with the deceased must be alert to the potential sequelae to the death. (Staff reactions are described later in the chapter.)

Kovansky (1989) reviewed the grief process for people who survive a suicide. This process is notably different from a typical grief reaction. Survivors usually have the following reactions:

- Reality distortion
- Massive guilt
- Disturbed self-concept
- Impotent rage with guilt and blaming
- Search for a meaning
- Denial

Families and other survivors of suicide may not receive the support that other bereaved people generally receive. People in the support network (often including other family members) are uncomfortable and embarrassed and are more likely to stay away than to help. Family members are often blamed for not preventing the suicide. Very often, suicide is denied or concealed. This secrecy further impedes grief work, because survivors cannot resolve the loss unless they discuss it openly. Suicide exacerbates dysfunctional family dynamics, such as scapegoating or blaming other family members. Besides making the usual preparations after death, families need to deal with police investigations, the media, and insurance companies. This can precipitate extreme stress, especially if only limited support is available.

Survivors rarely seek assistance from mental health professionals. They are much more likely to be furious with the group that "should have prevented this" and need to project their impotent rage on the professionals. A nurse working with survivors must be prepared for this reaction. Families and all significant others who survive a suicide need nursing intervention, but it is especially warranted for the following:

- Surviving children. Children of parents who commit suicide are at high risk for developing psychopathology in the future, both suicidal behavior and depression.

- Families who lack support from usual sources.

- Dysfunctional families who react by blaming, scapegoating, or covering up the death as an accident.

Therefore, nurses should plan outreach services for these groups. A typical plan might include telephoning the family immediately after the suicide and periodically until the first anniversary of the death and providing for staff or a staff representative to attend services, if appropriate. The family sometimes welcomes the assistance, but sometimes the family is angry and unable to relate to mental health professionals. The health care team must work together to formulate the most appropriate plan.

Staff Response to a Client's Suicide

One of the most significant professional crises that a nurse or a therapist will ever experience is a client's suicide. Staff members also need to resolve the loss and find meaning in it. Kottler and Blau (1989) have developed a multiple-stage model for resolving the loss of a client by suicide.

1. Denial. Seeking to blame someone other than oneself.

2. Self-confrontation. Assuming total responsibility for what went wrong and painfully confronting the situation head-on. This usually results in self-doubt and self-deprecating thoughts.

3. The search. Seeking to find out what really happened by discovering some significant dimension of the experience and putting the situation in a more realistic light.

4. Resolution. Gaining new information and insight about the event by virtue of having opened up oneself to discovery; recognizing and accepting one's part in the entire process.

5. Application. Transferring new learning to future clinical work, being open to learning, and having a strong desire to work more effectively.

These stages are neither sequential nor time-limited. Staff members work through the process at their own speed.

When a client commits suicide as an in-patient, the staff needs help to reduce the pain and keep functioning. Other interventions that will help the staff of an in-patient unit to deal with the suicide of a client are to:

- Immediately after the suicide, hold a staff meeting to provide accurate information and make necessary decisions.

- Assign one person the duty of dealing with police and reporters.

- Hold ward meetings to inform other clients, answer questions, and assure clients of staff availability.

- Assess clients individually and decide on changes in treatment plans.

- Unit leadership should meet with the treatment team to review their work with the deceased client.

- Encourage all to seek peer support and to attend funeral services.

- Some months after the event, hold a conference to review the suicide.

Those staff members who have little medical training or experience suffer more than those who have previously encountered illness and death. These workers need extra attention.

CHAPTER HIGHLIGHTS

• Suicide is a maladaptive response to a crisis.

• Nurses are in key positions to help clients resolve crises that lead to suicidal behavior.

• Suicidal behavior is affected by a number of social, demographic, and clinical variables.

• All suicide ideation, threats, and gestures need to be taken seriously and evaluated.

• A lethality assessment is the first step in helping self-destructive persons. The nurse uses this assessment to formulate a plan of care.

• The no-suicide contract is a useful tool for certain clients.

• Adolescents attempt suicide approximately 200 times as often as they complete a suicide.

• The elderly are the age group at highest risk for suicide.

• To work effectively with self-destructive people, nurses must examine their own experiences and feelings.

• Suicide survivors are in need of special grief counseling but are unlikely to receive it.

REFERENCES

Adam KS: Attempted suicide. *Psychiatr Clin North Am* 1985;8(2):183–203.

Aguilera DC, Messick D: *Crisis Intervention: Theory and Methodology,* ed 6. Mosby, 1990.

American Psychiatric Association: *Diagnostic and Statistical Manual of Mental Disorders,* ed 3, revised. APA, 1987.

Boxwell AO: Geriatric suicide: The preventable death. *Nurse Pract* 1988;13(6):10–19.

Capadanno AE: Assessment of suicide risk. *J Psychosoc Nurs Ment Health* 1983;21(5):11–14.

Clayton PJ: Suicide. *Psychiatr Clin North Am* 1985;8 (2):183–203.

Coid J, Allolio B, Rees LH: Raised plasma metenkephalin in patients who habitually mutilate themselves. *Lancet* 1983;2:545–546.

Cotton PG et al.: Dealing with suicide on a psychiatric inpatient unit. *Hosp Community Psychiatry* 1983; 34:55–59.

Curran DK: *Adolescent Suicidal Behavior.* Hemisphere Publishing, 1987.

Deykin EY: Adolescent suicidal and self-destructive behavior: An intervention study, in Klerman GL (ed): *Suicide and Depression among Adolescents and Young Adults.* American Psychiatric Press, 1986.

Dunn J: Psychiatric intervention in the community hospital emergency room. *J Nurs Admin* 1989;19(10):36–40.

Dunne-Maxim K: Survivors of suicide. *J Psychosoc Nurs* 1986;24(12):31–35.

Durkheim E: *Suicide.* The Free Press, 1951.

Erikson EH: *Identity, Youth and Crisis.* W. W. Norton, 1966.

Estes NJ, Heinemann ME: *Alcoholism: Development, Consequences, and Interventions.* Mosby, 1986.

Farazza AR et al.: Self-mutilation and eating disorders. *Suicide Life Threat Behav* 1989;19(4):352–361.

Farberow NL: Indirect self-destructive behavior: Classification and characteristics, in Farberow NL (ed): *The Many Faces of Suicide.* McGraw-Hill, 1980.

Finigan J: Assessment of childhood and adolescent depression and suicide. *J Emerg Nurs* 1986;12(1):35–38.

Freud S: *New Introductory Lectures on Psycho Analysis: Lecture XXXII: Anxiety and Instinctual Life.* Hogarth, 1964 (originally published 1933).

Gardner DL, Cowdry RW: Suicidal and parasuicidal behavior in borderline personality disorder. *Psychiatr Clin North Am* 1985;8(2):389–404.

Hawton K: *Suicide and Attempted Suicide among Children and Adolescents.* Sage Publications, 1986.

Hoff LA: *People in Crisis: Understanding and Helping,* ed 3. Addison-Wesley, 1989.

Kottler JA, Blau DS: *The Imperfect Therapist: Learning from Failure in Therapeutic Practice.* Jossey-Bass, 1989.

Kovansky RS: Loneliness and disturbed grief: A comparison of parents who lost a child to suicide or accidental death. *Arch Psychiatr Nurs* 1989;3(2):86–96.

Lichtenstein E, Bernstein DA: Cigarette smoking as indirect self-destructive behavior, in Farberow NL (ed): *The Many Faces of Suicide.* McGraw-Hill, 1980.

Linehan MM: Suicidal people: One population or two? in Mann J, Stanley M (Eds): *Psycho Biology of Suicidal Behavior.* New York Academy of Sciences, 1986.

Litman RE: Psychodynamics of indirect self-destructive behavior, in Farberow, NL (ed): *The Many Faces of Suicide.* Mc-Graw-Hill, 1980.

Maris RW: *Pathways to Suicide: A Survey of Self-Destructive Behaviors.* Johns Hopkins University Press, 1981.

Menninger A: *Man against Himself.* Harcourt, Brace, 1938.

Nkongho NO: Suicide in the elderly: A beginning investigation. *J Nurs Admin* 1988;2(2):47–57.

Orbach I: Personality characteristics, life circumstances, and dynamics of suicidal children. *Death Ed* 1984;8:37–52.

Pallikkathayil L, Morgan SA: Emergency department nurses' encounters with suicide attempters: A qualitative investigation. *Schol Inquiry Nurs Pract Int* 1988;2(3): 237–253.

Parker SD: Accident or suicide?: Do life change events lead to adolescent suicide? *J Psychosoc Nurs* 1988; 26(6): 15–19.

Raczek SW et al.: Suicidal behavior and personality traits. *J Pers Disord* 1989;3(4):345–351.

Reed PG, Leonard VE: An analysis of the concept of self-neglect. *Adv Nurs Sci* 1989;12(1):39–53.

Roberts J, McFarland L: Assessment of suicide risk in the elderly. *Caring* 1986;5(7):20–23.

Roy A: Suicide and psychiatric patients. *Psychiatr Clin North Am* 1985;8(2):227–242.

Saunders JM, Valente SM: Cancer and suicide. *Oncol Nurs Forum* 1988;15(5):575–581.

Schneider SG, Farberow NL, Kruks GN: Suicidal behavior in adolescent and young adult gay men. *Suicide Life Threat Behav* 1989;19(4):381–395.

Shneidman ES: *Definition of Suicide.* Wiley, 1985.

Simpson MA: Self-mutilation as indirect self-destructive behavior: "Nothing to get so cut up about . . .", in Farberow NL (ed): *The Many Faces of Suicide.* Mc-Graw-Hill, 1980.

Thompson J, Brooks S: When a colleague commits suicide: How the staff reacts. *J Psychosoc Nurs* 1990;28(10): 6–11.

U.S. Bureau of the Census: *Statistical Abstract of the United States: 1989,* ed 109. Washington DC, 1989.

Valente S: Suicide in school-aged children: Theory and assessment. *Pediatr Nurs* 1983;9(1):25–29.

Van der Kolk BA: The trauma spectrum: The interaction of biological and social events in the genesis of the trauma response. *J Traumatic Stress* 1988;1(3):273–290.

Walsh BW, Rosen PM: *Self-Mutilation: Theory, Research and Treatment.* Guilford Press, 1988.

Walters SM: Para suicide, crisis intervention and family therapy. *Nurs Times* 1983;79(2):17–20.

Wood KA et al.: Drug-induced psychosis and depression in the elderly. *Psychiatric Clin North Am* 1988;11(1): 167–195.

Codependence

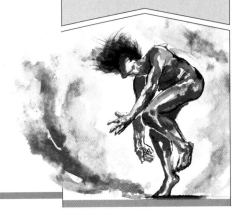

LEARNING OBJECTIVES

- Identify the characteristics of codependence
- Relate codependence to a theoretic model
- Apply a theoretic framework of codependence to a practical situation
- Formulate a response to an individual behaving in a codependent mindset
- Organize a healing-focused interaction

Maryruth Morris
Eileen Trigoboff

CROSS REFERENCES

Other topics relevant to this content are: Family therapy, Chapter 30; Personal integration, Chapter 2; Psychoactive substance use disorders, Chapter 11.

IMAGINE YOU HAVE JUST finished this day: You ran errands, made some phone calls about your significant other's car insurance, organized the budget (because it needs to be done and you are so good at it), and then called your family, giving some diplomatic excuse to cancel, again, the evening's activities—when in reality your significant other came home and fell on the bed, incoherent and not capable of socializing. There could be numerous reasons for this scenario. But, if this scenario typifies your day-to-day life, you are in a codependent relationship. Notice the following:

- The person doing all the work has not done anything for himself or herself.

- Tasks are taken care of only if that person does it.

Caring about others is a worthy enterprise, but taking care of other adults at the expense of meeting one's personal needs is draining, codependent behavior.

Definition of Codependence

What does cordependence mean? The definition is still being formulated and differs slightly from source to source. The basic version is that **codependence** is the dependence of one adult on a second adult, who is usually an addict of some sort. Here the term *addict* is defined broadly to include physical and/or psychologic dependence on a substance or behavior. Different types of addictions are included, such as alcoholism (a substance addiction), "rage-aholism" (an emotion addiction), and "workaholism" (a behavior addiction). A codependent person "needs" the significant other to be an addict. The codependent individual is a highly organized achiever who works continuously to maintain stability in the present situation. This behavior pattern emerges after routine exposure, usually in one's family of origin, to a set of rules that prevents open expression of feelings and direct discussion of problems. It is an effective coping pattern developed after years of reacting to crises.

Although codependence is effective in controlling the crisis situation, it is an unhealthy life-style because the exclusive focus on others promotes the neglect of self. One of the "rules" of this life-style is to deny the existence of a problem, to deny one's feelings, and to adhere to a code of silence about the situation. There is an expectation that negative feelings are not to be voiced. The origin of these codependent styles is believed to be a dysfunctional family system (Woititz 1985). Codependent behavior has its roots in what the person learned as a child (meeting everyone else's needs) and what the family failed to model (the give-and-take of a healthy relationship).

Codependence, as defined in this chapter, is a group of learned behaviors that prevents individuals from taking care of themselves and has at its core a preoccupation with the thoughts and feelings of others. Codependent people gear their behavior toward helping others or taking charge of situations that appear to be out of control. Because codependents assume responsibility for others' lives, codependent relationships require the participation of at least one other dysfunctional person.

Codependence is learned early in life. In a dysfunctional family, the child, to maintain some level of stability in the family, tries to sense what the adults need and want. Both the adults and the child see the child's needs, wants, feelings, and desires as unacceptable. Therefore, the child learns to ignore his or her own life.

Characteristics of Codependence

Characteristics of codependence, as expressed not only in the client population but also in everyday life, vary from the mild to the extreme. Mild traits can contribute to discomfort. Extreme codependence interferes with functioning, forcing individuals into awkward and untenable activities in which they totally ignore their own needs. Intermediate levels of these traits and symptoms can also occur.

The diagnostic grouping of individuals whose codependence symptoms greatly conflict with a healthy life-style may be specified in DSM-IV. The possibility that these behaviors constitute a specific and discernible entity has only recently been considered. Controversy surrounds this entry in the DSM-IV. The issue about including codependence as a diagnostic category revolves around the assertion of some that codependence is a set of behaviors characteristic of a distinct personality disorder. This assertion has not been demonstrated adequately in current research. Also, codependence as a diagnostic category may not describe the client any more accurately than other diagnostic categories already in existence. According to Cermak (1986), the suggested criteria for Codependent Personality Disorder (the most intense expression of these behaviors) are those identified in the accompanying box.

Codependence is not restricted to relationships and situations in one's personal life; these behaviors can be seen in the workplace as well. Some jobs require the person to assume the role of helper to others, focusing on details, minimizing mistakes, and rigidly adhering to technical policies and procedures. These job traits reinforce codependence. Being in an occupa-

Suggested DSM-IV Criteria for Codependent Personality Disorder

1. Continued investment of self-esteem in the ability to control both oneself and others in the face of serious adverse consequences

2. Assumption of responsibility for meeting others' needs to the exclusion of acknowledging one's own

3. Anxiety and boundary distortions in situations of intimacy and separation

4. Enmeshment in relationships with personality disordered, drug dependent, other codependent, and/or impulse disordered individuals

5. Exhibits three or more of the following:

- Excessive reliance on denial
- Substance abuse
- Constriction of emotions (with or without dramatic outbursts)
- Stress-related medical illnesses
- Depression
- Hypervigilance
- Compulsions
- Anxiety
- Has been (or is) the victim of recurrent abuse
- Has remained in a primary relationship with an active substance abuser for at least two years without seeking outside help

tion or profession that promotes codependence is unhealthy and debilitating for codependents. Because the choice of jobs is under the control of the individual, unlike the family of origin where these behaviors were likely instilled, there are options and alternatives. Persons with codependent traits must carefully examine an attraction to an occupation or profession that promotes or encourages codependence. If the person is already manifesting codependent behaviors on the job, or if the person sees tendencies to codependence inherent in it, several steps can be taken. First and foremost is to be aware of the problem. The next step is to obtain training to stop bearing responsibility for others and "fixing" other people's problems. Placing priority on oneself and choosing to have the freedom to meet one's own needs in the work situation are powerful tools for career advancement.

History of the Codependence Movement

The term *codependence* has its roots in the alcohol/addiction treatment movement. This term, coined in the 1970s, arises from the older idea of **co-alcoholic**, a term used in Al-Anon for the spouses and families of the alcoholic. Another phrase utilized during the formative years of alcoholism treatment was **co-ism**, a concept that implies that everybody in an alcoholic's family is emotionally impaired. Various authors estimate that the incidence of codependence in our culture ranges from approximately 33 percent to approximately 100 percent of the population. The latter estimate reflects a liberal and encompassing interpretation of codependent behavior.

An interesting (and controversial, for professionals) aspect of this movement is the commercial success of codependence-focused best sellers and treatment groups. There are rehabilitation centers, books, manuals, calendars, notepads, and wall plaques with inspiring messages on how to recover from codependence. Melody Beattie's book *Codependent No More* (1987) has, to date, sold over 1.5 million copies.

Another rapidly growing part of the codependence movement is the focus on the Adult Children of Alcoholics (ACoA or ACA). Therapeutic endeavors in this area have been extensive, and many peer-support groups or therapist-led groups are available in most communities. Similar formative stages characterize the ACoA and the codependent styles of interacting.

Nurses must keep in mind that this movement is relatively new and that the literature is based on mostly anecdotal data. Detailed descriptions of experiences of individuals and small groups, while interesting and extremely helpful in opening a new field of study, do not constitute research. Therefore, nurses must be wary of labeling anyone a codependent, especially considering the scarcity of controlled studies regarding personality theory development and treatment strategies.

Theories of Codependence

There are numerous theoretic bases for codependence. The following sections give an overview of current theories of codependence.

ACoA Perspective

Claudia Black (1987, 1990) well known for the treatment of children of alcoholics, has identified the characteristics of people who grew up in dysfunctional families. Although Black does not focus entirely on the codependent individual, her identification of the background common to codependent persons and recommendations for intervention are frequently cited in the treatment of codependence. In Black's perspective, the children of alcoholics learned that having feelings only makes things more of a problem—speaking about feelings usually makes situations worse rather than solving them. The child's solution is to stifle the feeling and say nothing. This ACoA becomes unable to recognize what feelings are, to articulate them, or to address them in a caring manner. Personal conduct centers on the rules "don't feel; don't talk; don't trust." These individuals have not learned how to take care of themselves in an adult relationship.

Codependent adults and ACoAs have strong needs to control others. This behavior originates, according to Black, in the child's need to have things done well and on time, before a parent or the neighbors see that things are not OK at home. The child hopes that being very good at everything will prevent awful consequences. Input from others is a nuisance and irrelevant when one knows how to do things the right way. As an adult, the person is not interested in hearing others' points of view. One manifestation of this attitude is cutting people off before they finish sentences. In addition, there are isolating repercussions from a childhood spent with an addict. Feeling cut off from people and perceiving oneself as alone in a crowd are telltale signs of the aftermath of growing up in an addiction-focused home.

According to Black's theoretic framework, healing involves verbalizing feelings and learning to trust oneself and others. Having the ACoA experience validated via therapy or peer-support groups breaks open the lock on talking about feelings.

Shame and Codependence

Shame as a major feature of codependence is the focus of John Bradshaw's (1988, 1990) work. In his view, the codependent is someone with a toxic form of shame. Toxic shame is a tremendous amount of shame that interferes with the ability to search outside of oneself for purpose and happiness.

Dysfunction in the family system is its basis. If a family does not meet each individual's needs and respond to the world in a healthy manner, unhealthy and dysfunctional patterns of response become ingrained. In Bradshaw's words, living a life that is **"other-aided"** is codependent because the person's concentration is always on someone else. Denial of one's own needs is one of the features of codependence. The goal of treatment is to return the focus to the self and work on breaking dysfunctional patterns of relating, for instance, by identifying one's needs and feelings and then making these needs and feelings a priority in one's life.

Proactive Approaches

John and Linda Friel, in a recent book *An Adult Child's Guide to What's "Normal"* (1990) define codependence, humorously but pointedly, as the "chase-your-spouse-around-the-room-with-the-self-help-book syndrome." The nurse can assess codependence by examining the amount of work each partner puts into a relationship. In a codependent relationship, one person routinely invests great energy keeping the relationship afloat, while the second person expends little or no effort. The Friels reinforce the idea that taking responsibility for another adult's life is not healthy caring. The move to health begins when codependents question whether they should continue, modify, or leave the relationship. Caring about others without being codependent involves paying attention to one's feelings and body, keeping one's identity, and undertaking a personal search that includes questioning the childhood styles of interacting that one learned along the way.

The Child Within Perspective

Charles Whitfield (1987, 1988) describes codependence as the result of the child growing up without nurturing or freedom of expression. He uses the term "our most common addiction" and describes it as a "disease of a lost self-hood." The unnurtured child still lives within the codependent adult, along with that unnurtured child's sense of the world. Adults who follow rules they made up when they were unnurtured children create a false-self, one that is not true to the genuine and spirited part of a human being. In other words, the false-self does not represent how a healthy adult interacts in the world.

To consider this further, speculate about what that unnurtured child inside the adult is feeling. It is frightening to see the world as a cold and critical place. Now imagine that grown-up person in situations that do not nurture or encourage freedom of expression. Old patterns start to play out. The person pretends to be strong—always—while in reality feeling vulnerable. Critical, perfectionistic, controlling self-righteousness becomes routine and prevents accepting oneself and others. The process of healing for the codependent person hinges on the healing of the child within. This healing addresses the needs of the child within, nurtures the child, and teaches the child healthy relating to others.

Feminism and Codependence

Feminism and the codependence model are inextricably entwined. *Feminism* is the focus on how being a woman influences, changes, and varies one's experiences. Feminism emphasizes what form these modified experiences take and how they can stultify or denigrate a woman. The women's movement has tended to confront directly the social and political inequities that may predispose a woman to a sense of powerlessness.

Nursing is predominantly a woman's field, and, while acknowledging the influence of men on nursing, anyone in a woman-dominated profession must carefully examine any theory or psychiatric label that defines women negatively. Codependence is one of the labels requiring feminist scrutiny because a codependent relationship is most likely to involve a male addict and a female significant other. Lerner (1989) addresses one such concern when she states "It's normal to want to help a family member or friend in trouble. The problem [of codependence] arises only when a woman becomes overinvolved with that trouble and becomes underfocused on herself." Keeping this distinction clear in our minds is paramount. Behavior that demonstrates caring about others, including mothering and competent caring in many areas, does not merit the label codependent. Applying the label in this way is, in effect, saying that involvement in the emotional health and growth of others—an activity that defines nursing—is a psychiatric problem. The stalwart, innovative woman who carries her family through trying times is to be admired, supported, and promoted as an ideal. To respond to this kind of strength with an automatic diagnosis of illness spuriously stigmatizes and denigrates such women.

Changing Codependent Behavior

The art of psychiatric nursing practice is to build a unique therapeutic approach on a theory-centered nursing relationship. This requires the integration of theory, the effort of self-examination, and the reinforcement of health in oneself.

The psychiatric nurse working with the codependent client must consider the client's readiness to change. Although many life-style patterns are unhealthy, individuals change their behavior only when they feel uncomfortable enough to want to learn something new. The analogy in the accompanying box illustrates the point at which most persons seek help with their codependence behavior.

Changing codependent behavior is a long process that often includes the following steps:

• Developing a desire to change how one looks at interpersonal relationships

• Developing an ability to learn functional rules of relationships

• Increasing an awareness of one's own thoughts, feelings, and desires

---

What Happened to My Boat?: An Analogy on Help-Seeking Behavior in Codependence

Think of two people in two boats equipped with oars. They are in a calm river. Their mission is to row upstream. Mary is in one boat, and John is in the other. Mary lovingly gazes over to see how John is doing. John is standing up in his boat, only one of his oars is in the water, and he is going nowhere. Mary, trying to be helpful, calls over to John, instructing him to sit down and row correctly. After observing for a period of time Mary sees that, although John has followed some of her directions, he continues to have only one oar in the water and has not gone anywhere. As time goes on, Mary feels she should be more helpful in her efforts to get John on his way upstream. She decides that the best way to help is to get into John's boat, to be closer to him and to be more available to him. While in his boat, she continues to tell him how to row and what to do. Finally, in frustration, Mary takes over the oars of John's boat, leaving her own boat adrift and going nowhere. Mary does not concern herself with her boat—she spends all her energy rowing John's boat. She notices that the load is quite heavy with two in the boat and that she is working very hard. As the boat progresses upstream, Mary begins to feel resentful watching John sit and ride. However, she still feels it is better for her to row. She thinks to herself, "If John would appreciate all my work, then I would not mind rowing for two." But as they progress upstream, John becomes critical, not complimentary, of Mary. Eventually he asks her to get out of his boat. At this point Mary is devastated as well as astonished by John's request. She argues with him, pointing out all that she has done for him, to no avail, and he again asks her to leave his boat. Mary now realizes that she does not know where her boat is and that she is completely confused about how to find it. Codependents like Mary often reach out for help at times like these.

• Learning to accept one's own thoughts, feelings, and desires

• Learning and using assertive interpersonal skills

The role of the nurse in the process of change is twofold. First, the nurse must be an appropriate role model of effective interpersonal relationships. Second, the nurse needs to be an effective teacher of functional relationship skills. Remember that codependent clients are most likely to seek help when they are feeling most vulnerable, confused, and angry that what they have learned to do in relationships does not work. Keeping this in mind helps the nurse maintain a therapeutic role when the codependent person requests or demands to be rescued from this dilemma. The nurse may wonder how best to help a client who, like Mary and John in the analogy, is struggling, confused, and somewhat helpless. Such clients may also repeatedly request more than support from the nurse. Clients may, out of confusion, ask the nurse, "What should I do?" or "What would you do if you were in my situation?" The nurse needs to model an independent position and convey confidence in the client's own ability to work out a problem-solving strategy. Possible encouraging responses include, "What alternatives have you already considered?" or "You seem unclear about what you want to do. I can appreciate how uncomfortable it is not knowing what to do." These responses redirect the codependent plea and reinforce the integrity of the client's self-concept while demonstrating concern and support during the client's struggle to learn new skills.

In teaching appropriate functional relationship skills, the nurse needs to be aware that at the core of codependence is the client's lack of functional personal boundaries. In simple terms, functional personal boundaries are limits indicating individuals' personal rights and preferences. Remember, as a child the codependent client learned to ignore and mistrust personal limits, feelings, needs, and wants. Such clients may react with anxiety to the unfamiliar concept that they have the right to set limits, to have and express feelings, and to acknowledge needs and express wants.

The nurse working with codependent clients must remember that they have established relationships with other dysfunctional people. The interpersonal systems in which these clients function often do not support the changes that they are struggling to make. A support group may encourage clients during the process of change. An alternative may be an ACoA group. Information about these groups is available through the local Alcoholics Anonymous organizations.

It is important to remember that the nurse-client relationship can be a difficult one. The codependent person has had years of experience and practice with dysfunctional patterns that work in the family of origin where they were initially established. The client is primarily confused and frustrated that the patterns that worked with the family do not work in healthy adult relationships. The establishment of new interactional patterns will cost the client some acceptance within the family of origin but will give the client a stronger, healthier sense of self.

Nursing Research in Codependence

There are many opportunities to examine questions, issues, and hypotheses relating to the concept of codependence and to the formulation of nursing interventions to address codependent behaviors. Unfortunately, few nursing researchers have taken advantage of these opportunities. A basic research question requiring immediate exploration is the validity of the concept. We need studies to determine whether or not codependent behaviors in fact make up an empirically discriminable clinical syndrome. The studies done to date have had major methodologic flaws. There is a need for methodologically sound studies to add to the body of knowledge on codependence, and there is an opportunity for nurse researchers to design these studies.

If codependence syndrome is verified, it is important to study which combination of treatment interventions is most effective in remediating these symptoms. Current literature addressing intervention strategies is largely anecdotal and/or case specific. It is therefore difficult to determine if the reported interventions can be generalized to apply to the codependent population. Unfortunately, it is possible that these reported interventions were effective only for those specific clients, or that those clients improved for reasons other than those suggested. The popular codependence movement has emphasized particular treatments. However, popularity is a poor substitute for sound research in developing effective treatments.

CHAPTER HIGHLIGHTS

• Codependence is a learned behavior that affects one's ability to meet personal needs because of overinvolvement in helping another adult.

• Codependence is a fairly new construct.

• Awareness of the definitions and implications of codependence requires a sensitivity to issues affecting women.

• Contemporary theories of codependence include dysfunction in the family, per the model Adult Children of Alcoholics, shame and codependence, proactive approaches, and the child-within perspective.

• Nursing interventions include role modeling of effective interpersonal relationships and teaching relationship skills.

• The inclusion in DSM-IV of codependence as a mental disorder is highly controversial.

• Nurses may be at risk by being in job situations that encourage codependent traits.

RESEARCH NOTE

Citation

Few studies of codependence have been reported in the health sciences literature. Therefore, this note outlines a study design to investigate codependence.

Study Problem/Purpose

The purpose of the proposed study is to validate codependence as a distinct syndrome, discriminable from dependence and other psychiatric syndromes.

Methods

Three groups of individuals are examined for behavioral and self-reported indications of codependence. Group A consists of diagnosed dependents. Group B consists of the significant others of group A. Group C consists of a sample of individuals already in psychiatric treatment, demographically matched to group B. The inclusion of group C rules out the possibility that the presence of other psychopathology might result in behavioral or self-report responses that mimic codependent behavior.

If codependence is truly different from dependence and from other psychiatric syndromes, then the presumed codependents (spouses or significant others of dependents) should differ on some criteria both from dependents and from other psychiatric clients. Informed consent would be obtained from all study participants. Two criteria would be used in this study, a behavioral measure and a self-report measure. The behavioral measure would consist of a contrived situation in which the research participant would be observed in a waiting room. An experimenter, one of several other people in the waiting room, would feign drunkenness and difficulty filling out forms. The response of the research participant would be catalogued for various attributes such as the extent to which the participant would take over and perform the task for the experimenter, the perfectionism with which the task is performed, and/or impatience, presumably codependent response tendencies. The self-report measure would consist of a well-known psychologic test such as the MMPI-2. Differences in response patterns might be expected for different syndromes.

Implications

If differences in either the behavioral or self-report data distinguish the codependent sample from the other samples, the results support the hypothesis that codependence is in fact a distinct clinical syndrome. If differences are not found, one interpretation is that codependence does not significantly vary from other clinical syndromes. Another possibility is that the measures used were not adequate to discriminate the syndrome. With an ongoing research program, it would be possible to determine the correct interpretation. One further direction for such a research program could be to investigate the hypothesis that codependence is merely a variety of dependence that is manifested only in the presence of an addicted significant other.

• Codependence may be treated once it is recognized and the desire to change is apparent in the client.

Adequate research on codependence is lacking, and nursing needs to focus on this problem.

REFERENCES

Beattie M: *Codependent No More*. Harper & Row, 1987.

Black C: *Double Duty*. Ballentine, 1990.

Black C: *It Will Never Happen to Me*. Hazelden, 1987.

Bradshaw J: *Healing the Shame That Binds You*. Health Communications, 1988.

Bradshaw J: *Homecoming: Reclaiming and Championing Your Inner Child*. Bantam, 1990.

Brown A, Harrison T, Palmer AP: *Dealing with Dependency Series* Boundaries, vol 2. Grindle Audio, Institute for Functional Behavior, 1990.

Brown A, Harrison T, Palmer AP: *Dealing with Dependency Series*, Me . . . codependent? vol 1. Grindle Audio, Institute for Functional Behavior, 1990.

Cauthorne-Lindstrom C, Hrabe D: Codependent behaviors in managers: A script for failure. *Nurs Management* 1990;21(2):35−39.

Cermak TL: Diagnostic criteria for codependency. *J Psychoactive Drugs* 1986;28(1):80.

Chesler P: *Women and Madness*, ed 2. Harcourt-Brace-Jovanovich, 1989.

Friel J, Friel L: *An Adult Child's Guide to What's "Normal."* Health Communications, 1990.

Haack M, Alim T: Anxiety and the adult child of an alcoholic: A co-morbid problem. *Fam Community Health* 1991;13(4):132–136.

Lerner HG: *The Dance of Intimacy.* Harper & Row, 1989.

McBride A: Developing a women's mental health research agenda. *Image* 1987;19:4–8.

Schaef AW: *Co-dependence: Misunderstood, mistreated.* Harper & Row, 1986.

Schaef AW, Fassel D: *The Addictive Organization.* Harper & Row, 1988.

Snow C, Willard D: *I'm Dying to Take Care of You . . . Nurses and Codependence: Breaking the Cycles.* Professional Counselor Books, 1989.

Subby R: Inside the chemically dependent marriage: Denial and manipulation, in *Codependency: An Emerging Issue.* Health Communications, 1984.

University of California at Berkeley *Wellness Letter.* 1990;1(7):7.

Webster D: Women and depression (alias codependency). *Fam Community Health* 1990;13(3):58.

Whitfield C: Co-dependence: Our most common addiction. *Wellness Associates Journal* Spring 1988:1.

Whitfield C: *Healing the Child Within.* Health Communications, 1987.

Woititz JG: *Struggle for Intimacy.* Health Communications, 1985.

HIV/AIDS:
A Mental Health Challenge

Carol Ren Kneisl
William G. Pheifer

LEARNING OBJECTIVES

- Explain why certain populations are at risk for acquired immune deficiency syndrome (AIDS)

- Discuss the incidence and geographic distribution of AIDS

- Describe the biologic, psychologic, developmental, social and cultural, economic, legal, political, and ethical impact of human immunodeficiency virus (HIV) infection

- Provide direct nursing care to persons with HIV disease in psychiatric settings

- Incorporate HIV risk reduction education and counseling regarding sexual behavior and substance abuse in work with clients and people in the community

- Identify the means by which psychiatric nurses can support caregivers of persons with HIV and AIDS

- Provide support to survivors of persons with AIDS (SOPWAs) and other individuals experiencing AIDS-related bereavements

- Suggest avenues of self-help for persons with HIV disease and their significant others

- Explain why continued nursing involvement in AIDS research is important

- Engage in advocacy and political activism related to the HIV epidemic

CROSS REFERENCES

Other topics relevant to this content are: Caring for clients with organic mental disorder, Chapter 10; Caring for depressed clients, Chapter 13; Caring for substance-abusing clients, Chapter 11; Visualization and stress management techniques for self-healing and pain and symptom control, Chapter 27.

THE CONTAGIOUS AND POTENTIALLY fatal condition of immune system depression known as **acquired immune deficiency syndrome (AIDS)** has no known cure and responds to limited treatments. It is of clinical concern to all nurses, but especially to psychiatric mental health nurses, who, by nature of their commitment and responsibility, become involved in human experiences. Clients with the **human immunodeficiency virus (HIV)** require care that promotes quality existence and personal growth in the face of serious illness.

Mental Health and the HIV Trajectory

The human experience associated with human immunodeficiency virus can be viewed as a trajectory (see Figure 25–1). The **HIV trajectory** describes the potential progression of HIV disease and provides a view of the individuals who are most directly affected by the virus. An understanding of the HIV trajectory can give psychiatric mental health nurses an increased awareness of the various needs that individuals affected by HIV may manifest at different points in their experience with the disease.

Individuals at Risk

The HIV trajectory begins with the category of **individuals at risk.** Other authors have sometimes described this group as the "worried well." Individuals at risk are those persons who are most likely to have or to contract HIV, due to past or current participation in high-risk activities (see the discussion later in this chapter). This specific group includes persons who have not been tested for HIV and those who have received negative HIV antibody test results but are considered to remain at risk.

Individuals at risk often experience anxiety, ineffective coping, and decisional conflicts related to HIV infection. These human responses may be manifested in many ways including fear of sexual expression related to risk of transmission, denial of risk as a primary defense, and conflict over whether to take the HIV antibody test. Maladaptive human responses in individuals at risk could result in self-destructive or irresponsible behaviors, such as suicide attempts or unsafe sexual practices. As the epidemic continues unabated, psychiatric mental health nurses should expect to see increasing numbers of persons struggling with issues related to HIV infections.

HIV Seropositive

The second category of individuals affected by HIV is **HIV seropositive (asymptomatic).** This group has received validation of HIV status through confirmatory diagnostic test results but as yet exhibits no symptoms associated with immune system suppression. It is not yet fully understood why some people pass through this stage in the disease progression fairly rapidly, while others may remain in this state indefinitely.

Persons who are HIV seropositive (asymptomatic) may experience many of the same responses as individuals at risk, in addition to problems of impaired adjustment and the development of a sense of powerlessness. This may be manifested in a variety of ways

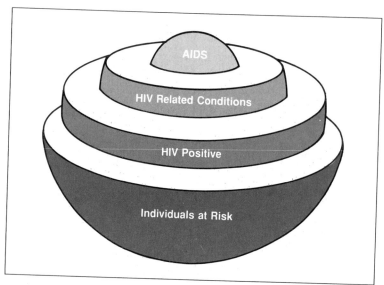

FIGURE 25–1 HIV trajectory.

including chronic depression and decreasing motivation.

As HIV seropositive people begin to deal with the reality of their condition, the nurse may be able to help them engage in health-seeking behaviors. Wellness activities not only promote physical health but also empower the individual, thus promoting mental health.

HIV-Related Conditions

The third category on the HIV trajectory includes individuals with **HIV-related conditions** (HRC). These persons are referred to in the Centers for Disease Control (CDC) classification system as *HIV seropositive (symptomatic)*. In the past, this diagnostic grouping was referred to as AIDS-related complex (ARC). The specific physiologic symptoms associated with HRC are discussed later in this chapter.

Individuals with HIV-related conditions have begun to experience the physical effects of immune system deterioration. In addition to having physical manifestations, these individuals may experience complicating psychosocial responses as well as the human responses previously discussed. These may include altered role performance and self-concept disturbance related to losses, and changes in their perceptions and abilities secondary to the development of physical symptoms and limitations.

Persons with AIDS

The fourth category of individuals on the HIV trajectory are those with a formal diagnosis of AIDS, as defined by CDC guidelines. These are characterized by the development of potentially life-threatening complications because of extensive immune system suppression.

Persons with AIDS (**PWAs**) may experience all of the human responses of individuals all along the trajectory. In addition, PWAs may also experience a sense of hopelessness, social isolation, impaired social interactions, or spiritual distress associated with the effects of a chronic life-threatening illness.

It is not yet fully understood why some individuals stay at an early point on the trajectory while others progress on to the development of HRC or AIDS. The face of the HIV epidemic is changing: AIDS initially presented as a terminal or fatal illness. HIV disease is now being recognized as a chronic potentially life-threatening illness.

Long-Term Survivors

A recent phenomenon in the HIV epidemic has been the identification of **long-term survivors**; people, who have outlived the generally expected lifespan for persons with HIV and AIDS. As more individuals with HIV infection are identified and treatments are discovered to slow or halt HIV progression in a predictable fashion, the number of long-term survivors will continue to increase. This has obvious implications for mental health professionals working with people affected by HIV infection.

Support Systems and Caregivers

One other category of persons affected by the HIV trajectory are the people who make up the support systems of persons with HIV infection. This includes significant others, friends, family, and caregivers of persons with HIV and AIDS. Experts predict that soon nearly everyone in the nation will know individuals affected by HIV disease. Psychiatric mental health professionals must recognize the effects this will have on people and be prepared to help them as they grapple with such diverse issues as ineffective family coping, altered family processes, traditional versus nontraditional definitions of family, and the grief process. The issue of bereavement associated with HIV and AIDS is addressed later in this chapter.

Overview of HIV Disease

HIV relentlessly disarms the immune system, preventing it from fighting infection. **Opportunistic diseases** normally warded off by a healthy immune system are given the opportunity to attack the body. Eventually weakened by the persistent and debilitating onslaught, the person with AIDS is vulnerable at any time to a final, all-out attack. Sometimes this happens within a few months, but often the progression of the disease runs for several years after symptoms appear.

What Causes HIV Disease?

An extremely tiny retrovirus (about 230 *million* would fit on the period at the end of this sentence), the human immunodeficiency virus (HIV), causes AIDS. It consists basically of a double-layered shell or envelope full of proteins, surrounding a bit of ribonucleic acid (RNA). HIV homes in on helper T-lymphocytes in much the same way that the hepatitis virus invades cells in the liver.

Like Greeks hidden inside the Trojan horse, HIV enters the body concealed inside a helper T-cell from an infected host. When the foreign T-cell meets a defending T-cell, the virus slips through the cell membrane into the defending cell and disables it. Once inside an inactive T-cell, the virus may remain dormant for months, even years.

Unlike true life forms, a virus cannot metabolize nutrients (in fact does not need them), does not grow, and cannot reproduce unless it has the assistance of a living host cell. Certain events are believed to shorten the latency period for the HIV-infected person. Repeated exposure to HIV, infections such as hepatitis B or tuberculosis, use of drugs that suppress the immune system (such as corticosteroids) and recreational drugs (such as marijuana, cocaine, or amyl nitrate "poppers"), poor nutrition, stress, or lack of sleep weaken the immune system and are thought to trigger the division of invaded T-cells. HIV begins to multiply by inserting its genes into the DNA of the host cell and ordering it to produce carbon copies of itself. The fact that it can clone itself a thousand times faster than any other known virus explains why HIV disease is such a rapidly progressive and devastating disease.

Who Is at Risk and Why?

The presence of HIV has been documented in blood, blood plasma, bone marrow, semen, cervical secretions, vaginal secretions, saliva, breast milk, lymph nodes, brain tissue, skin, tears, and cerebrospinal fluid. The presence of the virus in so many body fluids and tissues is one reason why the general public fears that HIV can be transmitted by casual contact. However, the research overwhelmingly indicates that the major modes of transmission of the virus are:

• Intimate unprotected sexual contact with an HIV-seropositive person

• Parenteral injection of blood or blood products infected with the HIV virus

• Transfer of the virus from an HIV-infected mother to a fetus or newborn infant in utero, during labor or delivery, or in the early newborn period

Because of the nature of these major modes of transmission and the epidemiology of the epidemic in the United States, several groups have been identified as being at *high risk* of contracting HIV.

• Homosexual/bisexual men (and their sexual partners)

• Intravenous drug users (and their sexual partners)

• Hemophiliacs (and their sexual partners)

• Children born to parents with HIV disease

• Prostitutes

Note that family members and friends in close contact with persons with HIV are not listed among the high-risk categories. In the one instance in which a mother apparently acquired the virus from her infant, she did not follow recommendations for handling her infant's secretions (Centers for Disease Control 1986). Research continues to confirm that there is little or no risk to those having long-standing household exposure to persons with HIV.

Health care providers are also not in the high-risk category. In addition to having close contact with persons with HIV, health care workers may be concerned about contracting HIV as the result of an accidental needlestick or being cut with a sharp instrument. A study of almost 1000 health care workers that documented parenteral or mucous membrane exposure to the blood or body fluids of persons with AIDS indicated that only two health care workers tested positive for HIV at a fifteen-month follow-up (McCray 1986). Three other health care workers identified in 1987 as infected with the HIV virus had been exposed to large amounts of infected blood (Centers for Disease Control 1987). Although later research has demonstrated other similar instances, the incidence among health care workers is extremely small.

Protection for health care workers and others in close contact with persons with HIV is discussed in more detail later in this chapter. Counseling others in strategies for preventing HIV transmission is also discussed later in this chapter.

Homosexual/Bisexual Men Homosexual/bisexual men continue to account for the highest percentage of reported cases in the U.S. and Europe. Studies of risk factors for homosexual/bisexual men indicate that having a large number of different sexual partners appears to be the most significant risk factor. Certain sexual practices, such as receptive anal intercourse, are more frequently associated with increased risk. Other studies have demonstrated the possibility of genetic susceptibility to the development of **Kaposi's sarcoma** (present in about 48 percent of homosexual men with AIDS) that may relate to an underlying immune defect (Krigel and Friedman-Kien 1985).

Intravenous Drug Users The second largest transmission category for HIV in the U.S. and Europe is intravenous drug users. The virus is believed to be transmitted among intravenous drug users through the transfer of small amounts of blood in shared needles or syringes. Intravenous drug users also constitute a bridge to others—their fetuses, newborns, and sexual partners—putting them at increased risk. It is believed that the category known as "heterosexual cases" is largely composed of the heterosexual partners of intravenous drug users.

Hemophiliacs The risk to hemophiliacs and persons with other coagulation disorders comes from receiving clotting factor concentrates. Pooled plasma that may obtain material from between 2500 and 25,000 blood or plasma donors is used to make clotting factor concentrates. As early as 1984 there was almost a total HIV seroconversion (the development of antibodies in response to infection) of hemophiliacs linked to the administration of factor concentrates contaminated with HIV. Hemophiliacs also constitute a bridge (although a much smaller one than intravenous drug users) to children and female sexual partners.

Blood Transfusion Recipients   The risk to blood or blood product transfusion recipients comes from receiving blood from an HIV-positive donor. Testing of potential donors by enzyme-linked immunoabsorbent assay (ELISA) and screening of potential donors at risk for HIV has been instituted to protect the blood supply. Although the number of persons who contract HIV in this way is low (2 percent), the possibility of contracting HIV from tainted blood remains. False negative reactions are possible because of the *window* that exists (the period of time between which a person becomes infected and the development of antibodies) or because of errors in testing. Although the window for most people is about 3 months in length, recent findings indicate that it can take up to 18 months for HIV seroconversion to occur. Researchers are working to develop new tests with a smaller window.

Incidence and Geographic Distribution

National   By early 1991, 174,890 cases of AIDS had been reported to the Centers for Disease Control (CDC), and the known deaths since records were first kept in early 1981 numbered 110,530, or 63 percent. The current incidence picture is illustrated in Figure 25–2A for adults and adolescents age 13 years and over and in Figure 25–2B for infants and children.

At the national level, AIDS has been reported in all fifty of the United States. New York, California, Florida, Texas, and New Jersey have the highest percentage of AIDS cases. The incidence in homosex-

ual men is highest in New York City, San Francisco, and Los Angeles. The incidence of AIDS among intravenous drug users is highest in the New York/New Jersey metropolitan area (where the incidence of AIDS among intravenous drug users has now surpassed the rate in homosexual men) and in neighboring Connecticut. Of heterosexuals whose only known exposure was through sex with a person at risk, approximately two-thirds are female partners of male intravenous drug users. In the undetermined category, slightly over half had heterosexual contact with a person with or at risk for AIDS, and slightly under half were born in countries in which heterosexual transmission is thought to play a major role (Haiti or central Africa). Approximately one-third of those who cannot be placed in a high-risk category had sexual contact with female prostitutes (among whom the incidence of HIV infection continues to rise).

Estimates of the number of people in this country infected with HIV range from 1 million to 3 million people. The epidemic is growing every day, partly because people who may not know they are infected are spreading the virus.

International   At the international level, AIDS has been reported in every continent of the world except for Antarctica. International statistics are not always reliable since there is no international law that requires the reporting of AIDS cases. It is unclear whether the scope of the problem is as well known in the rest of the world as it is in the Americas. In the Americas, the countries with the highest number of reported cases are the United States, Brazil, Canada, and Haiti. The European countries of France, West Germany, Denmark, Switzerland, and Belgium report a high number of cases. Most of the AIDS cases in Africa are from what has become known as the "AIDS belt"—Zaire, Zambia, Rwanda, Burundi, Kenya, Uganda, and Tanzania. It is estimated that one out of every twenty people in these African nations is infected with HIV.

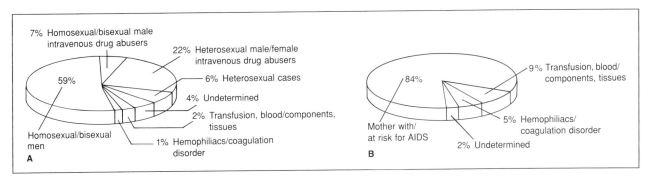

FIGURE 25–2   A. Incidence of AIDS among adults and adolescents age 13 and older. B. Incidence of AIDS among infants and children.   *SOURCE: Centers for Disease Control. HIV/AIDS Surveillance Report. July, 1991.*

The Biopsychosocial Impact of HIV Disease

HIV does not discriminate in its effects on the individual or society. It affects the biologic, psychologic, developmental, social, cultural, economic, political, legal, and ethical spheres.

Biologic

The extent of the symptoms and signs associated with HIV infection can vary from none, through nonspecific manifestations, to a variety of opportunistic infections and malignancies. Some people, although infected with HIV, remain healthy and never develop AIDS. They can, however, transmit the virus to others.

Symptoms and Signs of HRC Some people have a mild immune deficiency but do not have any life-threatening disease. These people are said to have HIV-related conditions (HRC). (For reporting purposes, the Centers for Disease Control uses a classification system that uses more specific and inclusive definitions than those presented here. However, for the purposes of this textbook, we are using the popular definition of HRC.)

Initially the symptoms associated with HRC may be the same as for any of a number of other conditions or illnesses; however, with HIV infection, they tend to be particularly prolonged. Persons with HRC may have symptoms and signs that include any combination of the following:

• Fatigue, possibly combined with headaches or lightheadedness

• Low-grade fever

• Night sweats

• Cervical, axillary, or femoral lymphadenopathy over several weeks

• Weight loss greater than 10 percent or 15 pounds not related to exercise or dieting

• Easy bruising or unexplained bleeding

• Chronic diarrhea

Symptoms and Signs of Aids The formal diagnosis of AIDS depends on whether the person can be diagnosed with one or more of the specific life-threatening opportunistic diseases the CDC has defined as indicative of AIDS (see the accompanying box).

The most serious opportunistic disease is **Pneumocystis carinii pneumonia (PCP)**, caused by the protozoan *Pneumocystis carinii,* the leading cause of death among persons with AIDS. It has symptoms similar to

---

Opportunistic Infections and Neoplasms Associated with AIDS

• Monilial infections of the mouth, trachea, esophagus, bronchi, or perineal and perianal areas caused by *Candida albicans*

• Cytomegalovirus infections

• Cryptococcal meningitis

• *Cryptosporidium* enterocolitis

• Herpes simplex virus and herpes zoster virus infections

• Kaposi's sarcoma

• *Pneumocystis carinii* pneumonia

• Primary lymphoma of the central nervous system

• Progressive multifocal leukoencephalopathy

• Toxoplasmosis

• Tuberculosis and other mycobacterial infections caused by *Mycobacterium avium* and *Mycobacterium intracellulare*

---

other severe forms of pneumonia, such as dry cough, difficulty breathing, and fever. This particular opportunistic disease has been implicated in more than half of the deaths from AIDS. One of the greatest advances in the medical treatment of HIV-infected persons has been the development of prophylactic treatments for PCP with drugs such as aerosolized pentamidine, sulfamethoxazole-trimethoprim (Bactrim, Septra), and dapsone (DDS). The use of aerosolized pentamidine has provided an effective treatment for PCP with fewer side effects than other drugs. The use of pentamidine as a prophylactic treatment for individuals with low T4 cell counts is expected to change these statistics over the next few years.

The most common malignancy is Kaposi's sarcoma. Usually appearing first on the legs as blue-violet or red-brown nodules or plaques, Kaposi's sarcoma can occur anywhere on the surface of the skin, in the mouth, or in the visceral organs such as the digestive tract and the lungs. Previously a rare malignancy of elderly men who survived for ten or more years after diagnosis, Kaposi's sarcoma is now the second most common cause of death among persons with AIDS. This malignancy was uncommon in North America and Europe until the AIDS epidemic. Currently, Kaposi's sarcoma has been implicated in more than 40 percent of the deaths from AIDS.

Neuropsychiatric Manifestations Neuropsychiatric manifestations represent one of the more complex aspects in the case of persons with HIV disease. Because the virus is able to invade central nervous system (CNS) tissue and because several of the opportunistic infections and neoplasms associated with AIDS also affect the CNS, significant numbers of persons with HIV experience neuropsychiatric manifestations.

Neuropsychiatric manifestations of HIV refer to a variety of disorders associated with physical or psychologic responses to HIV infection and/or HIV-related opportunistic processes. These can range from anxiety and depressive symptoms to delirium, dementia, and coma.

Psychologic HIV disease threatens psychologic integrity as well as physiologic integrity. The concept of loss is central to an understanding of the psychologic impact of HIV and the depression, anxiety, and suicidal ideation that often accompany it. HIV disease is frequently linked with several different loss experiences. These include loss of the following:

• Energy, appetite, strength, and physical stamina

• Control of body functions such as elimination, mobility, speech, sight, hearing, and tactile sensations

• Control of body appearance because of dramatic weight loss, oozing wounds, skin breakdown, hair loss, skin lesions, and so on

• Self-worth

• Mental clarity and cognitive ability

• Privacy

• Self-sufficiency and self-determination

• Employment, health insurance, salary

• Personal competency

• Physical intimacy, including sexual expression

• Friends and lovers to earlier deaths from AIDS

• Social support

• Hope

• Peace of mind and spirit

• Life itself

Persons with HIV and their families, friends, and caregivers experience these losses or fears. One psychiatric nurse (McEnany 1987) is concerned with the mental health effects that such an overwhelming number of losses will have on the increasing numbers of people being touched personally by AIDS as friends, loved ones, or colleagues die from it. McEnany predicts an increase in the numbers of people with the psychiatric diagnosis of post-traumatic stress disorder as more people face such overwhelming losses.

Psychiatric disorders in persons with HIV disease are probably grossly underdiagnosed. The reason may be that many health care providers often consider the overwhelming physical needs to take precedence.

Psychologic syndromes associated with HIV infection are generally related to initial diagnosis of HIV, crisis points along the HIV trajectory, or adjustment to the experience of chronic illness. The inherent lack of predictability and control, the fear of rejection and abandonment, and problems such as memory deficit and confusion play a role. Common psychiatric disorders frequently seen in people with HIV and AIDS are anxiety disorders, panic attacks, adjustment disorders with depressed mood, and major depression.

Neurologic Studies suggest that approximately 40 percent of PWAs develop physiologically based clinical neuropsychiatric manifestations or disorders (Levy and Bredesen 1987). Autopsy results suggest that about 70 percent of PWAs have CNS disease at the time of death (Moskowitz et al. 1984). It is estimated that about 10 percent of PWAs develop neurologic syndromes as the first clinical manifestation of HIV disease (Navia and Price 1987, So et al. 1987).

These may be seen as focal brain processes, such as **toxoplasmosis** (a parasitic opportunistic infection), cryptococcal meningitis (a fungal opportunistic infection), **cytomegalovirus** (CMV) encephalitis (a viral opportunistic infection), and CNS lymphoma (a neoplastic process). Signs and symptoms associated with these processes are focal deficits, altered level of consciousness, confusion, memory disturbances, headaches, and seizures.

An increasingly common neuropsychiatric disorder is HIV dementia (Massie et al. 1987, Navia et al. 1986). HIV dementia, a syndrome caused by direct HIV infection of the CNS, is characterized as a progressive dementia. It presents as a slowing and loss of precision in both cognitive and motor function. HIV dementia is now included in the CDC diagnostic criteria for AIDS. At different times during the epidemic this syndrome has been called subacute encephalitis, AIDS encephalopathy, and AIDS dementia complex. HIV dementia is generally manifested as a progressive cognitive impairment with accompanying motor and behavioral disturbances. The signs and symptoms of HIV dementia include the following:

• Cognitive indications: forgetfulness, loss of concentration, confusion, and slowness of thought

• Motor deficiencies: loss of balance, muscle weakness, and deterioration in fine motor skills such as handwriting

• Behavioral indications: apathy, withdrawal, dysphoric mood, organic psychosis, and regressed behavior

RESEARCH NOTE

Citation
Korniewicz DM, O'Brien ME, Larson E: Coping with AIDS and HIV: Psychosocial adaptation. J Psychosoc Nurs 1990;28(3):14–16, 19–21.

Study Problem/Purpose
The purpose of this study was to compare selected aspects of psychosocial adaptation—self-concept, self-esteem, alienation, and social functioning—among HIV-infected persons at various stages of the disease and among persons not known to be infected but in an identified high-risk group.

Method
Goffman's theory of stigma and social identity provided the theoretic basis for this study. Study subjects included four groups: (1) an HIV risk group ($n = 24$) of persons not known to be HIV-seropositive, but at high risk; (2) an HIV-infected asymptomatic group ($n = 10$) of seropositive persons who had not experienced any serious physiologic symptoms; (3) an early stage AIDS group ($n = 10$) of persons with early symptoms of AIDS who had been hospitalized no more than two times; and (4) a late stage AIDS group ($n = 19$) of persons who were severely ill with one or more identified AIDS-related conditions who had been hospitalized on multiple occasions for long periods. The following instruments were used to measure psychosocial adaptation: Sherwood's Self-Concept Inventory, Rosenberg's Self-Esteem Scale, the Dean Alienation Scale, and the Inventory of Social Functioning. Data were collected in the outpatient AIDS clinic and a designated twelve-bed inpatient AIDS unit of a large medical center in the middle Atlantic region of the USA, and in several community settings. The four paper-and-pencil tests took about 20 minutes to complete.

Findings
There were no significant differences among the four groups in self-concept, self-esteem, and social functioning across the spectrum of infection. However, infected but asymptomatic subjects and subjects at high risk for HIV infection had significantly higher alienation scores, particularly in powerlessness. Asymptomatic individuals experienced greater feelings of powerlessness as compared with the other three groups. Females evidenced more alienation than males, and blacks evidenced more alienation than whites.

Implications
It is possible that being identified as belonging to a high-risk group places an individual at risk for greater feelings of alienation and lack of control. Asymptomatic individuals, newly diagnosed with HIV, may be in an initial state of crisis in which they feel powerless and isolate themselves from friends, family, and partners. Many homosexual males are involved in community organizations that support gay life-styles, whereas infected women are more often heterosexuals without strong identification with a group or community organization. Greater levels of alienation among blacks is consistent with other studies that report that, as a community, black Americans exhibit negative attitudes toward homosexuality and often are rejected by family and friends if they become infected with HIV.

The results of this study raise several psychosocial issues relevant to nursing practice. It suggests that nurses should initiate psychosocial interventions with newly diagnosed persons before symptoms of AIDS become apparent. Nurses should also focus on or incorporate crisis intervention and psychoeducational methodologies and pay particular attention to women and black Americans. The early creation of psychosocial support groups is indicated because newly infected individuals experience greater alienation.

In addition, persons with HIV dementia may experience other symptoms such as headaches or seizures.

HIV dementia is often initially confused with psychiatric depression but generally progresses in a period of months to the point at which the affected individual is bedridden. Individuals with HIV dementia may quickly succumb to opportunistic infections due to an inability to engage in self-care activities.

The person with neuropsychiatric manifestations of HIV represents a tremendous challenge to both the professional and nonprofessional caregiver. Working with this population requires participation as a client advocate, effective multidisciplinary collaboration, and the ability to make appropriate referrals. To address the needs of this group adequately, one needs the ability to empathize with the individual with HIV and with **primary caregivers** (PCGs) and to act on the basis of that empathy. A primary caregiver is a person who is generally responsible for providing or coordinating daily care for a PWA who cannot perform self-care activities. Usually, a primary caregiver is a nonprofessional who is a significant other (life partner, spouse, family member, or close friend) of the person with AIDS.

Psychoneuroimmunology   Recently, there has been increased emphasis in the scientific literature on the study of psychoneuroimmunology. A growing body of evidence has demonstrated the interrelatedness of the body-mind-spirit connection and the immune system (Lovejoy and Sisson 1989). (See the Psychobiology box on page 594.) The implication is that nurses need to be more aware of psychologic and neurologic system impact on immune system disorders. There is widespread support for the use of holistic nursing practices and complementary treatment approaches to boost the immune system, in accordance with the findings in the growing field of psychoneuroimmunology.

Developmental

Most persons with HIV disease are young adults or adults in their middle years. The period known as young adulthood is normally the healthiest and is characterized by peaks in muscular strength. Cognitive development should be completed and cognitive abilities should be refined at this stage. Recall that the psychosocial task of identity consolidation is the major developmental task of young adulthood. HIV disease may disrupt the person's ability to negotiate this challenge successfully.

Typically, the middle years are very productive in the arenas of work and family. During this period, adults typically consolidate relationships and occupational status and goals. HIV disease may interfere with the individual's ability to accept the responsibilities inherent in such roles as parent, worker, mate or partner, and so on. Questions of dependence and independence, thought to have been resolved previously, are reawakened as illness forces a return to earlier developmental phases.

Children and adolescents with HIV infection face delays or changes in skills on all developmental fronts—physical, cognitive, and psychosocial—as they meet acute life-threatening illness and chronic disability. Failure to thrive is a striking feature of this illness in children, some of whom have been diagnosed with AIDS as early as 4 months of age (Boland 1987).

Sociocultural and Economic

Sociocultural Hostility   The social and cultural environments of most persons affected by HIV are generally hostile to them. Several factors seem to account for this sociocultural hostility. Strawn (1987) notes that the majority of persons with HIV, or affected by HIV ". . . are members of groups whose skin color, ethnic and cultural background, and/or life-style habits are regarded by many in the mainstream of American life with repugnance, fear, and moral condemnation."

The majority of persons with HIV are in two risk categories—homosexual/bisexual men and intravenous drug users—that engender fear, anger, and prejudice. **Homophobia** is the term used to describe unrealistic fear of homosexuality and homosexuals based on myths and stereotypes associated with homosexuality. According to Hughes, Martin, and Franks (1987, pp 107–108), homophobia may exist on both overt and covert levels and may be internalized, externalized, or institutional:

• Internalized homophobia is the self-rejection (feelings of shame, fear, guilt, and wrongdoing) that gay people may experience.

• Externalized homophobia is the rejection gay persons experience from others.

• Institutional homophobia is evident in the rules and regulations of hospitals, churches, employers, and other institutions, which invalidate the gay life-style by, for example, restricting hospital visitors in intensive care units to blood relatives only or denying gay people the right to worship.

Moral indignation is a frequent response to both gay people and to intravenous drug users. Many people consider homosexuality, bisexuality, and substance use evidence of lack of character, criminal behavior, or a sinful life-style. The two risk groups share other common characteristics (Hughes et al. 1987):

• Friends and partners (or lovers) are nontraditional support systems. Families of origin may be unaware of, or may reject, the individual's life-style and thus may be unable or unwilling to provide support.

• Persons in both risk categories may be estranged from institutions, such as organized religion, that view their life-style as sinful or immoral.

• Both groups may be set apart from the mainstream because of differences in norms, values, and language.

• The caregivers and support systems of persons in either of these groups may be members of the same high-risk groups, with which the nurse may not have had much previous contact.

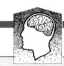

PSYCHOBIOLOGY: THE MIND/BODY CONNECTION

Psychoneuroimmunology: Communication between Mind and Cell in HIV Disease

Wars wage within our bodies every minute of every day. Most of the time we are unaware of the battles that go on within us. We have evolved legions of defenders—specialized cells that silently rout the unseen enemy. Their victories go unheralded. When our defenses are penetrated, our defenders are caught unprepared, or our defenders are routed and we've lost the battle, then we develop a cold, the flu, or even worse. Why did I catch a cold from the sick toddler on the plane when the woman next to me did not? Why didn't you come down with the flu when your roommate was sick? Why do only some of the people exposed to the HIV virus develop the disease? Why do some people with HIV disease die within a year or two while others have survived, or even thrived, for five, ten, or more years? We don't, as yet, have all the answers to these questions.

One particularly exciting field of research that has contributed toward answering these questions is *psychoneuroimmunology* (PNI), the study of the communication between the mind, the brain, the endocrine system, and the immune system. How does this communication occur? Certain messenger chemicals—neuroendocrines, neurotransmitters, and immunotransmitters— are released by the immune and neurologic systems. In this multiple-process communication system, the brain serves as the central post for these messengers that carry instructions to body organs along heavily trafficked electrochemical pathways. The messages are actually picked up at the cellular level by cell receptors.

Believing in the interconnectedness of mind, body, and spirit has long been a tradition of nursing. Recent scientific advances in PNI are important to nurses because they support the mind-body-spirit connection. They demonstrate the way in which emotions register on the body and the way in which the mind is influenced by the body, and suggest the role of attitudes and emotions in combating serious illness such as AIDS.

Perhaps the most important common characteristics of people with AIDS who live long past the time predicted for them is their refusal to accept the diagnosis of HIV disease as a death sentence. They do not deny the diagnosis, but *they do defy the fatal outcome* that is supposed to be connected to it. Long-term survivors are extremely goal-oriented and social. They treat their symptoms as if they were minor impediments in their lives; they are determined to prevail. Their immune systems seem to function better. They have higher T-cell counts and, in many cases, other immune system cells compensate for the ravaged T-cells. Emotional distress, on the other hand, has been found to accompany negative immune function factors in HIV-infected persons.

The highest incidence of illness and death occur in persons who experience stress after infection with HIV. This suggests that HIV-seropositive persons should reduce their exposure to stressful events. Assertive coping, less stress, more self-nurturing, and regular exercise have been associated with a better immune status, suggesting that stress-reduction behaviors may be effective in slowing the progression of HIV disease.

The research describing the relationship between PNI and HIV disease is investigational and has not been controlled for factors such as mutational changes in the HIV, the amount of virus in the body, or the number and frequency of opportunistic diseases the person has experienced. This means that we cannot promote the idea that clients are in total control of the disease process and the state of their health, or that the mind can cure AIDS. However, nurses can and should teach clients the self-care behaviors that long-term survivors are using to maintain their health. Nurses should also assess the level of stress, quality of social support, and mood, factors that influence the quality and quantity of life of persons with HIV disease. Standard and experimental drug therapies (especially psychotropic drugs) may bring about unexpected immunologic and neuroendocrine toxicities because of HIV-related defects in the person's cellular PNI communication system. For this reason, nurses

▶

PSYCHOBIOLOGY: THE MIND/BODY CONNECTION (continued)

need to monitor these systems very carefully and teach their clients to do the same. Nursing interventions to help clients enhance neurologic, immunologic, and cognitive functioning should focus on improved nutrition, adequate sleep-wake patterns, hygiene, stress reduction, and social support. Case management of clients caught in stressful family, financial, or emotional situations should be directed toward supportive problem solving.

It was Norman Cousins who suggested that *positive attitudes are not merely "moods," but biochemical realities.* We need to learn more about the effects of mental events on the immune system. Lovejoy and Sisson (1989) propose the following nursing research questions related to PNI:

- Do state personality characteristics (those that are transitory) or trait personality characteristics (those that are stable individual differences) influence the incidence, severity, or course of immunologically resisted and autoimmune diseases, including HIV disease?

- Do early life experiences modulate the PNI systems of adults with HIV disease?

- Is longevity among persons with HIV disease associated with superior psychologic defenses, interpersonal skills, and coping mechanisms?

- Are individuals who are out of touch with, unaware of, or unable to express emotions (particularly negative ones) most at risk for increased HIV progression rates?

- Are happiness, security, sense of control, relaxation, and other positive emotions accompanied by immune enhancement?

- Is onset of AIDS preceded by emotional distress or failure of coping mechanisms or psychologic defenses?

- What is the effect of chronic versus short-term stress on the HIV trajectory?

Answers to these questions will help clients learn how to minimize the challenge of living with HIV disease and maximize the quality of their lives.

—*Carol Ren Kneisl*

On one hand, children with HIV disease or persons who have contracted HIV from transfusion of blood or a blood product are usually perceived as "innocents" rather than sinners. On the other hand, they may be as feared and subject to discrimination as gays and drug users.

In her book *Illness as Metaphor* (1977) Susan Sontag suggests that people with illnesses that evoke feelings of apprehension and vulnerability in others become objects of that dread. This is especially true of HIV and AIDS. The well fear contamination by the sick with an illness for which there is no known cure.

Economic Factors   For the individual, HIV disease can mean an unstable financial situation. Days lost from work because of illness may cost people with HRC or AIDS their jobs and insurance benefits. Some insurers are avoiding or reducing claims by isolating high-risk applicants with HIV antibody tests, denying new policies to those at risk, and aggressively fighting existing policyholders' claims in court. Family and friends may be unable or unwilling to assist financially. Young adults, many in their early thirties, find themselves having to seek public assistance such as Medicaid for help in meeting health costs associated with HIV disease. The price of zidovudine (AZT; marketed as Retrovir), despite several price reductions since it

was first developed, ranges from $7000 to $8000 a year, a cost that by itself places HIV treatment beyond most persons' means.

Experts predict that in the 1990s AIDS care will cost the nation more than kidney dialysis or cancer of the lung, breast, or colon. Only care for cardiac clients and auto accident casualties is expected to cost more. Federal authorities estimate that about 40 percent of all persons with AIDS will eventually be without means or insurance and will need to rely on Medicaid.

Volunteer programs such as San Francisco's Shanti Project, a private organization of volunteers who donate their time, provides a lifeline for persons with AIDS. Shanti provides emotional support counselors to the dying and their families; sends out workers to clean, cook, shop, and provide transportation; runs several low-cost residences; and shuttles persons with AIDS back and forth to hospital and clinic appointments. Programs such as these have helped to lessen the financial impact. Unquestionably, HIV infection presents an economic problem of severe proportions.

Homelessness   A growing and critical problem is the lack of decent, appropriate housing for the growing number of persons with HIV disease. HIV disease is disproportionately high in persons already at the economic edge and in persons who are targets of discrimination in housing and medical care: persons of color, homosexuals, intravenous drug users, and homeless and runaway youth. In many communities around the country, available housing and services fall short of the need for appropriate residential care for thousands of people who have been made homeless by HIV-related illnesses, or whose struggle to survive on the streets has been worsened by the disease (National Coalition for the Homeless 1990). Fatigue, repeated hospitalization, and recurring illnesses all require time off from work, resulting first in the loss of employment, and then in the loss of housing. The lack of effective risk-reduction education programs among the homeless has led to predictable and dramatic increases in HIV-seropositivity among them.

Although most persons with impaired immune systems can live independently, they require a safe environment that helps them avoid exposure to infectious disease, get adequate rest, meet their special nutritional needs, and have access to support services and home help when necessary. Many shelters for the homeless refuse to accept persons with HIV or at risk for HIV infection. Consequently, many homeless persons are kept in hospital beds longer than necessary because they have no place to go. Others are discharged from hospitals without appropriate arrangements for residential care and find themselves on the street, where they are at high risk for infection and violence.

Legal

Law on HIV and AIDS is still in the formative stage. Several legal questions have not yet been answered. Some recommend legislation to ban discrimination against people infected with HIV, while others urge legislation to require mandatory testing and quarantine as two measures to protect the general public. Testing will probably not become common until people do not have to worry that they will lose their jobs or insurance if they test positive for HIV. The dilemma has to do with the violation of individual rights (by such activities as mandatory premarital or antepartal testing or mandatory testing of persons at high risk) as opposed to violation of the concept of societal good.

Bompey (1986) has reached the following conclusions on the direction of law related to employment rights and HIV disease based on recent court decisions:

• HIV disease is a "protected handicap."

• An employer cannot deny employment to an applicant with HIV unless the disease is far advanced and renders the applicant incapable of performing the duties of the job.

• Segregation of persons with HIV in the workplace is without medical justification and would probably violate prohibitions against discrimination on the basis of disability.

• Other employees generally cannot refuse to work with people who have HIV unless a claim can be substantiated that a dangerous work condition exists; such employees, after educational interventions, may be subject to discipline or dismissal if they still refuse to work with affected persons.

• Employers may not discharge an employee with HIV merely because they believe that individual will soon become incapacitated.

• Employers may not generally ask job applicants if they have HIV or have been exposed to the virus.

• Employers can probably require blood tests as part of the preemployment physical examination, but the employer would be limited in using the test results. Disclosure of such information to others would be highly inadvisable.

• Employers cannot force employees with HIV disease to take a medical leave unless they are unable to perform their jobs.

There are several cases in the courts over denied HIV-related medical insurance claims and life insurance policy claims. Insurance companies have been accused of using legal tactics to delay the resolution of litigation on the theory that the life of a person with AIDS is shorter than the life of a lawsuit. The wills of people who have died from AIDS and bequeathed their estates to gay partners are also being contested by estranged blood relatives.

Because cognitive impairment is common in persons with AIDS, decision-making regarding treatment, investments, and other financial matters is often transferred to another person with power of attorney.

Political

HIV activists have been concerned about the slow pace of the Food and Drug Administration (FDA) in approving new drugs for the treatment of HIV infection and argue that the FDA should be far more liberal in allowing use of untested drugs by those who have no hope of cure. The lack of easy access to drugs has encouraged the development of guerrilla AIDS clinics. These informal clinics, in living rooms and kitchens throughout the United States, provide a variety of medicines. Some are readily available prescription drugs. Others are more exotic mixtures of nutritional additives or items such as Brazilian tree bark and Chinese mushrooms. Still others are chemicals such as DNCB (a photographic solvent readily available at chemical supply houses, and traditionally used to treat warts), which is painted on Kaposi's sarcoma lesions with cotton-tipped applicators. Those who are desperate travel to Mexico and Europe to obtain drugs not yet approved for sale in this country.

The political climate also affects potential legislation to ensure confidentiality and to ban discrimination. For example, it may not be politically feasible for a legislator seeking reelection by a conservative, frightened, or unknowledgeable constituency to advocate measures the electorate would see as contrary to their best interests. Some politicians point to the HIV epidemic as graphically illustrating huge gaps in the health care system and the need for a comprehensive federal medical care program.

Ethical

According to Durham (1987), the mysterious nature of AIDS, the lack of an effective cure, and its highly lethal outcome combine to stigmatize persons with HIV disease. Durham also suggests that persons with HIV are doubly stigmatized because most of them are already members of other stigmatized groups—homosexuals, bisexuals, drug abusers, blacks, and Hispanics. The statistics for homosexuals, bisexuals, and drug users have been discussed earlier in this chapter and illustrated in Figure 25–2. The CDC reports that 45 percent of the reported adult and adolescent cases of AIDS are among blacks (29 percent) and Hispanics (16 percent), and 78 percent of the infant and child cases are also among blacks and Hispanics.

Breaches of confidentiality, such as reporting the results of testing to government agencies, employers, and insurance companies, or tattooing individuals who test HIV positive so that potential sex partners would be aware the individual has been exposed to the virus, would further stigmatize persons with HIV.

The ethical issues surrounding AIDS probably prompt most emotional responses. Some of the ethical questions that have arisen are:

• Should HIV antibody testing be made mandatory? If so, who should be tested—gay men, intravenous drug abusers, pregnant women, persons admitted to hospitals, prisoners, couples applying for marriage licenses, food handlers, health care workers, child care workers, people applying for health and life insurance, everyone?

• Is it in the public interest to identify, report, and make public the names of persons with AIDS or at risk for HIV?

• To what extent would the undertaking of preventive health measures be a matter of public health responsibility?

• Should persons infected with the virus be tattooed to protect potential sex partners from infection?

• Should persons with HIV and AIDS be placed in quarantine for the public good?

• Can or should employers suspend, terminate, or refuse to hire persons with HIV? If they are teachers? Food handlers? Health care workers?

• Should people who have had sexual contact with persons with HIV or received infected blood products be traced and informed by public health authorities?

• Do health care workers have a duty to inform those at risk when a person with HIV does not modify high-risk behavior?

• Is it appropriate to make experimental drugs and treatments that are not yet proven safe and effective available to persons with HIV disease?

• Should research protocols that call for administering placebos to some persons (who thus remain untreated) and experimental drugs to others be allowed?

• Can nurses or other health care professionals refuse to provide care to persons with HIV disease?

Engaging in the process of ethical reflectiveness discussed in Chapter 7 can be used to analyze these and other issues and resolve the ethical dilemmas inherent in them.

In 1985 the American Nurses' Association (ANA) reaffirmed its specific commitment to nursing care for persons with AIDS (ANA 1985b). In addition to this specific commitment to nursing care for persons with AIDS, the first two statements in ANA's code of ethics (ANA 1985a) provide guidance to nurses with respect to these nursing care dilemmas:

1. The nurse provides services with respect for human dignity and the uniqueness of the client unrestricted by considerations of social or economic status, personal attributes, or the nature of health problems.

2. The nurse safeguards the client's right to privacy by judiciously protecting information of a confidential nature.

Both the New York State Nurses Association (1983) and the California Nurses Association (1985) have published statements relative to nursing practice that make clear the professional nurse's responsibility in relation to the care of persons with AIDS. These statements address the need to provide appropriate care (both direct and indirect), health teaching, and advocacy.

Roles for Psychiatric Mental Health Nurses

Psychiatric mental health nurses will work with clients all along the continuum of HIV infection and disability. Schietinger (1986) has proposed the following continuum for describing the impact of HIV in terms of the person's functional ability. It conceptualizes four levels of disability:

1. *Apparently well.* The apparently well person has HIV disease but requires little or no medical intervention. Examples are a functionally independent gay man with a skin lesion diagnosed as Kaposi's sarcoma or the person who is HIV seropositive (asymptomatic).

2. *Acutely ill.* The acutely ill person may be experiencing HRC or an opportunistic infection. Hospitalization may be required for treatment to stabilize the condition.

3. *Chronically ill.* The chronically ill person has experienced HRC or a relapse of an opportunistic disease, has received a diagnosis of a new opportunistic disease, or has a progression or deterioration in physical or mental condition.

4. *Terminally ill.* The terminally ill person has a prognosis of six months or less to live.

Psychiatric mental health nurses may be involved in working with persons with HIV disease in in-patient settings in psychiatric hospitals, psychiatric units in general hospitals, mental health clinics, community health agencies, hospices or homes, private practice, industry, or schools and as citizens and neighbors. In addition to working with people at the four levels of disability listed above, psychiatric nurses have active roles with well people, with the family and friends of persons with HIV, and with bereaved survivors.

Direct Nursing Care in Psychiatric Mental Health Settings

Milieu Concerns Education of staff and clients is best begun before the first client with HIV disease is admitted to a unit. Generally, this is not the case. After-the-fact education about HIV is complicated by the surprise of the experience. Often it is wise to access outside resources, such as a community based **AIDS service organization (ASO)**, to provide education at the appropriate level for staff and clients. They give the most up-to-date information in a setting where people may feel most comfortable revealing their feelings and biases.

Evans et al. (1990) emphasize the importance of proactive preparation and programming in allaying the anxiety of both staff and clients when incorporating people with HIV disease into a psychiatric mental health milieu. Both staff and clients may have concerns about disease transmission, inadequate knowledge regarding HIV and AIDS, and lack of understanding of the unique needs of the person with HIV disease.

Special arrangements may need to be made about the scheduling of activities, visiting policies, and provision of physical treatments, depending on the physical and neuropsychiatric manifestations of the disease and the extent of HIV disease progression (Baer et al. 1987). Staff will need to make individual decisions on a case-by-case basis. Clear communication with staff and other clients is thus necessary to promote consistency and to prevent disruption of the milieu as a result of perceived inequities.

Clients with neuropsychiatric manifestations of HIV may present a special challenge to the staff and to the milieu. Their behavior may be erratic, frightening, and unlike that of the usual psychiatric client. This may require modification of generally accepted milieu standards. For example, a client who is frequently incontinent may disrupt meal times and other community activities. It may become necessary to exclude some clients (e.g., the client with HIV dementia) from certain activities. To prevent other clients from perceiving that the client with HIV disease is receiving special treatment, nurses should openly discuss these issues with the community while continuing to ensure individual client confidentiality, as appropriate.

The use of universal infection control precautions (see the accompanying Intervention box) in a psychiatric-mental health setting can also help to decrease staff and client anxiety (Evans et al. 1990). Not all persons with HIV (both staff and clients) are aware of their status or feel comfortable disclosing the information even if they are aware. Universal precautions, as prescribed by the CDC, will protect *all* staff and clients from transmission of HIV. This approach promotes confidentiality, since appropriate precautions are taken in the care of all clients. Therefore, it is unnecessary to identify HIV-infected individuals to the general community.

Persons with HIV Disease Several authorities have predicted that increasing numbers of persons with HIV will require hospitalization in a psychiatric setting. Psychiatric hospitalization may be needed because the client is depressed, suicidal, or psychotic or has an AIDS-related behavior disturbance, probably because of organic mental disorder.

Psychiatric nurses caring for clients with HRC or AIDS on in-patient units encounter a number of issues that are uncommon in psychiatric settings:

• The client may have a multitude of physical problems.

INTERVENTION

General Infection Control Precautions*

- Handle the blood of *all* clients as potentially infectious.
- Wash hands before and after all client contact and all specimen contact. (This is the single most important means of preventing infection.)
- Wear gloves for potential contact with blood and body fluids, including instances when the health care provider has a cut, scratch, or dermatologic lesion on the hands.
- Wear a gown when contact with blood or body fluids is anticipated.
- Wear a mask only if tuberculosis is a possibility or the client is coughing or likely to cough.
- Wear protective eyewear and mask if splatter with blood or body fluids is possible (e.g., bronchoscopy, oral surgery, other invasive procedures).
- Place used syringes immediately in a nearby specially designated impermeable container; do not recap, bend, clip, or manipulate the needle in any way.
- Treat all linen soiled with blood or body fluids as infectious.
- Discard all disposable supplies and equipment in a specially designated container.
- Label all soiled, reusable equipment and supplies and place them in an impervious bag before sending for decontamination and reprocessing.
- Process all laboratory specimens as potentially infectious.
- Place mouth pieces and resuscitation equipment where resuscitation is predictable.
- Clean all blood and body fluid spills with an appropriate disinfectant (seek advice from your health care facility's infection control practitioner).

---

*Infection control guidelines may change as more is known about AIDS. Be sure to contact an appropriate source for up-to-date guidelines (the infection control practitioner in your health care facility or the Centers for Disease Control in Atlanta, Georgia).

- The client has a condition that calls for infection control precautions (see the Intervention box earlier in this chapter).
- The quality of the nurse-client relationship is intensified through the additional contact required in giving physical care.
- The psychiatric nurse must confront the issue of caring for clients with life-threatening illnesses.

A necessary modification has to do with the use of touch. The physical care needs of AIDS clients require modifying the usual psychiatric injunction of limiting physical contact with clients. Because AIDS is such an isolating and stigmatizing condition, giving a massage or holding the client's hand has therapeutic value.

The psychiatric nurse caring for clients with a dual diagnosis that includes HIV disease faces a challenge that requires creative modification. Nursing care for clients with depression, suicidal ideation, psychosis, or organic mental disorder has been discussed in earlier chapters in this text. In persons with AIDS, it is important not to mistake delirium for depression.

The clinical example below (from Baer et al. 1987) illustrates the complexities of caring for a dual-diagnosis client in an in-patient psychiatric setting.

John was a 38-year-old gay white man with no psychiatric history except episodic binge drinking and a two-month history of AIDS (*Pneumocystis carinii* pneumonia). He was admitted after he became disruptive in an alcohol treatment program. Clinically, he appeared to be suffering an episode of bipolar disorder (mania) and exhibited insomnia, hyperactivity, pressured speech, flight of ideas, lability, grandiose and religious delusions, auditory and visual hallucinations, markedly impaired judgment, and complete denial of his AIDS diagnosis. It was unclear if his symptoms were directly caused by HIV infection of his brain or were part of a reactive or "functional" disorder. A negative CT scan and lumbar puncture suggested the latter was the case. John improved moderately after treatment with antipsychotic medication; lithium was not used as John had recent renal complications of AIDS. He was released ten days after admission, following a successful challenge of his mental health held in Superior Court.

John was readmitted ten days later after increasing fatigue and severely impaired judgment rendered him unable to obtain food, clothing, and shelter. Treatment with antipsychotic medication was reinstituted. At first he continued to exhibit manic symptoms. On one occasion he became threatening and required seclusion. He repeatedly abused the telephone, dialing 911 to get the police to rescue him, badgering friends, and trying to order everything from plane tickets to brass bands.

After a few weeks, John's clinical status began to change. Many of his "manic" symptoms diminished or disappeared; for the most part, he maintained his grandiose denial of his prognosis although this was punctuated by periodic lucidity and acknowledgment of his illness. He began to show signs of dementia; decreased attention to grooming and common etiquette, disorientation, failing short-term memory, wandering, and visual-spatial recognition deficits. He had a number of medication complications, although he was able to tolerate a neuroleptic and gradually required less of this. His dementia progressed rapidly, and he grew weaker and more in need of nursing assistance with basic activities.

John was placed on permanent conservatorship and no longer required acute psychiatric hospitalization after approximately two months, although he remained on the unit for nearly six months until he could be placed in a residential program with twenty-four-hour care. He died ten days after discharge.

It may be beneficial to set up a separate support group for people with HIV disease, where they can discuss issues specific to HIV in a supportive setting. If there aren't enough HIV clients for a group, then an ASO might provide support group services. An ASO can also be an important resource for the HIV client after discharge. The range of services available depends on the structure of the ASO but frequently includes support groups, buddy programs, educational programs, financial assistance, housing referral, legal aid, and client advocacy.

Clients with neuropsychiatric manifestations (NPM) of HIV, such as HIV dementia, may offer the greatest challenge to the inpatient unit staff. Nursing diagnoses common to persons with NPM are listed in the accompanying Nursing Diagnosis box. Three important but frequently ignored nursing diagnoses that apply to clients with NPM are **Impaired communication, Spiritual distress,** and **Impaired home maintenance management.** Clients with neuropsychiatric manifestations of HIV disease often have special discharge planning needs or experience placement problems. Intervention strategies appropriate to these three selected nursing diagnoses are discussed in the following sections.

Intervening with Clients Having Impaired Communication Because a client's symptoms are generally progressive, interventions do not reverse the dementia but may enhance the quality of life for both the client and the primary caregiver. Here are several strategies:

• Convey unconditional positive regard; maintain a relationship; maintain a sense of normality in interactions.

• Make verbal communication clear, concise, and unhurried; be sure to have the person's attention before starting; encourage the person to communicate; be comfortable with periods of silence; be aware of tone and volume of voice (this may prevent misperceptions).

• Use brief, direct statements: "Mike, eat this pudding" rather than "Why don't you and I have some pudding for dessert?"

• Ask questions that require only simple yes or no answers, and make only one request at a time.

• Be sensitive to the need to restate statements or questions at intervals.

• Continue to communicate with the person; don't stop communicating.

• The client may have memory loss; therefore, reintroduce yourself as often as necessary.

• Remember that nonverbal communication and touch are important; nonverbal communication may eventually become the primary communication mode between the client and the nurse or the client and the primary caregiver.

• Remember who the person was in the past, reminiscence and validation are important; provide familiar stimuli.

• Be sure not to equate aphasia or flat affect with absence of feelings; use empathy and interpretation of behaviors/statements to understand what is happening (for example, when a person who is at home says, "I want to go home"); support the person's feelings.

• Provide an environment of sheltered freedom, that is, the least restrictive level that is safe (unhurried, consistent, structured, with decreased external stimulation).

• Avoid mechanical or chemical restraints as much as possible.

• Avoid infantalizing the person, but remember that you may need to set firm limits.

• Be flexible; try different approaches; share information.

Intervening with the Client in Spiritual Distress Spiritual distress is usually evidenced by guilt, recriminations and self-blame, hyper-religiosity, rejection of significant others, and expressions of despair. The following list provides some helpful guidelines for working with clients experiencing spiritual distress:

• Give the person permission to experience personal feelings, no matter what they are, and encourage appropriate expression of these feelings.

• Accept the fact that primary caregivers may not be able to listen to the client's feelings. If the primary caregiver delegates this job, recognize the distress this may cause.

NURSING DIAGNOSIS

Neuropsychiatric Manifestations (NPM) of HIV Infection

General Nursing Diagnosis

- Activity intolerance (related to physical and psychologic impact of chronic HIV infection)
- Altered health maintenance (related to chronic HIV infection and NPM of HIV infection)
- Fatigue (related to chronic HIV infection and NPM of HIV infection)
- High risk for infection (related to compromised immune system and NPM of HIV infection)
- Impaired home maintenance management (related to NPM of HIV infection)
- Impaired tissue integrity (related to chronic HIV infection and NPM of HIV infection)
- Noncompliance (related to NPM of HIV infection)
- Self-care deficit (related to NPM of HIV infection)
- Sleep pattern disturbance (related to NPM of HIV infection)

Psychosocial Nursing Diagnoses

- Altered sexuality patterns (related to NPM of HIV infection)
- Altered thought processes (related to NPM of HIV infection)
- Anticipatory grieving (related to issues associated with HIV infection and NPM of HIV infection)
- Anxiety (related to actual or perceived threats, losses, and/or changes associated with HIV diagnosis)
- Decisional conflict (related to ethical dilemmas—e.g., quality of life, life-support measures—and NPM of HIV infection)
- Fear (related to actual or perceived threats, losses, and/or changes associated with HIV diagnosis)
- High risk for violence: Self-directed (Related to NPM of HIV infection)
- Hopelessness (related to chronic HIV infection and NPM of HIV infection)

- Ineffective individual coping (related to physiologic, situational, and/or maturational factors associated with HIV infection)
- Powerlessness (related to chronic HIV infection and NPM of HIV infection)
- Self-esteem disturbance (related to actual or perceived threats, losses, and/or changes associated with HIV diagnosis and/or NPM of HIV infection)
- Social isolation (related to NPM of HIV infection)
- Spiritual distress (related to NPM of HIV infection, diagnosis of HIV infection, unresolved identity crisis, confrontation of mortality)

Neurologic Nursing Diagnoses

- Acute pain or chronic pain (related to chronic HIV infection, immobility, neuropathy)
- Altered body temperature (related to CNS infection and/or increased intracranial pressure, chronic HIV infection, and opportunistic infections)
- Altered nutrition: Less than body requirements (related to altered level of consciousness or NPM of HIV infection)
- Altered urinary elimination (related to NPM of HIV infection)
- Bowel incontinence, or Colonic constipation, or Diarrhea (related to chronic HIV infection, opportunistic infections, immobility, and/or NPM of HIV infection)
- High risk for injury (related to sensory or motor deficits such as neuropathy, gait disturbance, and dyskinesia associated with HIV infection)
- Impaired physical mobility (related to NPM of HIV infection)
- Impaired verbal communication (related to memory loss and/or decreased ability to process information, or related to CNS changes in function and motor control such as aphasia, echolalia, and dysphagia)
- Sensory perceptual alterations (related to NPM of HIV infection)

• Recognize the stages of grieving and allow people to progress at their own rate; don't push the client into a stage that you think is necessary.

• Share spiritual resources as appropriate; encourage the person to find comforting spiritual outlets (poetry or other literature may be used to encourage reflection).

Enhancing Home Maintenance Management If clients return to the homes to be cared for by a nonprofessional, special preparations may be necessary. Impairment of home maintenance management is evidenced in several ways. The primary caregiver may verbalize difficulty with maintaining the home environment or caring for the person with HIV. Other situations to look for are evidence of poor hygiene in the home, an impaired caregiver, or an unavailable support system. The following list gives guidelines for discharge planning and placement:

• Begin planning for discharge when the client is admitted to the hospital.

• Assess the client's abilities to function in the home, the family's or primary caregiver's abilities to function in the home, and the housing or home environment itself.

• Make referrals to home care professionals and other community agencies.

• Help the primary caregiver to determine the appropriate level of care and to realistically assess his or her own ability to provide home care; explore all role responsibilities and related factors; assist in redefining and prioritizing roles and functions.

• Determine the primary caregiver's learning needs and facilitate the development of skills by identifying specific symptoms (e.g., memory loss) and developing strategies to address those symptoms.

• Provide respite care for primary caregivers.

• Provide emotional support to clients and primary caregivers and refer them to additional support systems.

Other Clients The staff and other clients on the unit will need health education to help them understand HIV infection and the behavior of persons with HIV in their midst. In their experience with AIDS clients on an in-patient psychiatric unit, Baer et al. (1987) noted that not all clients react favorably to the presence of persons with AIDS. They found that clients with paranoid disorders had the greatest difficulty accepting persons with AIDS. Among the behaviors they observed were hostility, incorporating AIDS into paranoid delusions, insisting on being transferred to an-

other unit, and insisting on the persons with AIDS being transferred to another unit.

Ways to help other clients include providing education, offering support, allowing the other clients to vent their fears and express their concerns, and emphasizing that the care of HIV clients is an important and normal part of the unit routine. The clients most vocal in their protests use the AIDS issue to avoid dealing with some of their own problems (Baer et al. 1987). Psychiatric mental health nurses should keep this in mind when developing individual nursing care plans or dealing with milieu issues.

Risk Reduction Education and Counseling

Taking a leading role in risk reduction education and counseling is a crucial role for all nurses during the HIV epidemic. Risk reduction education is directed toward three broad goals:

1. Educating clients, the public, other professionals, colleagues, friends, and neighbors in strategies to reduce the risk of contracting HIV

2. Counteracting the myths, stereotypes, and hysteria that surround HIV and AIDS

3. Correcting misinformation

Because more is being learned about HIV and appropriate and effective risk reduction and prevention, *readers should consult current CDC guidelines before implementing programs for persons at risk for contracting HIV.*

Teaching risk reduction can best be accomplished by listening, informing, and supporting clients in making choices that reduce their risk. Bjorklund (1987) suggests that, to motivate clients to reduce their risks, nurses need to understand the following principles:

• Risk reduction education is important for members of high-risk groups and their sexual contacts since a large percentage of members of high-risk groups have already been exposed to the HIV virus.

• An HIV-positive person is at risk for (1) developing AIDS, and (2) transmitting the virus even if healthy.

• The role of reexposure to HIV or other infectious organisms is not completely understood; reexposure may be implicated in the progression from either an asymptomatic state or HRC to AIDS.

• The change to low-risk behaviors for high-risk individuals may necessitate lifelong change. Lifelong change can be more effectively maintained if sexual activities that incorporate risk-reduction techniques are also satisfying.

- Clients need support to maintain low-risk behavior in an environment that reinforces high-risk behavior.

Sexual Behavior Many experts fear that educating persons about **"safer sex" practices** generates a false sense of security. In this AIDS era, these experts say, the only safe sex is no sex. Realistically, however, abstinence is not a lifelong change that will be maintained by many. Counseling persons about high-

risk sexual behaviors, low-risk sexual behaviors, and risk-free sexual behaviors makes more sense especially in terms of the principles outlined in the list above. High-risk sexual behaviors are those in which there is an exchange of blood or body fluids. Receptive anal intercourse is thought to be of highest risk because of the trauma caused to the mucous membranes of the rectum. Guidelines for counseling in terms of safer sex are given in the accompanying Client/Family Teaching box.

It is evident that the use of **condoms** (a barrier protection placed on the penis to prevent the transmission of body fluids during sexual activity) is important

---

CLIENT/FAMILY TEACHING

HIV Risk Reduction Guidelines

Sexual Behavior

Risk-Free Behaviors *Most of these behaviors involve skin-to-skin contact only. The virus is unlikely to be transmitted from one person to another unless breaks in the skin exist.*

- Mutual masturbation (male or female)
- Body massage, hugging
- Frottage (body-to-body rubbing without penetration)
- Dry (social) kissing
- Using one's own sex toys (dildos or vibrators) that are not shared
- Light S and M (sadism and masochism) activities (without bruising or bleeding)

Low-Risk Behaviors (Possibly Safe) *Small amounts of some body fluids may be exchanged during these activities. The risk of transmitting the virus is thought to be increased in proportion to the number of contacts.*

- Anal intercourse with condom (if used properly)
- Vaginal intercourse with condom (if used properly)
- Fellatio (oral sex) without ingestion of seminal fluid or semen
- Wet kissing (also called French kissing)
- Cunnilingus (oral-vaginal contact; risk is probably enhanced during menstruation)
- Using shared sex toys that are cleaned between uses and covered with a condom

- Urine contact (also called watersports) when skin is unbroken and urine is not taken by mouth or by rectum

High-Risk Behaviors (Unsafe) *These activities involve tissue trauma or exchange of blood or body fluids that may transmit HIV or other microbes.*

- Anal intercourse without condom (both receptive and insertive)
- Vaginal intercourse without condom
- Fisting (manual-anal contact)
- Fellatio with ingestion of semen
- Rimming (oral-anal contact)
- Using unclean, unprotected sex toys
- Piercing or drawing blood

Substance Abuse

- Remember that people who look healthy can carry the AIDS virus.
- Never share intravenous drugs or works (equipment).
- If a new needle and syringe are not available or equipment must be shared, remember to clean the works.
- Prevent sexual transmission.
- Avoid alcohol, marijuana, amphetamines, cocaine, and poppers.
- If you want to have children but have shared needles or may have been exposed to AIDS through sexual contact with someone who has, get medical advice.

in decreasing risk. However, condoms must be used effectively to decrease risk. Remember to include the following information about condoms in any risk reduction program:

• Latex condoms are probably safer to use than natural or lambskin condoms since the HIV may be small enough to be able to pass through the pores in natural condoms.

• Condoms with reservoir tips are safer than those without. (A reservoir tip provides space for the semen and helps to prevent breakage.)

• Condom packages should not be opened until use. Packages should be opened carefully. (This helps prevent damage that might result from rough handling or jagged fingernails).

• Condoms should be stored in a dark, cool, dry place. (Excessive heat or cold, sunlight, and moisture can damage the latex.)

• The condom should be applied before any genital contact. (Semen and seminal fluid may be discharged in advance of ejaculation.)

• The condom should be placed at the tip of the erect penis, and the air should be gently pressed out of the condom tip. (Air bubbles can cause condoms to break.)

• The condom should be held at the tip and rolled down and smoothed over the entire erect penis. Uncircumcised men should pull back the foreskin before applying the condom. (This provides a more effective seal.)

• A water-based product such as lubricating jelly or spermicidal jelly should be added before penetration. (Insufficient lubrication can cause condoms to tear or pull off. Oil-based lubricants such as petroleum jelly, baby oil, vegetable oil, mineral oil, cold cream, or hand lotion may cause the latex to disintegrate.)

• Spermicidal foams, creams, or jellies containing **nonoxynol-9** can be used in conjunction with condoms. (Nonoxynol-9 may inactivate the virus if the condom should break.)

• After ejaculating, but before losing the erection, the man should hold the base of the condom firmly while gently withdrawing the penis. (This prevents the escape of semen from the condom.) The used condom should be safely discarded and never reused.

Since HIV is most commonly transmitted through sex, being sexually active without taking proper precautions is definitely high-risk behavior. In this AIDS era, a person does not simply go to bed with one other person. When one calculates the possible length of the HIV latency period, a person goes to bed with the other person's entire sex history for approximately the past ten years.

Substance Use The transmission of HIV and intravenous drug use are linked in the following ways:

• Direct transmission of the virus through the sharing of intravenous drugs and equipment for injecting drugs (the most obvious link)

• Sexual transmission by infected intravenous drug users to their sexual partners

• Neonatal transmission by infected women who are themselves intravenous drug users or the sexual partners of intravenous drug users

While these modes of transmission address intravenous drug users, there are other less well known links to nonintravenous substance use and HIV. The use of **poppers** (volatile amyl and butyl nitrates in breakable glass capsules inhaled to enhance sexual pleasure) may be a cofactor in the development of AIDS and Kaposi's sarcoma because they are thought to lead to a generalized suppression of the immune system. Alcohol, as well as drugs such as amphetamines, cocaine, and marijuana, are also thought to damage the immune system. Another factor is lessened inhibition. That is, with loss of inhibition, a person under the influence of alcohol or drugs is more likely to engage in high-risk activities.

Realistic approaches to HIV risk-reduction education for intravenous drug users consist of more than information about, and encouragement to obtain treatment for, substance abuse. Those who are not ready for treatment must be counseled on how to reduce the risk to themselves and to others. Risk reduction guidelines for intravenous drug users are included in the Client/Family Teaching box, earlier. A counseling plan for clients with a dual diagnosis of HIV disease and substance use is given in the accompanying Intervention box.

Clients' risks to themselves derive from the practice of sharing drug use equipment with others. Clients should be instructed to never share intravenous drugs, needles, syringes, or other drug paraphernalia with others. If a new needle and syringe are not available, it is important that clients clean their **works** (syringe and needle) as recommended in Figure 25–3 on page 606. Bleach kills HIV.

Risks to sexual partners are the same as those discussed earlier in this chapter. Prevention of risk to sexual partners is important because intravenous drug users serve as a bridge for transmitting HIV to their sexual partners or to fetuses and newborns. Women who are intravenous drug users or the sexual partners of intravenous drug users are urged to postpone pregnancy until more is known about the significance of a positive antibody test for a pregnant woman, the

INTERVENTION

Counseling Plan for Clients with a Dual Diagnosis of HIV and Substance Use

- Check the level of understanding of basic HIV information and develop an education plan based on client needs.

- Confront denial or lack of commitment to minimize risk behavior.

- Offer hope for stabilization of health through positive health care measures.

- Check the need for and depth of motivation for referral to chemical dependency or alcohol treatment programs.

- Encourage joining or continuing commitment to the recovery process in treatment for chemical or alcohol dependency.

- Check the need for and refer to medical follow-up, emotional or sexual counseling, support groups, and other self-help programs.

- Help client verbalize feelings of anger, grief, and loss generated by the diagnosis; the need for change in sexual and drug use behavior; or possible delay in child bearing.

- Reinforce the fact that taking action now may help stabilize the client's health and slow further deterioration.

- Discuss "contagion" issues with client and family members to allay fears of spread by casual contact.

- Encourage and support client verbalization of such feelings as:

1. Fear of dying of AIDS
2. Fear of having exposed others to HIV or doing so through continued risk behavior
3. Feelings of guilt over risk behavior in the past
4. Feelings of loss over necessary behavior changes and possible postponement of childbearing
5. Fear of what others will think or do, or fear of being isolated and rejected

- Compile and distribute a list of community resources to serve people with HIV concerns or AIDS/HRC diagnosis.

- Stress the use of tools learned in recovering from chemical dependency and alcoholism in coping with this life crisis.

- Continue to confront the drug abuse as you would with other clients not diagnosed with HIV.

- Emphasize positive things the client can do to maximize health.

- Extend hope that, with continued attention to health matters, the client may live longer, possibly extending life until more effective treatments become available.

SOURCE: Adapted from O'Neil M: Aids and Bereavement: Partners, Families, Friends, in Hughes AM, Martin JP, Franks P: AIDS Home Care and Hospice Manual, 1987, p 137. By permission of the Visiting Nurses Association of San Francisco.

---

relationship between pregnancy and the onset of symptoms associated with HIV infection, and the risk of transmission to fetuses and infants (Centers for Disease Control 1985a).

Support for Caregivers

Psychiatric mental health nurses can be a vital support link for the wide spectrum of people who are caregivers of persons with HIV disease. This spectrum includes nurses and other health care professionals; the family members, friends, and partners (those to whom gay persons are committed in a long-term relationship) of persons with HIV; firefighters, police officers, and correction officers; and community volunteers. Nurses are now and will continue to be the health care professionals who are the frontline workers in providing health care to increasing numbers of persons with HIV disease.

Special emotional stamina is needed to care for persons with AIDS. Not only must nurses and other caregivers care for and comfort those who face great suffering and death, they also care for those infected with the virus who fear they will develop the disease. At the same time they provide help, nurses must cope with their fears for their own and their family's health (especially if the nurses themselves are members of a risk group) and their own pain in caring for persons who do not get well or whose future is uncertain.

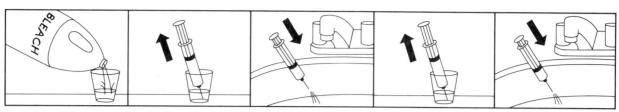

1. *Flush with bleach.* Pour bleach into glass. Fill syringe with bleach. Empty bleach from syringe. *Repeat.*

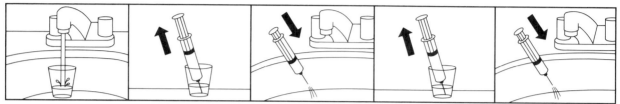

2. *Flush with water.* Fill a glass with clean water. Fill syringe with water. Empty water from syringe. *Repeat.* (Caution: Be sure the client knows not to omit this important step.)

FIGURE 25–3   Cleaning the works.

Specifically, the skills and knowledge of psychiatric mental health nurses make them particularly appropriate people to:

• Facilitate caregivers' expression of fears and concerns

• Help caregivers acknowledge their susceptibility to increased stress and burnout in AIDS work

• Instruct caregivers in stress management strategies and relaxation techniques

• Identify what needs to be reorganized and renegotiated in the work milieu to maintain the health of caregivers and clients such as (1) staff support groups, (2) networking with AIDS providers in other agencies and communities, (3) respite time for staff, (4) time off to attend funerals or memorial services, (5) rearranging staff assignments to avoid overloading or overburdening particular staff members, (6) creating getaway space for staff in the work setting

• Provide help to caregivers unused to dealing with delirium and dementia, who may have unrealistic expectations about the client's ability to adhere to procedures and treatment as mental capacities diminish

• Encourage administration to arrange time off and fund attendance at conferences and meetings that provide support and facilitate networking among people engaged in AIDS work

Successful stress management is particularly important because neither a cure nor a vaccine is in sight. This means that increased numbers of people (those who are currently infected with the virus and have yet to develop HRC or AIDS) will need nursing care in the coming years.

Bereavement Support

By the year 2000, millions of people will have experienced AIDS-related bereavements (Pheifer and Houseman 1988). There are several groups of people to whom the psychiatric mental health nurse can provide bereavement support. The most obvious is the person with AIDS who grieves over a potentially fatal diagnosis, the loss of other friends or family to the disease, or any of the several other losses discussed earlier in this chapter in the section on the biopsychosocial impact of HIV.

Bereavement support to family, friends, and caregivers should continue after death has occurred. Home visits to friends, lovers, and family members demonstrate the nurse's continuing interest and concern for the survivor's well-being. Bereavement support groups and individual and family counseling can all be helpful, depending on individual situations and the availability of volunteers and professionals.

To provide adequate bereavement support to the survivors of people with AIDS (SOPWAs), the nurse must consider a number of factors. SOPWAs represent a diverse segment of society: gay and bisexual men, IV drug users, people who have received transfusions of blood or blood products, sexual partners of PWAs, children of PWAs, parents and siblings of PWAs. Some SOPWAs may be in high-risk groups or may have HIV disease themselves, while some may have been unaware of the significant other's sexuality or life-style until diagnosis or death. Some survivors may have been responsible for the transmission of HIV, and many are members of minority groups and have few resources.

SOPWAs are often characterized by several factors that place them at high risk for complicated grief reactions (Geis et al. 1986). These include:

- Perceived inability to share the loss with others
- Lack of social recognition for the loss
- Ambivalent relationships prior to the death
- Traumatic circumstances of the death
- Concurrent life crises at the time of the loss

It is important to assess survivors for the presence of these factors, which can interfere with adaptive grieving. The high-risk bereavement factors are discussed in the accompanying Assessment box.

Worden's Principles of Bereavement Intervention have been described as appropriate to guide psychiatric mental health nurses in providing support to the

SOPWA (Pheifer and Houseman 1988). These principles include:

- Assisting survivors to actualize the loss by accepting its reality and finality. Helpful measures include encouraging survivors to talk about the death and the grieving rituals that they participated in, and assisting survivors to develop meaningful grieving rituals in the absence of socially sanctioned opportunities.

- Assisting survivors in identifying and expressing feelings by: acknowledging their loss, validating their feelings and their right to express these feelings, and encouraging them to express their feelings in an atmosphere of understanding, relatedness, and acceptance.

- Assisting survivors to continue living without the deceased by: identifying areas of their own lives that have been affected, and encouraging problem solving to promote independent functioning.

- Facilitating survivors in the process of emotional withdrawal by: encouraging the survivor, in time, to

ASSESSMENT

High Risk Bereavement Factors for SOPWAs

Stigma

Sources
- Discomfort with illness, death, and grief
- Sexuality and drug use often associated with AIDS
- Confusion and hysteria associated with AIDS

Results for SOPWAs
- May perceive need to mask cause of death
- May experience failure of community to recognize significance of relationship to deceased
- May perceive no support to facilitate mourning the loss or expressing feelings associated with this bereavement

Ambivalence

Sources
- Relationships strained due to life-style choices

Results for SOPWAs
- Guilt related to bereavement may arise
- Progress in grief process may be blocked

Untimely Nature of Death

Sources
- Faced with issues of mortality
- Generally young age of people with AIDS

Results for SOPWAs
- Anxiety, despair
- Lack of time for preparation to accept death

Concurrent Life Crises

Sources
- Fear of possibly having been exposed to a fatal illness
- Guilt if survivor feels he or she may have transmitted virus

Results for SOPWAs
- Anger and helplessness associated with being a SOPWA

Other Complicating Factors

- Lack of knowledge about HIV
- Lack of effective treatments, absence of a cure
- Paucity of health and social resources

form new relationships (a particular issue for survivors who have been in spousal or lover relationships with a PWA); accepting the feelings of the survivor; being informed about HIV, AIDS, safer sex practices, and other topics that the SOPWA may need to discuss; referring to support groups that offer a forum for those with common concerns; and helping survivors to recognize the benefits of relating to other persons in their lives.

• Providing survivors with time to grieve by: providing support for taking the time to grieve; allowing survivors to grieve at their own pace; and referring the survivor to counseling or support groups.

• Identifying and interpreting normal behavior for survivors by: recognizing and identifying for the bereaved the normal behaviors associated with grief (distractibility, forgetfulness, ruminations about the deceased, preoccupation with their own health, mood swings) and validating these as manifestations of grief.

• Considering the individuality of survivors by: recognizing the broad spectrum of human responses to loss; supporting individual expressions of mourning; helping support systems to recognize the individual's right to mourn in his or her own fashion.

• Providing ongoing support for survivors by: allowing for support during critical periods, and encouraging SOPWAs to use bereavement groups.

• Analyzing survivors' defenses and coping mechanisms by: recognizing that each survivor has his or her own defenses and coping mechanisms; exploring the effectiveness and adaptability of these coping mechanisms; pointing out the maladaptive nature of any negative or self-destructive strategies; and assisting the survivor in exploring more adaptive means of coping.

• Assessing survivors for pathologic grief responses by: assessing for depression, manic episodes, bizarre or acting-out behaviors, or suicidal ideation; and referring them to appropriate resources when the problems are beyond one's scope of practice.

The potential for dysfunctional grieving exists because multiple high-risk bereavement factors are characteristic of SOPWAs. Individual or group bereavement interventions can help survivors to engage in the grief process in an adaptive fashion.

Self-Help Support

Self-help is one way in which persons with HIV disease can move to reestablish a sense of self-control and reduce feelings of helplessness and powerlessness. Self-help can occur on several levels depending on the client's physical and mental abilities and motivation.

Clients should participate as much as possible in their own care and in decision making that affects them. Nurses can encourage clients to join peer support groups and engage in AIDS advocacy activities in their communities.

Clients may benefit from such activities as nutritional counseling and psychologic counseling. Boosting the immune system also helps keep people healthy. Stress management techniques and visualization and imagery for self-healing and pain and symptom control (such as those discussed in Chapter 27) are believed to boost the immune system by reducing stress.

Research

Not enough is known about HIV infection as an illness; the common nursing diagnoses in AIDS, HRC, and HIV seropositivity; or the strategies that help people cope when HIV affects them or their loved ones. Psychiatric mental health nurses have a direct role in research and an indirect role in supporting ongoing research and encouraging the undertaking and funding of new research. Being knowledgeable about the current research and incorporating it into clinical practice enables the psychiatric nurse to act on the basis of what is currently known or supposed.

Advocacy and Political Activism

Persons with HIV disease and their loved ones need advocates. Psychiatric mental health nurses can be effective advocates by speaking out against dehumanizing measures that threaten the well-being of persons with HIV.

A proposition was introduced in California that could have forced public health officials to establish camps to quarantine persons with AIDS, as well as anyone infected by the virus, whether healthy or unhealthy. This measure would also have flatly banned HIV-seropositive people from attending or teaching in public schools or holding jobs that involve food handling. The California Nurses Association was among the groups that actively spoke against the proposition and contributed to its failure.

As citizens and as advocates, nurses should be politically aware of pending legislation and move to influence it in a positive direction.

Earlier in this chapter, brief mention was made of state nurses' associations with published statements about the care of persons with AIDS and nursing's role. Other state nurses' associations and national specialty groups are also active in mobilizing the professional and political resources of the nursing community. It is each nurse's responsibility to find out what nursing groups are accomplishing or not accomplishing on local, state, and national levels. Beginning at the local level by becoming involved in local AIDS councils, self-help groups, and nursing organizations is a good way to start. Local involvement is a bridge to state and national involvement. Nurses can and should be part of a nationwide effort to lobby for adequate public and private funding for research, education, prevention, treatment, and cure for HIV.

CHAPTER HIGHLIGHTS

• AIDS, a contagious and potentially fatal condition of immune system depression, is a clinical issue of concern to all nurses, including psychiatric mental health nurses.

• Homosexual/bisexual men (and their sexual partners), intravenous drug abusers (and their sexual partners), hemophiliacs (and their sexual partners), children born to parents with HIV or at risk for HIV, and prostitutes are groups of people who have been identified as being at high risk of developing AIDS.

• HIV threatens the biopsychosocial integrity of individuals and of society.

• Persons with HIV and AIDS experience several different losses, may have neurologic or neuropsychiatric involvement because the virus invades the central and peripheral nervous systems, and find that their ability to successfully negotiate age-appropriate developmental tasks is disrupted.

• Persons with HIV and AIDS may experience social and familial rejection; discrimination in employment, housing, and health insurance; estrangement from institutions such as organized religion; and financial losses.

• Several ethical issues surround HIV and AIDS. Many of them revolve around questions of individual rights versus the public good.

• Psychiatric mental health nurses can anticipate the need to care for increasing numbers of persons with HIV disease in psychiatric mental health settings and in other community settings.

• Psychiatric hospitalization may be needed if the client is depressed, suicidal, psychotic, or has an AIDS-related behavior disturbance, probably because of organic mental disorder. The psychiatric mental health nurse will have to creatively combine and modify the nursing care for clients with a dual diagnosis that includes HIV disease.

• Taking a leading role in risk reduction education and counseling is a crucial role for all nurses during the HIV epidemic.

• Psychiatric mental health nurses can be a vital support link for the wide spectrum of people who are caregivers of persons with HIV disease.

• Psychiatric mental health nurses have direct roles in AIDS research and indirect roles in supporting ongoing research and encouraging the undertaking and funding of new research.

• Psychiatric mental health nurses can be effective advocates by speaking out against dehumanizing measures that threaten the well-being of persons with HIV; influencing legislation in a positive direction; and becoming part of a nationwide effort by lobbying for adequate private and public funding for research, education, prevention, treatment, and cure.

• Nurses are now and will continue to be the health care professionals who are the frontline workers in providing health care to increasing numbers of persons with HIV disease.

REFERENCES

Amchin J, Polan J: A longitudinal account of staff adaptation to AIDS patients on a psychiatric unit. *Hosp Community Psychiatry* 1986;37(12):1235–1238.

American Nurses' Association. *Code for Nurses.* ANA, 1985a.

American Nurses Association. *Nursing and the Human Immunodeficiency Virus.* ANA, 1988.

American Nurses' Association. Nursing profession urges health care community to step up efforts on AIDS (news release). ANA, 1985b.

Baer J, Hall J, Holm K, Lewitter-Koehler S: Challenges in developing an inpatient psychiatric program for patients with AIDS and ARC. *Hosp Community Psychiatry* 1987;38(12):1299–1303.

Baer J, Holm K, Lewitter-Koehler S: Treatment of AIDS/ARC patients on an inpatient psychiatric unit. *Focus: A Review of AIDS Research* 1987;2(2):1–3.

Binder R: AIDS antibody test on inpatient psychiatric units. *Am J Psychiatry* 1987;144(2):176–180.

Bjorklund E: Prevention: Reducing the risk of AIDS, in Durham JD, Cohen FL: *The Person with AIDS: Nursing Perspectives.* Springer, 1987, pp 178–191.

Boland MG: The child with AIDS: Special concerns, in Durham JD, Cohen FL: *The Person with AIDS: Nursing Perspectives.* Springer, 1987, pp 192–210.

Bompey S: AIDS—An employment issue for the eighties. *Digest Publication of International Foundation of Employee Benefit Plan* 1986;23(2):6–10.

California Nurses Association. Resolution on mobilization of nurses for care of AIDS patients. CNA, 1985.

Centers for Disease Control: *AIDS Weekly Surveillance Report.* September 14, 1987. Department of Health and Human Services.

Centers for Disease Control: Apparent transmission of human T-lymphotropic virus type III/lymphadenopathy-associated virus from a child to a mother providing health care. *MMWR* 1986;35:76–79.

Centers for Disease Control: Recommendations for assisting in the prevention of perinatal transmission of human T-lymphotropic virus type III/lymphadenopathy-associated virus and acquired immunodeficiency syndrome. *MMWR* 1985a;34:721–732.

Centers for Disease Control: Recommendations for preventing transmission of infection with HTLV-III/LAV in the workplace. *MMWR* 1985b;34(45):681–695.

Centers for Disease Control: Revision of the CDC surveillance case definition for acquired immunodeficiency syndrome. *MMWR* 1985c;36(1S):3S–15S.

Dilley JW: Diagnosis and treatment of major depression in AIDS. *AIDSfile* 1987;2(1):6–7.

Durham JD: The ethical dimensions of AIDS, in Durham JD, Cohen FL: *The Person with AIDS: Nursing Perspectives.* Springer, 1987, pp 229–252.

Evans C, Kassof M, Beckman E, Handel-Kindred J: Reducing AIDS anxiety on the unit with preventive infection control. *J Psychosoc Nurs* 1990;28(1):36–39.

Faltz B, Rinaldi G: *AIDS and Substance Abuse: A Training Manual for Health Care Professionals.* University of California, 1987.

Faultisch M: Psychiatric aspects of AIDS: *Am J Psychiatry* 1987;144(5):551–556.

Fetter MS, Larson E: Preventing and treating human immunodeficiency virus infection in the homeless. *Arch Psychiatr Nurs* 1990;4(6):379–383.

Frierson RL, Lippmann SB, Johnson J: AIDS: Psychosocial stresses on the family. *Psychosomatics* 1987;28(2):65–68.

Geis SB, Fuller RL, Rush J: Lovers of AIDS victims: Psychosocial stresses and counseling needs. *Death Studies* 1986;10:43–53.

Gottlieb M et al.: *AMFAR Directory Experimental Treatments for AIDS and ARC.* Mary Ann Liebert, 1987.

Grady C: Ethical issues in providing nursing care to HIV-infected populations. *Nurs Clin North Am* 1989;24(2):523–34.

Hughes A, Martin JP, Franks P: *AIDS Home Care and Hospice Manual.* AIDS Home care and Hospice Program, VNA of San Francisco, 1987.

Kemppainen JK: Imogene King's theory: A nursing case study of a psychotic client with human immunodeficiency virus infection. *Arch Psychiatr Nurs* 1990; 4(6):384–388.

Korniewicz DM, O'Brien ME, Larson E: Coping with AIDS and HIV: Psychosocial adaptation. *J Psychosoc Nurs* 1990;28(3):14–16, 19–21.

Krigel RL, Friedman-Kien AE: Kaposi's sarcoma in AIDS, in DeVita VT Jr, Hellman S, Rosenberg SA (eds): *AIDS: Etiology, Diagnosis, Treatment, and Prevention.* Lippincott, 1985, pp 185–211.

Lederman MM: Transmission of the acquired immunodeficiency syndrome through heterosexual activity. *Ann Intern Med* 1986;104:115–117.

Levy R, Bredesen D: Central nervous syndromes associated with AIDS, in Rosenblum M, Levy R, Bredesen D (eds): *AIDS and the Central Nervous System.* Raven, 1987.

Lovejoy N, Sisson R: Psychoneuroimmunology and AIDS. *Holistic Nurs Pract* 1989;3(4):1–15.

Massie M, Tross S, Price R, Holland J, Redd W: Neuropsychological and psychosocial sequelae of AIDS. *Antibiot Chemother* 1987;38:132–140.

McCray E: Occupational risk of the acquired immunodeficiency syndrome among health care workers. *N Engl J Med* 1986;314:1127–1132.

McEnany G: Personal communication, September 25, 1987.

Moskowitz L, Hensley G, Chan J, Gregorios J, Conley F: The neuropathology of the acquired immunodeficiency syndrome. *Arch Pathol Lab Med* 1984;108:867–872.

National Academy of Sciences. *Confront AIDS: Directions for Public Health, Health Care and Research.* National Academy Press, 1986.

National Coalition for the Homeless. *Fighting to Live: Homeless People with AIDS.* The Coalition, March, 1990.

Navia B, Jordan B, Price R: The AIDS dementia complex: I. Clinical features. *Ann Neurol* 1986;19:517–524.

Navia B, Price R: The acquired immunodeficiency syndrome dementia complex as the presenting or sole manifestation of human immunodeficiency virus infection. *Arch Neurol* 1987;44:65–69.

New York State Nurses Association. *The Role of the Nursing Practitioner Re: Acquired Immunodeficiency Syndrome (AIDS).* NYSNA, 1983.

Nokes KM, Kendrew J: Loneliness in veterans with AIDS and its relationship to the development of infections. *Arch Psychiatr Nurs* 1990;4(4):271–277.

Perry SW: Organic mental disorders caused by HIV: Update on early diagnosis and treatment 1990. *Am J Psychiatry* 1990;147(6):696–711.

Perry S, Markowitz J: Psychiatric interventions for AIDS-spectrum disorders. *Hosp Community Psychiatry* 1986; 37(10):1001–1006.

Pheifer W, Houseman C: Bereavement and AIDS: A framework for intervention. *J Psychosoc Nurs* 1988; 26(10):21–26.

Rich CL, Fowler RC, Young D, Blenkush M: San Diego suicide study: Comparison of gay to straight males. *Suicide Life Threat Behav* 1986;16(4):448–457.

Saunders JM, Valente SM: Gay and lesbian suicide: A review. *Death Studies* 1987;11:1–23.

Scherer P: How AIDS attacks the brain. *Amer J Nurs* 1990;90(1):44–52.

Schietinger H: A home care plan for AIDS. *Am J Nurs* 1986;86:1021–1028.

Schliefer SJ, Keller SE, Franklin JE, LaFarge S, Miller SI: HIV seropositivity in inner-city alcoholics. *Hosp Community Psychiatry* 1990;41(23):248–249.

Schmitz D: When IV drug abuse complicates AIDS. *RN* January 1990;53(1):60–66.

Serinus J: *Psychoimmunity and the Healing Process.* Celestial Arts, 1986.

Shilts R: *And the Band Played On.* St. Martin's Press, 1987.

So Y, Choucair A, Davis R: Neoplasms of the central nervous system in the acquired immunodeficiency syndrome, in Rosenblum J, Levy R, Bredesen D (eds): *AIDS and the Nervous System.* Raven, 1987.

Sontag S: *Illness as Metaphor.* Vintage Books, 1977.

Strawn J: The psychosocial consequences of AIDS, in Durham JD, Cohen FL: *The Person with AIDS: Nursing Perspectives.* Springer, 1987, pp 126–149.

Swanson B, Cronin-Stubbs D, Colletti MA: Dementia and depression in persons with AIDS: Causes and care. *J Psychosoc Nurs* 1990;28(10):33–39.

Torres RA, Mani S, Altholz J, Bricker PW: Human immunodeficiency virus infection among homeless men in a New York City shelter. *Arch Intern Med* 1990; 150:2030–2036.

van Servellen G, Nyamathi AM, Mannion W: Coping with a crisis: Evaluation of psychological risks of patients with AIDS. *J Psychosoc Nurs* 1989;27(12):16–21.

Psychobiology Box References

Cousins N: *Head First: The Biology of Hope.* Dutton, 1989.

Gorman JR, Locke SE: Neural, endocrine and immune interactions, in Kaplan HI, Sadock BJ (eds): *Comprehensive Textbook of Psychiatry/V.* Williams and Wilkins, 1989.

Lloyd R: *Explorations in Psychoneuroimmunology.* Grune and Stratton, 1987.

Locke SE, Gorman JR: Behavior and immunity, in Kaplan HI, Sadock BJ (eds): *Comprehensive Textbook of Psychiatry/V.* Williams and Wilkins, 1989.

Lovejoy NC, Sisson R: Psychoneuroimmunology and AIDS. *Holistic Nurs Pract* 1989;3(4):1–15.

PART FIVE

Intervention Modes

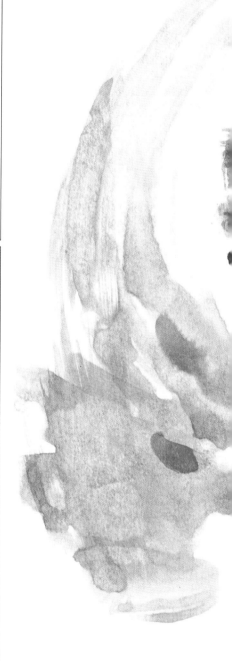

CONTENTS

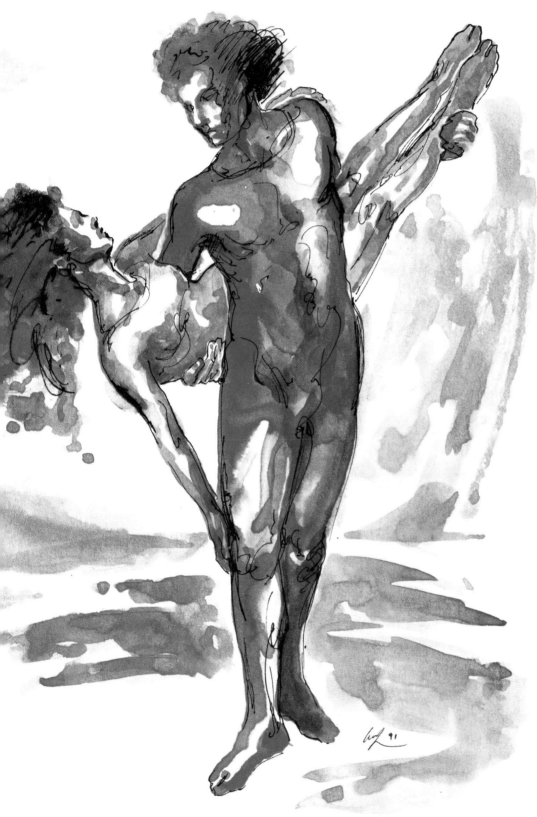

The instrument through which life is lived—the human body—is often a metaphor for human emotion.

The One-to-One Relationship

Beth Moscato

LEARNING OBJECTIVES

- Identify common characteristics of one-to-one relationships

- Recognize humanistic interactionist aspects of one-to-one relationships in a psychobiologic age

- Describe the interpersonal skills of the nurse that facilitate one-to-one relationships, including therapeutic use of self

- Delineate the client abilities and behaviors most often associated with growth-producing outcomes

- Analyze the following special concerns as these relate to psychiatric nurses: critical distance, self-disclosure, gifts, use of touch, and values

- Discuss the concept of resistance in one-to-one relationships, including its definition, possible manifestations, and general intervention strategies

- Specify the normal and troublesome aspects of transference and counter-transference in one-to-one relationships

- Explain the three phases of therapeutic relationships, high-lighting main objectives and therapeutic tasks of each phase

- Apply the nursing process in establishing and maintaining one-to-one relationships

CROSS REFERENCES

Other topics relevant to this content are: Assessment, Chapter 9; Communication skills, Chapter 8; Cultural considerations, Chapter 36; Facilitative personal characteristics of the nurse, Chapter 2; Historical aspects, Chapter 1; Self-disclosure, Chapter 2; Therapeutic use of self, Chapter 2; Values, Chapter 2.

THE PSYCHIATRIC NURSE WHO enters into a one-to-one relationship with a client finds that the invitation to any individual relationship is at once intriguing, challenging, and anxiety provoking.

A one-to-one relationship may evolve in any nursing situation: between a nurse who makes home visits and an ailing client, between a hospital nurse and a child intermittently hospitalized with leukemia, or between a nurse-counselor and a high-risk pregnant woman. Of particular relevance is the one-to-one relationship that evolves between the psychiatric nurse and the client. This may occur in medical facilities, psychiatric institutions, community mental health centers, and private practice settings. The individual psychiatric nurse-client relationship is the cornerstone of psychiatric nursing theory and practice.

How is it possible to define, initiate, and effectively use a one-to-one relationship? This chapter demystifies the characteristics, processes, phases, and problems of one-to-one relationships so that beginning psychiatric nurses can approach these relationships with increased awareness of their own interpersonal effectiveness. Practical guidelines on how to facilitate interpersonal effectiveness with clients are included. The principles, processes, and phases discussed in this chapter also apply to family, group, and community interventions or therapies.

Common Characteristics of One-to-One Relationships

The **one-to-one relationship** between psychiatric nurse and client is a mutually defined, collaborative, and goal-oriented professional relationship.

Professional

One-to-one relationships reflect a professional, rather than social, relationship. Psychiatric nurses use their personalities, interpersonal skills and techniques, and theoretic knowledge of psychiatric nursing practice in a purposeful, goal-directed manner to facilitate a useful change in their client's lives. This professional relationship differs from a social relationship in several significant ways. Table 26–1 summarizes the major differences between professional and social relationships.

The one-to-one relationship may also be differentiated from the nurse-client interaction. An interaction is some segment of actual behavior that takes place between the psychiatric nurse and the client. The one-to-one relationship may be viewed as a planned series of sequential nurse-client interactions with the following additional elements:

• The interactions occur over a designated period of time (daily, weekly, monthly).

• The interactions take place in a unique nurse-client structure, characterized by specific phases, processes, and problems.

• The interactions occur in a designated setting that tends to remain stable over time (home, private-practice office, mental health clinic, in-patient psychiatric unit, medical unit).

A professional one-to-one relationship can be either informal or formal. Spontaneous, informal nurse-client relationships are at one end of the continuum, and formal individual counseling or psychotherapy is at the other end.

TABLE 26–1   Differences between Professional and Social Relationships

Characteristic	Professional Relationship	Social Relationship
Purpose	Systematic working-through of troublesome thoughts, feelings, and behaviors	Companionship, pleasure, sharing of interests
	Planned evaluation (through stages)	Evolves spontaneously
Role delineation	Roles for psychiatric nurse and client with explicit use of psychiatric nursing skills and interventions	Generally not present, except for broad social norms governing the particular type of relationship (friend versus lover)
Satisfaction of needs	Client encouraged to identify, develop, and assess ways to meet own needs more effectively	Mutual sharing and satisfaction of personal and interpersonal needs
	Does not address personal needs of psychiatric nurse	
Time frame	Usually time-limited interactions with an expected termination	Usually not time limited, either in duration or frequency of contact
		No planned termination is planned

TABLE 26–2 **Similarities and Differences of Informal and Formal One-to-One Relationships**

Characteristic	Nature of Relationship	
	Informal	*Formal*
Setting	Varied	Generally psychiatric settings
Frequency and duration of contact	Flexible, depending on client need or tolerance. Example: short, frequent intervals on daily basis	Structured. Example: once weekly, with possible crisis sessions. Duration usually set at thirty minutes or one hour
Duration of relationship	May or may not involve time commitment. Generally a few days to a few weeks	Involves time commitment: weeks to months, for short-term work; months to years, for long-term work
Type of dysfunction	In general, more effective with severe dysfunction	In severe dysfunction, may be useful after client is stabilized on medication
Use of therapeutic contract	May involve simple therapeutic contract	Utilizes therapeutic contract; the more specific, the better
Fees	Usually not relevant	May be relevant. May be part of therapeutic contract
Degree of skill required	Nursing student or psychiatric nurse	Advanced degree beneficial, but not essential
Degree of supervision	Some degree and type of supervision always necessary	Consistent supervision or consultation usually necessary
Degree of effectiveness	For both, depends on client's level of functioning, skills of the psychiatric nurse, and time allotment	

Informal Informal nurse-client relationships may be prearranged and planned, but more often they occur spontaneously. They consist of a set of interactions limited in time. There is minimum structure and a sense of immediacy. These relationships occur in numerous medical and nonmedical settings and are particularly common in psychiatric institutions and community mental health settings.

Formal The more formal one-to-one relationship is used in crisis intervention, counseling, or individual psychotherapy. It requires more planning, structure, consistency, nursing expertise, and time. It occurs in various psychiatric settings, including psychiatric institutions, community mental health centers, and private practice.

The choice and effectiveness of informal or formal relationships depend upon:

• The client's level of functioning

• The psychiatric nurse's current abilities and skills

• To some degree, the time available to both participants

It is crucial to note that the principles, phases, processes, and problems of an informal relationship parallel those of a formal one. A comprehensive overview of all aspects of therapeutic relationships guides the nurse in applying principles to practice, even if the nurse is not directly involved in individual psychotherapy.

Table 26–2 highlights the similarities and differences of informal and formal relationship work. The differences between informal and formal relationships are discussed throughout this chapter.

Mutually Defined

A one-to-one relationship is mutually defined by the two participants. Both psychiatric nurse and client voluntarily enter the relationship and specify the conditions under which it is to evolve. For example, the client may seek immediate alleviation of symptoms rather than long-term individual psychotherapy. Nurse and client identify together where and when they will meet and other conditions of their participation. This contractual aspect of the one-to-one relationship is explored further in the discussion of the beginning (orientation) phase of therapy later in this chapter. Once the relationship is established, its maintenance depends on the commitment of both participants.

Collaborative

Both participants enter a relationship in which goals, strategies, and outcomes evolve within the context of the therapeutic work together. Mutual collaboration implies that each participant brings personal abilities, capabilities, and power to the relationship. Thus, the psychiatric nurse does not assume responsibility for client behaviors but actively works with the client to assess the self-defeating and growth-promoting aspects of specific behaviors. Mutual collaboration also means that the psychiatric nurses assess and are accountable for their own behavior with clients. Ongoing supervision often helps the nurse meet these particular goals.

Goal Directed

A one-to-one relationship is always goal-directed. The client is expected to identify and achieve specific physical, emotional, and social goals within the context of the relationship. Client goals vary widely in type and depth. For example, in informal relationship work, a client's goal may be to initiate one peer relationship within an in-patient psychiatric unit. Other examples include resolution of a divorce involving children and shared personal possessions, or coming to terms with the client's impending death. Often the client's initial goal is to solve an immediate problem, and this serves as a basis for establishing more extensive psychosocial goals. The psychiatric nurse also formulates personal therapeutic goals to enhance the growth-producing elements of the relationship.

Historical and Theoretic Foundations

The one-to-one relationship between psychiatric nurse and client has evolved as the cornerstone of psychiatric nursing theory and practice. In this century, nurses have moved from being primarily responsible for observing, reporting, and maintaining ward order to functioning members of an interdisciplinary treatment team. Although psychiatric nursing has expanded to include group, family, milieu, and a host of other therapies, one-to-one relationships remain the cornerstone.

Sound theoretic foundations are of critical importance. Peplau contends that psychiatric nursing is in a state of transition, moving from medical to nursing models for practice (Fitzpatrick et al. 1982, p vii). Nurses are no longer required to rely solely on theoretic foundations from outside sources (medicine, psychology, sociology, and communication sciences) as they participate in therapeutic relationships. Nursing conceptual models have emerged that characterize the psychiatric-mental health nursing approach.

Humanistic Interactionist Framework in a Psychobiologic Age

Humanistic philosophy in one-to-one relationships involves viewing humanness not as a static condition but as an evolving, active process unique to each person.

Openness   Humanistic interactionist philosophy stresses openness and honesty in human relations. Within a humanistic framework, the one-to-one relationship between nurse and client may be viewed as an experience in *shared dignity*. The psychiatric nurse adapts to allow clients to reveal their humanness freely and openly to the nurse. Each aspect of the nurse's verbal and nonverbal behavior encourages or inhibits clients from further revealing humanness.

Negotiation   The humanistic interactionist views the client as exercising free will, as an active decision maker. In addition, humanism stresses the client's uniqueness and the subjectiveness of the experiences underlying personal actions. In the one-to-one relationship, the client determines the type and length of involvement and is personally accountable for the work. The atmosphere of give and take within the relationship emphasizes mutuality, reciprocity, and interpersonal fairness. Establishment of a clearly defined, mutually agreed-on therapeutic contract represents a prime example of negotiation in one-to-one work. (The therapeutic contract is covered later in this chapter.)

Commitment   Commitment is based on the therapeutic contract between nurse and client. The contract establishes the limits of the relationship as well as the time and energy allotted to it. At some point in the relationship, the psychiatric nurse is confronted by the reality of the client's dysfunction. The beginning psychiatric nurse may respond by actively colluding with the client to deny or ignore the dysfunction and remain on a superficial, social level of communication. This collusion protects the nurse from having to address the client's helplessness, desperation, hostility, or raw grief. The nurse who does not let the client express these feelings is not sufficiently committed to the client. The opposite is also nontherapeutic. The overcommitted psychiatric nurse may assume an omnipotent or rescuer role to "cure" the client. This role robs the client of active decision-making power and accountability. The client will test the nurse's commitment in some phase of the relationship. Both nurse and client need to deal with this test explicitly on verbal and nonverbal levels.

Responsibility   Personal responsibility for the one-to-one relationship is also based on the therapeutic contract between nurse and client, and it, too, will be tested by the client in some phase of the relationship. Beginning psychiatric nurses usually encounter responsibility problems as they begin to perceive unattractive, dysfunctional, or blatantly offending interpersonal behavioral patterns or habits in their clients. Both nurse and client must deal explicitly with "who is responsible for what." In addition, the nurse should avoid making any agreements with a client that the nurse may be unable to fulfill.

Authenticity The appreciation of spontaneity and authenticity is another aspect of humanistic interactionist philosophy that applies particularly to one-to-one relationships. Psychiatric nurses need to create an atmosphere that conveys permission to express pain and pleasure. Expressions of joy and assessments of client abilities, talents, and capabilities are an often-neglected, yet essential, aspect of relationship work.

Search for Meaning Within the humanistic interactionist philosophy, the psychiatric nurse works with clients in a search for meaning in their lives. It is essential that nurses establish their own personal meaning and integration of self, for these are key resources in treatment. For psychiatric nurses to be effective, they must already possess the personal skills to deal with the client's symptoms. They must have personally worked through any problems that resemble those of the client. For example, nurses who cannot cope with their own feelings of depression cannot be effective with severely depressed clients.

Overview of Current One-to-One Therapies

Psychotherapeutic treatment in recent years has moved from intensive psychoanalysis to diversified techniques and systems of psychotherapy.

Recent systems of psychotherapy include transactional analysis, reality therapy, rational-emotive therapy, gestalt therapy, primal therapy, and logotherapy. A critical discussion of these popular approaches is beyond the scope of this chapter. The development of a new approach to one-to-one work, namely, short-term dynamic psychotherapy (STDP), is highlighted here. Concerns regarding a decrease in the availability of long-term psychotherapy are discussed. Other systems of psychotherapy are addressed elsewhere in this text (see Chapters 28–30).

Short-Term Dynamic Psychotherapy *Short-term dynamic psychotherapy* (STDP) is the synthesis of several approaches. STDP has evolved to treat a maximum number of clients with numerous issues in a minimum amount of time. This has gained increasing importance since clients are now seen for briefer periods of time. Characteristics of STDP include brief duration (usually sixteen to twenty hour-long sessions), a very active therapist role, identification of a central issue or "core conflict," limited goals that address the specific problems for which the client seeks treatment, and a wide range of therapeutic techniques. Transference is a concept basic to STDP.

Prospective clients are carefully assessed for their potential to benefit from STDP. The following clients would generally be excluded from participation in STDP (Davanloo 1985; Heber et al. 1984):

- Persons with chronic obsessions or phobias
- Persons with organic or functional psychoses
- Persons with poor impulse control
- Persons with a history of substance abuse
- Persons who are highly self-destructive
- Persons who seek symptom relief rather than change
- Persons who cannot choose a major life problem and maintain this focus throughout treatment
- Persons who cannot tolerate the very active role of the therapist
- Persons who need extensive long-term psychotherapy

A high degree of motivation for change on the part of the client is critical for selection.

Long-Term Psychotherapy The recent emphasis on efficiency in client selection and therapeutic outcome has decreased the emphasis on long-term psychotherapy. The extensive exclusion criteria for STDP may leave the severely dysfunctional client with minimal programs in today's mental health care delivery system. As we discuss in Chapters 1, 17, and 38, the staggering increase in the number of street people across the United States is a symptom of our nation's inefficiency in providing comprehensive programs to meet the needs of people with chronic and complex problems.

In addition to formal long-term psychotherapy, specific skill training can address the chronic problems of long-term psychiatric clients. Such training may include communication skills, skills needed in activities of daily life, community living skills, stress management skills, problem-solving skills, and medication education. The nurse-client relationship is just as crucial in these approaches as in STDP with more acutely ill clients.

Phenomena Occurring in One-to-One Relationships

Sometimes the nurse may initially sense confusion about what is happening in the nurse-client therapeutic relationship. This uneasiness may be difficult for the nurse to identify, describe, and explore. Keep the following phenomena in mind when attempting to "make sense" of a one-to-one relationship.

Resistance   Resistance inevitably surfaces in the course of one-to-one work. It most often occurs as the client begins to address self-defeating thoughts, feelings, and behaviors.

Definition   Resistance refers to all the phenomena that interfere with and disrupt the smooth flow of feelings, memories, and thoughts. Resistance in the traditional psychoanalytic sense means anything that inhibits the client from producing material from the unconscious. Conscious phenomena (feelings, memories, thoughts) may be forceful or weak, significant or unimportant. The same is true of unconscious material. However, in the psychoanalytic view, some unconscious productions may be intense forces under pressure to be discharged (archaic sexual and aggressive impulses), regardless of whether they are unrealistic, inappropriately timed, or illogical. These intense forces can be controlled only by another force equal in strength, which is labeled resistance.

Resistance is often mistakenly seen as the client's struggle against the nurse. Instead, the client is struggling against change, against self-awareness, and against responsibility for actions. Although the client's behavior patterns may have self-defeating aspects, they have also provided some satisfaction or prevented some discomfort. The client may also resist giving up a defense that offered protection from the anxiety associated with unbearable thoughts and impulses. Thus, resistance in therapeutic relationships is best understood as the client's struggle against change.

Resistance occurs in varied situations and settings. It may surface as a primary concern in the following examples: during therapeutic work of any kind (one-to-one, group, family) in community liaison services, home visitation programs, or consultative activities.

Manifestations   In general, the nurse may suspect resistance when the client's behavior appears to block the progress of the relationship. There are innumerable ways to express resistance. The following may be examples of resistance:

- Forgetting events

- Focusing on the past to avoid talking about the present (or vice versa)

- Consistently avoiding certain topics or inquiries

- Expressing antagonism toward the nurse

- Falling in love with the nurse

- Acting out (discussed later in this chapter)

Some manifestations of resistance are more subtle. For example, a client may introduce an abrupt crisis, an alarming childhood memory, or an intense new relationship whenever a certain topic is approached.

Likewise, a client may use flirtatious or seductive behaviors that embarrass the nurse to avoid working on a particular problem. Silence may indicate resistance, and so may an invigorating clinical discussion intended as a filibuster or "smoke screen" to avoid emotive expression or problem resolution.

The nurse must exercise caution in evaluating a client's behavior as resistive. The client's silence may indicate pensiveness, a pause before emotive expression, or a sense of completion. The client who is habitually late may have real difficulties adjusting a full personal schedule to accommodate the sessions. Resistance to specific topics or concerns may indicate that the client is not ready for investigative work at the time. Likewise, the client may resist giving up a defense that is desperately needed to keep anxiety about a present situation at manageable levels.

The humanistic stance is that the client has a right to assume a genuine and legitimate position of resisting one aspect of or the entire therapeutic process, as a matter of choice. The client's resistive behavior should be openly discussed, rather than ignored. The humanistic nurse views the client as exercising free will—as an active participant in decisions that shape the client's well-being, including the one-to-one relationship.

Acting Out   Acting out is a particularly destructive form of resistance in which the client puts into action (that is, "acts out") a memory that has been forgotten or repressed. It is important to recognize that the client is externalizing an inner conflict to people in the immediate environment. Rather than verbalizing conflicts or feelings, the client displays inappropriate behaviors. Examples of acting out include forcefully slamming a door, dressing provocatively, or slapping someone. In acting out, the client acts toward a mate, friend, relative, or other person those feelings and attitudes that the client does not express toward the nurse. An example of acting out is the development of third-person relationships to absorb the emotions and fantasies that belong in the therapeutic relationship. Exaggerated feelings of intense hostility toward the nurse may lead to violence or physical harm to the client, nurse, or the third person. Intense feelings of love for the nurse or therapist many precipitate an affair or marriage with the third person.

Acting out is difficult to deal with because the client does not talk about the feelings that precipitate the behavior and later tends to conceal or rationalize the behavior. Acting out can abruptly break up treatment, unless it is identified and dealt with explicitly. Specific nursing interventions regarding acting out include the following:

- Bring acting out to the attention of the client.

- Encourage the client to *talk about* impulses rather than to act them out.

• Encourage identification of feelings *before* putting them into action.

• Increase frequency of contact.

• Look for evidence of transference phenomena toward the nurse.

• With repeated dangerous acting out, consider withdrawing from the relationship unless the client sets limits on these personal behaviors.

The following clinical example illustrates acting out in a clinical setting:

Sharon is a 15-year-old with a history of self-abusive behavior. She had been the victim of repeated incestuous experiences with her stepfather over several years, despite her mother's knowledge of such activity. On an inpatient adolescent evaluation unit, she met daily in an informal one-to-one relationship with a nursing student, of whom she seemed fond. One day Sharon received a message from the team leader stating that the student had the flu and was unable to meet with Sharon that day but planned to meet again the following day. When the team leaders asked Sharon's reactions to this, Sharon refused to speak. She rushed out of the dayroom area, ran to her room, and pounded her fist into the cement wall numerous times, fracturing her right hand in two places.

The next day, the nursing student approached Sharon. Sharon offered no comment. The student's inquiry regarding the previous day's message also met with no comment. The student stated her concern for Sharon's welfare and her confusion regarding Sharon's injury. Sharon remained silent. The student stated her wish to sort things out together as they had done in the past and then sat quietly with Sharon. After two minutes, Sharon began crying, and talked about feeling alone.

The nonverbal behaviors of nurses affect clients. Acting out can be demonstrated by the nurse who manifests parental, erotic, sexual, or hostile behaviors. Examples of acting out by the nurse include the following:

• Placing the hands on hips or pointing a finger while setting limits on a client's behavior (parental)

• Patting a client on the shoulder and offering reassurance (parental)

• Blushing and giggling when a client makes a sexual remark (sexual)

These behaviors by the nurse encourage gross acting out by the client.

Parental or caretaker behaviors are the most common among beginning psychiatric nurses. They express the nurse's need to nurture and feed the client. These behaviors may indicate a countertransference problem for the nurse and discount the clients' ability to ensure their well-being. Recognition of acting out by the psychiatric nurse is essential and reinforces the need for formal supervision.

General Intervention Strategies Several consecutive approaches are used as general nursing intervention strategies for resistance. They begin with the psychiatric nurse's awareness of the resistance. Helpful intervention strategies include the following:

• Labeling the resistant behavior with the client. The psychiatric nurse may allow the resistance to occur several times to demonstrate its presence to the client. It is as if the psychiatric nurse were holding up a mirror for the client, reflecting and clarifying the specific resistant behavior.

• Exploring the accompanying emotion and history of its development.

• Exploring what function the resistance may serve, especially any self-defeating aspects.

• Facilitating working through the resistance by fully understanding and appreciating its implications in the client's life.

This sequence may occur repeatedly before a resistant behavior is resolved. Many examples of specific interventions are presented later in this chapter.

Transference Transference is a normal phenomenon that may surface and inhibit effectiveness in any phase of one-to-one relationship work. The term *transference* originated in psychoanalytic theory. Transference is the result of unresolved childhood experiences with significant others. Instead of remembering the past, the client "transfers" these unresolved feelings, attitudes, and wishes into present significant relationships in an attempt to resolve these in a more satisfying manner. Thus, the client misunderstands the present according to the unresolved problems of the past. The client is unaware of the nature of this action.

It is important to understand that transference is a form of resistance. The client unknowingly resists any recollection of childhood conflicts. Instead, the client transfers these conflicts to present relationships, including the nurse-client relationship.

A humanistic interactionist may view transference phenomena as distortions of meaning between psychiatric nurse and client. The nurse may suspect that a client is in transference when the client repeatedly assigns meanings to the nurse-client relationship that belong to one or more of the client's past relationships. It is as if the client's ability to assess the nurse-client interactions becomes confused and thwarted by the unfinished conflicts belonging to past interactions with significant others. Thus, the psychiatric nurse may be viewed as parent, sibling, lover, or friend.

The development of transference offers the psychiatric nurse an opportunity, by direct observation, to understand the development of the client's past conflicts. The appearance of highly emotional responses that do not "fit" the current therapeutic situation may indicate client transference. In traditional psychoanalytic work, handling the transference becomes the core of treatment. In the humanistic interactionist approach to transference, the psychiatric nurse explores the meaning of individual words, gestures, events, and situations in the current one-to-one relationship to determine how these reflect or replay distortions in past relationships. The therapeutic task is to separate feelings, thoughts, and behaviors that belong to the current one-to-one relationship from those that represent unresolved conflicts in past relationships.

Increasing awareness of the transference process often frees the client to work through past conflicts and explore the more creative, self-actualizing aspects of personal identity as they evolve in the current relationship. The psychiatric nurse must not behave as the client's parent or other transference figure has behaved. Rather, the nurse helps the client bring an unconscious event into consciousness, to examine its cause and meaning. The following example illustrates how transference may surface in a clinical setting:

Conrad Wilson is a 40-year-old married man hospitalized with moderate depression, which is manifested by restless agitation, inability to complete tasks, and subjective feelings of hopelessness. Conrad was assigned to a primary counselor, a male psychiatric nurse. Over the course of several meetings with his counselor, Conrad assumed a cowering, ingratiating manner. He seemed to resemble a little boy awaiting punishment from an intimidating, punitive father. This interpersonal orientation was observed by other male staff who informally initiated interaction with Conrad on the unit. In this instance, the transference figure appeared to be a father figure.

The counselor chose not to explore Conrad's past relationships. The aim of short-term work was to focus on concrete ways to decrease depressed feelings in Conrad's present life situation. The counselor addressed ingratiating behaviors in the nurse-client relationship only when they appeared to have an adverse effect on their short-term work together.

In the clinical example, the primary counselor chose to focus on present rather than past relationships in an effort to stabilize the hospitalized client. Transference may be dealt with in many ways, depending upon the client's functioning, the counselor's theoretic orientation, and the type of therapy.

Transference may be positive or negative. **Positive transference,** that is, positive feelings for the therapist, occurs when the client generally has had satisfying past relationships with significant others during childhood. The therapeutic relationship is usually able to progress in this instance. Negative transference is discussed shortly.

Countertransference While transference involves the client's reactions to the psychiatric nurse, **countertransference** involves the nurse's reactions to the client. The psychiatric nurse may develop powerful counterproductive fantasies, feelings, and attitudes in response to the client's transference or personality. A humanistic interactionist may also view countertransference as a distortion of meaning between psychiatric nurse and client in one-to-one relationship work.

Countertransference is suspected when the psychiatric nurse repeatedly assigns meaning to the nurse-client relationship that belongs to the nurse's other past relationships. In countertransference the psychiatric nurse's ability to assess the nurse-client interactions becomes confused or thwarted by unresolved past conflicts. Thus, the nurse may unconsciously employ behaviors (as parent, sibling, lover, or friend) that attempt to replay in the current situation some past identity with significant others. Countertransference indicates unresolved conflict in the psychiatric nurse. This conflict may be expressed in acts of omission or commission and in irrational friendliness or annoyance. These expressions may be covert or overt.

Countertransference is a normal occurrence, requiring supervision or consultation to prevent degeneration of the one-to-one relationship. Supervision may enable the psychiatric nurse to separate feelings, thoughts, and behaviors that belong to the current relationship from those that represent unfinished conflicts in past relationships. Awareness of the existence of countertransference is crucial. The nurse may act out unrecognized countertransference, confusing the client. Unrecognized countertransference can undermine the entire psychotherapeutic process.

Intervening in Problems with Transference and Countertransference

Negative Transference In **negative transference,** the client shows a number of reactions based on forms of hate (hostility, loathing, bitterness, contempt, annoyance). Although there are both positive and negative aspects to every transference, a predominantly negative transference is uncomfortable for client and nurse alike. The client does not like to be aware of and express this hate, and the nurse does not like to be the target of it. When negative transference appears unresolvable, it may be advisable to terminate relationship work rather than run the risk of further client dysfunction.

It is important to note that negative transference responses that seem related to deep-seated depression or paranoia are usually not dealt with in relationship work. The reason is that exploration may stir up issues and intense emotions that cannot be dealt with in a limited time span (Arieti 1974–1981).

Psychotic Transference In psychotic transference, or transference psychosis, the relationship with the psychiatric nurse supersedes all other relationships, although the client has no insight into the existence of the transference and denies its presence. Psychotic transference requires repetitive, concrete reality testing to separate the nurse from significant others in the client's life. In addition, psychotic transference may be minimized by decreasing the frequency and/or duration of contact with the client. Both negative transference and psychotic transference problems require consistent supervision and cautious management.

Unanalyzed Countertransference Unanalyzed countertransference is almost always a problem, because it inhibits client understanding and may be acted out. One purpose of clinical supervision is to help the mental health professional develop awareness of individual countertransference reactions. Chessick (1974) highlights the following signs of countertransference in waking life or while dreaming:

- Anxiety reactions

- Reactions of irrational concern about and irrational kindness toward the client

- Reactions of irrational hostility toward the client

The following are more specific signals that countertransference may be a problem:

- Uneasy feelings during or after meetings

- Being late or extending the agreed-on duration of meetings for no apparent reason

- Dreaming about the client

- Preoccupation with the client during the nurse's leisure time

It is reassuring that most countertransference problems can be resolved by self-assessment with professional supervision. Once the countertransference process is identified, the nurse can consciously develop therapeutic, goal-directed responses. In rare instances, however, referral to another nurse is appropriate when the first nurse cannot control the disturbed attitudes and emotions.

Interpersonal Skills in Therapeutic Relationships

The effectiveness of psychiatric nurses has often been subjectively assumed, unquestioned, or discounted without a scientific data base for evaluation. This discussion of their therapeutic effectiveness includes a brief exploration of the conflict between caretaker and therapist roles, and of personal characteristics known to facilitate therapeutic effectiveness.

Conflict between Caretaker and Therapist Roles

Traditional nursing education may keep the psychiatric nurse from developing therapeutic effectiveness if it stresses the denial of personal feelings and the need for a caretaker role. Nurses may erect rigid defenses aimed at denying their feelings because of the emotional demands of nursing. For example, some procedures actually require the nurse to violate a client's emotional or physical state (injections, dressings). Defending against feelings becomes one way for the nurse to cope with inflicting pain on another person. Yet psychiatric nurses can deal effectively with the feelings of clients only to the extent that they explore their own personal feelings.

Continued assumption of the caretaker role also undermines the therapeutic effectiveness of psychiatric nurses. The caretaker role tends to involve sympathy rather than empathy. The difference between these two responses is significant to therapeutic outcomes.

A one-to-one relationship requires the psychiatric nurse to help the client actively explore the meaning underlying the client's personal pain, distress, or discomfort. Nurses must avoid the caretaker role in which they alleviate pain. Rather, they must encourage clients to develop ways to do so for themselves. Similarly, the caretaker role requires nurses to make decisions for clients. It does not encourage clients to be accountable for their own decisions.

Therapeutic Use of Self

Psychiatric nurses may increase their therapeutic effectiveness by knowledge and practice of specific interpersonal skills in therapeutic relationships. Research repeatedly indicates that interpersonal skills may be acquired, increased, and refined through education, workshops, and human relations laboratories.

Therapeutic use of self involves a pulling together of several important personal elements to bring to any one-to-one relationship work:

- Development of healthy self-awareness

- Exploration of the growth-facilitating, humanistic self and personal impact on others

- Thorough use of theoretic and experiential knowledge in mental health

Therapeutic use of self is discussed in Chapter 2.

The goal is to develop commitment, therapeutic processes, and a therapeutic relationship between client and nurse. Sometimes the nurse may feel uneasy, awkward, or offended if the client unexpectedly asks personal questions, presents a gift, discusses values such as religion, or seeks physical contact. Although these experiences may happen during any phase of

RESEARCH NOTE

Citation

Hardin SB, Durham JD: First rate: Exploring the structure, process, and effectiveness of nurse psychotherapy. J Psychosoc Nurs Ment Health Serv 1985;23:9–15.

Study Problem/Purpose

This descriptive study was designed to explore nurse psychotherapy as perceived by nurse therapists and their clients. Purposes of the study were to determine the structural parameters of therapy, characteristics of the nurse-client relationship, and therapeutic effectiveness of treatment.

Methods

The study included eighty-two nurse therapists throughout the United States. Each was a psychiatric nurse prepared at the master's level and was a primary psychotherapist for individual clients. Thirty-eight nurse therapists (46 percent) agreed to send questionnaires to former clients. The ninety-five clients in the study had been treated for at least six sessions in the previous year by a nurse therapist cooperating in the study. A major limitation of the study was that nurse therapists selected the client sample.

The measure utilized by nurse therapists was a nurse psychotherapist questionnaire. Measures for clients were a client attitude scale and a client questionnaire to measure general satisfaction with psychotherapy. These questionnaires from both groups provided demographic, quantitative, and qualitative data. Measures were based on previously used research tools.

Findings

Nurse therapists were predominantly female, had extensive psychotherapy experience, and were highly educated (some held doctorates or were enrolled in doctoral programs). Fifty-four percent worked alone, while others identified psy-

chiatrists, psychologists, social workers, and other nurses as their coworkers. Clients were generally unmarried, well-educated females between 20 and 40 years of age. They most often sought treatment for depression or for problems in coping with separation and divorce. Nurse therapists tended to screen acting out, psychotic, and chemically addicted clients from their practices.

The structure of practice typically consisted of verbal psychotherapy on a weekly basis. The average duration of treatment was fourteen months at an average charge of $37 per session.

Nurse therapists rated highest as empathic, warm, and excellent listeners. Other helping actions with clients included increasing insight, imparting skill in problem solving, improving self-esteem, validating feelings, and increasing independence.

Both nurse therapists and clients viewed psychotherapy as a satisfying and successful experience. Ninety percent of clients expressed satisfaction regarding an overall evaluation of their psychotherapy experience. Seventy percent of clients claimed extreme satisfaction. Ten percent of clients reported dissatisfaction with therapy.

Implications

This descriptive study is noteworthy, since there is little systematic research regarding nurse therapists, i.e., whom they treat, how they conduct treatment, and how desirable this treatment is. The authors view the study sample as effective, self-directed therapists. They further suggest that nurse therapists will probably not attain true autonomy without additional powers. These powers may include hospital privileges and prescriptive authority. The authors also urge nurses to continue their organized efforts to bring about third-party payment, based on the findings of this study.

---

therapeutic work, they frequently occur during the working phase. During this phase, the client slowly gets to know the psychiatric nurse as a separate, concerned person. Critical distance is an additional concern from the moment that the nurse attempts interpersonal contact. Each of these concerns requires ongoing nursing assessment and evaluation so that positive therapeutic outcome may be maximized.

Critical Distance It is important for the nurse to observe how the client uses physical space. Hall (1966) asserts that people need to keep a critical distance between themselves and others to maintain their well-being. That specific distance depends on the relationship between the individuals. Nurses may allow physical distance between themselves and clients, especially early in therapy. This distance promotes verbal communication and reduces any existing anxiety and hostility. Moving rapidly toward closeness, especially in establishing the nurse-client relationship, may overwhelm the client and increase anxiety.

The physical distance between the psychiatric nurse and the client can be indicative of other therapeutic processes. For example, a client may sit in a chair at a great distance from the nurse during initial meetings but move closer and closer as the working relationship is established. The psychiatric nurse needs to assess the possible interpersonal implications of proximity (nearness) for each client. As the relationship progresses, the nurse must assess whether physical distance or proximity reduces client anxiety. The client's need for distance usually increases as the client experiences panic or near-panic levels of anxiety.

Self-Disclosure Self-disclosure means being open to personal feelings and experiences, being "real" as opposed to hiding behind a professional facade or being a technician of various communication skills. If the nurse reveals personal feelings when appropriate, the client learns that it is OK to explore feelings in the therapeutic setting. How much should a nurse share with a client? Under what circumstances?

It may be helpful to view self-disclosure on a continuum. One end represents underdisclosure; the other, overdisclosure. When evaluating any self-disclosure at a given time, nurses should ask themselves two essential questions. First, what is the purpose of the revelation, i.e., who is this self-disclosure for? Does this self-disclosure meet the client's therapeutic goals or does it meet the nurse's needs? Second, does this self-disclosure foster the development of a more productive therapeutic relationship?

Facilitative self-disclosure must be used within the context of the therapeutic relationship, where attention is given to its timing, appropriateness, and degree. For example, the nurse must use self-disclosure cautiously with a severely dysfunctional client with poor ego boundaries. This client may not be able to separate thoughts and feelings that belong to the client from those that belong to the nurse. The client might misinterpret the nurse's self-disclosure or might not be able to make sense of the disclosure. The client may also fear engulfment by the nurse, i.e., the nurse's feelings might be perceived as so threatening that they overwhelm the client. Facilitative self-disclosure fosters the development of the therapeutic relationship rather than threatening its continuance.

When the nurse chooses to disclose personal information in a given instance, nursing evaluation must follow. If the "flow" of the work together was enhanced, then the nurse suspects that the self-revelation was facilitative. If the psychiatric nurse is unsure of the outcome, a frank inquiry may be in order. For example, "How did you feel when I told you my age?" The client's reaction and subsequent exploration together can be a gauge for measuring how this client perceives and responds to self-disclosures by the nurse. As the nurse expresses feelings about the evolving relationship, the client may feel free to reciprocate. At times, the psychiatric nurse may choose to role model emotive expression.

When the psychiatric nurse chooses to avoid self-disclosure in a given instance, several communication techniques may be helpful. For instance, a client might ask the nurse to disclose marital status, home address, religious affiliation, or a pressing personal problem. Auvil and Silver (1984) offer the following ways to deflect a request for self-disclosure:

- *Use honesty.* "I don't want to share my home address with you."

- *Use benign curiosity.* "I wonder why you're asking me this today?"

- *Use refocusing.* "You were talking about how your father treats you. I wonder why you changed the topic? You were saying that . . ."

- *Use interpretation.* "I notice that every time you talk about your father, you change the subject and ask me a question." (pause)

- *Seek clarification.* "You keep asking me my home address. I wonder what concerns you might have about me today and as we work together?"

- *Respond with feedback and limit-setting.* "I'm really uncomfortable when you ask me who pays my tuition. Talking about my finances isn't part of our agreement to work together." Adding "the last time we met, you were deciding if you were going to call your boss on the phone . . ." helps to restructure the situation.

The nurse uses these communication techniques in the context of the therapeutic relationship, where the nurse assesses and evaluates the client response in an ongoing manner.

Gift Giving The giving of gifts may be a special concern in therapeutic relationships. Gift giving may take various forms: a fleeting social amenity (e.g., the purchase of a cup of coffee), a gesture (e.g., the loan of a favorite book), or the present of a valued object (e.g., the giving of an original painting). Like self-disclosure, gift giving in any instance must be met with ongoing nursing assessment and evaluation to determine its form, intent, appropriateness, and meaning in the context of the therapeutic relationship. No rule covers all instances of gift giving. Rather, several broad guidelines can help the nurse evaluate the particular situation.

The Client as Gift Giver During the orientation phase of a therapeutic relationship, the client may overtly offer or ask for a gift. This gesture may be as incidental as offering the nurse (or asking for) a cigarette. The psychiatric nurse examines this overture, keeping in mind several possible motivations. The client may seek to bribe or manipulate the nurse, thereby seeking to control the direction of the therapeutic relationship. The client may seek to "buy" the nurse's time and attention. The client may ask for small gifts to reinforce a helpless, "take-care-of-me" interpersonal stance. Of course, the client may have no covert intent and may simply need a cigarette. In the orientation phase, it may be helpful for nurses not to accept or give any gift they feel uncomfortable giving. Rather the nurse should explore the client's intent. Often this mutual exploration not only clarifies the client's intent but also helps to define the parameters of the evolving relationship and models the exploratory process for the client.

During the working phase, particularly after the client has implemented positive growth, the client may offer a gift in the form of a craft or skill. As in the orientation phase, the intent of the gift needs to be made explicit. The nurse can encourage this exploration by making statements such as "How is it that you're sharing this gift with me?" or "What feelings might you want to share with this gift?" A client might give a gift during the working phase for several reasons. The client may wish to acknowledge the mutual work that has taken place. The client may wish to show appreciation for being allowed to share concerns with another person. A gift may be a "smoke screen" to block further exploration of a major dynamic. A gift may outwardly cover up anger or frustration felt inwardly. Finally, a gift may indicate the client's perception that the therapeutic work is finished. In every instance, the nurse must assess the intent of the gift, as well as its timing and appropriateness, in the context of the therapeutic relationship.

Gifts are most often given during the termination phase of one-to-one relationships. In this phase, a gift may have several overt and covert meanings. The client may wish to give a token of appreciation for any positive personal growth that occurred in this mutual learning endeavor. The client may desire to change the therapeutic relationship into a social one. The client may wish to prolong sessions to avoid the final good-bye. Some nurses accept a small gift from a client at the time of termination if feelings regarding the gift have been explored and clarified. (The gift may be an appropriate remembrance of a mutual and positive growth experience.) The nurse may find receiving a gift at times awkward and "artificial." Yet such a situation gives the nurse the opportunity to help the client toward further self-expression and self-knowledge.

The Nurse as Gift Giver The nurse is an infrequent and judicious gift giver. Most often, the psychiatric nurse relates to the client by therapeutic use of self rather than through objects, such as gifts. There are possible exceptions. For instance a psychiatric nurse may give a gift to establish initial contact with a severely dysfunctional client in a ward setting. During the working phase, the nurse may share a resource (e.g., a book or article) about some facet of the client's therapy or growth. During termination, the nurse may give the client a small gift to acknowledge mutual growth during therapeutic work. In every instance, the psychiatric nurse evaluates the client's response and the meaning assigned to this gift. The nurse also evaluates personal motives and the personal meaning of the gift.

Use of Touch Physical contact is used cautiously in therapeutic work. It is best to avoid unplanned physical contact without therapeutic rationale. Clients with poor ego boundaries may become intensely threatened and feel overwhelmed by physical contact. For example, a client may lose the ability to distinguish self from the nurse during simple hand contact. Such contact may be perceived as a hostile or sexual gesture, although not intended as such by the nurse. In contrast, an acutely grief-stricken client, too distraught to focus on words, might receive needed support from being held.

The psychiatric nurse employs the nursing process when considering any use of touch. The nurse must ask: First, does touch meet the client's therapeutic goals or does it meet the nurse's needs? Second, does touch foster a more productive therapeutic relationship? The nurse evaluates the use of touch, like self-disclosure, in the context of the therapeutic relationship, paying attention to its timing, appropriateness, and type. For example, a client is thrilled to achieve an employment goal that has taken much personal time and effort. The psychiatric nurse determines that a firm handshake and a statement of congratulations are facilitative in this instance and at this working phase of the relationship. If the nurse is unsure of the effect of such a gesture, a frank inquiry may be in order: "How did you feel when I shook your hand a few moments ago?" Again, the client's reaction and subsequent exploration can be a gauge for measuring how the client perceives and responds to the use of touch. Chapter 16 deals with manipulation.

Values It is crucial for psychiatric nurses to be aware of their personal value system, since the therapeutic relationship may be a vehicle for value transmission. In this process, the client may change cultural, religious, and personal values, usually in the direction of the nurse's value system. Such transmission may be helpful or detrimental, and it requires consistent nursing assessment and evaluation (Herron and Rouslin 1982).

Nurses must also address client values and beliefs that interfere with adaptive functioning. The following people hold cultural values and beliefs that may interfere with constructive change:

• The abusive spouse who believes the partner should be subservient and, conversely, the partner who defers personal needs to preserve the relationship

• The abusive parent who believes that to "spare the rod" is to "spoil the child"

• The child, raised with the family injunction that family problems should not be discussed outside the home, who may view the nurse's actions as an invasion of privacy

Religious beliefs, too, may become delusions or at least interfere with change:

• The client who believes that God takes care of His people, and so there is no need to solve personal problems

• The client who believes that divorce is a sin and therefore will never be forgiven (or forgive self)

Initially, the nurse should become aware of the specific values and beliefs that influence the immediate relationship work. It is often useful to label the value or belief with the client, exploring its history, importance, and impact. Nonjudgmental, alternative values may be discussed if the client initiates such an exploration. Competent and consistent supervision is useful to the nurse regarding the issue of values. The humanistic nurse respects the client's values and beliefs, and the client's ultimate choices regarding personal value systems.

Client Abilities

The psychiatric nurse can increase the chances of success by knowing the client's abilities. Schuable and Pierce (1974) have demonstrated that the following client characteristics are conducive to effective relationship work:

• The nurse-client relationship is more effective if clients are aware of and show willingness to assume responsibility for their feelings and actions. In contrast, some clients act as if their problems are entirely external and beyond their control.

• Clients must admit their feelings and show awareness that the feelings are tied to specific behaviors. By contrast, clients who avoid accepting their personal feelings and view them as belonging to others or as situational and outside themselves are not likely to benefit from relationship work.

• Clients need to express a clear desire to change and cooperate with the nurse as opposed to resisting involvement.

• Clients must show willingness to learn how to differentiate feelings, concerns, and problems and must recognize their unique reactions and individuality.

Only an ideal client has all these abilities. Such a client is not typically found in the long-term public facilities in which many psychiatric nurses have their clinical experiences. Nurses who work with chronic, resistant, long-term clients may learn that clients can make concrete improvements if both the client and nurse work specifically with one client ability over time. Awareness of client abilities conducive to one-to-one relationships is essential regardless of the setting.

The Therapeutic Alliance

The **therapeutic alliance** is a conscious relationship between a helping person and a client. In this process, the nurse forms a mature alliance with the growth-facilitating aspects of the client. Each implicitly agrees that they need to work together to help the client with personal problems and concerns. More specifically, the nurse identifies and provides feedback regarding the client's patterns of reaction, abilities, and potentials. The client can use these assets to handle unresolved problems constructively. The establishment of the therapeutic alliance enhances informal one-to-one relationships. It is essential in formal one-to-one relationships. Such a binding alliance between nurse and client allows the one-to-one relationship to continue, especially when the client experiences increased anxiety and resistance to change.

Nursing Process and the Three Phases of Therapeutic Relationships

A one-to-one relationship has three distinct phases:

1. The **orientation** (beginning) **phase,** characterized by the establishment of contact with the client

2. The **working** (middle) **phase,** characterized by maintenance and analysis of contact

3. The **termination** (end) **phase,** characterized by the termination of contact with the client

Each phase of a one-to-one relationship is distinguished by important goals and therapeutic tasks.

The time required for each phase depends on the severity of client dysfunction, the psychiatric nurse's skills, the number and types of problems surfacing during treatment, and the type of therapeutic contract negotiated between psychiatric nurse and client. Although these phases are presented here in their entirety to develop a comprehensive theoretic framework, nurses rarely experience them in such detail and sequence. Nurses are more likely to experience the development of several short-term goals and to experiment with several subsequent interventions in any phase of relationship work. Nevertheless, an exploration of each phase increases the nurse's familiarity with the flow—that is, "what comes next"—and may also provide a framework in which the psychiatric nurse can see client and nurse behaviors as partial expressions of a specific phase. Finally, an understanding of each phase of a one-to-one relationship may help the nurse select interventions appropriate to that phase. Nursing interventions appropriate in the beginning phase may be very different from those appropriate in the working phase.

In addition to needing familiarity with significant phases of one-to-one relationships, the psychiatric nurse needs to develop awareness of and effectiveness in using numerous processes that occur in any one-to-one relationship work. The beginning nurse often attends carefully to the *content* of the client sessions—i.e., what the client says—and only after considerable experience becomes actively attuned to *process*. Process here does not mean nursing process but rather a complex communication skill that allows the nurse to focus on several aspects of the nurse-client relationship at the same time. Process involves attention to all nonverbal and verbal client behaviors. It involves responding to client "themes," e.g., anger, hopelessness, and powerlessness. The experienced nurse is simultaneously aware of both content and process, interweaving both for maximum therapeutic effectiveness.

Orientation (Beginning) Phase: Establishing Contact

The primary goal of the beginning phase is to establish contact, or a working relationship with the client. The phase of establishing contact includes the initial encounters between psychiatric nurse and client—how they approach and interact with each other, both verbally and nonverbally. The nurse and the client meet to discuss how they will work together toward a common goal. The nurse is aware of having impact on the client and acknowledges the client's personal impact as a unique individual.

In informal relationships, contact usually begins when the psychiatric nurse seeks out the client in an in-patient psychiatric setting. Establishment of contact may involve developing client awareness of the nurse's presence, followed by working to communicate with the client on a verbal level.

In formal relationships, contact may begin when the client inquires about services or when the psychiatric nurse contacts the client following referral. Settings may include an in-patient unit, an outpatient clinic, or community settings, including the home and private practice facilities. In formal relationships, the sense of working together in a therapeutic alliance enables the client to endure anxiety and deal with resistance to change, which inevitably surface during the course of one-to-one relationships. This phase of the therapeutic relationship concludes with mutual agreement on a therapeutic contract, which may be verbal and quite simple. The contract spells out the client's goals for treatment and the nurse's professional responsibilities.

Issues of trust and confidentiality arise during the orientation phase, both for the client and the nurse. Another concern for the nurse is how best to develop a verbal contract with the client. Initial verbal therapeutic contracts are discussed below. More formal (sometimes written) therapeutic contracts are explored in the section on the working phase.

Issues During the Orientation Phase

Trust   Concerns about trust surface in this first phase of the relationship. Trust between psychiatric nurse and client evolves over time as the client tests the emotional climate of sessions, risks self-disclosure, and observes nurse follow-through on responsibilities delineated in the therapeutic contract. The nurse can promote trust by responding to all the client's feeling states without being judgmental or attempting to control emotive expression. The following interventions enhance initial trust:

- Listen attentively to client feelings

- Respond to client feelings

- Exhibit consistency, especially regarding appointment times

- View situations from the client's world view

Self-awareness of personal feeling states on the part of the nurse also enhances trust. It allows the client to disclose uncomfortable, even forbidden, feelings in safety. A common failing among those learning relationship skills is focusing on technique. This produces mechanical, unfeeling responses. It is also important to avoid giving premature reassurances about trust, which may inhibit exploration of this vital therapeutic issue and create distance between therapist and client. The verbatim example in Table 26–3 illustrates the emergence of trust as an initial therapeutic issue.

Confidentiality   Client concerns about the level of **confidentiality** also surface in this first phase of the therapeutic relationship. Like the issue of trust, the

TABLE 26-3   Verbatim Example, Orientation Phase

Verbatim Interaction	Nursing Intervention	Rationale
Client: It's so difficult for me to talk . . . to let you know about me.		
(Thirty-second pause.)	None	To allow client space to proceed at own pace; if silence is uncomfortably long to client in first few contacts, nurse may use reflection, e.g.: "I sense how difficult talking is for you."
Client: Every time I start to tell anybody about myself, they usually end up laughing at me.		
Nurse: Can you give an example of this?	Encourage elaboration	To explore meaning of this statement to client
Client: Well, just last week I started talking to my neighbor. I told him that I was laid off from work again. Next thing you know, he's laughing, slapping my back, and saying "Hey, hard times, eh?"		
(Shifts in chair, poor eye contact.)		
Nurse: What was this like for you?	Explore client's personal reaction, especially accompanying feelings	To further explore meaning of this specific incident as perceived by the client
Client: Awful . . . lousy . . . that's all.		
(Pause.)		
Nurse: I wonder if you're concerned that the same might happen here—that you'll be laughed at?	To apply concern regarding "external" issue to here-and-now, i.e., one-to-one relationship	Issues concerning client's immediate life situations often reflect parallel issues in nurse-client relationship
Client: Well, maybe. . . . I don't know you, so how do I know what you might do? You don't look like the type, but then again—how do I know?		
Nurse: It sounds like you're wondering if it's safe to trust me.	Move to what appears to be the *metamessage* or underlying central concern (theme)	Reflection of what appears to be the central concern (theme) encourages client assessment by validation or correction
Client: Yeah . . . no offense though.		
Nurse: Let's talk about how safe you feel today and as we continue to work together.	Underline trust as an issue for further exploration; stress evolving working relationship	Avoid premature reassurances so that trust can evolve and be assessed periodically

issue of confidentiality must be explicitly addressed when the client makes even vague reference to it. The psychiatric nurse should state explicitly which persons will have access to client revelations (clinical instructor, case supervisor, consultant, colleague) and explore how the client feels in response to this information.

Initial Therapeutic Contract   A simple verbal therapeutic contract between client and nurse is helpful at the beginning of the orientation phase. It may simply involve the client's definition of goals to work on (however simple), some determination of time and place for meeting together, and a delineation of the nurse's responsibilities.

In informal relationships, the nurse may begin by saying: "I'd like to talk with you to get to know you better" or "I'd like to talk to you to see if there is anything we can discuss together." An initial verbal contract helps to build trust, convey empathy, and develop rapport. This contract is crucial in an in-

patient setting, where clients may be suspicious or withdrawn.

Even a simple therapeutic contract may take several meetings to formulate. For example, an elderly in-patient with organic mental disorder agrees to meet with a nursing student every Wednesday when she visits his unit. He wants to learn ways to deal with isolation after his discharge. The nursing student agrees to telephone the client if she is unable to meet with him on any specific Wednesday.

Carefully and thoroughly attending to a mutual agreement on an initial verbal contract precedes, and has priority over, data collection. Comprehensive client assessment is not possible unless the client at least agrees to talk with the nurse regularly for a definite purpose. Even in formal relationships, the agreement to meet the first time can be viewed as an initial contract. Provisions for the contract can be flexible and dynamic. These provisions may be renegotiated according to changing needs or circumstances. The contract is redefined, i.e., more formal goals and responsibilities are established, as the orientation phase progresses.

Assessing   Client assessment begins at the first moment of contact. Assessment continues throughout the therapeutic relationship but is particularly important during the orientation phase. The client is the primary source of data. It is very important to repeat or "replay" important data for the client. This replay gives the client ample time to identify, articulate, and adjust data so that the nurse gets the closest approximation to the "real picture" of the client's world. Also, it is essential to note any factors that may influence data collection, such as cultural or language differences.

The degree of collaboration depends on client ability. In the ideal situation, the client participates fully with the psychiatric nurse in all aspects of data collection. In real situations, depending on the functioning ability of the client at initial assessment, part of the assessment data may come from significant others who have known the client for some time. For example, a very suspicious client may not tolerate a comprehensive assessment during the initial interview. Family may be asked to help the nurse develop a "beginning picture" of the client's overall level of functioning. After the client stabilizes, the psychiatric nurse may choose to validate important data with the client. In long-term in-patient settings, data collection may be incomplete due to client dysfunction and lack of other data sources.

Observation   Observation, a process long regarded as essential to clinical nursing practice, is of particular importance in one-to-one relationship work. Observation is an intensive process requiring concentration and practice to gather data through the use of all the senses. It includes attention to verbal, nonverbal, and environmental cues. The observer strives to develop simultaneous sensitivity to vision, hearing, smell, taste, and touch in nurse-client interactions. The observer also needs to check out personal distortions, biases, or unreality. In addition to observing what elements are present, the nurse notes elements in the nurse-client interaction that are missing, distorted, or imbalanced. What the client avoids discussing is often more crucial than what is shared. See Peplau's seminal works regarding observation (Peplau 1952, 1962, 1989) as well as Chapter 9 of this text for more information on observation.

Examination   Data collection by examination ideally includes the following: mental status examination, complete physical examination, nursing history, and psychologic testing, as needed. Which examinations are done and by whom are generally determined by the agency or institution in which the psychiatric

nurse works, and by the psychiatric nurse's expertise in these specific areas. (See Chapter 9 for a comprehensive discussion of examination.) To address practical matters, Robitaille-Tremblay (1984) offers a data-collection tool for nurses seeking to take nursing histories. She incorporates the following helpful suggestions:

• Respect the client's pace. When questions appear threatening, do not insist. Return to them later.

• Rearrange the order of questions if the client appears defensive or distrustful.

• Take into consideration all of the information the client gives.

• Avoid an inquisitive attitude so that the client does not feel interrogated.

• Adapt questions to the client's abilities, using examples as necessary.

Interview   Interviewing is a process that generally occurs in the beginning (orientation) phase of one-to-one relationships. Although a psychiatric nurse may use the structured initial interview in formal one-to-one work, it is rarely used in informal relationships. Nevertheless, it is important for beginning nurses to familiarize themselves with the kinds of background data collection useful in mental health work. They can incorporate various elements of the initial interview as appropriate for specific clients over an extended time span. The initial interview has the following purposes:

• To initiate trust building

• To establish rapport with the client

• To obtain pertinent client data

• To initiate client assessment

• To make practical arrangements for treatment

The initial interview is crucial because it sets the stage for subsequent therapeutic contact.

Amount of Structuring   The psychiatric nurse must structure the initial interview to establish rapport, decrease anxiety, and convey willingness to address the client's suffering. The psychiatric nurse may begin the interview by introducing herself or himself, inviting the client to be seated, and making a statement about information thus far known about the client's seeking of services. An open-ended question, such as "How is it that you are here today?" provides an opportunity for the client to talk about concerns. The psychiatric nurse may inform the client that the purpose of the initial interview is to get an overview of the client's current situation and then determine the availability of appropriate services.

Essential Data One primary purpose of structuring the initial interview is to collect essential data. Chapter 9 details essential and helpful client data to obtain. In in-patient settings, it is unusual for students to collect all data from the hospitalized client. Students may rely on chart data more than independent practitioners do.

The psychiatric nurse needs to address client resistance if it surfaces during the initial interview. This resistance may occur when the client has initiated services at someone else's request or insistence, has fears and misconceptions about therapy, or has had an unsatisfactory therapeutic experience in the past. Nursing intervention calls for explicit exploration of the specific resistance before further data collection. Refer to the earlier discussion regarding general intervention strategies for resistance. Clients with moderate to high anxiety levels may be confused about or misinterpret information given during the initial interview. Most clients experience some degree of anxiety at the beginning of therapy. Manifestations of anxiety must be differentiated from manifestations of resistance. The nurse may need to repeat information several times or in subsequent meetings.

Areas to Avoid Wolberg (1988) offers the following list of practices for the psychiatric nurse to avoid during the initial interview. These apply to informal, as well as more formal, one-to-one relationships.

• Do not argue with, minimize, or challenge the client.

• Do not praise the client or give false reassurance.

• Do not make false promises.

• Do not interpret to the client or speculate on the dynamics of the client's problem.

• Do not offer a diagnosis even if the client insists on it.

• Do not question the client on sensitive areas.

• Do not try to "sell" the client on accepting treatment.

• Do not join in attacks the client launches on parents, mate, friends, or associates.

• Do not participate in criticism of another therapist.

Remember that shortcuts taken in assessment procedures almost always jeopardize the ultimate quality of care. Crucial areas of concern may go unaddressed or be treated superficially.

Diagnosing Following a comprehensive assessment of the client in one-to-one relationships, the psychiatric nurse gathers and organizes all the data collected during the assessment phase to formulate preliminary nursing diagnoses. The word *preliminary* is used to imply the ongoing potential for revision as client behaviors unfold during the course of the relationship.

The goal in organizing the data is to understand the data as they reflect the client's unique, private world. Data are scientifically and systematically grouped into categories that reflect the client's potential problems, actual problems, strengths, and abilities. The nurse attempts to look for dominant themes or central issues in the client's response to the environment.

When the assessment in the beginning phase is comprehensive, organized, and analyzed, then the nursing diagnoses seem to "flow" from the data. Nursing diagnoses should be prioritized, with the most pressing and detrimental pattern listed first, followed by others of decreasing significance. It is then easier for the nurse to identify goals and determine appropriate intervention strategies.

Implementing Interventions

Making a Therapeutic Contract Client assessment and nursing diagnosis are the basis on which the psychiatric nurse formulates a plan of action. This plan is a **therapeutic contract** negotiated in a one-to-one relationship. The therapeutic contract evolves to become the client's definition of personal goals for treatment plus the nurse's professional responsibilities. The goal of the beginning phase of one-to-one work is to establish contact and begin a working relationship with the client. The therapeutic contract is a concrete, detailed, and mutually negotiated expression of this working relationship. The therapeutic contract may be modified over time but always serves as a tool for evaluating the benefit to the client and the effectiveness of the nurse. In an informal therapeutic relationship, the therapeutic contract may differ from the usual care plan often developed in outpatient and in-patient settings. For example, an initial contract may begin as a very simple agreement concerning the time and place of subsequent meetings together.

Planning is achieved by arriving at client-centered therapeutic goals, which represent the client's personal goals for treatment. These may be long-term or short-term goals, but they always specify detailed, observable outcomes. The nurse strives for the most concise, detailed, and accurate description of client goals in the beginning phase. Clearly stated goals facilitate subsequent mutual evaluation during the middle and end phases of one-to-one work. Goals may focus on:

• Decreasing or eliminating troublesome behaviors

• Increasing socialization

• Increasing living skills

A frequently overlooked area of goal formation is preventive health education. For example, the psychiatric nurse may provide a client with information or literature regarding health precautions for HIV disease when the client has indicated concern or fear.

In both settings, the client participates in the formation of a therapeutic contract by determining personal goals. At times, client goals may be long term or even inappropriate. In this situation, the psychiatric nurse may help the client define initial steps toward the long-term goal. For example, a readmitted chronic client may pinpoint discharge as an important goal. The nurse may then work with this client to determine the steps needed to achieve this goal. One step may be to maintain self-care in the area of bathing/hygiene. When severe dysfunction limits client input into planning, the nursing staff may supplement goals that are determined to be beneficial to the client.

In a formal therapeutic relationship, as in individual psychotherapy, the therapeutic contract is more detailed and generally includes three practical matters:

1. Determination of the place, duration, and time of therapy

2. Establishment of fees and payment intervals, if any

3. Consideration of optional referral sources, should the client be unable to negotiate an agreement on the first two matters

The most essential aspect of the therapeutic contract is the client's definition of goals for treatment. Client goals most often contribute to the establishment of a working relationship when they are specific, address intrapersonal or interpersonal behavior patterns, and delineate the degree of change necessary for client self-satisfaction.

In formal therapeutic relationships, the therapeutic contract may not reflect client problems and strengths in their entirety. At that moment, the client may not determine that an area is, in fact, a problem. Thus, the therapeutic contract in formal relationship work reflects the *client's* definition of personal goals at one moment in time. The psychiatric nurse, in this instance, remains aware of other probable problem areas and assesses these areas with the client in an ongoing manner, as appropriate.

Some nurses advocate the use of immediate, intermediate, and ultimate objectives in delineation of therapeutic goals. The nurse and client mutually determine the ultimate therapeutic goal and then work backward, determining the intermediate and finally the immediate goals (Ward 1984).

Regardless of the form that goal delineation takes, the therapeutic contract serves the following functions:

• Facilitates humanistic involvement with the client as an individual

• Involves the client as a full partner in the therapeutic process

• Serves as a basis for communication in the therapeutic process

• Provides continuity for the client and everyone involved with the client

The initial goals of the therapeutic contract may be modified or deleted in subsequent phases of the one-to-one relationship as appropriate or necessary.

The therapeutic contract should also reflect the nurse's professional responsibilities, i.e., independent, interdependent, or dependent nursing functions. Psychiatric nursing students are most likely to be limited by institution policies to concrete independent functions, such as problem solving, skill training, and teaching. Although students may attend team meetings and collaborate with staff in designing plans, they are not likely to take over nursing functions, such as conducting an intake interview by themselves.

At the independent level, the nurse and client work together in assessment, diagnosis, planning of care, and its full implementation. At the interdependent level, the nurse is part of a health team. At the dependent level, the nurse carries out direct orders of a physician or follows a treatment protocol, e.g., giving emergency treatment for a drug overdose, as defined in a specific setting.

Addressing the Client's Suffering   Interventions during the orientation phase are valid and important, even if the nurse does not reach the working phase with a particular client (e.g., because of time limitations or because the client is unable to agree on goals). The psychiatric nurse intervenes by directly addressing the client's suffering. This intervention allows clients to share how they perceive, experience, and manifest the problem. The following verbatim example illustrates how the nurse encourages a client to "move outside himself" and begin to assess the interpersonal impact as one aspect of his suffering. Assessment has already occurred regarding the severity of the client's depression on the "inside," i.e., how it feels to the client in relation to sleep, appetite, and activity level.

Client: This depression is like a big log weighing on my chest.

Nurse: How might I, or someone else, know that you are suffering in this way?

Client: Well . . . I sigh a lot . . . I don't move a lot, only when I have to . . . I wouldn't look at you, or bother to talk to you. I guess when I feel like this, I close people out. Yeah, I close everyone out, even my wife.

Nurse: So when you suffer in this way, you "close people out." And what is this like for you?

Client: I'm alone and lonely. Not a soul on earth cares for me.

Clarifying Purpose, Roles, and Responsibilities   An additional therapeutic task is for the nurse to intervene directly in clarifying the purpose of the relationship work, the role of the nurse, and the responsibilities of the client. When this preliminary exploration of purpose, roles, and responsibilities is explicit and detailed, each participant better understands how to move within the relationship. It also decreases anxiety and the chance that a client may use the relationship to obtain special privileges. From the first meeting the nurse also intervenes to reinforce effective coping skills and increase client self-esteem. The accompanying Intervention box summarizes the important goal, therapeutic tasks, and subsequent nursing interventions in the orientation phase of one-to-one relationships.

INTERVENTION

Goals, Tasks, and Interventions in the Orientation Phase

Goal	Therapeutic Tasks	Nursing Interventions
Establishment of contact in the form of a working relationship with the client	Clarification of purpose of relationship work, role of nurse, and responsibilities of client	Educative. Provide information regarding purpose, roles, and responsibilities in relationship work to alleviate initial client anxiety
		Immediately and explicitly address any misconceptions, fantasies, and fears regarding relationship work and/or nurse
	Addressing client suffering directly, and offering to work with the client toward its alleviation	Use facilitative characteristics, especially empathic understanding
		Avoid premature reassurance (allow trust to evolve)
		Be explicit about who has access to client's revelations (degree of confidentiality)
	Negotiation of therapeutic contract (client's definition of personal goals for treatment and nurse's professional responsibilities)	Whenever possible, encourage delineation of goals that are specific, address intrapersonal and interpersonal behavioral patterns, and designate degree of change necessary for client self-satisfaction
		In informal relationship work, contract generally includes determination of time and place for working together to the extent that client function permits
		In formal relationship work, the contract generally includes place, duration, and time of therapy; fees and payment intervals, if any; and optional referral sources

TABLE 26–4   **Signs of a Working Relationship**

For Nurse	*For Client*
Sense of making contact with the client	Nonverbal and verbal evidences of liking the nurse
Sense that client is responding well to the relationship	Sense of relaxation with nurse
Sense that nurse can facilitate client growth regardless of severity of client dysfunction	Sense of confidence in nurse
Sense of commitment to address client problems	Nonsuperficial (in nature and depth) problems addressed

Evaluating   In the orientation phase, evaluation includes the nurse's initial comprehensive evaluation of client behaviors, any initial steps toward the development of client self-evaluation, and the psychiatric nurse's ongoing self-evaluation. The more specific and goal-oriented the therapeutic contract, the easier it is for the client and nurse to evaluate the effectiveness of the therapeutic relationship.

In addition to evaluating the effectiveness of each therapeutic task, the psychiatric nurse needs to evaluate the important goal of the orientation phase: Has a working relationship evolved between the client and nurse, and, if so, to what degree? The **working relationship** in this initial phase is the framework on which the client constructs behavioral change in the next phase. Table 26–4 highlights common signs of a working relationship. These signs are predicated on trust and a sense that the nurse can be helpful.

Evaluation of specific goals and outcome criteria generally occurs in the working and resolution phases. Crucial to any evaluation is the need for the nurse to engage in consistent clinical supervision to maximize therapeutic use of self and constructive outcomes. Clinical supervision is addressed later in this chapter.

Working (Middle) Phase: Maintenance and Analysis of Contact

Once contact is established, attention turns to maintenance and analysis of contact in the working or middle phase. *Analysis of contact* refers to an in-depth exploration of how the client relates to others as manifested in the nurse-client relationship. In this working phase, the client may address developmental and situational problems, as well as interpersonal problems. This is called the working phase because during this phase the nurse and client actively and systematically identify, explore, link, modify, and evaluate specific behaviors, especially those determined to be dysfunctional for the client.

The client's clearly stated goals in the therapeutic contract are now explored with the nurse. The nurse has the following two therapeutic goals in this working phase:

• *Behavioral analysis.* The nurse and client determine the dynamics of the client's response patterns, especially those considered to be dysfunctional. Such analysis also addresses dysfunctional thought and emotive patterns, because these inevitably alter the client's behavior. This analysis flows from the therapeutic contract, in which the client identified specific goals for the one-to-one relationship.

• *Constructive change in behavior,* especially in dysfunctional response patterns.

Thus, the psychiatric nurse and client work together to analyze behavior and institute behavioral change in this essential phase of the one-to-one relationship.

Assessing   Assessment is continued, detailed, and expanded upon. The nurse builds on the data obtained during the orientation phase. The nurse's observations of nonverbal, verbal, and environmental responses continue to have vital importance as the client begins to address personal response patterns. In addition, the nurse continues to assess emotive, cognitive, and behavioral aspects. The nurse seeks to fill gaps of information not obtained in the orientation phase. The nurse may just now acquire a detailed assessment about a subject that the client was unable to share or ignored in the orientation phase. The following clinical example illustrates that what was not said (that is, what was avoided, blocked, rejected) by the client may have more significance than what the client shared.

During initial sessions, 18-year-old Maureen avoided any inquiries about her parents, other than to say that she lived alone. She negotiated to work on fear associated with recent, short-term employment.

After several sessions, the nurse again asked about the parents. Maureen replied softly with tears welling in her eyes. "They're dead. They died in a car crash two years ago." She slowly related how, since their deaths, she has spent so much energy trying to survive that she has barely felt much of anything. Subsequent sessions dealt with her apparent delayed grief reaction.

The new data caused the nurse to revise and update the tentative nursing diagnoses and make a marked change in the direction of the sessions. Such shifting is not uncommon in one-to-one relationships. When a change in direction occurs, the nurse assesses if the sudden change indicates the need to avoid a certain topic, or indicates a move toward a deeper level of emotive expression.

In the working phase, the nurse facilitates many aspects of assessment with the client. First, the psychiatric nurse collaborates with the client in identifying important behavioral trends and patterns. Once a pattern is identified, it is explored in elaborate detail to determine its origin, causes, operation, and effects on the client and the people in the client's world. Environmental factors (familial, political, economic, or cultural) are separated from intrapersonal factors (e.g., depression or anxiety) contributing to the pattern. The client figuratively holds the pattern to the light to examine and make sense of its every aspect. The elements of one pattern will inevitably link with others, so that the major life patterns gradually unfold. The verbatim example in Table 26–5 from the middle (working) phase demonstrates how elements of one behavioral pattern are linked to others and gradually reveal central life patterns. In this case, the client's initial anger in reaction to concerned relatives led to awareness of the need to avoid contact in several additional situations. The nurse may now help the client explore what appears to be a central life pattern of interpersonal isolation devoid of intimacy. The first part of the accompanying Intervention box summarizes the therapeutic tasks undertaken to achieve this objective and offers specific nursing approaches to helping the client.

There are two noteworthy considerations regarding therapeutic tasks of the first objective:

1. As clients begin to describe and reexperience conflict, they consciously or unconsciously use defenses to ward off the anxiety this awakens. The development of a good working relationship enables clients to tolerate increased anxiety in the working phase.

2. As clients become familiar with self-assessment, they may modify original personal goals, or develop additional goals, in keeping with what they have learned.

It is important in the working phase for the psychiatric nurse to encourage client self-assessment of growth-facilitating and growth-inhibiting behaviors. After assessing one specific response, the client is often able to transfer this skill to begin assessing other aspects of life as well. A realistic self-assessment process is perhaps the most valuable skill that the client can "take home." It is often thrilling for the nurse to experience the client "taking over" and further applying realistic assessment skills developed in one-to-one work. As the above discussion indicates,

TABLE 26–5 Verbatim Example, Working Phase

Verbatim Interaction	Nursing Intervention	Rationale
Client: My nosy relatives are at it again. Since my mother died and I'm living alone, they keep phoning me to see if I'm all right.		
Nurse: You sound irritated. . . .	Reflection of feeling tone to explore client's reaction to this situation	Reflection of feeling tone encourages client to validate or clarify emotive response to situation
Client: Not irritated—mad! Those phonies don't care about me. Why should they! Why should they?!? They don't.		
Nurse: What do you think motivates them to call?	Seeking clarification about how client perceives the immediate situation	Clarifying statements help explore the meaning of this specific situation as perceived by the client
Client: To pester me. People do it all the time. That one woman at work that I told you about last week—she does the same thing. She smiles and says good morning. She's concerned . . . but I don't want anything to do with her either.		
Nurse: You're talking about two situations where you don't want to deal with people: your relatives and the woman at work. I remember your description of how you wanted to avoid an old classmate last month. Is there something common to all these situations?	Actively linking elements of several behavioral patterns accumulated over time (current session, last session, last month) to search for commonality	Elements of one pattern may link to others with a gradual unfolding of central life patterns
Client: I can't see anything—except that I go out of my way to avoid people. I avoid everyone. I live alone and want to stay alone.		

INTERVENTION

Goals, Tasks, and Interventions in the Working (Middle) Phase

Goals	Therapeutic Tasks	Nursing Interventions
Behavioral analysis (mutual determination of dynamics of response patterns identified by client, especially those considered dysfunctional)	Identification and detailed exploration of important response patterns	Explore response pattern in depth, including origin, causes, operation, and effect of pattern (intrapersonally and interpersonally)
		Separate environmental factors (familial, political, economic, cultural) from intrapersonal factors
		Link elements of one response pattern to other patterns as appropriate, for a gradual unfolding of central life patterns
	Analysis of client's mode of conflict resolution	Encourage detailed exploration of how client reacts to reduce anxiety associated with conflict
		Increase awareness of defenses employed to ward off anxiety awakened by such exploration
	Facilitation of client self-assessment of growth-producing and growth-inhibiting response patterns	Encourage client to evaluate each response pattern to determine which are self-defeating and/or thwart gratification of basic needs
Constructive change in behavior, especially in dysfunctional response patterns identified by client	Address forces that inhibit desired change (troublesome thoughts, feelings, and behaviors)	Assist client in challenging client's personal resistance to change
		Use problem-solving strategies, active decision making, and personal accountability
		Assist client to learn and apply problem-solving strategies
		Encourage client to assert own needs when external environmental conditions (group, agency, institution) are an inhibiting force
	Create an atmosphere offering permission for active experimentation to test and assess effectiveness of new behaviors	Allow freedom to make and assess mistakes and blunders
		Avoid parental judgment of any behavioral experimentation—encourage client self-assessment instead

▶

INTERVENTION (continued)

Goals, Tasks, and Interventions in the Working (Middle) Phase

Goals	Therapeutic Tasks	Nursing Interventions
	Facilitate development of coping skills to deal with anxiety associated with constructive changes in behavior	Address, rather than avoid, anxiety and its manifestations
		Strengthen existing growth-promoting coping skills, especially regarding unalterable conditions (e.g., terminal illness, physical deformity, loss of significant other by death)
		Encourage development of new coping skills and their application of actual life experiences

assessment is an ongoing process for both the client and the nurse in the working phase.

The initial goal of behavioral analysis of client's response patterns continues throughout the working phase. The goal is achieved when the client has awareness of, understanding of, and insight into the causes and manifestations of patterns in the current personality structure and can assess these major trends.

Diagnosing In the working phase, nursing diagnoses may be revised, expanded, or deleted to more accurately reflect a central pattern of concern in the evolving one-to-one relationship. In the previous clinical example, the nurse made a tentative diagnosis of fear related to employment. An additional nursing diagnosis of dysfunctional grieving was added later. This second diagnosis was given higher priority because, as the client indicates, it is related to difficulty in overall functioning ability.

As the working phase proceeds, the priority assigned to a nursing diagnosis may change, e.g., when the client is able to implement positive change in some areas. Those nursing diagnoses designated as "potential problems" may move up or down on the priority list, depending on what interventions, if any, have been effective. A potential diagnosis may decrease in priority after preventive health education, if both the client and the nurse evaluate this intervention as beneficial.

Implementing Interventions   In the working phase, planning is ideally done collaboratively between

client and nurse. Such planning involves frequent consideration of the client's initial goals. When planning has been systematic and thorough, there is hardly a moment to worry about "what to do." The short-term and long-term treatment goals in the form of the therapeutic contract are a map indicating the direction, momentum, and steps needed to reach a designated point.

There is, however, a potential danger in the implementation of the planning component: moving too quickly and incompletely through an exploration of the client's feelings and thoughts in an attempt to fulfill a designated goal. *Slowness* and *thoroughness* are all-important here. Change needs to take place in the client's feelings, thoughts, and behaviors. If change does not occur in all aspects, then it is destined to be short-lived and ineffectual in the long run and may contribute to client discouragement.

When the client is working on an issue that is unresolved at the end of a meeting, it is often helpful to summarize the unfinished work for the next meeting. This technique may help the client anticipate, plan, or prepare to tackle this area of concern again. Personal experiments, such as trying out new behaviors in real situations, may be encouraged between sessions. Some clients may be able to continue working through a problem on their own between meetings.

Active intervention is especially important to achieve the second goal of the working phase. This goal is the initiation of constructive changes in behavior, particularly in self-defeating, growth-inhibiting behavior patterns. Establishing behavioral change flows from the first goal of behavioral analysis. The objectives are interrelated and essential for successful therapeutic work. Understanding and insight need to be complemented by behavioral implementation. This statement deserves much attention, since particular clients may consistently generate and thrive on sophisticated insights while continuing to assume a powerless stance about implementing constructive change in their condition. The Intervention box on page 635 also highlights therapeutic tasks and specific nursing interventions for the second goal.

The psychiatric nurse also uses active experimentation to test the effect of new behaviors. The introverted male client who resolved to establish relationships with women may assume various postures (cavalier, paternal, seductive) with a female psychiatric nurse to determine the appropriateness of these behaviors before displaying them outside of sessions. Permission to "try on" or role play new ways of being must also include freedom to make mistakes. Errors and blunders are rich sources of additional learning and occasional fun. A client who is able to see humor in errors in a nondefeatist manner has acquired a new skill. The client can be encouraged to apply this skill, and any other coping skills learned in relationship work, to normal maturational and situational crises encountered throughout life.

In in-patient settings, the nurse must work with other members of the staff to make all members of the team aware of the meaning of the client's behavior as positive actions that may be exaggerated at first. For example, some staff members may encourage a depressed client to verbalize anger and begin by shouting. If there is no staff collaboration, the client may receive negative feedback (e.g., room restrictions) for testing out new coping skills.

Problem-Solving Strategies   **Problem-solving strategies,** as a mode of intervention, are particularly important in the working phase. Problem-solving strategies are essential after the client has identified, explored, and assessed important behavioral patterns. The psychiatric nurse can help the client use the sequential problem-solving strategies discussed below.

Observation   Observation as a problem-solving strategy involves gathering and analyzing facts about a potential problem area. It eliminates opinions and impressions and emphasizes facts. Observation, as an aspect of assessment, is discussed earlier in this chapter.

Definition   Definition is perhaps the most significant and far-reaching problem-solving strategy. It involves an initial specification of a problem, followed by a question. Starting a problem-solving exploration with the word "How" (for example, How is it? How

does it manifest itself? How has this come about?) focuses on the process regarding a specific problem. It is generally more useful than asking "Why," which emphasizes rationale. ("Why" questions are explored in Chapter 8.)

Next, it is helpful to determine whether the problem involves fact finding (calling for data answers), judgment or decision, or creative exploration. In dealing with problems requiring creative exploration, all the ideas that imagination can produce may be helpful. Thus, evaluation is temporarily deferred or suspended to allow for the consideration of numerous alternatives.

The following clinical material illustrates definition of the most basic form of a problem:

Fern is a 19-year-old, single female seeking individual counseling at a local university counseling center. She was referred because she felt depressed following a split with her boyfriend over the summer. Emotional concerns included a marked feeling of depression, plus verbalized feelings of guilt, loneliness, and confusion. Physical concerns involved sleep disturbance (difficulty falling asleep with resultant sense of fatigue), eating disturbance (increased compulsive eating when under stress, with subsequent sudden weight gain), and minor self-mutilation (picking skin around fingernails and scratching face). Fern denied suicidal ideation and appeared to be a minimal suicide risk. She showed a general flatness of affect, characterized by very slow and monotonous speech, minimal facial or body gestures, and periodic silences and quiet weeping. She lives in an apartment with three female roommates and maintains a 3.8 academic average as a junior student majoring in biology. She negotiated for weekly one-hour sessions of individual psychotherapy for the duration of the school year. The following exchanges occurred in the final ten minutes of the third session:

Fern: This weekend will be a long weekend. I don't know what to do.

Nurse: I'd like to hear more about this long weekend.

Fern: Well, Marc might want to go out with someone else, so I don't want to take up his time. My three roommates are busy. . . . I don't want to call Marty. . . . My friend Judy won't be home.

Nurse: Which of these is most troublesome for you?

Fern: Well, I don't care about Marc anymore. . . . My roommates are always busy. . . . Sometimes Judy gets on my nerves.

Nurse: What do you suppose is the problem about all this?

Fern: I feel that I'm not going to have a good time. I won't study. Usually no one is home, and I'll be lonely. Yeah, . . . I'll be lonely again.

Nurse: The problem with this long weekend seems to be more loneliness for you.

Fern (Sighs): That sums it up.

In this example, the client moved from identifying several subproblems to the more basic problem of loneliness. The nurse assisted the client by encouraging definition and reflecting the probable central theme back to the client.

Preparation   Preparation involves collecting additional pertinent data related to the basic problem that may prove useful in later stages of problem-solving strategies. This aspect of problem-solving enables the nurse and client to anticipate which data might be most useful.

Analysis   As a problem-solving strategy, analysis involves breaking down the relevant material into subproblems so that each subproblem may be assessed separately.

Ideation   Ideation involves accumulating alternative ideas on how to resolve the basic problem. The following clinical material illustrates Fern's initial use of ideation as a problem-solving strategy in the beginning of the fourth session:

Fern: My weekend wasn't that bad. (Laughs mildly.)

Nurse: Let's hear about it.

Fern: Well, Saturday night I went out to dinner with my roommate, and Friday night I went to the movies.

Nurse: I wonder what were the "good" and "bad" parts of this.

Fern: Well, I can honestly say that I enjoyed the movie, and dinner with Sara (roommate) was OK, too.

Nurse: What did you do to make your weekend "not that bad"?

Fern: Well, I planned my time, so I wasn't always alone. I had some studying to do for one exam.

Fern changed the topic to discuss one teacher who added requirements to his course. When she mentioned the weekend again, the nurse tried to refocus.

Nurse: Fern, are you aware of any steps involved in dealing with loneliness over the weekend?

Fern: Yeah. I actively sought out doing things. I made sure that I was doing things.

Nurse: Can you be more specific?

Fern: I kept busy. I had to study. I went to the library on Saturday so I wasn't home alone. I told you about going out to dinner and the movie.

Incubation   Incubation is used when the problem-solving process or one aspect of it is set aside for a period of time to allow for illumination.

Synthesis   As a problem-solving strategy, synthesis involves putting together all elements of the basic problem, subproblems, and possible alternatives.

Evaluation   Evaluation consists of making judgments about the resultant ideas.

Development   As a final problem-solving strategy, development involves planning the implementation of these ideas.

Problem-solving abilities may improve with time and experience. During the eighth session, Fern and the nurse were skilled enough to piece together Fern's definition of her current problem: how to handle angry feelings without feeling trapped by them.

The situation precipitating that exploration was that Fern's roommate repeatedly left dishes in the sink for days, after having agreed to clean them nightly. Fern identified two problem-solving alternatives in this session. First, Fern could set the dirty dishes aside for her roommate to see. She evaluated this activity to be a less satisfactory solution, since her roommate might then avoid the kitchen area. Second, Fern might directly share her anger with the roommate. Fern previously avoided sharing anger directly with anyone. She anticipated that she could maintain her assertive position by justifying that everyone has to help with housework. Fern judged that if her roommate washed the dishes, then the outcome would be satisfactory for her.

Fern used preparation and incubation as problem-solving strategies in the interim between the seventh and eighth sessions. Synthesis was apparent in Fern's integration of known subproblems of an identified problem and active seeking of alternatives. She used ideation and evaluation in her identification of problem-solving alternatives and evaluation of the potential outcome of each. In informal relationship work, some or all elements may be used in a similar manner.

Challenging the Client's Resistance to Change

The nurse also assists the client by challenging the client's resistance to change. There are two major categories of forces that inhibit desired change:

1. Intrapersonal forces, which may arise from troublesome thoughts, feelings, or behaviors. Examples include thoughts that hamper the client's sense of worth, the client's inability to control and express emotion appropriately, or the client's inability to relate to others in a meaningful manner.

2. The client's personal resistance to change, which is the greatest inhibiting force. In fact, the client's challenge to this resistance constitutes the major work in one-to-one relationships.

Problems of resistance and general intervention strategies are discussed earlier in this chapter. Of equal significance is the previous discussion of transference and countertransference phenomena, as these may require careful, planned nursing interventions. Sometimes transference and countertransference are so intense that they become a problem for the beginning psychiatric nurse.

Evaluating Several levels of evaluation occur simultaneously in the working phase. First, the nurse does an ongoing evaluation of the client's various levels of intrapersonal and interpersonal functioning. Feedback from family, community agencies, or the client's employer may enhance any current comprehensive evaluation. For example, does the client seem to be facing an impending crisis? If so, the nurse may choose to switch from intrapersonal exploration to a crisis intervention strategy. Second, the nurse encourages client self-evaluation, as explored in previous discussion. Finally, the nurse constantly performs self-evaluation as a helping person growing in skill and experience. Nursing self-evaluation is done by informal discussions with staff and other mental health personnel and by formal clinical supervision.

"On-the-spot" evaluations of relevant short-term and long-term goals can occur during any meeting with the client. For example, as the client talks about increasing socialization skills, the nurse may reflect: "Let's look at our contract together. You originally wanted to date a girl of your choice for two hours during an evening without leaving the situation. How do you think this compares with what you're now saying has happened?" The nurse supports any effort at evaluation on the part of the client and explores what else needs to happen for the client to achieve the short-term goal. An additional area of evaluation involves the client's "trying on" alternative behaviors to determine if these new behaviors may work for the client.

The client and nurse should mutually evaluate the appropriateness of goals in any one of the following areas in the light of current functioning: degree of client success in achieving specific goals, client's growth-producing and growth-inhibiting behavior patterns, and unfinished business that must be resolved to achieve a desired goal. In addition, the working phase may also involve ongoing evaluations of the status, characteristics, and depth of the nurse-client relationship. The client may view the nurse in different ways (parent, sibling, friend) at various times. It is only when the client makes these views explicit that the nurse may intervene to clarify roles and responsibilities in a facilitative manner.

The psychiatric nurse and the client have moved through the first two phases of therapeutic relationships when:

- They have established a working relationship

- They have analyzed the dynamics of the client's behavioral patterns

- The client has effectively instituted behavioral changes in keeping with the therapeutic contract

In informal relationship work, the nurse may touch on only one or two aspects of the middle (working) phase. Even the advanced psychiatric nurse rarely addresses all therapeutic tasks in this phase of relationship work.

Termination (End) Phase

During the termination (end) phase of one-to-one relationships, the psychiatric nurse and client discontinue contact. This phase is as important as the previous two phases, although both the nurse and client frequently avoid it because of past difficulties with separation.

The goal of the end phase is termination of the one-to-one relationship in a mutually planned, satisfying manner. The nurse should remind the client that termination was first addressed in the orientation phase, when the duration of the relationship was discussed. The nurse also needs to emphasize the growth and positive aspects of the relationship, rather than focus exclusively on separation.

A smooth and complete termination sometimes occurs in actual practice. In informal relationship work in in-patient settings, termination more often occurs with the client's abrupt departure or planned medical discharge. Even in formal relationship work in community settings, contact often ceases without explanation after a series of missed appointments, or with a phone call by the client to inform the therapist of the client's decision to terminate, or with the client abruptly leaving a session and failing to resume subsequent contact. In these instances, the nurse can call or write the client and suggest an additional session to deal with either the therapeutic good-bye or a willingness to continue the relationship work. Termination requires careful preparation, adequate time for the client to work through the feelings about ending, and an opportunity for the psychiatric nurse to explore personal reactions with a clinical instructor, colleague, supervisor, or consultant.

Assessing Assessment as a component of the nursing process in the resolution phase deals primarily with determining when the client may be ready to terminate, how the client deals with termination, and how the nurse deals with termination. The following criteria may be useful to determine whether the client is ready to terminate:

- *Relief from the presenting problem.* Symptoms no longer interfere with the client's comfort.

• *Achievement of treatment goals.* These ideally are planned goals included in the therapeutic contract between the nurse and client.

• *Improvement in social functioning.* The client experiences increased satisfaction in interpersonal relationships.

• *Acquisition of adaptive coping strategies.* Ideally, these strategies include the client's use of effective problem-solving strategies on a daily basis.

• *Acquisition of more effective defense mechanisms.* A client who cannot achieve adaptive coping strategies should develop more effective defense mechanisms to ensure stabilization.

• *Attainment of identity.* The client experiences self-satisfaction and no longer needs to depend on the nurse for a sense of well-being.

• *Disruption due to a major impasse in the one-to-one relationship.* Stubborn resistances may surface and persist on the part of the client. Uncontrollable countertransference may develop on the part of the nurse.

Many factors influence how the client reacts to termination. These factors include:

• *Degree of client involvement.* The greater the involvement, the more intense the client's reaction to termination.

• *Length of treatment.* In general, the longer the nurse-client relationship lasts, the more time should be spent in exploring all aspects of termination.

• *Client's past history of significant losses.* A client who has lost significant others may reexperience past conflicts and emotional responses.

• *Ability to separate from others.* The reaction to termination is influenced by how well the client has mastered the early separation-individuation phase of development.

• *Degree of success achieved.* Reaction to termination depends on how successful and satisfying the relationship has been for the client.

• *Degree of transference in the relationship.* The greater the transference in the nurse-client relationship, the more intense the client's reaction to termination.

The psychiatric nurse must be alert to client responses during termination. Any number of client responses (e.g., repression, regression, anger, denial, sadness, withdrawal, avoidance, acceptance, or joy) may surface. It is not unusual for several to surface at once. When repressing, the client shows no emotional response. Regression on the part of the client is an extremely common response to termination. Regressive behavior may range from statements of abandonment and hopelessness to inability to tend to personal hygiene. The central message conveyed is: "See? I can't make it without you!"

Finally, assessment involves how the nurse personally manages separation in the one-to-one relationship. Like the client, the nurse can have any number of responses. Some common responses are:

• Regret that the client did not achieve more than the client actually did

• Hesitation to give up the dependency elements of the relationship

• Collusion with the client to prolong sessions to avoid the inevitability of separation

Diagnosing   Nursing diagnoses during termination should reflect the termination behaviors manifested by the client. A wide variety of nursing diagnoses may be relevant. Potential nursing diagnoses that stem from regression during the termination phase may be: self-care deficit, hopelessness, powerlessness, and ineffective individual coping. These and other nursing diagnoses should be modified as necessary as the client moves through the termination experience.

Implementing Interventions   Planning involves the preparing for the final good-bye and making any needed referrals (to another nurse or therapist, self-help group, community agency, or job-training program). When a referral is made, it is often wise for the client to have an initial contact with the referred person or agency before termination. In this way, the nurse can immediately deal with any initial misconceptions. Termination should include mutual planning about where the client may seek future help if the need arises. Options most frequently include returning to the nurse, referral to crisis services, or referral to other community agencies. The shift to dependence on other support systems (referrals, family, friends) is a therapeutic task requiring the psychiatric nurse's awareness of planning and intervention strategy.

Intervention strategies vary according to the behaviors manifested by the client. The nurse may respond to the client who is repressing the reality of termination by repeatedly observing that the client is not addressing the issue of the impending separation. The nurse may then attempt to explore this avoidance with the client. Useful interventions for clients who are regressing in response to termination include the following:

• Address the possible underlying fears of abandonment

- Emphasize the growth achieved by the client

- Continue to focus on the realities of separation

The acting-out client may protest termination in numerous ways (suicide gestures or attempts, psychiatric hospitalization, terminating employment, rejection of therapist) before the termination date. In general, the underlying feelings, fears, and fantasies need ventilation, exploration, and working through. The client reactions of anger, depression, or grief require the same. An exception to this general guideline is the client who uses distraction maneuvers, such as introducing explosive new material in final sessions. The following clinical example illustrates a client's manipulative attempts to prevent termination by using acting-out behaviors. The psychiatric nurse used limit setting rather than exploration because of time constraints specific to this one-to-one work. The example also illustrates that there may be "unfinished business" despite planning and effort.

Kim was a 19-year-old, single female who was self-referred to a local university student counseling center. Her chief complaint was an inability to maintain relationships with both female and male peers. her history included excessive experimentation with drugs and frequent superficial sexual encounters with males who subsequently mistreated and left her.

Kim negotiated for two semesters of individual psychotherapy and was informed that after that time, the psychiatric nurse would not be available because she was being relocated. Kim's behavior in the sessions was characterized by attempts to trap the nurse, displace and project anger onto others, and avoid accountability for her presenting problem. Although termination was carefully planned and referral sources considered, Kim resisted by offering money, crying, and leaving sessions early. She resisted exploration of any thoughts or feelings regarding termination and refused to consider referral.

During the last session, she eagerly reported having her first homosexual experience with a woman who resembled the nurse. She then asked how the one-to-one relationship could end without exploring this new behavior. The nurse was aware of the far-reaching implications of this final issue in terms of Kim's psychodynamics as well as its impact on the one-to-one work. The nurse was also aware of Kim's challenging attitude associated with another attempt, this time regarding sexual acting out, to prolong sessions. The nurse emphasized that this explosive issue needed further exploration, again discussed and encouraged use of referrals, and addressed the issue of good-bye. Both nurse and client were dissatisfied with the time limitation in this case. A sense of mutual termination was not realized.

The nurse has the final task of participating in an explicit and therapeutic good-bye with the client. Nursing responsibilities in this final phase include anticipating the nurse's personal reaction to separation and, optionally, expressing this reaction in a manner that does not burden the client. In addition, the nurse may share a special wish for the client, based on the client's particular assets within the therapeutic relationship. A therapeutic good-bye gives the client a sense of freedom to move on to other relationships. The end phase may take from one meeting to several months of meetings, depending on the duration of the one-to-one relationship. In general, the longer the duration of the relationship, the longer the time needed to deal explicitly with termination of contact. The Intervention box on page 642 summarizes the goal, therapeutic tasks, and specific nursing interventions of the end phase. Ideally, the client can completely work through feelings regarding separation so that there is no unfinished business between the psychiatric nurse and client. The nurse-client relationship has given the client the opportunity to depend on another in a realistic and mature manner. Assessment of the experience helps the client practice self-assessment skills and may help set the stage for additional relationship work in the future. The direct, explicit good-bye is frequently the first such experience for the client. It is usually a moment of unique humanness for both the psychiatric nurse and client.

Evaluating   Evaluation is a vital component of the nursing process during the resolution phase. The psychiatric nurse has the task of helping the client evaluate the therapeutic contract. The criteria for evaluation are the goals formulated in the orientation and working phases of the one-to-one relationship. Each goal is evaluated in terms of measurable, observable behavior. Were the goals appropriate, practical, and specific to the client? Did the goals actually help evaluate motivation and effort? Did the goals enable the client and nurse to evaluate progress and outcome? What are the therapeutic gains? What are the areas for possible further therapeutic work? How does the client evaluate motivation, effort, progress, and outcome?

The psychiatric nurse also assists client evaluation of the therapeutic experience in general. Evaluation of the experience may help set the stage for future psychotherapeutic work. Would the client seek a similar experience in the future, if deemed necessary? The nurse may also invite feedback from the client about the nurse's impact on the client. In certain clinical settings, the nurse also has the therapeutic task of evaluating the effectiveness of the psychiatric treatment service in relation to this particular client (Stanley 1984).

The nurse's personal ongoing self-evaluation also warrants emphasis here. It is essential that the psychiatric nurse continuously evaluate which personal

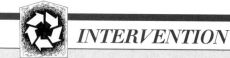

INTERVENTION

Goals, Tasks, and Interventions in the Termination (End) Phase

Goal	Therapeutic Tasks	Nursing Interventions
Termination of contact in a mutually planned, satisfying manner	Assist client evaluation of therapeutic contract and of therapeutic experience in general	Encourage client's realistic appraisal of personal therapeutic goals (motivation, effort, progress, outcome) as these evolved in treatment
		Provide appropriate feedback regarding appraisal of goals
		Review client's assets and therapeutic gains
		Review areas for further therapeutic work
	Encourage transference of dependence to other support systems	Encourage client to develop reliance on others in client's immediate environment (spouse, relative, employer, neighbor, friend) for empathic, emotional support
	Participate in explicit therapeutic good-bye with client	Be alert to surfacing of any behavior arising on termination (repression, regression, acting out, anger, withdrawal, acceptance)
		Assist client in working through feelings associated with these behaviors
		Anticipate own reaction to separation and share in a manner that does not burden client
		Allow "time" and "space" for termination; the longer the duration of the one-to-one relationship, the more time is needed for the termination phase

behaviors consciously or unconsciously promote, inhibit, and actively block growth-producing client abilities.

Supervision is essential if the one-to-one relationship is to be effective. Professional supervision helps the psychiatric nurse use transference effectively and recognize countertransference phenomena. The supportive function of supervision may be used to monitor the personal needs of the nurse and decrease the likelihood of severe clinical stress and burnout. There are various methods of evaluation: interpersonal process recordings, videotapes, client evaluations, audiotapes, didactic instruction, and referral to specific clinical readings. There are several kinds of supervision available, such as intradisciplinary supervision with a psychiatric clinical nurse specialist, or interdisciplinary supervision by another mental health professional (psychologist, psychiatrist, psychiatric social worker). All can be helpful, depending on the skills and availability of supervisors or consultants. Supervision helps the psychiatric nurse effectively define, initiate, use, and evaluate client and self in any therapeutic relationship.

CHAPTER HIGHLIGHTS

• A therapeutic one-to-one relationship may evolve in any nursing situation.

• The one-to-one relationship between psychiatric nurse and client is a mutually defined, mutually collaborative, goal-oriented professional relationship.

• Characteristics of a humanistic one-to-one relationship include openness, negotiation, commitment, responsibility, and authenticity.

• Client abilities that tend toward successful therapy outcomes include awareness and ownership of feelings, desire to change, and ability to differentiate feelings, concerns, and problems.

• The establishment of a therapeutic alliance is an essential ingredient of formal one-to-one relationship work.

• Psychiatric nurses need to be aware of both content and process in a one-to-one relationship.

• Resistance is best understood as the client's struggle against change; the humanistic stance is that the client has a right to resist the therapeutic process.

• One-to-one relationships may be organized around the nursing process.

• Phases of a therapeutic relationship include the orientation (beginning), working (middle), and termination (end).

• The orientation (beginning) phase of therapeutic relationships is characterized by the establishment of contact and the formation of a working relationship. This phase focuses on establishing rapport, obtaining pertinent information, initiating client assessment, developing a therapeutic contract between the client and nurse, and making practical arrangements for treatment.

• The working (middle) phase of the relationship is characterized by behavioral analysis and constructive behavioral change.

• The termination (end) phase of the therapeutic relationship is characterized by the termination of the relationship in a mutually planned, satisfying manner.

• Evaluation is an ongoing psychotherapeutic process as well as a step in the nursing process, and includes continuous evaluation of client behaviors, development of client self-evaluation, mutual evaluation of the relationship, and the nurse's self-evaluation in each one-to-one relationship.

REFERENCES

Arieti S (ed): *American Handbook of Psychiatry*, vols 1–7. Basic Books, 1974–1981.

Carter EW: Psychiatric nursing, in Kaplan HI, Sadock BJ: *Comprehensive Textbook of Psychiatry*, ed 4. Williams and Wilkins, 1985, pp 1936–1939.

Chessick R: *The Technique and Practice of Intensive Psychotherapy*. Jason Aronson, 1974.

Davanloo H: Short-term dynamic psychotherapy, in Kaplan HI, Sadock BJ: *Comprehensive Textbook of Psychiatry*, ed 4. Williams and Wilkins, 1985, pp 1460–1467.

deShazer S: *Clues: Investigating Solutions in Brief Therapy*. Norton, 1988.

Emrich K: Helping or hurting? Interacting in the psychiatric milieu. *J Psychosoc Nurs* 1989;27(12):26–29.

Fitzpatrick J et al.: *Nursing Models and Their Psychiatric Mental Health Applications*. Brady, 1982.

Forchuk C, Brown B: Establishing a nurse-client relationship. *J Psychosoc Nurs* 1989;27:30–34.

Hall E: *The Hidden Dimension*. Doubleday Anchor Books, 1966.

Hardin SB, Durham JD: First rate: Exploring the structure, process, and effectiveness of nurse psychotherapy. *J Psychosoc Nurs Ment Health Serv* 1985;23:9–15.

Heber S, Levin S, Sookram S: The nurse as short-term psychotherapist. *Can Nurse* 1984;80:32–35.

Herron WG, Rouslin S: *Issues in Psychotherapy*. Brady, 1982.

Hoeffer B, Murphy S: The unfinished task: Development of nursing theory for psychiatric and mental health nursing practice. *J Psychosoc Nurs Ment Health Serv* 1982;20:9–14.

Kaplan HI, Sadock BJ: *Comprehensive Textbook of Psychiatry*, ed 5. Williams and Wilkins, 1989.

Lakovics M: Classification of countertransference for utilization in supervision. *Am J Psychother* 1983;37:245–256.

Lamb H: One to one relationships with the long-term mentally ill: Issues in training professionals. *Comm Mental Health J* 1988;24(2):328–337.

Lego S: The one-to-one nurse-patient relationship, in Huey F (ed): *Psychiatric Nursing 1946–1974: A Report on the State of the Art*. American Journal of Nursing, 1975.

Lego S: Point/counterpoint: A psychotherapist is a psychotherapist . . ." *Perspect Psychiatr Care* 1980;18:27,39.

Leibenluft E, Goldberg R: Guidelines for short-term inpatient psychotherapies *Am J Psychiatry* 1986;143(12):1507–1517.

Loomis M: Levels of contracting. *J Psychosoc Nurs* 1985;23(3):8–14.

Pasquali E: Learning to laugh: Humor and therapy. *J Psychosoc Nurs* 1990;28(3):31–38.

Peplau H: Future directions in psychiatric nursing from the perspective of history. *J Psychosoc Nurs* 1989:27(2):18–21, 25–28, 39–40.

Peplau H: *Interpersonal Relations in Nursing.* Putnam, 1952.

Peplau H: Interpersonal techniques: The crux of psychiatric nursing. *Am J Nurs* 1962;62:50–54.

Robitaille-Tremblay M: A data collection tool for the psychiatric nurse. *Can Nurse* 1984;81:26–31.

Schuable P, Pierce R: Client in therapy behavior: A therapist guide to progress. *Psychotherapy* 1974;11:229–234.

Stanley R: Evaluation of treatment goals: The use of goal attainment scaling. *J Adv Nurs* 1984;9(4):351–356.

Strupp HH, Blackwood GL: Recent methods of psychother-apy, in Kaplan HI, Sadock BJ: *Comprehensive Textbook of Psychiatry,* ed 4. Williams and Wilkins, 1985.

Ursano R, Hales R: A review of brief individual psychotherapies. *Am J Psychiatry* 1986;143(12):1507–1517.

Ward M: The nursing process in psychiatry. I. The teachers' dilemma. *Nurs Times* 1984;80(24):37–39.

Witherspoon V: Using Lakovic's system. Countertransference classifications. *J Psychosoc Nurs Mental Health Serv* 1985;23:30–34.

Wolberg L: *The Technique of Psychotherapy,* vols 1 and 2. Grune and Stratton, 1988.

Stress Management

LEARNING OBJECTIVES

- Discuss the bases on which stress-management techniques appear to be effective

- Enumerate the therapeutic uses of each of the stress-management techniques discussed in this chapter

- Describe the stress-management techniques discussed in this chapter

- Practice stress-management strategies before using them with clients

- Apply stress-management strategies to the care of clients in any health care or community setting

- Apply stress-management techniques at a personal level to enhance personal and professional functioning

- Teach clients and their families how to use stress-management techniques to promote, maintain, and restore emotional well-being

Carol Ren Kneisl

CROSS REFERENCES

Other topics relevant to this content are: Anxiety disorders, Chapter 14; Psychophysiologic disorders, Chapter 18; Psychotropic medications that may cause hypotension during stress-reduction exercises, Chapter 32; Role of stress, anxiety, and coping, Chapter 5.

HELPING CLIENTS TO MANAGE stress creatively and helping nurses to manage their own stress creatively are the subjects of this chapter. Although no one can escape all the stresses of life completely, one can learn to counteract habitual counterproductive responses to them. Being able to relax decreases the alarm response to stress and returns the body to a more normal or balanced state.

Although we do not know exactly how stress-reduction techniques work, research shows that most persons find them helpful. These techniques help people gain control of their lives and ease tension before it becomes unmanageable. As a result, the quality of their lives is enhanced.

Nurses in any setting can use the techniques described in this chapter. Other techniques, such as autogenic training, self-hypnosis, and biofeedback, require additional training or equipment and are discussed only briefly in this chapter. To learn more about them, refer to the references at the end of this chapter. This chapter explores stress-reduction techniques that go beyond the everyday ways to cope with stress discussed in Chapter 5.

The Nursing Role in the Creative Management of Stress

Stress management is a creative and powerful tool as long as clients learn to use the methods properly. Unfortunately, many clients do not reduce the stresses in their lives because they do not realize that they are at the mercy of involuntary *fight-or-flight* responses. Many fail to identify environmental, physiologic, or cognitive sources of stress.

Like clients in any other health care setting, psychiatric clients must endure time pressures, weather, noise, crowds, interpersonal demands, job performance demands, and various threats to security and self-esteem. Genetics, developmental changes, biochemical makeup, aging, illness, nutrition, and sleep patterns are some of the physiologic factors influencing how well people cope with stress. The accompanying Psychobiology box focuses on the connection between stress and sleep disorders. And, perhaps more than clients in many of the other settings in which nurses practice, psychiatric clients experience cognitive stress because of how they interpret and label their experiences. For instance, a client might interpret the boss's facial expression as amused rather than pleased or as disgruntled rather than quizzical. This interpretation is likely to provoke anxiety. Dwelling on one's concerns and anxieties causes physical tension in the body, which in turn creates the subjective feeling of uneasiness and leads to more anxious thoughts.

The nurse should begin with the assessment phase of the nursing process to identify clients who might benefit from stress-management techniques. Assessment of stress and anxiety are discussed in Chapters 5 and 14. Once assessment has been accomplished, nurses can play a significant role in making clients aware of these methods and facilitating their effective use. Of course, if planning to use these techniques to help others who are experiencing stress, nurses must first develop personal familiarity with them.

Monitoring Physical Problems

Anyone undergoing a stress-reduction program should first discuss the program with the health care provider monitoring any physical problems. Because these techniques lower the blood pressure, decrease the heart rate, and reduce pain and anxiety, persons beginning a stress-reduction program should have their medications closely monitored. Monitoring is particularly important for psychiatric clients receiving psychotropic medications that may cause hypotension.

Experimenting with What Works

It is not necessary to use every suggestion or technique in this chapter. If a particular technique for stress reduction or relaxation doesn't seem to help, move on to another one. What is important is to give each a fair trial and experiment to find out what works in each person's individual situation.

Enhancing Chances of Success

Stress management is not magical; one has to work at it and enhance chances of success through regular practice. It is unrealistic to expect that simply reading about these techniques is all that is required to use them in times of stress or that everyone will be able to make a commitment to daily practice. The following nursing actions help clients to make the commitment and to follow through:

• Recommending stress-reduction strategies to clients and their families

• Providing information about stress-reduction strategies that are likely to meet clients' specific needs

• Encouraging clients to make the decision to practice relaxation

• Encouraging clients to devote this time to themselves alone

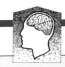

PSYCHOBIOLOGY: THE MIND/BODY CONNECTION

Troubled Sleep for Troubled People

Sleep is a mystery, and the stuff of which myths are made. Rip Van Winkle, so Washington Irving's story goes, fell asleep one evening in the Catskill Mountains, only to awaken befuddled and stooped with age twenty years later. According to the Greek legend, the Romans killed Perseus by depriving him of sleep. While it is highly unlikely that any of us will sleep for twenty years or die from lack of sleep, one in three of us, or as many as 100 million Americans, is sleep-deprived or has problems with falling asleep, staying asleep, or getting enough restful sleep. Sleep deprived persons have more accidents, are more irritable, and have problems with memory, concentration, and learning.

Sleep disturbance is one of the earliest symptoms of impending psychosis and of an impending suicide attempt, and insomnia is one of the most common concerns of psychiatric clients. Depressed persons have several abnormal sleep patterns. Their insomnia is more likely to be a difficulty in remaining asleep rather than a difficulty in falling asleep. Depressed persons may also have frequent awakenings during the night, early-morning awakenings, and hypersomnia (increased total sleep time). Persons with schizophrenia, anxiety disorders, and post-traumatic stress disorder experience disturbances of sleep, most probably an effect of extreme anxiety. An increasing incidence and severity of nightmares can signal a schizophrenic episode. Alcoholics and persons with post-traumatic stress disorder are particularly prone to sleep-disturbing dreams.

Scientists have learned much about the mysterious process of sleep. Although the basic question—Why do we sleep?—has not yet been answered, we do know that sleep has value for the entire body, especially the brain. Sleep helps to repair the wear and tear of consciousness on the brain, aids in taking in information, and enhances memory.

The study of the biology of sleep has yielded several interesting bits of information. Electroencephalograms of the brain's electrical activity show that sleep alternates through two major states. The first stage, *non-REM sleep*, is a quiescent state of both light and deep sleep that occupies about three-quarters of our sleep time. Non-REM sleep offers restorative rest—the muscles relax, blood pressure and body temperature drop, and the heart rate and metabolism slow down. *REM (rapid eye movement) sleep*, sometimes called dream sleep, occurs at intervals and resembles wakefulness in many ways. The muscles move, eyes twitch, blood pressure rises and falls, and the heart rate speeds up and slows down. REM sleep occurs about every ninety minutes and lasts from five to twenty minutes at a time. Most of our dreaming occurs during REM sleep.

The natural cycle between sleep and wakefulness is regulated by two body mechanisms—the biologic clock and homeostasis. Located in the hypothalamus of the brain, *the biologic clock*, a bundle of 10,000 nerve cells about the size of a pinhead, controls both sleeping and waking up times. The biologic clock actually runs on solar energy—variations in the amount of sunlight that enters the eye, hits the retina, and sends messages from the optic nerve fibers of the retina to the brain. Recent research suggests that homeostasis, the body's natural tendency to seek equilibrium, provides the primary push toward sleep through an as yet unidentified sleep-inducing chemical that accumulates while a person is awake. The urge to sleep grows stronger and stronger as the amount of this chemical in the body increases.

Try some of the following very simple measures to help your clients fall asleep, fall back asleep if they awaken during the night, and sleep more soundly and more restfully:

Count sheep. This old-fashioned remedy is not a myth. It actually works by distracting both the left brain and the right brain. While the left hemisphere does the counting, the right hemisphere conjures up the images, boring the person to sleep.

Meditate. Some of the early experiments on the relaxation response to meditation showed that the body's metabolism drops further during a twenty-minute meditation than it does during eight hours of sleep. The restful hypometabolic physiology of the relaxation response substitutes for some of the lost sleep by converting useless time to a chance to rest very deeply. Counting

▶

PSYCHOBIOLOGY: THE MIND/BODY CONNECTION (continued)

sheep is a form of meditation, as are the deep-breathing exercises outlined in this chapter.

Eat a carbohydrate nightcap. Carbohydrates stimulate the secretion of insulin. Insulin then washes all amino acids except tryptophan from the blood. This allows tryptophan to reach the brain in larger quantities, where it stimulates the production of *serotonin*, a brain chemical that calms and focuses the mind and induces sleep. Try a few crackers, some pasta, or a piece of toast with jelly or jam. Avoid protein foods because they introduce the amino acid tyrosine into the body. *Tyrosine* stimulates the production of dopamine and norepinephrine, the brain's alertness chemicals and mental energizers. The traditional glass of warm milk, while a natural source of tryptophan, is *not* a good nightcap because of its high protein content.

Avoid coffee and other beverages, food, and medications that contain caffeine (caffeine is chemically related to amphetamines and is a powerful central nervous system stimulant). Some of these are, ranked in order of caffeine content: one Dexatrim tablet (200 mg), two Excedrin tablets (130 mg), one NoDoz tablet (100 mg), a cup of instant coffee (50-75 mg), a can of Diet Coke (46 mg), a cup of tea (35-46 mg), a can of Pepsi (36 mg), one Midol tablet (32 mg), a cup of hot cocoa (5-10 mg), a one-ounce chocolate bar (1-15 mg). Because caffeine's "buzz" usually peaks two to four hours after it is taken, it is best to avoid caffeine in the evening hours.

Avoid using alcoholic beverages to make yourself drowsy. A rebound phase of excitement of the sympathetic nervous system, similar to the fight-flight response discussed in Chapter 5, occurs a few hours after a drink. People often awaken feeling anxious and restless because of this nervous system shift. Alcohol also suppresses REM sleep. Because the body naturally tries to make up lost REM sleep, a person's sleep the night *after* a night of drinking is likely to contain more dreams. This explains why alcoholics often experience nightmares and disturbed sleep for weeks and even months after becoming sober.

Use sleeping pills only as a temporary measure. People become quickly habituated to most sleeping medications and require increasing amounts of the medication to achieve the same result. In this case, more is not better. Withdrawal from sleeping pills should be gradual and supervised by a physician. Sleep induced by sleeping pills is usually of poorer quality, and marked by less REM sleep and less deep sleep. The person often wakes up feeling tired and lethargic.

Investigate your client's medication regimen. Many prescription and over-the-counter drugs interfere with sleep.

Avoid going to sleep while listening to the radio or the television. Because our bodies can't tell the difference between what is actually happening and what we imagine is happening in our dreams, restless, tense, or disturbing dreams will affect how we feel upon awakening. We have enough to do in contending with what our own mind manufactures without adding the fantasies of others on television or radio. We are particularly open to disturbing influences at the time of falling asleep.

Avoid using nicotine. Nicotine is a powerful stimulant that can also interfere with sleep. Heavy smokers have more trouble falling asleep, wake up more often during the night, and have less deep and REM sleep than nonsmokers.

If all else fails, suggest that your client try a sleep disorders clinic.

—*Carol Ren Kneisl*

• Enlisting the support of family members, fellow workers, and friends in meeting clients' need for uninterrupted time in a quiet setting

• Encouraging family members, fellow workers, and friends to lend verbal support to the client

• Reminding family members, fellow workers, and friends that because they are also under stress, they too may find relaxation techniques helpful

Enhancing Relaxation with Music

Many persons find that listening to certain kinds of music is relaxing. Dentists have used music to help their clients relax and to mask the sounds of the drill. Several health care facilities use soothing music in conjunction with guided visualizations on audiotape or videotape as a substitute for or adjunct to pain medication and tranquilizers when the client chooses.

Sometimes the tapes are prescribed before or during surgery, during chemotherapy or kidney dialysis, and during recovery from spinal injury or burns.

The therapeutic use of music has led to a new health-related career. Music therapists use a combination of visual imagery and music to teach clients to lower their blood pressure ten to twenty points. Music with sixty beats per minute can help those with cardiac dysrhythmias achieve a more relaxed heart rate.

How does music achieve its relaxing effect? One theory is that music produces endorphins in the brain—the same "feel-good" chemicals that running and meditation produce. These natural opiates, secreted by the hypothalamus, reduce the intensity with which pain is felt.

Because persons vary in their response to music, encourage clients to experiment with different kinds of music to discover which has positive effects and then to develop their own personal library. A quicker way is for clients to purchase tapes and records specifically for stress reduction sold in bookstores and through catalogs. They are often available through the public library. Recommend that clients pay attention to their breathing as they listen to music. Slow and deep breathing enhances the relaxing effect of music.

Assessing Body Tension

Many persons fail to recognize stress in themselves. They direct their attention externally rather than internally. Because stress and body tension are simultaneous, one of the first steps in recognizing stress is to recognize tension in the body. Recognizing body tension helps people recognize stress and anxiety. **Body scanning** helps increase awareness of muscular tension.

Make sure that the spine is straight before beginning body scanning or any of the other exercises described in this chapter. Stand, sit, or lie on the floor—whichever is most comfortable—while maintaining a good posture.

Begin by closing your eyes and turning your attention to your own internal world by focusing on your body. Focus on your toes and move up slowly. As you do this, ask yourself: Where am I tense? Become aware of all of the muscles in your body and especially of the parts of your body that feel tense or tight. Note the location of the tenseness and talk to yourself about it, reminding yourself that muscular tension is self-produced. Perhaps you might say: "The muscles in the back of my neck feel tight. This means that I'm creating tension in my body. Tension causes me problems."

Body scanning should be a prelude to the stress-reduction techniques that follow. Use the body-scanning method to determine where tension collects in your body.

The importance of body states and their relationship to stress have been emphasized by Eastern philosophies such as yoga and zen. In this century, Western psychiatrists were persuaded to study this interaction by Wilhelm Reich, originally a student of Freud. Two contemporary therapies that focus on the body and its relationship to emotional stress are the bioenergetic therapy of Alexander Lowen and the gestalt therapy of Fritz Perls. Both emphasize the notion that the body registers stress long before the conscious mind does.

According to Lowen, body tension is an inevitable response to stress. Once stress is removed, tension goes away. In Lowen's theory, specific muscle groups are tightened by specific attitudes. For example, chronic neck tension and pain can occur in a person who believes that it is bad to express anger.

According to Perls, it is important to differentiate between external awareness (stimulation of the five senses from the outside world) and internal awareness (physical sensations or emotional discomfort or comfort within the body). This distinction helps people separate the world from one's physical reaction to it. Perls believes that we fail to feel the tension in our bodies because we direct most of our awareness to the outside world. Recognizing the tension in our bodies is the first step in reducing stress.

Keeping a Stress-Awareness Diary

Most people find that some parts of the day are more stressful than others and that some events produce more physical and emotional symptoms than others. Keeping a stress-awareness diary helps people identify how particular stresses result in predictable symptoms. Some persons react to interpersonal confrontations with a stomach upset or with diarrhea. Feeling rushed or overloaded with tasks or responsibilities may result in vasoconstriction and cause a headache or hypertension.

Clients can keep a stress-awareness diary to discover and chart their own personal stressful events and characteristic reactions. In the sample stress-awareness diary in Figure 27–1, a gasoline station manager records the events of a Friday. Note that it indicates the time that a stressful event took place as well as any physical or emotional reactions that could be related to the stressful event. Clients should keep a stress-awareness diary for at least two weeks, tracking this information daily.

Stress-Management Techniques

The stress-management techniques that follow are based on the belief that mind and body are interrelated and that the condition of one will eventually affect the

Stress Awareness Diary

Date _5/6/92_   Day of the week _Friday_

Time	Stressful Event	Physical and Emotional Reactions
6⁵⁰ AM	Alarm didn't go off; rushing to get to work	
7⁴⁵ AM	Late to relieve night clerk; he threatened to quit	
9³⁰		Slight headache; took aspirin
10⁰⁰		Headache pounding; aspirin not helping
11⁰⁰	Customer backs into gas pump & dents pump	Anger
2³⁰	Teenager drives away without paying for gas	Anger
3³⁰		Headache back
4⁰⁰	Employee calls in sick; have to call in relief worker	
5³⁰	Commute traffic heavy; twice as long to get home	Indigestion
7⁰⁰	Argument with son	
7⁰⁵	Wife defends son	
7¹⁰	Argument with wife	
7³⁰		Indigestion worse
8³⁰		Went to bed

FIGURE 27–1   Stress-awareness diary.

condition of the other. A relaxed body is incompatible with anxiety. If the body is relaxed, the mind will feel relaxed as well. These stress-management techniques teach you how to relax in order to enhance your personal life and your professional life as a nurse. You can then teach these relaxation techniques to clients in any type of health care setting.

Breathing Exercises

Under most circumstances, people take breathing for granted as an automatic body function. They usually become aware of their pattern of breathing only when it has gone awry, such as when they are out of breath. Nurses notice the apneic client or the client with Cheyne-Stokes respirations because they know something has gone wrong and that breathing is essential to life. Breathing properly can, by itself, reduce stress. Psychiatric nurses and maternal health nurses who prepare expectant women for labor have long recognized that breathing exercises can reduce tension. Unfortunately, breathing techniques are virtually ignored in other clinical areas.

Breathing calmly and deeply keeps the blood well oxygenated and purified. It helps to remove waste materials from the blood and clears thinking. Poorly oxygenated blood may contribute to fatigue, mental confusion, anxiety, muscular tension, and feelings of depression. The following exercises are designed to facilitate proper breathing.

Awareness of Breathing Do you breathe properly or does your breathing actually deprive you of oxygen? Take time to pay attention to your own breathing.

Begin by placing one hand just below your rib cage and taking a deep breath. Note what happened when you inhaled. Did your hand move in? Did your hand move out? Did your hand move at all? If your hand moved out, you were breathing properly. But if your hand moved in or didn't move at all it was probably because you learned, as most did, to hold your stomach in and push your chest out while breathing. People who breathe this way do not fill the lungs to full capacity; they fill only the top third or top half.

Deep Breathing During **deep breathing**, you move the diaphragm downward and fill the lower part of the lungs with air. The chest expands as the middle part fills with air, and the shoulders move upward as the upper part fills. To teach yourself or a client how to take deep, healthful breaths follow the directions in the accompanying Client/Family Teaching box.

Deep breathing becomes easier with practice. It may become almost automatic. This is an exercise few resist—it is easy to do, it is inconspicuous, and it gives fast results.

Ten-to-One Count This exercise is also quick and simple. Inhale, taking a deep breath, while saying the number 10 to yourself. Then exhale slowly, letting out all the air in your lungs. Inhale again saying the number 9 to yourself. As you exhale, tell yourself: "I feel more relaxed than I did at number 10." With your next breath, say the number 8 to yourself. As you exhale remind yourself: "I feel more relaxed than I did at number 9." Continue counting down and experience increasing calmness as you approach the number 1. Some persons use an abbreviated version and begin

---

CLIENT/FAMILY TEACHING

Deep-Breathing Guidelines

- Sit, stand, or lie with your spine straight.
- Scan for body tension.
- Place one hand on your chest and the other on your abdomen.
- Inhale slowly and deeply so that your abdomen pushes up your hand.
- Visualize your lungs slowly filling with air. Your chest should move only slightly as you inhale, but you should be aware of the movement of your abdomen.
- Exhale through your mouth, making a soft, whooshing sound by blowing gently. Keep your face, mouth, and jaw relaxed.

- Be aware of what it feels like and what you sound like when you breathe properly.
- Continue to take long, slow, deep breaths for at least ten minutes at a time, once or twice a day.
- Increase the frequency if you wish once you have mastered the technique.
- Scan your body for tension again, comparing the tension to what it was like before you began the deep-breathing exercise.

counting at the number 5; others require the full count of 10 to feel calm.

Alternate-Nostril Breathing Although somewhat more difficult, **alternate-nostril breathing** also helps to reduce tension and sinus headaches. First, close off your right nostril by lightly pressing it with your right thumb. Now inhale through your left nostril as slowly and quietly as possible. Remove your thumb from the right nostril and use your forefinger to close off the left nostril. Now exhale slowly through your right nostril. Inhale through your right nostril as slowly and quietly as possible and follow the same procedure outlined above, closing your right nostril with your right thumb while exhaling through your left nostril.

The basic cycle for alternate-nostril breathing should begin with ten breaths and can be increased up to twenty-five breaths. It may be easier to breathe through the right nostril at certain times of the day and through the left nostril at other times. The reason is that people breathe primarily through one nostril for approximately four hours, then breathe primarily through the other for the next four hours.

Progressive Relaxation

Progressive relaxation has its roots in a theory developed in 1929 by Chicago physician Edmund Jacobsen. The technique of progressive relaxation is based on the premise that muscle tension is the body's physiologic response to anxiety-provoking thoughts. Muscular tension increases the feeling of anxiety and reinforces it. Deep muscle relaxation, by contrast, decreases physiologic tension and blocks anxiety.

Progressive relaxation decreases pulse and respiratory rates, blood pressure, and perspiration. In addition, it helps to reduce anxiety. Clients with muscle spasms, low back pain, tension headaches, insomnia, anxiety, depression, fatigue, irritable bowel, hypertension, or mild phobias are among those who can achieve positive results using this technique.

It may take longer to master progressive relaxation than the deep breathing stress-reduction techniques discussed earlier. With practice, one can learn to relax faster and easier.

Active Progressive Relaxation **Active progressive relaxation** helps people identify which muscles or muscle groups are chronically tense by distinguishing between sensations of tension (purposeful muscle tensing) and deep relaxation (a conscious relaxing of the muscles). Each muscle or muscle grouping is tensed for five to seven seconds and then relaxed for twenty or thirty seconds. This cycle is repeated. Four major muscle groups are covered—hands, forearms, and biceps; head, face, throat, and shoulders; chest, abdomen, and lower back; thighs, buttocks, calves, and

feet. Use the instructions in the accompanying Client/Family Teaching box as a guide to a typical exercise. This guide was written by a nurse (Flynn 1980) who uses these principles in her clinical practice.

Counsel clients to observe some cautions while carrying out this technique. The muscles of the neck and back should not be excessively tightened to avoid soft-tissue and spinal injury. Tightening the muscles of the toes and feet too vigorously could also result in uncomfortable muscle cramps.

Practice progressive relaxation while lying down or seated in a chair with a head support. Remember to check for muscle groups that are only partially relaxed and return to them to bring about deeper relaxation.

Passive Progressive Relaxation In **passive progressive relaxation,** the muscles are not tensed. The goal is to relax the muscles without first tightening them. The sequence in which body parts are relaxed differs from that of the active progressive method. Begin with muscles easiest to relax (in the toes) and progress to muscles most difficult to relax (in the head). The sequence is as follows:

- Feet
- Lower legs
- Knees and upper legs
- Hips and buttocks
- Lower back
- Lower arms and hands
- Chest and diaphragm
- Abdomen
- Pelvis and genitals
- Neck
- Forehead and upper face
- Mouth and jaw

Some report feeling less alert after either active or passive progressive relaxation. When alertness is important, one of the other exercises is probably better.

Visualization

A French pharmacist, Emil Coue, began to use the power of imagination with clients around the turn of the century. Carl Jung used it in his psychiatric practice in the early part of the century. Most recently, Carl Simonton and Stephanie Matthews Simonton have had remarkable success in the use of visualization to treat cancer clients. Author Norman Cousins has written of his control over serious illness by using the healing power of his own imagination.

CLIENT/FAMILY TEACHING

Active Progressive Relaxation Exercise

Sit or lie in a comfortable position and let your eyes close.

I take a moment to be here (allow time).

I focus my attention on my right hand, and I make a fist.

Slowly and steadily, I clench my fist and study the tension.

Now I let go and feel the difference.

I repeat that.

I clench my fist, tightly, feeling the tension.

I let go and enjoy the contrast in my feelings.

Now I tense my right forearm.

Studying the tension.

And let go and notice the difference.

Now I tense my biceps—tighten.

And let go.

I stretch my arm straight out and feel the tension in my arm and shoulder.

I let go and appreciate the difference.

Now I focus my attention on my left hand, and I make a fist.

Slowly and steadily, I clench my fist and study the tension.

Now I let go and feel the difference.

I do that again.

Clenching my fist, tightly, feeling the tension.

And let go and enjoy the contrast in my feelings.

Now I tense my left forearm.

Studying the tension.

And let go and notice the difference.

Now I tense my biceps—tighten.

And let go.

I stretch my arm straight out and feel the tension in my arm and shoulder.

I let go and appreciate the difference.

I focus my attention on my scalp.

I tighten it.

And now I smooth it out.

I pay attention to the muscles of my forehead—I frown.

And study the tension as I frown.

I let go and notice the difference.

I raise my eyebrows and hold them for a few seconds.

And let go.

Now the muscles around my eyes—I tense and tighten them.

And let go.

The muscles of my cheeks, I tighten them.

And release, acknowledging the difference.

Now I tighten my jaw muscles, tighter—

And let go.

I bring my tongue to the roof of my mouth and tighten it.

And let go.

I let it relax.

And now the muscles in the back of my neck—I tighten those.

I feel the tension, and now I let it go.

I pull my shoulders back and up and tighten the muscles between my shoulders.

Tighten and notice the tension.

And let go.

Now I tighten the muscles of my upper back.

Tighten—and let go.

I focus my attention now on the muscles of my lower back.

I tighten them and notice the tension and

Let go.

Now the muscles of my buttocks.

Tighten—feel the tension.

And let go.

Breathing easily and calmly, deeply and efficiently.

I bring my attention to the muscles of the front of my neck.

I tighten them, bringing my chin up.

And let go.

Now I tighten my chest muscles—tighten.

And let go.

I let myself take in a good deep breath and hold it, feeling all my muscles expand.

And now I let go—letting all the breath out.

I repeat this and notice my feelings.

▶

CLIENT/FAMILY TEACHING *(continued)*

I tense the muscles of my abdomen.

I tighten them and notice the tension.

And let go and appreciate the relaxation.

And my pelvic muscles—I tighten them—tight.

And let go.

My thighs—I tighten those muscles.

And let go, noticing the difference.

Now the muscles of my calves and lower legs.

I tense them tighter and note the tension.

And let go.

And the muscles of my feet—tighten them.

Letting go and appreciating the difference.

And now I take a moment to scan my

body—noticing any part of my body that still needs relaxation.

And I tense that part and let go.

Any other muscles—I take a moment to tense them.

And let go.

And now feeling the pleasure of this relaxation, I take a few moments to bring my attention back to this time and this place, and filled with energy and peace I open my eyes, stretch, and get up.

SOURCE: *Flynn PAR: Holistic Health: The Art and Science of Care. Brady, 1980, pp. 165–167. By permission of Appleton & Lange.*

Positive **visualizations** use a person's own imagination and positive thinking to reduce stress or promote healing. It was Coue who asked his clients to repeat this now-famous phrase twenty times to themselves on awakening: *"Every day in every way I am getting better and better."* He believed that predicting failure or success in advance was bound to make it happen. Thus, positive visualizations anticipating success reduce stress. Visualization should be used in conjunction with the body-scanning and deep-breathing exercises discussed earlier.

Not everyone finds using the imagination in this way easy, and the technique may not work for everyone. Constructing a detailed, effective visualization requires time, patience, and practice.

Visualization for Relaxation Relaxing through visualizing is enhanced by constructing in one's own mind a relaxing environment. Some find the soothing sounds of a seashore calming; others prefer to imagine themselves floating above the world on a soft cloud or a magic carpet. Still others relax as they imagine themselves descending on a slow-moving escalator into a calmer and more relaxed state.

If visualization seems difficult (and if a warm bath, hot tub, or swimming pool is relaxing) try constructing a visualization while in warm water, combining the physiologic effects of the warm water with the products of the imagination (see the accompanying Client/Family Teaching box).

Visualization for Symptom Control or Healing Although visualization techniques for symptom control or healing are practiced in a variety of health care settings around the country, they should be part of a well-rounded health program. For example, visualization can be used with conventional medical treatment for cancer clients and with preoperative clients to control postoperative pain and enhance tissue healing. Persons with vascular problems—migraine headache, hypertension, or Raynaud's disease—benefit from visualization. Allergies, asthma, rheumatoid arthritis, gastritis, colitis, peptic ulcer, insomnia, depression, and chronic pain all respond to visualization. See the Client/Family Teaching box on page 656 for two sample visualizations for the reduction of pain.

Meditation

Meditation is a kind of self-discipline that helps one to achieve inner peace and harmony by focusing uncritically on one thing at a time. Meditation has been associated with various religious doctrines and philosophies for thousands of years. It is seen as a way of becoming one with God or the universe, finding enlightenment, and achieving such virtues as selflessness. However, the person who practices meditation need not associate it with religion or philosophy. It can be practiced as a means of reducing inner discord and increasing self-knowledge.

CLIENT/FAMILY TEACHING

Visualization for the Bath

In a warm bath, it is difficult to worry or to sustain an anxiety attack. The body feels lighter, muscles are relaxed by the heat and movement of the water, and circulation is increased. Being in warm water for a half hour will lower the blood pressure and slow down your breathing. Though the effects will be the opposite for the first two minutes and you may feel stimulated, the calming properties of warm water will soon soothe you.

This visualization can be used in a bathtub, hot tub, heated swimming pool, or any warm body of water. The temperature should not be over 103°F, and you should not stay in the water for longer than thirty minutes. If you are alone, ask someone to call you on the phone after one-half hour or set a music alarm to rouse you. Turn out the lights and light a candle or use a small night light.

Get into a comfortable position, either reclining or sitting. Be sure that your back is supported and your breathing unconstricted. Take a full, deep breath and exhale fully and completely. Slowly close your eyes and feel your heart beating strongly and then begin to slow down. Let your thoughts just drift through your consciousness, as you allow them to leave with the warm air. Imagine that with each and every breath, you can breathe away tension or anxiety, as you allow yourself to relax more and more. All the day's burdens, worries, and expectations are leaving your consciousness and evaporating with the hot, moist steam. Feel your arms floating on the water, and the warm, soothing water gently lifting and caressing your body. As you continue to breathe slowly and naturally, let go of any thoughts still remaining in your mind. Watch as your thoughts flow through you and out of you, and see them disappear into the air, leaving your mind clear and calm.

Gently turn your attention to your body, and scan your body for any tension that you might still be holding. Allow it to leave with the next exhalation, as the warm water evaporates into steam. As you continue to breathe slowly and calmly, turn your awareness to your feet and to your legs. The water tenderly massages your legs and your feet, as the tension flows through you and out of you. With your next breath, breathe away any tightness still remaining in your feet. Move your attention to your abdomen and your chest, allowing the muscles to just let go, and the tension to melt away from your body. Feel your abdomen and your chest relax, as you gently loosen all the muscles and just breathe away any remaining tension. Focus on relaxing your arms and your hands, letting the muscles go completely loose and limp. Relax your fingers, and your hands, and let the feeling of deep relaxation spread up into your arms. Breathe away any tension still remaining.

Now, relax the muscles of your shoulders and your neck, and feel the heaviness gradually increase throughout your musculature, as all your muscles just let go. The muscles in your back go loose and limp, as the water gently supports your whole body. Allow the relaxation to spread to your head and your face, and the muscles around your eyes, in your jaw, your tongue, and in your forehead. Let yourself drift deeper into a dreamlike state of calm relaxation.

Imagine that the blue water becomes the sky, and the soft clouds gently support you as you drift up above the trees. You no longer feel the weight of your head upon your shoulders, and gravity no longer ties you to the earth. The warm, soft, billowy, pink clouds support you as the sun's gentle heat penetrates through any remaining tension. As you peacefully float through the warm air, the golden sun fills your body with warming heat and light. This golden light penetrates through any tension still remaining in your body. As you free-float in space, your body is becoming lighter and lighter.

When you have floated as high as you wish, you become still, and the clouds gently cradle you in the warmth of the sun's golden rays. The golden sun finds any tension still remaining in your body, and dissolves it in the warm, glowing light. Whenever you are ready, you may return. Feel the warm, pink clouds transform into water, and become aware of the water gently cradling you. Take a few, deep breaths, becoming more and more aware of your surroundings. When you are ready to become fully alert, take a full, deep breath and gently open your eyes on the exhalation. Take a few more deep breaths, and slowly get out of the water, gently drying yourself and feeling the relaxation throughout your body.

SOURCE: *Reprinted with permission from Mason LJ:* Guide to Stress Reduction. *Celestial Arts, 1986, pp 61–63. © 1980, 1986, Celestial Arts, Box 7327, Berkeley, CA 94707.*

CLIENT/FAMILY TEACHING

Visualization for Relief from Pain

Alternative I

Imagine that your body is filled with orange and blue lights.

The orange lights signify areas of pain or tension.

The blue lights signify pain-free or calm areas.

Imagine changing the orange lights to blue lights.

Note that the pain is going away and that you're feeling more and more relaxed.

Alternative II

Concentrate on the part of your body where the pain exists.

Attach a symbolic visual image to the pain (a knot in your stomach, a hammer pounding your head).

Imagine the symbol being relaxed, becoming looser, getting smaller or weaker as you feel your pain becoming less and less.

SOURCE: *Kneisl CR, Ames SW: Adult Health Nursing: A Biopsychosocial Approach. Addison-Wesley, 1986, p 71.*

The state of meditation is equivalent to a state of deep rest. The heart rate slows, the body uses less oxygen, and blood lactate—a waste product of metabolism—decreases sharply. Alpha waves, which characterize brain activity during states of calm alertness, increase.

Meditation seems to have long-standing effects as well. Stress-related problems such as insomnia and asthma diminish. It has been used successfully in the prevention and treatment of hypertension, heart disease, and stroke. Meditation has also helped people decrease their consumption of food, alcohol, tobacco, and drugs and curtail obsessive thinking, anxiety, depression, and hostility. It also improves concentration and attention.

Some theorists believe that meditation quiets the brain, as the person makes contact with more orderly and coherent levels of the mind. The left hemisphere, thought to be responsible for rational and logical thinking, comes into electrical balance with the underdeveloped right hemisphere, thought to modulate intuition, holistic comprehension, and artistic qualities.

Meditation exercises can be relatively easy to learn. Some people experience immediate relief and pleasure in only one session. To experience deeper effects, the person needs to practice meditation regularly for at least a month.

These are the four major requirements of meditation:

1. A quiet place

2. A comfortable position

3. An object or thought to dwell on

4. A passive attitude

The environment for meditation should be one that minimizes distractions—a quiet place set aside as a haven from the urgencies of everyday life. A comfortable position that can be held for twenty minutes without stress facilitates meditation. Some possible positions are the yoga lotus position or sitting tailor-fashion or Japanese-fashion (sitting back on one's heels). Avoid meditating within two hours of a heavy meal since digestion interferes with the ability to relax. Something to dwell on—e.g., a repeated word, an object or symbol to look at or think about, or a specific thought or feeling—helps keep distracting thoughts from entering the mind. A passive attitude requires understanding that thoughts and distractions will occur and can be cleared from the mind. If they occur, they should be noted and let go without concern about their interference. It is counterproductive to worry about how well you are doing at meditating.

Some of the stress-management techniques discussed earlier—body scanning, the breathing ten-to-one count, and visualization—can satisfy the requirement of an object to dwell on. Many people who meditate prefer to use a **mantra,** a syllable, word, or name that is repeatedly chanted aloud. Some teachers of meditation insist that each person have a special mantra with a specific meaning and vibration to achieve individual effects. Others recommend the use of any word or phrase the individual is drawn to, e.g., *peace, love,* or *calm.* Some popular eastern mantras are *om* (I am), *so-ham* (I am he), and *sa-ham* (I am she). Avoid chanting too loudly or too vigorously. After about five minutes, shift to whispering the mantra as you relax more deeply. When it is not possible to chant aloud, some people chant silently.

The best results from meditation are achieved by persons who meditate for fifteen minutes a day, five to seven days a week for two weeks. After this period of time, the length of the sessions may be increased to thirty minutes if desired.

Therapeutic Touch

Therapeutic touch was developed by Dolores Krieger (1979) as a nursing activity, although the "laying on of hands" to help heal is as old as history. It is defined as the specific transfer of energy in a therapeutic manner; that is, some of the excess energies of the healer are directed to the client, or energy is transferred from one place to another within the body of the client. This technique is based on the concept of illness as an imbalance of energies in the body. *Prana* is the subsystem of energy that Krieger believes is the basis of the energy transfer in therapeutic touch. Healthy people usually have an excess of prana, and since each person is an open system, energy can be transferred to another person. This transfer of energy is not a cure but provides an infusion of energy for people depleted by struggles with illness. This energy benefits them until their own healing processes take over.

Therapeutic touch is a conscious, deliberate act composed of three steps called centering, scanning, and rebalancing. The healer first prepares for the procedure through *centering*, the discovery of an inner physical and psychologic stability in which the healer achieves a sense that all faculties are under command. This gathers and focuses the healer's energies on the client and excludes extraneous thoughts from the mind, a process akin to meditation.

The healer then *scans* the client from head to foot without actually touching the client's body, attempting to sense temperature changes or feelings of pressure. These areas indicate a static condition, an imbalance, or congestion in the client's energy field.

Intervention consists of mobilizing or *rebalancing* these congested areas. The healer places the hands, with palms facing away from the client, in the area where pressure is felt and moves the hands away from the client's body in a sweeping gesture while consciously directing a flow of energy to the client, a process called *unruffling the field*. Therapists report relief of the sense of pressure they feel in problem areas of the client's body and consider the treatment complete when they no longer perceive an imbalance in the person's symmetry.

Clients report a sense of relaxation and relief from pain. Krieger (1979) has demonstrated experimentally that therapeutic touch has produced a significant change in the hemoglobin component of red blood cells. Advocates of therapeutic touch have found that, although the freeing of bound energy is not long lasting, it does seem to facilitate the repatterning of energy necessary for healing. However, the published

---

RESEARCH NOTE

Citation
Carter MA: An experimental trial of therapeutic touch in the treatment of arthritis. West J Nurs Res 1983;5(3):56–64.

Study Problem/Purpose
The purpose of this study was to see if the use of therapeutic touch by nurses would increase the range of motion of joints and decrease pain in persons with arthritis.

Methods
This study used an experimental design. Subjects were drawn from a convenience group of clients from an ambulatory, senior citizen practice of nurse faculty. Twenty-eight subjects (14 control and 14 experimental) were selected from subjects who volunteered for the study. All subjects had a diagnosis of arthritis and were taking at least one drug for arthritis daily. The range of motion of shoulders, knees, and hips was measured for each subject. Level of pain was assessed by a linear scale from 0 = no pain to 10 = the worst pain ever experienced. The experimental group then received 15 minutes of therapeutic touch from a nurse experienced in this modality. The pulses of the control group were taken in their wrists, ankles, and knees by the same nurse who performed therapeutic touch for the experimental group. The pulse-taking procedures also took 15 minutes. All subjects were remeasured for range of motion and level of pain. Data were analyzed by use of repeated measures ANOVA.

Findings
No significant differences were found between pretest and posttest or between experimental and control groups for range of motion or level of pain.

Conclusions and Implications
Therapeutic touch did not produce an immediate effect measured by changes in range of motion or levels of pain. Of interest were subjects who said that therapeutic touch made them "feel better" and yet showed no changes in range of motion or pain levels.

---

research literature indicates that empirical support for the practice of therapeutic touch is, at best, weak (Clark and Clark 1984).

Rolfing

Rolfing, or structural integration, is based on the belief that psychologic conflicts are recorded and perpetuated in the body. Ida Rolf (1977), the founder of this therapy, viewed the body as an area of energy within the earth's gravitational field. To function properly, a person must be in correct alignment with the forces of gravity. When the body is in an incorrect position, the myofascia or connective tissue that supports the body weight shortens and undergoes metabolic changes that decrease its energy and interfere with free movement.

Many people are not in proper relationship to the field of gravity because they have become alienated from their own bodily sensations. At different points in their development, they have responded to inner and outer threats by turning off their responses. They have inhibited those responses by contracting the muscles that are related to the impulse that is being blocked. For example, if the impulse is aggressive, they may contract arm muscles. Repeated inhibition and the resulting muscular contractions produce chronically spastic muscles that inhibit motility. The musculature acts as a repository of stored feelings. Energy that would otherwise be available for conscious use is expended internally to keep these muscles tense.

As people age, their posture becomes a reflection of accumulated unresolved feelings. When people become aware of how they contract their muscles in traumatic situations, they can begin to take responsibilty for their own physical structure by experimenting with alternative responses. Gracefulness and unitary movement are signs of personal integration. When a body is coordinated and balanced physically, there is a corresponding emotional balance.

Rolfing is a method of working with the body to achieve a realignment of the body structure. The basic therapy consists of ten one-hour sessions. The rolfer massages and manipulates the client's deep connective tissue. Once this tissue is freed, the body is able to realign itself with gravitational forces. The emotional release and physical healing that often accompany rolfing are not the major goal of therapy. However, they are proof that emotional and physical problems are related to the body's misalignment. Many clients who have been rolfed report they have changed so much that they have difficulty relating to their past environment and must alter their work, interpersonal relationships, and values.

Bioenergetics

Alexander Lowen (1967a, 1967b, 1976), founder of the Institute for Bioenergetics, also emphasizes body work. **Bioenergetics** offers techniques for reducing muscular tension through the release of feelings. It makes less use of direct body contact (between client and therapist) than other body therapies, guiding the client instead through a series of exercises and verbal techniques. Stressor and releaser exercises are used to increase the client's awareness of body defenses. The exercises begin with deep breathing and progress to stretching and kicking the limbs. This enables the client to break through muscular rigidity and express feelings previously trapped in habitual postural modes. These modes, which are called *muscular armoring,* prevent the free flow of energy. The theory is comparable to that of other body-mind therapists.

If the body is relatively unalive, perceptions and responses are diminished. People in this situation are often depressed. According to Lowen, depressed people were denied the mother love they needed. Now they have no faith in themselves or in life. They cannot pursue the goals they really wish to achieve, and they are usually unaware of the reasons for their lifelessness. During bioenergetic therapy, these people are encouraged to make deep contact with their feelings of sadness. Lowen discusses a client with chronic depression who benefited by a session of screaming and kicking. Her depression lifted as she went through this series of exercises and was able to release her emotional controls. The intense energy that had previously been immobilized in depression became available to her. Lowen emphasizes that clients must break through frozen emotions by themselves and thus become able to care for themselves in the way their parents failed to do.

Lowen also thinks that the study of *auras,* or energy fields around the body, can be used to diagnose disturbances in body functioning. In the energy field of a person with schizophrenia, for example, a trained observer can see characteristic alterations, such as interruptions of energy flow or color changes. Different parts of each person's body radiate different kinds of feelings. When chronic muscle tension blocks energy, negative feelings result. The head, neck, and shoulders can radiate openness and affirmation or express hostility and holding back. The belly can radiate pleasure and laughter or suffering. The legs can radiate security and balance or instability. When there are no constrictions that disturb energy flow, the feeling is positive, the personality is integrated, and the aura is bright and intense.

People excite and depress each other through their energy fields. People with strong energy fields influence others in a positive way. We are in touch with others only when our energy contacts and excites their energy. Bioenergetics attempts to facilitate this free flow of energy through exercises.

Autogenic Training

Autogenic training is used across the country in stress-reduction and holistic health centers to teach self-regulation of the autonomic nervous system. It has its origins in the research done by Oskar Vogt, a brain physiologist who worked in Berlin in the last decade of the nineteenth century. Johannes Schutz, a Berlin psychiatrist, combined Vogt's research into the effects of hypnosis on the brain with some yoga techniques and published his first work on autogenic training in 1932. Wolfgang Luthe brought autogenic training to the United States in 1969. In its contemporary form, autogenic training does not require a hypnotist. Most individuals can learn autogenic exercises in four to ten months through a systematic training program or a written course of study.

Autogenic training is based on the achievement of six physiologic outcomes:

1. Heaviness in the extremities

2. Warmth in the extremities

3. Regulation of the heartbeat

4. Regulation of breathing

5. Abdominal warmth

6. Cooling of the forehead

Once clients learn to perform the six standard exercises designed to achieve these results, they may go on to learn meditative exercises specifically developed for each client or neutralization exercises to promote abreaction and verbalization.

Autogenic training has proved helpful for the following problems:

- Hyperventilation and asthma

- Gastrointestinal problems, e.g., constipation, diarrhea, gastritis, ulcer, and gastrointestinal spasm

- Cardiovascular problems, e.g., cardiac dysrhythmias and hypertension

- Some thyroid conditions

- Headaches and insufficient circulation to the extremities

- Anxiety, irritability, and fatigue

- Pain

- Sleep disorders

It is not recommended for children under five years of age or for psychotic persons. Persons with serious physical health problems should be under the supervision of a health care provider while in autogenic training. Any trainees who experience distress, uncomfortable symptoms, or changes in blood pressure during autogenic training should continue only under the supervision of a qualified instructor.

Self-Hypnosis

Milton Erickson is generally recognized as a leading proponent of the use of hypnosis in medical and psychotherapeutic contexts. Erickson redefined hypnosis as an experience originating in the client in order to cope with a problem overwhelming to the conscious mind.

People practice **self-hypnosis** to achieve significant relaxation, to make positive suggestions for change (e.g., to lose weight, to stop smoking, to overcome fear of the dark, or insomnia), to increase learning and remembering, and to uncover significant but forgotten events. Table 27–1 gives examples of some life problems and hypnotic suggestions that can be used to overcome them. Contrary to popular belief, even the most inexperienced of self-hypnosis practitioners cannot harm themselves.

Most people can achieve significant relaxation within two days with self-hypnosis. Self-hypnosis can be self-taught through books on the subject (see the references at the end of this chapter). Community adult education programs or holistic health centers often offer courses on self-hypnosis. Self-hypnosis is clinically effective in relieving insomnia, low to moderate levels of chronic pain, tics and tremors, and low to moderate levels of anxiety. It is a well-established treatment for chronic fatigue.

Thought Stopping

Thought stopping is a behavior therapy technique that is particularly useful in helping a person control obsessive and phobic thoughts. It involves concentrating on the unwanted thoughts and, after a short time, suddenly interrupting the thought and emptying the mind. Thought stopping is based on the belief that negative and frightening thoughts invariably precede negative and frightening emotions. Controlling these thoughts can reduce stress. Some of the obsessive and phobic thought processes that can be interrupted by thought stopping are color naming, counting, rechecking, hypochondriasis, sexual preoccupation, recurring thoughts of failure, and simple phobias among others. Thought stopping is more successful with phobias than it is with compulsive ritualistic behavior.

Thought stopping begins by using the command "stop," a loud noise, or a distracter such as pinching oneself or pressing the fingernails into the palm of the hand to interrupt the unpleasant thoughts. Once the

TABLE 27-1 Life Problems and Related Hypnotic Suggestions

Life Problem	Hypnotic Suggestion
Fear of coming into the dark house at night	I can come in tonight feeling relaxed and glad to be home.
Anxiety that prevents working or studying to meet deadlines	I can work steadily and calmly. My concentration is improving as I become more relaxed.
Insomnia	I will gradually become more and more drowsy. In just a few minutes I will be able to fall asleep, and sleep peacefully all night.
Chronic fatigue	I can waken feeling refreshed and rested.
Obsessive and fearful thoughts about death	I am full of life now. I will enjoy today.
Minor chronic headache or backache	As I become more relaxed, my headache (backache) lessens. In just a few minutes, it will go away. Soon my head will be cool and relaxed. Gradually I will feel the muscles in my back loosen, In an hour, they will be completely relaxed. Whenever these symptoms come back, I will simply turn my ring a quarter of a turn to the right and the pain will relax away.
Feelings of inferiority	The next time I see ____, I can feel secure in myself. I can feel relaxed and at ease because I am perfectly all right.
Anxiety about an upcoming evaluation or test	Whenever I feel nervous, I can say to myself . . . (insert your own special key word or phrase here) . . . and relax.
Chronic anger (or chronic guilt)	I can turn off anger (guilt) because I am the one who turns it on. I will relax my body and breathe deeply.
Worry about interpersonal rejection	Whenever I lace my fingers together, I will feel confidence flowing through me.
Chronic tension in a particular part of the body.	I will think about my ____ every hour and let it relax.

individual has mastered interrupting the unpleasant thought, the next step involves *thought substitution* (replacing the obsessive or phobic thought with a positive assertive statement that is appropriate to the situation). For example, the person who is afraid to drive across a bridge might say to himself or herself, "This is a gorgeous view from up here."

To be effective, thought stopping should be practiced conscientiously throughout the day for three days to one week. At first the thought will return, but with practice it returns less frequently, and in many instances, eventually ceases to recur.

Refuting Irrational Self-Talk

Self-talk is intrapersonal communication, the thoughts with which we describe and interpret the world to ourselves. Irrational or untrue self-talk causes stress and mental disorder. Two common forms of **irrational self-talk** are statements that "awfulize" (catastrophic, nightmarish interpretations of an event or experience) or "absolutize" (words such as *should, must, always,* etc. that imply the need to live up to a standard). These ideas are based on the rational-emotive therapy formulated by Albert Ellis (1975).

Rational-emotive therapy emphasizes human values as the important component of personality. Healthy functioning is possible only when the values we believe in are rational ones. Absolutist, perfectionist attitudes are irrational. Ten basic irrational ideas described by Ellis are discussed in the accompanying Theory box.

According to Ellis, emotional reactions are not caused by events or by our emotional reaction to events but by belief systems. Being insulted, for instance, does not cause us to withdraw from others.

THEORY

Albert Ellis' Ten Basic Irrational Ideas

1. It is an absolute necessity for an adult to have love and approval from peers, family, and friends. In fact, it is impossible to please all the people in your life. Even those who basically like and approve of you will be turned off by some behaviors and qualities. This irrational belief is probably the single greatest cause of unhappiness.

2. You must be unfailingly competent and almost perfect in all you undertake. The results of believing you must behave perfectly are self-blame for inevitable failure, lowered self-esteem, perfectionistic standards applied to mate and friends, and paralysis and fear at attempting anything.

3. Certain people are evil, wicked, and villainous, and should be punished. A more realistic position is that they are behaving in ways that are antisocial or inappropriate. They are perhaps stupid, ignorant, or neurotic, and it would be well if their behavior could be changed.

4. It is horrible when people and things are not the way you would like them to be. This might be described as the spoiled-child syndrome. As soon as the tire goes flat the self-talk starts: "Why does this happen to me? Damn, I can't take this. It's awful, I'll get all filthy." Any inconvenience, problem, or failure to get your way is likely to be met with such awfulizing self-statements. The result is intense irritation and stress.

5. External events cause most human misery—people simply react as events trigger their emotions. A logical extension of this belief is that you must control the external events in order to create happiness or avoid sorrow. Since such control has limitations and we are at a loss to completely manipulate the wills of others, there results a sense of helplessness and chronic anxiety. Ascribing unhappiness to events is a way of avoiding reality. Self-statements *interpreting* the event caused the unhappiness. While you may have only limited control over others, you have enormous control over your emotions.

6. You should feel fear or anxiety about anything that is unknown, uncertain, or potentially dangerous. Many describe this as, "a little bell that goes off and I think I ought to start worrying." They begin to rehearse their scenarios of catastrophe. Increasing the fear of anxiety in the face of uncertainty makes coping more difficult and adds to stress. Saving the fear response for actual, perceived danger allows you to enjoy uncertainty as a novel and exciting experience.

7. It is easier to avoid than to face life's difficulties and responsibilities. There are many ways of ducking responsibilities: "I should tell him/her I'm no longer interested—but not tonight . . . I'd like to get another job, but I'm just too tired on my days off to look . . . A leaky faucet won't hurt anything . . . We could shop today, but the car is making a sort of funny sound."

8. You need something other or stronger or greater than yourself to rely on. This belief becomes a psychologic trap in which your independent judgment, and the awareness of your particular needs are undermined by a reliance on higher authority.

9. The past has a lot to do with determining the present. Just because you were once strongly affected by something, that does not mean that you must continue the habits you formed to cope with the original situation. Those old patterns and ways of responding are just decisions made so many times they have become nearly automatic. You can identify those old decisions and start changing them *right now*. You can learn from past experience, but you don't have to be overly attached to it.

10. Happiness can be achieved by inaction, passivity, and endless leisure. This is called the Elysian Fields syndrome. There is more to happiness than perfect relaxation.

SOURCE: *Adapted from Davis M, Eshelman ER, McKay M: The Relaxation and Stress Reduction Workbook. ed. 2. New Harbinger Publications, 1982, pp 106–107.*

Our *beliefs* about being insulted are what cause us to withdraw. Though it is rational to feel angry about insults, since they are destructive, withdrawal is irrational because it indicates that an individual has defined being insulted as a frightening event to be avoided. Ellis defines beliefs as rational when they help the individual accept reality, live in intimate relationships with others, work productively, and enjoy recreational pursuits. Irrationality is self-destructive behavior.

Both emotions and behavior depend on the cognitive mediating process that occurs in relation to every experience. Rational-emotive therapy helps people dispel their disturbing beliefs by explaining what irrational beliefs are and how they cause emotional difficulty. After they have logically analyzed their irrational beliefs, clients see how unnecessary they are and eliminate them.

Rational-emotive therapy frequently uses reinforcing techniques to help people change. Clients are taught to reward themselves for working on self-defeating ideas and to penalize themselves if they do not. Clients are also shown how to speak and think more objectively and give up the use of vague terms and overgeneralizations in order to define their own problems in specific terms. For example, the client is shown that the statement "I have some characteristics that are irritating to others" is more precise than "I am an irritating person."

Rational-emotive therapy narrows the focus for change to specific traits and behavior. Because people create most of their own psychologic symptoms, they can eliminate these symptoms by changing their values.

Biofeedback

Biofeedback, or visceral learning, is a technique for gaining conscious control over such involuntary body functions as blood pressure and heartbeat, which are mediated by the autonomic nervous system. The clinical application of biofeedback was pioneered by Alyce and Elmer Green of the Menninger Foundation in the late 1960s. Many other researchers have followed them in exploring this method of treatment. Certified biofeedback practitioners can be found in almost any large city, and training is available at most large universities.

Biofeedback treatment is based on the ability to voluntarily control some autonomic functions to a degree once thought impossible. It has been shown, for instance, that migraine headaches can be relieved by increasing blood flow to the hands.

The technique is based on giving continuous feedback about the results of each consecutive attempt at control. In a typical session, a person might be given this feedback by equipment that amplifies body signals and translates them into a flashing light or a steady tone. Once people can "see" a heartbeat, for instance, and observe when it slows down or speeds up, they have the information they need to control their heart rate. They are instructed to change the signal as they observe it. They are not told to slow the heartbeat, but to slow the flashing light. If they can do this, their heart rate will be modified.

Inexpensive monitoring equipment for home use has been developed within the past few years. The drawback is that these systems usually measure only temperature, heart rate, or the alpha activity of the brain, thus giving feedback on only a single system. Single-system feedback often isn't enough to achieve total relaxation.

Biofeedback has been found useful in treating a variety of problems, e.g., tension or migraine headaches, insomnia, muscle or colon spasm, pain, hypertension, anxiety, phobias, asthma, stuttering, bruxism (grinding of the teeth), and epilepsy. The psychologic states achieved through biofeedback can be beneficial in decreasing tension and reactions to unpleasant stimuli.

CHAPTER HIGHLIGHTS

• There are environmental, physiologic, and cognitive sources of stress. Psychiatric clients may experience more cognitive stress than most other persons do because of how they interpret and label their experiences.

• Most persons, including clients and nurses, find stress-reduction techniques helpful in counteracting habitual and counterproductive responses to the stresses of life.

• Nurses who plan to use stress-management techniques with clients must first develop personal familiarity with them.

• Anyone participating in a stress-reduction program should be sure that any physical problems and medications are closely monitored by a health care provider.

• Psychiatric clients taking psychotropic medications that may cause hypotension should be closely monitored when they do stress-reduction exercises.

• Regular practice enhances the chances of successfully using stress-management techniques.

• People should use the relaxation and stress-management techniques that work best in their individual situations.

• Body tension is an inevitable response to stress; once stress is removed, tension goes away.

• Keeping a stress-awareness diary helps people identify how particular stresses result in predictable symptoms.

• Breathing calmly and deeply keeps the blood well oxygenated and purified. Breathing properly can, by itself, reduce stress.

• Progressive relaxation teaches clients to decrease physiologic tension and block anxiety by achieving deep muscle relaxation.

• Positive visualizations use a person's own imagination and positive thinking to reduce stress or promote healing.

• The state of meditation is equivalent to a state of deep rest. It helps a person to focus uncritically on one thing at a time to achieve inner peace and harmony.

• Therapeutic touch is the "laying on of hands" to help or heal. It is based on the ability of a healer to transfer excess energy to a client, or to transfer energy from one part of the client's body to another.

• In rolfing, the structural realignment of the body to the field of gravity is accompanied by a corresponding emotional balance.

• Bioenergetics offers techniques for reducing muscular tension by releasing feelings through physical exercises and verbal techniques.

• Autogenic training is a structured program of exercises that have been found to be effective in the treatment of numerous physical symptoms. It is also used to reduce anxiety, irritability, and fatigue; to modify the reaction to pain; and to reduce or eliminate sleep disorders.

• Self-hypnosis is clinically effective in relieving insomnia, low to moderate levels of chronic pain, tics and tremors, and low to moderate levels of anxiety. It is a well-established treatment for chronic fatigue.

• A behavior therapy technique, thought stopping helps to control phobic and obsessional thoughts.

• Irrational self-talk creates stress and mental disorder. Changing irrational beliefs can reduce or eliminate emotional difficulty.

• People can learn to control involuntary body functions through biofeedback and reduce or eliminate stress-related conditions.

REFERENCES

Bandler R, Grinder J: *Patterns of the Hypnotic Techniques of Milton H. Erickson*, vol 1. Meta Publications, 1975.

Borysenko J: *Guilt Is the Teacher, Love Is the Lesson.* Warner, 1989.

Borysenko J: *Minding the Body, Mending the Mind.* Addison-Wesley, 1987.

Bramson RM, Bramson S: *The Stressless Home: A Step-by-Step Guide to Turning Your Home into the Haven You Desire.* Doubleday, 1985.

Clark PE, Clark MJ: Therapeutic touch: Is there a scientific basis for the practice? *Nurs Res* 1984;33(1):37–41.

Cousins N: *Head First: The Biology of Hope.* Dutton, 1990.

Dawkins JE, Depp FC, Selzer NE: Stress and the psychiatric nurse. *J Psychosoc Nurs* 1985;23:8–15.

Ellis A: *A New Guide to Rational Living.* Prentice-Hall, 1975.

Flynn, PAR: *Holistic Health: The Art and Science of Care.* Brady, 1980.

Hamilton JM: Effective ways to relieve stress. *Nurs Life* 1984;4:24–27.

Hoover RM, Parnell PK: An inpatient education group on stress and coping. *J Psychosoc Nurs* 1984;22(6):16–23.

Jacobson E: *Progressive Relaxation.* University of Chicago Press, Midway Reprint, 1974.

Krieger D: *The Therapeutic Touch.* Prentice-Hall, 1979.

Lachman VD: *Stress Management: A Manual for Nurses.* Grune and Stratton, 1983.

Larson D: Helper secrets: Internal stressors in nursing. *J Psychosoc Nurs* 1987;25(4):20–27.

LeCron L (ed): *Techniques of Hypnotherapy.* Julian Press, 1961.

LeShan L: *How to Meditate.* Bantam Books, 1974.

Lowen A: *The Betrayal of the Body.* Macmillan, 1967a.

Lowen A: *Bioenergetics.* Penguin Books, 1976.

Lowen A: *Depression and the Body.* Macmillan, 1967b.

Luthe W (ed): *Autogenic Therapy,* 6 vols. New York: Grune and Stratton, 1969.

Mason LJ: *Guide to Stress Reduction.* Celestial Arts, 1986.

Meichenbaum D, Jaremko M (eds): *Stress Reduction and Prevention.* Plenum Press, 1983.

Miller J: *States of Mind.* Pantheon Books, 1983.

Miller NE: Rx: Biofeedback. *Psychol Today* 1985:19:54–59.

Morris F: *Self-Hypnosis in Two Days.* Intergalactic, 1974.

Pelletier KR: *Mind As Healer, Mind As Slayer.* Dell, 1977.

Randolph GL: Therapeutic and physical touch: Physiological response to stressful stimuli. *Nurs Res* 1984;33(1):33–36.

Rolf I: *Rolfing: The Structural Integration of Human Structure.* Rolf Institute, 1977.

Spreads C: *Breathing—The ABC's.* Harper & Row, 1978.

Sterman MB: Biofeedback and epilepsy. *Hum Nature* 1978;23:50–57.

Stokols D: A congruence analysis of human stress. *Issues Ment Health Nurs* 1985:7:35–41.

Stroebel CF: Biofeedback and behavioral medicine, in Kaplan HI, Sadock BJ (eds): *Comprehensive Textbook of Psychiatry,* ed 4. Williams and Wilkins, 1985.

Stroebel CF: *The Quieting Reflex: A Six-Second Technique for Coping with Stress Anytime, Anywhere.* G.P. Putnam's Sons, 1982.

Sutterley DC, Donnelley GF (eds): *Coping with Stress: A Nursing Perspective.* Aspen, 1982.

Tache J, Selye J: On stress and coping mechanisms. *Issues Ment Health Nurs* 1985;7:3–24.

Tolman R, Rose SD: Coping with stress. A multimodal approach. *Social Work* 1985;30:151–158

Turin AC: *No More Headaches! Practical, Effective Methods for Relief.* Houghton Mifflin, 1981.

Vandereycken W, et al.: Body-oriented therapy for anorexia nervosa patients. *Am J Psychother* 1987;41(2): 252–259.

Wilson LK: High-gear nursing: How it can run you down and what you can do about it. *Nurs Life* 1986;6: 44–47.

Wollert R, Levy L, Knight B: Help-giving in behavioral control and stress coping self-help groups. *Small Group Behav* 1982;13:204–218.

Wolpe J: *The Practice of Behavior Therapy.* Pergamon Press, 1969.

Psychobiology Box References

Borysenko J: *Minding the Body, Mending the Mind.* Addison-Wesley, 1987.

Hales D: *Invitation to Health,* ed 4. Addison-Wesley, 1989.

Perry S, Dawson J: *The Secrets Our Body Clocks Reveal.* Ballantine, 1990.

Raymond CA: Sleep patterns scrutinized as depression therapy. *J Am Med Assoc* February 19, 1988; 265(6)212–213.

Toufexis A: Drowsy America. *Time* December 17, 1990.

Crisis Intervention

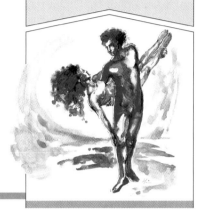

Carol Ren Kneisl
Elizabeth A. Riley

LEARNING OBJECTIVES

• Trace the crisis sequence and relate its significance for nursing care of clients in crisis

• Define the types of crisis a person may encounter

• Discuss the major crisis intervention modes

• Develop a plan for nursing intervention for clients experiencing a crisis

• Discuss the importance of crisis origins and balancing factors in the assessment phase of crisis management

CROSS REFERENCES

Other topics relevant to this content are: Anxiety, stress, and coping, Chapter 5; Depression, Chapter 13; Ethics, Chapter 7; Nursing intervention in anxiety and panic, Chapter 14; Post-traumatic stress disorder, Chapter 14; Stress management, Chapter 27; Suicide and lethality assessment, Chapter 23; Violence and abuse, Chapters 21 and 22.

THIS CHAPTER EXPLORES THOSE extremely difficult points in a person's life when circumstances produce an unbearable situation. Under such pressure, a person may make unsound decisions, may become mentally disordered, or may commit or attempt suicide. It is an intriguing puzzle to understand what constitutes a crisis for an individual and how that individual behaves in response to it. This inquiry into the cause and effect of crisis is the focus of crisis theory.

Humanism is the basis of crisis theory in that individuals are recognized as having their own unique view of the word. Crisis points are as unique as the individual's responses to the crisis. Humanism also promotes the individual's ability to reason and choose freely. In accordance with these concepts, the task of the person who intervenes in the crisis is (a) to help the individual understand what combination of events led to the crisis and (b) to guide the individual toward a resolution that will meet the client's unique needs and foster future growth and strength.

Early writers have described crisis in Western culture since writing about Adam and Eve leaving the Garden of Eden. In findings ways to cope with this first crisis, Adam and Eve engaged in what must have been the first example of crisis intervention. We have since come to a better understanding of just what a crisis is, why people behave the way they do in crisis situations, and how to help people in crisis.

Nurses are in a unique position to intervene in crises. Clients and families in crisis come to their attention in the multitude of health care settings in which nurses work. However, crisis intervention is not the specialty of any one professional group. People who intervene in crises come from the fields of nursing, medicine, psychology, social work, and theology. Police officers, teachers, school guidance counselors, rescue workers, and bartenders, among others, are often on the spot in moments of crisis. Crisis intervention can be the business of many different persons.

Historical and Theoretic Foundations

Two events in the 1940s can be said to have provided the starting point for contemporary crisis theory and intervention. One was the report by psychiatrist Erich Lindemann (see Cobb and Lindemann 1943, Lindemann 1944) of the crisis response many people had in their direct or indirect experience with the tragic Cocoanut Grove nightclub fire in Boston, in which hundreds of people lost their lives. Lindemann's observations and theoretic developments were a landmark in understanding the behavior of people facing emergency situations and the grieving behavior of people who lose loved ones in such situations.

The other event was the observation and treatment by military psychiatrists of battle-weary and emotionally upset military men. In most instances, men who received immediate help at the front lines were able to return to duty rather than being sent to in-patient psychiatric facilities. This immediate front-line treatment was therefore the preferred mode. Later studies and observations during the Korean War added to the knowledge of the behavior of people under stress.

James Tyhurst (1957) contributed further to the understanding of people's responses to natural disasters. He also studied transition states such as parenthood and retirement. Gerald Caplan (1965), who is best known for his work in preventive psychiatry and anticipatory guidance, had similar interests. Many of his methods were tested in the early days of the Peace Corps.

The report of the Joint Commission on Mental Illness and Health (1961) was an important development in crisis work. Its far-reaching mental health recommendations have been discussed in other chapters. The following conclusions of the Joint Commission apply specifically to this chapter:

• People in crisis did not receive immediate help but instead were put on lengthy waiting lists.

• When they did receive attention, it was often through lengthy and expensive psychotherapy.

• Extended and/or late psychotherapy is often not helpful to people in crisis.

• When people in crisis needed help, almost 50 percent sought out their clergyman, family physician, or other non-mental-health professional.

• Interested persons with minimal training could be helpful to people in trouble.

• A large group of interested persons in the community had been neglected as a resource for helping people in crisis.

Soon after the publication of the Joint Commission report, large amounts of federal funding were made available for community-based mental health programs. One result was the establishment of suicide prevention and crisis services throughout the country. These were spearheaded by the efforts of mental health professionals on the West Coast. Crisis telephone counseling services, known popularly as **hot lines,** became common. So did the use of both paid and volunteer nonprofessional crisis workers. As community-based mental health programs became more firmly established and organized, many of them took on these crisis intervention functions.

Norris Hansell (1976) has developed a contemporary approach to people in crisis. Hansell's work with those in distress is based on findings of the theorists and researchers discussed earlier. In Hansell's social framework approach, the reestablishment of severed social attachments is necessary for successful crisis resolution. In this view, the emphasis is on social factors as the sources of problems. Other individuals whose work has influenced modern-day crisis intervention are Abraham Maslow (1970) and Erik Erikson (1963).

Crisis Defined

The word *crisis* stems from the Greek *krinein*, "to decide." In Chinese two characters are used to write the word *crisis*—one is the character for *danger* and the other the character for *opportunity*. A **crisis** is an acute, time-limited state of disequilibrium resulting from situational, developmental, or societal sources of stress. A person in this state is temporarily unable to cope with or adapt to the stressor by utilizing previous methods of problem solving. To understand the concept fully, we must differentiate among levels of distress to illustrate what a crisis is not. Stress is not crisis. Everyone feels stress at various times, in a variety of forms. Stress is pressure and tension. Stressful situations may demand our attention and may be exhausting; however, stress is not a crisis. An emergency is a situation that often demands an immediate response to ensure the survival of an individual. Although an emergency is not itself a crisis, an emergency can ultimately precipitate a crisis. A crisis is not a mental disorder. A crisis can happen to someone who never had a mental disorder or to someone who is currently experiencing a mental disorder. See Table 28–1 for additional information differentiating levels of distress.

Crisis situations are turning points or junctures in the life of an individual. Successful negotiation of a crisis leads either to a return to the precrisis state or to psychologic growth and increased competence. Unsuccessful negotiation of the crisis leaves the person feeling anxious, threatened, and ineffective. Persons may also respond to a crisis event with disturbed personal coping or frankly psychotic behavior.

Because a state of disequilibrium is so uncomfortable, a crisis is self-limiting. However, the person who experiences a crisis alone is more vulnerable to unsuccessful negotiation than the person who works through a crisis with help. Working with a helping person increases the likelihood that the person in crisis will resolve it in a positive way.

All crises have these factors in common:

- All crises are experienced as sudden. Often, the person is not aware of a warning signal, whether or not others could "see it coming." The individual or family feels that they have little or no preparation for the event or trauma.

- The crisis is often experienced as ultimately life-threatening, whether this perception is realistic or not.

- Often, communication with significant others is decreased or cut off.

- There may be perceived or real displacement from familiar surroundings or significant loved ones.

- All crises have an aspect of loss, whether actual or perceived. The losses can include an object, person, a hope, a dream, or any significant factor for that individual.

The next section addresses origins of crises. Natural, accidental, and man-made disasters are discussed later in this chapter. Other kinds of crises are covered in appropriate chapters.

Crisis types have been a traditional focus of study. In the contemporary view, the origins of crises are as important as the types of crises. Hoff (1989) points out that if we know how the crisis began, we have a better opportunity to intervene effectively. These are the three categories of crisis origins:

1. Situational (traditional term: unanticipated)

2. Transitional (traditional term: anticipated)

3. Cultural/Social

Situational Crisis

Situational crises can originate from three sources: material or environmental (e.g., fire or natural disaster), personal or physical (e.g., heart attack, diagnosis of fatal illness, bodily disfigurement), and interpersonal or social (death of a loved one or divorce). These situations are usually unplanned and unexpected. Because the event leading to the crisis is usually unexpected, one generally cannot do anything directly to prevent it. In a more indirect sense, an individual can attempt to keep healthy and focus on the most effective methods of interacting with others. However, the complexity of the experience influences the resolution of the trauma. For instance, an individual coping with one traumatic incident is more likely to resolve the experience than the individual faced with multiple traumas or factors.

TABLE 28–1 Distress Differentiation

Type of Distress or Problem	Origins	Possible Manifestations
Stress (acute)	Hazardous life events (such as heart attack, accident, death of loved one, violent attack, sudden job loss, natural disaster)	Emotional crisis General adaptation syndrome
	Invasion by microorganisms	General adaptation syndrome Disease process
	Man-made disaster	Annihilation of present civilization
Stress (chronic)	Strain in social relationships (such as marriage)	Burnout
	Position in social structure (age, sex, race, class)	Psychosomatic or "stress-related" illness Emotional or mental breakdown
	Socioeconomic problems (such as unemployment)	
	Chronic ill health	Emotional ⎫
	Developmental transition states	Behavioral ⎬ Changes Cognitive Biophysical ⎭
Crisis	Traumatic situations (material, personal/physical, interpersonal)	
	Transition states (developmental and other)	
	Cultural values, social structure	
Emotional or mental breakdown	Failure of positive response to acute stress and/or crisis	Neurotic and/or psychotic symptoms (such as learned helplessness or self-denigration of a battered woman)
	Continuation of chronic stress from various sources	

Transitional Crisis

This category consists of two types, universal and nonuniversal transition states. Universal transition states are those life cycle changes or normal transitions of human development. These are the traditional stages of human development that include infancy, childhood, puberty, adolescence, adulthood, middle age, and old age. During each stage, the individual is subject to unique stressors. Each stage of development is characterized by developmental tasks that the individual must accomplish to progress to the next level. A failure at any one level compromises the next stage of development.

People in transition usually experience increased anxiety and tension as they move through each successive stage. For every stage, there are changes in expectations, roles, sense of self, body image, and attitudes toward others. Thus, the stages are predictable, and the nurse can assist by preventive, educative techniques.

The second category of transition states, termed nonuniversal transition states, includes such changes as marriage, retirement, and the transition from student to worker. Crises associated with these states arise when the individual enters a new area of development or functioning and cannot adapt to function at that level. Crises originating from these sources differ from situational crises. Nonuniversal transition states are like developmental transition states in that they can usually be anticipated and planned and prepared for. Unlike developmental events or transitions, however, they are not experi-

Possible Responses		Duration
Positive	**Negative**	**Duration**
Grief work	Failure to ask for and accept help	Brief
Adaptation, emotional and social growth through healthy coping	Suicide, assault, addiction, emotional/ mental breakdown	
Medical treatment, rest, exercise	Refusal of treatment, complications, possible death	
Prevention: Political action	Denial	
Life-style changes (such as diet, rest, exercise, leisure)	Exacerbation of burnout	Weeks, months, years, or lifetime
Social change strategies	All of the above, and mystification by and response to *symptoms vs. sources* of chronic stress	
Transition state preparation	Inability to accomplish new role tasks	
Grief work	Same as for acute stress	Few days to 6 weeks
Crisis coping and management by use of personal, social, and material resources		
Prevention: Education about sources of crisis and appropriate preventive action (such as contemporary rites of passage, action to reduce social disparity)		
Reorganization or change of ineffective emotional, cognitive, and behavioral response to stress and crisis (usually with help of therapy)	Same as all of above, and increased vulnerability to crisis and inability to cope with acute and chronic stress	Weeks, months, years, or lifetime
Action to change social sources of chronic stress		

SOURCE: Hoff LA: *People in Crisis: Understanding and Helping,* ed. 3. Addison-Wesley, 1989, pp 52–53.

enced by everyone. An individual in a transitional state is at risk of experiencing a crisis. If the individual experiences additional trauma or change, the risk increases. Whenever individuals experience more than two life changes or traumatic events, their coping capacity may be strained, and the potential for crisis becomes greater. Crises that originate from situational and transitional states are generally less complex and more easily treated than cultural/social crises.

Cultural/Social Crisis

Crises with cultural and social sources include job loss stemming from discrimination, deviant acts of others, and behavior that violates accepted social norms such as robbery, rape, incest, marital infidelity, and physical abuse. These crises are never expected, but they are still somewhat predictable. Crises arising from sociocultural sources are less amenable to control by individuals. There is often a stronger component of community control or influence. Very often, cultural views or government action may be a component of either the identification or resolution of these crises.

Crisis Sequencing

A crisis can be thought of as having these three stages: precrisis, crisis, and postcrisis. One assumption in crisis theory is that all individuals are in a state of

Myths and Realities about Crisis

Myth	Reality
People in crisis are suffering from a form of mental illness.	Not everyone who is in crisis is "mentally ill"; however, people who are in crisis may have had a prior emotional problem. Inadequate resolution of a crisis may result in more chronic emotional problems.
People in crisis cannot help themselves.	Many who work with people in crisis mistakenly believe this myth. This belief often leads to an incomplete or compromised resolution of the crisis. It also leaves people who work with those in crisis at a risk for rescue fantasies, feeling overwhelmed and burned out.
Only psychiatrists or highly trained therapists can effectively help people in crisis.	A great deal of crisis work has been done by volunteers, police, ministers, and front-line workers. Many mental health professionals have not completed courses in crisis training.
Crisis intervention is merely a stopgap or Band-Aid and is a trivial approach in comparison with "real therapy" given by professionals.	This myth is slowly fading as more people become acquainted with crisis intervention techniques. Crisis intervention may be the preferred treatment, especially if the individual was functioning at a high level prior to the crisis.
Crisis intervention is a form of psychotherapy.	While crisis intervention is not a Band-Aid, it is also not psychotherapy.
Crisis intervention happens only as a "one-time shot" and produces changes for a short time.	Crisis intervention is often done in two to eight sessions over a six-week period. Crisis intervention has been shown to have long-lasting benefits.

SOURCE: Adapted from Hoff LA: *People in Crisis: Understanding and Helping,* ed. 3. Addison-Wesley, 1989, pp 6–8.

dynamic equilibrium with their environment. An individual strives to maintain this state of equilibrium by adapting or coping with events of daily living.

At times in everyone's life, situations occur that have the potential to disrupt the equilibrium and may result in a crisis. Factors that influence whether or not an individual enters a crisis state are called balancing factors. These are described in a later section. Myths about crisis are contrasted with realities about crisis in the accompanying box.

Precrisis

The *precrisis stage* is the stage of maintaining or attempting to maintain equilibrium. If the individual's problem-solving methods are successful, the person avoids a crisis and reverts to a state of dynamic equilibrium. If the problem(s) are too severe or if the balancing factors are inadequate, equilibrium is not maintained, the problem is not solved, and a crisis results.

Crisis

The *crisis stage* is the reaction to the event, problem, or trauma, not the event itself. Reactions to such events or traumas are highly individual. In this phase, the balancing factors have failed and the individual is in a full crisis state. In this state of disequilibrium, the individual cannot apply previous methods of reducing tension and anxiety. Inner turmoil and intrapersonal

Citation

Williams JS, Siegel JP: Marital disruption and physical illness: The impact of divorce and spouse death on illness. J Traumatic Stress 1989;2(4):555–562.

Study Problem/Purpose

The purpose of this study was to examine the relationship between the incidence of life stresses and the occurrence of illness in the general population. It was hypothesized that people who experienced spouse death or divorce in the preceding five years would have a higher rate of illness than those who did not experience these stressful events.

Methods

The sample for this study was chosen from the total noninstitutionalized English-speaking population of the United States aged 18 and older. A full probability sampling procedure was utilized. The data for the analysis were taken from the General Social Survey of the National Data Program for Social Science gathered in 1986 and 1987 by the National Opinion Research Center. All information was obtained by personal interviews. The authors of the survey chose to accept the presence of any debilitating disease as representative of illness. The reporting of illness constituted their measurement of illness. Survey respondents were asked (a) if they had been hospitalized for any reason other than child delivery during the last five years and (b) if they had been disabled or unable to carry on regular life activities for one month or longer due to illness in the last five years.

The sample was divided into four groups: respondents whose spouse had died during the last five years ($n=52$), those who had been divorced during the last five years ($n=263$), those who had married or remarried in the last five years ($n=1741$), and those who had never married. (This last group was not included in the survey because spouse death and divorce did not apply to them). Two surveys were combined (1986 and 1987) for a total sample of 2802. Of those, 5.4 percent had lost a spouse, 9.4 percent had been divorced, 62.1 percent were married, and 23.1 percent were single. The sample was also classified according to age group, income level, and educational preparation.

Findings

The findings from the study suggest that both divorce and loss of a spouse are meaningful predictors of increased illness. It is also evident that people respond to divorce and spouse death differently, depending on the individual's age, sex, income, and level of education.

The relationship between the loss of a spouse and increased incidence of illness is strongly affected by age, with the younger age group having the strongest relationship. The authors speculate that the increased responsibilities of raising a young family may result in cumulative stress, an effect that has been speculated to occur in studies of low socioeconomic single-parent families. The relationship between loss of spouse and increased physical illness is not as evident among the older group. Because the incidence of spouse death increases with age, the older group may be better prepared psychologically for the likelihood of losing a spouse.

Other findings include:

- Within the five year age span, females had a healthier adjustment to divorce.

- Middle income earners showed the highest incidence of illness related to spouse death, while this group had the lowest incidence among divorced responders.

- Higher education was found to have a mitigating effect on the relationship between loss of spouse and incident of illness. The opposite was found in regard to divorce; responders with highest levels of education who had been divorced were found to have the highest incidence of illness.

Implications

This study reinforces some of the current data suggesting that divorce and death of spouse are significant life crises for many people. The variables associated with these factors point out additional factors that will alert a nurse to evaluate who is at high risk for crisis. Since physiologic distress might indicate an incomplete resolution of a stressful event, these factors are additional "red flags" to help the nurse identify and assist people at risk. The most important finding is that this study gives further credibility to the establishment of links between these life crises and illness. In addition, the authors suggest additional research into other variables associated with this phenomenon.

conflict are great, as are anxiety and tension. Often the individual makes erratic attempts to solve the problem. Significant others may observe a disorganization uncharacteristic of that person.

The crisis state is so disruptive that an individual cannot maintain this state for long. Crisis states are time limited and do not last longer than six weeks.

Postcrisis

Because the crisis phase is time limited, everyone who experiences a crisis enters the postcrisis phase. During this phase, the individual arrives at or develops a new equilibrium. This new equilibrium may be close to that of the precrisis state, or it may be a more positive or more negative state. If the new equilibrium is more positive, the person experiences growth and may now have a better social network, newfound problem-solving abilities, or an improved self-image. If the new equilibrium is more negative, the individual may lose skills, adopt a regressive stance, or develop socially unacceptable behaviors. An example of all three crisis phases follows.

Mike is a 62-year-old man. For the last 40 years of his life he has carried a diagnosis of Schizophrenia, Paranoid Type. For the last 20 years, he has avoided repeated hospitalizations and exacerbations of his illness because he and his wife have been alert for beginning signs of problems and he has continued to take his medication. In October of last year, their apartment caught fire and burned. He and his wife were upset but thankful that they and their dog had escaped without injury.

Neighbors rallied around them and helped Mike and his wife find and furnish a new apartment. For two months things appeared to return to normal. Then in December Mike's wife died after a stroke. Mike was very sad but continued to live in the new apartment. He increased his visits to the mental health clinic, and his widowed sister visited daily. Mike's medication remained at the same level, and he did not experience additional symptoms. In February of this year, Mike's dog died. Shortly after that, he experienced a mild heart attack. Mike felt lost and alone. Because of the cardiac problems, Mike's former medication—which he believed kept him from hallucinating—was now contraindicated. Mike became increasingly depressed and stated that he had nothing to live for. He began to experience auditory hallucinations, which were not immediately controlled by the new medications. In March, Mike took an overdose of cardiac and neuroleptic medications and was found dead by his sister the next day.

Not all people who are exposed to stress (even extreme stress) experience serious or prolonged disorders. Approximately 80 percent of all people who are confronted with serious life experiences are able to work through these situations themselves with support from significant others. The remaining 20 percent have difficulties that require intervention and assistance.

Although not every person experiencing a life change needs psychotherapy, most people benefit from information, support, and advice. An individual's resiliency and vulnerability to stress are important. See Chapter 5 for additional information on stress and the stress adaptation syndrome.

Who will enter a crisis state, since not everyone does? Many factors determine whether a person faced with a life change or traumatic event will enter a crisis period. These balancing factors are discussed in the following section.

Balancing Factors

The nature of the trauma or experience is one influence on the resolution of the crisis. In addition, the greater the number of balancing factors in the crisis equation, the more effective the resolution. Aguilera (1990) indicates that these three balancing factors are important to the successful resolution of a crisis:

• *Perception of the event*—how individuals perceive and understand the event/crisis in their lives. Are they being punished? Is this happening only to them and never to anyone else? How will the event affect their future? Do they see the situation realistically, or is it distorted?

• *Situational supports*—the availability of people who can help individuals in crisis solve the problem. Meaningful relationships with others give support and assistance during the crisis. Individuals with inadequate support are likely to experience a decrease in self-esteem. In turn, lowered self-esteem may make an event appear more threatening.

• *Coping mechanisms.* All people use mechanisms to cope with anxiety and tension. Because the individual has used these coping mechanisms with success in the past, they become part of the individual's coping repertoire. These tension-relieving mechanisms can be obvious or subtle. They are not considered pathologic unless they interfere with the activities of daily living or the individual's ability to cope, e.g., an alcoholic who utilizes denial about his alcohol intake to decrease his anxiety about it.

If all these balancing factors are present when an individual experiences a state of disequilibrium, it is unlikely that a crisis will result. Figure 28–1 illustrates how these balancing factors affect the outcome of a stressful event.

The Nursing Process and Crisis Intervention

Crisis intervention as a therapeutic strategy is strongly

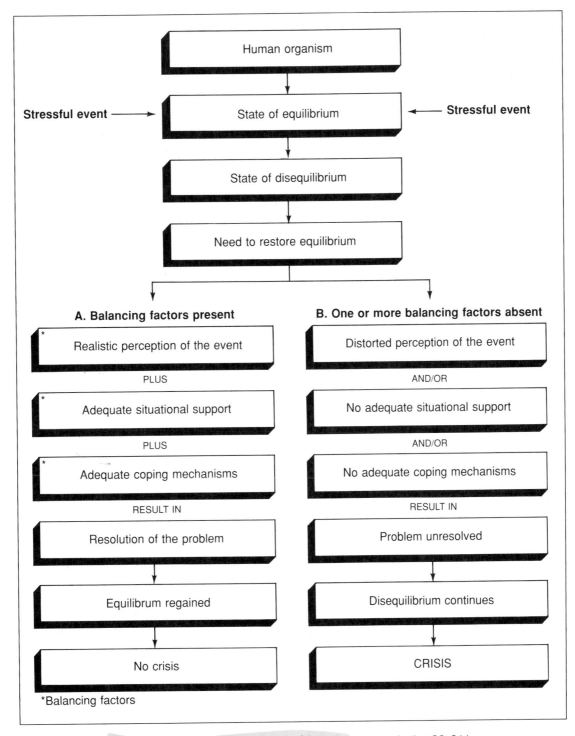

FIGURE 28–1   The effect of balancing factors in a stressful event.   *SOURCE: Aguilera DC: Crisis Intervention: Theory and Methodology, ed 6. Mosby, 1990, p 66.*

humanistic. People are viewed as capable of personal growth and as having the ability to influence and control their own lives. During the acute stage of a crisis, the goal of crisis intervention is to restore the survivor to the pretrauma level of functioning as quickly as possible. This can be accomplished by taking advantage of rapid therapeutic gains that are possible when the person's normal defenses are rela-

tively permeable or weakened. As the disequilibrium subsides, reorganization takes place. This state is generally seen as adaptive and integrative. However, it can also be maladaptive, and if so it might result in further crises or even be destructive. Intervention prior to a maladaptive response is the goal of crisis intervention. The traditional steps of the nursing process correspond closely to the steps of crisis intervention.

Assessing

Assessment of the individual is the first phase of crisis intervention. The nurse or helper must focus on the person and the problem. The nurse gathers data about the client, the client's coping style, the precipitating event, the situational supports, the client's perception of the crisis, and the client's ability to handle the problem. This is an essential and critical step of crisis intervention. This information is the basis for later decisions about how and when to intervene, and whom to call.

The nurse needs to assess and evaluate the client's suicide potential. (See Chapter 23 for lethality assessment.) During this time, a client may need to be hospitalized to ensure safety, and a referral to the psychiatrist or emergency room of the local hospital may be necessary. Part of the overall assessment is to determine what is necessary to return this client to a state of equilibrium; this may be different from what is necessary to solve the problem.

Often the "symptom bearer" or "identified patient" may really be seeking assistance for the entire family. The crisis may be a response to a family problem.

Kristen, age 13, was referred to the school nurse after talking openly in the classroom about suicide. Kristen lived with her mother, and she had changed schools three times in this school year because of her mother's recent hospitalization. Initially, it appeared that Kristen was reacting to the multiple moves and her mother's hospitalization. However, after further interviews with both mother and Kristen, the problem became much clearer. Kristen's father had not been able to see her despite her recent attempts to connect with him. He had been a source of support during her mother's absence. Kristen later said she was frightened that her mother would be rehospitalized and that no one would be there for her. Her parents continued to have a stormy relationship after their divorce, and often arguments would end in cold silences. Kristen said she was frightened and that she wanted and needed some attention. She mentioned being "terrified that I might be all alone." She thought her talk of suicide might make her parents stop fighting and bring them back together.

Some common family crises are death of a family member, terminal illness of a family member, single parenting, divorce, drug/alcohol dependence, family violence, infidelity, remarriage, mental illness, incest, and "empty nest syndrome." These usually come under the heading of situational or transitional crises. To intervene effectively, the nurse should meet with as many family members as possible to assess family resources, coping skills, and interpersonal styles. Very often these crises accompany role changes or additional stress in families that do not have the resources to meet the challenge.

Diagnosing

Which nursing diagnoses apply to people in crisis depends on the individual's response to the situation. These are among the nursing diagnoses that might apply:

- Anxiety

- Impaired verbal communication

- Ineffective individual coping

- Hopelessness

- Social isolation

- Ineffective family coping: Compromised or Disabling

- Impaired social interaction

- Altered thought processes

- Chronic (or Situational) low self-esteem

- Rape-trauma syndrome

- Dysfunctional grieving

- High risk for self-directed violence

- Sleep pattern disturbance

- Spiritual distress

Planning and Implementing Interventions

Effective planning for crisis intervention must be:

- Based on careful assessment

- Developed in active collaboration with the person in crisis and the significant people in that person's life

- Focused on immediate, concrete, contributing problems

- Based on an understanding of human dependence needs

- Appropriate to the person's level of thinking, feeling, and behaving

- Consistent with the person's life-style and culture

- Time limited, concrete, and realistic

- Mutually negotiated and renegotiated

- Organized to provide for follow-up

Crisis intervention as a treatment modality is quite different from other kinds of mental health interventions. See Table 28–2 on pages 676–677 for additional information on these distinctions.

Types of Crisis Intervention Modes

Crisis Counseling   Crisis counseling is a type of brief therapy. Unlike therapies that focus on bringing about major personality changes, crisis counseling focuses on solving immediate problems. It lasts from five to six sessions and involves individuals, groups, or families. The following techniques are used:

- Listen actively and with concern

- Encourage the open expression of feelings

- Help the client gain an understanding of the crisis

- Help the client gradually accept reality

- Help the client explore new ways of coping with problems

- Link the client to a social network

- Engage in decision counseling or problem solving with the client

- Reinforce newly learned coping devices

- Follow up the case after resolution of the crisis

Telephone Counseling   Suicide prevention and crisis intervention centers rely heavily on telephone counseling by volunteers who have professional consultation available to them. Sometimes called *hot lines* and often available round-the-clock, they allow the caller to remain anonymous and test what it is like to ask for help. No appointment, travel, or money is necessary, and help of some kind is immediate. The volunteers usually work within a protocol that indicates what information they need from the client to assess the crisis. Their goal is to plan steps to provide immediate relief and then long-term follow-up, if necessary.

The following interventions are important in telephone counseling:

- If the caller is reluctant to give a name and location, do not press for this information. The caller may feel threatened and hang up.

- Listen for background noises that may give clues to the caller's location.

- Use a note pad to write messages to coworkers so that the conversation is not interrupted.

- Keep the caller talking. This gives the nurse time to begin to develop a relationship, to trace the call, or to contact relatives or police if necessary.

- Allow the caller to ventilate all feelings. The nurse should accept anger, manipulation, etc., in order to keep contact.

- Emphasize that the nurse is available to talk as long as the caller needs to do so.

- Reinforce positive responses and actions, such as the fact that the caller is talking instead of acting out hopeless feelings.

- Acknowledge that the caller feels distress but explain that the caller does not need to inflict self-harm to emphasize it.

- Do not overuse reflection of feelings, which, in this setting, may sound uncaring or superficial. Instead, offer direction and solutions to problems

- If the caller is threatening immediate harm to self or to others, notify the police, an area mental health crisis unit, or family members to intervene with the caller. Most hot lines have the ability to trace phone calls.

- To fully assess the caller for risk of suicide, perform a lethality assessment (see Chapter 23).

- If the nurse is knowledgeable about making a no-suicide contract, this can ease the transition from telephone to in-person treatment.

This type of intervention can be very stressful for the nurse/counselor. Remember that despite our efforts to communicate concern, the ultimate decision maker is the caller.

Home Crisis Visits   Home visits are made when telephone counseling does not suffice or when the intervenors need to obtain additional information by direct observation or to reach a client who is unobtainable by telephone. Home visits are appropriate when the intervenors need to initiate contacts rather than waiting for clients to come to them—e.g., when a telephone caller is assessed to be highly suicidal or when a concerned neighbor, physician, or clergyman informs the agency of clients in potential crisis.

Often these clients are too disorganized or distraught to seek help by themselves. The police may arrange for a home crisis visit to avoid imprisoning or hospitalizing a client. Problems commonly encountered are spouse battering, child abuse, psychiatric emergencies, and medical emergencies.

The crisis intervenors are usually a male-female team who are highly skilled and experienced in crisis intervention. The male-female team might be perceived as less threatening than two men, two women, or a single person. Their goal is to defuse the situation with as little disruption and violence as possible and to engage the clients in longer-term treatment.

There are others who intervene in community crises as well. The public health nurse is in an excellent position to identify, assess, and intervene with clients experiencing a life crisis. They often have access to community resources as well as informal communication lines, and they usually maintain contact with families and clients for longer periods of time than nurses in other settings. Public health nurses are often

TABLE 28-2 Differential Aspects: Crisis, Mental Health, and Social Service Models

	Psychotherapy	Medical-Institutional	Crisis Intervention	Social-Rehabilitation
Type of People Served	Those who wish to correct neurotic personality or behavior patterns	People with serious mental or emotional breakdowns	Individuals and families in crisis or precrisis states	Those who are chronically disabled
Service Goals	Work through unconscious conflicts Reconstruct behavior and personality patterns Personal and social growth	Control, adjust Recover from acute disturbance	Growth-promoting Personal and social integration	Return to normal functioning in society as far as possible
Service Methods	Introspection Catharsis Interpretation Free association (Use of additional techniques depends on philosophy and training of therapist)	Medication Behavior modification Electric shock Group activities (Use of additional techniques depends on philosophy of institution)	Social and environmental manipulation Focus on feelings and problem solving May use medication to promote goals Decision counseling	Work training Resocialization Training in activities of daily living

recognized by the community as knowledgeable experts who are available for immediate assistance.

Emily, age 78, and her sister Frances, age 84, lived in a run-down part of town. Frances became seriously ill with pneumonia and became progressively weaker. Emily became more anxious about Frances's health when her sister refused to see a doctor. She was sure her sister would need to go to a nursing home. When the visiting nurse came by to visit Emily's neighbor, Emily asked the nurse to see Frances. Together they were able to persuade Frances to get medical care so that she could stay home.

Other Interventions One-to-one interventions are important to an individual in crisis. However, the nurse who works with people in crisis often needs to use many nontraditional interventions, which can be as important as any verbal interventions. The nurse who works successfully with people in crisis must have a flexible, open view of what may be therapeutic with different individuals. This nurse needs a full repertoire of skills and interventions that can be individualized to assist all types of clients in crisis. Some examples of these interventions follow.

Assisting with Environmental Changes

• Finding shelter for a homeless person

• Obtaining shelter for a battered woman and her children

• Evacuating a family when a hurricane warning has been posted

Assisting with Planned Events

• Discussing methods of contraception with adolescents or young men and women

• Preparing a child for a tonsillectomy

• Arranging for a volunteer from the Reach for Recovery Program to visit a woman who has had a mastectomy

Helping Develop Social Supports

• Introducing a woman whose husband is an alcoholic to Al-Anon groups in her community

• Referring a family with a terminally ill member to a local hospice

TABLE 28–2 *(continued)*

	Psychotherapy	*Medical-Institutional*	*Crisis Intervention*	*Social-Rehabilitation*
Activity of Workers	Exploratory Nondirective Interpretive	Direct, noninvolved or indirect	Active/direct (depends on functional level of client)	Structured less than in crisis intervention
Length of Service	Usually long-term	Short or long (depends on degree of disability and approach of psychiatrist) High repeat rate	Short—usually six sessions or less	Long-term—a few months to 2–3 years
Beliefs about People	Individualistic or social (depends on philosophy of therapist)	Individualistic—social aspect secondary Institution and order often more important than people	Social—people are capable of growth and self-control	People can change Mental disability or a diagnosis should not spell hopelessness
Attitudes toward Service	Emphasis on wisdom of therapist and fifty-minute hour Flexibility varies with individual therapist	Scheduled Staff attitudes may become rigid and institutionalized	Flexible, any hour	Willingness to stick with it and observe only slow change Hopefulness and expectation of goal achievement

SOURCE: Hoff LA: *People in Crisis: Understanding and Helping,* ed. 3. Addison-Wesley, 1989, pp 21–22.

• Giving a rape victim the telephone number of the rape crisis hotline

Confidentiality Confidentiality is a concern to many people seeking crisis assistance, as the accompanying case study of Ms B shows. Ms B experienced extreme anxiety when she thought her husband would find out where she was and come to hurt her or the children. It is important for anyone working with clients in crisis to understand and maintain confidentiality.

Evaluating

Nurses in acute care or short-term settings may not see the long-term effects of their interventions. Typically, nurses in these settings need to evaluate the crisis, set up the plan, and begin implementing it.

In long-term settings, the nurse can evaluate the client or family response to the intervention by determining if clients have resumed their precrisis level of functioning or evidence increased functioning (growth) in the area. A nurse in either a long- or short-term setting may also have an opportunity to evaluate if a similar problem might lead to another crisis for the client.

Natural and Accidental Disasters

We have only recently begun to understand crisis intervention in disaster situations. Federal aid for reconstruction of communities devastated by natural disasters has been available for many years, and the provision of crisis intervention services through the National Institute of Mental Health (NIMH) was organized in 1972. Before then, a community in crisis depended on the voluntary help of social service and religious groups.

Nurses are often at the scene of natural disasters.

A number of nurses were in the newest hotel in Kansas City, Missouri, in July 1981 when two skywalks in the four-story lobby collapsed, killing 111 and injuring 188 persons. These nurses, along with others who responded to calls for emergency personnel, assisted the injured and provided crisis intervention services. Some of the same nurses provided counseling services for people in the community, such as a fireman who was terrified to go on to the next emergency call and 200 people from the community who attended a session to understand their re-

Text continues on p. 683

CASE STUDY

A Client in Crisis

Identifying information

Ms B is a 28-year-old black woman who has recently separated from her husband. Until seven days ago, she resided with her 38-year-old husband and their three children in their apartment. She is employed as a cashier at the local supermarket, but has called in sick the last few days. She is referred to you after the police have found her and her three children living in her car and when they attempted to talk with her, she was confused, disoriented and unable to answer questions. The police have sent her and her three children to the waiting room of the emergency room.

Client's Definition of Present Problem, Precipitating Stressors, Coping Strategies, and Goals for Care

At the point of initial contact, Ms B was unable to discuss her problem. After spending a few hours in a "crisis holding" bed and having a meal, she is able to speak more coherently. Provisions had been made for her children (they were placed with social services for the night). Ms B was able to say "I know I need some help . . . I'm so afraid and I'm falling apart. I just can't do it by myself." Her speech then rambles and she talks of being afraid.

History of Present Problem

Ms B's current problems began approximately two months ago when her husband lost his job at the electric company. The termination was not sudden, and Mr B had been ruminating about it for some time. Since that time, Mr B has been drinking heavily and become increasingly physically and verbally abusive. Two weeks ago, the physical attacks became a daily occurrence, and he began to hit the children as well. Seven nights ago, Ms B took the car and did not return. She parked near her home, and she and her children slept in the car. In the morning, she awakened to her husband pounding on the car with a bat. She became frightened and drove away. Since that time, she has been driving and parking for short periods of time while she naps. She admits she has not had more than two hours of sleep for the last forty-eight hours. She was unable to go to her neighbors or seek out any other assistance and is afraid her husband will kill her or their children because "he's just not himself."

Psychiatric History

Ms B denies any previous psychiatric history, but does state she has attempted to convince her husband to receive treatment for alcoholism. He refused, and she has not pursued this herself. She is embarrassed that she is in a psychiatric facility now and states "I can't believe this is happening to me. I don't even believe in psychiatrists."

Family History

Ms B's parents have died within the last three years. She states she did not know her father well, but she and her mother were close. The family "always" had financial trouble "so that's nothing new," and her parents had separated numerous times in the past. There had often been physical violence in her home. Her mother was usually the target, but she and her sister also were frequently slapped and excessively punished. Her sister has lived out of state for the past six years. Ms B has kept in contact with her, and they were "quite close" as children. When Ms B discusses her sister, she smiles for the first time and states "she's probably the only one who still cares."

Social History

Ms B describes herself as a hard worker. She and her husband have been married for the last eight years, and she describes most of the relationship as a "good one." "He only started this slapping thing after he started drinking." She believes she caused this behavior by making her husband angry. She has

▶

CASE STUDY (continued)

had trouble leaving home when these situations happen. She describes their three children—Peter, 9; Michael, 8; and Marilyn, 7—as "really good kids" and tells many stories about how they "help out." She says that tension and conflict began about two years ago with the death of her parents. Ms B felt increasingly alone. About one year ago, after hearing rumors about layoffs in the electric company, her husband began drinking more heavily. There were more physical fights with injuries. After this last one, Ms B decided she "couldn't take it any longer" and left. She was afraid to go to any of her neighbors and couldn't think of anywhere else to go, so she stayed in the car with her children.

Significant Health History

Ms B states she has no ongoing physical problems. She does not have allergies or illnesses. Her health history is unremarkable except for a tubal ligation a few years ago. However, today on physical examination, there is clear evidence of multiple contusions about her face and upper torso. There are several superficial abrasions on her hands and face that are in various stages of healing. She has significant discomfort in her rib area, which X-ray examination later determines is a fractured rib. Also, her lips and skin are cracked and dry, and she evidences signs of dehydration.

Current Mental Status (after three hours in holding bed)

Ms B is casually dressed, but not well groomed. Her hygiene is poor, and her clothes are rumpled. She is calmer now and speaks in a soft tone that is without energy or anger. However, over the last few hours she has had periods of mood lability and is, at times, incoherent.

Sensorium

Client is oriented to place and person. She continues to have questions about the "real time," and is disbelieving that it is a week later than she thought. She can be articulate, but also at times her thoughts wander and become quite circumstantial. Her speech becomes so disjointed as to be incoherent. Her remote memory is intact and retrievable; however, she cannot remember many details of the last week. Her judgment is impaired, her insight is compromised at this time.

Feelings

Affect was at times incongruent with mood or topics discussed. She would discuss abuse without anger and sad situations without any affect. At other times, her mood is more labile: she could initially discuss a concern in a calm manner and within minutes be crying loudly, denouncing herself and her situation.

Voice and Speech

Initially, Ms B's speech was pressured and disorganized. She had great difficulty concentrating on the topic. Progressively, over the next few hours, she was able to speak more coherently with less rambling.

Motor Behavior

Initially, Ms B was agitated and unable to sit for more than five minutes. She would pace the length of the room. As the staff stayed with her, she was able to relax more and was able to sleep for short intervals.

Thought Content

There was extreme anxiety and worry about her safety and the children's safety. She was distraught that she may be homeless with no place to go. She denied suicidal thoughts ("someone has to take care of the kids") and homicidal thoughts ("I know what it's like to be hurt. I don't want to hurt anyone else"). She is embarrassed that she now finds herself in a situation "like you see others on TV" (meaning being homeless).

CASE STUDY *(continued)*

Thought Processes	Ms B initially had trouble with concentration and was unable to focus on any concern for more than a few minutes. Her associations were loose. There is expressed content that sounds paranoid, e.g., wondering if people on the street will tell her husband where she is, or if others may also be out to harm her. However, given the major disruption on her life, it is not clear if this is a delusion. Overall she is disorganized and states "I just can't think right now."
Defenses	Ms B is currently utilizing these defense mechanisms: avoidance, denial, and intellectualization.
Insight	She has minimal insight into the nature of her current problems.
Other Significant Subjective or Objective Clinical Data	Ms B appeared during her initial stay to be more relaxed with women than with men. She would become tense and not speak when a male staff member was in the room. In a telephone call with her sister, staff gathered this additional information: She and her sister are frequently in touch; there has been episodic violence in Ms B's home for years; Ms B's sister is willing to have Ms B and the children come to live with her but is unable to pay for their fares or to transport them there.
Diagnostic Impression Nursing Diagnoses	Ineffective family coping: Disabling Ineffective individual coping Altered thought processes Post-trauma response Anxiety Sleep pattern disturbance
DSM-III-R Multiaxial Diagnosis	Axis I: Brief Reactive Psychosis, 298.80 Axis II: Post-Traumatic Stress Disorder, 309.89. Axis III: Status post trauma: injuries with contusions, fractured rib. Axis IV: Psychosocial Stressors: Severity = 4 (severe) husband's loss of a job, violence directed at her and children, homelessness, lack of financial resources. Axis V: Current GAF = 30. Highest GAF past year = 78.

NURSING CARE PLAN

Nursing Planning/Intervention		Evaluation

Nursing Diagnosis: *Ineffective family coping: Disabling*

Client will identify the current problem and the resulting violence as a family crisis.	Meet with as many of family as possible, e.g., sister or husband if this is clinically indicated. Help family to identify the true etiology of the current problem—that it is a family crisis and is multiply determined.	Client evaluates the ability of the family to resolve this difficulty now or in the future.

▶

Client Care Goals	Nursing Planning/ Intervention	Evaluation
	Assist family to set goals and identify alternatives to problems.	
	Give information to family on how to operate as a unit while also recognizing individual differences and individual needs.	

Nursing Diagnosis: *Ineffective individual coping*

The client will verbalize an awareness of her own coping style and skills. Client will express current needs and utilize needed community resources.	Encourage client to verbalize feelings about her current problems.	Client evaluates her current needs and makes plans to utilize a support network and available community resources.
	Encourage client to be accepting of the full range of her feelings.	
	Help client to take an inventory of her skills and match against current needs.	
	Help client review available support network.	
	Give information about community resources.	

Nursing Diagnosis: *Altered thought processes*

Client's thinking will be clear; client will be oriented.	Provide for basic needs (nutrition, sleep) for next 48 hours.	Client discusses her concerns in a coherent manner and can formulate a plan for herself and children.
	Reassure client frequently.	
	Allow client to verbalize all feelings without restriction. Discuss with her that anxiety, ambivalence and fear are normal responses at this time. If thought disorganization persists for more than 48 hours refer to psychiatrist for evaluation.	

Nursing Diagnosis: *Post-trauma response*

Client will be less anxious and discuss problem-solving skills to intervene in current crisis.	After developing rapport with client:	Client verbalizes understanding in her response to this crisis.
	Identify and assess the degree of fear, anxiety that are connected with the threat perceived by the client.	Client identifies methods to manage anxiety.
	Assist client in realistic decision-making and problem-solving methods to resolve her current problem.	

NURSING CARE PLAN (continued)

Client Care Goals	Nursing Planning/ Intervention	Evaluation
	Discuss usual responses to trauma, e.g., helplessness, powerlessness, feelings of guilt, tension, and anxiety.	Client verbalizes understanding in her response to this crisis.
	Encourage client to review situation without utilizing self-deprecating thoughts.	Client identifies methods to manage anxiety.

Nursing Diagnosis: *Anxiety*

Client will be able to discuss her feelings and problems with nursing staff.	Provide a safe environment:	Client verbalizes decreasing anxiety and increased feelings of comfort.
	Make safety a first priority.	
	Do not leave client alone, especially if she is very anxious.	
	Provide a room with minimal stimulation.	
	Remain calm when approaching the client.	
	Use simple, clear, direct, short statements. Avoid unclear language.	
	Use of antianxiety medications should be considered.	

Nursing Diagnosis: *Sleep pattern disturbance*

Client will reestablish precrisis sleep patterns.	Assess client's sleep patterns now and in the past. Discuss possible strategies to aid in sleep promotion, then draw up a plan to assist client to implement these.	Client sleeps 6–7 hours during the next 36 hours.
	Consider use of hypnotic agent for brief period if client is unable to sleep for another 24 hours.	
	It may be useful during the first 24 hours to stay with client or assure her that others are available should she reexperience increasing anxiety.	

sponses and reactions. Some of the nurses themselves reported that since the disaster they have experienced shock, helplessness, nightmares, and difficulty in relaxing and concentrating.

The Dunlap article (1981) about the Kansas City disaster makes it clear that helpers on the scene may have many of the same responses to a disaster as its victims do. These responses are delineated more specifically below.

Assessing

James Tyhurst (1951, 1957) identifies three overlapping phases in response to disaster. The first stage, *impact*, is stimulated by the catastrophe. The victims recognize what is happening to them and are concerned mainly with the present. During this acute phase, the victim's major concern may be staying alive. According to Tyhurst, about 75 percent of the victims experience shock and confusion. Although they appear dazed, they also exhibit the physical signs of fear. Another group of people, up to 25 percent, are "together." They logically and rationally assess the situation and develop and implement a plan for dealing with the immediate problems brought on by the catastrophe. A third group, also up to 25 percent, may panic or become immobilized with fear. They may behave hysterically, or they may be overlooked because they sit and silently stare into space.

In *recoil*, the second stage, the initial stress of the disaster has passed, and victims may no longer find their lives in immediate danger, although injuries and other discomforts come to their awareness. Emergency shelter, food, and clothing become available. Behavior of victims is usually dependent—they want to be taken care of. Weeping is common as survivors begin to realize all that has happened to them.

The full impact of the losses the victims have experienced comes in the third, or *post-trauma* period. Grief is a predominant response to the losses in their lives. Disturbed and psychotic responses may occur.

Many people essentially "relive" the experience in their dreams by having recurrent nightmares. Other sleep disturbances, including insomnia, often occur. Victims may feel a psychic numbing or emotional anesthesia in relationship to other people, previously enjoyed activities, and feelings of intimacy, tenderness, and sexuality. They may have difficulty in concentrating and remembering. The survivors of mass trauma may also feel guilty about having survived or about behavior that helped them survive. When victims are exposed to situations that resemble or in some way symbolize the traumatic event, their symptoms may increase and they may feel even greater distress.

Interventions to address the longer-lasting effects of a traumatic incident are more complicated than interventions in the acute phase of crisis intervention. These principles are indicated for treatment of delayed or chronic post-traumatic stress disorder reactions:

- Establishment of the therapeutic trust relationship
- Education regarding the stress recovery process
- Stress management and stress reduction
- Regression back to or a re-experiencing of the trauma
- Integration of the trauma experience

The brief examples below illustrate the post-trauma experience.

On December 21, 1988, Pan Am flight 103 crashed over Lockerbie, Scotland. All 259 people on the plane, as well as 11 people on the ground, were killed. Family members of those on the flight, as well as the community of Lockerbie, were shocked and grief-stricken. During the search for clues to the cause of the crash, many personal items were recovered. Each item that was found renewed the families' torment.

At Cape Canaveral, Florida, on January 28, 1986, the space shuttle *Challenger* exploded seconds after launching. All seven astronauts aboard were killed. The entire nation grieved. Each replaying of the videotape of the explosion renewed the grief of the families and of the nation.

In a freak upstate New York snowstorm, over one hundred people were involved in a sixty-car pile up on a major interstate highway. Ten people died as a result of injuries sustained during the crash. One month later, people who live nearby are startled whenever they hear car brakes or horns. Eight people involved in the crash still will not drive.

Diagnosing

The nursing diagnoses determined for these persons depend on their individual responses. The nursing diagnoses listed earlier in this chapter on page 674 are also appropriate in natural disasters.

Planning and Implementing Interventions

The type of help needed by disaster victims changes as the disaster unfolds. Initially, people need information about evacuation plans, rescue efforts, locations of food, shelter, and medical care. The media can provide this information, especially when there is time to plan and anticipate need (as with floods or hurricanes). Table 28–3 outlines assistance needed during natural disasters.

TABLE 28–3   **Assistance during Three Phases of Natural Disaster**

	Help Needed	Help Provided by	Possible Outcomes if Help Unavailable
Phase I: **Impact**	Information on source and degree of danger Escape and rescue from immediate source of danger	Communication network: radio, TV, public address system Community rescue resources: police and fire departments, Red Cross, National Guard	Physical injury or death
Phase II: **Recoil**	Shelter, food, drink, clothing, medical care	Red Cross Salvation Army Voluntary agencies such as colleges used as mass shelters Local health and welfare agencies Mental health and social service agencies skilled in crisis intervention Pastoral counselors State and federal assistance for all of the above services	Physical injury Delayed grief reactions Later emotional or mental disturbance
Phase III: **Post Trauma**	Physical reconstruction Social reestablishment Psychologic support concerning aftereffects of the event itself; bereavement counseling concerning loss of loved ones, home, and personal property	State and federal resources for physical reconstruction Social welfare agencies Crisis and mental health services Pastoral counselors	Financial hardship Social instability Long-lasting mental, emotional, or physical health problems

SOURCE: Hoff LA: *People in Crisis: Understanding and Helping,* ed. 3. Addison-Wesley, 1989, pp 316–317.

After acute needs are met at the disaster scene, in makeshift hospitals, or in emergency rooms, morgues, and shelters, more far-reaching interventions are necessary. People need housing, jobs, and help in reconstructing their emotional lives. These are the psychologic needs of victims both during and after a disaster:

• To talk out the experience and express their feelings of fear, panic, loss, and grief

• To become fully aware and accepting of what has happened to them

• To resume concrete activity and reconstruct their lives with the social, physical, and emotional resources available

To assist victims through the crisis, crisis workers should:

• Listen with concern and sympathy and ease the way for the victims to tell their tragic story, weep, express feelings of anger, loss, frustration, and despair.

• Help the victims of disaster accept in small doses the tragic reality of what has happened. This means staying with them during the initial stages of shock and denial. It also may mean accompanying them back to the scene of the tragedy and being available for support when they are faced with the full impact of their loss.

• Assist them to make contact with relatives, friends, and other resources needed to begin the process of social and physical reconstruction. This could mean making telephone calls to locate relatives, accompanying someone to apply for financial aid, or giving information about social and mental health agencies for follow-up services.

People who are hysterical or panicked should receive prompt attention to avoid the contagion of panic that sometimes occurs in large groups. It sometimes helps hysterical or panic-stricken persons to perform a small but structured task that focuses their energies constructively. Nurses should remember, however, that assigning tasks beyond the person's capabilities at that time will add to the person's anxiety and feeling of helplessness. Nurses in disaster situations incorporate concepts and intervention strategies related to death and loss.

Immediate and effective community responses to disaster or crisis situations help victims and survivors resolve their experiences satisfactorily. The example below demonstrates how a community crisis or disaster can be managed.

In November 1989, a tornado strikes an elementary school in a small Northern community. Twelve students are killed when an external wall collapses on them. The community is devastated. A group of concerned counselors from a nearby community begins meeting with groups of students, family members, faculty members, and others. The community holds a memorial service at the church, and area businesses close for the day so that all may attend. One month later, an investigation begins to determine how this could have happened. There is much energy behind the group—all are determined to find the cause so that nothing like this happens ever again.

Evaluating

It is difficult to evaluate the effectiveness of disaster intervention because of the large numbers of people involved and the innately disruptive nature of a disaster. Evaluation can take place at many different levels: Nurses can evaluate their work with individual clients; mental health agencies can monitor statistics on groups of clients; government agencies can assess the numbers of unemployed and homeless; public health departments can measure the extent of disease and disability. The most important aspect of evaluation is the opportunity it gives for reflection on the nature of the disaster. Some catastrophes are accidents, some are clearly avoidable, some are caused by human greed and insensitivity. All afford the survivors the chance to be better prepared for future crises.

Effect of Crisis Work on Nurses

Crisis intervention is stressful work. Nurses who work with victims of abuse, incest, violence, or other trauma of human origin see the results of humankind at its worst. To remain effective in their work, nurses should:

• Be aware of the impact of repeatedly hearing accounts of traumatic stories

• Strive for a balance between their professional and personal lives

• Formulate supportive networks both professionally and socially

• Talk about their feelings with coworkers

• Receive regular supervision

• Stay updated on new information

• Involve administrative/supervisory people when making extensive intervention plans that call for more than the usual effort

• Develop realistic expectations of what might be accomplished with clients, who are always in charge of the plan

• Develop realistic expectations of what staff can or should do

CHAPTER HIGHLIGHTS

• Everyday living brings desirable and undesirable changes that result in stresses and tensions with the potential for becoming crises.

• A crisis is a self-limiting situation in which usual problem-solving or decision-making methods are not adequate.

• A crisis offers the opportunity for renewal and growth.

• Working with a helping person increases the likelihood that a crisis will be solved in a positive way.

• Nurses are often in key positions to help clients grow through the crisis experience.

• Crises may originate from three sources: transitional states (usually developmental or maturational experiences), situational experiences (stressful life events that are usually not anticipated), and cultural/societal sources (such as discrimination).

• The crisis episode may be understood as a sequence that involves three time periods—precrisis, crisis, and postcrisis.

• Crisis intervention as a therapeutic strategy is strongly humanistic in that people are viewed as capable of personal growth and able to control their own lives.

• Intervention strategies such as individual crisis counseling, crisis groups, family crisis counseling, telephone counseling, and home crisis visits are appropriate modes for dealing with either internal or external crisis.

REFERENCES

Aguilera DC: *Crisis Intervention: Theory and Methodology,* ed 6. Mosby, 1990.

Bartelo S: The aftermath of suicide on the psychiatric inpatient unit. *Gen Hosp Psychiatry* 1987; 9(3):189–197.

Britton JG, Mattson-Melcher DM: The crisis home: Sheltering patients in emotional crisis. *J Psychosoc Nurs* 1985;23(12):18–23.

Burgess AW, Hartman CR, Wolbert WA, Grant CA: Child molestation: Assessing impact in multiple victims (part 1). *Arch Psychiatr Nurs* 1987;1(1):33–39.

Caplan G: *Principles of Preventive Psychiatry.* Basic Books, 1965.

Cobb S, Lindemann E: Neuropsychiatric observations after the Cocoanut Grove fire. *Ann Surg* 1943;117:814.

Crisis intervention. *Adv Nurs Sci* 1984;6:entire issue.

Disasters and Mental Health. National Institute of Mental Health. American Psychiatric Press, 1986.

Dunlap MJ: Nurses assist injured at Hyatt disaster. *Am Nurse* 1981;13:1.

Erikson E: *Childhood and Society,* ed. 2. W. W. Norton, 1963.

Everstine DL, Everstine L: *People in Crisis: Strategic Therapeutic Interventions.* Brunner/Mazel, 1983.

Gil T et al.: Cognitive functioning in post-traumatic stress disorder. *J Traumatic Stress Disord* 1990:3(1)29–45.

Gilbert CM: Sexual abuse and group therapy. *J Psychosoc Nurs Ment Health Serv* 1988;26(5):19–23.

Hall JM, Stevens PE: AIDS: A guide to suicide assessment. *Arch Psych Nurs* 1988;1(2):116–120.

Hansell N: *The Person in Distress.* Human Services Press, 1976.

Hayes G, Goodwin T, Miors B: After disaster: A crisis support team at work. *Am J Nurs* 1990;90(2):61–64.

Heinrich LB: Care of the female rape victim. *Nurs Pract* 1987;12(11):9–19.

Herman JL, Perry JC, Van der Kolk B: Childhood trauma in borderline personality disorder. *Am J Psychiatry* 1989; 146(4):490–495.

Hoff LA: *People in Crisis: Understanding and Helping,* ed 3. Addison-Wesley, 1989.

Joint Commission on Mental Illness and Health. *Action for Mental Health.* Basic Books, 1961.

Janosik EH: *Crisis Counseling: A Contemporary Approach.* Wadsworth, 1984.

Karl, GT: Survival skills for psychic trauma. *J Psychosoc Nurs Ment Health Serv* 1989;27(4):15–19.

Kolk BA: *Psychological Trauma.* American Psychiatric Press, 1986.

Kovansky RS: Loneliness and disturbed grief: A comparison of parents who lost a child to suicide or accidental death. *Arch Psychiatr Nurs* 1989;3(2):86–96.

Kus RJ: Crises intervention, In Bulechek GM, McCloskey JC (eds): *Nursing Interventions: Treatments for Nursing Diagnoses.* Saunders, 1985.

Lindemann E: Symptomatology and management of acute grief. *Am J Psychiatry* 1944;101:101–148.

Maslow A: *Motivation and Personality,* ed 2. Harper & Row, 1970.

McCann IL, Pearlmann LA: Vicarious traumatization: A framework for understanding the psychological effects of working with victims. *J Traumatic Stress* 1990; 3(1):131–149.

Merker MS: Psychiatric emergency evaluation. *Nurs Clin North Am* 1986;21:387–396.

Michael S et al.: Rapid response mutual aid groups: A new response to social crises and natural disasters. *Social Work* 1985;30(3):245–252.

Minrath M: Breaking the race barrier. *J Psychosoc Nurs* 1985;23(8):19–24.

Mullis M: Vietnam: The human fallout. *J Psychosoc Nurs* 1984;22(2):27–32.

Mitchell J, Bray G: *Emergency Services Stress: Guidelines for Preserving the Health and Careers of Emergency Services Personnel.* Prentice-Hall, 1990.

Murphy SA: Perceptions of stress, coping, and recovery one and three years after a natural disaster. *Issues Ment Health Nurs* 1986;8:63–77.

Newberger CM, DeVos E: Abuse and victimization: A life span developmental perspective. *Am J Psychiatry* 1989; 146(5):667–669.

Parad HJ, Resnick HLP: A crisis intervention framework, in Resnick HLP, Ruben HL (eds): *Emergency Psychiatric Care.* Charles Press, 1975, pp 3–7.

Parker SD: Accident or suicide: Do life changes/events lead to adolescent suicide? *J Psychosoc Nurs* 1988;26(6): 15–19.

Patten SB et al.: Post-traumatic stress disorder and the treatment of sexual abuse. *Social Work* 1989;5:197–202.

Puskar KR, Obus NL: Management of the psychiatric emergency. *Nurs Pract* 1989;14(7):9–15.

Smith KA: Victims of abuse: Learning to appreciate the life force. *Focus* 1990;1:37–46.

Sullivan-Taylor L: Policemen and nursing students: Crisis intervention team. *J Psychosoc Nurs* 1985;23: 31–33.

Tyhurst JS: Individual reactions to community disaster. *Am J Psychiatry* 1951;107:764–769.

Tyhrust JS: The role of transition states—including disasters—in mental illness. Paper read at the Symposium on Preventative and Social Psychiatry, Walter Reed Army Institute of Research and the National Research Council, Washington, D.C., April 15–17, 1957.

Van der Kolk BA: *Psychological Trauma*. American Psychiatric Press, 1987.

van Servellen G, Nyamathi AM, Mannion W: Coping with a crisis: Evaluating psychological risks of patients with AIDS. *J Psychosoc Nurs* 1989;27(12):16–21.

Waigandt A et al.: The impact of sexual assault on physical health status. *J Traumatic Stress* 1990;3(1):93–102.

Weinrich S, Harden SB, Johnson M: Nurses respond to Hurricane Hugo victims' disaster stress. *Arch Psychiatr Nurs* 1990;4(3):195–205.

Group Process and Group Therapy

LEARNING OBJECTIVES

- Develop an appreciation for the influence of group dynamics in the lives of people

- Explain the importance of physical environment, leadership approach, decision making, trust, cohesion, and power in group functioning

- Apply knowledge of group process in work with groups of clients and groups of colleagues

- Describe four frameworks for the assessment and understanding of therapy groups

- Assess small groups in terms of their functional, structural, and interactional characteristics

- Relate the egalitarian cotherapy approach to humanistic psychiatric nursing practice in interactional group therapy

- Describe the process of creating and maintaining a group

- Identify the stages in therapy group development

- Discuss the application of here-and-now activation and process illumination to psychotherapy groups

- Describe other related group therapies and therapeutic groups

Carol Ren Kneisl

CROSS REFERENCES

Other topics related to this content are: Client government groups and milieu, Chapter 31; Group therapy with adolescents, Chapter 34; Group therapy with children, Chapter 33.

People live most of their lives in groups. They depend on others for much of their sense of personal fulfillment and achievement. The activities they undertake toward personal fulfillment are, more often than not, activities that they carry out in the company of others.

Why are groups so important? Human beings are born into a group—the family—and their survival from the moment of birth depends on relationships formed with other human beings. The sense of self, of being, of personal identity derives from the ways in which people are perceived and responded to by the other members of the groups to which they belong. People interact with others at all stages of their lives in various groups—family groups, peer groups, work groups, play groups, worship groups.

Many of the goals people set for themselves cannot be achieved without membership in groups. Other people are important to each of us, just as we are important to others. Through cooperation and coordination in groups, we can achieve objectives and reach goals that we could not through individual effort alone. In this way groups help us improve the quality of our lives.

Much of the nurse's professional life is spent in groups—groups of clients and groups of colleagues with whom the nurse plans and implements the delivery of health care services. To use groups rationally and effectively, nurses must understand the forces that underlie small group interactional processes and recognize their own patterns of participation. Group intervention is one way that psychiatric nurses can provide humanistic care for their clients. Therapy through the group process gives clients the opportunity to seek validation, give and receive interpersonal feedback, and test new and different ways of being that may improve quality of life. Groups influence a person's psychologic well-being. Mental well-being can be preserved, maintained, and restored through interaction with others in productive groups.

Historical Perspectives

Joseph Hersey Pratt, a Boston physician, began to work with tubercular persons in groups in the United States in 1906. His learning groups were organized as weekly classes of twenty to twenty-five people to whom he lectured on the importance of strict hygiene, diet, and rest in the treatment of tuberculosis. Pratt also offered support and encouragement to his clients, whose long course of illness was discouraging at best. By 1930 he had established a clinic at the Boston Dispensary in which the group method was the central therapeutic focus. His writings throughout more than fifty years of work with groups of tubercular clients demonstrate his increasing awareness of the group dynamics of this style of treatment. He is usually recognized as the founder of group psychotherapy.

Just before World War I, some physicians in the United States began to use group approaches in the treatment of psychiatric clients. E. W. Lazell (1921), one of the better-known physicians, published the first contribution to the literature on use of group treatment with psychotic (especially schizophrenic) individuals. Like Pratt, he used the lecture method. During this period, the emphasis was on encouraging, inspiring, and persuading group members, while providing information designed to educate and influence them. At about the same time, a minister named L. C. Marsh (1935), who became a psychiatrist, began to use other techniques such as art and dance classes in his work with groups.

Joshua Bierer (1942) began his work in 1939 in Great Britain, where he established social clubs for the treatment of the mentally disordered. His methods included discussion, writing, painting, and entertainment. Bierer believed that it was best to discuss individual problems in an impersonal way. He often disguised the problems for discussion to keep members of the group from realizing that their particular problems were under consideration. Bierer attempted to help persons solve the problems of daily living and make their attitudes toward life more positive. His methods were based on those of Alfred Adler, who was using group psychotherapy in his child guidance work. Adler, a socialist and one of Sigmund Freud's first students, had established clinics to provide a variety of services and resource persons to large groups of workingclass people with emotional problems. Social clubs like Bierer's gained importance in the United States over the years. Social clubs for the rehabilitation of "nervous persons" are still popular and can now be found throughout the United States. Perhaps the best known is Recovery, Inc.

A Viennese psychiatrist, Jacob L. Moreno (1946), introduced the term **group therapy** into the clinical literature in 1932. His interest in drama led him to formulate a group psychotherapy called **psychodrama.** He used dramatic techniques and the language and settings of theatrical productions to achieve psychotherapeutic goals. Moreno founded the first professional journal concerned with group psychotherapy and the first professional organization of group psychotherapists—known today as the American Society of Group Psychotherapy and Psychodrama.

During the late 1920s and early 1930s, Trigent Burrows (1927), another pupil of Freud, became interested in applying psychoanalytic principles of treatment in group settings. An American psychoanalyst,

Alexander Wolff (1949, 1950), began to apply these principles in groups. In his psychoanalytic group, Wolff analyzed the individual in interaction with other individuals instead of treating a group. He took the position that it is not valuable, and may be detrimental, to attend to group dynamics in group analysis. At about the same time that Wolff was establishing psychoanalytic groups in the United States, S. H. Foulkes began a similar practice in Great Britain (Foulkes and Anthony 1957). Both Wolff and Foulkes implemented their techniques with the armed forces in the United States and Great Britain.

Samuel R. Slavson, who is best known for developing activity group therapy for children, was also active in using psychoanalytic concepts in therapy groups (Slavson 1947). He was a prime mover in establishing the American Group Psychotherapy Association and was the first editor of the *International Journal of Group Psychotherapy.*

During World War II, group psychotherapy grew extensively in the United States. It was hailed for its economic advantages, since a large number of clients could be treated by the relatively few available psychotherapists. It was also popular among military psychiatric personnel, who found themselves overwhelmed with the number of soldiers experiencing post-traumatic stress disorder and needing some form of psychotherapy.

Since World War II there has been a tremendous growth in the group movement and a corresponding increase in the variety of group methods and group approaches in existence. In addition to the recreation groups, educational groups, and therapy groups that gained acceptance after the war, growth groups have become popular. These are oriented to understanding the self and the experience of membership by analyzing interactions with others in groups. Sadock (1985) proposes that an important factor that accounts for this growth is the waning influence of such natural groupings as the family and organized religion. Because human beings are gregarious animals with a strong desire to belong, small groups can provide the social network to help satisfy our strong desires to belong. There are similarities and differences among the characteristics of various types of groups. e.g., task groups, self-awareness/growth groups, therapy groups, and social groups. Their characteristics are compared in Table 29–1.

Although small groups have been around for as long as history itself, scientific interest in the operation and dynamics of small groups can be traced to the work of sociologists and social psychologists in the 1940s and 1950s. Notable among these early theorists was Kurt Lewin, who introduced the notion that a group was different from the simple sum of its parts. Lewin theorized that the behavior of an individual in a group cannot be based on an understanding of the psychodynamics of that individual alone but must be understood in relation to the group itself.

The small-group theories that resulted from these early studies form the base for understanding **group dynamics,** Lewin's term for the total of all the interactions among members of a group. Although there is as yet no one theory that adequately explains why people behave the way they do when in groups, several theoretic constructs help to explain the forces that modify and shape groups. Among these are decision-making processes, leadership, and power. These explanations are discussed later in this chapter.

Nurses have long been involved in working with clients and their families in small groups brought together for health teaching or supportive purposes. The role of the psychiatric nurse as group therapist, however, is relatively recent. It first received professional endorsement by the American Nurses' Association (ANA) in 1967. Qualifications of the group therapist are identified later in this chapter.

Theoretic Perspectives

To be effective, any group must accomplish three main functions:

1. Accomplishing its designated goals

2. Maintaining its own cohesion

3. Developing and modifying its structure to improve its effectiveness

Table 29–2 on page 693 lists some factors that influence these functions. These are useful in evaluating the effectiveness of a given group. They constitute the major characteristics generally observable in effective and ineffective groups and illustrate different ways of dealing with the dynamic forces in every group.

Several forces modify and shape groups, influencing their effectiveness. These forces, as well as several frameworks for analyzing and understanding group process, are discussed in the following sections.

Physical Environment

Groups exist in complex environmental settings that strongly influence the group process. The building, room, and chair and table arrangements are aspects of the environmental setting that influence the operation of the group. Superimposed on the physical structure are the influences of territoriality, personal space, and cultural background. As you read about these influences, try to visualize the specific and peculiar features of hospital units, nurses' stations, and ward versus private accommodations for hospitalized clients.

TABLE 29–1   Differences in Characteristics of Types of Groups

Characteristic	Task Groups	Self-Awareness/ Growth Groups	Therapy Groups	Social Groups
Purpose, goals	Performance of specific job or task explicitly agreed on by all members at initiation of group. Member participation is determined by task.	Development or use of interpersonal strengths. Broad objectives, such as to study group process, communcation patterns, or problemsolving are usually apparent at initiation of group.	Clearly defined: to do the work of therapy. Individual works toward seif-understanding, more satisfactory ways of relating, handling stress, and so on.	Recreation, relaxation, and comfort promoted through mutual pleasure and enjoyment among friends and acquaintances in a social situation such as a party at someone's home.
Shared aim	To achieve group's task goal.	To improve functioning of group one returns to (job, family, community) through translation of one's own interpersonal strengths or to improve perception of members.	To improve perception of members and to improve individual health.	To experience fun, companionship, and satisfying relationships with friends.
Format	Defined at outset by leader and/or members. Method is specific to task to be performed.	Specific format, if any, and methods defined throughout group process by all members and leader/trainer. Lack of agenda and structure may produce some difficulty.	Defined by therapist within context of some psychotherapeutic orientation. Definition is apparent through implementation of therapeutic principles.	Usually spontaneous. May be defined by members in case of planned recreational activities.
Focus	Completion of specific task.	Interpersonal concerns around current situations.	Member-centered. Past experiences may be just as relevant as current concerns depending on therapist's orientation.	Member-centered toward enjoyment and mutual meeting of needs.
Role of leader	To establish exchange of information among members and direct group toward task accomplishment, adhering to agenda.	To establish group interaction at emotional level among group members, and to serve as resource person guiding group by calling attention to certain events or processes and facilitating problem solving, mutual understanding, communication.	To establish group interaction between self and individual members and among group members. To facilitate members' interactions in work of therapy.	To meet basic requirements for social companionship, providing place, planning activity, preparing food, drink, etc.
Title of leader	Usually called chairperson.	Usually called trainer.	Usually called therapist.	Usually called host or hostess.
How leader differs from members	Chairperson identifies specific task, clarifies communication, and assists in expressing opinions and offering solutions.	Trainer differs from members by having superior skills in specialized area (understanding and facilitating group process). Trainer's superiority diminishes as group continues and members learn and implement similar skills.	Therapist differs from members by having superior skills in specialized area (group psychotherapy). Therapist never truly becomes member but may at times take on members' roles.	Host or hostess is member of group and works toward own as well as others' pleasure and enjoyment.
Requirements of leader	Qualified background and expertise in area of task emphasis. Must be accepted by members as an appropriate leader.	Sufficient preparation, experience, and skill to maintain effective control of interpersonal tensions.	Sufficient preparation and skill to undertake psychotherapy within context of situation.	Willingness to take steps to initiate social interaction.

▶

TABLE 29–1 *(continued)*

Characteristic	Task Groups	Self-Awareness/ Growth Groups	Therapy Groups	Social Groups
Orientation of group work	Reality oriented in terms of adhering to explicit work goal. If group deviates into interpersonal realm, task is not accomplished most efficiently.	Reality testing with here-and-now emphasis. Assumption is that members can correct inefficient patterns of relating and communicating with each other. Members learn group process experientially through participation and involvement.	Oriented toward having members gain insight as basis for changing patterns of behavior toward health.	Oriented toward having fun, seeking pleasure and relaxation, releasing tension.
Selection of members	Selection made possibly in terms of individual's functional role, not usually in terms of personal characteristics, often in terms of employment status.	Selection criteria range from simply expressed desire to become more self-aware to mixture of criteria based on personality characteristics.	Selection usually based on extensive consideration of constellation of personalities, behaviors, and needs and identification of group therapy as treatment of choice.	Selection based on considerations of friendship or social obligation. Host or hostess chooses whom to invite.
Title of members	Known as committee members.	May be called trainees.	Known as clients or, in some settings, patients.	Known as guests.
Interviewing of prospective members	Usually not interviewed before entry into group.	May or may not be interviewed and/or requested to complete questionnaires on personal data and personality characteristics before entry into group.	Extensive selection interview(s) required before entry into group.	Not interviewed. Usually known through prior social acquaintance.
Length of group life	Target date usually set in advance.	Tends to be short term, with target date set in advance.	Usually not set. Termination date usually determined mutually by therapist and members.	May be set in advance or spontaneously determined.

Territoriality   Most people at some time have experienced violating an unspoken and unwritten rule by sitting in someone else's chosen seat. The violator may be treated to some form of protest—a direct one in which the "proprietor" of the seat points out the transgression, or a less direct one in which the proprietor may complain of the behavior to others and/or send darting glances of hostility in the violator's direction.

This assumption of proprietary rights to space is but one example of the notion of territoriality. **Territoriality** is the assumption of a proprietary attitude toward a geographic area by a person or a group. People defend their right to the designated territory against invasion by others despite the lack of legal sanction. People do not really "own" their territory but rather occupy it, permanently or intermittently, and act as if the property belonged to them.

Avoidance of intragroup conflict depends in part on the degree to which group members respect one another's territorial rights. Intergroup conflict may result when one group fails to respect the territorial

rights of another group; in fact, this is how most wars between nations begin. In addition, territoriality provides a modicum of privacy for the individual or the group. It may also serve as a method of dominance by an individual or a group over others. The head nurse's chair, or the unit chief's chair at the head of the conference table, are concrete examples.

Personal Space   **Personal space** is an invisible bubble of territory around a person's body into which intruders may not come. It differs from territoriality in that it is space maintained and carried around with the person, rather than a specific geographic location. Robert Sommer (1969), a psychologist who studied the effects of physical setting on attitudes and behavior, has stated that the best way to learn the location of the invisible boundary of personal space is to keep walking toward a person until he or she complains.

A common defensive response to unwanted intrusion is selecting a position that is as inaccessible as possible. Another common response is flight. The need to defend personal space may also interfere with group

TABLE 29–2   **Comparative Features of Effective and Ineffective Groups**

Factor	Effective Groups	Ineffective Groups
Atmosphere	Informal, comfortable, and relaxed. It is a working atmosphere in which people demonstrate their interest and involvement.	Obviously tense. Signs of boredom may appear.
Goal setting	Goals, tasks, and objectives are clarified, understood, and modified so that members of the group can commit themselves to cooperatively structured goals.	Unclear, misunderstood, or imposed goals may be accepted by members. The goals are competitively structured
Leadership and member participation	Shift from time to time, depending on the circumstances. Different members assume leadership at various times, because of their knowledge or experience.	Delegated and based on authority. The chairperson may dominate the group, or the members may defer unduly. Member participation is unequal, with high-authority members dominating.
Goal emphasis	All three functions of groups—goal accomplishment, internal maintenance, and developmental change—are emphasized.	One or more functions may not be emphasized.
Communication	Open and two-way. Ideas and feelings are encouraged, both about the problem and about the group's operation.	Closed or one-way. Only the production of ideas is encouraged. Feelings are ignored or taboo. Members may be tentative or reluctant to be open and have "hidden agendas" (personal goals at cross-purposes with group goals).
Decision making	By consensus, although various decison-making procedures appropriate to the situation may be instituted.	By the highest authority in the group with minimal involvement by members, or an inflexible style is imposed.
Cohesion	Facilitated through high levels of inclusion, trust, liking, and support.	Either ignored or used as a means of controlling members, thus promoting rigid conformity.
Conflict tolerance	The reason for disagreements or conflicts are carefully examined and the group seeks to resolve them. The group accepts basic disagreements that cannot be resolved and lives with them.	Attempts may be made to ignore, deny, avoid, suppress, or override controversy by premature group action.
Power	Determined by the members' abilities and the information they posses. Power is shared. The issue is how to get the job done.	Determined by position in the group. Obedience to authority is strong. The issue is who controls.
Problem-solving ability	High. Constructive criticism is frequent, frank, relatively comfortable, and oriented toward removing obstacles to problem solving.	Low. Criticism may be destructive, taking the form of either overt or covert personal attacks. It prevents the group from getting the job done.
Self-evaluation as a group	Frequent. All members participate in evaluation and decisions about how to improve the group's functioning.	Minimal. What little evaluation there is may be done by the highest authority in the group, rather than by the membership as a whole.
Creativity	Encouraged. There is room within the group for members to become self-actualized and interpersonally effective.	Discouraged. People are afraid of appearing foolish if they put forth a creative thought.

functioning. Unwanted intrusion of one member into another's personal space creates discomfort, unease, and other negative feelings. These feelings affect the group dynamics and interfere with group progress.

Cultural Background   Cultural background is a strong influence on territoriality and personal space. An American who wants to be alone goes into a room and shuts the door, relying on architectural features for screening. English people have never developed the habit of using space to protect themselves from others. They use other barriers, such as "the silent treatment,"

which they expect others to recognize and respect. When an Englishman becomes silent in the company of an American man, the American is likely to expend extra effort to break through the barrier to assure himself that all is well.

Americans believe that propinquity (geographic nearness) is an acceptable basis for interaction. Living next door to a family entitles a neighbor family to socialize with the members, borrow a cup of flour from them, and have its children play with theirs. To others, propinquity it not enough, especially when social status rather than space governs relationships.

Most Europeans perceive Americans as loud. They see this as an intrusive trait, because being overheard interferes with the privacy of others. Americans perceive their "loudness" as an expression of openness or having nothing to hide. They perceive the quiet or hushed conversations of others as sly or secretive.

Conditions that people in the United States perceive as crowded, others (Latin Americans and those from Mediterranean cultures) may perceive as spacious. A North American in Latin America or the Middle East is likely to feel crowded and hemmed in. In this person's view, people come too close and touch too much. The Middle Eastern or Latin American may experience the North American as cold. But, in English and Scandinavian cultures, it is the North American who perceives the others as aloof.

Influences from the various cultures carry over from generation to generation. For satisfactory functioning, a group must pay attention to the cultural factors that influence the individual member. In a large hospital or metropolitan mental health center, where members of many cultures come together, these differences may lead to misunderstandings and thwart effective group functioning.

Material Aspects of the Setting

The material aspects of the physical environment influence the functioning of groups in interesting ways. Students in social science courses generally learn of the classic studies of worker productivity conducted at Western Electric Company (Roethlisberger and Dickson 1939). The investigators found that workers at first were more productive when the intensity of lighting was increased. However, after a period of weeks, production fell. This time the researchers decreased the lighting intensity and found the same effect—productivity increased again—even though this environmental change was directly opposite to the first one. This phenomenon, called the *Hawthorne effect,* spurred a host of other studies. Similar results were reported in studies that introduced music, coffee breaks, and so on. The primary variable seemed to be the workers' perception of the situation; if they believed that someone cared enough about them to be concerned about the conditions under which they worked, they responded by working harder and/or more effectively than when they believed no one cared about them.

Color and noise have been found to influence people's perceptions and performance. Workers complain of feeling uncomfortably cold in a room painted a cool blue. The same workers feel too warm at the same temperature when the room is painted in warm yellows and restful greens. Recent research indicates that a specific shade of pink initially decreases aggressive behavior. In response, some prison administrators have painted their jail cells pink. Unpredictable noise has been found to evoke feelings of frustration and lead to a decrease in performance. Sound conditioning of work areas has been found to reduce worker discomfort and annoyance.

Likewise, workers in an ugly room report more headaches, monotony, fatigue, hostility, discontent, and room avoidance than workers in a beautiful room. Studies about the material aspects of a setting indicate that elements of the environment are important in determining group and individual behavior. Productivity, interpersonal behavior, and intrapsychic experiences are all affected.

Spatial Arrangements

Seating arrangements have been methodically studied since Bernard Steinzor first wrote about the face-to-face discussion groups he was conducting in 1950. His interest was piqued by the behavior of one of his group members—a man who changed his seat in order to sit directly opposite another man with whom he had previously had an argument. Since that time, researchers have found that adults prefer a side-by-side arrangement for cooperation and a direct face-to-face arrangement for competition. This knowledge can be helpful in understanding the interaction among members of a psychotherapy group, a nursing team conference, or an interdisciplinary clinical conference at a community mental health agency.

People also select positions according to their perceived status in the group. Studies of twelve-person jury tables have demonstrated that jurors holding managerial or professional status frequently select the chair at the head of the table. Jurors seated at the end positions of the rectangular jury table tended to be more influential and to participate more than persons who chose side positions (Strodtbeck and Hook 1961).

There is also a relationship between spatial arrangement and leadership. Because the person who sits at the head of the table is usually perceived as the leader, the spatial position a person occupies in a group has important consequences for that person's chances of emerging as a group leader or for undertaking significant leadership responsibilities. Round tables tend to enhance the development of leadership traits among the membership rather than to invest certain members with authority because of their spatial position.

There are many other fascinating facets to the influence of space and environment on groups and individuals. This presentation provides only a starting point for further study by interested readers.

Leadership

Leadership functions within a group can be fulfilled (a) by the person designated as the leader, and (b) by members who engage in leadership behavior. This distinction is an important one for understanding the emergence of leadership within groups.

Leadership is an influence relationship that occurs among mutually dependent group members attempting to achieve the group's goals. Because all group members influence other members, at times, each member exerts leadership at some time in the group's life. This approach to understanding leadership behavior is called the *distributed functions approach*. Other approaches are also considered in this section.

Distributed Functions Approach The functional approach to group leadership is based on two major beliefs:

1. Any member of a group may become a leader by taking actions that serve group functions.

2. Different members may fulfill various functions.

Each member may enact more than one role during a meeting of the group and a wide range of roles in successive participations. Any member may play any or all of the roles. The various functional roles may be grouped in two categories:

1. **Task roles** are related to the task of the group. The job of people assuming these roles is to facilitate and coordinate group efforts in the selection, definition, and solution of a group problem. Examples of task roles are *information seeker, information giver, elaborator, procedural technician, coordinator, opinion seeker*, and *opinion giver*, among others.

2. **Maintenance roles** are oriented toward building group-centered attitudes among the members and maintaining and perpetuating group-centered behavior. Members who function as *encourager, compromiser, standard setter, follower, group observer*, or *harmonizer* carry out some of the maintenance roles possible in groups.

Sometimes members of a group satisfy individual needs that are irrelevant to the group task. These *self-serving roles* (the *recognition seeker, blocker, aggressor, dominator, self-confessor*, and *playboy*, for example) may also be negatively oriented to group maintenance functions. If a group is to function effectively, it must perform a self-diagnosis to determine what the needs of the group are, and how they can be met, so that the self-serving roles no longer present obstacles to effective functioning.

The functional theory of group leadership emphasizes the importance of distributing leadership functions among the group members. Distributed leadership is the most effective approach because it teaches people the diagnostic skills and behaviors needed to accomplish the group task and maintain good interpersonal relationships. The distributed functions approach can be best described through its main assumption: *Responsible membership is the same thing as responsible leadership*. Of course, in psychotherapy groups, some functions or activities may be largely, or even solely, the province of the therapist.

Trait Approach The trait approach is essentially a "great person" theory. It is based on the belief that a leader is a charismatic person who possesses unique, inborn leadership traits. Its central thesis is that leaders are born, not made; discovered, not trained. However, researchers have found similar traits both in leaders and in followers, so this theory does not explain what makes one person assume a leadership role while another does not. The assumption can be made, however, that people who are energetic, self-confident, determined, and motivated to succeed will become leaders, because they work hard to reach positions of leadership.

Position Approach In the position approach, leadership is seen as a position of authority in the formal role system that defines the authority hierarchy. Although this approach can certainly explain who has the designated title of leader at a drug-abuse outreach center, for example, it does not take into account the fact that other members beside the designated leader influence the group's activities.

Style Approach This classic theory of leadership behavior developed in 1939 by Lewin, Lippitt, and White identified three leadership styles: democratic, autocratic, and laissez faire. In the *democratic* style, the leader functions as a facilitator who encourages group discussion in decision making. The *autocratic* leader is one who determines policies unilaterally and gives orders and directions to the group members. The *laissez-faire* condition is characterized by a hands-off style in which the leader participates at a minimal level.

The democratic style has proved the most effective. However, under some conditions each of the other two styles seems to be the most effective. For example, when an urgent decision is necessary, the autocratic style may be the most effective. A laissez-faire style facilitates group functioning best when a group has made an effective decision, is committed to it, and is able to implement it.

Decision Making

A group that makes sound decisions is a group that functions effectively. The purpose of group decision making is to construct well-conceived, well-understood, and well-accepted realistic actions toward the goals agreed on by the group.

Effective Decisions These are the five major characteristics of effective decisions:

1. The resources of the group members are well used. The group listens to any member who has ideas or input that helps them make decisions.

2. The group's time is well used. The group concentrates on the task at hand and keeps interruptions and sidetracks to a minimum.

3. The decision is correct or of high quality. The alternative the group picks to execute is appropriate, reasonable, and error free.

4. The decision is put into effect fully by group members. Members feel committed to the decision and responsible for its implementation.

5. The problem-solving ability of the group is enhanced. Members feel satisfied with their participation, and the positive group atmosphere increases the members' perception of themselves as adequate problem solvers.

Decision Methods A group can arrive at decisions in several ways:

• When decisions are reached by *consensus,* the group arrives at a collective opinion after each member has had a fair chance to exert influence. Consensus decisions are not always unanimous. However, members support the decision and are willing to give it a try.

• Sometimes group decisions are made by the person selected as the *group expert.*

• *Averaging members' opinions* is another method for arriving at decisions. It means that the most popular opinion becomes the group decision. Nonetheless, fewer than half the members may hold that opinion.

• *Decision by majority vote,* 51 percent or more of the members, is the most common method used.

• Decisions can be made through *minority control* of a group. Executive committees of groups with many members exercise minority control over the whole group. A small minority may also quickly and forcefully "railroad" decisions (force the group to accept them by exerting intense pressure).

• In decision making by an *authority after discussion* with the members, the designated leader makes the final decision but first discusses the issue with the members to get their ideas and views.

• In decisions by *authority rule without discussion,* the designated leader makes decisions without consulting the group.

Each of these decision-making methods is appropriate at certain times. In psychotherapy groups, certain decisions (such as whether to add a new member, for example) should be made by the group expert—in this instance the group therapist—who has the clinical expertise. A group that has to make a decision must take several factors into account before selecting a method. Questions such as these should be raised: What type of decision has to be made? How much time can be spent in the decision-making process? What resources are available to the group? What is the past history of the group? What is the task to be worked on? How does the setting influence the method that should be chosen? What are the consequences of the particular method for the group's future operation? These questions are answered for each of the seven decision-making methods in Table 29–3.

Risk Taking in Group Decisions Decisions made by a group are riskier than members' private decisions. This phenomenon, called a *risky shift,* has profound implications, particularly when the decision of a group affects a large number of people.

Three major explanations for the risky shift have been given. The first is that high risk takers are more influential and persuasive than low risk takers. Thus, in a group decision the high risk takers' position tends to win out over less risky alternatives. The second hypothesis is that in group decision-making, responsibility is diffused. Any cost or imagined loss that might result from a risky decision is borne by all rather than just one individual. The final explanation is that decision making gives group members information about peer norms. They learn the value attached to being risky in the process. Members then attempt to meet the group norm in relation to both risk and caution.

Indecisiveness Sometimes a group has a hard time making decisions. Members cannot agree about what the decision should be. These are some reasons for indecisiveness:

• Fear of the consequences of the decision

• Conflicts among members that make cooperative activity difficult

• Choice of a decision-making method inappropriate to the immediate situation

• Member loyalty to other groups that makes it difficult to commit themselves to making good decisions in this group

Once the reasons for indecisiveness have been identified and put on the table, a group can work to remove the obstacles in its way. It may be necessary for the

TABLE 29–3   **Strengths and Limitations of Decision-Making Methods**

Method	Strengths	Limitations
Consensus	Produces innovative, creative, and high-quality decision; elicits commitment by all members to implement decison; uses the resources of all members; enhances future decision-making ability of group; is useful in making serious, important, and complex decisions requiring commitment from all members.	Takes great deal of time and psychologic energy and high level of member skill; can be used only when time pressure is minimal and no emergency is in progress.
Expert	Is useful when expertise of one person is so far superior to that of all other group members that little is to be gained by discussion; should be used when need for membership action in implementing decision is slight.	Can be ineffective when it is difficult to determine who is expert; does not build commitment for implementing decision; loses advantages of group interaction; may result in resentment and disagreement that can sabotage group effectiveness; does not use resources of other members.
Average of members' opinions	Is useful when it is difficult to get group members together to talk, when decision is so urgent that there is no time for group discussion, when member commitment is not necessary for implementing decision, and when group members lack skills and information to make decision any other way; is applicable to simple, routine decisions.	Does not allow enough interaction among group members for them to gain from each other's resources and to get benefits of group discussion; does not build commitment for implementing decision; leaves unresolved conflict and controversy that may damage future group effectiveness.
Majority vote	Can be used when sufficient time is lacking for decision by consensus or when decision is not so important that consensus needs to be used, and when complete member commitment is not necessary for implementing decision; closes discussion on issues that are not highly important for group.	Usually leaves an alienated minority, which damages future group effectiveness; may lose relevant resources of many group members; does not build total commitment for implementing decision; does not obtain full benefit of group interaction.
Minority control	Can be used when everyone cannot meet to make decision, when group is under such time pressure that it must delegate responsibility to committee, when only few members have any relevant resources, when broad member commitment is not needed to implement decision; is useful for simple, routine decisions.	Does not use resources of many group members; does not establish widespread commitment for implementing decision; can leave unresolved conflict and controversy that may damage future group effectiveness; does not obtain much benefit from group interaction.
Authority rule after discussion	Like consensus, uses resources of group members more than other methods; gains some benefits of group discussion.	Does not develop commitment for implementing decision; does not resolve controversies and conflicts among group members; tends to create situations in which group members either compete to impress designated leader or tell leader what they think leader wants to hear.
Authority rule without discussion	Applies more to administrative needs than to member needs; is useful for simple, routine decisions; should be used when very little time is available to make decision, when group members expect designated leader to make decision, and when group members lack skills and information to make decision any other way.	Uses only one person as resource for every decision; loses advantages of group interaction; develops no commitment among other group members for implementing decision; can produce resentment and disagreement that may sabotage and reduce group effectiveness; does not use resources of other members.

SOURCE: Johnson DW, Johnson FP: Joining Together: Group Theory and Group Skills, ed 3, © 1987; pp 104–105. Adapted by permission of Prentice-Hall, Inc., Englewood Cliffs, New Jersey.

group to rearrange its membership, redefine its task, select another decision-making method, or work at resolving the conflicts among its members before continuing its work on the identified task.

Trust

Many theorists and researchers have studied the complex phenomenon of **trust**. Some of the better-known work is by Morton Deutsch (1949, 1958). In this view, trusting behavior comes about through the following four steps:

1. The person realizes that the decision to trust another may result in either positive or negative consequences for the self. The person realizes the risk involved in trusting another.

2. The person realizes that the future behavior of the other determines whether trusting will bring positive or negative consequences for the self.

3. The person will suffer more if the trust is violated than the person will gain if the trust is fulfilled.

4. The person feels reasonably confident that the other will behave in ways that will bring the beneficial consequences.

The person who decides to have minor elective surgery of little consequence is engaging in the four steps of trusting behavior. The client: (a) recognizes that the choice could lead to either beneficial or harmful consequences, (b) realizes that the consequences of the choice depend on the behavior of the surgeon, (c) would suffer much more if the trust is violated and the surgeon does a bad job, and (d) feels relatively confident that the surgeon will make sure that beneficial consequences result.

Trust develops in relationships when people disclose more and more of their thoughts, perceptions, attitudes, and reactions to one another. The group member who makes a suggestion; discloses an attitude, feeling, experience, or perception; gives feedback; or confronts another also engages in trusting behavior and assumes the risks inherent in trusting. Trusting and being trusted are intimately linked to risk taking. The level of trust among the members of a group determines the extent of risk-taking behavior in the group.

Cohesion

"Hanging together" is the aspect of group life generally referred to as group **cohesion**. Groups that hang together or cohere possess a certain spirit of common purpose. The members have a yen for mutual association. Groups in which cohesion is minimal seem always on the verge of breaking up or falling apart. Cohesion is the primary factor keeping a group in existence and working effectively.

The Need for Attraction   A group is cohesive when its members are attracted to it. People are attracted to a group for a wide variety of reasons. The group may meet their needs for affiliation, interpersonal security, or financial security. It may have admired members who not only are available for human interaction but also have important shared attitudes, values, interests, and beliefs. An attractive group has explicit, mutual, and attainable group goals with clear paths to goal attainment. Its members engage in an interdependence that is cooperative rather than competitive. The activities the group undertakes are satisfying and successful, and there is a high degree of member participation in a democratic structure. Communication networks are open, central, and flexible in a warm and friendly atmosphere.

This implies that cohesive groups are not born but developed. Although some features of attraction may account for a "love-at-first-sight" phenomenon, others do not become evident until the group has come together long enough to have shared experiences that provide the basis for attraction.

Evaluating Cohesion   What indicates that the spirit of cohesion exists in a given group? How do groups with sufficient cohesion differ from groups with minimal cohesion? The accompanying Assessment box identifies the characteristics of highly cohesive groups and compares them to those of minimally cohesive groups.

Building Cohesion   How can a group's tendency to cohere be enhanced? Some methods are increasing the trusting and trustworthy behavior of members; the affection expressed among members; the expressions of inclusion and acceptance among members; and the influence that members have on one another. Two other methods for building cohesion are promoting group norms and structuring cooperative relationships among group members.

Promoting Group Norms   Norms are the set of unwritten rules of conduct or prescriptions of behavior established by members of a group. They derive from the common beliefs of the group about appropriate behavior. In other words, they tell how members are expected to behave. Norms prevent chaos because they lay out the expectations of members. They help members predict the behavior of others and anticipate the actions that they should take themselves.

Norms are evaluative. They tell members what ought and ought not be done. They represent value judgments that establish accepted standards for behav-

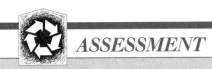

ASSESSMENT

Group Cohesion

Characteristics of High-Cohesion Groups	Characteristics of Low-Cohesion Groups	Characteristics of High-Cohesion Groups	Characteristics of Low-Cohesion Groups
Members like one another.	Members seem uncaring or may actively dislike one another.	Group goals are consistent with goals of individuals.	Group goals and individual goals are not consistent.
Members are friendly and willing to interact.	Member seem unfriendly and unwilling to become involved.	Group goals can best be handled by group action.	Goals can best be handled by individual action.
Members enjoy interacting with one another and interact readily.	Members get little pleasure from interaction and interact reluctantly.	Group goals difficult to achieve are met by persistent efforts.	Group goals difficult to achieve are given up.
Members receive support on issues from one another.	Members do not give one another active support.	Attendance is high, and members arrive on time.	Attendance is low or uneven, and members may arrive late or leave early.
Members praise one another for accomplishments.	Members do not acknowledge one another's accomplishments or belittle them.	Efforts are directed toward maintaining, strengthening, and regulating group.	Efforts are not directed toward maintaining, strengthening, and regulating group.
		Risk taking is high.	Risk taking is low.
Members share similar opinions and attitudes.	Members have dissimilar or mutually exclusive opinions and attitudes.	Participation is high.	Participation is low.
		Commitment to group goals increases.	Commitment to group goals is minimal.
Members are likely to influence one another and are willing to be influenced by other members.	Members make few influence attempts and are unwilling to be influenced by other members.	Communication is high.	Communication is low.
		"We" is frequently heard in discussions.	"I" is frequently heard in discussions.
		Leadership is democratic.	Leadership is autocratic.
Members accept assigned tasks and roles readily.	Members are reluctant or refuse to accept assigned tasks and roles.	Group action is interdependent and cooperative.	Group action is independent and competitive.
Members trust one another.	Members do not trust one another.	Group output and productivity are high.	Group output and productivity are low.
Members are loyal to group and defend it against external criticism and attack.	Members do not defend group and may criticize it to others.	Group norms are adhered to and protected.	Group norms are violated.
Members stay in group.	Members drop out.	Members experience increase in security and self-esteem and reduction in anxiety.	Members experience decrease in security and self-esteem and increase in anxiety.
Group goals are valued.	Group goals are not valued.	Satisfaction with members and work of group is high.	Satisfaction with members and work of group is low.

ior. The following characteristics of norms influence group behavior:

- Norms are developed about situations that are important to the group. Groups do not establish norms for every conceivable situation.

- Norms may apply to every member of a group, or to certain members in specific roles only. For example, skiers are expected to wait their turn in the chair lift line, but a member of the National Ski Patrol may cut in at the head of the line without challenge.

- Norms vary in the degree to which they are accepted by group members. Most persons accept the norm that the driver of a vehicle should not pass a stopped school bus, but many violate the norm that drivers of slow-moving vehicles should stay in the right lane.

- Norms vary in the extent to which people can permissibly deviate from them. Violating a norm that members arrive for the meetings on time is a more acceptable transgression than violating the norm against physically attacking another group member.

- Norms differ in the sanctions applied for their violation. Members who arrive late may be subjected to mild disapproval, whereas the member who slaps or hits another member may be barred from the group for continuing the behavior.

The importance of norms in the power, influence, and conformity aspects of group life is discussed more completely later in this chapter.

Structuring Cooperative Relationships It takes cooperative action on the part of members to meet group goals. In addition to group goals, members have individual goals. When the personal or individual goals of group members differ from the group goals, competitive relationships may develop that destroy the effectiveness of group relationships. For example, it is common for members who are in disagreement with the group goals to acquire hidden agendas that interfere with group functioning. A **hidden agenda** may be defined as a personal goal, unknown to the other group members, which is at cross-purposes with the dominant group goals.

To structure cooperative relationships around group and individual goals, members need to review and discuss group goals thoroughly when the group is formed, even though goals may have been prescribed for the group by others. Discussion clarifies members' understanding of the goals and the tasks necessary to reach them. The group goals should be recognized and rephrased during the discussion, encouraging members to feel a sense of "ownership" toward the goals. The accompanying Intervention box provides suggestions for dealing with hidden agendas.

Cooperative relationships to meet goals are extremely important for group effectiveness. When hidden agendas structure a group competitively, members strive for individual goal accomplishment in a way that blocks others from obtaining the group goal.

Groupthink: A Special Case of Cohesion

Groups that "hang together" can sometimes be easily hanged. Irving Janis (1971a, 1971b) has coined the term **groupthink**, a word reminiscent of George Orwell's *1984* society, to refer to the mode of thinking of a highly cohesive in-group in which uniformity and agreement are given such high priority that critical thinking is impossible or unacceptable. Groups infected with groupthink have developed group norms around the maintenance of unity and loyalty, no matter what the cost.

How can one tell if a group is obsessed with the need for concurrence that characterizes groupthink? Janis (1971a, p 44) lists the following main symptoms of groupthink:

- *Invulnerability*. Most or all members of the in-group share an *illusion* of invulnerability that gives them some degree of reassurance about obvious dangers. It makes them overoptimistic and willing to take extraordinary risks. It also makes them ignore clear warnings of danger.

- *Rationalization*. Victims of groupthink collectively construct rationalizations to discount warnings and other forms of negative feedback that, taken seriously, might lead the group members to reconsider their assumptions each time they recommit themselves to past decisions.

- *Morality*. Victims of groupthink believe unquestioningly in the inherent morality of their group. This belief inclines the members to ignore the ethical or moral consequences of their decisions.

- *Stereotypes*. Victims of groupthink hold stereotyped views of outsiders. These stereotyped views are usually negative ones.

- *Pressure*. Victims of groupthink apply direct pressure to any individual who momentarily expresses doubts about any of the group's shared illusions or questions the validity of the arguments supporting an alternative favored by the majority. This gambit reinforces the concurrence-seeking norm that loyal members are expected to maintain.

- *Self-censorship*. Victims of groupthink avoid deviating from what appears to be a group consensus. They keep silent about their misgivings and minimize even to themselves the importance of their doubts.

- *Unanimity*. Victims of groupthink share an *illusion* of unanimity within the group about almost all

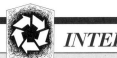

INTERVENTION

Steps for Dealing with Hidden Agendas

Suggestion	Rationale
Look for the presence of hidden agendas.	The group cannot diagnose or solve a problem until its presence it recognized.
Once the presence of hidden agendas has been pinpointed, judge whether or not they should be brought to the surface and rectified.	Sometimes hidden agendas should be left undisturbed, if the consequences of bringing them to the attention of the entire group may be negative, rather than facilitating the work of the group.
Determine whether group members are willing and able to deal with hidden agendas. Suggest that perhaps not all there is to say has been said, but do not force members to disclose their hidden agendas.	Disclosing hidden agendas may be harmful to group attempts to reach cohesion and may result in the premature ouster of the member with the hidden agenda.
Accept members whose hidden agendas have been revealed, without rejecting or criticizing them.	Hidden agendas are common and legitimate group occurrences. They should be worked on in the same way that group tasks are.
Devote group time to working on the hidden agendas of members.	Hidden agendas impede group progress. The attention given to hidden agendas should be determined by the extent of the effect on group effectiveness.
As a group, evaluate the group's ability to deal with hidden agendas.	Learning better ways of handling agendas more openly will result from evaluation and reduce the need for keeping agendas hidden.

judgments. This is expressed by members who speak in favor of the majority vote.

• *Mindguards.* Victims of groupthink sometimes appoint themselves as mindguards to protect the leader and fellow members from adverse information that might break the confidence they share in the effectiveness and morality of past decisions.

Members afflicted with groupthink behave in characteristic ways, according to Janis (1971a, p 75).

• They limit group discussions to a few alternative courses of action (often only two) without an initial survey of all worthwhile alternatives.

• Members fail to reexamine the course of action initially preferred by the majority after they learn of risks and drawbacks they had not considered originally.

• Members spend little or no time discussing whether there are gains they may have overlooked in a rejected alternative or ways of reducing the seemingly

prohibitive costs that made a rejected alternative appear undesirable to them.

• Members make little or no attempt to obtain information from experts within their own organizations who might be able to supply more precise estimates of potential losses and gains.

• Members show positive interest in facts and opinions that support their preferred policy. They tend to ignore facts and opinions that do not.

• The group spends little time deliberating about how the chosen decision might be hindered by bureaucratic inertia, sabotaged by opponents, or temporarily derailed by common accidents. It fails to work out contingency plans to cope with foreseeable setbacks that could endanger the overall success of the chosen course.

How can groupthink be prevented? The Intervention box on page 702 identifies goals that prevent or remedy groupthink and suggests constructive behaviors a group may undertake to correct its functioning.

INTERVENTION

Preventing Groupthink

Goal	Preventive and Remedial Behaviors	Goal	Preventive and Remedial Behaviors
Discouraging members from soft-pedaling their disagreements; not allowing their striving for agreement to inhibit critical thinking.	Each member should be assigned the role of critical evaluator to encourage the group to assign high priority to open airing of objections and doubts. This practice needs to be reinforced by the leader's acceptance of criticism.	Challenging the majority position.	Whenever the agenda of the group calls for an evaluation of policy alternatives, at least one member should take on the "devil's advocate" role, functioning as a good lawyer would in challenging the testimony of those who favor the majority position.
Encouraging open inquiry and imparital probing of a wide range of alternatives.	An impartial stance, rather than a statement of preferences and expectations at the beginning, should be adopted by the key members of a hierarchy when they assign a policy-planning task to any group within their organization.	Discouraging stereotyped views of other groups.	When the issue involves relations with a rival group, the group should devote a sizable block of time to surveying the signals and cues from the other group and writing alternative scenarios on the rivals' intentions.
Preventing the insulation of an in-group.	Several outside policy-planning and evaluation groups with different leaders should be set up to work on the same policy question.	Encouraging alternative plans.	The group should, from time to time, break up into two or more subgroups that meet separately, with different leaders, develop separate plans, and then come back together to negotiate differences.
Preventing the establishment of desire for "unity at all costs."	Each member should be asked at intervals to check out group conclusions with trusted associates and to report their reactions back to the group.	Rethinking the entire issue.	After reaching a preliminary consensus, the group should hold a "second chance" meeting, encouraging each member to express residual doubts before making a final choice.
Discouraging members from accepting unchallenged the views of core members.	One or more outside experts should be invited to each meeting, on a staggered basis, and encouraged to challenge the views of core members.		

SOURCE: *Compiled from Janis IL: Groupthink.* Psychology Today, *November 1971, p 76. By permission of Ziff Davis Publishing Company.*

Groupthink has a negative influence on the quality of the decisions made by a group. The groupthink decision is less reliable than decisions by consensus. Too much cohesiveness leads members to pat each other on the back even while headed toward disaster.

Power and Influence

Power is a potent force that explains a good deal about the nature, operation, and patterns of interpersonal behavior. It is impossible to discuss group dynamics without discussing power because it is impossible to interact without influencing, and being influenced by, others. This process constantly occurs within groups, forcing members to adjust to one another and modify their behavior. In some instances, attitudes and beliefs are modified as well. Ferguson (1985) defines *power* as the ability to do or act, to have possession of command or control over others, to achieve the desired result. The terms *power* and *influence* are used interchangeably in this chapter.

There is a definite process by which power is mobilized to help accomplish goals. Powerful people:

• Determine and clarify their personal goals

• Affirm the resources or informational level they bring to the group (what they can contribute toward the accomplishment of their goals and the goals of group members)

• Determine what coalitions are necessary to secure the information and resources needed to accomplish the goals

• Develop the necessary coalitions so that the resources can be applied (i.e., find out what they want from the others, what the others want from them, and what they can exchange so that everyone can accomplish the goals)

• Carry out the necessary activities for reaching the goals

Some people perceive power and influence as negative forces. These people are frequently unaware of the influence they themselves exert on others, or they confuse the judicious use of power in building effective groups with the use of power to control, manage, and manipulate others. Nurses are only now becoming aware of how they might employ power and influence in the service of their clients and their profession.

Power Sources

According to power theorists, there are six possible sources of a person's power. These are: reward power, coercive power, legitimate power, referent power, expert power, and informational power. People have *reward power* if they can deliver positive consequences or remove negative ones in response to the behavior of group members. They have *coercive power* if they can deliver negative consequences or remove positive ones in response to the behavior of group members. When group members believe a person ought to have influence over them because of the person's position in the group or organization, that person can be said to have *legitimate power*. A person has *referent power* when group members identify with or want to be like that person. Members do what that person wants out of liking, respect, and the desire to be liked themselves. The person with *expert power* is seen by the group as trustworthy and having some special knowledge or skill. When a person has *informational power,* group members believe that this person has access to information not available elsewhere that will be useful in accomplishing their goal.

The Problem of Unequal Power

A group in which certain members have much power and others have little power is likely to be in trouble. The unequal distribution of power affects both the task and the maintenance functions of a group. Members who believe they have little influence within the group are unlikely to feel committed to group goals and to implementation of group decisions. Their dissatisfaction with the group decreases its attractiveness and reduces its cohesion.

High-power people often are the most popular or have the most authority. Neither circumstance is satisfactory for high-quality decision making. High-quality decision making results when power is based on expertise, competence, and relevant information, not on popularity or authority.

Destructive Obedience to Authority

Stanley Milgram (1963, 1964) conducted an absorbing and rather frightening series of social science experiments on obedience to authority. Milgram became interested in the obedience phenomenon that occurred during World War II, which formed the defense of many accused war criminals during the Nuremberg trials. He set up experiments in which subjects were to administer increasingly high doses of electric shocks to others who failed to memorize a given sequence of words. Subjects believed they were administering mild to severe (up to 300-volt) shocks that could have damaging physical consequences. Despite the possible severe consequences, 62 percent of the subjects administered the most extreme level of electrical shock under no compulsion other than the repeated verbal requests of the experimenter. Such unquestioning obedience to authority may prevent rational and humane decision-making behavior. Group members should assess and critique suggestions from the authority to avoid the consequences of uncritical obedience.

Because much of the role socialization of the nurse emphasizes "following orders," nurses must be especially critical of an unquestioning tendency to behave in concert with the wishes of persons in authority. Psychiatric nurses need to find a balance between a submissive role and an autocratic role, seeking instead to temper autonomy with reason and sensitivity. The autocratic and powerful personas of such motion picture nurse figures as the icily dictatorial Miss Davis in *The Snake Pit* and the ruthlessly punitive Nurse Ratched in *One Flew Over the Cuckoo's Nest* are examples of misdirected autonomy.

FIRO: The Interpersonal Needs Approach

The Fundamental Interpersonal Relationship Orientation (FIRO) is a popular approach developed by William Schutz (1958a, 1958b). Some of his ideas were generated during his work for the Department of the Navy. The Navy was concerned with interpersonal problems experienced by the crews of nuclear submarines during their long-term cruises beneath the polar ice cap. While some crews functioned effectively and were satisfied with one another, others performed ineffectively and voiced their dissatisfactions. Schutz set out to learn how to predict which people were compatible with which other people. Theoretically, nuclear submarine crews could be composed of compatible individuals who would be more likely to perform effectively together and would find their lengthy enforced togetherness, if not totally pleasurable, at least tolerable.

The basic assumption of Schutz's theory is that people need people. In addition, people need to establish some equilibrium between themselves and the people in their environment. This equilibrium is determined by the interaction of certain interpersonal needs, and it appears to be synonymous with interpersonal compatibility.

Three Basic Interpersonal Needs   An interpersonal need is one that can be satisfied only through relationships with people. Schutz reasoned that every individual has three interpersonal needs: inclusion, control, and affection.

Inclusion   The interpersonal **need for inclusion** is the need to establish and maintain relationships with others that offer interactions and associations satisfying to the individual. The following characterize a satisfying position in terms of inclusion:

• A psychologically comfortable relation with people somewhere on a continuum that ranges from initiating or originating interaction with all people to not initiating interaction with anyone. In other words, this dimension is *expressed* toward others.

• A psychologically comfortable relation with people in regard to wanting others to initiate interaction somewhere on a continuum that ranges from always initiating interaction with you to never initiating interaction with you. In other words, this dimension is *wanted* from others.

To put this another way, *expressed inclusion* is the ability to take an interest in others to a satisfactory degree, and *wanted inclusion* is the ability to allow other people to take an interest in you to a satisfying degree to yourself.

Connotative terms that point to a positive inclusion relation are: *associate, interact, mingle, communicate, belong, companion, comrade, attend to, member, togetherness, join, extrovert.* At the other end of the scale are terms that connote lack of inclusion, such as: *exclusion, isolate, outsider, outcast, lonely, detached, withdrawn, abandoned, ignored.* This need determines whether a person is outgoing or prefers privacy.

Control   The interpersonal **need for control** is the need to establish and maintain a satisfactory relation between oneself and other people with regard to power and influence. The following characterize a satisfactory position in terms of control:

• A psychologically comfortable relation with people somewhere on a continuum that ranges from controlling all the behavior of other people to not controlling any behavior of others

• A psychologically comfortable relation with people in regard to their control behavior on a continuum that ranges from always wanting to be controlled by them to never wanting to be controlled by them

To put this another way, *expressed control* is the ability to take charge to a satisfactory degree, and *wanted control* is the ability to establish and maintain a feeling of respect for the competence and responsibleness of others to a satisfying degree to yourself.

Connotative terms for primarily positive control are: *power, authority, dominance, influence, control, ruler, superior officer, leader.* At the other end of the scale are terms that connote lack of control, or negative control: *rebellion, resistance, follower, anarchy, submissive, Milquetoast.*

Affection   The interpersonal **need for affection** is the need to establish and maintain a satisfactory relation between the self and other people with regard to love and affection. The following characterize a satisfactory position in terms of affection:

• A psychologically comfortable relation with others somewhere on a continuum that ranges from initiating close, personal relations with everyone to originating close, personal relations with no one

• A psychologically comfortable relation with people in regard to their affection behavior on a continuum that ranges from wanting everyone to originate close, personal relations toward you, to wanting no one to originate close, personal relations toward you

To put this another way, *expressed affection* is being able to love other people or to be close and intimate to a satisfactory degree, and *wanted affection* is having others love you or to be close and intimate with you to a satisfactory degree.

Connotative terms for an affection relation that is primarily positive are: *love, like, emotionally close, positive feelings, personal, friendship.* At the other end of the scale are terms that connote lack of affection or negative affection: *hate, dislike, cool, emotionally distant.*

Figure 29–1 illustrates the dimensions of the FIRO theory.

Group Development The interpersonal needs theory asserts that any group, given enough time, moves through three interpersonal phases—inclusion, control, and affection, in that order—that correspond to the three basic interpersonal needs.

Inclusion Phase The first or inclusion phase is concerned with the problem of *in or out.* People attempt to find their place in the group and are concerned with learning whether they will be acknowledged as individuals or left behind and ignored. Because these concerns give rise to anxiety, this phase is dominated by behavior centered around the self.

Overtalking, withdrawal, exhibitionism, and sharing other group experiences and biographies are some examples.

Frequently, *goblet issues* predominate. These are issues of minor importance to the group that help people get to know one another and test each other. They are a vehicle for sizing up people. Goblet issues may revolve around the weather, the World Series, rules of procedure, and so on.

Control Phase The second or control phase is concerned with the problem of *top or bottom,* which becomes salient after problems of inclusion have been resolved. Concern about decision-making procedures predominates, and the problems that emerge involve the sharing of responsiblity and the distribution of power and influence. This phase is dominated by competitive behavior. There are struggles for leadership and about the structure, rules of procedure, and methods of decision making. Members are attempting to establish comfortable positions for themselves in terms of responsibility and influence.

Affection Phase The third or affection phase is concerned with the problem of *near or far,* and it follows satisfactory resolution of the preceding two phases. Individual members are now faced with the problem of becoming emotionally integrated. Concerns about not being liked by, being too close to, or not being close enough to others become relevant. The behavior in this phase is generally characterized by high emotion—positive feelings, jealousy, hostility, and pairing are some examples. Schutz (1958a) de-

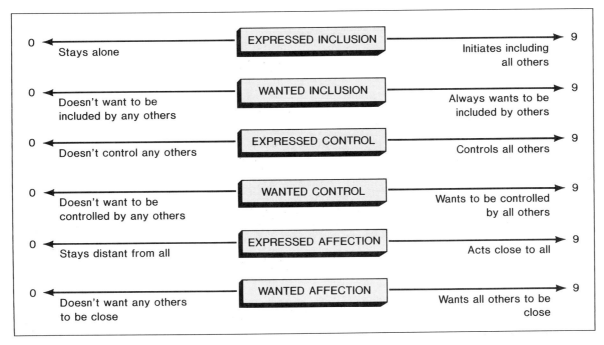

FIGURE 29–1 Dimensions of the FIRO theory.

scribes this phase as one in which, like porcupines, people attempt to get close enough to receive warmth, yet avoid the pain of sharp quills.

Interweaving of Phases None of these phases is distinct, since all three problem areas are present at all times, even though only one predominates. Schutz (1958a, p 130) uses a tire-changing analogy, what he calls *tightening the bolts,* to describe the sequence of the phases:

When a person changes a tire and replaces the wheel, he first sets the wheel in place and secures it by tightening the bolts one after another just so the wheel is in place and the next step can be taken. Then the bolts are tightened further, usually in the same sequence, until the wheel is firmly in place. Finally each bolt is gone over separately to secure it.

The leader helps the group work on all three interpersonal need areas in similar fashion, returning to and working over each area to a more satisfactory level than was reached the last time.

Applying the Theory *Clearing the air* by making covert interpersonal difficulties overt is a major step in applying the FIRO theory. Although this step is initially uncomfortable, the final result is rewarding. The following interpersonal difficulties can be made overt:

- Withdrawal or silence by members

- Inactivity and unintegrated behavior by members

- Overactivity and destructive behavior by members

- Power struggles between members

- Battles for attention among members

- Dissatisfaction with the leadership

- Dissatisfaction with the amount of recognition a member receives for contributions

- Dissatisfaction with the amount of affection and warmth demonstrated in the group

A group that is relatively compatible can function smoothly with minimal discussion of its problems. Groups in which the interpersonal problems are extremely minor can usually ignore them (or, if problems exist between two members, work them out outside the group) without hampering group effectiveness. A group that is basically incompatible has to spend much time and energy resolving its interpersonal problems so that it can function effectively.

The interpersonal needs approach of Schutz is based on the belief that the way to attack problems within groups is by investigating what is going on among the individuals in the group and attempting to improve their interpersonal relations.

The Authority Relations/Personal Relations Approach

Two major areas of internal uncertainty or stress in groups, according to the theory developed by Warren Bennis and Herbert A. Shepard (1956), are dependence (authority relations) and interdependence (personal relations). The first area has to do with group members' orientations toward authority—the handling and distribution of power within the group. The second area has to do with group members' orientations toward one another. A central assumption in this theory is that the principal obstacles to a valid group communication (and hence to group effectiveness) derive from the members' orientations toward authority and intimacy.

A new group is highly concerned with authority and power. Earlier experiences with authority influence and partially determine members' orientations toward other members. Bennis and Shepard have called this Phase I. As the group develops, it moves away from its preoccupation with authority toward a preoccupation with personal relations. This constitutes the second major phase in group development, called Phase II. These major phases, and their subphases, are summarized in the accompanying Theory box.

Relevant Aspects of Member Personality Bennis and Shepard view members as either conflicted or unconflicted about the dependence and personal aspects of group life. A **conflicted member** is one whose posture toward dependence or intimacy may be viewed as inflexible, rigid, or compulsive. These members insist on adopting certain roles despite the situation. Conflicted members are responsible for confused communication within groups. An **unconflicted member,** also called an *independent,* is better able to assess situations and alter roles or behavior as appropriate.

There are two ways in which persons can be conflicted around authority relations. Members who are comforted by rules of procedure and agendas and rely on the decisions of others (who are viewed as experts) are said to be *dependent.* Members who are uncomfortable with structure and authority are *counterdependent.* Counterdependents manifest their dissatisfaction with authority by opposing it regardless of its style or intent. Nothing the authority or leader does is acceptable. The counterdependent views failure to design an agenda as evidence of the authority's lack of ability. Paradoxically, designing an agenda may be viewed as too controlling. The counterdependent takes a "damned if you do, and damned if you don't" stance toward authority.

Members can be conflicted about personal relations in two ways as well. People who direct uninterrupted efforts toward reaching a high degree of

THEORY

The Bennis and Shepard Model

Phase I (Dependence-Power Relations)

Subphase 1: Dependence-Submission This subphase is characterized by dependency and flight. Members discuss problems external to the group. Assertive or aggressive members play dominant roles. Self-oriented behavior and subgrouping are evident.

Subphase 2: Counterdependence This subphase is characterized by counterdependence and fight. Members discuss the organization and structure of the group. Assertive counterdependent and dependent members play dominant roles. Group searches for what to talk about and how to make decisions. Uncertainty causes anxiety.

Subphase 3: Resolution This subphase is characterized by involvement in the group tasks. Assertive independents play dominant roles. The group unifies to pursue the task and members take over some leadship roles.

Phase II (Interdependence-Personal Relations)

Subphase 4: Enchantment This subphase is characterized by a high level of solidarity, fusion, camaraderie, and suggestibility. Members talk about the positive aspects of the group and its members. For the first time in its history, there is general distribution of participation. Overpersonals play dominant roles. Laughter and joking are common, as is planning social events outside of the group.

Subphase 5: Disenchantment This subphase is characterized by fight-flight evidenced in distrust and suspicion of various group members. The content themes in Subphase 1 are revived. The most assertive counterpersonal members play dominant roles; overpersonal members are also active. The group may divide on the basis of shared attitudes toward intimacy. The group may be disparaged by the members in a variety of ways.

Subphase 6: Consensual Validation This subphase is characterized by understanding and acceptance. Assertive independents play dominant roles. The group views itself and its accomplishments in realistic terms. Consensus on important issues is easier to achieve.

intimacy with all other group members are termed *overpersonal*. Members who expend great amounts of energy in avoiding intimacy and maintaining distance are said to be *counterpersonal*.

Persons unconflicted in terms of either the authority relations or the personal relations in the group are responsible for major movements in the group's development toward valid communication. These unconflicted members who move the group on to the next phase are called **catalysts**. They reduce the internal uncertainty or stress in the group. Actions of these unconflicted members that move the group forward into the next phase are called *barometric events*. Figure 29-2 presents a grid of these aspects of member personality.

Relationship to Group Strategies   The Bennis and Shepard model demonstrates group development along a continuum from the emphasis on power to the emphasis on affection. The activities of Phase I are concerned with such things as social class, ethnic background, and personal and professional interests. Concern with personality and reaction of feelings, such as warmth, anger, love, and anxiety, arise in Phase II. Bennis and Shepard believe that group therapies should be based on an adequate understanding of the group dynamic barriers to communication.

The Therapeutic Problem Approach

The final approach to the analysis of groups considered in this chapter describes group development—specifically, theory group development—in six discrete phases. E. A. Martin and William F. Hill (1957) formulated this theory of group development from the basic assumption that distinct and common growth patterns exist in therapy groups and can be described, observed, and predicted. The major therapeutic problem encountered is the focal point for describing each phase. In this model, transitional stages between the

	CONFLICTED	UNCONFLICTED
AUTHORITY RELATIONS	Dependent Counterdependent	Independent (catalyst)
PERSONAL RELATIONS	Overpersonal Counterpersonal	Independent (catalyst)

FIGURE 29-2   Member personality categories.

developmental plateaus indicate potentials for movement from one phase to another. These are the six phases of therapy group development, according to Martin and Hill:

- *Phase I.* Individual unshared behavior in an imposed structure

- *Phase II.* Reactivation of fixed interpersonal stereotypes

- *Phase III.* Exploration of interpersonal potential within the group

- *Phase IV.* Awareness of interrelationships, subgrouping, and power structure

- *Phase V.* Responsiveness to group dynamic and group process problems

- *Phase VI.* The group as an integrative-creative social instrument

Like the other theorists discussed above, Martin and Hill see groups as passing along a developmental continuum from minimal to optimal effectiveness. Groups differ in the time they spend in any phase and the problems they face. Most groups disband before reaching the sixth, or ultimate, phase of development.

Phase I—Individual Behavior The group in Phase I is best described as an aggregate of social isolates held together loosely by vague perceptions of the therapist and his or her role. Imposed structure, such as regularity of meeting time and place, consistency of membership, and a group seating arrangement encourage "groupness," slight though it may be. Because of a lack of interpersonal, group-relevant structure, esprit de corps and cooperative ventures are latent but not yet realized. There is little justification for calling the aggregate of individuals in Phase I a group.

Transition from Phase I to Phase II The major characteristic of the first transitional phase is that the therapist emerges as the leader of the group and is publicly acknowledged by the members. Autistic behavior diminishes. It is replaced by an *asyndetic* mode of interaction, a form of interpersonal interaction in which elements in a statement by one speaker function as a cue for the next speaker. A third, fourth, or fifth speaker may similarly be cued by the preceding speaker. It is a chain reaction that seems highly autistic, in that the material evoked by the cues is highly personal and does not enhance or elaborate the productions of the earlier speaker. There is some group relevance, however, in that the remarks indicate that members have paid at least some attention to each other. They thus establish indirect social contacts. The

therapist can help the group move on to the next phase through modeling behavior that is not asyndetic but rather recognizes the members as social beings.

Phase II—Fixed Stereotypes In the second phase, members' perceptions of one another are based on previously learned stereotypes. Although members publicly acknowledge one another's existence, the acknowledgment is in terms of "ghosts" of earlier interpersonal experiences. These stereotyped perceptions or ghosts fail to acknowledge the uniqueness of each member. The perception of a member as a "redneck," "sweet," or "macho," may reflect the assigned stereotype rather than any real trait. The leader is frequently typecast in some sort of omniscient role, and dependence on the leader emerges. It is the socialization aspects of this phase that provide therapeutic value.

Transition from Phase II to Phase III Social stereotypes break down during this transition period. Members openly express resentment about being stereotyped and insist on their own rights and views. Appraisals of one another become more realistic. The members' idiosyncratic perceptions of the leader begin to give way to a group view. The therapist assists the group by helping members become more aware of the discrepancies in their views of the therapist.

Phase III—Exploration of Potential This phase is characterized by active emotional exchange geared to giving group members recognition as individuals. Although many asyndetic processes and autisms still occur, the group begins to deal with the here-and-now events in the group and with their perceptions of one another. A group norm appears that places high value on individual importance. It may be demonstrated by the devotion of one or more entire sessions to the problems or personality of one member or by a rapidly shifting give-and-take. Because the individual is of paramount importance, membership is valued, and absences, tardiness, or dropping out are grave concerns. In this phase, members learn to give emotional feedback to one another and become more aware of their effects on one another. The experience of being valued gives one a sense of purpose and promotes self-worth.

Transition from Phase III to Phase IV At the third transition point, the group becomes restless, finding the detailed analysis of one another's personalities boring and repetitive. The excitement and novelty of exploration diminish, and group discussions turn to consideration of the relationships that have developed among group members. The therapist can help the group transcend this feeling of "same old faces and same old problems" by making members aware of their boredom and encouraging their exploration of the relationships among members.

Phase IV—Awareness of Interrelationships

Growing awareness of certain relationships between and among members surfaces during Phase IV. Pairing relationships and hierarchical relationships are among those that emerge. Member skill at identifying relationship dynamics encourages them to consider their attempts to structure specific relationships with the therapist. "Teacher's pets" and "junior therapists" may be identified at this time. The group becomes divided, as opinion leaders and emotional attitude leaders begin to surface and subgroups form around them. Consequently, rivalries also develop, and subgroups struggle for power. The therapist's task is to help the members identify subgroup leaders and supporters and consider the potential consequences of a power struggle.

Transition from Phase IV to Phase V   Much tension exists within the group, and there is decreasing tolerance for the tension in the transition stage. Members may attempt, usually unsuccessfully, to replace subgroup operation with a total group orientation. To help the group attain a level of total group orientation, the therapist should make the group aware of the source of its dissatisfaction and provide helpful techniques, such as role playing, to identify and highlight the subgroup problems that have emerged.

Phase V—Responsiveness to Group

mics Individual and subgroup problems become reinterpreted as group problems in the fifth phase. The group becomes process oriented and attuned to the group dynamics. It demonstrates its awareness of silences, difficulty in getting started, taboo topics, and similar phenomena. The group seems to be concerned about learning how it functions. The therapist can help by providing expertise in the description and comprehension of dynamics and processes. Because it is difficult for a group to remain for long at this sophisticated level of operation, regression to earlier behaviors is common.

Transition from Phase V to Phase VI   After experiencing process analysis as a rewarding endeavor, the group attempts to remedy or take care of unwanted or undesirable features that came to light in the analysis. However, the desire to remedy does not always ensure the ability to remedy. The group finds itself frustrated in its problem-solving attempts and may need to rely on the skills of the therapist.

Phase VI—The Group as Social Instrument

The sixth phase constitutes the ideal phase of group life. The group becomes superbly effective at engaging in cooperative problem solving, diagnosing process and dynamics, and making acceptable and appropriate decisions. In short, this group is characterized by competence. Leadership is fully distributed among the members, and the therapist becomes a resource person. Martin and Hill (1957, p 28) describe the members of such groups as "masters of their fate."

Interactional Group Therapy

There is a great diversity and flux in the field of group therapy. Many types of groups are found in mental health settings or in communities at large. People may belong to encounter groups, sensitivity training groups, gestalt groups, transactional analysis groups, psychodrama groups, psychoanalytic groups, nonverbal groups, body movement groups, nude swimming therapy groups, and so on. This list is certainly incomplete—a wide and bewildering array of group approaches is available to the willing.

Certain common principles seem to apply to all therapeutic groups, although specific methods and techniques may vary according to the purpose of the group or the skills and theoretic orientation of the therapist. Irvin Yalom (1985) uses the term *interactional group therapy* to describe a process of group therapy in which member interaction plays a crucial role. The common principles that apply to interactional group therapy are discussed below.

Advantages of Group over Individual Therapy

The advantages of group therapy stem from one major factor—the presence of many people, rather than a solitary therapist, who participate in the therapeutic experience. Specifically, group therapy provides the following:

• Stimuli from multiple sources, revealing distortions in interpersonal relationships so that they can be examined and resolved

• Multiple sources of feedback

• An interpersonal testing ground that allows members to try out old and new ways of being in an environment specifically structured for that purpose

Qualified Group Therapists

Mental health professionals may believe, in error, that group therapy is less complex and therefore "easier" than individual therapy, for example, because the

RESEARCH NOTE

Citation

Selander JM, Miller WC: Prolixin group: Can nursing intervention groups lower recidivism rates? J Psychosoc Nurs Ment Health Serv 1985;23:16–20.

Study Problem/Purpose

The purpose of this study was to answer the research question: Does receiving fluphenazine (Prolixin) in a nursing intervention group versus receiving neuroleptics in a variety of settings reduce the relapse rate of the group members?

Methods

The number of psychiatric admissions and the duration of hospitalizations of clients after they became members of a Prolixin group were compared to the number of admissions and the duration of hospitalizations before they entered the group. During each meeting, members had fifty minutes of group discussion; ten minutes were spent on fluphenazine injection. For each subject, the ratio of the total time spent in the hospital divided by the total number of admissions to the hospital was computed both over the total number of months in the Prolixin group and over a matching number of months prior to membership in the Prolixin group. Correlated *t*-tests were then computed.

Findings

The mean number of admissions was reduced from 2.6 before treatment to 1.0 after treatment. The mean of the total duration of hospitalization in days was 133.7 before treatment compared to 30.8 after treatment. The mean average duration of each hospitalization was 71.4 days before treatment compared to 13.2 days after treatment.

Implications

A Prolixin group can reduce the relapse rate of its members as evidenced by fewer and shorter hospitalizations. In these days of decreased funding and increased accountability, this method offers nursing an opportunity to demonstrate that it can cost effectively combine nursing intervention though the group process with medication surveillance and medication administration. The group is also a way to teach clients group process, the target symptoms of schizophrenia, and the effects and side effects of medications.

---

presence of more people makes interactions between therapist and client less intense. Although it is true that the interactions between any one member and the therapist may be less intense because interactions are dispersed among others, it *does not follow* that anyone can be an effective group therapist.

To be effective, the group therapist should have the following special preparation:

- Education in small group dynamics

- Education in group therapy theory

- Clinical practice with groups

- Expert supervision of the clinical practice (with ongoing supervision and/or consultation, depending on level of expertise)

The ANA Standards (see Chapter 2) identify the group psychotherapy role as appropriate for clinical specialists prepared at the master's level. Competent therapists report that it is also valuable to be a member of a therapy or sensitivity training group, before becoming a group leader.

The Curative Factors

Yalom (1985) contends that eleven interdependent curative factors or mechanisms of change in group therapy help people. These factors are the framework for an effective approach to therapy, because they constitute a rational basis for the therapist's choices of tactics and strategies. They are identified and defined in Table 29–4.

Types of Group Leadership

Groups can be led by a therapist working alone or by cotherapists working together in a variety of ways. Leaderless groups are another possibility. Each approach is described and evaluated in the sections that follow.

The Single Therapist Approach Groups led by a single therapist are common. They have an economic advantage in that only one therapist need be involved. A disadvantage is that the therapist cannot compare analyses of the group process with a cotherapist or get

TABLE 29–4   **Curative Factors of Group Therapy**

Factor	Definition
THERAPIST	
Instilling of hope	Imbuing the client with optimism for the success of the group therapy experience
Universality	Disconfirming the client's sense of aloneness or uniqueness in misery or hurt
Imparting of information	Giving instruction, advice, or suggestions
Altruism	Finding that the client can be of importance to others; having something of value to give
CLIENT	
Corrective recapitulation of the primary family group	Reviewing and correctively reliving early familial conflicts and growth-inhibiting relationships
Development of socializing techniques	Acquiring sophisticated social skills, e.g., being attuned to process, resolving conflicts, and being facilitative toward others
Imitative behavior	Trying out bits and pieces of the behavior of others and experimenting with those that fit well
Interpersonal learning	Learning that one authors one's interpersonal world and moving to alter it
Group cohesiveness	Being attracted to the group and the other members with a sense of "we"-ness rather than "I"-ness
Catharsis	Being able to express feelings
Existential factors	Being able to "be" with others; to be a part of a group

instant feedback or validation from a peer. Therapists working alone, however, do not have to direct their energies toward creating and maintaining a relationship with a colleague.

Recorders or observers may be used to help the solitary therapist be aware of the multiple complexities of any one group session. Nonparticipant observer/recorders are especially useful when they give the therapist feedback and focus on the nonverbal aspects of the session. If they are truly to be nonparticipants, recorder/observers must be very careful not to react on a nonverbal level to the content or process of the session.

The Cotherapy Approach   Groups led by two therapists, who share responsibility for leadership of the group to varying degrees, are gaining in popularity. The two models seen most often are the junior-senior and the egalitarian styles of cotherapy.

The Junior-Senior Position   In the junior-senior approach, the therapists have unequal responsibilities toward the group. The senior member of the team is usually the more experienced or educated. Besides having major responsibility for the success of the group, the senior therapist is responsible for training the junior member of the team. This approach is commonly used in agency settings, because it provides in-service training of new personnel and nonprofessionals under the guidance and watchful eye of an experienced group leader. However, relationship problems frequently surface when the roles of the leaders are not clear, or when one or both leaders are unable, or unwilling, to remain in the designated roles. The members of the group may also be unclear about the subordinate/superordinate roles and unsure of how to deal with and respond to leaders of unequal abilities and responsibilities.

The Egalitarian Position   In the egalitarian approach to cotherapy, two therapists of relatively equal skill, ability, and status share equally in responsibility for the group. The method is also used for training, with both cotherapists working under clinical supervision. It is preferable to the junior-senior approach for many reasons, which are set forth in Table 29–5. The egalitarian position is not without certain potential disadvantages, however. These are listed in Table 29–6. Overall, the advantages of the egalitarian approach outweigh its potential disadvantages. Cotherapists who arrange for supervision or consultation for themselves find that potential disadvantages can be turned in their favor. Identification and analysis of disadvantages that arise can lead to learning and behavior change in the cotherapists.

Nurses considering an egalitarian cotherapy relationship with one another need to engage in preliminary work to determine whether such a relationship is feasible for them. Exploration should include a discussion of each therapist's theoretic approaches, intervention styles, past experiences with groups, background, and personality characteristics. The therapists should consider and resolve such issues as how and when feedback is to be given, how disagreements between them are to be handled in the session, and the general conditions under which they will work together.

Decisions on client selection, length and number of sessions, time, and place are made together. Decisions of an emergency nature made by one therapist in the absence of the other should be based on mutually agreed procedures for just such situations.

Obviously egalitarian cotherapists must establish and maintain clear channels of communication. Not

TABLE 29-5   Advantages of Egalitarian Cotherapist Approach

Advantage	Rationale
Facilitates group development	Two therapists of similar abilities can monitor and facilitate group development better than one alone.
Facilitates dealing with heightened affect	One therapist can relate more directly to the member experiencing heightened affect, while the other therapist assumes responsibility for assisting the group members with their responses. When one therapist is involved in an interaction with a member or members, the other can take an observer stance, helping those involved to become more aware of the interaction and their participation in it.
Enhances therapists' personal and professional development	Egalitarian cotherapists can provide one another with corrective feedback and help one another analyze group process and plan intervention strategies.
Provides a synergistic effect	This is another way of saying "two heads are better than one." It is likely that two persons working together will make better decisions than one person working alone. The synergistic effect is similar to that of making decisions by consensus.
Provides an opportunity for modeling	Group members observe the acceptance and respect for one another that egalitarian cotherapists demonstrate. The therapists tolerate differences and disagreements between them in an atmosphere of mutual trust.
Reduces dependence	Because leadership is shared, the problem of dependence is somewhat dissipated.
Promotes appropriate pacing	Cotherapists check one another's timing, thus allowing the process to emerge. The presence of a cotherapist provides a respite from being continually "on guard" in relation to group process.

TABLE 29-6   Potential Disadvantages of Egalitarian Cotherapist Approach

Potential Disadvantage	Rationale
Creates conflict if therapists have different orientations	Although there is room for uniqueness and difference, radically different styles or beliefs about group therapy between cotherapists may hinder therapeutic work within the group.
Requires extra energy and time	Each therapist must spend time and energy maintaining an effective working relationship with the other, since the quality of the relationship between them determines their effectiveness in the group setting.
May make members feel overloaded	If the style of the therapists turns out to be "two-on-one" (both working at once with one group member), members may feel overwhelmed or "overtherapized."
May suffer from the fact that the therapists share blind spots	Therapists who are very similar in style and personality may have the same blind spots and fail to give one another corrective feedback.
May provide the opportunity for misleading modeling	The model the therapists provide may be negative if their relationship is tense, mistrustful, closed, competitive, or threatening.

only must they expend a great deal of time and energy in preparation for the group experience, but they must also plan for presession and postsession meetings, joint analysis of data, and joint supervision or consultation.

The Leaderless Approach   There is increasing interest in leaderless groups in two common forms—the occasional or regularly scheduled leaderless meeting as part of the structure of a group that is basically led by a therapist, and the leaderless group structured in some programmed format, usually through audiotapes.

Leaderless meetings in a therapist-led group should not be scheduled until the group has become cohesive and has established productive norms. Then the process can foster a sense of autonomy and responsibility. However, therapists should identify and examine their rationale for planning leaderless meetings. The repercussions of leaderless meetings are varied and complex and require an experienced group therapist to deal with them.

Other leaderless groups may be structured totally around following directions in a booklet and on tape. Encounter group or sensitivity training tapes are common. For example, members listen to a tape explaining the exercises assigned for that session. The members participate as instructed on the tape and spend the remainder of the session discussing the exercise and their reactions to it.

Creating the Group

The effectiveness of a group depends greatly on the conditions under which it is created. Much as architects design buildings, therapists design groups with certain functions and characteristics in mind.

Selecting Members Selecting the members is one of the most important functions of the therapists, since the quality of the interpersonal relationships among the members constitutes the core of successful group treatment. This is one of the major differences between group and individual therapy.

Inclusion Criteria It is more difficult to identify the characteristics of people who make good candidates for group therapy than those of people who do not make good candidates. We know that a person's motivation for therapy in general, and group therapy in particular, is of primary importance. Inclusion in a therapy group should also be at least partially determined by the effect a prospective member will have on the others, in terms of the prospective member's ability to bring the curative factors into play. Inclusion is also determined by the balance, in terms of behavior or characteristics, a prospective member will bring to the group. Will the person's subdued presentation prevent a member with similar behavior from being marginal and alone in the group? Does the person's age, occupation, or sex match another's so that the member will not feel singled out as different or deviant? The factor that appears to be most important, however, is that members be homogeneous in terms of their vulnerability or ego strength. Highly vulnerable members retard the progress of the less vulnerable, and vice versa.

Exclusion Criteria There have been a number of studies of group therapy dropouts. Dropouts significantly reduce the effectiveness of a group. They tend to have a demoralizing effect on the remaining group members. Group members see the act of dropping out as a comment on the worth of the group. For this reason, therapists should gear selection to avoid taking on members who are likely to terminate prematurely. Irvin Yalom (1985) identified several reasons given for premature termination. They are detailed in Table 29–7. Yalom's research has also demonstrated that people who drop out are likely to have some of the following characteristics:

- They use denial to a significant extent.
- They somatize frequently.
- They are less well motivated than those who continue.

TABLE 29–7 Client Reasons for Premature Termination of Group Therapy

Reason	Rationale
External factors	
Physical reasons	Distance, commuting, transportation, or scheduling problems may arise.
High external stress	An extremely stressful life may make it difficult or impossible for a client to expend energy participating in the group.
Group deviance	Members who differ significantly from others may wish to terminate; however, deviance that is unrelated to the group task is irrelevant.
Problems of intimacy	Isolated and withdrawn persons, or those with a pervasive dread of self-disclosure, are threatened by group therapy.
Fear of emotional contagion	Members may find they become highly upset on hearing the problems of others.
Early provocateurs	Members may create a nonviable role for themselves in the group; they plunge in with behavior that provides the main focus, are furiously active, then wish to withdraw.
Problems in orientation to group therapy	If pretherapy tasks have not been properly undertaken, the member may not be realistically prepared for the group.
Complications arising from subgrouping	Subunits that split up the group may disrupt therapeutic work if not understood and handled appropriately.
Complications arising from concurrent individual and group therapy	The member's two therapies may work at cross-purposes; members may "save" their affect and experiences in the group for exploration in an individual session.

- They are less psychologically oriented than those who continue.
- They have more severe psychiatric pathology.
- They are less likable (by group therapists).
- They are lower in socioeconomic status than those who continue.

- They are less effective socially than those who continue.

- They have lower IQs than those who continue.

It is also not uncommon to find that group therapy dropouts are persons who used the group for crisis resolution. They drop out once the crisis has passed.

The Selection Interview The pregroup interview session has two major purposes: selecting the members and establishing the initial contract. Cotherapists should always interview potential members jointly, and both should make all decisions regarding membership. The interview session gives members and therapists the opportunity to be exposed to one another. The therapists should accomplish the following tasks in the selection interview:

- Determine the motivation of the potential member

- Determine the presence and extent of any exclusion criteria

- Identify the presence of any external crisis that may have propelled the person into treatment

- Encourage the client to ask questions about the group

- Correct erroneous prejudgments or misinformation the client has about group therapy

- Inquire about any major pending life changes that may prevent the client's full and continued participation in the group

- Inquire about what hurts; what the client sees as a need to work on

- Establish and clarify the initial group contract

During this period, therapists and members have a chance to decide whether they can work together in the specific group under consideration. Clients as well as therapists can choose whether they will participate or not.

The Group Contract The group contract identifies the shared rights and responsibilities of therapists and members. It is a negotiated set of rules or arrangements for the structure and functioning of the group. It may be written or verbal, and it should cover the following elements:

- Goals and purposes of the group

- Time and length of meetings

- Place of meetings

- Starting and ending dates

- Addition of new members

- Attendance

- Confidentiality

- Roles of members and therapists

- Fees

Goals and Purposes The purpose of the group must be clear to all persons involved. In interactive group psychotherapy, the purpose is to bring about enduring behavioral and character change. The interactive group psychotherapy experience takes place largely in the here-and-now.

Goals may be long term or short term and are both group oriented and individualized. Some goals may be identified as early as the selection interview, and others may be added as they emerge during the life of the group. Goals may be altered as appropriate.

Time, Length, and Frequency of Meetings Time of meetings may be mutually determined by the participants. The length and frequency of meetings should be determined by the therapists after consideration of the clients' needs. Most outpatient clients find one eighty- to ninety-minute session per week useful. Shorter periods may not allow adequate time for discussion. Longer periods generally tax the endurance and alertness of both members and therapists. Inpatient groups are generally held more than once per week and frequently last for fifty to sixty minutes, although they may be longer or shorter depending on the anxiety and tolerance levels of the particular clients.

Place of Meetings The physical environment is important and influences the interaction among members. It is best to choose a pleasant room with comfortable chairs, preferably placed in a circle. The room should be private and free from external distractions.

Starting and Ending Dates If the group has a predetermined life span and the inclusive dates are known, members should be told the dates. Groups without fixed termination dates usually plan termination individually as each member is ready to move away from the group.

Addition of New Members Open groups accept members after the first session; closed groups begin with a certain number of members and do not add new members. Open groups maintain their size by replacing members who leave the group. They may continue indefinitely or have a predetermined life span. Closed groups are more common in settings where stability of membership is likely. Such settings include residential facilities of various types, long-term psychiatric in-patient settings, and prisons. A major problem with the closed group is that it runs the risk of extinction as members leave the group for various reasons.

Attendance It is important that members make a commitment to attend every session. Absences hinder the establishment of cohesion and have a demoralizing effect, especially when perceived as evidence that a member lacks interest or that the group is not attractive and valuable to its members. Stability of membership and high attendance have been demonstrated to be critical factors in the successful outcome of group therapy.

Confidentiality Some rules regarding confidentiality should be established, and client's concerns about which people will have access to information concerning them should be explored. Many therapists like to use tape recorders so that their work can be evaluated afterward by supervisors. They must obtain the clients' agreement to use of a tape recorder.

Rules about confidentially and access may be determined by the therapists' employing agency. In some instances, therapists may be required to make regular notes concerning each member's participation. Therapists may also wish to establish with group members guidelines on confidentiality that allow the therapists to share content with professionals when clients are dangerous to themselves or others. A good rule of thumb is: *Promise only what you can safely deliver.* Members should also be held accountable to maintain the confidentiality of the group.

Roles of Members and Therapists Therapists and clients should reach an understanding about the responsibilities of participants. Humanistic psychotherapy involves the full and informed participation of the client in the therapeutic process. Participants should share their expectations about the behavior and functions of clients and therapists and should clearly understand the modes of participation.

Fees Fees should be determined in advance and arrangements for payment made. Most mental health agencies have a sliding fee scale determined by the client's income and ability to pay. Clients should know whether fees will be charged for missed sessions.

Stages in Therapy Group Development

There is comfort in being able to predict, to some extent, the behavior of members at specific points in the group's life. Therapists organize predictions around stages or phases in the therapeutic experience, hoping to be prepared for expressions of behavior. They must bear in mind, however, that human experiences are dynamic and fluid and do not always progress as neatly as predicted.

The Schutz, Bennis and Shepard, and Martin and Hill frameworks, presented earlier in this chapter, give clear indications of how group life develops. This section focuses on the characteristics of member behavior and therapist interventions in the beginning, middle, and termination phases of interactional group therapy. As members' problems in living are revealed, the group life becomes richer and more complex. Therefore, there is no "cookbook" method that a therapist can follow to respond to every situation. The Intervention box on page 716 is presented simply as a guide for identifying some common member behaviors and therapist interventions at various points in the life of the group.

The Here-and-Now Emphasis

The core of interactional group therapy is the here-and-now. According to Irvin Yalom (1985, p 136), the here-and-now work of the interactional group therapist occurs on two levels:

1. Focusing attention on the member's feelings toward other group members, the therapists, and the group

2. Illuminating the process (the relationship implications of interpersonal transactions)

Thus, group members need to become aware of the here-and-now events—i.e., *what* happened—and then reflect back on them—i.e., *why* it happened. Yalom has called this the *self-reflective loop.*

The first task of the therapist is to steer the group into the here-and-now. As the group progresses and becomes comfortable with awareness of the here-and-now, much of the work is taken on by the members. Initially, however, the therapist actively steers group discourse in an *ahistoric* direction. In other words, events in the session take precedence over those that occur outside or have occurred outside.

If the group is to engage in interpersonal learning, the therapist must illuminate process. This is the second task of prime importance. The group must move beyond a focus on content toward a focus on process—the how and the why of an interaction. The process can be considered from any number of perspectives. The perspective chosen should be determined by the mood and needs of the group at that particular time. The group must recognize, examine, and understand process. The task of illuminating it belongs mainly to the therapist.

Process commentary is anxiety-producing, because there are so many injunctions against it in social situations. For example, commenting on someone's nervousness at a cocktail party is generally taboo. It not only makes the nervous person uncomfortable but also puts the process commentator in a high-risk situation. The comment may well be taken as criticism or viewed as inappropriate to the social context, and

INTERVENTION

Characteristic Member Behaviors and Nursing Interventions in Phases of Group Therapy

Member Behavior	Nursing Interventions	Member Behavior	Nursing Interventions
BEGINNING PHASE Anxiety is high.	Move to reduce anxiety; avoid making demands until group anxiety has abated.	Self-disclosure increases.	Encourage exploration and move to problem solving.
Members are unsure of what to do or say; need to be included.	Be active and provide some structure and direction; suggest members introduce themselves; work to sustain therapeutic rather than social role; include all members and encourage sharing but limit monopolizing.	Members are more aware of interpersonal interactions in the here-and-now.	Encourage members to participate in observing and commenting on here-and-now; make process comments.
Members are unclear about contract.	Clarify contract; give information to dispel confusion or misunderstandings.	Additions and losses of members evoke strong reactions.	Prepare members for additions and losses where possible; provide opportunity to talk about addition and loss experience.
Members test therapists and other members in terms of trustworthiness, value stances, etc., often through goblet issues.	Capitalize on opportunity to "pass" tests by proving trustworthy and by being open to and accepting the values of others.	Ability to maintain focus on one topic increases.	Encourage exploration of topic area in depth.
Beginning attempts at self-disclosure and problem identification are made.	Focus on related themes; begin exploration; begin to focus on here-and-now experiences in session.	**TERMINATION PHASE** Feelings about separation may run gamut (anger, sadness, indifference, joy, etc.)	Provide adequate time in as many sessions as necessary to work through affective responses; be sure members know termation date in advance; help members leave with positive feelings by identifying positive changes that have occurred in individual members and in group.
Members have sense of "I"-ness, little sense of "we"-ness.	Encourage involvement with others through curative factor of *universality*.		
MIDDLE PHASE Sense of "I"-ness is replaced by "we"-ness.	Encourage cohesion; provide opportunity for expression of warm feelings.	Members may feel lost and rudderless.	Explore support systems available to individual members; bridge gap where possible (to another agency, another therapist, etc.); keep in focus task of resolving loss.

the commentator is then vulnerable to retaliation from others.

Focus on the here-and-now experience differentiates interactive group psychotherapy from many other group therapies or therapeutic groups. The following section discusses some of these other approaches.

Other Group Therapies and Therapeutic Groups

Analytic Group Psychotherapy

Analytic group psychotherapy stems from psychoanalysis and shares its goal of personality reconstruction. In this process, there is an intensive analytic focus on the individuals in the group. It is sometimes described as treatment of one person in front of an audience of many. Dream material and fantasies are explored in the group, and the technique of free association is used. The interpersonal interactions of the members are of secondary importance and are explored in terms of how they demonstrate unresolved conflicts in the individual members' earlier relationships.

Psychodrama

Psychodrama is chiefly concerned with problems unique to the individual. It provides a medium through which catharsis can be achieved on both the nonverbal action and gesture level and the verbal level. In psychodrama groups, members act out real or imagined situations, while alter egos (other members) attempt to add what they think the actor may be feeling or thinking. The participants are encouraged to change roles. The practice of role reversal offers them the opportunity to "get into the other person's skin." The psychodramatist (therapist) is called a "director" whose responsibility is to direct the drama toward the goal of achieving catharsis and reaching for insight.

The psychodramatic stage may be quite complex. It sometimes consists of a series of tiers where different parts of the drama are acted out. Complex lighting and mood music may also be used to achieve the desired effect.

Self-Help Groups

The major operating principle in self-help groups is that the help given to members comes from members. A professional mental health worker is viewed as unnecessary. In fact, many of these groups were developed because of the failure of programs planned and implemented by professionals. In most, leaders are former members. Alcoholics Anonymous is a relatively well-known example.

There are a wide variety of self-help groups. Some are:

- Recovery Incorporated, Schizophrenics Anonymous, and Neurotics Anonymous, concerned with mental illness

- TOPS, Weight Watchers, Diet Workshop, and Overeater's Anonymous, concerned with obesity

- Gamblers Anonymous and Gam-Anon, concerned with compulsive gambling

- Five-Day Plan and Smoke Watchers Anonymous, concerned with smoking

- Child Abuse Listening Mediation, Inc. (CALM) and Parents Anonymous, concerned with child abuse

- La Leche League, concerned with breast-feeding

- Al-Anon and Al-a-Teen, concerned with the families of alcoholics

Self-help groups are proliferating rapidly. Groups for divorced, widowed, or single persons, for parents of runaways and troubled adolescents, for parents who abuse their children, and for the recently bereaved are a common part of the scene in most major cities throughout the world. Client clubs for persons having had a colostomy, ileostomy, laryngectomy, mastectomy, or amputation are also popular.

The role of the nurse in self-help groups is that of a resource person. Nurses need to be informed about such groups so that they can refer potential members to groups appropriate to their needs or to provide consultation when invited to do so.

Remotivation and Reeducation Groups

Remotivation and reeducation groups were developed to help persons who had undergone long-term institutionalization become less isolated and more socially adept. Long-term institutionalization produces apathy and isolation. Clients ready for release are often unaware of accepted norms or socially appropriate behavior and therefore are ill equipped to live outside a totally protected environment. Remotivation and reeducation groups help prepare these people to live beyond the confines of the institution. The groups bring members up to date with contemporary society. They can be led effectively by people with minimal preparation in group work. In many psychiatric hospitals, this role falls to the psychiatric aide. Nurses are more likely to supervise than to lead remotivation groups.

Client Government Groups

Most therapeutic milieus have numerous group activities. One common activity is some form of client government. Client governments take many forms, but in most cases staff and clients meet together once or twice a week to discuss and resolve day-to-day issues on the ward. Generally, these are key principles in client government:

• The client government should actually make and enforce most of the ward rules.

• The client government should organize and execute most of the routine ward tasks.

• No staff member should attempt to solve a problem if it can be delegated to the client government.

Among the problems the client government considers are the tidiness of the unit, late-night use of the television, the decision to have or not to have a Christmas tree, and individual clients' disruptive behavior. To make client government work, staff members must consciously refrain from making unilateral decisions that override client prerogatives. This strategy produces power relationships unlike those in the traditional medical model, in which it is believed that doctors and nurses are the experts and clients do not know what is best for them. Client government does not require that staff sit silently by, however. Rather, staff members should offer their perspective while agreeing to abide by the group's decision. Obviously, client government raises many thorny issues. Decisions about the granting of leave or the issuing of medications have legal implications that sometimes make client government impractical. In many cases the real decisions on these subjects are made in a substructure of separate staff meetings. It is often preferable for staff members to discuss issues that present problems for them in the open forum of the client government meeting. Otherwise, clients have no way of knowing how the system really operates, how decisions are made, or what their place is in the overall structure. A client government usually:

• Has a constitution with bylaws, holds regular meetings, and elects officers

• Votes on complaints and suggestions and presents the outcome to hospital authorities as the collective wishes of the group rather than of one individual

• Organizes ward rules

• Recommends changes in ward rules

• Arranges, organizes, conducts, and assumes responsibility for social activities

• Originates, plans, and carries through a variety of special activity programs, such as mural painting or writing and editing a newspaper

Proponents of client government as a strategy of milieu therapy argue that it is a logical and effective way of permitting clients to provide themselves with a more creative and wholesome hospital life. Ideally, instead of experiencing hospitalization as a combination of idleness, inactivity, boredom, and regimentation, they will learn democratic living and acquire more versatile social skills. The success of this approach, however, depends on the willingness of hospital administrators and psychiatric professionals to be receptive to clients' ideas and suggestions. If they do not accept as valid the clients' definitions of their hospital experience, nothing can be accomplished.

Client government has many advantages. It offers:

• A way of making life in a mental hospital resemble life in the external community

• A way of controlling deviant behavior with group pressure

• Group support for very disturbed clients

• A way of increasing recreational activities

• An opportunity for clients to understand administrative policy and help formulate it

• A way of increasing clients' self-esteem

• An opportunity for clients to express annoyances and resentments

• A channel of communication between clients and staff members

• A way to improve morale through the free interchange of ideas and feelings

• A way to uncover and work out tensions between staff and clients

The psychiatric staff nurse often serves as a resource person to client government groups, attending meetings to discuss issues of concern to clients and staff.

Activity Therapy Groups

Activity therapies are manual, recreational, and creative techniques to facilitate personal experiences and increase social responses and self-esteem. Although nurses may participate, activity therapies are generally the province of health and recreation specialists specifically educated to perform these roles.

Some activity therapies, such as the creative arts therapies discussed below, are organized and conducted in groups. Although there are specifically educated creative arts therapists, their numbers are small. Nurses may participate in these groups or use their principles to reach beyond the ordinary realm of verbal communication with clients.

Poetry Therapy Groups   The goal of poetry therapy groups is to help members get in touch with feelings and emotions through the use of poetry. Poems that are read aloud provide the stimulus for understanding and catharsis. They are selected as the therapeutic medium because they are powerful but not explicit avenues of communication. It is not necessary to be able to write poetry to be a member or leader of a poetry therapy group, although some members or leaders may be stimulated to write poems of their own.

Art Therapy Groups   Painting offers many people a comfortable opportunity for social exchange. In art therapy groups, the art produced by each member gives the art therapist a personal insight into the artist's personality. The art is produced during the session and is used as the basis for discussion and for exploring the members' feelings.

Music Therapy Groups   Music therapy consists of singing, rhythm, body movement, and listening. It is designed to increase the group members' concentration, memory retention, conceptual development, rhythmic behavior, movement behavior, verbal and nonverbal retention, and auditory discrimination. It is also used to stimulate the member's expression and discussion of affect.

Dance Therapy Groups   Dance as a therapeutic mode combines movement and verbal modes. In dance, members find it easier to express nonverbally the feelings and emotions that are a part of them but have been difficult to realize and communicate by other means. The person's inner sense is often reflected in body movements, and dance therapists work to help members integrate their experiences on the verbal level as well as the nonverbal one.

Bibliotherapy Groups   In bibliotherapy, literature is the means for achieving a therapeutic goal. The purpose of a bibliotherapy group is to assimilate the psychologic, sociologic, and aesthetic insights books give into human character, personality, and behavior. Literature provides the stimulus for the members to compare events and characters with their own interpersonal and intrapsychic experiences.

Groups of Medical-Surgical Clients and Their Families

Groups composed of medical-surgical clients are increasingly common, as psychiatric nurses move into general hospital settings offering liaison and consultation services to clients and hospital staff. Group work is useful for chronically ill or disabled persons, preoperative and postoperative clients, clients with regulative medical problems (such as diabetes, cardiac disease, or kidney disease), dying clients, the aged, and clients with psychophysiologic disorders, among others.

Such groups generally focus on the stress of hospitalization and illness and have as their goal the reduction of stress. Groups may be composed of clients alone, family members alone, or a combination.

Community Client Groups

Psychiatric nurses in community settings are involved with different kinds of community groups. These settings include schools, youth centers, industries, neighborhood centers, churches, prisons, summer camps, single-room occupancy boarding houses, transitional facilities (halfway houses), apartments for the elderly, and residential facilities for delinquent youths, runaways, and unwed mothers. The clients may also be persons who have direct contact with these groups, such as teachers, youth counselors, prison guards, police officers, and camp counselors.

Groups with Nurse Colleagues

There is increasing interest among nurses who work together in forming discussion and counseling groups to help reduce their job-related stress and to help them deal with problems of interpersonal relationships in more satisfying ways. Nurses in various intensive care and other high-pressure settings identify with increasing frequency the need for group work services that the psychiatric nurse can provide. The psychiatric nurse may also identify the need and offer this opportunity to colleagues.

CHAPTER HIGHLIGHTS

• Most people's lives are spent interacting with other human beings in groups. An individual's sense of being arises through membership in groups that help achieve goals they set for themselves.

• Nurses interact with groups of clients and colleagues in a wide variety of settings. To use groups rationally and effectively, nurses must understand the forces that underlie small group interactional processes and recognize their own patterns of participation.

• Effective groups accomplish their goals, maintain cohesion, and develop and modify their structure in ways that improve effectiveness.

• Regardless of setting or composition, several forces shape and modify the structure and functioning of groups. They include space and seating arrangements, material aspects of the physical environment, leadership styles and roles, methods of decision making, trust, risk-taking, cohesion and conformity, interpersonal attraction, and power and influence.

• The most effective group leadership is based on the assumption that responsible membership is the same thing as responsible leadership. In this distributed-functions approach, both the leader and the members engage in leadership behavior.

• Sound decision making that leads to well-conceived, well-understood, and well-accepted realistic actions toward the goals agreed on by the group is the hallmark of a group that functions effectively.

• The existence of trust in groups allows members to make suggestions; disclose attitudes, feelings, experiences, and perceptions; give feedback; and confront one another.

• Cohesion in groups is the spirit of "we-ness' that develops when a group has had shared experiences that provide a basis for attraction—the primary factor keeping a group in existence and working effectively. Too much cohesiveness (groupthink) may have a negative influence on the quality of a group's decisions.

• Power and influence in groups operate constantly and force members to adjust to one another and modify their behavior.

• Nurses can provide humanistic care to clients in a variety of settings through the mode of group intervention by offering them opportunities to seek validation, give and receive interpersonal feedback, and test new and different ways of being that may increase their quality of life.

• According to Schutz's FIRO approach, groups move through three interpersonal phases: inclusion, control, and affection.

• According to the Bennis and Shepard theory (authority relations/personal relations), obstacles to communication in groups stem from the orientations of the group members toward authority and intimacy.

• The theory of Martin and Hill (therapeutic problem approach) is that therapy groups have distinct and common growth patterns that can be described, observed, and predicted.

• A commonality among all four frameworks is the notion that group development occurs in identifiable stages and has implications for member behavior and therapist intervention.

• Curative factors, or mechanisms of change that constitute a rational basis for the therapist's choices of tactics and strategies, are unique to the group therapy process.

• The most advantageous leadership style in interactional therapy groups is the egalitarian cotherapy approach in which leadership is shared by two therapists of relatively equal skill, ability, and status.

• Critical considerations in designing a group are the selection of members and the establishment of a group contract.

• In interactive groups, member interaction plays a crucial role in change, which is achieved through the use of the here-and-now to illuminate group process.

REFERENCES

Alfonso DD: Therapeutic support during inpatient group therapy. *J Psychosoc Nurs* 1985;23(11):21–25.

Beeber LS, Schmitt MH: Cohesiveness in groups: A concept in search of a definition. *Adv Nurs Sci* 1986;9:1–11.

Bennis W, Shepard HA: A theory of group development. *Hum Relations* 1956;9:415–437.

Bierer J: Group psychotherapy. *Br Med J* 1942;1:214–217.

Birckhead LM: The nurse as leader: Group psychotherapy with psychotic patients. *J Psychosoc Nus* 1984;22:6–11.

Burrows T: The group method of analysis. *Psychoanal Rev* 1927;19:268–280.

Collison CR: Grappling with group resistance. *J Psychosoc Nurs* 1984;22(8):6–12.

Deutsch M: Conflicts: Productive and destructive. *J Soc Issues* 1969;25:7–41.

Deutsch M: The effects of cooperation and competition upon group process. *Hum Relations* 1949;2:129–152, 199–231.

Deutsch M: Trust and suspicion. *J Conflict Resolution* 1958;2:265–279.

Echternacht MR: Day treatment transition groups. *J Psychosoc Nurs* 1984;22(10)11–16.

Eklof M: The termination phase in group therapy: Implications for geriatric groups. *Small Group Behav* 1984;15:4–9.

Erickson RC: *Inpatient Small Group Psychotherapy: A Pragmatic Approach.* Charles C Thomas, 1984.

Fisher DW: Guidelines to effective group functioning. *Point View* 1985;22:6–8.

Foulkes SH, Anthony EJ: *Group Psychotherapy.* Penguin Books, 1957.

Gans JS: Hostility in group psychotherapy. *Int J Group Psychother* 1989;39:4–11.

Gilbert CM: Sexual abuse and group therapy. *J Psychosoc Nurs* 1988;26(5):19–23.

Gordon VC, Gordon EM: Short-term group treatment of depressed women: A replication study in Great Britian. *Arch Psychiatric Nurs* 1987;1(2):111–124.

Hierholzer R, Liberman R: Successful living: A social skills and problem-solving group for the chronically mentally ill. *Hosp Community Psychiatry* 1986;37(9):913–918.

Hunka CD. O'Toole AW, O'Toole RW: Self-help therapy in parents anonymous. *J Psychosoc Nurs* 1985;23(7):24–32.

Jacobs BC, Rosenthal TT: Managing effective meetings. *Nurs Econ* 1984;2:137–141.

Janis I: Groupthink. *Psychology Today.* November 1971a, p 43.

Janis I: Groupthink among policy makers, in Sanford N (ed): *Sanctions for Evil.* Jossey-Bass, 1971b, pp 71–89.

Johnson DW, Johnson FP: *Joining Together: Group Theory and Group Skills,* ed 3. Prentice-Hall, 1987.

Kahn EM: The choice of therapist self-disclosure in psychotherapy groups: Contextual considerations. *Arch Psychiatr Nurs* 1987;1(1):62–67.

Kanas N: Inpatient and outpatient group therapy for schizophrenic patients. *Am J Psychother* 1985;39:212–218.

Kane CF, DiMartino E, Jimenez M: A comparison of short-term psychoeducational and support groups for relatives coping with chronic schizophrenia. *Arch Psychiatr Nurs* 1990;4(6):343–353.

Kaplan KL: *Directive Group Therapy: Innovative Mental Health Treatment.* Slack, 1988.

Kelly KK, Sautter F, Tugrul K, Weaver MD: Fostering self-help on an inpatient unit. *Arch Psychiatr Nurs* 1990;4(3):161–165.

Lazell EW: The group treatment of dementia praecox. *Psychoanal Rev* 1921;8:168–179.

Lettieri-Marks D: Research in short-term inpatient group psychotherapy: A critical review. *Arch Psychiatr Nurs* 1987;1(6):407–421.

Marsh LC: Group therapy and the psychiatric clinic. *J Nerv Ment Dis* 1935;32:381–390.

Martin EA Jr, Hill WF: Toward a theory of group development. *Int J Group Psychother* 1957;7:20–30.

Maves PA, Schulz JW: Inpatient group treatment on short-term acute care units. *Hosp Community Psychiatry* 1985;36:27–34.

McHale M: Getting the joke: Interpreting humor in group therapy. *J Psychosoc Nurs* 1989;27(9):24–28.

Milgram S: Behavioral study of obedience. *J Abnorm Soc Psychol* 1963;67:371–378.

Milgram S: Group pressure and action against a person. *J Abnorm Soc Psychol* 1964;59:137–143.

Moreno JL: *Psychodrama.* Beacon Press, 1946.

Newton G: Self-help groups: Can they help? *J Psychosoc Nurs* 1984;22:(7):27–31.

Pollack LE: Improving relationships: Groups for inpatients with bipolar disorder. *J Psychosoc Nurs* 1990;28(5):17–22.

Prehn RA, Thomas P: Does it make a difference? The effect of a women's issues group on female psychiatric inpatients. *J Psychosoc Nurs* 1990;28(11):34–38.

Reed G, Sech ES: Bulimia: A conceptual model for group treatment. *J Psychosoc Nurs* 1985;23(5):16–22.

Roback H, Smith M: Patient attrition in dynamically oriented treatment groups. *Am J Psychiatry* 1987;144(4):426–431.

Roethlisberger FJ, Dickson WJ: *Management and the Worker.* Harvard University Press, 1939.

Rose L., Finestone K, Bass J: Group support for families of psychiatric patients. *J Psychosoc Nurs* 1985;23(12):24–29.

Sadock BJ: Group psychotherapy, combined individual and group psychotherapy, and psychodrama, in Kaplan HI, Sadock BJ: *Comprehensive Textbook of Psychiatry,* ed 4. Williams and Wilkins, 1985, pp 1403–1427.

Schutz WC: Interpersonal underworld. *Harvard Business Review* 1958a;36:123–135.

Schutz WC: *The Interpersonal Underworld: FIRO.* Science and Behavior Books, 1958b.

Selander JM, Miller WC: Prolixin group: Can nursing intervention groups lower recidivism rates? *J Psychosoc Nurs* 1985;23(11):16–20.

Shoham H, Neuschatz S: Group therapy with senile patients. *Soc Work* 1985;30:69–72.

Slavson SR: *The Practice of Group Psychotherapy.* International Universities Press, 1947.

Sommer R: *Personal Space: The Behavioral Basis of Design.* Prentice-Hall. 1969.

Steinzor B: The spatial factor in face-to-face discussion groups. *J Abnorm Soc Psychol* 1950;45:552–555.

Strodtbeck FL, Hook LH: The social dimensions of a twelve man jury table. *Sociometry* 1961;24:397–415.

Urbancic JC: Resolving incest experiences through group therapy. *J Psychosoc Nurs* 1989;27(9):4–10.

Vannicelli M: *Group Psychotherapy with Adult Children of Alcoholics.* Guilford Press, 1989.

Vinogradov S, Yalom ID: *A Concise Guide to Group Psychotherapy.* American Psychiatric Association Press, 1989.

Wolff A: The psychoanalysis of groups. *Am J Psychother* 1949;3:525–558 and 1950;4:16–50.

Yalom ID: *Inpatient Group Psychotherapy.* Basic Books, 1983.

Yalom ID: *The Theory and Practice of Group Psychotherapy,* ed 3. Basic Books, 1985.

Family Process and Family Therapy

LEARNING OBJECTIVES

- Identify the existing diverse forms of family life

- Identify the developmental tasks that confront couples and families

- Describe the family in terms of the relationships, associations, and connections that occur in a dynamic, interacting whole

- Describe relationship and communication complexities in functional families and families in difficulty

- Discuss strategies for family assessment and intervention

- Identify primary, secondary, and tertiary prevention approaches that may be used to provide for family mental health

- Describe some of the important factors in the counseling of couples

- Apply understandings of family process and family therapy in promoting and maintaining family mental health

Carol Ren Kneisl

CROSS REFERENCES

Other topics relevant to this content are: Codependence, Chapter 24; Communication skills, Chapter 8; Cultural considerations in families, Chapter 36; Intrafamily physical and sexual abuse, Chapter 22.

THE FAMILY IS THE context in which people develop their first relationships with other people. Their view of the larger social world outside their own unique family is molded by the events that happen within families and that influence the development of the individual.

Nurses encounter families in many areas of their practice—in the emergency room, the intensive care unit, the school, the cancer hospital, the community health setting, and the mental health setting, among others. Preventive approaches to family mental health, assessment of families in trouble, and intervention on their behalf must be based on an understanding of how families grow and interact and how family coping patterns develop. This chapter describes those processes and offers strategies for intervention into dysfunctional family systems.

Historical Foundations

Today's family is:

- Mom, dad, and 2.4 kids

- A couple with eight kids—three of hers, three of his, and two of theirs

- A 32-year-old electrical engineer and his three foster children

- A divorced woman and her infant child

- A widowed man, his two children, and his parents

- A grandmother raising her two grandchildren

- Two lesbian mothers and their children

- Two couples sharing an apartment neither could afford alone

- Three gay men who live and work together

- Four couples and their children in a remote commune

The nuclear family—mom, dad, and 2.4 kids—is the family structure people refer to when they speak of "strengthening the family."

Is it true that the family is dying out or needs strengthening? Actually, constant transformation or change is the one permanent quality of the family. Many family forms have appeared, disappeared, reappeared, and coexisted within and across cultures. Families have been defined by blood relationships, tribes, households, kinship systems, clans, and language alliances. They have been called *blended, extended, conjugal,* and *communal.* The American family is changing, but not dying: It is simply becoming different. Sensitive psychiatric nurses reject a narrow definition of family and adapt their clinical practice to the wide variety of family constellations that exist in contemporary society.

The Traditional Nuclear Family

The traditional **nuclear family** is a two-parent, time-limited, two-generation family consisting of a married couple and their children by birth or adoption. Despite its name, it is a relatively recent development in human history. It evolved as societies became more urban and industrialized in the move away from agrarianism. It is time-limited because, in most instances, the members of the younger generation begin their own families soon after they are 20 years of age.

Soon after its development, the traditional nuclear family became known as the *isolated nuclear family.* Ties to the **extended family**—all persons related by birth, marriage, or adoption to the nuclear family—were weakened. This diminished the basic support system that formerly surrounded families. The isolated nuclear family had less contact with the adults' **families of origin** (the families from which they came).

The Single-Parent Family

A *single-parent family* is also two-generational and occurs when a lone parent and offspring live together as a nucleus. It is a more common family form than most people believe. The number of single-parent families has been steadily increasing since 1970. The current prevalence in the United States is one in five.

Although most single-parent families result from death or divorce, increasing numbers of women are bearing children with the intention of rearing them alone. Single women and men are also adopting children with increasing frequency, something that was not done or even permitted only a few years ago. And more often than ever before, single parent families are headed by men.

The Blended Family

The **blended family,** an increasingly common phenomenon, is one in which one or both marital partners have previously been divorced or widowed, and bring with them their children from a former relationship. Various types of blended families exist. The loosest structure is a weekend blending that occurs when the children from one parent's previous marriage visit that parent's later family for a brief time. In a more permanent blend, the children from a previous marriage live with one parent and a later spouse, forming the new nucleus. In a third type of blended family, the children from previous marriages of both spouses are included in the same household. A "mine, yours, and ours" variety also includes children who are the offspring of the new marriage.

Alternative Family Forms

Alternative families consist of persons with or without blood or conjugal (marriage) ties who live and interact together to achieve common goals. Two or more adults, of the same or opposite sexes, and their children, or adults without children, may choose to live together. Unlike the family constellations described earlier, alternative families may be one-generational, consisting of adult members of a single generation.

Communal families, in which many people band together, are found both in sophisticated metropolitan centers and in more remote agricultural areas. The commune is further defined by how members have negotiated the privileges and responsibilities associated with their roles, material possessions, economic concerns, sexual expressions, and parenting activities. The Israeli kibbutzim are among the best known of the communes. Another type of communal arrangement is that of the religious cult.

Households of homosexual (gay) people are another alternative family form. Gay people who live together in the same household are choosing to be open about their life-style. Not all segments of society recognize this life-style as an acceptable alternative, and gays still face restrictions that often prevent them from adopting children or gaining custody of children from their previous heterosexual marriages that ended in divorce.

Even the well-known phrase, "You can choose your friends but you can't choose your relatives," is becoming obsolete, according to Lindsey (1982), who has written a book on chosen kin. In her view, two factors in contemporary life are important. The first is economics. Because many singles and the elderly can no longer afford to live alone, there is a trend toward communal, familial living among these groups. The second is geography. Because the average American moves once every three years, an individual who lives in the East may have family on the West Coast. Friends, chosen to re-create the extended family, become kin.

Evolution of Family Therapy

Professionals doing psychotherapy were bound by commitment and theoretic orientation to the practice of one-to-one work with clients until the early 1940s. In those early years, Freud's psychoanalytic theory was the dominating force in psychotherapeutic work with clients. The child-guidance movement, which began in the 1940s, is credited with including the client's family

in the thinking and activities of therapists. However, family thinking at this time was an extension of psychoanalytic theory. Generally, the child was seen by the psychiatrist and the family by the social worker. Child guidance workers saw no reason to work with the child and the parents or other family members together.

The psychoanalytic theory of personality development continued to be tremendously influential in the 1940s. Although most theorists and clinicians were aware of the effects of family relationships, they resisted active involvement of the family in treatment. To do so would have been viewed as a violation of the sacred analyst-client relationship.

In the early 1950s, some therapists began to experiment somewhat secretly with family therapy. Many therapists who were seeing families did not talk or write about their work. They had to refrain from alienating the psychiatric establishment, which considered family members irrelevant to the nature and treatment of psychopathology. Because these therapists earned their living in the mental health field, they cautiously avoided incurring the wrath of their professional groups.

The family therapy movement gained momentum and began to be acknowledged openly by the mid-1950s. Some theorists and clinicians began to publish their views, experiences, and research and learn of the work of others.

Since that time, the family therapy movement has flourished. There are now several different schools or approaches, each with its own style.

Theoretic Foundations

Developmental Tasks Confronting Families

Families, like individuals and groups, are confronted with developmental tasks. The family sociologist Evelyn Duvall (1985) lists the following developmental tasks of American families:

- *Physical maintenance*—providing food, shelter, clothing, health care

- *Resource allocation (both physical and emotional)*—meeting family expenses; apportioning material goods, space, and facilities; and apportioning emotional goods, such as affection, respect, and authority

- *Division of labor*—deciding who does what in relation to earning money, managing the household, caring for family members, and so on

- *Socialization of family members*—guiding members in mature patterns of controlling aggression, elimination, food intake, sexual drives, sleep, and so on

• *Reproduction, recruitment, and release of family members*—giving birth to or adopting children, rearing them for release from the family at maturity, incorporating new members, and establishing policies for including others, such as in-laws, stepparents, and friends

• *Maintenance of order*—ensuring conformity to family and/or societal norms

• *Placement of members in the larger society*—interacting with the community, school, church, and economic and political systems to protect family members from undesirable outside influences

• *Maintenance of motivation and morale*—rewarding members for achievements; developing a life philosophy and sense of family loyalty through rituals and celebrations; satisfying personal needs for acceptance, encouragement, and affection; meeting personal and family crises

These developmental tasks are a considerable undertaking. It is the families who do not succeed very well at accomplishing them who come to the psychiatric nurse's attention most often.

The Family As a System

In a general systems theory framework, a family can be seen as a system of interrelated parts forming a whole. A family system includes not only the family members but also their relationships, their communication with one another, and their interactions with the environment.

Wholeness   Because a system functions as a whole, its parts are interdependent, and a change or movement in any part of the system affects all other parts. For example, an accomplishment by one member of the family affects all the other members in the family system. Dysfunction in one member also changes the whole system. This concept of *wholeness* is important in understanding families. It means that counseling one family member will change all members in some way.

Homeostasis   Another important characteristic of a system is that it strives to maintain a dynamic equilibrium, or balance, among the various forces that operate within and on it. This process is referred to as *homeostasis*. All systems need to balance themselves within a range of functioning in which the work of the system can be accomplished. The mental image of a seesaw may help show what happens in the attempt to achieve balance. Too much weight on one end brings it to the ground. It is no longer in balance. However,

before that point, balance can be achieved at any of several points, even though the seesaw is not perfectly horizontal. When a family member behaves in a way not prescribed within the family system, other members react with attempts to minimize the disruption, always trying to maintain a steady state. Don D. Jackson (1957) introduced the concept of *family homeostasis* based on his observations that the families of psychiatric clients often experienced depression or psychophysiologic disorders when the client improved. He postulated that these behaviors of family members and the psychologic disruptions of the client were homeostatic mechanisms that operated to bring the disturbed system back into its delicate balance. When a family has to use most of its energy to maintain balance, little energy is left for the growth of the family or its individual members.

Subsystems   Elements in the system may also be parts of another system. Billy may be simultaneously the oldest child in the family, a catcher for the Little League baseball team, and a member of the debate team. Billy's family is a member of other larger systems as well—the extended family, the city, the nation, and so on. The family itself has *subsystems,* such as dyads (Billy and his father), triads (Billy, his brother, and his sister), or other groups of members who are linked together in some special association.

Openness   Systems can also be viewed as *open* or *closed,* although these are actually the extremes of a continuum. Some family systems are more open than others, while some are more closed. Openness requires that a system be flexible in adapting to the changes demanded by the environment. Adaptation takes energy to maintain homeostasis in the face of outside information or new input. Families whose systems are more closed tend to shut out or distort information from the environment so as not to upset their balance.

Boundaries   Family systems have *boundaries* as well. Boundaries define who participates in the system. They also tell family members the extent of differentiation permitted (among members and between members and outsiders), the amount or intensity of emotional investment in the system, the amount and kind of experiences available outside the system, and particular ways to evaluate experiences in terms of the family system. Boundaries may be clear, rigid, diffuse, or conflicting. These critical factors in family systems are referred to throughout this chapter.

Relationship Strains or Conflicts   Relationship strains or conflicts can occur between subsystems in the family or between various systems in the family or outside of it. A strain can exist between the individual members of a family, for instance, between two

RESEARCH NOTE

Citation

Lund K, Ostwald S: Dual-earner families' stress levels and personal and life-style–related variables. Nurs Res 1985(Nov–Dec);34:357–361.

Study Problem/Purpose

Dual-earner families with young children are a steadily growing population. Yet little is known about the effect of dual-earner life-styles on family stress levels or the health of the family. This study examined the relationship between personal and life-style–related factors and family stress levels in dual-earner families with young children.

Method

The study was a cross-sectional survey conducted in six day-care centers operated by a major day-care provider in a large metropolitan area. Subjects were 200 dual-earner families with children 6 years old or younger. The instrument used in the study was a closed-ended questionnaire with 103 items that measured family stress levels and personal and life-style–related variables. Family stress level was measured by the Family Inventory of Life Events and Changes (FILE). Availability of support systems and planning and organizing of family life were measured by adaptation of items from the Dual-Employed Coping Scales (DECS). The investigators developed additional questions to measure personal and life-style–related variables.

Findings

This study found that the majority of dual-earner families (76 percent) had a moderate level of family stress compared to national stress-level norms calculated for families in the preschool stage of development. This finding contradicts the commonly held belief that dual-earner families have increased stress due to the mother's employment outside the home. Thus, the study data indicate that the dual-earner life-style may not, in itself, predispose families to a high level of stress. The authors hypothesized that the advantages that result from a dual-earner life-style may serve to mediate stress and help maintain equilibrium within the family.

Variables that correlated significantly with the family stress score included parental age, age of the children, family income, satisfaction with the income, flexibility in vacation, necessity of separate vacations, and satisfaction with child care. The older the couple and the older the average age of the children, the lower the family stress score. The higher the income and the greater the satisfaction with income, the lower the family stress score. The more flexibility parents had in planning vacation, the lower the family stress score, and the more satisfied the parents were with child care, the lower the family stress score.

Implications

The major changes occurring in family and community life due to dual-earner family life-style demand attention from the health care system. Nurses are in a pivotal position to enhance family coping and reduce stress through education, planning, and providing direct service to support these families. Community health and industrial nurses can advocate to increase flexibility in the workplace, thus further reducing stress on the dual-earner family. Preventive health care for children and their families has always been a focus for nurses and can be expanded to include attention to the need for quality day care.

---

siblings with differing views on an issue. Conflict or strain can also occur between a member of the family and the rest of the family, or between a minority of family members and the other members. This commonly occurs when a previously and unanimously held family view is challenged by one or more members. Strain can also exist between a family and the community when a family view differs from that of the community at large. On a broader level, strain can exist between communities when one community's priorities differ from those of another.

Family Characteristics and Dynamics

Whether they are functional or dysfunctional, families have certain characteristics and dynamics. The functional family is distinguished from the dysfunctional one by the amount and quality of the energy used to maintain the family system.

Family Roles   Members of a family must determine how to accomplish the family developmental tasks listed earlier in this chapter. They do so by establishing roles, patterns of behavior sanctioned by the culture. Don D. Jackson (1965) believes that families set roles by operating as a rule-governed system—an ordered format designed so that members may be aware of their positions in relation to one another. Although a family system engages in a multitude of behaviors, a relatively small set of rules is sufficient to govern family life. Roles are assigned according to family rules. Families decide which roles will exist within the system, socialize members into the roles, and then expend energy maintaining members within their roles.

When members are unable or unwilling to perform assigned roles, the family experiences stress. For example, the roles of mother and father have long been stereotyped in American society. Mothers were the family nurturers and caretakers, whereas fathers were the family decision makers and wage earners. These roles are not completely satisfying to all American families, and many women and men have moved to negotiate their roles differently. The trend in society is now toward dual-earner families with two working parents and families in which fathers share, or assume, the nurturing role. For the health of the family system, roles often must be negotiated in other than stereotyped ways. When the roles are not negotiated satisfactorily, family disequilibrium results.

Power Structure Most families have a hierarchical power structure in which the adults wield power, usually in an authoritarian manner. The power structure is often developed in this way because it creates a safe environment in which young children can grow and develop, and because it is easy to operate. However, stress develops when disagreements exist about who holds the power.

Tom, the 17-year-old son in the M family, always used the family car without permission. Although some serious arguments ensued between Tom and his father, no restrictions were placed on Tom's behavior, and the car keys continued to hang on a key rack in the front hall. Tom's paternal grandfather, who lived with the M family, took Tom's side in his arguments with his father. Grandfather M adopted a fond "boys-will-be-boys" stance. One evening when the family car was in an auto repair shop for some minor work, Tom "borrowed" his grandfather's new car. Tom was involved in a collision about an hour later. Although no one was injured, Grandfather M's car had to be towed away, extensively damaged. Later that night, the adults of the M family managed to come together to agree on a stance that they could mutually support.

Once the adults in the M family were able to acknowledge their internal power struggle and come to an agreement on what rules were to be set and by whom, the system was less stressed.

Grandparents residing with a family are not the only causes of disagreements. Disagreements between husband and wife about who holds the power are also common. In some dysfunctional families, there is chronic discord about power.

When children mature and become capable of assuming greater responsibility for their own functioning, power is often diffused among all members of a family system in a more democratic fashion. Certain families, however, do not allow power to be redistributed, thus hindering the individual development of the members who have less power.

Family System Behavior In the systems view of a family, the family interaction system has four important qualities. The first, *wholeness,* is discussed earlier in this chapter. It refers to the interrelationship of all the elements in the system.

Synergy, the second characteristic, refers to the fact that the whole is greater than the sum of its parts. In other words, combined efforts produce a greater effect than the sum of individual actions. Two young children at play in their mother's cosmetics exemplify the effects of synergy. They encourage one another gleefully and enthusiastically to open and use the various jars, pots, and tubes they have discovered. Before long, the children and the environment have been thoroughly decorated. To their angry mother, each child blames the other, believing that without the other they would not have been in trouble. The effects of synergy can also be seen in families distinguished by open affection. Open affection stimulates more open affection, which cycles back into the system to stimulate even more of this particular distinguishing characteristic.

Circularity and *feedback* also characterize family system behavior. Each member engages in behavior that influences the other members. The process has been described as an uninterrupted sequence of interchanges. The usual way people think about relationships does not allow for circularity. In a teenage daughter's view, for example, if her mother would only trust her, they would get along better. The mother's view is that the problem lies with the teen's uncooperativeness. Both mother and daughter are stopping the circular process by seeing one behavior as a cause and the other as an effect. The circular view is that each person's behavior is both cause and effect at the same time. Mother and daughter are caught up in a cycle, as they monitor and influence one another.

Family Therapy

Nurses in the past have worked with families and family problems in many different settings. Most often, nurses encountered family members while in a health teaching role. While caring for the diabetic client, the client who has undergone major surgery, or the client who has had a myocardial infarction, the nurse taught the client's family how to care for that person physically and what life-style changes the illness might impose on the family. Psychiatric nurses have a psychoeducation role with families. The family therapy role, however, is still a relatively new one for nurses. Nurse family therapists should be prepared at the master's level.

Family therapy is a different way of viewing problems. In general, family therapists believe that the emotional symptoms or problems of an individual are an expression of emotional symptoms or problems in a family. Therefore, family therapists view the family system as the unit of treatment. Their concerns are basically with the relationships between the family members, not with the intrapsychic functioning of Mom, Dad, Kevin, or Susan.

Various therapeutic strategies have emerged from these shared beliefs. Family therapists do not have as fixed a set of procedures for intervention as psychoanalysts do. However, certain intervention strategies and therapeutic postures seem to flow naturally from the basic beliefs family therapists hold.

Approaches to Family Therapy

Rather than identify family therapy approaches by the names of the family therapists who developed them, we will briefly discuss the approaches according to the seven categories proposed by Jones (1980):

1. The integrative approach is represented by the work of Nathan Ackerman (1958). Ackerman emphasized the need to take individual as well as family dynamics into account. Although his approach is the only one that does not rely heavily on systems concepts, it does bridge the gap between the psychoanalytic approach and approaches that focus on interpersonal and transactional phenomena.

2. The psychoanalytic approach is based directly on Freudian psychoanalytic theory and conforms to an illness model of family therapy. According to this model, one or more disturbed marital partners account for the dysfunctions experienced in the family. An emphasis is placed on the reconstruction of the personality of the disturbed mate(s). The names of Boszormenyi-Nagy and Framo (1965) are linked with the psychoanalytic approach.

3. Bowen thought of the family as a system combining both emotional and social relationships. Bowen (1960, 1978) developed his approach into specifics that can be easily taught. Some of his concepts, such as family triangles and multigenerational transmission

processes, are discussed later. This approach is an extremely popular one, probably because it is so specific.

4. The structural approach describes the family as an open system governed by rules or boundaries that define who participates with whom, and how (Minuchin 1974). There are two types of dysfunctional patterns—enmeshment and disengagement—both of which are discussed later. The goal of the family therapist in this approach is to transform the family structure in the interest of creating clear boundaries.

5. The interactional approach is called a communicational approach in some of the literature. The unit of analysis for therapy is the behavior and communication among and between family members. These concepts were developed in the 1950s and 1960s through research on the possible relationship between the double-bind concept and schizophrenia and on dysfunctional communication in families (see Bateson et al. 1956; Haley 1987; Jackson 1957, 1968a, 1968b; Lidz et al. 1957; and Satir 1967). Many of these concepts are discussed later in this chapter.

6. The social network approach includes the persons—friends, neighbors, relatives, fellow workers—with whom the family in crisis has a social relationship (Speck 1967). Social network therapy resembles extended group therapy with the goal of bringing together as many people of a family's social network as possible. It takes place in the home and involves large groups of people (from 40 to 100 is not uncommon). It has been found particularly helpful in crisis and disaster situations and has been compared to the tribal meetings for healing purposes that occur in other cultures (Speck and Attneave 1973).

7. The behavioral approach is based on Skinner's theories of learning. It consists of adapting principles and techniques of behavior modification for use with families. Gerald Patterson (1976) is one of the most prominent authors and theorists concerned with the behavioral approach to family therapy.

Qualifications of Family Therapists

Family therapists should be specially educated in the practice of family therapy and strongly committed to a belief in the importance of the family. Increasing numbers of psychiatric nurse clinical specialists are being prepared in graduate programs that provide both theory and supervised clinical practice in this specialized area. Although undergraduate nursing programs focus on the importance of relating to families in all settings, they (rightfully) do not prepare nurses as family therapists.

Relationship and Communication Intricacies in Families

People negotiate their views of themselves and others according to their perceptions. Perceptions also influence how people interact with one another on both content and relationship levels. In a family system, each person's behavior is contingent on the behavior of the others. This creates some interesting and complex turns in family relationships.

Functional families allow for individuation and growth-producing experiences. Rigidity within a family system makes it difficult for the family to adapt to change and easier for the family to become dysfunctional. Some of the relationship complexities described below exist in all families, but dysfunctional families handle them differently than functional families do. Other factors arise only in family systems that are dysfunctional.

Although some of the factors discussed below may be easily categorized as communicational, it is important to recognize their relational aspects. Other communication factors (discounting, disconfirming, disqualifying, symmetry, complementarity, congruity, and incongruity) are discussed in Chapter 8.

The Self-Fulfilling Prophecy and Life Scripts

A **self-fulfilling prophecy** is an idea or expectation that is acted out, largely unconsciously, thus "proving" itself. In families, self-fulfilling prophecies are often seen in the guise of family **life scripts.** Claude Steiner (1974, p 51) calls a script "the blueprint for a life course." It is a plan decided not by the fates, but by experiences early in life. In Steiner's words (p 54), "Human beings are deeply affected by and submissive to the will of the specific divinities of their household—their parents—whose injunctions they are impotent against as they blindly follow them through life, sometimes to their self-destruction." People with life scripts are following forced, premature, early childhood decisions. Steiner notes that, although not everyone has a script, script-free living is the exception rather than the rule.

There is an endless variety among life scripts. The Miss America script is decided for the 5-year-old girl whose parents enroll her in the Little Miss New York State (or Kansas or Colorado) competition. There are My Son the Doctor, Delinquent, Alcoholic, and Drug Addict scripts. A person with a script, either "good" or "bad," is terribly disadvantaged in terms of autonomy or life potentials. Unless people recognize what the script is and take steps to change it, they are prevented from living to the fullest human potential.

Family Myths, Life-Styles, and Themes

Family myths, life-styles, and themes help families maintain balance by permitting them to resist change. **Family myths** are well-integrated beliefs, shared by all family members, about each other and their positions in family life. The beliefs are unchallenged, even though family members may have to resort to distortions to maintain the myth. The family myth is related to the family's inner image—how the family appears to its members. For example, one family myth was that the father had the ability to make wise decisions. Individual members in this family participated to maintain the myth of the father as a Solomon by gearing interactions with him in such a way that he appeared to make high-level family decisions single-handedly.

The concepts of family theme (Hess and Handel 1959) and family life-style (Deutsch 1967) are alike in their focus on the family's ways of relating to the outside world. The **family theme** is the family's perception of its development and history. One family had a theme constructed around second-generation grandparents of Austrian descent, who were able to provide their oldest son with a law school education through their hard work. This family conceived of persons on welfare as "lazy," thus reaffirming its view of the value of working hard and becoming educated. Determining the salient themes in a family's life is important because they shape the fates of individual members and determine the pressures with which each person must contend.

The **family-life-style** has to do with the family's biased perception of the outside world and its automated means of coping with this world. Family life-styles are designed to uphold particular images of the family—as the most popular, talented, financially successful, nonconformist, or whatever. The life-style is the front or facade the family strives to present to others.

Coalitions, Dyads, and Triangles

Of all the forms of communicative exchange, dyadic communication is the most common. In fact, a family begins with a dyad, the marital couple. The natural alliance, or coalition, of this dyad presents a united front to the world—to deal with one member, people have to deal with them both. However, if one partner does not actively support the other, severe strain results.

The presence of a third person always has an effect on an existing dyad. When the marital couple gives birth to a child, the relationship becomes triadic. A triad is not a stable social situation, since it actually consists of a dyad plus one. Shifting alliances characterize triads—mother and father may unite to discipline the child, mother and child may unite to argue for a family vacation, or father and child may join forces to go fishing together. The process of forming a triad is called **triangulation.** Triangulation becomes dysfunctional when issues are solved in families by shifting the intimacy among members, rather than by working the actual issue through. Such coalitions always result in someone feeling "left out." Triangulation is a major concept in the Bowen approach to family therapy.

Coalitions arise basically to affect the distribution of power. By joining forces, two persons can increase their influence over a third. A husband and wife frequently pair up to discipline their child better. However, the child may also attempt to pair up with one parent to avoid discipline. In families with a number of children, typical coalitions involve children closest in age, or children of the same sex.

Pseudomutuality and Pseudohostility A family in which pseudomutuality occurs functions as if it were a close, happy family. According to Lyman Wynne and his associates (1958), who use the interactional approach to family therapy, this pattern of relating has the following characteristics:

- Persistent sameness in the structuring of roles

- Insistence on the desirability and appropriateness of the role structure, despite evidence to the contrary

- Intense concern over deviations from the role structure or emerging autonomy

- Marked absence of spontaneity, enthusiasm, and humor in participating together

In these families, the members do not form intimate bonds with one another as individuals. Instead, an inordinate amount of energy is expended in maintaining ritualized and stereotyped ways of behaving and relating. There is a desperate struggle to maintain harmony. Wynne and associates (1958) give a perfect example in one mother who said: "We are all peaceful. I like peace if I have to kill someone to get it." Such a family requires its members to give up their sense of personal identity.

Pseudohostility exists in families characterized by chronic conflict, alienation, tension, and inappropriate remoteness. As in pseudomutuality, family members deny the problems in an attempt to negate the hostility. Family members view their differences as only minor ones. Both pseudomutual and pseudohostile family environments are stifling milieus.

Deviations in the Parental Coalition In some families, problems develop from the parents' inability to form a satisfying coalition in terms of intimacy and control. Several common deviations are examined in the sections below.

Schism Theodore Lidz and his associates (1957), who also advocate the interactional approach, have identified two types of families with parental coalition problems. They result from marital schism and marital skew. **Schismatic families** are those in which the children are forced to join one or the other camp of two warring spouses. Lidz et al. believe that the constant fighting in these families is a defense against intimacy or closeness. In schismatic families, the spouses devalue and undercut one another. This makes it difficult for the children to want to be like either of them.

Skew **Skewed families** are those in which one spouse is severely dysfunctional. The other spouse, who is usually aware of the dysfunction of the partner, assumes a passive, peace-making, submissive stance to preserve the marriage. The passive partner is caught between effectively responding to the view of "reality" of the outside world and giving up this view within the home, accepting the dysfunctional mate's view. On the surface, a skewed couple may appear to be complementary. Their relationship is actually lopsided and unsuited to many basic family tasks, however.

Enmeshment Other family patterns are enmeshment and disengagement, as described by Salvador Minuchin (1974), who advocates a structural approach to family therapy. **Enmeshed families** are characterized by a fast tempo of interpersonal exchange. Interactions within the family are of high intensity and are directed more toward issues of power than toward issues of affection. In enmeshed families, one parent, usually the mother, is often found to be overcontrolling and becomes anxious over the possibility of losing control over the children. The mother appears to be trying to prevent herself from becoming helpless. Adult males are often absent in these families, or, if present, are controlled in much the same way the children are.

Disengagement **Disengaged families** move to the other extreme from enmeshment—abandonment. Family members seem oblivious to the effects of their actions on one another. They are unresponsive and unconnected to each other. Structure, order, or authority in the family may be weak or nonexistent. Assuming control and guidance increases the anxiety of the parent, who may feel overwhelmed and depressed. In these families, a child often assumes the parental role.

Scapegoating Scapegoating is a social process that has been written and talked about since the time of the ancient Greeks. A scapegoat is one who is made to bear the blame for others or to suffer in their place. In families, a disturbed member may play the role of family scapegoat, thus acting out the conflicts in the system and stabilizing it. For example, one or both parents may blame the child when things go wrong rather than blame themselves or one another. This allows the parent to declare "our marriage would be fine if it weren't for that kid."

According to Nathan Ackerman (1971) the following constellation of roles occurs:

• The *scapegoat*, or victim, who best symbolizes the conflicts

• The *family persecutor*, who uses a special prejudice as the vehicle of attack

• The *family healer*, who intervenes to neutralize the attack and rescue the victim

Children are not the only persons who are scapegoated. Adults, or whole groups of people, may also be scapegoated.

Paradoxes and Double Binds A **paradox** is a self-contradictory communication. An example is the paradoxical bumper sticker: "Individualists Unite!" Paradoxes are common in everyday communication. The client who says: "Tell me what to do, so I can be independent," creates a paradox for the nurse. The nurse who says: "I think you should find a new job, but it's not my place to say so," creates a paradox for the client.

The **double bind** is a complex series of paradoxes. The example of a double-bind situation classically cited is from Gregory Bateson and his associates (1956, p 259):

> A young man who had fairly well recovered from an acute schizophrenic episode was visited in the hospital by his mother. He was glad to see her and impulsively put his arm around her shoulders, whereupon she stiffened. He withdrew his arm and she asked, "Don't you love me anymore?" He then blushed, and she said, "Dear, you must not be so easily embarrassed and afraid of your feelings." The client was able to stay with her only a few minutes more and following her departure he assaulted an aide and was put in the tubs.

The conditions necessary to produce the double bind are present in this example:

• Two persons, one of whom is the victim (the young man)

• A repeated experience, so that the double bind becomes a habitual expectation

• A primary negative injunction, carrying a threat of punishment (mother stiffens)

• A secondary injunction conflicting with the first injunction, but at a more abstract level. Like the primary injunction, the second threatens punishment ("Don't you love me anymore?")

• A tertiary negative injunction prohibiting the victim from escaping from the field ("Dear, you must not be so easily embarrassed and afraid of your feelings.")

It is theorized that repeated exposure to double binds in families produces schizophrenia. The evidence, however, is not convincing. Although people labeled schizophrenic are victims of double binds, not all victims of double binds are, or become, schizophrenic. In addition, the theory does not allow for a biologic basis.

The Treatment Unit and the Treatment Setting

Most family therapists recommend that all persons in the family constellation participate in the assessment phase of family therapy. Not all agree on what persons make up the family constellation or the treatment unit. Some include all members of the nuclear family; others include members of the extended family; and still others, large numbers of people in the family's social network. Different coalitions may be seen together at different times to accomplish specific purposes. For example, the mates are often seen together for the first few sessions.

Children 4 years of age and younger are often not included in ongoing family therapy sessions. They may misinterpret, or be frightened by, the dialogue. In addition, small children tend to be disruptive. Some therapists, however, make it a point to bring all the children into therapy for at least two sessions to see how the family as a whole operates.

Family therapists often reverse the traditional territorial control of the professional by engaging the family system in therapy in its own milieu—the home. There are several reasons these therapists see families on their own ground:

• The interactions of the family system are more natural in their usual environment.

• Customary roles are more spontaneously played out on home ground.

• Family members reluctant to participate in therapy tend to be less so in the home than in a formal office or mental health agency setting.

Family Assessment

Family therapy consists of three major components—assessment, contract or goal negotiation, and intervention. The first phase of a therapeutic process involves the initial assessment of the family. According to Bross (1983), family assessment involves gathering data in the following three areas:

1. Demographic information—data pertaining to gender, age, occupation, religion, ethnicity, and family income

2. Substantive information—data pertaining to past treatment, history, pertinent medical facts, identity of the "identified patient," information regarding sensitive topics or recent events

3. Interactional data—information pertaining to family rules, alignments, coalitions, subsystems (marital, parental, sibling), hierarchy, patterns of behavior, cultural differences

Compton and Galaway (1979, pp 251–252) suggest that a thorough family assessment should include the following:

1. *Family as a social system*

   a. Family as responsive and contributing unit within network of other social units
      (1) Family boundaries—permeability or rigidity
      (2) Nature of input from other social units
      (3) Extent to which family fits into cultural mold and expectations of larger system
      (4) Degree to which family is considered deviant

   b. Roles of family members
      (1) Formal roles and role performance (father, child, and so on)
      (2) Informal roles and role performance (scapegoat, controller, follower, decision maker)
      (3) Degree of family agreement on assignment of roles and their performance
      (4) Interrelationship of various roles—degree of "fit" within total family

   c. Family rules
      (1) Family rules that foster stability and maintenance
      (2) Family rules that foster maladaptation
      (3) Conformity of rules to family's life-style
      (4) How rules are modified; respect for difference

   d. Communication network
      (1) How family communicates and provides information to members
      (2) Channels of communication—who speaks to whom
      (3) Quality of messages—clarity or ambiguity

2. *Developmental stage of family*

   a. Chronologic stage of family

   b. Problems and adaptations of transition

   c. Shifts in role responsibility over time

   d. Ways and means of solving problems at earlier stages

3. *Subsystems operating within family*

   a. Function of family alliances in family stability

   b. Conflict or support of other family subsystems and family as a whole

4. *Physical and emotional needs*

   a. Level at which family meets essential physical needs

   b. Level at which family meets social and emotional needs

   c. Resources within family to meet physical and emotional needs

   d. Disparities between individual needs and family's willingness or ability to meet them

5. *Goals, values, and aspirations*

   a. Extent to which family member's goals and values are articulated and understood by all members

   b. Extent to which family values reflect resignation or compromise

   c. Extent to which family permits pursuit of individual goals and values

6. *Socioeconomic factors*

   a. Economic factors—level of income, adequacy of subsistence; how this affects life-style, sense of adequacy, self-worth

   b. Employment and attitudes about it

   c. Racial, cultural, and ethnic identification: sense of identity and belonging

   d. Religious identification and link to significant value systems, norms, and practices

Family assessments may be accomplished in a variety of ways. Some suggestions are given below. Others are discussed in the later section on intervention.

Taking a Family Life Chronology   Virginia Satir (1967) suggests that the family therapist should structure at least the first two sessions of therapy by taking a family life chronology. Her rationale is based on the following factors:

• The family therapist enters a session knowing little more than who the "identified patient" (IP) is and what symptoms that person manifests. The therapist does not have clues about the meaning of the symptoms—how the pain that exists in the marital relationship is expressed, how the mates have attempted to cope with their problems, or what models have influenced each mate's expectations about being a mate or parent.

• The therapist knows that the family has a history but does not know what the history is—what events have occurred and which members were influenced (directly or indirectly) by those events.

• Family members are fearful about embarking on family therapy. Structuring early sessions with a family life chronology helps decrease the threat. Members can answer relatively nonthreatening questions, and they tend to relax as the therapist demonstrates ability to take charge and keep things under control.

• Family members are often despairing when they enter therapy. The therapist's structure tells the family that they can take specified directions to accomplish goals. The questions also provide family members with the opportunity to review successes as well as failures.

• The family life chronology is a nonthreatening way to change the focus from a "sick" family member to the family system and marital relationship.

• Taking the chronology gives the family therapist the opportunity to be a model of effective communication and provides the framework within which change can take place.

Figure 30–1 shows the structure of the family life chronology recommended by Satir.

Family Genealogy or Time Line   Walter Toman's family constellation theory (1976), which uses generational transmission concepts, is a useful basis for constructing a family genealogy or time line.

From the study of families in detail, it becomes apparent that patterns are spread over generations. At first Bowen believed that a schizophrenic child could be produced after psychologic impairment in 3 generations. He now believes that the level of impairment in schizophrenia is the result of 8 to 10 generations of impairment. An intrinsic difficulty in analyzing generational transmission is that only a minute slice of a family generation—3 generations out of at least 4000—can be studied. Few people are able to do what one university professor can. He can trace his paternal ancestry in China back to 2255 B.C.—an incredible 4000 years and 131 generations.

Each generation, according to Laing (1972, p 77), projects onto the next the following elements:

• What was projected onto it by prior generations

• What was induced in it by prior generations

• Its response to this projection and induction

This process, which Laing calls *mapping,* is endless. Since it is impractical and impossible to understand the effect of 4000 earlier generations on a family, the time line can serve a therapist and a family as a more limited means for understanding the family's roots.

The time line is highly effective as a visual representation. By drawing it on a long, narrow piece

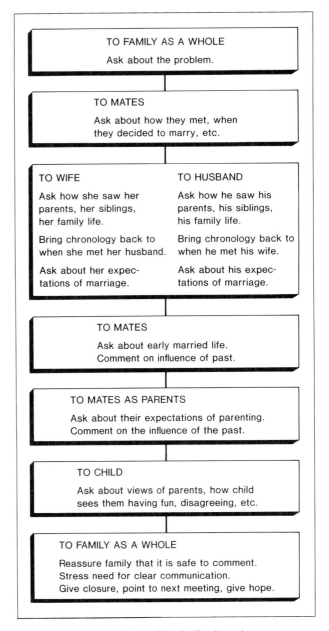

FIGURE 30–1 Main flow of family life chronology.   *SOURCE: Adapted from Satir V: Conjoint Family Therapy, rev ed. Science and Behavior Books, 1967.*

of paper and taping it to the wall during the family's sessions, the therapist can use it repeatedly as family therapy progresses. Colored lines can differentiate individual family members. Colored flags, pins, or asterisks can identify and call attention to significant events in the family history. Births, deaths, marriages, and leavetakings should be noted. The family therapist can use any of several family tree or genealogic tracings for the family time line.

The Structured Family Interview A structured family interview (Watzlawick 1966) has elements similar to Satir's family life chronology. In addition, the family members are asked to participate in demonstrating the system's operation. The structured interview is composed of the following segments:

• *The main problems:* Each member is asked separately to identify what he or she considers the main problems in the family. The therapist assures the family member that the answer will not be divulged. Family members are then brought together to discuss this topic. The therapist leaves the room after telling the family members that their conversation will be recorded and they will be observed through a one-way screen. This task undermines the myth that the IP is the only "problem" in the family and paves the way for future work.

• *Planning something together:* The family is asked to plan something together, as a family, in the five minutes during which the therapist leaves the room. The important things to notice are whether and how a decision was reached. The content, while revealing, is of secondary importance.

• *How the mates met:* This task is for the mates only. With the children in another room, the mates are asked how, out of all the millions of people in the world, they got together. The parents share their views of the past and reveal their predominant patterns of interacting in the present.

• *The meaning of a proverb:* The parents are asked to discuss the meaning of the proverb "A rolling stone gathers no moss." At the end of five minutes, they are to call the children in and teach them the meaning of the proverb. This proverb has two valid but mutually exclusive interpretations—that *moss* (roots, stability, friends) is valuable, or that *rolling* (not stagnating, being alert, moving) is desirable. This task reveals how the mates handle disagreements and how they explain things to their offspring.

• *Blaming:* The entire family and the therapist are together for this task. The father sits to the left of the therapist followed at his left by the mother and the children, from the oldest to the youngest, in a clockwise direction around the table. Each family member is asked to write down, on a three-by-five card, the main fault of the person to the left. (The youngest child writes what he or she sees as the main fault of the father.) The therapist writes two cards, which state "too good" and "too weak." The therapist collects the cards and reads them out loud, beginning with the two the therapist has written. The therapist then asks to which two family members these cards apply. The other cards are read aloud in random order,

and the authors are not revealed. This task reveals such processes as scapegoating, favoritism, and self-blame. This assessment tool may actually serve a therapeutic function and be used as an intervention technique if it helps family members achieve spontaneous understanding of the patterns and relationships in their family.

Contract or Goal Negotiation

The negotiation phase of family therapy is begun by identifying what each member would like changed in the family. When each family member and the therapist have identified what they see as important goals, work begins on negotiating a set of attainable goals that everyone is willing to work on. Compromise is needed to achieve a working goal. At this time, the family therapist may also identify the means—tasks, strategies, and so on—that will be used to reach the negotiated goals.

Written and verbal contracts for work with individuals are discussed in Chapter 26.

Intervention

Therapy for a family system involves understanding and use of the here-and-now, of the basic processes that occur in the system. General guidelines for using the here-and-now process with families are given below. Some of the wide variety of specific strategies and tasks are also discussed.

Role of the Family Therapist Virginia Satir (1967, pp 160–176) offers the following classic guidelines for the role of the family therapist:

1. Creating a setting in which members can risk looking at themselves and their actions

   a. Reducing their fears

   b. Giving direction

   c. Helping them feel comfortable and hopeful about the therapy process

   d. Accepting the "expert" label and being comfortable in the role

   e. Structuring questions to gain important data

2. Being unafraid but open

   a. Framing questions to help members be less afraid

   b. Validating members' assumptions and questioning personal assumptions

   c. Eliciting the facts about planning processes, loopholes in planning, perceptions of self and others, perceptions of roles, communication patterns and techniques, sexual feelings and activities

   d. Responding with a belief in the integrity of the members

3. Helping members see how they look to others

   a. Sharing observations of how members manifest themselves

   b. Teaching members how to share their observations with one another

   c. Playing back tape recordings (or video tapes)

4. Asking for and giving information in a matter-of-fact, nonjudgmental, light, congruent way

   a. Verbally recreating situations (with imagination) in order to collect pertinent facts

   b. Being easy about giving and receiving information and thereby making it easier for family members to do so

5. Building self-esteem

   a. Making constant "I value you" comments

   b. Labeling assets

   c. Asking questions that family members can answer

   d. Emphasizing that the therapist and family members are equals in learning from therapy

   e. Responding as a person whose meaning or intent can be checked on

   f. Noting past achievements

   g. Accentuating the family's "good" intentions but "bad" communication

   h. Asking each family member what he or she can do to bring pleasure to another family member

   i. Being human, clear, and direct (and recognizing that warmth and good intentions are not enough in themselves)

6. Decreasing threat by setting rules for interaction

   a. Seeing to it that all members participate

   b. Making it clear that interruptions are not tolerated

   c. Emphasizing that acting out or making it impossible to converse is not allowed

   d. Making sure that no one speaks for anyone else

   e. Helping everyone speak out clearly so that each can be heard

   f. Using humor appropriately

   g. Connecting silence to covert control

7. Decreasing threat by structuring sessions

   a. Announcing concrete goals and a definite end to the therapy or deadlines for reevaluation

   b. Viewing the family as a family and not taking sides

   c. Seeing units or subsystems of the family alone to accomplish specific work or because this is feasible or practical (e.g., other members are not available), with the knowledge and understanding of all members

8. Decreasing threat by reducing the need for defenses

   a. Discussing anger and hurt openly, thus decreasing fears about showing anger or hurt

   b. Interpreting anger as hurt

   c. Acknowledging anger as a defense and dealing with the hurt

   d. Showing that pain and the "forbidden" are safe to look at

   e. Burlesquing basic fears—painting a picture exaggerated to the point of absurdity—to decrease overprotectiveness and feelings of omnipotence

9. Decreasing threat by handling loaded material with care

   a. Using careful timing

   b. Moving from the least loaded to the most loaded

   c. Switching to less loaded material when things get hot (to another subject or to the past rather than the present)

   d. Generalizing about what a therapist expects to see in families (hurt, anger, fear, fighting, and so on)

   e. Relating feelings to facts (events, circumstances)

   f. Using personal idioms, slang, profanity, or vulgarity when appropriate, and avoiding pedantic words and psychiatric jargon

   g. Preventing closure on episodes or complaints; assuring that things will become clearer as learning continues

10. Reeducating members to be accountable

a. Reminding members of their ability to be in charge of themselves

b. Identifying global pronouns

c. Dealing openly with tattletales, spokespersons, and acting-out members

d. Highlighting problems of accountability in the relationship with the therapist

11. Helping members see the influence of past models on their expectations and behavior

a. Reminding members that they are acting from past models

b. Openly challenging expectations

c. Highlighting expectations by helping members verbalize the unspoken

d. Highlighting expectations by exaggerating them

12. Delineating family roles and functions

a. Recognizing roles by calling the parents "Mom" and "Dad" when referring to them as parents and "Jane" and "Bill" when addressing them as individuals or as husband and wife

b. Including members in history taking in the order of their entrance into the family

c. Questioning members about their roles

d. Teaching explicitly about role responses and role choices

13. Completing gaps in communication and interpreting messages

a. Clarifying the content and relationship aspects of messages

b. Separating comments about the self from comments about others

c. Pointing out significant discrepancies, incongruities, or double-level messages

d. Spelling out nonverbal communication

Structured Family Tasks   Structured family tasks are used for joint assessment and intervention purposes. They provide historical data and, in some cases, relate the data to present behavior. They offer family members the opportunity to collaborate actively in changing the family system.

In her practice, Virginia Satir (1967) uses *role playing* with families. The simulated family experience is used to teach families about themselves. Family members may simulate each other's behavior or their

conceptions of it. They may also play themselves in a simulated situation. Videotape feedback helps family members become acquainted with their own behavior. In addition, systems games and communication games are used to help families communicate more effectively and congruently. These role-playing experiences are also effective educational tools in the preparation of family therapists.

Rae Sedgwick (1978) suggests *photostudy of the family album* as a means of providing tangible, longitudinal evidence to raise questions, validate or invalidate hunches, and developmentally examine the individual and the family. Sedgwick suggests that the family picture album is one of the most obvious, and most overlooked, tools for understanding family dynamics. The photographs and the process of selecting them give insights into decision making, themes, interaction patterns, patterns of development, and power and influence relationships within the family. The therapist and family discuss and analyze the photographs together.

Other interesting *family tasks* suggested by Sedgwick include writing a family autobiography; comparing and contrasting family members with one another and with selected families from the neighborhood, the school, or the church; drawing a family picture; writing a family news article or a family epitaph; dispelling a family myth; weaving a family dream; or writing a family play. Such tools are helpful in examining histories, prophecies, scripts, and myths. They are limited only by the imagination and ingenuity of the therapist.

Therapeutic rituals can help families mobilize their resources for healing, growth, and change. The rationale for the creation of a family ritual is that family rituals facilitate life-cycle transitions. Conversely, their lack inhibits family development. Bright (1990) constructs therapeutic rituals to help families resolve conflicts or resentments, to negotiate new roles or relationship boundaries, and to develop new, shared meanings about their life together. She cautions that rituals must be constructed around an understanding of the family's culture, values, and needs; for example, a healing forgiveness ritual constructed in the language of a sacramental rite for a couple from a strong Roman Catholic background, or a celebration ritual to mark a family transition such as a birth or adoption, a graduation, or an anniversary.

Interestingly, the brief ecstatic change that occurs during a ritual results from changes in neurologic activity. Routinely, either the sympathetic or the parasympathetic nervous system is in a state of excitation. This excitation of the one system inhibits the other. During rituals, however, both sides of the central nervous system are simultaneously stimulated (Bright 1990). This neurobiologic event is responsible for the release of the intensely pleasurable experience of ecstasy, and the sense of union and oneness with others and life itself that occurs during a ritual.

Criteria for Terminating Treatment

Reid (1985) suggests that termination in family therapy should occur in a flexible way, helping families achieve realistic goals and end service with a feeling of accomplishment. Satir (1967, p 176) has developed criteria for determining when to terminate family therapy. Termination is appropriate when family members can

- Complete transactions, check, and ask

- Interpret hostility

- See how others see them

- Tell one another how they appear

- Tell one another their hopes, fears, and expectations

- Disagree

- Make choices

- Learn through practice

- Free themselves from the harmful influences of past models

- Give clear messages

The Nursing Process and Family Counseling

The following case study of the Wilson family (Black 1983) demonstrates a humanistic psychiatric nursing approach to family counseling. It shows how a nurse applied an understanding of family process and dynamics (elaborated on in this chapter) and used the covert rehearsal phase of the symbolic interaction model (illustrated in Figure 8–5) and general communication principles (Chapter 8) along with principles of relationship building (Chapter 26).

Case Example[*]

John, a graduate student in psychiatric-mental health nursing, is assigned to work with the Wilson family during his final clinical placement. The arrangement is

---

made by his instructor in cooperation with the family clinic of the local community mental health center. The family is selected by the staff team that John has joined as a member. The team includes a social worker, a psychiatrist, a psychologist, and a clinical nurse specialist. On each of his clinical days, John attends the daily team meeting in which the group shares their progress in working with their families, exchanges insights, and provides each other with mutual support as family problems are worked through. John's instructor attends several of the meetings on John's clinical days.

The intake report provides the team with information on which to base John's assignment. Mr and Mrs Wilson applied to the center as a result of a referral made by a local police official. Ross Wilson, their 10-year-old son, had been brought home by an officer following his fifth runaway episode in as many weeks.

At the request of the team, the intake worker makes a first appointment for John to meet with Ross and his parents at the center. Ross's younger brother and sister are left at home with their aunt. They can be expected to share in the benefits resulting from favorable behavioral and role changes brought about in a significant part of the family system. The assignment of this particular family to John is made mainly because the dysfunction seems to be of recent origin and essentially located within the triangle formed by Ross and his parents. This limits the complexity of the interrelationships that John will be called on to deal with.

Initiating the Relationship John prepares himself for his first interview with the family by engaging in an inner rehearsal. He anticipates that the parents will be anxious and embarrassed at having to explain their problem to yet another stranger. Their anxiety will be compounded by the prospect of being required to incorporate an outsider into the family's functional system. This, John reasons, might be offset to some extent by the fact that a state of psychologic crisis tends to create an unusual openness in its victims to accepting outside help.

John sees his immediate task as twofold: (a) to build the foundation of a relationship of mutual trust with the client family and (b) to work with them in defining the problem or problems that precipitated the present family crisis. Recognizing that his sensitivity to his clients' feelings will enable him to express genuine concern and a sincere desire to help, he also determines to keep the meetings family centered throughout. He plans to clarify his own role as catalytic but peripheral to the family's identification and implementation of new methods of coping. By these measures he hopes to reinforce the family's potential to function as a complete, interdependent system of mutual support.

Ross proves, on acquaintance, to be the least self-conscious of any in the group. He is an outgoing child, not overtly concerned about his problem behavior, but obviously eager to please his parents in other ways. When John issues a general invitation to all three to fill him in on the details of the problem that brought them to the center, all three participate about equally in the response. The parents tell of their worry over what might happen to Ross during his absence from home. Ross speaks sheepishly, but with a touch of pride, about having been repeatedly picked up in various public places by uniformed police officers late at night. John reflects the parental concern as inevitable under the circumstances, then to Ross his fascination with the police uniform.

Ross responds boastfully that his father also has a uniform and drives a truck. This leads to a description of the family's general life-style and, from that, to the particular events connected with the runaway episodes. The remainder of the first meeting and most of the next is taken up with the family's story. At first, John keeps it moving comfortably with only an occasional continuing response.

It develops that Mr Wilson, who is employed to drive locally for a department store, is becoming increasingly discontent with the duties the job entails. At this point in the narrative, he and Mrs Wilson engage in an argument that is a replay of one that, they admit, frequently breaks out at home. The husband says that he wants to transfer to a long-distance assignment, whereupon his wife complains to John that her husband's transfer would leave her with night and day responsibility for the home and family much of the time. Also addressing John, Mr Wilson raises his voice in angry frustration at not being given an opportunity to explain how much better off the family would be if he could only take a better-paying job.

Mindful of the principles he has studied, John is alert to the danger of being triangled into the family conflict. He reflects Mrs Wilson's apprehension directly to her and Mr Wilson's anger to him, and he gently calls their attention to the fact that they are reliving feelings aroused in the past in the midst of the group's present information-gathering task.

With only an occasional outburst centering on the same theme, the sequence of events that typically precedes and follows Ross's leaving home is elicited as follows:

1. The argument about Mr Wilson's proposed transfer begins in the course of a work-day evening meal.

2. Mr Wilson shouts in frustration; Mrs Wilson voices her fears and finally leaves the room in tears with the two younger children to put them to bed.

3. Ross remains with his father, who tells him of the joys of long-distance trucking.

4. On returning, Mrs Wilson scolds Ross and her husband for lack of consideration for her and sends Ross to do his homework.

5. Mr and Mrs Wilson are uncommunicative with each other and with Ross for the next day or two.

6. One evening soon after, Mrs Wilson prepares her husband's favorite dishes for supper. When Ross is again banished to do his homework, it is obvious to him that his parents are averse to having him present during their reconciliation.

7. Ross wanders off instead of going to school the next morning.

8. The police bring him home late in the evening.

9. His mother cries and scolds Ross, his father whips him with a belt, and he is sent to bed without any supper.

10. At supper the next evening, Mr Wilson casually asks Ross where he went and what happened on the day that he missed school. He listens to the account with interest. Mrs Wilson does not participate and, before long, suggests that Mr Wilson would probably like to run away from the family too. The argument about the transfer begins again.

John recognizes that Ross, without being fully aware of it, picks up the metacommunicative approval and empathy in his father's questions about his escapades and identifies with his father's desire to see new places. Although Mrs Wilson has come close to recognizing the command aspect of her husband's transactions, her feedback conveys criticism rather than understanding. With John's help, the three family members are able—the parents grudgingly at first—to identify the meanings that are thinly covered in their pattern of interaction.

Team discussion corroborates John's opinion that the family pattern currently displays a typically dysfunctional family triangle: a repetitive cycle of conflict, distance, and closeness; scapegoating to a minor degree; and the feedback cycle that Weakland describes. These insights are not communicated to the family. The team is in agreement that the maladaptive pattern will be broken up and reassembled as family members move to assume the group task of defining their goals and accepting responsibility for each other in a unified effort at planning and implementation.

Nursing Assessment and Planning   At his third meeting with the family, it is evident to John that Mr and Mrs Wilson have done some homework between meetings. Mr Wilson announces that, although Ross's running away from home is in no way excusable, he and his wife feel that their quarreling has made the child's home too hellish at times for him to want to stay there. Mrs Wilson adds that the two younger children have been unusually fractious in the worrisome home atmosphere. She perceives her own impatience as both causing and resulting from the family's general state of disorder. Not to be outdone, Mr Wilson says then that because his job is his own responsibility, he will see what he can do about it without bothering anyone else.

John observes, while Mr Wilson is speaking, that Mrs Wilson is becoming flushed and Ross is beginning to squirm. John briefly reinforces the starts the parents have made toward defining their feelings about their present situation. He then points out in matter-of-fact terms the body language he noted, and he makes the connection between it and Mr Wilson's statement about solving a significant family problem alone. Mrs Wilson says emphatically that the problem concerns all of them and that she would like to have some say in how it is solved. Her husband concedes that she has that right, and they begin to discuss the pros and cons of the transfer.

This time, the parents address one another rather than attempting to involve John. Their argument is less heated than at the previous meeting. When they tend to move to positions at extreme ends of the issue, John helps them identify gray areas and calls attention to connections between judgmental opposites. Tendencies to blame or to dwell on the past are diverted into making plans to cope with present and foreseeable circumstances.

Ross's fist attempt to contribute to the discussion is disregarded until John breaks in to reflect its underlying feeling. It shows that the boy is beginning to identify more evenly now and is trying to find ways of supporting his mother's point of view as well as his father's. John's response, although directed to Ross, serves to remind the parents that Ross's feelings are a significant factor in the problem as a whole. Thereafter they try, sometimes with John's help, to integrate Ross's comments into their overall assessment.

During the remainder of this meeting and the next, the family group is involved in action planning that is divided between the improvement of family relationships and a solution to the question of Mr Wilson's transfer. The problem of Mrs Wilson being left to cope alone while her husband is out of town brings a response from Ross that signifies that, as the man of the house, he is quite able to protect her. It also leads to an assessment of resources outside the immediate family. Grandparents, an uncle, and two aunts who live nearby are identified as being closely concerned with the family's welfare. The parents admit that the relatives' interest in the children has recently been neglected.

As discussion proceeds, John continues to be aware of the importance of modeling clear and accurate communication in his own statements. He also gives and elicits feedback when necessary to clarify the contributions of the other three participants. Generalizations that the parents tend to make on the basis of untested assumptions are exposed and called into question, and interdependent, supportive interactions are strongly reinforced. Frequent summary evaluations of progress serve to reassure, as well as reinforce, the family as an effectively functioning unit.

Implementation   By the fifth meeting, a compromise plan has been reached on the question of the transfer. Implementation of the plan is clearly a family responsibility. The family agrees that Mr Wilson will postpone making a change until both of the younger children attend school for a full-day session. Mrs Wilson feels that she will be better able to cope with intercurrent difficulties when they are in someone else's care for a few hours a day. Mr and Mrs Wilson resolve to keep in closer touch with the relatives on whom Mrs Wilson can depend for moral support. Ross promises to stay near his home and to spend some of his free time each day with the younger children.

Evaluation and Termination   John is able to utilize evaluation both as an ongoing impetus to the process of intervention and as a learning experience for himself. The three Wilsons soon participate with pleasure in the reviews, which highlight the steps of their progress in family collaboration as well as in problem solving. At staff team meetings, John reports each day's interaction with as much verbatim content as he can remember, and he joins the other team members in an evaluative exchange of questions, interpretations, and suggestions.

The team discusses the matter of termination midway in the series of six meetings. Progress to date gives every indication that the family will soon be functioning at a somewhat higher level than they achieved before lapsing into dysfunction. The shared prediction is that, if they agree to termination by the sixth meeting, it will be effected at that point without referral or planned follow-up.

Much of the fifth meeting is taken up by the members of the now-functional triangle in telling John how well things are going at home. John periodically expresses his observation of their sensitivity to each other's feelings and their supportiveness of one another. As the meeting ends, he indicates that they are now working together so effectively that there is little need for any help he can give. They assent willingly to his suggestion that the sixth meeting be the last and that it be used as a general windup. When his mother remarks that the children's aunt will be relieved to hear that her babysitting chore is nearly over, Ross suggests that the other two children come along for the last meeting so that John can meet them.

With the two children aged five and six present, the sixth meeting turns out be a little boisterous. John notes that Ross now identifies with his parents in monitoring the behavior of the younger children in keeping with his parents' commands. When he takes the others to explore a courtyard that can be seen from the window of the meeting room, the parents thank John for all his help, saying that they wish they had known sooner of the work of the family clinic. John uses this opportunity to reinforce their consciousness of new-found strength in their unified approach to problems, adding that there are sure to be more problems as time goes on. He assures them of the continuing availability of the clinic as a community resource. Ross proffers a gruff thank you when the children gather to add their farewells to those of their parents.

CHAPTER HIGHLIGHTS

• The family is the context in which people develop their first relationships with others. How one views the world is molded by the events that happen within the family.

• Family forms in the United States are changing and becoming more diverse; a wide variety of family constellations exists in contemporary society.

• The family can be viewed as a system in terms if the relationships, associations, and connections that occur in a dynamic, interacting whole.

• The family system includes not only family members but their relationships, communications, and interaction with the environment.

• A change or movement in any part of the family system affects all other parts of the family system.

• The family seeks to maintain a dynamic balance, or homeostasis, among various forces that operate within and upon it.

• Just as individuals and groups are confronted with developmental tasks, so are families.

• The functional family is distinguished from the dysfunctional one by the amount and quality of energy used to maintain the family system and to achieve the developmental tasks.

• Family therapists believe that emotional symptoms or problems of an individual are an expression of emotional symptoms or problems in a family. In family therapy work, the family system is the unit of treatment.

• Nurses at all levels and in all areas of nursing work with families and family problems in many settings. To function as a family therapist, however, the psychiatric nurse needs graduate-level preparation.

• The following affect the functioning of the family and its members: life scripts, family myths, life-styles, and themes; coalitions, dyads, and triangles; pseudo-mutuality and pseudohostility; marital schism and skew; enmeshment and disengagement; scapegoating; and double binds.

• Contemporary approaches to family therapy include the integrative approach, psychoanalytic approach, Bowen approach, structural approach, interactional approach, social network approach, and the behavioral approach.

• The milieu for family therapy often is the family's own home.

• Major components of family therapy include assessment, contract negotiation, and intervention.

• It is best for all family members to participate in the assessment phase of family therapy.

• The family therapist may use structured family tasks and therapeutic strategies for both assessment and intervention.

• The family therapist helps family members look at themselves in the here-and-now and recognize the influence of past models on their behavior and expectations.

REFERENCES

Ackerman NW: Prejudicial scapegoating and neutralizing forces in the family group with special reference to the role "family healer," in Howells JG (ed): *Theory and Practice of Family Psychiatry*. Brunner/Mazel, 1971, pp 626–634.

Ackerman NW: *The Psychodynamics of Family Life*. Basic Books, 1958.

Aponte H: If I don't get simple, I cry. *Family Process* 1986;25(4):531–548.

Bateson G, Jackson DD, Haley J, Weakland, JH: Toward a theory of schizophrenia. *Behav Sci* 1956;1:251–264.

Bishop SM: *Family Psychiatric Nursing*. Mosby, 1991.

Black K: *Short-Term Counseling: A Humanistic Approach for the Helping Professions*. Addison-Wesley, 1983.

Boscolo L, Cecchin G, Hoffman L, Penn P: *Milan Systemic Family Therapy*. Basic Books, 1987.

Boszormenyi-Nagy I, Framo J (eds): *Intensive Family Therapy*. Harper and Row, 1965.

Bowen M: A family concept of schizophrenia, in Jackson DD (ed): *The Etiology of Schizophrenia*. Basic Books, 1960, pp 346–372.

Bowen M: *Family Therapy in Clinical Practice*. Jason Aronson, 1978.

Bright MA: Therapeutic ritual: Helping families grow. *J Psychosoc Nurs* 1990;28(12):24–29.

Brock G, Barnard C: *Procedures in Family Therapy*. Allyn & Bacon, 1988.

Bross A: *Family Therapy*. Guilford Press, 1983.

Carter B, McGoldrick J: *The Changing Family Life Cycle*. Gardiner Press, 1988.

Compton BR, Galaway B: *Social Work Processes,* ed 2. Dorsey Press, 1979.

Deutsch D: Family therapy and family life-style. *Individual Psychol* 1967;23:217–223.

Doherty W, Burge S: Attending to the context of family treatment: Pitfalls and prospects. *J Marriage Fam Ther* 1987;13(1):37–47.

Drake R, Oscher F: Using family psychoeducation when there is no family. *Hosp Community Psychiatry* 1987; 38(3):274–277.

Duvall E: *Family Development.* Lippincott, 1985.

Griffith J: Employing the God-family relationship in therapy with religious families. *Fam Process* 1986;25(4):609–618.

Griffith J, Griffith M: Structural family therapy in chronic illness. *Psychosomatics* 1987;28(4):202–205.

Haber J: A family systems model for divorce and the loss of self. *Arch Psychiatr Nurs* 1990; 4(4):228–234.

Haley J; *Problem Solving Therapy.* Jossey-Bass, 1987.

Hess RD, Handel G: *Family Worlds: A Psychosocial Approach to Family Life.* University of Chicago Press, 1959.

Imber-Black E: *Families and Larger Systems.* Guilford Press, 1988.

Jackson DD (ed): *Communication, Family, and Marriage.* Science and Behavior Books, 1968a.

Jackson DD: Family rules: Marital quid pro quo. *Arch Gen Psychiatry* 1965;12:589–594.

Jackson DD: The question of family homeostasis. *Psychiatr Q* 1957;[Suppl]:79–90.

Jackson DD (ed): *Therapy, Communication, and Change.* Science and Behavior Books, 1968b.

Jones SL: *Family Therapy: A Comparison of Approaches.* Robert J. Brady, 1980.

Kanter J et al.: Expressed emotion in families: A critical review. *Hosp Community Psychiatry* 1987;38(4):374–380.

Kiecolt-Glaser J et al.: Marital quality, marital disruption, and immune function. *Psychosom Med* 1987; 49(1):13–34.

Kunzer MB: Marital adjustment of headache sufferers and their spouses. *J Psychosoc Nurs* 1987;25(5):12–17.

Laing RD: *The Politics of the Family.* Vintage Books, 1972.

Lesser E, Comet J: Help and hindrance: Parents of divorcing children. *J Marriage Fam Ther* 1987;13(2):197–202.

Lidz T, Cornelison AR, Terry D: The intrafamilial environment of the schizophrenic patient: Marital schism and marital skew. *Am J Psychiatry* 1957;114:241–248.

Lindsey K: *Friends or Family.* Beacon Press, 1982.

McGoldrick M, Gerson R: *Genograms in Family Assessment.* Norton, 1985.

McGoldrick K, Rohrbaugh M: Researching ethnic family stereotypes. *Fam Process* 1987;26(1):89–99.

Minuchin S: *Families and Family Therapy.* Harvard University Press, 1974.

Palazzoli MS, Cirillo S, Selvini M, et al.: *Family Games: General Models of Psychotic Processes in the Family.* W. W. Norton, 1989.

Patterson G: *Living with Children: New Methods for Parents and Teachers.* Research Press, 1976.

Reid W: *Family Problem Solving.* Columbia University Press, 1985.

Satir V: *Conjoint Family Therapy,* rev ed. Science and Behavior Books, 1967.

Sedgwick R: Photostudy as a diagnostic tool in working with families, in Kneisl CR, Wilson HS (eds): *Current Perspectives in Psychiatric Nursing: Issues and Trends.* Mosby, 1978, vol 2, pp 60–69.

Speck RV: Psychotherapy of the social network of a schizophrenic family. *Fam Process* 1967;6:208–214.

Speck RV, Attneave L: *Family Networks.* Pantheon Books, 1973.

Steiner C: *Scripts People Live.* Grove Press, 1974.

Toman W: *Family Constellation,* ed 3. Springer Publishing, 1976.

Watzlawick P: A structured family interview. *Fam Process* 1966;5:256–271.

Watzlawick P, Beavin JH, Jackson DD: *The Pragmatics of Human Communication.* W. W. Norton, 1967.

Worthington E: Treatment of families during life transitions: Matching treatment to family response. *Fam Process* 1987;26(2):295–308.

Wynne L, Ryckoff IM, Day J, Hirsch SI: Pseudo-mutuality in the family relationships of schizophrenics. *Psychiatry* 1958;21:205–220.

Milieu Therapy

LEARNING OBJECTIVES

- Define milieu therapy

- Describe three historical events that have affected the current status of milieu therapy

- Discuss Wiedenbach's nursing theory and its application to humanistic psychiatric nursing practice

- Describe two physical structures and two social issues that influence the characteristics of the milieu

- Apply the nursing process to intervention techniques based on manipulation of inanimate qualities of the environment

- Identify three social interaction therapy principles

- Apply the nursing process to intervention techniques based on social interaction

- Identify three behavior modification principles

- Apply the nursing process to intervention techniques based on behavior modification principles

Susan Hunn Garritson

CROSS REFERENCES

Other topics related to this chapter are: Behaviorism, Chapter 4; Community mental health and deinstitutionalization, Chapter 38; Era of moral treatment, Chapter 1; Ethics, Chapter 7; Group therapy, Chapter 29; Legal issues, Chapter 37; Violence and victimatology, Chapter 21.

In THIS CHAPTER, **milieu therapy** is defined as the purposeful use of people, resources, and events in the client's immediate environment to promote optimal functioning in the activities of daily living, development or improvement of interpersonal skills, and ability to manage outside the institutional setting.

This definition of milieu therapy incorporates the important concepts of social influences (people) and physical setting (resources) considered so essential during the revolutionary changes in psychiatric care of the 1800s. This definition has also been influenced by more recent events in the history of psychiatry, including the following:

- The decline of the state mental hospital

- The emergence of psychiatric theories that emphasize the significance of disturbed interpersonal relations and the curative potential of therapeutic interpersonal encounters

- The influence of legal concepts and decisions on clinical management techniques and philosophy

- Deinstitutionalization

- Knowledge of biologic factors in psychiatry

These historical influences and the importance of the external environment to psychiatric care are discussed in the "Historical Overview" section of this chapter. Wiedenbach's nursing model is presented in the "Theoretic Foundations" section as a framework to implement milieu therapy in humanistic psychiatric nursing. Physical structure and social issues that affect the milieu are described in the section "Context for Nursing Practice." Assessment and manipulation of these factors can indirectly influence client behavior. Interaction and behavior modification principles and techniques are described in the section "Professional Treatment Techniques." Case examples and nurse-client dialogues are used throughout the chapter to illustrate specific issues.

Historical Overview

Ideas about mental illness and human nature have always influenced approaches to client care and management. During the 1600s, madness was thought to be caused by man's "animal nature" because the insane were perceived to act like wild beasts. Men and women were chained in their cells, as one might chain a dog, when they were violent. Blankets, clothes, and food were withheld, since the lunatic was considered to be insensitive to cold and hunger. People were burned at the stake or confined to dungeons to remove

their evil nature. The external environment was used cruelly and harshly to manage the behavior of the mentally ill.

During the 1800s, ideas about human nature began to change, and the importance of the individual began to be emphasized. This focus on the individual, combined with a growing spirit of social reform, drew attention to the inhumanity of the lunatic's surroundings. Philippe Pinel (1745–1826) released the inmates of the Bicêtre and Salpêtrière from their chains and provided food, clothing, fresh air, and kind treatment. William Tuke (1732–1822) established the York Retreat in England as a refuge for those suffering from lunacy, "the greatest of human afflictions" (Rosenblatt 1984, p 246). Tuke considered bleedings and purges—then common medical treatment for the insane—inadequate to relieve human suffering. The philosophy of the retreat emphasized hearty meals; warm and clean clothes; beautiful countryside; and the distractions of walk, readings, music, and conversation.

Moral Treatment

Humanitarian approaches to care of the mentally ill ushered in the era of moral treatment. During the 1800s, the term *moral* was equivalent to *emotional* or *psychologic*. The world *moral* was associated with *morale* and implied hope, spirit, and confidence. **Moral treatment** was considered to be a mandate on those more fortunate to provide compassionate and understanding care to sufferers.

Benjamin Rush (1746–1813) stimulated the interest of American physicians in humanitarian treatment of the mentally ill. Moral treatment became a principal technique in the growing number of mental institutions in America during the 1800s. Although the physician-client relationship was gaining importance, the greatest benefit of moral treatment was the attention it focused on the value of the physical setting and social influences of hospital life as curative agents (Bockoven 1963). The philosophy and techniques of moral treatment were the forerunners of modern-day milieu therapy.

Decline of State Mental Hospitals

The early success of moral treatment led to continued expansion of state mental facilities. Vast numbers of people were hospitalized despite the original tenet of moral therapy to treat no more clients than the psychiatrist could know intimately. During the second half of the nineteenth century, major population shifts from rural to urban settings and the influx of poverty-stricken immigrants resulted in a tremendous demand for mental hospital services. Day rooms were converted to dormitories to meet requirements for more beds, but nothing replaced dwindling recreational rooms. Ethnic prejudice obscured clinical judgment and human kindness, and insane immigrants were assumed to be incapable of appreciating comfortable surroundings. The standard of living in mental hospitals and the ratio of attendants and physicians to clients severely deteriorated. Finally, the original proponents of moral treatment failed to train sufficient successors, and by 1870 most moral treatment leaders had died or retired.

Public Concern for Conditions in Mental Hospitals

As early as 1900, professional reports documented the miserable state of mental hospitals (Figure 31–1). In 1908, Clifford Beers published *A Mind That Found Itself,* in which he described the abuses and suffering experienced by clients in mental institutions. Although critics questioned any form of institutional care, numerous social factors hindered early efforts to close mental institutions. These factors included lingering influence of the belief in humanistic care, investment of great sums of money in the asylum system, strong public opposition to community treatment, lack of any other social structure to provide for the indigent, and growing professionalization of medicine and efforts by institutional superintendents to identify themselves as a medical specialty, thereby limiting public interference with their professional domain (Schull 1977).

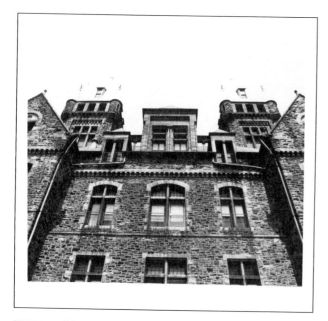

FIGURE 31–1 Confinement in imposing structures such as this public mental hospital often meant condemning a person to life within the walls of an asylum. Wrongful confinement and loss of personal liberty play a significant part in the history of legal issues that concern psychiatric nurses.

Finally, the public's opinion that mental illness was incurable made organizational change and improved treatment seem futile.

Therapeutic Potential of Interpersonal Relations

Following World War II, several factors contributed to renewed interest in mental health services. Large numbers of men had been rejected from military service because of psychiatric symptoms, and other veterans developed psychiatric problems during military duty. Traditional psychiatric treatment in the context of a one-to-one relationship was inadequate to deal with the volume of new clients, and further institutional expansion was out of the question.

At the same time, psychodynamic perspectives were increasingly influenced by the social sciences. The focus of attention shifted from forces within the individual to interpersonal relations and events in the social context. In 1931 Harry Stack Sullivan reported on an intensive interpersonal treatment approach with a small group of schizophrenic clients and a variety of hospital personnel. Other extended interpersonal techniques to *prescribe attitudes* specific to each client's symptoms and to define clients as responsible participants in the recovery process. Bettleheim applied therapeutic environment approaches in a facility for severely disturbed children. Maxwell Jones applied similar ideas to launch the **therapeutic community** movement in England. "The concept of the therapeutic community draws attention to the need to make optimal use of the potential in trained staff, volunteers, clients, their relatives, and any other people with a contribution to make mental health" (Devine 1981, p 20). As Maxwell Jones refined his techniques and ideas of therapeutic community, traditional roles among staff members and between staff and clients became blurred. His ideas emphasized a decline in hierarchical organizational structures, shared decision making, and equal distribution of authority (APA 1984). The recognized interaction between environment and mental illness added a new dimension to psychiatric thinking.

Impact on Nursing Therapeutic concepts were applied in numerous settings and were incorporated into the professional roles of various disciplines. Nurses described both the theoretic relevance and the practical significance of interpersonal and environmental perspectives in nursing practice. In her 1952 book, *Interpersonal Relations in Nursing,* Hildegard Peplau described nursing as a "significant therapeutic interpersonal process." She discussed various roles the nurse assumes, including teacher, resource, counselor, leader, technical expert, and surrogate (Belcher and Fish 1980). She noted that both the nurse's and client's culture, religion, race, education, past experiences, and preconceived ideas influenced their interpersonal interaction (Belcher and Fish 1980).

Gwen Tudor (1962) critically analyzed the interactive nurse-client relationships in her discussion of mutual withdrawal. The problem of mutual withdrawal involves reciprocal avoidance between staff and client, resulting in a limited and stable though stagnant pattern of interaction. Staff may rationalize their avoidance through labels such as "hopeless," "unresponsive," or "assaultive" and thereby discourage new approaches to interaction. Such labeling and routinized staff behaviors reinforce the client's behavior, and the interaction cycle is perpetuated.

Influence of Legal Concepts

Legal involvement in commitment hearings was informal during the first half of the 1900s. Court involvement in social welfare cases gradually increased during the 1960s and 1970s, and the civil rights movement had repercussions for psychiatric clients. Clients' rights, free choice, self-determination, and privacy became important concerns. Numerous court decisions extended the principle of the **least restrictive alternative** to psychiatric issues. As a legal doctrine, the least restrictive alternative represents the perspective that government actions should be those that least interfere with individual liberties. When applied to psychiatric care issues, the principle was used to protect clients' rights against infringement of unwarranted or unproved psychiatric treatments. Between 1966 and 1979, the courts' application of the least restrictive alternative became increasingly specific and included location of treatment, environment in which treatment occurs, development of alternative facilities, and rankings of treatment. The least restrictive alternative concept has been incorporated into psychiatric ideology and is routinely considered in the evaluation of treatment environments.

Deinstitutionalization

Deinstitutionalization refers to the closing of state mental hospitals and discharge of thousands of mentally ill inmates. Proponents of deinstitutionalization were motivated by a humanitarian philosophy and were committed to the notion that clients should receive treatment in their own communities. Many social, economic, and psychiatric treatment factors influenced the public's receptiveness to community care.

Custodial Care in State Hospitals The concept of the therapeutic potential of the environment was slow to reach state mental hospitals. Personnel continued to pay minimal attention to the basic needs of clients. This **custodial care** contrasted sharply with advances in psychiatric treatment outside the state hospitals.

Numerous discussions and critiques of state hospital treatment have been published. Stanton and Schwartz (1954) contrasted the low prestige of the twenty-three hours of the day devoted to daily living activities with the status of the psychotherapy hour. They also described the impact of the hospital environment and staff actions (e.g., staff conflict and poor communication) on client behavior.

Strauss et al. (1981) contrasted three treatment environments: (1) the chronic services of a state hospital, (2) the treatment services of a state hospital, and (3) a private psychiatric research and training hospital. They found that chronic services staff lacked knowledge of psychotherapy and provided hydrotherapy, work therapy, good food, and medical care—techniques consistent with a belief that mental illness has a physical origin. The treatment services at both the state and private hospitals provided psychodynamic treatments. At the private hospital the psychotherapeutic treatment was individually oriented. However, because the treatment services at the state hospital dealt with large numbers of clients with fewer staff, milieu therapy was the principal psychodynamic treatment. The study concluded that treatment philosophy, professional identity, and type of institution are critical determinants of psychiatric treatment.

Goffman (1961) was influential in raising awareness about institutional environments. He described the restrictive institutional atmosphere as derived from regulations and judgments by staff and from sanctions for activities from outside the client group. Staff move clients in blocks to manage large groups of people in the institution. Free movement is restricted because it increases the difficulty of overall surveillance. Contact with the outside becomes a privilege. Clients are separated from their outside roles and identities via limitations on visitors, confiscation of personal property, and lack of private space. Contact is largely confined to other inmates. Telephone use, cigarette smoking, and communication with a physician may be controlled by staff. Goffman described clients as "institutionalized" when they exhibit dependence on the institution, apathy about discharge, lack of interest and competence in outside activities, and resignation toward institutional life.

Gruenberg (1974) used the term *social breakdown syndrome* to refer to behavior that was once thought to stem from psychosis but that seems to resolve when environmental restrictions are removed. Social breakdown syndrome may be caused by conflict between what the client is capable of doing and what the institution demands or requires. It is manifested by danger of self-damage and self-destructive acts, disturbing noisiness, and inability to manage daily living activities such as eating, dressing, toileting, and going to bed (Gruenberg 1974, p 702).

Cost of Institutional Care

In addition to legal challenges and criticisms about institutional care, other social and economic forces increased public receptivity to the closing of state mental hospital systems. The rate of institutional hospitalization was growing at a rate disproportionate to general population growth. The original asylums needed massive repair, and construction of new facilities was tremendously costly. Other sources of expense stemmed from the unionization of state hospital employees, the forty-hour week, and the results of class-action suits, which had limited the use of clients as unpaid employees and established the client's legal right to treatment. The growing welfare system provided a way to support clients in the community more cheaply than in an institution. There was less opposition from organized psychiatry since new areas of specialization could be developed in community care. Other events that accelerated this process included availability of social security (at federal expense) to noninstitutionalized clients, financial inducements to the counties to avoid sending clients to state hospitals, growth of privately owned and community-based "institutions," and tightening of the eligibility for involuntary commitments (Schull 1977, p 140). By 1975 approximately two-thirds of state hospital clients had been discharged back to their communities.

 Biologic Factors in Psychiatry   New knowledge in psychobiology and pharmacology has led to the development of a range of highly specific psychopharmacologic agents. The use of medications to control behavior provided significant momentum to the deinstitutionalization movement and has played a major role in shortening acute psychiatric hospitalizations. Biologic explanations of behavior have seriously challenged the basic tenet of milieu therapy—that behavior is the product of social forces. Shortened hospital stays have decreased the significance of milieu therapy as a principal treatment modality. Rationales for acute psychiatric hospitalization currently emphasize intensive assessment, behavior management, and medication administration. A long-term group experience to accomplish emotional growth and increase responsibility for oneself is available in only a few acute care facilities. The requirements for a stable, cohesive group that provides a therapeutic experience through open communication are more likely to be met in a subacute or rehabilitative setting, where lengths of stay and consistent group makeup promote the establishment of a milieu culture.

The declining significance of traditional milieu therapy in acute psychiatric care and the simultaneous emergence of biologic interventions may overemphasize a biomedical perspective of treatment. The traditional biomedical model, in which the physician is responsible for determining the nature of the client's distress and proposing a cure while the client assumes a "sick role" contrasts with the milieu therapy model, in which organizational hierarchy is flattened, therapeutic potential is seen in multiple relationships, and client assumes personal responsibility for behavior. Psychiatric nursing's challenge in the current decade is to synthesize a new model that includes the best aspects of both the biologic and milieu therapy models.

Current Ideas about Milieu Therapy

Current concerns of milieu therapists include general atmosphere and restrictiveness, extent of the client's utilization of treatment resources, and a framework for applying milieu techniques during brief, acute treatment.

Moos' Ward Atmosphere tool has been used extensively to describe treatment environments. The **Moos Ward Atmosphere Scale** describes dimensions of atmosphere as involvement, support, spontaneity, autonomy, practical focus, personal focus, order, clarity, control, and expression of anger. Moos has demonstrated that these factors vary with treatment setting, client needs, unit philosophy, and life cycle of the unit, and he supports research to link the treatment environment to client outcomes (Kahn and Fredrick 1988).

The restrictiveness of the treatment environment has been characterized according to physical, psychologic, and social dimensions. The physical environment includes the nature of the setting, such as location in the community, security, and options for behavior control (e.g., seclusion). The psychologic environment is composed of staff and client backgrounds, behavior, attitudes, and values. The social environment consists of the rules and regulations that govern the operation of the setting as well as the treatment standards for managing client behavior (Garritson 1987).

Allen et al. (1988) extend the concept of the **therapeutic alliance** in the psychotherapy relationship to hospital treatment. Alliance in hospital treatment is primarily characterized by the client's collaboration in the treatment process. Collaboration is the extent to which the client actively utilizes treatment opportunities as resources for constructive change. The collaboration concept has three dimensions:

• Goal orientation—thoughtful, reflective and purposeful participation in hospital treatment

• Involvement—communication with staff

• Use of structure—utilization of the prescribed treatment program

Collaboration is highly correlated with severity of psychopathology as well as treatment outcome. In in-patient treatment, collaboration is multidimensional and facilitated or impeded by the variety of treatment relationships characteristic of milieu therapy.

Kahn and White (1989) propose a framework for acute, short-term treatment programs that incorporates biologic and psychosocial perspectives with milieu techniques to achieve an intensely supportive treatment environment. This environment maximizes utilization of multidisciplinary therapeutic opportunities. These are the principles of this acute care milieu framework:

• Establish a consistent, caring environment characterized by (a) safety, (b) structure, (c) support, (d) socialization, and (e) self-understanding. These elements are fostered through the philosophy, policies, and procedures that define the treatment program. Staff promotes safety by stating expectations for conduct clearly and maintains it through such interventions as suicide precautions, time-outs, seclusion, and restraint. Structure is established through client orientation, activity schedules, and methods to address noncompliance. Staff establishes a positive social climate by observing the ward atmosphere, assessing staff attitudes and parallel issues, establishing clear goals and accountability, promoting communication, and intervening in disruptive events.

• Provide graduated therapy with levels individualized to the client's phase of illness, resources, and support systems. A graduated therapy program involves: (a) orientation to the program and development of goals, (b) education about the illness, treatment, and coping skills, and (c) integration of the illness and hospital experience into the client's self-concept and postdischarge plans.

• Emphasize commonalities between clients' experiences to instill hope, promote interpersonal feedback, achieve mastery over a crisis, and regain social connectedness.

Kahn and White's dimensions provide a framework for establishing a therapeutic milieu in an acute psychiatric hospital setting. The factors of the Ward Atmosphere Scale and the concept of restrictiveness offer a means to describe the milieu and to influence the therapeutic environment by altering aspects of its physical, psychologic, or social structure. Assessment of collaboration offers a method to evaluate the efficacy of the therapeutic alliance and progress of overall hospital treatment. Together, these allow the nurse to establish a therapeutic milieu, prescribe and manipulate milieu interventions, and evaluate the client's progress to promote a positive outcome.

Various terms such as *therapeutic milieu, therapeutic environment, therapeutic community,* and *milieu therapy* have been applied to discussions of the treatment environment. While some argue that different strategies and theoretic perspectives are associated with these labels, they are frequently used interchangeably and are based on the general premise that resources in the environment can be used therapeutically on behalf of the client. The term *milieu therapy* was defined in the introduction to this chapter and will be used throughout the remaining sections to refer to the therapeutic potential of the hospital setting. By addressing the entire context within which the management and care of the client takes place, milieu therapy incorporates an endless array of human and inanimate variables. Specific techniques have evolved from the manipulation of environmental factors, and these are equally linked to milieu therapy. The remaining sections describe further theoretic aspects of milieu therapy and demonstrate how the nurse employs the milieu to accomplish the nursing process.

Theoretic Foundations

Nurse-Client-Environment Interactive Model

In 1969 Ernestine Wiedenbach published a theory of nursing based on three factors (Bennett and Foster 1980):

1. Central purpose of the discipline

2. Activities to fulfill the central purpose

3. Realities in the immediate situation

These key factors provide a useful framework for understanding and implementing milieu therapy in humanistic biopsychosocial psychiatric nursing practice.

Wiedenbach describes the central purpose of nursing as reverence for the gift of life; respect for the dignity, value, autonomy, and individuality of each human being; and resolution to act on these beliefs. Wiedenbach develops the concepts of individuality and autonomy. Among her beliefs are the following (Bennett and Foster 1980):

• Each human being is endowed with unique potential to develop self-sustaining resources

• The human being basically strives toward self-direction and relative independence and desires to use personal capabilities and potentialities and to fulfill responsibilities.

• The human being needs stimulation to make best use of personal capabilities and to realize self-worth.

• Current behavior represents the individual's best judgment at the moment.

Using this humanistic philosophy, the nurse works with the client to develop a plan for care. The care plan is mutually understood and agreed on and may be carried out by either the client or the nurse.

The nurse recognizes and deals with the realities of the situation in which nursing care is provided. According to Bennett and Foster, these are the realities of the nursing care situation:

• Nurse (or delegate): personal characteristics, competence, capabilities

• Client: personal characteristics, problems, capacities, and ability to cope with current experiences

• Goal: the desired result to be attained through nursing care

• Means: method (based on application of knowledge and spiritual and material resources)

• Framework: human, environmental, professional, and organizational facilities that make up the context (and provide limits) within which nursing is practiced

The central purpose, care plan activities, and realities are interdependent and interactive. The nurse's beliefs about human beings influence the selection of nursing interventions. The facility within which the nurse and client find themselves further limits and guides potential nursing actions. Finally, the nurse's interventions are specific to the client's unique behavior.

These interacting beliefs, interventions, and realities affect the individual's capacity to think, plan, relate to others and experience a sense of self apart from others. "An environment that subverts, interferes with, or prevents the use of these qualities threatens human dignity" (Proshansky 1973, p 2). Nurses' philosophies about client autonomy and the growth-enhancing potential of the environment also influence the more informal expectations and operational procedures that involve both staff and clients. Rules, routines, and procedures that negate client input and are controlled by staff also control staff and increasingly restrict the milieu.

Selecting interventions in the in-patient psychiatric treatment environment presents unique challenges to the nurse who values the autonomy and individuality of the client. The following nursing concerns are examples.

Privacy Individuals routinely vary their contact and withdrawal from others as well as the information they share about themselves. The very nature of psychiatric hospitalization clashes with the need for privacy.

Intimate personal details are examined and discussed, and there may be no opportunities to escape staff surveillance or social contact. Nurses respect clients' privacy by keeping surveillance and monitoring to the minimum necessary for client safety, respecting the confidentiality of personal information, and maintaining routine social practices such as knocking on doors and waiting for an answer before entering bedrooms or bathrooms.

Autonomy The rules and schedules that characterize psychiatric treatment settings usually promote the management of groups of people and may interfere with the personal decision making and autonomy of the individual client. Although the ability of mentally ill clients to carry out age-appropriate roles may be significantly impaired, the therapeutic milieu provides opportunities for normal functioning according to each client's abilities.

Safety Mentally ill clients may pose significant safety hazards to themselves or others because of suicidal or assaultive behaviors, poor judgment, or confusion. Nurses' efforts to maintain client's safety may deprive clients of privacy and autonomy. For example, clients requiring close surveillance have little or no privacy; nurses may intervene to override decisions made by clients whose judgment is impaired.

Group Well-Being A client's behavior may be disruptive or detrimental to the overall well-being of other clients. Nurses may need to monitor or manage certain clients to maximize the common good. As with the concept of safety, the individual's privacy and autonomy may be violated when group well-being is considered primary. (Some philosophers, however, consider that the group's well-being enhances the individual's autonomy.) Individual autonomy, individual well-being and group well-being are often conflicting issues. Nurses must be sensitive to situations in which clashes occur.

Ellis and Krch-Cole (1987) analyzed staff responses to a client with AIDS. Their study is an excellent example of the impact of staff values and attitudes on client care and the atmosphere of the milieu. Staff's reactions to the client with AIDS were negative, as demonstrated by comments that an infectious client does not belong on a psychiatric unit and that other patients or staff members might contract the disease. These reactions influenced all aspects of the milieu, including the environment, communication, and social integration.

Environment

• The client's use of the shower, bathroom, and laundry was restricted to times when other clients had finished using them. The areas were thoroughly cleaned after use by the client with AIDS.

• The client was not allowed access to community meal areas and the kitchen; meals and snacks were provided with disposable utensils.

• A separate telephone and ashtray were provided.

• The client had a private room that was marked with a bright orange isolation tag. Isolation linen was kept outside the door.

A client, who had been admitted for paranoid and psychotic symptoms, responded by always wearing a red headband, using tape to mark all his belongings with crosses, and taping his closet and bathroom doors closed. The client said the taping would "ward off all those who could come into contact" with him.

Communication   The client, staff, and other clients never mentioned the AIDS diagnosis. During the client's twelve-week stay, no one questioned the client's nonparticipation in unit activities or the special procedures related to his self-care regime. The diagnosis became the "unit secret" and was rationalized by the need to maintain confidentiality.

Social Integration   Although the client's physical needs were provided for and one-to-one precautions were maintained, verbal interactions were minimal. Limits were loose and inconsistent because staff wished to avoid any confrontation in which the client might require physical restraint. The client, sensing staff's fear of close contact, acted out by threatening to bite, spit, and scratch. Other clients maintained their distance by leaving living areas when the identified client appeared.

Using the Nursing Process

The nurse uses the nursing process to assess the client's behavior in the context of the treatment environment and to assess characteristics of the environment that may influence the client's behavior. Thus the familiar components of the nursing process—assessment, planning, intervention, and evaluation—are also performed on aspects of the milieu. For example, the nurse considers subjective and objective data about a client and develops a nursing diagnosis. Next the nurse considers behaviors of staff and other clients and characteristics of the environment to determine whether any of these contextual areas contribute to the client's diagnosed problem. The nurse implements a milieu-therapy–based intervention by manipulating the aspect of the environment that seems to contribute (either by its presence or absence) to the client's behavior. The nurse evaluates the results by reassessing the client's behavior and assessing the overall environment for unanticipated or unintended changes. In this

interactive model, the nurse considers the impact of environmental interventions on the behavior of other clients and staff. The therapeutic environment must promote basic safety and group well-being, which sometimes conflicts with efforts to promote an individual's autonomy. A central task in creating and managing milieu therapy is to achieve a balance between attention to the needs of the group and promotion of individuality. Thus many philosophic, technical, and situational forces influence the nursing process.

Humanistic Interactionist Implications

In this chapter, milieu therapy is broadly interpreted to reflect the therapeutic potential of people, resources, and events. Wiedenbach's nursing framework provides the humanistic and interactionist perspectives that make milieu therapy an effective and versatile technique in psychiatric nursing practice. Nurses' twenty-four-hour-a-day contact with clients affords a unique opportunity to claim the creation and management of the therapeutic milieu as a special domain for nursing. No other discipline literally shares with clients the living space of the ward. Nurses individually influence the milieu through their presence, by providing human contact, support, and direction and by sharing philosophy and values, establishing collaborative work relationships, and exhibiting professionalism.

Using the nurse-client interaction process as a medium, nurses introduce various techniques, such as activities, expectations, or contracts, to help clients learn new behaviors. Group activities are also a successful forum in which to learn new behavior. Groups provide opportunities to experience membership, cooperation, compromise, and leadership. These here-and-now nursing interventions provide opportunities for immediate observation, feedback, and learning (see the Intervention box on page 750). When these new experiences occur within a comfortable, humane setting, clients may experience a new sense of self-worth and dignity.

Legal and regulatory agencies have established criteria for the structural environment, yet staff often become insensitive to simple environmental impediments that they could change. Locked doors to bedrooms, bathrooms, kitchen, or laundry interfere with normal aspects of daily living. Simple readjustments of staffing assignments, improved client-staff communication, or use of behavior contracts may allow necessary monitoring and behavior management without restricting the environment. These alternative interventions are based on the therapeutic use of individuals, communication, and client participation to create an environment that promotes human achievement.

INTERVENTION

Guidelines for Working with Clients in the Therapeutic Milieu

- Provide for basic needs of the client, including safety, privacy, activities of daily living, and shelter.
- Make resources necessary for self-care available to clients.
- Enhance the normality of the environment through the use of clocks, calendars, ramps, railings, furniture, and other resources.
- Maintain visibility and availability (i.e., presence) to guide and supervise clients' activities.
- Offer organization and structure, including boundaries (e.g., limits, schedules, and expectations), supervision and assistance, and a routine allowing participation in activities that promote growth and release tensions.
- Give support and aid personal growth by helping clients use personal time, encouraging them to accomplish treatment goals, and intervening in emergency and crisis situations.
- Help clients gain interpersonal and interactional skills by promoting new ways to interact, giving validation and feedback, or redirecting clients who cannot tolerate the stimulation of group activity.
- Promote coping skills such as decision making, practical living skills, and activities that prepare for return to the community.
- Maintain open communication with nurses, other professionals, and staff.
- Include clients in decisions about their own care.
- Support formal and informal group activities to promote sharing, cooperation, compromise, and leadership.
- Examine personal attitudes toward issues of clients' rights, self-determination, social control, and deviance.

The therapeutic milieu is more than locker space, square footage requirements, and assorted group experiences, although these are important components. The therapeutic milieu includes the belief in the dignity of all people, and this philosophy pervades the structure, interactions, and interventions that in turn reinforce the therapeutic atmosphere.

Context for Nursing Practice

Physical Environment

Psychiatric treatment takes place in a variety of settings. Krauss and Slavinsky (1982) have ranked these settings according to their restrictiveness or interference with the client's independence.

1. Total institutions (e.g., state hospitals)—*most restrictive*

2. Nearly total institutions (e.g., nursing homes)

3. Institutions with partially independent residents (e.g., halfway homes)

4. Institutions with independent but isolated residents (e.g., single-room-occupancy hotels)

5. Family of origin, friends, other relatives

6. Family of orientation (i.e., family resulting from marriage or other relationship)—*least restrictive*

The physical structure of many institutions—e.g., locked doors, communal living arrangements, and limited access to community resources—interferes with clients' freedom of movement and individuality. Thus, facilities located in huge hospital complexes, which do not interface with the community's shopping, religious, or entertainment activities or provide for clients' privacy, have a more restrictive milieu than community-based settings.

The physical structure of mental institutions has been linked to the problem of **institutionalization,** in which the client's ability to function declines. "Institutionalized" clients become apathetic about discharge, resigned toward institutional life, and dependent on the setting for their total care. Goffman (1961) theorized that clients grew unable to negotiate and manage daily living activities outside institutions that provided for all aspects of their lives and prevented access to the community by high walls, barred windows, or geographic isolation.

Physical structure also has an immediate impact on the milieu. Structural characteristics influence social interaction and clients' opportunities to carry out activities associated with adult roles. Removal of personal property, lack of personal space, and regulation of adult activities (e.g., smoking, using the telephone, and receiving visitors) diminish privacy and self-control and thereby decrease individuality and autonomy.

Acutely psychotic and chronically mentally ill men and women are admitted to a twenty-bed locked unit in a large county hospital. Nurses on this unit seem rushed and complain of having no time to discuss nursing care issues or write nursing care plans. A nurse consultant observed work patterns for several days and noted that the staff were involved (frequently unnecessarily) in intimate details of the clients' daily activities. This involvement extended to lighting matches for cigarettes and squeezing toothpaste onto toothbrushes. Simple routines that interfered with client autonomy also controlled staff by preventing professional performance and relationships.

Nursing Process

• *Assessment:* Staff complains of excessive workload; staff controls clients' daily activities.

• *Diagnosis:* Self-Care Deficits: Bathing/hygiene, Dressing/grooming, Feeding, Toileting

• *Intervention:* Increase client self-care according to actual abilities.

• *Evaluation:* Professional performance and relationships of nurses improve, client self-care increases

Changes in the security of the environment, such as unlocking the door of a normally locked unit or locking the door of a normally unlocked unit, have been noted to increase client agitation.

Mrs A is a 72-year-old woman hospitalized for evaluation of a sudden onset of confusion and forgetfulness. Nurses locked the unit's main door to keep Mrs A from inadvertently wandering off the ward. Other clients were free to come and go but were inconvenienced by relying on staff to unlock the door.

Staff noticed an increase in irritability and demanding behavior of several clients soon after the door was locked. Small cliques of clients collected near the door, while others paced nearby.

Staff decided that the impact of the locked door on the overall milieu was detrimental. A nurse was assigned to keep Mrs A within eye contact at all times to ensure her safety, and the unit door was unlocked. The ward atmosphere soon returned to normal.

Nursing Process

• *Assessment:* Client is confused and forgetful.

• *Diagnosis:* Altered thought processes

• *Intervention:* Lock main door to protect client safety.

• *Evaluation:* Client safety is maintained, but other clients show increased irritability and demanding behavior.

• *Intervention:* Begin one-to-one nursing care of Mrs A

Seclusion and restraint represent interventions that use structure to control client behavior. Studies indicate that seclusion and restraint are frequently used

within a few hours of admission, possibly to control behavior until medications take effect or to intervene in agitated behavior before it escalates (Kirkpatrick 1989). Other factors linked to use of seclusion are unit philosophy, staff attitudes and education, client-staff ratios, and level of unit disturbance. Because seclusion and restraint are highly restrictive interventions that interfere with client autonomy and freedom of movement, it is important to implement alternative steps whenever possible (see Chapter 21.)

Nurses at one psychiatric hospital were able to drastically reduce seclusion and restraint hours (Craig et al. 1989). A multivariate program was undertaken with hospital administration and interdisciplinary staff involvement. This included structural renovation of the seclusion-restraint rooms to maximize staff access, reduce external stimulation, and ensure client privacy. A conceptual nursing model was developed that defined seclusion and restraint as intensive care, and interactions to reduce fear and helplessness were identified. Registered nurse staffing was improved, and nurses used alternative interventions such as flexible barriers (e.g., opened and closed doors), personal distance, and selected interactions to provide intensive care. All staff received training in assaultiveness management, crisis theory, and alternative interventions. Staff of other disciplines were involved in recommending behavior interventions for management problems and in reviewing restrictive treatment lasting longer than twelve hours. During the first twelve months of this program, restraint decreased more than 600 hours per month. There was a combined seclusion-restraint decrease of over 950 hours per month.

Wilson (1982) studied "infracontrol" phenomena at Soteria House, an experimental personal growth community for schizophrenics. Conventional control mechanisms such as locked doors, medications, and strict regulation of activity or property are avoided in this setting. Soteria's ideology emphasizes self-regulation, tolerance for deviance, and group cohesiveness. However, an ideology of eliminating structural control does not eliminate the need to maintain safety or the problem of social control of psychotic clients' behavior. Wilson studied how problems of social control are solved in the absence of conventional psychiatric control structures. The process of *presencing* was identified as a key mechanism to manage resident behavior. Staff and residents spend a great deal of daily living time together, and the basic *presence* of people with individual patterns of tolerance and interaction guides and limits behavior. Such a milieu might well be characterized as "low EE" or low *expressed emotion.* Nurses frequently use the presencing technique by sitting with or listening to clients, although they are apt to describe it as "providing support" or "the therapeutic use of self." The last example illustrated how the use of presencing not only kept Mrs A safe but also improved the environment by allowing the unit door to remain unlocked.

Structural controls may not always be obvious, of course, and staff can become oblivious over time to controls that were instituted for a specific purpose that no longer applies.

A fifteen-bed unlocked ward had laundry facilities so that clients could care for their own clothes. A psychotic and confused client put a potted plant through a wash cycle, causing major damage to the washing machine. Staff locked the laundry facilities to prevent future damage to the machines. The doors remained locked even after this client was discharged, preventing any independent client access to the facilities. Preventing possible future damage to machines became a predominant staff concern.

Nursing Process

- *Assessment:* Client is psychotic and confused.

- *Diagnosis:* Altered thought processes

- *Plan:* Maintain client safety and avoid damage to environment.

- *Intervention:* Lock laundry facilities.

- *Evaluation:* Damage is avoided, but independence and self-care of other clients declines.

- *Intervention:* Unlock doors.

A voluntary, unlocked unit has a progressive nursing philosophy emphasizing client self-care, autonomy, and independence. The clients' dining room has a small kitchenette, and clients frequently prepare their own snacks. The clients' refrigerator had always been located in the locked medication room. Thus, any independent meal preparation or simple decision to have a glass of juice required the client request access to the refrigerator. Despite the inconvenience of having to unlock the door, staff were initially reluctant to move the refrigerator. They rationalized that they could better monitor clients' intake by controlling access to the refrigerator. Once the refrigerator was moved to the kitchenette, however, staff were more likely to discuss food and fluid intake with their clients. This elimination of a structural control provided an opportunity for client-staff communication and improved staff's counseling and education related to clients' diets.

Nursing Process

- *Assessment:* Clients frequently approach staff for juice and snacks.

- *Diagnosis:* Altered health maintenance

- *Intervention:* Move refrigerator to community area.

- *Evaluation:* Clients have better access to necessary resources for self-care and health maintenance, and staff-client communication improves.

The structural environment should not *dehumanize* its inhabitants; moreover, it should actively contribute to their improved functioning and comfort. Reality-orientation resources such as the following contribute to a sense of normality:

- Clocks and calendars to promote time orientation

- Newspapers to encourage awareness of social events

- Ramps and rails to promote movement

- Furniture arranged to promote interaction

Healthy people may take these for granted, but yet they are critical resources to the impaired client.

Mrs T is a 47-year-old woman with severe depression. She is very agitated and is having trouble sleeping. Although sleep medication has been ordered, Mrs T has been in and out of bed and is pacing. As a result of her restlessness, the sheets and blankets are strewn about and the plastic mattress cover is exposed. The rumpled bedding and cold mattress further contribute to Mrs T's discomfort. Nurses order a mattress pad and contoured sheets to promote Mrs T's comfort until her symptoms respond to medication.

Nursing Process

- *Assessment:* Client is agitated, restless, and not able to stay in bed.

- *Diagnosis:* Sleep pattern disturbance

- *Intervention:* Decrease discomfort by providing padding and contoured sheets and thereby promote client's rest

- *Evaluation:* The distractions and discomfort created by the environment (e.g., bedding) are removed.

Deinstitutionalization has changed the location of psychiatric treatment, and walled institutions with barred windows are less common today than they were forty years ago. However, structural controls remain in community psychiatric settings. Lack of access to rooms, equipment, or pleasantries of normal life perpetuate the restricted atmosphere of institutions. The previous examples demonstrate how staff may justify structural controls, how structural controls interfere with client autonomy, and how elimination of structural controls can improve client-staff communication and the ward atmosphere.

Social Environment

Social norms affect the environment by creating both overt and covert rules governing actions and relations to others. Social norms are derived from:

• Public influences such as clients' rights groups, professional practice standards, regulatory agencies, or court decisions

• Styles of interaction among staff (Schatzman and Strauss 1966)

Public Influences *Wyatt v Stickney,* 1972, a landmark mental health court case, upheld clients' rights to treatment as opposed to mere custodial care (see the accompanying Advocacy box). The decision also established standards for the treatment environment. The standards specified minimum square footage per client in bedrooms, dayrooms, and dining facilities; maximum number of clients per bedroom, toilet, and shower; and requirements for personal storage space, basic furniture, dayrooms with outside windows, and bathroom facilities with curtains and doors.

ADVOCACY

Wyatt v Stickney, 1972: An Overview

Bryce State Hospital, the first public institution for the mentally ill in Alabama, opened in 1861 in response to the efforts of Dorothea Dix to have the mentally ill hospitalized rather than left to wander the streets. Over the next 100 years the buildings were inadequately maintained and overcrowded. Treatment for the mentally ill stagnated.

In 1970 the Alabama Department of Mental Health faced a tremendous budget deficit due to a decline in tobacco tax revenues and an across-the-board salary increase. The department decided to lay off 120 professional staff at Bryce, both to manage the fiscal crisis and to dramatize to the legislature the need for more funding. Several employees and a client, Ricky Wyatt, filed a complaint in federal court charging that the layoffs would effectively end all treatment programs and only custodial care would be provided. The federal court agreed to hear the portion of the case concerned with clients' rights to treatment and ordered the state to produce an adequate treatment program. Without treatment, the court said, involuntary hospitalization would result in confinement without due process of law.

The state produced a vague program found inadequate by the court. The court ultimately adopted staffing and physical plant standards deemed to provide a humane physical and psychologic environment.

The Joint Commission on Accreditation of Hospitals (1987) has also specified criteria for the therapeutic environment (see the box on page 754). These standards address requirements for lighting; ventilation; furnishings; storage; general aesthetic appeal of clients' living area; and eating, bathing, and toileting facilities. (These standards currently apply only to non-hospital-based psychiatric facilities and are no longer requirements for hospital-based psychiatric services.)

The Joint Commission and *Wyatt v Stickney* criteria are similar, and both illustrate the impact of social norms and expectations for care on the physical features of the hospital setting. Although the court's standards applied only to Bryce State Hospital in Alabama, the court's willingness to hear the *Wyatt v Stickney* case demonstrated concern for the plight and rights of the mentally ill. The Joint Commission's regulatory authority extends these standards to multiple facilities. Furthermore, enforcement of environmental requirements by the Joint Commission has legislative support because reimbursement for Medicare clients depends on accreditation status.

The therapeutic environment as a nursing intervention modality is described in the professional psychiatric nursing practice standards (ANA 1982) (see the Intervention box on page 757). These standards include structure, process, and outcome criteria. Structure criteria, which include safety, cleanliness, and attractiveness, are consistent with the more detailed Joint Commission standards. Structure criteria also emphasize implementation of seclusion and restraint according to written policies and procedures and the general use of environment to facilitate client gains. Process criteria identify the use of the nursing process to analyze and intervene according to milieu principles. Process criteria also emphasize communication to orient clients, corroborate with others, teach, and continually evaluate the impact of the milieu. Outcome criteria reflect measureable goals such as time frames for completing orientation, behavior change, or articulation of new knowledge. Standards of practice are statements of professional consensus regarding performance, responsibilities, and competence, and they establish what the public can expect from the professional nurse.

Staff Interaction: Communication Staff interaction patterns influence the ward milieu and may mirror client interaction patterns.

A consulting clinical nurse specialist met with a group of staff nurses from an adolescent treatment unit to discuss an increase in staff absences due to illness. Several staff complained that administrators' rules limited their ability to make independent decisions. The next day in a group meeting, clients discussed their anger about not receiving weekend passes. That evening two clients left the unit without passes.

Criteria for the Therapeutic Environment

1. The facility establishes an environment that enhances the positive self-image of patients and preserves their human dignity.

2. The grounds of the facility have adequate space for the facility to carry out its stated goals.

2.1. When patient needs or facility goals involve outdoor activities, areas appropriate to the ages and clinical needs of the patients are provided.

3. The facility is accessible to handicapped individuals or the facility has written policies and procedures that describe how handicapped individuals can gain access to the facility for necessary services.

4. Waiting or reception areas are comfortable, and their design, location, and furnishings accommodate the characteristics of patients and visitors, the anticipated waiting time, the need for privacy and/or support from staff, and the goals of the facility.

4.1. Appropriate staff are available in waiting or reception areas to address the needs of patients and visitors.

4.2. Rest rooms are available for patients and visitors.

4.3. A telephone is available for private conversations.

4.4. An adequate number of drinking units are accessible at appropriate heights.

4.4.1. If drinking units employ cups, only single-use, disposable cups are used.

5. Facilities that do not have emergency medical care resources have first-aid kits available in appropriate places.

5.1. All supervisory staff are familiar with the locations, contents, and use of the first-aid kits.

6. Programs providing partial-hospital or 24-hour care services provide an environment appropriate to the needs of patients.

6.1. The design, structure, furnishing, and lighting of the patient environment promote clear perceptions of people and functions.

6.2. When appropriate, lighting is controlled by patients.

6.3. Where possible, the environment provides views of the outdoors.

6.4. Areas that are used primarily by patients have windows or skylights.

6.5. Appropriate types of mirrors that distort as little as possible are placed at reasonable heights in appropriate places to aid in grooming and to enhance patients' self-awareness.

6.6. Clocks and calendars are provided in at least major use areas to promote awareness of time and season.

7. Ventilation contributes to the habitability of the environment.

7.1. Direct outside air ventilation is provided to each patient's room by air-conditioning or operable windows.

7.2. Ventilation is sufficient to remove undesirable odors.

8. All areas and surfaces shall be free of undesirable odors.

9. Door locks and other structural restraints are used minimally.

9.1. The use of door locks or closed sections is approved by the professional staff and the governing body.

10. The facility has written policies and procedures to facilitate staff-patient interaction, particularly when structural barriers in the therapeutic environment separate staff from patients.

10.1. Staff respect a patient's right to privacy by knocking on the door of the patient's room before entering.

11. Areas with the following characteristics are available to meet the needs of patients:

11.1. Areas that accommodate a full range of social activities, from two-person conversations to group activities.

11.2. Attractively furnished areas in which a patient can be alone, when appropriate.

11.3. Attractively furnished areas for private conversations with other patients, family members, or friends.

12. Appropriate furnishings and equipment are available.

12.1. Furnishings are clean and in good repair.

12.2. Furnishings are appropriate to the ages and physical conditions of the patients.

12.3. All furnishings, equipment, and appliances are maintained in good operating order.

12.4. Broken furnishings and equipment are repaired promptly.

Criteria for the Therapeutic Environment (continued)

13. Dining areas are comfortable, attractive, and conducive to pleasant living.

13.1. Dining arrangements are based on a logical plan that meets the needs of the patients and the requirements of the facility.

13.2. Dining tables seat small groups of patients, unless other arrangements are justified on the basis of patient needs.

13.3. When staff members do not eat with the patients, the dining rooms are adequately supervised and staffed to provide assistance to patients when needed and to assure that each patient receives an adequate amount and variety of food.

14. Sleeping areas have doors for privacy.

14.1. In rooms containing more than four patients, privacy is provided by partitioning or the placement of furniture.

14.2. The number of patients in a room is appropriate to the goals of the facility and to the ages, developmental levels, and clinical needs of the patients.

14.3 Except when clinically justified in writing on the basis of program requirements, no more than eight patients sleep in a room.

14.4. Sleeping areas are assigned on the basis of the patient's need for group support, privacy, or independence.

    14.4.1. Patients who need extra sleep, whose sleep is easily disturbed, or who need greater privacy because of age, emotional disturbance, or adjustment problems are assigned to bedrooms in which no more than two persons sleep.

15. Areas are provided for personal hygiene.

15.1 The areas for personal hygiene provide privacy.

15.2. Bathrooms and toilets have partitions and doors.

15.3. Toilets have seats.

16. Good standards of personal hygiene and grooming are taught and maintained, particularly in regard to bathing, brushing teeth, caring for hair and nails, and using the toilet.

16.1 Patients have the personal help needed to perform these activities and, when indicated, to assume responsibility for self-care.

16.2 Incontinent patients are cleaned and/or bathed immediately upon voiding or soiling, with due regard for privacy.

16.3 The services of a barber and/or beautician are available to patients either in the facility or in the community.

17. Articles for grooming and personal hygiene that are appropriate to the patient's age, developmental level, and clinical status are readily available in a space reserved near the patient's sleeping area.

17.1. If clinically indicated, a patient's personal articles may be kept under lock and key by staff.

18. Ample closet and drawer space are provided for storing personal property and property provided for patients' use.

18.1. Lockable storage space is provided.

19. Patients are allowed to keep and display personal belongings and to add personal touches to the decoration of their rooms.

19.1. The facility has written rules to govern the appropriateness of such decorative display.

19.2 If access to potentially dangerous grooming aids or other personal articles is contraindicated for clinical reasons, a member of the professional staff explains to the patient the conditions under which the articles may be used.

    19.2.1. The clinical rationale for these conditions is documented in the patient record.

19.3 If the hanging of pictures on walls and similar activities are privileges to be earned for treatment purposes, a member of the professional staff explains to the patient the conditions under which the privileges may be granted.

    19.3.1. The treatment and granting of privileges are documented in the patient record.

20. Patients are encouraged to take responsibility for maintaining their own living quarters and for day-to-day housekeeping activities of the program, as appropriate to their clinical status.

20.1. Such responsibilities are clearly defined in writing, and staff assistance and equipment are provided as needed.

►

Criteria for the Therapeutic Environment (continued)

20.2. Descriptions of such responsibilities are included in the patient's orientation program.

20.3. Documentation that these responsibilities have been incorporated in the patient's treatment plan is provided.

21. Patients are allowed to wear their own clothing.

21.1. If clothing is provided by the program, it is appropriate and is not dehumanizing.

21.2. Training and help in the selection and proper care of clothing are available as appropriate.

21.3. Clothing is suited to the climate.

21.4. Clothing is becoming, in good repair, of proper size, and similar to the clothing worn by patients' peers in the community.

21.5. An adequate amount of clothing is available to permit laundering, cleaning, and repair.

22. A laundry room is accessible so patients may wash their clothing.

23. The use and location of noise-producing equipment and appliances, such as television sets, radios, and record players, do not interfere with other therapeutic activities.

24. A place and equipment are provided for table games and individual hobbies.

24.1. Toys, equipment, and games are stored on shelves that are accessible to patients as appropriate.

25. Books, magazines, and arts and crafts materials are available in accordance with patients' recreational, cultural, and educational backgrounds and needs.

26. The facility formulates its own policy regarding the availability and care of pets and other animals, consistent with the goals of the facility and the requirements of good health and sanitation.

27. Depending on the size of the program, facilities are available for serving snacks and preparing meals for special occasions and for recreational activities.

27.1. The facilities permit patient participation.

28. Unless contraindicated for therapeutic reasons, the facility accommodates patients' need to be outdoors through the use of nearby parks and playgrounds, adjacent countryside, and facility grounds.

28.1. Recreational facilities and equipment are available, consistent with patient's needs and the therapeutic program.

28.2. Recreational equipment is maintained in working order.

SOURCE *Joint Commission on Accreditation of Hospitals: Consolidated Standards Manual for Child, Adolescent, and Adult Psychiatric, Alcoholism, and Drug Abuse Facilities and Facilities Serving the Mentally Retarded/Developmentally Disabled, 1990.*

Nursing Process

• *Assessment:* Staff absences are increasing, and staff complains about limited independence. Clients are angry about pass restrictions, and two clients go AWOL.

• *Diagnosis:* Impaired social interaction

• *Plan:* Decrease avoidance behavior of staff and clients

• *Intervention:* Discuss perceptions of decreased autonomy with all involved. Increase opportunities for independent decision making for both staff and clients.

• *Evaluation:* Parallel avoidance behavior declines.

In this example, the parallel issues for staff and clients are related to self-control and autonomous decision making. Both groups acted out tension through avoidance (use of sick leave and AWOL).

Mrs L, 48 years old, has a history of bipolar mood disorder. She is demanding, loud, argumentative, and irritable and has been admitted to an unlocked unit. There has been a recent change in the unit's chief physician administor. The previous chief recommended rapid medication to calm agitated clients and maintain a quiet environment. The replacement chief physician prefers several medication-free days to evaluate clients' behaviors. Staff are not completely comfortable with managing unmedicated clients, and the ward has been hectic with several psychotic clients under evaluation. In addition, the head nurse has been on vacation for several weeks, and her replacement is much less experienced with staff conflict management. Mrs L's admission triggered bitter staff complaints about the new chief physician and the ward philosophy. Several individuals inquired into transfers to other units, and others joked about career changes. Absenteeism increased, and several medication errors were made. Two clients became embroiled in an altercation, and others expressed concern about their care. When the head nurse

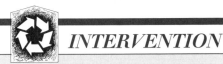

INTERVENTION

ANA Guidelines for a Therapeutic Environment

The nurse provides, structures, and maintains a therapeutic environment in collaboration with the client and other health care providers.

Rationale

The nurse works with clients in a variety of environmental settings such as inpatient, residential, day care, and home. The environment contributes in positive and negative ways to the state of health or illness of the client. When it serves the interest of the client as an inherent part of the overall nursing care plan, the setting is structured and/or altered.

Structure Criteria

1. Mechanisms exist within the practice setting that govern the establishment and maintenance of settings that are clean, safe, humane, and attractive.

2. Written policies and procedures that govern the safe use of seclusion, restraint, or aversive measures are utilized when staff institute such activity.

3. The environment is characterized by features that facilitate therapeutic gains on the part of clients.

Process Criteria

The nurse:

1. assures that clients are adequately oriented to the milieu and are familiar with scheduled activities and rules that govern behavior and daily living.

2. observes, analyzes, interprets, and records the effects of environmental forces upon the client.

3. assesses and develops the therapeutic potential of the practice setting on behalf of clients through consideration of the physical environment, the social structure, and the culture of the setting.

4. fosters communications in the environment that are congruent with therapeutic goals.

5. collaborates with others in the development and institution of milieu activities specific to the client's physical and mental health needs.

6. articulates to the client and staff the justification for use of limit setting, restraint, or seclusion and the conditions necessary for release from restriction.

7. participates in ongoing evaluation of the effectiveness of the therapeutic milieu.

8. assists clients living at home to achieve and maintain an environment that supports and maintains health.

Outcome Criteria

1. Within 24 hours after admission to a psychiatric setting, the client has been oriented to the milieu, including scheduled activities and rules governing behavior, unless unusual client circumstances interfere with the orientation process.

2. If restrained or secluded, the client can state the reason for such action and the conditions necessary for release, unless unusual client circumstances prevail.

3. The client demonstrates an awareness of the effects of environment on his health and incorporates that knowledge into self-care.

SOURCE: Standards of Psychiatric and Mental Health Nursing Practice, *American Nurses Association, 1982.*

---

returned from vacation, the ward milieu was tense, and the signs of disintegration were obvious. The head nurse met with both staff and the chief to identify their concerns. The chief believed that clients were being medicated too quickly and that a period of reconsideration of their symptoms might lead to alternative approaches. The nurses were concerned about safety. The head nurse suggested the following approach, which was acceptable to both the nurse and physician staff:

1. Teach assaultiveness management theory and skills to all staff.

2. Teach staff alternative interventions to use before medication.

3. Limit the number of unmedicated psychotic clients at any time through controlled admissions and varying lengths of medication-free trials.

Staff also agreed to discuss the ward milieu specifically during their treatment planning meetings. The overall social environment improved when the head nurse's plan was carried out.

RESEARCH NOTE

Citation

Emrich K: Helping or hurting? Interacting in the psychiatric milieu. J Psychosoc Nurs Ment Health Serv 1989;27:26–29.

Study Problem/Purpose

- Is there a relationship between interactions classified according to transactional models and those classified according to confirming/disconfirming communication models?

- Is there a relationship between the type of interaction and the participant (e.g., nurse or client)?

Methods

One hundred twenty-seven observations of spontaneous interactions were made over a seventeen-week period in a single setting. Written verbatim records and descriptions of nonverbal behavior served as the units of analysis. A panel of experts reviewed and categorized the data according to predetermined criteria that reflected two communication models.

Findings

Seventy-six observations were of nurse-client interactions and fifty-nine were of client-client interactions. Nurse-client interactions were more frequently classified as parental and disconfirming. Client-client interactions had a similar frequency of adult-adult and child-child categories and were more likely to be confirming.

Implications

Nurses' interactions in a psychiatric milieu may not promote client dignity, responsibility, or positive therapeutic outcome. This "parent" style may be the result of the nurse's role in an authoritarian organizational structure, efficiency in managing the work setting, lack of value for client autonomy, and an overall paternalistic attitude toward clients. Milieu therapy interventions that promote more positive interaction include client involvement in treatment planning and unit government, and decreased emphasis on the order and organization of the setting.

Nursing Process

- *Assessment:* Assessment reveals staff complaints, absenteeism, medication errors, client assaultiveness, and client complaints.

- *Diagnosis:* Impaired social interaction

- *Plan:* Decrease tension and increase milieu stability

- *Intervention:* Discuss concerns with all group members. Provide in-service education to enhance nurses' skills with unmedicated clients. Achieve milieu management through controlled admissions and varied lengths of medication-free trials. Improve communication through ward milieu discussions.

- *Evaluation:* The supportive atmosphere of the milieu increased, aggressive behaviors decreased.

Professional Treatment Techniques

Interaction Methods

A variety of interaction techniques have been developed from efforts to control the environment and prescribe therapeutic activities. Some techniques, such as community meetings, client government, and speciality theme groups (e.g., movement or work groups), promote normal functioning through the use of social interaction, group activities, group pressure, and peer expectations. Clients are considered responsible people able to take action and adjust their behavior in a purposeful manner. Social interaction interventions are based on the following principles (Paul and Lentz 1977, pp 49–51):

- *Expectations* for behavior are clearly communicated in order to maintain or change behavior.

- The acquisition and maintenance of new behaviors depend on the degree of *personal participation* and *involvement* in learning the necessary new skills.

- The occurrence of a behavior depends on the *sense of being a member* of the group. Group expectations and sanctions have significant influence on behavior.

Community Meeting Groups provide an opportunity for clients to solve problems of conflicting interests, experience cooperation with others, share responsibility, and experience leadership in the group. The most common milieu-oriented group is the community meeting. Its functions include:

- Welcoming new members

- Identifying and discussing unit rules (i.e., expectations)

• Discussing aspects of the unit environment such as cleanliness, privacy, radio and television use, or other interpersonal problems that may interfere with the quality of life for the group

• Planning activities

Clients usually chair the community meeting and report on assignments, such as checking for cleanliness of areas of responsibility (e.g., kitchen or bedrooms).

Unit Rules   All clients should be given the regulations of the setting either before or as soon after admission as possible. Although written expectations do not automatically ensure acceptable behavior or prevent harmful behavior, they provide a clear baseline, serve as reminders, and provide structure for clients.

Two written documents—the no-harm contract (Figure 31–2) and basic expectations (see the accompanying box)—establish behavioral requirements for all clients. These rules reinforce staff's commitment to basic safety and specify obligations for all members of the setting. Written expectations may be presented to clients at the time of admission, discussed in community meetings, and used as a reference if a client violates a rule.

A 45-year-old depressed and suicidal man is admitted to a voluntary unit. This conversation takes place after the nurse greets the client at the time of admission:

Nurse: Dr K informed me that you have been very depressed. Have you thought about harming yourself?

I agree that I am in control of my behavior. I understand that intended injury to myself, others, or property is grounds for discharge from this unit or commitment to another psychiatric setting as an involuntary patient.

If I have impulses to harm myself or others, I agree to talk with a staff member, whom I can expect to assist me in controlling my own behavior.

_____   _____
Date   Client

                               _____
                               Witness

FIGURE 31–2   An example of a no-harm contract.
SOURCE: Langley Porter Psychiatric Hospital and Clinics, Nursing Staff, Behavioral Neurosciences Service.

Mr L: Sometimes I wake up in the middle of the night and I think I can't go on. I just want to sleep, but I am tormented by my thoughts.

Nurse: Do you want to kill yourself now?

Mr L: Not this minute. The middle of the night is the hardest time for me.

Nurse: Nursing staff can sit with you or talk to you when you want to hurt yourself—even during the night. It is important that you tell your nurse when you feel suicidal. You are in control of your behavior even though life seems bleak right now.

Mr L: All right.

Nurse: Nursing staff have a written agreement to be available to keep you, and all other clients here, safe. (Hands Mr L the no-harm contract.) Do you feel able to make this commitment to control your behavior?

Mr L: Yes. (Signs contract.)

(Later, in a community meeting)

Nurse: I would like to introduce and welcome Mr L. (Group members introduce themselves.)

Nurse: Since several new members have come to the unit this week, this might be a good time to discuss the unit's rules.

Mrs A: We all came here for help, but sometimes that means we have to take charge of ourselves.

Nurse: What does "take charge" mean?

Mrs A: I am ultimately responsible for what I do to myself. I know I can't stay here if I cut myself like I did at home. I asked my nurse to sit with me when I first came in.

Group Living   The community meeting is also used to solve problems related to living with a large group of people or living in the hospital unit.

Clients on a 25-bed unlocked unit had access to two pay telephones. Both telephones, however, were near the nurses' station, and conversations could be overheard easily. Clients complained in community meeting of the lack of privacy, and a nurse intervened to help them write a letter to the hospital administration. The administration purchased a new cordless telephone, which allowed clients to make and receive calls in any area of the unit.

Client Government   Some client community groups also grant clients privileges for completing ward jobs or for demonstrating certain behaviors in the community living groups. Clients are expected to take responsibility for themselves and each other and to learn the consequences of their actions. Involving clients in the management of the unit and receiving therapy with other clients provide opportunities for participation, corrective learning experiences, and development of new behavior patterns. Feedback is an essential technique to increase insight and promote learning. This type of community group, known as

client government, may be most suitable to intermediate and long-term care settings, where the client group is stable and a group culture evolves over time.

The community meeting group of a twenty-bed adolescent program bases recommendations for weekend passes on members' requests and the individual's functioning in the client community. Lisa, 14 years old, has a history of running away from home, lying, drug and alcohol abuse, prostitution, and suicide threats. She requested a Saturday day pass although she did not have specific plans for how she would spend the time. Other clients commented that Lisa had not completed her ward job of checking the cleanliness of the kitchen, and staff noted that she continued to withdraw from social contacts. The group agreed that Lisa should not receive a pass until she could demonstrate some improved ability to structure her time and interact with others.

Nursing Process

- *Assessment:* Lisa is withdrawn and has failed to complete her ward job.

- *Diagnosis:* Social isolation (Withdrawal)

- *Plan:* Help Lisa improve her ability to structure her time and interact with others

- *Intervention:* Client group and staff provide feedback to Lisa regarding her behavior and group expectations for performance of responsibilities.

- *Evaluation:* Lisa's pass privileges are withheld.

Basic Expectations   Nurses have developed written basic expectations (see the accompanying box) to help clients take care of themselves. When Lisa complained about not receiving a pass, the following conversation ensued:

Nurse: Perhaps we should review the expectations for how you should act so that you can earn a pass. Do you have your copy? (Lisa finds her copy of the written basic expectations in the back of her nightstand drawer.)

Nurse: The expectations are like directions. They explain what you should do to earn pass privileges.

Lisa: I act OK. I should have gotten a pass. I didn't know I was supposed to check the kitchen to get a pass.

Nurse: The directions say you are expected to complete your ward job. The directions also tell you to participate in the activity program.

Lisa: I lost my schedule for the activities.

Nurse: Let's write a new schedule out together so we can talk about what activities you enjoy doing.

Individualized Written Expectations: Contracts   McEnany and Tescher (1985) describe the use of individualized written expectations for clients. They

recommend that this technique be used only with carefully selected clients. Clients must have the intellectual capacity to follow through with the contract negotiation process and the motivation to stick with a plan that works toward specific goals. The nurse should be knowledgeable about the client's disorder and its behavioral manifestations, change theory, and teaching-learning principles.

The goals of individualized contracting are to:

- Provide a consistent behavioral approach to the client by all staff

- Give the client an opportunity to use personality strengths by making decisions related to hospital care and discharge

- Give the client an opportunity to learn behaviors that enhance coping skills and ability to function

The following case example illustrates an intervention using individualized behavioral contracting:

Beverly is a 30-year-old white female admitted to an inpatient psychiatric unit following an overdose of trifluoperazine. This twice-married, twice-divorced woman has two children in foster homes. She has a long history of alcohol, marijuana, and cocaine use; multiple psychiatric hospitalizations; and treatment with antipsychotic drugs. On admission, Beverly was poorly groomed, pale, and thin. She denied hallucinations, delusions, or dramatic mood shifts, and her reality testing was intact. She said that after her boyfriend left her alone recently, she experienced her body as disjointed and "falling apart," and she feared leaving her hotel room. She described feeling "suffocated" by her relationships, yet she also described her sense of emptiness. She had no long-term relationships. During hospitalization Beverly was emotionally labile, had difficulty following her schedule, and was easily frustrated by the limits and compromises of living in the hospital. She demanded medication, threatened suicide, and complained of paranoia and various somatic symptoms. Beverly's primary nurse proposed that they work together to identify goals and behaviors for improved personal and interpersonal functioning. Beverly identified problems of emptiness, poor relationships, and anger and chose to focus on the goal of improved social skills. Beverly agreed to the following expectations:

- I will participate in group therapy and psychodrama to express my feelings verbally.
- I will participate in movement therapy to express my feelings physically and learn to control my body.
- I will identify uncomfortable situations with other people and discuss the interactions with my nurse at appointed times.
- I will continue my routine activities until the appropriate time to meet with my nurse.

Nursing Process

- *Assessment:* Client's behaviors are labile and

Basic Expectations

1. Food and Fluid
I agree to:
   A. Eat all meals in the dining room with the client group.
   Exception: ———
   B. Report problems with food/fluid intake to primary care nurse.

2. Elimination
I agree to:
   A. Maintain positive elimination habits.
   B. Report problems with elimination promptly to assigned nurse.

3. Personal Hygiene and Body Temperature
I agree to:
   A. Keep myself and my room area (including laundry and linen) clean.
   B. Complete my assigned ward job.
   C. Report problems with body temperature or hygiene to assigned nurse.

4. Rest/Activity
   A. Rest
   I agree to:
      1. Get up by 8:00 A.M. and remain up during the daytime.
      Exception: Scheduled nap time after lunch from _____ P.M. to _____ P.M.
      2. Retire to bed no sooner than 9:00 P.M. or later than 12:00 (midnight).
      Exception: ———
      3. Remain in bed until 7:00 A.M. "wake-up" except to get water or use the bathroom.
      4. Notify staff if I cannot sleep and work with them, according to the care plan, to try to sleep.
   B. Activity
   I agree to:
      1. Attend all scheduled R.T. activities, group therapy meetings, Thursday R.T. outings, community meetings, and weekend outings.
      2. Accept nursing staff referral to my personal schedule if I have a question about my participation in activities.
      3. Use no alcohol or nonprescribed drugs while on the unit or on passes.

5. Solitude and Socialization
If I have suicidal or self destructive ideas or feelings, I agree to:

   A. Discuss my ideas or feelings only in therapy sessions (individual, group, or family) or with the nurse assigned to my care and not with other clients.
   B. Accept reminders from nursing staff that I have signed the no-harm contract.
   C. Accept assistance from the nurse assigned to my care to learn new ways to manage my feelings and behavior to remain safe.

I can expect the nurse assigned to my care to assist me by:

   A. Discussing my immediate feelings and behavior and identifying alternative activities to maintain my safety.
   or B. Going to my room with me and sitting with me quietly for five to ten minutes, and then assisting me to get involved in a game (cards, pool) or with other clients in a group situation (television, living room).
   or C. Teaching me new coping behaviors such as relaxation techniques, deep-breathing exercises, or writing my thoughts.
   or D. Referring me to my primary therapist.

I also agree to discuss other problems—including concerns about medication—in therapy sessions (individual, group, or family).

———

SOURCE: *Adapted from Langley Porter Psychiatric Hospital and Clinics, 1985. Nursing Staff, Behavioral Neurosciences Service.*

manipulative. Client has difficulty maintaining a routine, and her interpersonal skills are poor.

• *Diagnosis:* Impaired social interaction

• *Plan:* Improve personal and interpersonal functioning.

• *Intervention:* Develop an individual behavior contract

• *Evaluation:* Client participates in ward activities, and her social skills improve.

Behavior Modification

The goal of behavior modification is also to bring about change in behavior through the use of the environment; however, emphasis is on consequences for actions rather than group pressure and encouragement. These are the key principles of behavior modification (Paul and Lentz 1977):

- The frequency of a behavior depends on positive or negative *consequences*.

- Events that occur together will come to be *associated*.

- New behaviors are developed through others' *teaching and role modeling*.

Positive Reinforcement   Positive reinforcement is an environmental consequence that encourages a behavior. For example, praising a client who expresses knowledge about medication encourages the client to demonstrate this knowledge. Praise is positive reinforcement. Sometimes staff actions may also inadvertently encourage a client's symptomatic behavior.

Gustavo becomes increasingly anxious about discharge. As the date approaches, his ability to follow the ward routine and take care of himself declines. Staff decide he is not ready for discharge. Gustavo's ability to care for himself then improves. A new discharge date is set and, again, Gustavo's behavior deteriorates as the date approaches. Staff again delay the discharge date. The staff's decision to delay discharge positively reinforces the client's anxious behavior as discharge approaches.

Tokens have also been used in behavior modification programs as positive reinforcement. Through acceptable behavior, clients earn tokens that they can exchange for desirable items.

Negative Reinforcement   Negative reinforcement is used to decrease or eliminate behavior. Examples of negative consequences include:

- Showing no response to undesirable behavior

- Removing something of value for undesirable behavior

- Removing the client from the situation in which undesirable behavior takes place (called "time out")

A young woman with no organic illness repeatedly collapses in front of the nurses' station. Initially staff rush to her assistance. Over time this reaction positively reinforces an undesirable behavior. Nursing staff agree to implement a behavior modification plan based on "no response to undesirable behavior." Subsequently, when the client falls to the floor at the nurses' station, all staff continue with their work.

In some token-based behavior modification programs, the client may not only earn tokens for desirable behavior but also lose tokens for unaccept-

able behavior. "Loss of tokens" illustrates a negative reinforcement technique based on removal of a valued item.

Negative reinforcement can also inadvertently discourage acceptable behavior. For example, a nurse who makes no response to a client exhibiting medication knowledge discourages the client from verbalizing this understanding.

An 18-year-old woman with gorging and vomiting behaviors was admitted voluntarily to an in-patient psychiatric unit. Karen was 5′7″ and weighted 90 pounds. She stated that she was fat and that she could not control her eating patterns. She had agreed to hospitalization only on the insistence of her family. The nurse's diagnoses were: Body image disturbance and Self-care deficit: Feeding. The nursing team agreed that Karen's physical status required stabilization, and a behavior modification plan was developed.

- Karen would receive a nutritionally balanced meal on a tray.
- She would eat the entire meal under the supervision of the nurse.
- If Karen did not eat the entire meal, she would be tube-fed the remaining food.
- Karen would be supervised by the nurse for 30 minutes following the meal to prevent vomiting.
- Karen would receive nursing supervision during toileting or showering to prevent vomiting.

Karen was weighed three times per week to determine if she was steadily gaining weight. The desired goal was 110 pounds, and an increase of 2 pounds per week was determined to be acceptable progress. Failure to maintain progress resulted in a loss of privileges to attend group outings and leisure activities. Progressive weight gain would result in increased privileges such as toileting, showering, and eating without nurse supervision.

This behavior modification plan uses both positive and negative consequences. For example, the possibility of tube feeding reinforced the adaptive behavior of eating the well-balanced meal. Increased independence (i.e., removal of nursing supervision at meals and toileting) was a reward (positive reinforcement) for progressive weight gain. Continued supervision and loss of privileges were negative reinforces designed to discourage and eliminate continued low weight.

The nurse and Karen reviewed her progress toward gaining weight on a weekly basis. Karen gained 3 pounds the first week, 2 pounds the second week, but nothing the third week. The nurse explored this lack of progress with Karen in the following conversation:

Nurse: You accomplished the expected weight goals the first two weeks, but there was no progress this third week.

Karen: (Crying) I don't want to gain any more weight.

Nurse: Are you concerned about being fat?

Karen: No. I enjoy having you sit with me, and I know you will stop when I have gained enough weight.

The nurse realized that close supervision, originally intended to eliminate low weight, actually reinforced it since Karen enjoyed the personal attention. The nurse, with Karen's agreement, revised the treatment plan.

- Other staff would supervise Karen's eating and toileting but would not engage in any discussion. This would allow staff to monitor Karen's eating and possible vomiting, but the "no response" technique would negatively reinforce (or eliminate) Karen's efforts to initiate a social relationship.
- Karen's primary nurse would meet with Karen three times a week, contingent upon successful weight gain. This meeting would act as additional positive reinforcement to gain weight since Karen enjoyed meetings with her nurse.

Reevaluation: Karen resumed her pattern of progressive weight gain, thus indicating that the revised intervention was successful.

In this example, the treatment-planning process is similar to that in the earlier example of individualized behavior contracting. In both cases the expected behaviors were identified and the client participated in the development of the plan. Karen's example illustrates selected principles of positive and negative reinforcement. Social interaction or no response might also be interpreted as components of a therapeutic interpersonal relation approach. This blurring of the boundaries between behavior modification and interpersonal techniques highlights the underlying principle common to both approaches: Milieu therapy is based on the purposeful use of people, resources, and events in the client's immediate environment to achieve optimal functioning.

Ethics Ethical principles underlying nursing care in milieu therapy include autonomy, beneficence, privacy, and distributive justice (see Chapter 7). These principles may, at times, pose conflicts in priority setting for the nurse. For example, a client's threats may necessitate nursing interventions to protect the client or others. Protective interventions such as one-to-one supervision or seclusion are based on the beneficence principle of preventing harm. This may have a higher priority than the principle of client autonomy. The principle of autonomy also conflicts with the conceptual framework underlying behavior modification techniques. Skinner's (1971) "science of behavior," based on the control of human functioning through environmental manipulation, creates doubt about the existence of free will and the possibility for personal autonomy.

The client's right to privacy and the nurse's obligation to maintain confidentiality may conflict with milieu principles of open communication, interpersonal feedback, and participative membership in a group. The right to privacy is the client's prerogative to reveal or not to reveal information, behavior, or beliefs and to be free of unreasonable intrusions by others. The nurse's obligation to maintain confidentiality protects against information disclosure without the client's consent. Client unwillingness and nurse inability to explore clinical issues in group situations may contribute to a climate of secrecy, which can be nontherapeutic in milieu treatment.

Although nurses' ethical dilemmas generally arise from the nurse-client relationship, the ethical problem of allocating scarce resources—distributive justice—is illustrated by the trend toward shorter hospital stays and diminished significance of milieu therapy.

Ethical criteria for resource distribution include equality, need, personal effort, societal contribution, and merit. Social productivity and equality do not take the inherent value of each individual into account. Needs-based criteria require determination of which needs will receive resources. Because current criteria for distribution of mental health care resources are based on severity of need, acute psychotic symptoms are most likely to receive resources. Individuals with less serious symptoms (needs) who might nevertheless benefit from a personal growth experience in long-term milieu therapy are unlikely to receive external financial assistance (e.g., third-party reimbursement) for this care. Different allocation schemes for existing mental health dollars or reallocation of resources from other areas such as education, social welfare, or general health care will ultimately reflect social values of what constitutes an acceptable human condition.

CHAPTER HIGHLIGHTS

- Milieu therapy is the purposeful use of people, resources, and events in the immediate environment to ensure safety, promote optimal functioning in daily activities, develop or improve interpersonal skills, and foster the capacity to manage outside the institutional setting.

- The humanistic interactionist perspective of milieu therapy stems from belief in the importance of the individual and human/environment interaction theories.

- Beliefs in the importance of humane physical surroundings proposed during the moral therapy era continue to be reflected in modern legal and regulatory standards.

- Milieu therapy provides a therapeutic (rather than custodial) role unique to psychiatric nursing.

• The nursing process is used to assess client behavior within the context of the treatment environment and to plan interventions that draw on the therapeutic potential of the individual nurse, other people, and environmental facilities.

• The nursing process can also be used to assess and intervene in characteristics of the environment that influence a client's behavior.

REFERENCES

Allen JG, Deering D, Buskirk JR, Coyne L: Assessment of therapeutic alliances in the psychiatric hospital milieu. *Psychiatry* 1988;51:291–299.

American Nurses' Association: *Standards of Psychiatric and Mental Health Nursing Practice*. ANA, 1982.

American Psychiatric Association: *The Psychiatric Therapies*. APA, 1984.

Belcher JR, Fish LJB: Hildegard Peplau, in *Nursing Theories: A Base for Professional Nursing Practice*. Prentice-Hall, 1980.

Bennett AM, Foster PC: Ernestine Wiedenbach, in *Nursing Theories: A Base for Professional Nursing Practice*. Prentice-Hall, 1980.

Bockoven JS: *Moral Treatment in American Psychiatry*. Springer Publishing, 1963.

Craig C, Ray F, Hix C: Seclusion and restraint: Decreasing the discomfort. *J Psychosoc Nurs Ment Health Serv* 1989;27(7):16–19.

Devine BA: Therapeutic milieu/milieu therapy: An overview. *J Psychosoc Nurs Ment Health Serv* 1981;19:20–24.

Ellis NK, Krch-Cole E: Providing a therapeutic milieu experience for a patient diagnosed with acquired immune deficiency syndrome. *Arch Psychiatr Nurs* 1987;1(6):436–440.

Emrich K: Helping or hurting? Interacting in the psychiatric milieu. *J Psychosoc Nurs Ment Health Serv* 1989;27(12):26–29.

Garritson SH: Characteristics of restrictiveness. *J Psychosoc Nurs Ment Health Serv* 1987;25(1):10–19.

Gerlock A, Solomons HC: Factors associated with the seclusion of psychiatric patients. *Perspect Psychiatr Care* 1984; 21(April–June):46–53.

Goffman E: *Asylums*. Aldine Publishing, 1961.

Gruenberg E: The social breakdown syndrome and its prevention, in Arieti S (ed): *American Handbook of Psychiatry*, ed 2. Basic Books, 1974.

Joint Commission on Accreditation of Hospitals: Therapeutic environment, in *Consolidated Standards Manual for Child, Adolescent, and Adult Psychiatric, Alcoholism, and Drug Abuse Facilities and Facilities Serving the Mentally Retarded/Developmentally Disabled*. Joint Commission on Accreditation of Hospitals, 1987, pp 177–182.

Kahn EM, Frederick N: Milieu-oriented management strategies on acute care units for the chronically mentally ill. *Arch Psychiatr Nurs* 1988;2(3):134–140.

Kahn EM, White EM: Adapting milieu approaches to acute inpatient care for schizophrenic patients. *Hosp Community Psychiatry* 1989;40(6):609–614.

Kirkpatrick H: A descriptive study of seclusion: The unit environment, patient behavior, and nursing interventions. *Arch Psychiatr Nurs* 1989;3(1):3–9.

Krauss, J, Slavinsky A: *The Chronically Ill Psychiatric Patient and the Community*. Blackwell Scientific Publications, 1982.

McEnany G, Tescher B: Contracting for care. *J Psychosoc Nurs Ment Health Serv* 1985;23:11–18.

Paul GL, Lentz RJ: *Psychosocial Treatment of Chronic Mental Patients: Milieu versus Social Learning Programs*. Harvard University Press, 1977.

Proshansky HM: The environmental crisis in human dignity. *J Soc Issues* 1973;29:1–20.

Richardson B: Psychiatric inpatients' perceptions of the seclusion room experience. *Nurs Res* 1987;36(4):234–238.

Rosenblatt A: Concepts of the asylum in the care of the mentally ill. *Hosp Community Psychiatry* 1984;35:244–250.

Schatzman L, Strauss A: A sociology of psychiatry: A perspective and some organizing foci. *Social Problems* 1966;14:3–16.

Schull AT: *Decarceration: Community Treatment and the Deviant: A Radical View*. Prentice-Hall, 1977.

Skinner BF: *Beyond Freedom and Dignity*. Alfred A. Knopf, 1971.

Stanton A, Schwartz M: *The Mental Hospital*. Basic Books, 1954.

Strauss A, Schatzman L, Bucher R, Ehrlich D. Sabshin M: *Psychiatric Ideologies and Institutions*, rev ed. Free Press of Glencoe, 1981.

Tudor GE: A sociopsychiatric nursing approach to intervention in a problem of mutual withdrawal on a mental hospital ward. *Perspect Psychiatr Care* 1970;8:11–35. (Reprinted from *Psychiatry: Journal for the Study of Interpersonal Processes* 1952;(May):15.)

Whitehead CC, Polsky RH, Crookshank C, Fik E: Objective and subjective evaluation of psychiatric ward redesign. *Am J Psychiatry* 1984;141(May):639–644.

Wilson HS: *Deinstitutionalized Residential Care for the Mentally Disabled—The Soteria House Approach*. Grune & Stratton, 1982.

Biologic Therapies

LEARNING OBJECTIVES

- Outline the historical foundations of biologic therapies

- Discuss two reasons for interest by psychiatric nurses in the biologic model of illness

- List and describe the classes, properties, uses, and side effects of the major psychotropic medications

- Identify four pieces of information concerning clients' drugs that must be included in client teaching

- Develop a teaching plan appropriate to clients being discharged from a hospital setting with psychotropic medications

- Discuss two indications for the use of electroconvulsive therapy

- Describe three different visual-imaging techniques used in psychiatry

- Discuss one appropriate indication for the use of psychosurgery

- List and describe two humanistic interactionist implications for biologic therapies in psychiatry

Geoffry McEnany

CROSS REFERENCE

Other topics related to this content are: Anxiety disorders, Chapter 14; Drugs, Appendix B; Historical perspectives, Chapter 1; Mood disorders, Chapter 13; Philosophic perspectives, Chapter 1; Psychobiology, Chapter 6; Recidivism among the chronically mental ill, Chapter 17; Schizophrenia, Chapter 12.

BIOLOGIC THERAPIES HAVE BEEN interwoven into the evolutionary fabric of psychiatry, and, more recently, psychiatric nursing. In Chapters 1 and 6 you read about the historical underpinnings of contemporary psychiatry and psychobiologic thought. Over time the philosophic pendulum has swung between fully biologic explanations of mental disorders to etiologic beliefs based fully on demonologic, magical, or spiritual reasoning. Treatment has largely depended on the philosophic and socially accepted attitudes of a given society during a specific era. For example, the ancient Greek and Roman civilizations maintained strong beliefs about the biologic substrates of mental disorders. A similar psychobiologic understanding of behavior and illness is emerging today in Western societies. However, the period between early civilizations and the twentieth century was characterized by a potpourri of approaches to and interventions for mental disorders. These approaches were mainly spiritual, moralistic, or psychodynamic in origin.

Historical Foundations of Biologic Therapies

Exploring the Biologic-Psychologic Linkage

From a biologic perspective all behavior is the result of neurochemical actions and reactions in the central nervous system. Of course, the systematized chemical reactions are influenced by many factors, such as the environment, interpersonal social exchanges, stress, and the idiosyncratic responses of one's body systems (e.g., endocrine, neurologic, immunologic). So, behavior is the holistic response of a set of body systems to a given stimulus.

Psychobiology and the biologic understanding of human behavior may eliminate dualism and a fragmented approach to client care. But if this is true, why have the nursing and medical sciences not revolutionized approaches to client care by fully adopting a psychobiologic framework in understanding illness? To answer that question, one must appreciate the influences of time, tradition, and the dominant philosophic viewpoints of caregivers today. The biological approach to mental disorders is not new, but it *is* undergoing a renewed interest by clinicians and researchers in different parts of the world. However, many professionals in nursing, psychiatry, and collaborative disciplines know little or nothing of psychobiologic mediation of behavior. Their training and philosophies may not support the perception of mental

disorder as a psychobiologic entity. Such dissonance between learned philosophies and advances in the biology of behavior make it difficult to take a fully unified approach to care for the mentally disordered.

Trends in Biologic Therapies Over Time

Chapter 1 addresses many of the biologic therapies used from preliterate times through to the twentieth century. In this chapter the goal is to review advancements in biologic therapies over the last 100 years, which have produced the most scientific and precise psychobiologic discoveries known to psychiatric care and have witnessed a revolution in the assessment of, and traditional approaches to, behavioral problems and mental disorders.

Perhaps a reasonable way to conceptualize the current changes in understanding the biologic underpinnings of behavior called mental disorder is to frame the biologic approaches as molecular rather than "psychologic," "social," or "cultural." In other words, biologic therapies often yield healing because they produce changes in the function of cells in the central nervous system. These changes permit the emergence of new behavior.

ECT   Probably the earliest "new" biologic intervention in the twentieth century was electroconvulsive therapy (ECT). Introduced in 1938, the then unrefined treatment was used for clients with unremitting or recurrent severe depression, some forms of schizophrenia, or bipolar disorder. Of course, lack of standardized nomenclature for diagnostic labeling during the first half of the twentieth century made it difficult to know *who* was being treated with ECT; what one diagnostician called "schizophrenia" may have been considered "depression with psychotic features" by another. This raised the question of whether schizophrenia and various forms of mood disorders might be part of the same continuum—a blasphemous thought in the opinion of some clinicians today! ECT will be more thoroughly discussed later in this chapter.

Drugs   Other biologic therapies that have revolutionized psychiatry include the various drugs developed and applied to clinical practice since the late 1940s. The earliest medication discovery was made in 1949 by an Australian physician, John Cade. Dr. Cade found that lithium worked to subdue wild behavior in animals. To the astonishment of his colleagues, Cade went one step further and gave lithium to humans. Since then, of course, lithium has become the drug of choice for the treatment of bipolar affective disorder.

This century has witnessed many other great pharmacologic discoveries, including most of the drugs used in psychiatry today. In the 1950s **antipsychotic, antidepressant,** and some **anxiolytic** medications were discovered. Until then the care of psychiatric clients had consisted mainly of behavioral interventions, seclusion, and various forms of restraint. Suddenly many clients were suffering less, getting better, and returning to the mainstream of life. However, for a variety of complex reasons, some clients found themselves lodged in the psychiatric system, unable to do much more than become permanent residents of the psychiatric community.

Psychobiology and Nursing Interventions

Other biologic therapies continue to unfold as time passes. While physicians continue to look for biologic markers or clear physical indices of mental illness, some nurses are trying to understand how select nursing interventions affect the psychobiology of clients. Subjects of such nursing research include:

- Specific types of dietary influences on behavior

- Ways to assess and "harness'" clients' normal circadian rhythms, with the goal of improving the specificity of nursing interventions and overall client care

- Effects of exposure to full-spectrum light during winter months as a preventive measure against seasonal cyclic depressive disorders

- Effects of limited sleep deprivation to reduce the response time of depressed clients to antidepressant medications

- Biologic effects of relaxation techniques

- Biologic effects of seclusion or restraint

Psychiatric-mental health nurses need to understand and remain abreast of current advances in psychobiology. By doing so nurses can maintain an updated knowledge based for clinical work with clients and therefore develop accurate and effective nursing interventions.

The biologic model is of particular interest to any nurse who administers medications and is involved in client teaching. According to this model, *the mind is not separate from the brain,* and there are underlying biologic reasons for all behavior. An understanding of biologic reasoning allows nurses to adopt a truly holistic approach to mental disorder while working with and teaching clients.

Psychotropic Medications and Nursing Responsibilities

The word *drugs* conjures a variety of powerful positive and negative images. Television coverage of the devastating effects of crack cocaine exemplifies the negative image. Another image leaps from the pages of nursing and medical journals; pharmaceutical advertisements show people leading productive lives or smiling nurses, allegedly grateful for a medication that controls psychiatric symptoms. Still another drug-related image is that of school children being inoculated against diphtheria, polio, and pertussis. All these images are powerful, and each is backed by truth.

Nurses' responsibilities to clients receiving psychotropic medications are very different from the responsibilities of nurses in other settings. A nurse working with clients having cardiac difficulties, for example, may have clear physiologic indices for the administration of drugs such as isosorbide dinitrate or nitroglycerin, but psychiatric nurses rarely have comparable consistent complexes of symptoms on which to base clinical judgments. In psychiatric work, nurses must often observe client behaviors closely to be aware of the sometimes subtle nature of the presenting symptom. Pacing, mild diaphoresis, slight increases in blood pressure or pulse, a heightened muscle tone, and hypervigilant posture may be indicative of escalating anxiety, but they may also point to other problems such as caffeine toxicity or excessive use of tobacco. Accurate nursing assessment of client behavior is crucial if medications are to be given effectively and appropriately. For example, over the last five or six years there has been an increasing trend among hospital psychiatrists to prescribe a class of drugs known as *benzodiazepines* (the diazepam/Valium family) more liberally in conjunction with low-dose antipsychotic drugs (also known as **neuroleptic** drugs). This minimizes the use of the neuroleptics and possibly diminishes the potential for tardive dyskinesia, an extreme side effect of neuroleptic use among some clients receiving this class of drugs. In light of this trend, nurses must be able to assess the finer differences between anxious and psychotic behavior. Sometimes the two are difficult to differentiate, especially when the client's anxiety is high and the client "covers" or "masks" the psychotic behavior.

Medication Teaching

In addition to assessment, nurses have the major responsibility of planning for client learning about medication. Compliance with medication regimens is often an issue for psychiatric clients, and nurses have explored the efficacy of teaching as a means to improve adherence to medication regimens after discharge.

Variables related to compliance include socioeconomic class, marital status, number of concurrent medications, diagnosis, side effects, health benefits, and health values. Although the data vary on the degrees of influence of these variables, compliance is thought to be better among people who are upper middle class, married, taking more than four types of medication, and diagnosed as having a bipolar disorder with reported mild or nonexistent side effects from medications. Clients' individual differences must be addressed in the course of the teaching-learning process.

An issue of great concern to many nurses involves the planning of teaching-learning experiences for clients who suffer from chronic mental illness. Although this population has learning needs concerning care and treatments, teaching is often difficult, depending on the severity and chronicity of the client's illness. Selander and Miller (1985) express concern over clients' **recidivism** and the learning needs of chronically mentally disordered people. Specific to the work of Selander and Miller, the term *recidivism* means a tendency to relapse into a previous mode of behavior. The target population of these authors included predominantly clients diagnosed as schizophrenic and receiving fluphenazine decanoate (Prolixin Decanoate) as part of their treatment. The authors hypothesized that recidivism rates would decline for the clients who were involved in the fluphenazine groups. Nurses organized the groups, incorporating group therapy, teaching, medication surveillance, and medication administration into a regular format. Selander and Miller found that admission rates dropped significantly and length of stay was significantly briefer.

Another concern for nurses working with mentally disordered clients is the need to assess the learning capacity of clients at different points in their disorders. For example, when clients are first admitted to an in-patient unit, they may be too disorganized to focus on specific learning tasks. Depressed clients may be so psychomotorally slowed, because of hormonal shifts and dysfunctional neurotransmitter activity at the synapses, that they may be unable to learn. Given appropriate treatment and care, however, the clients' psychobiologic disequilibrium may be corrected, making learning possible.

Even when a nurse perceives that a client is ready to learn (i.e., cognitive abilities are intact), learning will not necessarily occur. Many nurses discuss medication groups on an acute psychiatric unit and address the importance of not only assessing cognitive abilities but also exploring affective and social issues that may contribute to effective learning experiences. Clients are no different in many ways from other learners. When presented with material that is clearly beneficial to them, they are likely to be more interested in the learning process.

Evaluation of teaching efforts is essential to complete the teaching-learning process. This part of the process can be as informal or formal as the nurse chooses or deems necessary to check the client's knowledge of information taught. The nurse cannot evaluate a client's understanding of information unless, at the least, the client verbally reiterates information or performs a return demonstration of the skill. A nurse desiring a more extensive evaluation may consider using a paper-and-pencil "pretest/posttest" format. In this case, the nurse develops a written test to cover the content of the teaching and has the client complete the test *before* the nurse begins teaching. This provides a written measure of the client's learning needs. After the nurse implements the teaching plan, the client completes the same examination (a posttest). Comparison of the pretest and posttest results yields a documented measure of how much learning has occurred as a result of the nurse's teaching intervention.

Antipsychotic Drugs

Background

The discovery of the first antipsychotic drug, chlorpromazine (Thorazine), is a prime example of the role chance has played in the history of psychopharmacology. Chlorpromazine was initially synthesized as an antihistamine and was not tried as a tranquilizer for schizophrenic persons until 1952. Its effects on the behavior, thinking, affect, and perception of schizophrenic persons were so profound that knowledge of its properties was rapidly disseminated, and it became widely used within three or four years. Chlorpromazine's effects on the hospital practice of psychiatry were staggering. Its use contributed to reversing a steadily increasing census in United States mental institutions, and the mental hospital population has progressively decreased ever since. One might say that chlorpromazine gave birth to the modern notions of psychiatric treatment—unlocked wards, milieu treatment, occupational and recreational therapy, and halfway houses. The entire field of community mental health is ultimately linked to its discovery, because it enabled clients to return to their homes.

Major Effects

The beneficial effects of antipsychotic medications in all psychotic states have been demonstrated beyond question. Multiple and varied criteria have been used to measure improvement. These drugs have been used successfully in clients with delusional thinking, confusion, motor agitation, and motor retardation. Antipsychotic drug treatment also decreases formal thought disorder, blunted affect, bizarre behavior, social withdrawal, hallucinations, belligerence, and uncooperativeness.

The most common disintegrative condition treated with antipsychotic drugs is the group of symptoms traditionally labeled schizophrenia. (See Chapter 12 for information on evaluating the schizophrenic client and the diagnostic criteria in DSM-III-R.) The problem of assessment is complicated by the fact that many diseases can cause organic brain syndromes with features like those of schizophrenia. For example, auditory hallucinations may indicate a variety of DSM-III-R conditions, including schizophrenia and organic brain syndrome. The finer points of differentiation between these two conditions include assessments of cognitive functioning and the client's presenting history. (Chapter 10 offers a more detailed delineation of organic brain syndrome and related disorders.) All clients manifesting psychotic symptoms should have a thorough medical history and physical examination to rule out treatable "medical" illnesses, many of which are accompanied by behaviors considered psychotic or "psychobiologic."

Choice of Specific Drug

There are many antipsychotic medications on the market. Claims are made for the greater effectiveness of one over another, especially by the respective drug companies. Controlled studies, however, have failed to demonstrate substantial differences in antipsychotic effects among the drugs. The choice of a particular medication, then, depends on knowledge of the vari-

ous pharmacologic properties and side effects, the client's or a family member's history of drug response, and the psychiatrist's experience with various compounds. Important client variables are past successes with specific drugs, history of allergies, and history of serious or intolerable side effects. Certain side effects can often be used beneficially with clients. A certain amount of trial and error is expected in each clinical application.

Table 32–1 summarizes the characteristics of the major antipsychotic drugs. The list of these drugs is extensive and growing, and it makes sense for each member of the treatment team to become familiar with just a few representative drugs, their predictable effects, and their common side effects. The characteristics covered in the table are discussed in sequence in the sections that follow (see also Appendix B).

There are now five distinct chemical classes of antipsychotic medications commonly used in the United States. (One class, the **phenothiazines**, can be broken down into three different types of medications.) This provides a broad choice in terms of side effects and potential client responsiveness. A client who is unresponsive to one class may well respond to another than circumvents a problem in absorption, accumulation at neurotransmitter receptor sites, or metabolism.

Table 32–1 shows the wide variety among these medications in milligram-per-milligram potency. This fact has most relevance when treating clients who require large doses. In such cases a potent medication is best.

Two new antipsychotic drugs—clozapine (Clozaril) and **pimozide** (Orap)—have been recently intro-

TABLE 32–1   Antipsychotic Drugs

Class	Generic Name	Trade Name	Potency (mg equivalent to 100 mg Chlorpromazine)	Usual Dosage Range (Mg/Day)	Sedative	SIDE EFFECTS Extra-pyramidal*	Anti-cholinergic*
Phenothiazines							
Aliphatic	Chlorpromazine	Thorazine	100	150–1500	Very strong	Moderate	Strong
Piperadine	Thioridazine	Mellaril	100	150–800	Moderate	Minimal	Moderate
Piperazine	Trifluoperazine	Stelazine	5	10–60	Weak	Strong	Weak
	Fluphenazine	Prolixin	2	3–45	Weak	Strong	Weak
	Perphenazine	Trilafon	10	12–60	Weak	Strong	Weak
Butyrophenones	Haloperidol	Haldol	2.5	2–40	Weak	Strong	Weak
Thioxanthenes	Thiothixene	Navane	5	10–60	Weak	Strong	Weak
	Chlorprothixene	Taractan	100	40–600	Strong	Moderate	Strong
Dihydroindolones	Molindone	Moban	10	15–225	Weak	Moderate	Weak
Dibenzoxazepines	Loxapine	Loxitane	20	10–100	Moderate	Strong	Moderate

*Extrapyramidal and anticholinergic side effects are discussed later in this chapter.

duced. Both of these drugs offer new options for the care and treatment of persons suffering from psychotic conditions.

According to Green and Salzman (1990), clozapine is an antipsychotic drug with an unusual pharmacologic and clinical profile. It has only recently been approved for use in the United States and is generally used for clients with a treatment-resistant psychosis, e.g., certain schizophrenics. Approximately one third of treatment-resistant schizophrenics who have taken clozapine have demonstrated improvement, although the degree of improvement varies from client to client. Despite its capacity to ameliorate symptoms of some very recalcitrant clients this drug has some serious side effects. The most serious is agranulocytosis, which occurs in approximately 1 to 2 percent of the population taking this medication. The risk period for the emergence of this side effect is anywhere from six weeks to six months, but it can occur later during the course of treatment. If a client experiences agranulocytosis as a result of the use of clozapine, the drug cannot be reinstituted. Other serious side effects include potential for seizure; such a side effect seems to be dose related. Less acute, but nonetheless important side effects include sedation, tachycardia, and hypotension.

Pimozide is used to ameliorate psychotic symptoms and seems to be particularly effective in the treatment of tactile hallucinations. Although this medication does not have as serious potential side effects as clozapine, its side effect profile is similar to that of other drugs in its class.

The emergence of new antipsychotic drugs raises issues about the care and treatment of clients who do not respond to customary measures, such as neuroleptics. According to Osser (1989), neuroleptic-resistant psychosis is a complex phenomenon that requires close assessment and careful intervention, including an evaluation of neuroleptic resistance and assessment of the client's **neuroleptic threshold** (the optimal dose at which the client responds, taking into consideration parkinsonian side effects). Osser points out that a relationship between neuroleptic-induced pseudoparkinsonism and clinical effects is expected when neuroleptics are administered, but this relationship is not linear.

Dosage

Dosage ranges vary widely among clients. Medications must be titrated against the psychotic target symptoms and the appearance of side effects. Most clients are initially given a relatively low dose (e.g., 20 to 50 mg orally or 25 mg intramuscularly [IM] of chlorpromazine) to test for adverse effects for one to two hours. Then the medication is typically given in a starting dose of 300 to 400 mg (or IM equivalent) per day, and

gradually increased by 25 to 50 percent a day until maximum improvement is noted or intolerable side effects are encountered.

The treatment setting frequently influences the drug regimen. In a crowded hospital emergency room, for example, hourly doses of medication may be given until a client is sedated. In more completely staffed, private in-patient units, a client may be observed for several days before medication is given. However, in terms of long-term outcome and length of eventual remission, neither approach can claim documented superiority.

Clients who are extremely agitated, violent, severely withdrawn, or **catatonic** require significant doses during the first few days of treatment, delivered by injection to ensure rapid relief. Chlorpromazine, 50 to 100 mg IM, may be used, particularly if sedation is required. The nurse must be aware that this is an irritating drug; injections must be deeply intramuscular in either the buttocks or upper arms, and sites must be rotated. Substantial IM doses of the more potent antipsychotics, such as haloperidol 10 mg or trifluoperazine 10 mg, may be given to agitated clients. This approach frequently avoids some of the more troublesome side effects while ameliorating behavioral and cognitive symptoms.

Because the antipsychotic medications have a rather long biologic half-life, and many have significant sedative effects, there is little reason to give divided doses of medication after the initial days of treatment. It is recommended that the drugs, particularly the sedative ones such as chlorpromazine, be given in substantial doses at bedtime. In addition to promoting sleep, decreasing the chances the client will forget to take a dose after discharge, and saving nursing time in the hospital, this method saves money because large-dose capsules or tablets cost less than an equivalent amount of medication prepared in smaller doses.

After maximum clinical improvement has been obtained, antipsychotic drugs are generally reduced gradually. Continuing to give a client modest doses of an antipsychotic medication following a psychotic episode lowers the chances of relapse and rehospitalization. Psychotherapy with schizophrenic clients may not be particularly effective without maintenance medications in conventional treatment settings, but it does improve psychosocial functioning in clients who are also taking maintenance medications. It is generally believed that clients should be kept on doses of antipsychotics sufficient to suppress symptoms for three months to one year following an acute episode. After such an interval, the particular client's course and life situation must be considered and treatment individualized. Some clients recover from a psychotic episode completely within six months. These clients, with schizophreniform disorder, should not receive long-term maintenance drug treatment. For individuals who have already experienced recurrent episodes and demonstrate a deteriorating course, it is clearly advantageous to prevent relapses with drugs if possible.

Decision to Use a Drug

Today, these general principles govern antipsychotic drug use:

• Drugs are given to treat target symptoms of schizophrenia or other psychotic disorders.

• Initial treatment may require parenteral doses. These are changed to oral pill or concentrate forms as the behavior disturbance subsides.

• Total dosages are tailored to individual needs; wide variations exist among clients.

• As soon as practical, divided doses are changed to a single dose given at bedtime to maximize use of the drugs' sedative properties.

• Most clients with a chronic course require maintenance doses for sustained improvement.

Special Considerations

These special considerations apply to the use of antipsychotic medication:

A Unique Route of Administration The phenothiazines fluphenazine (Prolixin) and haloperidol (Haldol) are available in long-acting intramuscular injectable forms that behave like sustained-release capsules. These medications are gradually released over a long period of time—two to three weeks. Long-acting fluphenazine and haloperidol are available in **decanoate** (long-acting depot injection) preparations. The main advantage of the long-acting injectable forms is that they reduce clients' ambivalence about taking medication and eliminate the need for constant pill taking. The treatment team must also honor the clients' civil liberties; truly involuntary treatment can be performed only according to due process, as required by a particular state's mental hygiene laws.

The psychiatric nurse in a community setting may frequently have occasion to administer the long-acting fluphenazine or haloperidol. A dose of regular fluphenazine or haloperidol is usually taken first to rule out the possibility of allergic reactions. Such reactions can be devastating if discovered after a two- or three-week supply of medicine has been given. If no adverse reactions are noted within one hour, the long-acting form is injected, usually in the upper, outer quadrant of the buttocks.

Medication Requirements of Certain Age Groups In elderly persons the agitation often associated with organic mental syndromes is markedly responsive to phenothiazines. Other sedatives, such as the barbiturates and the benzodiazepines, may further compromise cerebral functioning (further depress the level of awareness and concentration) and thus worsen such syndromes. Doses of phenothiazines are generally reduced for the geriatric population. Trifluoperazine (Stelazine) 5–20 mg per day, or haloperidol, 1–6 mg per day, might constitute adequate treatment.

Antipsychotic medications are effective in treating childhood psychoses and in managing the behavior problems associated with mental retardation. The general principle of reduced dosage is again applicable. The upper limit of the usual daily dosage for children under twelve might be 200 mg per day of chlorpromazine (Thorazine) or thioridazine (Mellaril) or 20 mg per day of trifluoperazine. Amounts of individual intramuscular injections must also be kept at 25 to 50 mg.

Potential Side Effects of the Antipsychotic Medications Their continuous contact with clients gives nurses an advantage over physicians, who may see a client only every other day or, at best, once every day at the same time. Both the dangerous and the more uncomfortable side effects frequently have a rapid onset and need attention promptly.

The side effects of antipsychotic medications that nurses must recognize can be divided into the following general classes:

• Autonomic nervous system

• Extrapyramidal

• Other central nervous system

• Allergic

• Blood

• Skin

• Eye

• Endocrine

Table 32–2 lists the side effects of various antipsychotic medications.

Autonomic Nervous System Effects The antipsychotics all possess **anticholinergic** and antiadrenergic side effects. That is, they interfere with the usual transmission of nerve impulses by acetylcholine and epinephrine, in both central and peripheral nerves. The most common side effects are the anticholinergic ones. These include dry mouth, blurred vision, constipation, urinary hesitance or retention, and, under rarer circumstances, paralytic ileus.

Postural hypotension is a common antiadrenergic effect. The primary danger here is injury from a fall.

TABLE 32-2   Side Effects of Antipsychotic Medication

Effect	Chlorpromazine (Thorazine)	Haloperidol (Haldol)	Loxapine (Loxitane)	Molindone (Moban)
Akathisia	Occasional	Frequent	Occasional	Frequent
Allergic skin reactions	Occasional	Rare	Rare	Rare
Anticholinergic effects	Frequent	Not reported	Rare	Occasional
Blood dyscrasia	Occasional	Occasional	Not reported	Rare
Cholestatic jaundice	Occasional	Rare	Not reported	Not reported
Dystonias	Occasional	Frequent	Rare	Occasional
Impotence	Occasional	Not reported	Not reported	Not reported
Parkinsonism	Occasional	Frequent	Frequent	Occasional
Photosensitivity	Occasional	Rare	Not reported	Not reported
Postural hypotension	Frequent	Occasional	Rare	Rare
Retinitis pigmentosa	Not reported	Not reported	Not reported	Not reported
Sedation	Frequent	Not reported	Occasional	Rare

▶

Clients receiving parenteral medications, such as chlorpromazine intramuscularly, must have their blood pressure monitored lying and standing before and a half hour after each dose. Clients should be advised to rise from a supine position gradually and to sit down if they feel faint. Support stockings and a large intake of fluids may be indicated. This problem is much less significant with oral administration of the drugs. However, nurses working with clients receiving oral antipsychotic medications should take both baseline and routine measures of vital sign readings at regular intervals. Such a practice establishes the client's tolerance for medications without the untoward side effects of orthostatic hypotension and subsequent falls. The accompanying box gives guidelines for measuring orthostatic blood pressure.

Extrapyramidal Effects   Another common and sometimes frightening group of adverse reactions results from the effects of antipsychotics on the extrapyramidal tracts of the central nervous system, which are involved in the production and control of involuntary movements. These **extrapyramidal side effects** (EPS) can be broken down into four types, each with distinguishing clinical characteristics and times of onset after the initiation of drug therapy.

The earliest and most dramatic reactions are the *acute dystonic reactions*. These occur in the first days of treatment, sometimes after a single dose of medication. They involve bizarre and severe muscle contractions usually of the tongue, face, or extraocular muscles, producing **torticollis, opisthotonos,** and **oculogyric crisis.** Of particular importance to the nurse is

that dystonic reactions may also lead to laryngeal spasm. This spasm may begin as a scratching feeling in the back of the client's throat, leading to a coughing fit, and advancing to respiratory distress. The respiratory distress may lead to respiratory arrest, which necessi-

Guidelines for Measuring Orthostatic Blood Pressure

1. Instruct the client to lie down for approximately five minutes. This allows for an equilibration of the blood pressure in the supine position and gives a precise supine reading. *Do not substitute a supine reading for a sitting reading!* Take the client's blood pressure and pulse.

2. Instruct the client to stand. Wait for approximately thirty seconds to one minute and retake the blood pressure and pulse. Waiting this brief period allows for a full evaluation of the initial orthostasis.

3. Wait two more minutes and retake the vital signs once again. This third set of measurements allows for an evaluation of the client's body mechanisms to compensate for the presence of any orthostasis that may be present.

Developed by the Nursing Service Division, Langley Porter Hospital, University of California, San Francisco.

TABLE 32–2 *(continued)*

Thioridazine *(Mellaril)*	*Thiothixene* *(Navane)*	*Trifluoperazine* *(Stelazine)*	*Fluphenazine* *(Prolixin)*
Occasional	Occasional	Frequent	Frequent
Not reported	Rare	Rare	Rare
Frequent	Occasional	Frequent	Frequent
Rare	Rare	Rare	Rare
Rare	Rare	Rare	Rare
Occasional	Occasional	Frequent	Frequent
Occasional	Not reported	Occasional	Occasional
Occasional	Occasional	Frequent	Frequent
Occasional	Rare	Occasional	Occasional
Frequent	Occasional	Rare	Rare
Occasional	Not reported	Not reported	Not reported
Frequent	Frequent	Not reported	Occasional

tates mechanical ventilation. These reactions can be physically painful and are almost always frightening to the individual. They are readily reversible with one of the antiparkinsonian agents—benztropine, 1 to 2 mg, or diphenhydramine, 20 to 50 mg, intravenously (for immediate relief), intramuscularly (for rapid action), or orally (for relief within hours). Table 32–3 summarizes useful information about the antiparkinsonian agents.

The **parkinsonian syndrome,** named because of its striking resemblance to true Parkinson's disease, commonly occurs after a week or two of the therapy. It is the result of dopamine blockade caused by the neuroleptic drugs. The hallmark signs include masklike facies, resting tremor, general rigidity of posture with slow voluntary movement, and a shuffling gait. This syndrome is treatable with the antiparkinsonian agents listed in Table 32–3. Oral medication is usually sufficient, since urgency is seldom a consideration in the management of this syndrome.

A third reversible extrapyramidal syndrome is known as **akathisia.** This characteristically is a motor restlessness perceived subjectively by the client and experienced as an urge to pace, a need to shift weight from one foot to another, or an inability to sit or stand still. Akathisia is generally a later complication of drug treatment, occurring weeks to months into the course of therapy. Nonetheless it responds to oral antiparkinsonian agents as well.

Accurate observation of the course of therapy by the psychiatric nurse can promote prompt recognition and proper interpretation of these syndromes. If care is

TABLE 32–3 **Antiparkinsonian Agents**

Trade Name	Generic Name	Maximum Daily Dosage	Available in Injectable Form
Symmetrel	Amantadine	300 mg	No
Cogentin	Benztropine	8 mg	Yes
Benadryl	Diphenhydramine	100 mg	Yes
Kemadrin	Procyclidine	15 mg	No
Artane	Trihexyphenidyl	15 mg	No
Akineton	Biperiden	8 mg	Yes

SOURCES: *Derogatis L: Clinical Psychopharmacology. Addison-Wesley, 1986; Appleton WS, Davis JM: Practical Clinical Psychopharmacology. MedCom, 1973.*

not taken, the health care provider may misinterpret the increasing withdrawal, emotional blunting, apathy, and lack of spontaneity as increasing schizophrenic behavior. This error in interpretation may lead to a mistaken increase in dosage of antipsychotic medication, which will aggravate the syndrome. Akathisia can also be confused with psychotic agitation, and this error also prompts an increase in medication. For a comparison of the two conditions, see the accompanying Assessment box. Clients with akathisia require a reduction in the dosage of phenothiazines or other offending agents and/or treatment with an antiparkinsonian drug. The nurse can save the client many uncomfortable and worrisome days by being aware of the frequency with which these syndromes complicate treatment and by reporting any suspicious sign or symptom to the physician, while reassuring the client of the reversibility of the syndrome in almost all cases.

Whether clients should be treated prophylactically with antiparkinsonian agents, in view of the relatively high incidence of these syndromes, is open to debate. Some argue that the use of antiparkinsonian agents eventually leads to relatively higher antipsychotic doses and thus increases the probability of serious side effects. Another argument is that antiparkinsonian agents also pose risks and thus should be used only to counteract extrapyramidal syndromes, not to guard against their possible emergence. Moreover, a great many clients never develop the syndromes. If the likelihood of an extrapyramidal reaction is high (if, for example, the client has a history of them) and the possible consequences significant (e.g., the client may discontinue medication or drop out of treatment altogether), antipsychotic and antiparkinsonian agents are frequently initiated simultaneously.

Nursing assessment of extrapyramidal side effects is important to the quality care of clients receiving psychotropic medications. One difficulty is *consistency* of assessment among caregivers. For example, nurses usually assess for the presence of cogwheeling or muscle rigidity in clients receiving psychotropic drugs. However, the reliability among those assessments is sorely lacking; what one nurse may consider moderate to severe side effects may be assessed as mild to moderate by another nurse.

Two assessment aids are the **Simpson Neurological Scale** for the assessment of extrapyramidal side effects and the **Abnormal Involuntary Movement Scale** (AIMS) for the assessment of iatrogenic movements resulting from particular psychotropic drugs. See Figures 32–1 and 32–2 on pages 776–779. They are helpful in quantifying EPS prior to administering a medication to counteract the side effect. Readministering the instruments after the medication is given helps the nurse assess the amelioration of the side effect. These data chart the course of a client's side effects and the effectiveness of medications to decrease them. This information is critical to quality nursing care planning.

The last extrapyramidal syndrome to emerge in the course of treatment is also the severest, since it can be largely irreversible. This is **tardive dyskinesia** (TD), a disorder characterized by involuntary movements of the face, jaw, and tongue that produce bizarre grimaces, lip smacking, and protrusion of the tongue. There may also be jerky choreiform movements of the upper extremities, slow writhing athetoid movements of the arms and the legs, and tense, tonic contractions of the neck and back. The symptoms are categorized in Table 32–4. The syndrome frequently appears after years of antipsychotic drug treatment, although it can occur earlier. It usually occurs after a maintenance dose is discontinued or reduced, and it can be masked—but not treated—by reinstituting the medication or the dosage or by switching to another drug. There is no known cure for the syndrome. The recommended intervention is to stop all medication to see if the syndrome resolves spontaneously. This course of action must be weighed against the client's need for medication and the likelihood of relapse into psychosis. Reserpine, deanol, and several other drugs have been used experimentally to treat tardive dyskinesia, with equivocal results.

Other Central Nervous System Effects

Other central nervous system side effects of antipsychotic medications are sedation and reduction of seizure threshold. Because antipsychotic drugs vary in their sedative effects, this side effect is troublesome,

ASSESSMENT

Comparison of Akathisia and Agitation or Psychotic Relapse

Akathisia	Agitation or Relapse
Relieved by reducing phenothiazine dosage	Worsened by reducing phenothiazine dosage
Worsened by increasing phenothiazine dosage	Improved by increasing phenothiazine dosage
Outside voluntary control	Controllable
Responsive to antiparkinsonian agents	Unresponsive to antiparkinsonian agents
Motor restlessness predominant	Verbalization predominant

TABLE 32–4 **Extrapyramidal Effects of Antipsychotic Medications**

Type	Timing	Symptoms	Treatment	Nursing Implications
Acute dystonic reaction	First days of treatment; possibly after the first dose	Physically painful, bizarre, and frightening symptoms; severe muscle contractions of the face, extraocular muscles, and tongue with torticollis, opisthotonos, and oculogyric crisis (eyes look upward, head is turned to one side.)	Antiparkinsonian agents such as benztropine (Cogentin), trihexyphenidyl (Artane), biperiden (Akineton), procyclidine (Kemadrin), diphenhydramine (Benadryl)	Secure order for p.r.n. antiparkinsonian agents when antipsychotic medications are first begun so client discomfort can be treated quickly. Respond immediately to any symptoms and administer antiparkinsonian medication. Reassure client that side effect is reversible. Remain with client until side effect abates.
Parkinsonian syndrome	After 1 to 2 weeks of treatment	Similar to Parkinson's disease; masklike face, shuffling gait, pill-rolling tremor of the hands, rigidity of posture, and slow movement.	Same	Reassure client that side effect is reversible. Administer antiparkinsonian medication.
Akathisia	Weeks to months into the course of treatment	Characterized by motor restlessness; pacing, shifting weight from one foot to another, foot tapping, inability to sit or stand still or rest. Results from injury to basal ganglion areas.	Same	Careful assessment is necessary to prevent confusing this extrapyramidal response with anxiety or agitation. Confusion may result in increasing the client's dose, thus worsening the extrapyramidal effects. Reassure client that side effect is reversible. Administer antiparkinsonian medication.
Tardive dyskinesia	Often after years of treatment when a maintenance dose is reduced or discontinued	Involuntary bizarre grimacing, lip smacking, and protrusion of the tongue; jerky choreiform movements of the upper extremities; slow, writhing athetoid movements of the arms and legs; tonic contractions of the neck and back.	No known cure. Medication may be discontinued. Otherwise, the symptoms can only be masked by reinstituting treatment.	Contact physician immediately for medical evaluation. Do not give antiparkinsonian medications—they only worsen the symptoms. Informed consent for continued treatment with antipsychotic medication should be obtained.

SOURCE: *Kneisl CR:* Wadsworth's Review of Nursing. *Reprinted by permission of Jones and Bartlett Publishers, 1983, p 131.*

but it can be managed by changing to a less sedative agent. Seizures are not a contraindication for the drugs, but they do require close client observation.

Allergic Effects The principal allergic manifestation of the antipsychotics is cholestatic jaundice, which arises with chlorpromazine treatment. This occurs much less commonly than in the early days of psychopharmacology, and it is usually a benign and self-limiting condition.

Blood, Skin, and Eye Effects Among the other side effects, agranulocytosis (that is, a marked decrease in granulated white blood cells, or leukocytes) is the most serious. It is both potentially fatal and, fortunately, extremely rare. Usually the person gets an infection and deteriorates rapidly or begins to bleed spontaneously. It requires emergency medical attention. Skin eruptions, photosensitivity leading to severe sunburn, blue-gray metallic discolorations over face and hands, and pigmentary changes in the eyes are all potential side effects of chlorpromazine. Clients are generally advised to avoid prolonged exposure to sunlight or to use a sunscreen agent when outdoors.

Text continues on page 780

DEPARTMENT OF HEALTH AND HUMAN SERVICES PUBLIC HEALTH SERVICE Alcohol, Drug Abuse, and Mental Health Administration NIMH Treatment Strategies in Schizophrenia Study	PATIENT NUMBER	DATA GROUP	EVALUATION DATE
NEUROLOGICAL RATING SCALE **(Simpson)**	___ ___ ___ ___	**eps**	__ __ . __ __ . __ __ M M D D Y Y

PATIENT NAME

RATER NAME

RATER NUMBER	EVALUATION TYPE *(Circle)*
___ ___ ___	1 Baseline 4 Start double-blind 7 Start open meds 10 Early termination 2 2-Week minor 5 Major evaluation 8 During open meds 11 Study completion 3 6 Other 9 Stop open meds

The examination should be conducted in a room where the patient can walk a sufficient distance to allow him/her to get into a natural rhythm, e.g., 15 paces.

Each side of the body should be examined; if one side shows more pronounced pathology than the other, record more severe pathology.

Cogwheel rigidity may be palpated when the examination is carried out for items 3, 4, 5, and 6. It is not rated separately and is merely another way to detect rigidity. It would indicate that a minimum score of 2 would be mandatory.

1. **GAIT:** The patient is examined as he walks into the examining room—his gait, the swing of his arms, his general posture, all form the basis for an overall score for this item.

    1 = Normal
    2 = Mild diminution in swing while the patient is walking
    3 = Obvious diminution in swing suggesting shoulder rigidity
    4 = Stiff gait with little or no armswing noticeable
    5 = Rigid gait with arms slightly pronated; or stooped-shuffling gait with propulsion and repropulsion
    9 = Not ratable

2. **ARM DROPPING:** The patient and the examiner both raise their arms to shoulder height and let them fall to their sides. In a normal subject, a stout slap is heard as the arms hit the sides. In the patient with extreme Parkinson's syndrome, the arms fall very slowly.

    1 = Normal, free fall with loud slap and rebound
    2 = Fall slowed slightly with less audible contact and little rebound
    3 = Fall slowed, no rebound
    4 = Marked slowing, no slap at all
    5 = Arms fall as though against resistance; as though through glue
    9 = Not ratable

3. **SHOULDER SHAKING:** The subject's arms are bent at a right angle at the elbow and are taken one at a time by the examiner who grasps one hand and also clasps the other around the patient's elbow. The subject's upper arm is pushed to and fro and the humerus is externally rotated. The degree of resistance from normal to extreme rigidity is scored as detailed. The procedure is repeated with one hand palpating the shoulder cuff while rotation takes place.

    1 = Normal
    2 = Slight stiffness and resistance
    3 = Moderate stiffness and resistance
    4 = Marked rigidity with difficulty in passive movement
    5 = Extreme stiffness and rigidity with almost a frozen joint
    9 = Not ratable

4. **ELBOW RIGIDITY:** The elbow joints are separately bent at right angles and passively extended and flexed, with the subject's biceps observed and simultaneously palpated. The resistance to this procedure is rated.

    1 = Normal
    2 = Slight stiffness and resistance
    3 = Moderate stiffness and resistance
    4 = Marked rigidity with difficulty in passive movement
    5 = Extreme stiffness and rigidity with almost a frozen joint
    9 = Not ratable

FIGURE 32–1 Simpson Neurological Rating Scale.

5. **WRIST RIGIDITY:** The wrist is held in one hand and the fingers held by the examiner's other hand, with the wrist moved to extension, flexion and ulner and radial deviation or the extended wrist is allowed to fall under its own weight, or the arm can be grasped above the wrist and shaken to and fro. A ''1'' score would be a hand that extends easily, falls loosely, or flaps easily upwards and downwards.

    1 = Normal
    2 = Slight stiffness and resistance
    3 = Moderate stiffness and resistance
    4 = Marked rigidity with difficulty in passive movement
    5 = Extreme stiffness and rigidity with almost a frozen wrist
    9 = Not ratable

6. **HEAD ROTATION:** The patient sits or stands and is told that you are going to move his head from side to side, that it will not hurt and that he should try and relax. (Questions about pain in the cervical area or difficulty in moving his head should be obtained to avoid causing any pain.) Clasp the patient's head between the two hands with the fingers on the back of the neck. Gently rotate the head in a circular motion 3 times and evaluate the muscular resistance to this movement.

    1 = Loose, no resistance
    2 = Slight resistance to movement although the time to rotate may be normal
    3 = Resistance is apparent and the time of rotation is shortened
    4 = Resistance is obvious and rotation is slowed
    5 = Head appears stiff and rotation is difficult to carry out
    9 = Not ratable

7. **GLABELLAR TAP:** Subject is told to open eyes wide and not to blink. The glabellar region is tapped at a steady, rapid speed. Note number of times patient blinks in succession. Take care to stand behind the subject so that he does not observe the movement of the tapping finger. A full blink need not be observed; there may be contraction of the infraorbital muscle producing a twitch each time a stimulus is delivered. Vary speed of tapping to assure that muscle contraction is related to the tap.

    1 = 0-5 blinks
    2 = 6-10 blinks
    3 = 11-15 blinks
    4 = 16-20 blinks
    5 = 21 and more blinks
    9 = Not ratable

8. **TREMOR:** Patient is observed walking into examining room and then is re-examined for this item with arms extended at right angles to the body and the fingers spread out as far as possible.

    1 = Normal
    2 = Mild finger tremor, obvious to sight and touch
    3 = Tremor of hand or arm occurring spasmodically
    4 = Persistent tremor of one or more limbs
    5 = Whole body tremor
    9 = Not ratable

9. **SALIVATION:** Patient is observed while talking and then asked to open his mouth and elevate his tongue.

    1 = Normal
    2 = Excess salivation so that pooling takes place if mouth is open and tongue raised
    3 = Excess salivation is present and might occasionally result in difficulty in speaking
    4 = Speaking with difficulty because of excess salivation
    5 = Frank drooling
    9 = Not ratable

10. **AKATHISIA:** Patient is observed for restlessness. If restlessness is noted, ask: ''Do you feel restless or jittery inside; is it difficult to sit still?'' Subjective response is not necessary for scoring but patient report can help make the assessment.

    1 = No restlessness reported or observed
    2 = Mild restlessness observed, e.g., occasional jiggling of the foot occurs when patient is seated
    3 = Moderate restlessness observed, e.g., on several occasions, jiggles foot, crosses and uncrosses legs or twists a part of the body
    4 = Restlessness is frequently observed, e.g., the foot or legs moving most of the time
    5 = Restlessness persistently observed, e.g., patient cannot sit still, may get up and walk
    9 = Not ratable

	DEPARTMENT OF HEALTH AND HUMAN SERVICES PUBLIC HEALTH SERVICE Alcohol, Drug Abuse, and Mental Health Administration NIMH Treatment Strategies in Schizophrenia Study	PATIENT NUMBER	DATA GROUP	EVALUATION DATE

DEPARTMENT OF HEALTH AND HUMAN SERVICES
PUBLIC HEALTH SERVICE
Alcohol, Drug Abuse, and Mental Health Administration
NIMH Treatment Strategies in Schizophrenia Study

ABNORMAL INVOLUNTARY MOVEMENT SCALE (AIMS)

PATIENT NUMBER _ _ _ _   DATA GROUP aims   EVALUATION DATE _ _ - _ _ - _ _ (M M - D D - Y Y)

PATIENT NAME

RATER NAME

RATER NUMBER _ _ _

EVALUATION TYPE (Circle)

1 Baseline   4 Start double-blind   7 Start open meds   10 Early termination
2 2-week minor   5 Major evaluation   8 During open meds   11 Study completion
3   6 Other   9 Stop open meds

INSTRUCTIONS: Complete Examination Procedure (reverse side) before making ratings.
MOVEMENT RATINGS: Rate highest severity observed.

Code:
1 = None
2 = Minimal, may be extreme normal
3 = Mild
4 = Moderate
5 = Severe

			(Circle One)			
FACIAL AND ORAL MOVEMENTS:	1. **Muscles of Facial Expression** e.g., movements of forehead, eyebrows, periorbital area, cheeks; include frowning, blinking, smiling, grimacing	1	2	3	4	5
	2. **Lips and Perioral Area** e.g., puckering, pouting, smacking	1	2	3	4	5
	3. **Jaw** e.g., biting, clenching, chewing, mouth opening, lateral movement	1	2	3	4	5
	4. **Tongue** Rate only increase in movement both in and out of mouth, NOT inability to sustain movement	1	2	3	4	5
EXTREMITY MOVEMENTS:	5. **Upper** (arms, wrists, hands, fingers) Include choreic movements, (i.e., rapid, objectively purposeless, irregular, spontaneous), athetoid movements (i.e., slow, irregular, complex, serpentine). Do NOT include tremor (i.e., repetitive, regular, rhythmic)	1	2	3	4	5
	6. **Lower** (legs, knees, ankles, toes) e.g., lateral knee movement, foot tapping, heel dropping, foot squirming, inversion and eversion of foot	1	2	3	4	5
TRUNK MOVEMENTS:	7. **Neck, shoulders, hips** e.g., rocking, twisting, squirming, pelvic gyrations	1	2	3	4	5

GLOBAL JUDGMENTS:	8. Severity of abnormal movements	None, normal	1
		Minimal	2
		Mild	3
		Moderate	4
		Severe	5
	9. Incapacitation due to abnormal movements	None, normal	1
		Minimal	2
		Mild	3
		Moderate	4
		Severe	5
	10. Patient's awareness of abnormal movements Rate only patient's report	No awareness	1
		Aware, no distress	2
		Aware, mild distress	3
		Aware, moderate distress	4
		Aware, severe distress	5
DENTAL STATUS:	11. Current problems with teeth and/or dentures	No	1
		Yes	2
	12. Does patient usually wear dentures?	No	1
		Yes	2

ADM 9-117
11-85

FIGURE 32-2   Abnormal Involuntary Movement Scale (AIMS).

EXAMINATION PROCEDURE

Either before or after completing the Examination Procedure observe the patient unobtrusively, at rest (e.g., in waiting room).

The chair to be used in this examination should be a hard, firm one without arms.

---

1. Ask patient to remove shoes and socks.

2. Ask patient whether there is anything in his/her mouth (i.e., gum, candy, etc.) and if there is, to remove it.

3. Ask patient about the <u>current</u> condition of his/her teeth. Ask patient if he/she wears dentures. Do teeth or dentures bother patient <u>now</u>?

4. Ask patient whether he/she notices any movements in mouth, face, hands, or feet. If yes, ask to describe and to what extent they <u>currently</u> bother patient or interfere with his/her activities.

5. Have patient sit in chair with hands on knees, legs slightly apart, and feet flat on floor. (Look at entire body for movements while in this position.)

6. Ask patient to sit with hands hanging unsupported. If male, between legs, if female and wearing a dress, hanging over knees. (Observe hands and other body areas.)

7. Ask patient to open mouth. (Observe tongue at rest within mouth.) Do this twice.

8. Ask patient to protrude tongue. (Observe abnormalities of tongue movement.) Do this twice.

9. Ask patient to tap thumb, with each finger, as rapidly as possible for 10-15 seconds; separately with right hand, then with left hand. (Observe facial and leg movements.)

10. Flex and extend patient's left and right arms (one at a time). (Note any rigidity.)

11. Ask patient to stand up. (Observe in profile. Observe all body areas again, hips included.)

12. Ask patient to extend both arms outstretched in front with palms down. (Observe trunk, legs, and mouth.)

13. Have patient walk a few paces, turn, and walk back to chair. (Observe hands and gait.) Do this twice.

These conditions usually remit. One serious and permanent eye change is retinitis pigmentosa, which may occur in persons on doses of thioridazine exceeding 800 mg a day. This reaction may lead to blindness. Therefore, doses exceeding 800 mg per day are contraindicated.

Endocrine Effects   Lactation in females and gynecomastia and impotence in males lead a list of endocrine changes that can occur with antipsychotic drug treatments. The nurse should be alert to any changes in body functions reported by clients receiving such drugs.

Psychobiologic Considerations

Understanding the psychobiology of antipsychotic medications requires a basic knowledge of the functions of the central nervous system. An extended discussion of how neuroleptics work to reduce symptoms is beyond the scope of this chapter. Here is a brief overview of basic mechanisms of action. According to Tamminga and Gerlach (1987), drugs that modify psychosis may be symptom or symptom-complex specific, not disease specific. The authors exemplify this point by pointing out the differences in both positive and negative signs of schizophrenia and the very different response of these two distinct entities to psychopharmacologic intervention.

Generally, neuroleptics work by blocking a variety of amine receptors in the central nervous system. In other words, drugs such as antipsychotics do not work on only the neurotransmitter system. Conversely, it is likely that several types of neurotransmitters and neuromodulators are affected by the administration of a single medication. While most neuroleptics have affinity for several types of neurochemicals (e.g., dopamine, serotonin, histamine, and acetylcholine), others are more specific and work more selectively on particular neurochemicals. These differences account for the effects of the various neuroleptic medications.

Clinical Implications

Nurses have many responsibilities to clients receiving neuroleptic drugs. A primary responsibility is to be aware of the incompatibilities between neuroleptics and of the problems with administering neuroleptics with certain juices or liquids. Kerr (1986) points out that oral liquid neuroleptics are often mixed with juices or syrups. Because of the acid-base characteristics of the drug, precipitates may form and adhere to the containers or cups. The danger is obvious: potential underdosing. Kerr also points out that coffee, tea, or cola beverages, because of their tannic acid content, may decrease the effectiveness of neuroleptics. Table 32–5 is a chart of compatibilities between different neuroleptics and liquids.

Neuroleptic Malignant Syndrome   Derogatis (1986) cites an infrequently noted complication of high-potency drugs (e.g., fluphenazine, thiothixene, haloperidol) known as **neuroleptic malignant syndrome.** This extreme condition occurs in clients who are severely ill and is believed to be the result of dopamine blockade in the hypothalamus. Nurses are in the best position to assess for this condition because it presents with symptoms of diaphoresis, muscle rigidity, and hyperpyrexia. Mutism is a prominent symptom of this condition. If cooling and rehydration are not achieved quickly, the client may die. Because neuroleptic malignant syndrome often occurs in persons whose presentations are already complex, the nursing assessment can be difficult. The clinical example below illustrates this serious side effect.

Alicia is a 22-year-old woman admitted to the in-patient psychiatric unit of a general hospital for treatment of bipolar disorder, manic. Prior to her admission, she had been taking 600 mg of lithium carbonate twice daily, which adequately controlled her symptoms. Two weeks ago her father was killed in an automobile accident. Since the funeral, Alicia has had a sleep disturbance evidenced by a need for only three hours of sleep per night. Her thoughts began racing five days prior to admission, and two days ago she began hearing the voice of her father "telling me to join him by jumping out of a fourth story window."

On admission to the unit, the physician prescribed lithium at the above noted dose, with orders for a lithium level to be drawn the next day. Additionally, the physician ordered haloperidol (Haldol), 5 mg by mouth twice daily, and alprazolam (Xanax), 0.5 mg every four hours by mouth as needed for agitation. On the fourth day of her hospitalization, Alicia began to demonstrate increasing agitation and psychotic thought. Nurses working with her administered the maximum number of doses of alprazolam allowed under the physician's orders. Recognizing that the psychotic agitation was becoming worse despite the medication, the physician increased the haloperidol dose to 8 mg twice daily. A day later the agitation was still worsening, and the haloperidol dose was again increased to 10 mg twice daily. On the eighth day of the hospitalization, nursing staff recognized that Alicia had extrapyramidal side effects. They reported this to the physician, who in turn ordered benztropine mesylate (Cogentin), 2 mg by mouth twice daily. The side effects worsened, as did the client's mental status. At this point, she rambled incoherently, drooled, was extremely diaphoretic, exhibited significant muscle rigidity, and had a fever of 39.5C (treated symptomatically). The hyperpyrexia led the treatment team to believe that Alicia had developed neuroleptic malignant syndrome.

All neuroleptic medications were stopped immediately. An intravenous line provided Alicia with needed hydration and some calories, as she was unable to cooperate with eating. She required total nursing care for 72 hours, at which time her mental status began improving and she re-engaged in her own care.

TABLE 32–5   Compatible Liquid Vehicles for the Common Neuroleptic Agents and Lithium Citrate

C = Generally compatible together
X = Incompatible: DO NOT MIX
Blank = No information available—chose "C" liquid to dilute

Oral Liquid Neuroleptics	Liquids					Fruit Juices												Carbonated Liquids					Oral Liquid Neuroleptics				
	Water	Saline	Milk	Coffee	Tea	Apple juice or cider	Apricot	Cranberry	Grape juice or drink	Grapefruit	Lemonade, reconst. frozen	Orange juice	Pineapple	Prune	Tang	Tomato	V-8	Cola (Coke, Pepsi, etc.)	Mellow-Yellow	Orange	7-Up, Sprite	Soups, Pudding	Chlorpromazine	Haloperidol	Lithium citrate	Thioridazine	Trifluoperazine
Chlorpromazine (generics, Thorazine)	C		C	C*	C*			X		C		C			X	X	C		C		C	C	C		X		
Fluphenazine (Prolixin)	C	C	C	X	X	X	C			C		C	C	C		C	C	X			C	C					
Haloperidol (Haldol)	C	X		X	X	C						C				C		C							X		
Lithium citrate (generic)	C	C	C	C	C	C	C	C	C	C	C	C	C	C	C	C	C	C	C	C	C	C	C	X	X	X	X
Loxapine (Loxitane)										C		C		C					C		C						
Perphenazine (Trilafon)	C	C	C	X	X	X	C			C		C	C	C		C	C	X			C	C					
Thioridazine 30 mg/mL (Mellaril)	X		X	X	X		C	X		C†	C	C**				X	X	X	C		C				X		
Thiothixene (Navane)	C		C			X	C	C		C		C	C	C		C	C	X									
Trifluoperazine (generic, Stelazine)	C		C	C	C					C		C	C	C		C	C	C	C	C	C	C			X		

*Data differs with brand—avoid if using generics.
† Canned only, not frozen concentrate.
** Canned OJ only.

SOURCE: From "Oral Liquid Neuroleptics" by Lisa E. Kerr as appeared in the Journal of Psychosocial Nursing and Mental Health Services, March, 1986.

Client Teaching As for any other medication, client teaching is essential for clients receiving neuroleptic medication. A medication teaching plan for antipsychotics is presented in the Client/Family Teaching Box on pages 782–783.

Antidepressant Drugs

Background

Like the antipsychotic drugs, the major antidepressant drugs were discovered accidentally. Two classes of antidepressants currently exist: tricyclic antidepressants and monoamine oxidase inhibitor antidepressants. In the case of imipramine (Tofranil), the first of the tricyclic antidepressants, investigators were actually searching for effective antipsychotics similar to chlorpromazine. Iproniazid, a monoamine oxidase inhibitor (MAOI), was discovered when tuberculous clients regularly treated with a similar drug, isoniazid, became less depressed. The antidepressants have shed considerable light on the biochemical mechanisms of the brain in both normal and abnormal emotional expression.

The initial distinction to be understood in the psychopharmacology of depression is between true antidepressants and stimulants or euphoriants. The tricyclic antidepressants (TCA) and the MAOI are not stimulants and will not induce euphoria in normal persons but, in a single dose, have a sedative effect. Amphetamines and methylphenidate (Ritalin), on the other hand, are stimulants but not antidepressants in the pharmacologic sense. They can induce an increased sense of well-being in certain individuals, but they do nothing to combat depression on a lasting basis.

MAOI are considered the "first generation" of antidepressant medications; that is, they were among the first medications identified as effective in the treatment of depression. Since these drugs appeared on the psychopharmacologic treatment horizon, yet another generation of antidepressant medications has become available (see Table 32–6). Although one of these drugs, nonifensine, is no longer available in the United States (due to documented, serious side effects), another drug, bupropion (Wellbutrin) is being used.

CLIENT/FAMILY TEACHING

Medication Teaching Plan: Antipsychotics

Brand Name: _____

Generic Name: _____

Administration: Your medication is taken by mouth or by injection.

Purpose: Your medication provides relief from your symptoms so you are able to participate in activities, use therapy more effectively, and take better care of yourself.

Target Symptoms: Your medication will decrease some symptoms you are having, such as: _____

Report any sore throat, fever, increased fatigue, vomiting, diarrhea, skin rash, or unusual body movements to your nurse and doctor. If you are pregnant, or think you may be pregnant, discuss this with your doctor. Sudden stoppage of your medication may result in a return of symptoms or other side effects. Discuss any decision about stopping medications with your doctor.

Other special instructions (if any): _____

_____

_____

_____

The material, on both sides of this form, has been presented to me and discussed with me by: _____

Client's Signature _____ Date _____

Air, Food, Fluid

Dry mouth — Rinse mouth with water.
Brush teeth more frequently.
Chew sugarless candy/gum.
Apply Chapstick to your lips and nostrils.

Nasal stuffiness — Avoid use of over-the-counter nasal sprays/drops.

Weight gain — Eat less sugar, starch, and fats.
Increase protein intake.
Exercise daily.
Follow a diet prescribed by your doctor.

Elimination

Difficulty urinating — Drink 6–8 glasses of fluid each day.
Notify your nurse and doctor.
Do relaxation exercises to promote urination.
Apply warm water to genital area.
Take a lukewarm shower.
Listen to running water.

Constipation — Drink 6–8 glasses of fluid each day.
Eat green vegetables and bran each day.
Exercise daily.
Eat prunes or raisins.
Take laxative medication only with your doctor's advice.
Notify your nurse and doctor.

Personal Hygiene and Body Temperature

Decrease of normal bacteria in mouth may result in infection — Avoid foods high in sugar.
Observe your tongue for signs of thick white coating.
Increase mouth care including brushing tongue and gargling with mouthwash.

Increased sensitivity to the heat and decreased sweating — Shower in lukewarm water.
Avoid exertion in hot weather.
Dress appropriately for environmental conditions.
Take own oral temperature.
Avoid temperature extremes such as hot tubs.

CLIENT/FAMILY TEACHING (continued)

Personal Hygiene and Body Temperature

Greater chance of a bad sunburn	Use sunscreen and Chapstick when out in the sun. Wear clothes that protect skin, including a hat. Wear sunglasses.
Vaginal dryness	Use lubricant such as K-Y jelly.
Menstrual period may stop	Notify your nurse and doctor. Continue to use birth control.
General changes in interest in sex	Notify your nurse and doctor.
Decreased moisture around eyes	Use extra caution if you wear contact lenses to avoid eye irritation.

Rest/Activity

Dizziness	Lie down and rest. Get up slowly from lying position; dangle legs over edge of bed. Have nurse check blood pressure.
Drowsiness	Drive your car or other vehicles with extra care. Avoid alcoholic beverages or street drugs.

	Plan for extra rest time. Avoid other medications unless approved by your doctor.
Muscle tightness/ cramping in arms, legs, neck, or face	Notify your nurse and doctor. Take medications for side effects.
Compulsion to keep moving and inability to sit down; restlessness	Notify your nurse and doctor. Take medication for side effects.
Blurred vision	Use a magnifying glass for reading.
Eye pain in sunlight	Wear sunglasses out of doors.

Solitude/Socialization

Understanding of illness and medications	Talk with your nurse and doctor to identify symptoms that are part of your illness or side effects from your medication.
Decreased interest in surroundings and usual activities	Discuss this feeling with your nurse and doctor.

SOURCE: Adapted from Langley Porter Psychiatric Institute Hospital and Clinics, 1984. University of California, San Francisco.

TABLE 32–6 Antidepressant "Generations"

First Generation	Second Generation
Imipramine (Tofranil)	Maprotiline (Ludiomil)
Amitriptyline (Elavil)	Amoxapine (Asendin)
Desipramine (Norpramin)	Trazodone (Desyrel)
Nortriptyline (Aventyl)	Bupropion (Wellbutrin)
Protriptyline (Vivactil)	Nonifensine* (Merital)

*Nonifensine, while still available in Europe and Canada, was completely recalled in the United States by the Food and Drug Administration. The reasons cited for the recall involved the reporting of untoward side effects related to the use of nonifensine.

Bupropion is a nonsedating drug (Massachusetts General Hospital 1985a). It also has few anticholinergic side effects and essentially no important cardiovascu-

lar effects and has not so far seemed to cause postural hypotension. Of note, however, is that this drug lowers the seizure threshold. This effect is dose related. Nurses must keep this in mind during assessment especially of clients with seizure disorders. Although this drug has not yet had the "test of time," it seems likely to be helpful for clients who are unable to tolerate other antidepressant medications.

A newcomer to the psychopharmacologic scene is the antidepressant medication fluoxetine (Prozac). This medication has received great attention both in the professional literature and in the common press. Fluoxetine is a potent and highly specific reuptake blocker of the neurotransmitter serotonin; the only other medication that is similar in action is trazodone (Desyrel) (Perry et al. 1989). Although the initial reports on the effectiveness of this medication are very promising, it too needs further investigation before it is fully established in the field of psychopharmacology. The advantage of this drug is its side-effect profile, which is quite low, making it an ideal drug for those who cannot tolerate the more severe side effects of the tricyclic antidepressants.

Nursing Responsibilities When Clients Receive Uncommon Drug Combinations

In the early 1980s, physicians began to prescribe combinations of antidepressants for clients who had received no relief of depressive symptoms with a single antidepressant medication. Unfortunately, some clients still did not respond, and these treatment-resistant clients received either TCA/MAOI combinations, antidepressant and stimulants, or combinations of all three classes of drugs, with predominant improvement (Massachusetts General Hospital 1985b). However, some clients experienced elevated blood pressure, while others experienced orthostatic hypotension. While no clients in this group experienced a hyptertensive crisis, the possibility existed. Other clinically significant side effects included dizziness, nausea, impaired memory, insomnia, confusion, and hypomania.

Several other unusual drug combinations are becoming more popular. For example, Pope et al. (1988) discuss the use of fluoxetine and lithium in those who have depressions that have been refractory to treatment with several types of medications, including fluoxetine alone. The authors found that lithium augmentation may represent a useful strategy in dealing with refractory depression. Additionally, it is not uncommon for physicians to augment neuroleptic use with medications from the benzodiazepine class, commonly alprazolam (Xanax). These combinations reduce anxiety and the discomfort associated with both positive and negative symptoms (Douyan et al. 1989). The client is not only potentially more comfortable but, with benzodiazepine supplementation rather than neuroleptic increase, also at lower risk for long-term effects, such as tardive dyskinesia.

As drug combinations and innovative psychobiologic therapies become more commonplace in the practice of psychiatry, psychiatric nurses are going to need to be more observant for idiosyncratic responses among clients. Planning and implementing care for this specialized subpopulation of clients are likely to be challenging, and nurses need to be aware of the underlying psychobiology to recognize potential drug-related behaviors among clients on multiple drug regimens.

Clinical Considerations in Use

The most important clinical consideration in the use of medications to treat depression is that antidepressant drugs are not effective in all cases of depressed mood. Evidence from research and clinical practice indicates that only a portion of depressive disorders respond to this class of drugs. For example, TCA, MAOI, and amphetamines are generally contraindicated in depression resulting from what commonly has been referred to as grief reaction or pathologic grief. Other types of depression, described in the DSM-III-R, may be more amenable to psychopharmacologic intervention. Thus, accurate diagnosis is necessary to ensure maximum effectiveness.

Persons for whom antidepressants are indicated usually suffer from characteristic symptoms: a severely depressed mood, loss of interests, inability to respond to normally pleasurable events or situations, a depression that is worst in the morning and lessens slightly as the day goes by, early morning awakening (and inability to fall asleep again), marked psychomotor retardation or agitation, significant anorexia and weight loss, and excessive or inappropriate guilt. DSM-III-R calls this melancholia. In fact, the symptoms of melancholia are the features that most reliably predict response to drug therapy. A significant, and commonly overlooked, clinical consideration is that antidepressants have a delayed reaction onset. A client will not show lessening of depressed mood until two to three weeks after the institution of an adequate dose of tricyclic antidepressants, for example.

Tricyclic Antidepressants

By far the most important and most commonly used class of antidepressant drugs is the tricyclics. These compounds are close in chemical structure to the phenothiazines and have many similar side effects, but they have profoundly different effects on mood, behavior, and cognition. Tricyclic antidepressants are not antipsychotic agents when given to schizophrenic persons and may in fact aggravate a disintegrative pattern or precipitate overt symptoms in a client with latent disintegrative behavior. Imipramine (Tofranil) and amitriptyline (Elavil) are the two prime representatives of tricyclic antidepressants. Desipramine (Norpramin, Pertofrane), nortriptyline (Pamelor), and protriptyline (Vivactil) are compounds prepared in simpler forms (similar to the conversions made in normal metabolism) that are reported to reduce the incidence of side effects.

Dosage What constitutes an adequate dose of tricyclics is a matter of debate, but most clinicians agree that the bulk of responsive clients with a major depression need doses of 150 to 250 mg per day. Some may respond to as little as 75 mg and some require 400 mg, but these are exceptional doses.

A client is ordinarily started on 25 mg of a tricyclic antidepressant three times a day for two days, and the dosage is increased by 25 to 50 percent every other day, until 200 or 250 mg is reached or intolerable side effects are encountered. Common clinical practice is to use imipramine in the presence of motor retardation and amitriptyline with agitated clients because it has a more sedative effect. Once the client's dosage is established, it can be converted to a single bed-time dose. This practice frequently precludes the need for insomnia medication. The onset of action takes seven to ten days. Although full improvement may take as long as four weeks, a gradual lessening of the symptoms will become apparent in those who are going to respond.

After remission of the symptoms, clients who are put on a reduced maintenance dose (perhaps 50 percent of the acute dosage) show less likelihood of relapse. Therefore, most clients are continued on treatment for six months to one year following a major depressive episode. Clients who have had repeated episodes may require longer drug maintenance or should be considered for lithium carbonate treatment because of its prophylactic effects on recurrent major depression and the depressive episodes of bipolar disorder.

Most depressive clients who do not respond to tricyclic antidepressants suffer from a form of illness that is not of the melancholic type. These may include so-called neurotic or characterologic depressions, termed *dysthymic disorder* in DSM-III-R. Other clients do not reach or maintain effective blood levels of the drugs even when given adequate daily doses because of idiosyncrasies in their metabolic processes. However, tricyclic blood levels can be measured and doses increased until an effective blood level is obtained.

Side Effects Many of the common side effects of the tricyclic drugs are autonomic due to the anticholinergic characteristics of the medications. These side effects include dry mouth, blurred vision, constipation, palpitations, and urinary retention. Clients with glaucoma must be treated with caution. Some allergic skin reactions have been observed. Tricyclics also cause changes in the normal electrical conduction of the heart, which is particularly significant in treating persons with a history of cardiovascular disease, especially heart block. Sudden death has occurred during tricyclic treatment. Clients with known heart disease and most elderly clients require electrocardiograms before, and periodically during, the course of tricyclic therapy. Several other central nervous system effects may occur, including tremor, twitching, paresthesias, ataxia, and convulsions.

Overdose Effects One aspect of tricyclic treatment that deserves attention is the consequences of an overdose. Significant overdoses may cause delirium; hyperthermia; convulsions; and even coma, shock, and respiratory failure. A lethal dose of an antidepressant such as amitriptyline is estimated at between ten and thirty times the usual daily therapeutic dose. Drug intake deserves close attention, since many of the clients treated with these drugs are severely suicidal. Serious overdosage is a medical emergency and may require heroic resuscitative measures. When the nurse reports delirium and peripheral autonomic symptoms of anticholinergic poisoning due to mild overdose, the psychiatrist can intervene with intravenous or intramuscular physostigmine (0.2 or 0.4 mg), an anticholinesterase that will reverse the delirium and other symptoms at lest transiently.

Client Teaching The Client/Family Teaching box on pages 786–787 outlines the main side effects of tricyclic antidepressants and self-care measures to counteract side effects experienced by the client.

Monoamine Oxidase Inhibitors

Clients who do not respond to tricyclic antidepressants may respond to the other major class, MAOI. These drugs generally are not as effective as tricyclics and are somewhat slower to act, sometimes requiring a month of treatment before improvement shows. Isocarboxazid (Marplan) is considered the most effective, with phenelzine (Nardil) and tranylcypromine (Parnate) slightly behind. Complicating the decision to use MAOI is their association with several very severe side effects. Hepatic necrosis, commonly fatal, and **hypertensive crisis** leading to intracranial bleeding are among the most threatening. The latter reaction, heralded by severe headache, stiff neck, nausea, vomiting, and sharply increased blood pressure, follows the ingestion of foods that contain the amino acid tyramine and of sympathomimetic medications.

Client Teaching The MAOI antidepressants require an especially strong, concerted teaching effort from nurses. These medications have many drawbacks that directly affect nursing intervention. For example, clients on MAOI antidepressants *must* avoid foods that contain even moderate amounts of tyramine; failure to do so results in hypertensive crisis. The Client/Family Teaching box on pages 788–790 outlines the low-tyramine diet and shows a teaching plan for the client receiving MAOI antidepressants.

The principles guiding the use of MAOI and TCA medications are as follows:

• Drug treatment does not preclude psychotherapy, electroconvulsive therapy, or behavioral treatments if they are also indicated.

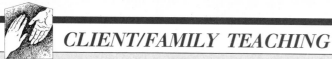

CLIENT/FAMILY TEACHING

Medication Teaching Plan: Tricyclic Antidepressants

Brand Name: _____

Generic Name: _____

Administration: Your medication is taken by mouth.

Purpose: Your medication provides relief from your symptoms so you are able to participate in activities, use therapy more effectively, and take better care of yourself. Initially you may experience some sedation. The antidepressant effects occur in about 7–28 days.

Target Symptoms: Your medication will decrease some symptoms you are having, such as: _____
_____

Report any sore throat, fever, increased fatigue, vomiting, diarrhea, skin rash, or unusual body movements to your nurse and doctor. If you are pregnant, or think you may be pregnant, discuss this with your doctor. Sudden stoppage of your medication may result in a return of symptoms or other side effects. Discuss any decision about stopping medications with your doctor.

Other special instructions (if any): _____
_____
_____
_____
_____

The material, on both sides of this form, has been presented to me and discussed with me by: _____

Client's Signature _____ Date _____

Air, Food, Fluid

Dry mouth	Rinse mouth with water. Brush teeth more frequently. Chew sugarless candy/gum. Apply Chapstick to your lips and nostrils.
Nausea, vomiting, poor appetite	Eat crackers, toast, drink tea. Drink protein supplement to maintain weight.
Weight gain	Eat less sugar, starch, and fats. Increase protein intake. Exercise daily. Follow a diet prescribed by your doctor.

Elimination

Difficulty urinating	Drink 6–8 glasses of fluid each day. Notify your nurse and doctor. Do relaxation exercises to promote urination. Apply warm water to genital area. Take lukewarm shower. Listen to running water.

Constipation	Drink 6–8 glasses of fluid each day. Eat green vegetables and bran each day. Exercise daily. Eat prunes or raisins. Take laxative medication only with your doctor's advice. Notify your nurse and doctor.

Personal Hygiene and Body Temperature

Decrease of normal bacteria in mouth may result in infection	Avoid foods high in sugar. Observe your tongue for signs of thick white coating. Increase mouth care including brushing tongue and gargling with mouthwash.
Increased sensitivity to the heat and decreased sweating	Shower in lukewarm water. Avoid exertion in hot weather. Dress appropriately for environmental conditions. Take own oral temperature.

CLIENT/FAMILY TEACHING (continued)

Personal Hygiene and Body Temperature

	Avoid temperature extremes such as hot tubs.
Greater chance of a bad sunburn	Use sunscreen and Chapstick when out in the sun.
	Wear clothes that protect skin, including a hat.
	Wear sunglasses.
Vaginal dryness	Use lubricant such as K-Y jelly.
Menstrual period may stop	Notify your nurse and doctor.
	Continue to use birth control.
General changes in interest in sex	Notify your nurse and doctor.
Decreased moisture around eyes	Use extra caution if you wear contact lenses to avoid eye irritation.

Rest/Activity

Dizziness	Lie down and rest.
	Get up slowly from lying position; dangle legs over edge of bed.
	Have nurse check blood pressure.
Drowsiness	Drive your car or other vehicles with extra care.
	Avoid alcoholic beverages or street drugs.
	Plan for extra rest time.

	Avoid other medications unless approved by your doctor.
Muscle tightness/ cramping in arms, legs, neck, or face	Notify your nurse and doctor.
	Take medications for side effects.
Compulsion to keep moving and inability to sit down; restlessness	Notify your nurse and doctor.
	Take medication for side effects.
Blurred vision	Use a magnifying glass for reading.
Eye pain in sunlight	Wear sunglasses out of doors.

Solitude/Socialization

Understanding of illness and medications	Talk with your nurse and doctor to identify symptoms that are part of your illness or side effects from your mediation.
Decreased interest in surroundings and usual activities	Discuss this feeling with your nurse and doctor.

SOURCE: Adapted from Langley Porter Psychiatric Institute Hospital and Clinics, 1984. University of California, San Francisco.

• Tricyclic treatment should be given first unless there are contraindications, clinical indications for MAOI, or a past history of unresponsiveness to tricyclic antidepressants.

• The usual therapeutic range is 150 to 300 mg per day. Dosage may vary and may be limited by significant side effects.

• A response is seen two or three weeks after the therapeutic dose is reached.

• Clients with recurrent major depressive episodes with melancholia may require long-term maintenance treatment, although doses are usually lower than those needed in acute episodes.

Nursing Considerations with "Second-Generation" Antidepressants

The second-generation antidepressants were the result of a scientific search for drugs with fewer toxic side effects and greater biologic predictability in the treatment of depression (Coccaro and Siever 1985). They are believed to be more neurotransmitter specific and better able to treat conditions related to dopamine, serotonin, or nonadrenergic dysfunctions. The following medications exemplify the new drug classification:

• Trazodone (Desyrel)—triazolopyridine derivative

• Maprotiline (Ludiomil)—tetracyclic

• Amoxapine (Asendin)—tricyclic dibenzoxazepine

Medication Teaching Plan: MAO Inhibitors

Brand Name: _____
Generic Name: _____
Administration: Your medication is taken by mouth.
Purpose: Your medication provides relief from your symptoms so you are able to participate in activities, use therapy more effectively, and take better care of yourself. It may take several days to a few weeks for you to feel less anxious, more optimistic, and more in control.
Target Symptoms: Your medication will decrease some symptoms you are having, such as: _____

Report the following symptoms to your doctor: rapid heartbeat, frequent headaches, yellowing of eyes or skin, severe increases or decreases in blood pressure. If you are pregnant or think you may become pregnant, report this to your doctor.

In general, tell any doctor who is prescribing medication for you that you are taking this medication and check over-the-counter medications with your therapist. If a severe, sudden, or unusual headache develops, it may be a symptom of a rise in blood pressure. Notify your doctor immediately.
Other special instructions (if any): _____
_____
_____
_____
_____

The material, on both sides of this form, has been presented to me and discussed with me by: _____
Client's Signature _____ Date _____

Air, Food, Fluid

Dry mouth	Rinse mouth with water. Brush teeth more frequently. Chew sugarless candy/gum. Apply Chapstick to your lips and nostrils.	Limitations on certain foods	Discuss diet limitations with nurse or doctor. Refer to the low-tyramine diet for foods to avoid. Determine substitute food choices. Continue food and drug limits for 10 days after stopping the medication.
Nausea, vomiting, poor appetite	Eat crackers, toast, drink tea. Drink protein supplement to maintain weight.		
Weight gain	Eat less sugar, starch, and fats. Increase protein intake. Exercise daily. Avoid over-the-counter reducing pills. Follow a diet prescribed by your doctor.	**Elimination**	
		Constipation	Drink 6–8 glasses of fluid each day. Eat green vegetables and bran every day. Exercise every day. Take laxative medications only with your doctor's advice. Notify your nurse and doctor.
Limitations on over-the-counter drug use	Avoid cold/hay fever medications. Avoid weight-reducing medications.		
Severe, sudden, or unusual headache due to increased blood pressure	Follow attached diet to prevent problem. Report headache to your doctor immediately.	**Personal Hygiene and Body Temperature**	
		Flushing/sweating	Take lukewarm showers.

▶

Rest/Activity

Dizziness	Lie down and rest.
	Get up slowly from lying position; dangle legs over edge of bed.
	Have nurse check blood pressure.
Drowsiness	Drive your car or other vehicles with extra care.
	Avoid alcoholic beverages or street drugs.
	Plan for extra rest time.
	Take medication at bedtime.

Swelling in legs or feet	Eat less salt, salty foods.
	Sit with feet raised.
	Practice careful skin care.

Solitude/Socialization

Confusion/poor memory	Discuss this with your doctor or nurse.
Understanding of your illness and medication	Talk with your nurse and doctor to identify symptoms that are part of your illness or side effects from your medication.

Low-Tyramine Diet

The MAO inhibitors combine with certain foods and medications to produce a significant increase in your blood pressure, which can be a health problem. In general, foods that can cause this reaction are ones that have been pickled, fermented, smoked, or aged. The list below includes the main foods and medications to avoid while you are taking this medication and for two weeks after discontinuing this medication.

Food and beverages to avoid completely:

Meats and fish:
  Pickled herring
  Dried fish
  Unrefrigerated fermented fish
  Liver
  Caviar
  Fermented sausage (bologna, salami, pepperoni summer sausage)

Sauce
  Hoisin (fermented oyster sauce used in Oriental dishes)

Vegetables:
  English broad beans
  Chinese pea pods
  Fava beans

Dairy products:
  Most cheeses (exceptions listed below)
  Yogurt

Beverages:
  Chianti, aged red wines
  Imported, aged beers

Combination foods
  Pizza
  Lasagna
  Souffles
  Macaroni and cheese
  Quiche
  Pate (liver)
  Caesar salad
  Eggplant parmesan

Also:
  All yeast extracts (e.g., Marmite) and all yeast preparations (e.g., brewer's yeast)

Food and beverages to avoid taking in large amounts:

Dairy products:
  Processed American Cheese

Fruits:
  Raisins
  Prunes
  Bananas
  Avocados
  Plums
  Canned figs

Caffeine sources:
  Coffee
  Chocolate
  Colas

Beverages:
  Domestic jug red wines
  Domestic beers, ales, and stouts
  Sherry

Food and beverages that may be taken without problems:

Diary products:
  Cottage cheese
  Cream cheese
  Milk, cream, and ice cream

▶

CLIENT/FAMILY TEACHING (continued)

Low-Tyramine diet (continued)

Food and beverages that may be taken without problems:
Beverages:
  White wines
Also:
  Any baked goods raised with yeast

Medications to avoid:
  Cold medications
  Nasal decongestants (tablets, drops, or sprays)
  Hay fever medications
  Weight-reducing preparations, "pep pills"
  Antiappetite medications
  Asthma inhalants

SOURCE: Adapted from Langley Porter Psychiatric Institute Hospital and Clinics, 1984. University of California, San Francisco.

Coccaro and Siever (1985) point out that the second-generation antidepressants are as efficient in decreasing depressive symptoms as imipramine or amitriptyline. The side effects of these medications are generally less than those of the first-generation antidepressants. However, nurses need to continue assessing signs of anticholinergic activity, cardiovascular effects, and effects on a given individual to perform psychomotor tasks.

Other Drugs

Stimulants, such as amphetamines and methylphenidate (Ritalin), and the phenothiazines are less commonly used antidepressants. Stimulants are not a proven treatment. Phenothiazines may be particularly useful in the presence of agitation. Some clinicians and researchers believe that major depressive episodes with psychotic features (delusional depressions) respond better to a combination of an antidepressant and an antipsychotic agent or to electroconvulsive therapy (ECT) than to antidepressants alone. Others simply recommend higher-than-usual doses of antidepressants.

Psychobiology of Depression

Chapter 13 gives an overview of the current psychobiologic theories of depression. Knowledge of the pharmacology of the antidepressants has led to a theory of the biochemistry of depression. Basically, all the true antidepressants make the neurotransmitter substances norepinephrine (NE) and serotonin (5-HT) more available to the synaptic receptors in the central nervous system. Tricyclics block the reuptake of these substances into the neuron after their release, thereby

postponing their degradation. The MAOI interfere with the enzymes responsible for the actual breakdown of the neurotransmitters. Since both are antidepressants, these observations have led to the theory that NE and 5-HT shortages in the brain cause depression, at least the type of depression that responds to drug therapy. Refer to Chapter 13 for a more detailed discussion of this topic. The accompanying Client/Family Teaching box details a teaching plan to be used with clients undergoing the dexamethasone suppression test, an examination of psychoendocrine function in light of depressive behavior.

The Antimania Drug (Lithium)

Background

The psychopharmacologic treatment of conditions labeled mania has become virtually synonymous with lithium carbonate therapy in the United States in the past ten years. Many well-controlled clinical studies indicate unequivocally that lithium is the most effective agent for treating the vast majority of acute manic and hypomanic episodes. In addition, because of the absence of sedative side effects, the client feels much more related to the environment and able to function normally while under the influence of lithium.

In the last few years, several drugs have been added to the list of pharmacologic treatments for bipolar disorder. Of special interest is the use of carbamazepine (Tegretol) as a treatment to control bipolar symptoms in people who either cannot take lithium or do not respond therapeutically to it. Approximately 30 percent of clients with bipolar

CLIENT/FAMILY TEACHING

Dexamethasone Suppression Test Information

For: _____ Date: _____

Therapists often order a test called the *Dexamethasone Suppression Test* (DST). The results of this test are useful to staff in making decisions about medications to control depressive symptoms. Some forms of depression are associated with a hormonal imbalance in the body that may respond favorably to certain antidepressant medications. Your therapist has ordered the DST for you. This sheet tells you what you can expect during the two-day period required to complete the test.

On the first day of the test, a technician will draw a small amount of your blood at 4:00 P.M. The purpose of this test is to measure a hormone in your blood known as *cortisol*. On the evening of the first day at 11:30 P.M., you will receive a very small dose (1 mg) of *dexamethasone*. The 1 mg of dexamethasone should not cause any side effects, but may cause a *decrease* in your blood level of *cortisol*. On the day after you receive the

dexamethasone, your blood level of cortisol will be measured two separate times—once at 4:00 P.M. and again at 11:00 P.M. The results of this test will be used, along with other information about you, by your therapist and the treatment team to plan your treatment with you.

If you have further questions about the DST or depression, ask your primary care nurse or primary therapist. Your primary therapist will let you know the results of your test.

1. *Cortisol test:* Blood drawn at 4:00 P.M. on (date) _____

2. *Dexamethasone:* 1 mg at 11:30 P.M. on (date) _____

3. *Cortisol test:* Blood drawn at 4:00 P.M. on (date) _____

4. *Cortisol test:* Blood drawn at 11:00 P.M. on (date) _____

This was explained to me by _____

SOURCE: *Adapted from Langley Porter Psychiatric Institute and Clinics, 1985. University of California, San Francisco.*

disorders do not respond to lithium, and up to 50 percent of responders may experience bipolar symptom relapses while taking maintenance doses of lithium (Massachusetts General Hospital 1985b).

Recent reports address a psychobiologic phenomenon known as kindling, and relate this process to aberrant activity in the limbic system, which is often called the emotional brain. Some psychobiologists believe that the characteristic behaviors of bipolar disorder are reflective of underlying limbic system dysfunction. Carbamazepine is chemically similar to the tricyclic imipramine, and it blocks the return of select neurotransmitters (norepinephrine). Such action may be the psychobiologic reason that carbamazepine has the potential effect on behaviors of the bipolar spectrum. Derogatis (1986) also points out that carbamazepine is used in the treatment of such conditions as alcohol withdrawal syndrome, explosive personality, and impulse disorders and in pain management and seizure control. One can only speculate on the underlying psychobiology of these disorders and wonder if the etiologies are similar, possibly involving a phenomenon such as limbic kindling.

Recognizing the potential effectiveness of carbamazepine in select mood disorders, other physicians prescribe another seizure medication, valproic acid amide, to treat clients with diagnoses of bipolar effective disorder or schizoaffective disorder. Valproic acid and verapamil, both calcium channel blockers, currently are also used to control affective symptoms. Possibly such innovative uses of various medications will yield valuable information concerning the underlying psychobiology of behavioral disturbances, especially effectively related conditions.

Despite these advances, lithium continues to be the first-line pharmacologic intervention for the treatment of bipolar affective disorder and, more recently, cyclic unipolar depressions or "rapid cycling," a condition in which bipolar cycles occur at unusually brief intervals.

Dosage

The management of an acute manic episode involves rapid initiation of lithium, increased to substantial doses during the first week of treatment. Usually between 1500 and 2100 mg per day are needed by the average-size client in an acute period. Lithium is available only in oral form in 250, 300, and 450 mg capsules and time-released tablets or as a liquid known as lithium citrate. Since lithium is an ion, its concentration can be measured in the blood. In the acute phase the blood level usually must attain a concentration of 1.0 to 1.5 mEq/L. After a week to ten days, as the bipolar symptoms subside, the dose can be decreased to 900 to 1200 mg per day, with the blood level maintained in the range of 0.6 to 1.2 mEq/L for continuing control.

The basic principles for antimania drug therapy are as follows:

• Lithium is indicated and effective in the treatment of acute manic episodes and in the prevention of recurrent manic or depressive episodes, cyclic unipolar depression, or "rapid cycling."

• Lithium is usually given in divided doses with increases in daily dose until the blood level reaches 1.0–1.5 mEq/L in acute stages of the disorder. Blood levels must be monitored after each increase.

• Antipsychotic medications may be necessary early in the course of treatment for behavior control.

• Blood levels are checked every two to three months or when there is a behavioral reason to suspect a change.

The following clinical example demonstrates the appropriate use of lithium in the case of a client suffering from bipolar disorder.

Walt, a 23-year-old musician, came for treatment after losing his job in a Broadway show. His producer had fired him because he was irritable and argumentative and seemed to refuse to concentrate on his pieces during rehearsals, instead roaming around the stage giving unsolicited advice to others. His wife had called the mental health center in desperation, claiming that Walt was pacing the apartment talking out of his head and that he seemed totally unconcerned about losing his job. The previous day he had been admitted and discharged against medical advice from a local hospital, where he had received chlorpromazine.

On observation, Walt exhibited pressured speech with grandiose ideas, an irritable mood, and inability to sit in the chair in the interviewing room. His family history revealed that his father had lost many jobs and had been taking lithium for the past five years. Walt was told that he had bipolar disorder with a genetic basis, and he was started on lithium carbonate 300 mg BID. This was raised by 300 mg every third day, with a blood level sample drawn and tested after each increase, until Walt was on 1500 mg per day and showed a level of 1.3 mEq/L. Walt was asymptomatic one week later, without hospitalization, and returned to work.

Side Effects

Lithium has a significant number of side effects that can be troublesome and, in some cases, quite dangerous. Significant side effects are usually correlated with blood levels of lithium above 1.5 mEq/L. Common side effects include tremor, nausea, thirst, and polyuria. Thyroid goiter has also been seen as a side effect. Severe lithium poisoning is a potential medical emergency. Early signs include vomiting and diarrhea, lethargy, and muscle twitching. These may progress to ataxia and slurred speech. The client may become semiconscious or comatose; seizures may occur; and electrolyte imbalances may lead to cardiac arrest. This syndrome of severe toxicity ordinarily occurs only when the client has a lithium level of 2 or 3 mEq/L. The client may have overdosed or severely restricted food or salt intake (or taken diuretics) to induce this state.

Occasionally very violent, agitated, or paranoid individuals with mania require phenothiazines or phenothiazine/benzodiazepine combinations at the beginning of their treatment. These can be started simultaneously with the lithium, raised to whatever level is required to control the disintegrative behavior, then gradually reduced, and eliminated after therapeutic lithium levels have been effective for approximately one week.

Client Teaching and Nursing Considerations

The accompanying Client/Family Teaching box outlines a teaching plan for the client receiving lithium therapy and the box on page 795 outlines an additional medication teaching plan for the client who is undergoing a trial of carbamazepine to control affective symptoms. The nursing care plan on pages 797–798 offers guidelines for the care of clients receiving lithium therapy.

In a review article on the uses of lithium in clients without major affective illness, Van der Kolk (1986) points out the effective treatment of the following disorders with lithium:

• Impulsive-aggressive disorder

• Post-traumatic stress disorder

• Cyclothymia

• Alcoholism

• Bulimia

CLIENT/FAMILY TEACHING

Medication Teaching Plan: Lithium Carbonate

Brand Name: _____

Generic Name: _____

Administration: This medication is taken by mouth.

Purpose: This medication should provide relief from symptoms so that you are able to participate in activities, use therapy more effectively, take better care of yourself and work more productively. It may take 1–3 weeks before improvement is felt.

Target Symptoms: This medication should decrease some symptoms you have, such as: _____

_____

Report the following symptoms to your physician or nurse: diarrhea, vomiting, chills, fever, infection, dizziness, slurred speech, weak muscles, unsteadiness when walking, twitching muscles, sleepiness and/or blurred vision. If you are pregnant, or think you may be, report this to your physician. Follow up with appointments for blood tests to check lithium levels. Do not discontinue taking this medication without the assistance and advice of your physician.

Other special instructions: _____

_____

_____

The material, on both sides of this form, has been presented to me and discussed with me by: _____

Client's Signature _____ Date _____

Air, Food, Fluid

Initial symptoms of nausea	Take lithium with meals or with food in the stomach. Drink tea or broth and eat soda crackers.
Worsening of symptoms of nausea or vomiting	Notify nurse and physician. Do not take your next dose of lithium until you speak with your nurse and physician.
Dry mouth	Rinse mouth with water. Brush teeth more frequently. Chew sugarless candy/gum. Apply Chapstick to lips and nostrils.
Need to maintain food/fluid intake	Drink 6–8 glasses fluid each day. Eat usual foods including foods containing salt (ie., ham, pickles, tomato juice). Do not diet unless specifically prescribed by your physician.

Elimination

Increased urination	Drink 6–8 glasses of fluid each day. Notify nurse and/or physician.

Diarrhea	Maintain fluid intake. Notify nurse and/or physician.

Personal Hygiene and Body Temperature

Skin Breakdown due to swelling	Elevate legs when swelling is present. Maintain good personal hygiene.
Sweating may affect the lithium level	Avoid exposure to changes in temperature. Wear clothes appropriate to the temperature. Maintain fluid and salt intake.

Rest/Activity

Increased sweating due to exercise	Wear clothes appropriate to the temperature. Maintain fluid and salt intake. Do not change exercise habits without discussion with nurse and physician.
Muscle weakness	Operate your car and other vehicles with care. Plan for extra rest time. Do not use alcoholic beverages or street drugs.

- Premenstrual tension
- Obsessive-compulsive disorder
- Borderline personality disorder
- Schizoaffective disorder

Perhaps the extensive list of uses for lithium will increase as more is learned about the psychobiologic effects of this drug, as well as the underlying biologic substrates for behavior.

Psychobiology of Lithium

Although the specifics of bipolar disorder are difficult to delineate, much can be said about the psychobiology of lithium. Lithium, not unlike the antidepressants, affects neurotransmitters, especially norepinephrine and serotonin. In short, lithium aids in the reduction of neurotransmitter release into the synapse and enhances its return, yielding a lower overall amount of the neurotransmitter in the synapse. Behaviorally, these biologic changes can be observed as an absence of mania or depression. What is unclear at this time is why lithium takes up to a few weeks to be fully effective, when the drug's effects can be observed on synaptic activity almost immediately. Also, why do some people with bipolar disorder *not* respond at all to lithium therapy? Many psychobiologists believe that lithium's effects are likely to be based on neurocellular changes that occur over weeks or months after a client begins lithium therapy. A similar explanation may hold true for the effectiveness of carbamazepine.

Anxiolytic Drugs

Effects

The antianxiety agents—sedatives and hypnotics—have very similar pharmacologic attributes. All can be used in small or modest doses to relieve anxiety and in larger doses to induce sleep. Although they share the major clinical effect of tranquilization or **disinhibition** of fear-induced behavior, their side effects, including their addictive potentials and overdose sequelae, make certain representations of this class more suitable for routine use and others better to reserve for limited, special circumstances.

The antianxiety agents are sometimes called "minor tranquilizers," but this is a misleading term, since their effects on anxiety are qualitatively, not quantitatively, different from those of the "major tranquilizers" or antipsychotic agents.

Drug Classification

Meprobamate Meprobamate (Miltown, Equanil) was the first antianxiety agent to gain popularity in the 1960s. The result of controlled studies of the effects of meprobamate compared to placebos are generally favorable but not overwhelmingly convincing. This, and the addictive and fatal overdose potentials of the drugs, prompted investigators to develop more effective and safer medications that have all but made meprobamate obsolete.

CLIENT/FAMILY TEACHING

Medication Teaching Plan: Carbamazepine

Brand Name: _____

Generic Name: _____

Administration: Your medication is taken by mouth.

Purpose: Your medication provides relief from symptoms so that you are able to participate in activities, use therapy more effectively, take better care of yourself.

Target Symptoms: Your medication will decrease some symptoms you are having, such as: _____

Other special instructions: The following drugs may cause increases or decreases in your blood level of carbamazepine: Troleandomycin (Tao), warfarin (Coumadin), erythromycin (Robimycin), phenytoin (Dilantin), isoniazid (INH), propoxyphene (Darvon, Wygesic, Unigesic), and nicotinic acid (Nicobid, Nicolar). Before taking any of these medications, be sure that the prescribing physician is aware that you are taking carbamazepine.

Do *NOT* stop taking this drug without the assistance or advice of your doctor. Carbamazepine is a medicine that must be slowly withdrawn.

If any of the following symptoms occur, report them immediately to your nurse or physician: fever, sore throat, mouth ulcers, easy bruising.

The material, on both sides of this form, has been presented to me and discussed with me by: _____

Client's Signature _____ Date _____

Air, Food, Fluid

Dry mouth — Rinse mouth with water. Brush teeth more frequently. Chew sugarless candy/gum. Apply Vaseline or Chapstick to your lips and nostrils.

Nausea/vomiting, poor appetite — Eat soda crackers, toast; drink tea. Notify your nurse or physician.

Elimination

Difficulty urinating or increase in frequency of urination — Notify your nurse or doctor. Drink 6–8 glasses of fluid each day. If you are having difficulty urinating, try the following: Apply warm water to genital area.

Diarrhea — Take a lukewarm shower. Listen to running water. Maintain fluid intake. Notify your physician and nurse.

Personal Hygiene and Body Temperature

Possible inflammation of the tongue and lining of the mouth — Notify your physician or nurse immediately. Use a soft bristle toothbrush. Rinse mouth frequently. Avoid foods that contain spices such as pepper, nutmeg, or vinegar.

Possible rash/itching skin — Notify your nurse or doctor. Apply lotions to skin. Do not use soaps that dry the skin.

CLIENT FAMILY TEACHING (continued)

Rest/Activity		Solitude/Socialization	
Dizziness	Lie down and rest. Get up slowly from a lying position; dangle legs over edge of bed for 5 minutes before standing up. Have nurse check your blood pressure.	Understanding your illness and medication	Talk with your nurse or physician to identify symptoms that are part of your illness or side effects of your medication.
Drowsiness	Drive car or other vehicles with extra care. Avoid alcoholic beverages or street drugs. Plan for extra rest time.		
Blurred vision	Notify your nurse or physician. Use a magnifying glass for reading.		

SOURCE: *Adapted from Langley Porter Psychiatric Institute Hospital and Clinics, 1984. University of California, San Francisco.*

 Benzodiazepines The major class of drugs today in the management of anxiety is the benzodiazepines. This group, represented by chlordiazepoxide (Librium), diazepam (Valium), and others, accounts for a very high percentage of all the psychoactive medications prescribed in the United States by psychiatrists and medical practitioners alike. This fact usually evokes a mixed response in professional circles. The easy distribution of drugs for such a ubiquitous human phenomenon as anxiety fosters the development of a pill-oriented and pill-dependent society, say critics. Sympathizers focus on the proved effectiveness of the drugs, which help people achieve higher levels of functioning, more pleasurable experiences, and even more productive psychotherapies in some instances.

 New Drugs In the last decade, the arena of anxiety-related research has expanded tremendously, and several new anxiolytic drugs have been introduced. Lorazepam (Ativan), alprazolam (Xanax), and clonazepam (Klonopin) are the newest introductions to the benzodiazepine family, but prazepam (Centrax) is a relatively new drug as well. The newer benzodiazepines give prescribers a wider range of therapies to target the often idiosyncratic manifestations of anxiety manifested by clients. Some of the new drugs have more rapid onsets and shorter half-lives (lorazepam, alprazolam), while others have a usual benzodiazepine onset time and an extended half-life (clonazepam).

With the psychobiologic knowledge explosion, a great variety of drugs has been used in the treatment of anxiety disorders. According to Derogatis (1986), the psychopharmacologic treatments of anxiety-related conditions include the following:

- Benzodiazepines (the Valium family)
- Antidepressants (especially for panic disorders)
- Beta-blockers (e.g., propranolol)
- Antihistamine sedatives (e.g., hydroxyzine)
- Major tranquilizers (e.g., neuroleptics)
- Sedatives with hypnotic effects (e.g., barbiturates)
- Propanediols (e.g., meprobamate)
- New drugs (e.g., buspirone)

Researchers are asking questions about the psychobiologic connections between conditions such as phobias and anxiety. For example, social phobia is not a well-studied behavioral complex, but its manifestations usually include fearfulness and anxiety. In a recent study, atenolol, a beta-adrenergic blocking agent was given to a group of clients with a diagnosis of social phobia (Gorman et al. 1985). The majority of clients in the study improved. This finding indicates autonomic nervous system innervation in social phobia, since atenolol affects that part of the central nervous system.

New drugs and new uses for existing drugs are accompanied by new side effects and the need for new teaching plans developed by nurses for use in client

NURSING CARE PLAN

A Client on Lithium

Client Care Goals	Nursing Planning/ Intervention	Evaluation
Nursing Diagnosis: *Altered Nutrition: Less than body requirements*		
Client will maintain balanced food and fluid intake.	Obtain diet history to determine usual intake.	Client is well hydrated and ingests sufficient amounts of food.
	Monitor intake of foods containing sodium.	
	Teach clients to avoid fluctuations of sodium intake.	
	Monitor fluid intake.	
	Encourage at least 6–8 glasses fluid per day.	
Client will have the least discomfort possible when experiencing unavoidable side effects.	Administer lithium spaced through the day (TID or QID).	Client reports that side effects are minimized.
	Give with meals or with food in the stomach.	
	Give tea and crackers for nausea.	
	Teach clients to rinse mouth frequently and practice oral hygiene when they experience dryness of the mouth.	
	Observe for persistence and exacerbations of GI side-effects.	
Nursing Diagnosis: *Altered urinary elimination*		
Client will maintain balanced intake and output.	Monitor bowel and bladder output.	Client reports satisfactory urinary elimination.
Client will have the least discomfort possible when experiencing unavoidable side effects.	Observe for persistence and exacerbations of GI side effects.	
	Assess for signs of diabetes insipidus.	
Nursing Diagnosis: *High risk for impaired skin integrity*		
Client will maintain physical hygiene and skin integrity.	Assess skin condition and hygiene needs.	Client's skin is healthy, well hydrated, and not swollen.
	Monitor symptoms of edema through measuring extremities with a tape measure.	
	Teach clients to elevate legs when edema is present.	

▶

NURSING CARE PLAN *(continued)*

Client Care Goals	Nursing Planning/ Intervention	Evaluation
	Teach and assist clients to perform routine personal hygiene.	
	Monitor skin condition and observe for signs of dehydration, pruritus, or hypothyroidism.	

Nursing Diagnosis: *Sleep pattern disturbance*

Client will achieve a healthy balance of rest and activity. If the client experiences side effects client will feel the least discomfort possible.	Assess rest/activity pattern.	Client gets adequate rest and sleep.
	Identify activity that may result in excessive perspiration.	
	Protect clients from exhaustion due to overactivity by providing a quiet room and limited stimulation.	
	Promote safety by teaching clients to avoid operating an automobile or smoking alone if they experience lethargy.	
	Assist clients to plan schedule for rest and activity.	

Nursing Diagnosis: *Impaired social interaction*

Client will maintain a balance of solitude and socialization and will demonstrate socialization skills.		Client participates in activities appropriately.

education. In a recent article, three case reports demonstrated acute paroxysmal excitement (disinhibition) in conjunction with alprazolam treatment (Strahan et al. 1985). Across the United States, hundreds of thousands of doses of alprazolam are probably being administered on a routine basis to anxious clients. The assessment skills of nurses must be finely tuned to detect unusual behaviors in relation to benzodiazepine therapy. The following symptoms are characteristic behaviors of paroxysmal excitement (disinhibition) associated with alprazolam treatment (Strahan et al. 1985):

- Insomnia

- Racing thoughts/persistent thoughts

- Increased energy

- Irritability/hostility

- Impulsiveness

- A feeling similar to that experienced with amphetamine use

- Acute onset

Use in Reducing Anxiety

There is no question that the benzodiazepine family offers a rapid, effective, and safe treatment for the emotional state commonly known as anxiety. In contrast to all other sedatives with proved effectiveness, the benzodiazepines do not interfere with or accelerate the metabolism of medications taken con-

RESEARCH NOTE

Citation

Garvey MJ, Tollefson GD: Prevalence of misuse of prescribed benzodiazepines in patients with primary anxiety disorder or major depression. Am J Psychiatry 1986;143(12):1601–1603.

Study Problem/Purpose

Misuse and abuse of benzodiazepines by psychiatric clients has been consistently documented in the professional literature and in clinical work. The authors of this study attempted to determine the prevalence of benzodiazepine misuse or abuse in specific psychiatric diagnostic groups. In addition, the investigators examined potential predictors of benzodiazepine misuse and abuse among study participants.

Methods

Participants in the study were seen in a psychiatric outpatient clinic over the course of 18 months. Any clinic client who received benzodiazepines was given a structured psychiatric interview that explored symptoms, course of illness, history of alcohol use, demographic characteristics, and family history of psychiatric illness. Clients were studied prospectively at one- and four-week intervals.

Three groups of clients who met DSM-III criteria for major depression received benzodiazepines: (1) those who switched to alprazolam (Xanax) after one or more failed trial(s) on tricyclic antidepressants; (2) those who received benzodiazepines (in addition to tricyclic antidepressants) to control symptoms of residual anxiety; and (3) those who received a benzodiazepine hypnotic for severe insomnia. Clients with drug or alcohol abuse or dependence were excluded from the study. Abuse was gauged according to DSM-III definition. Benzodiazepine misuse occurred if: (1) the benzodiazepine was used in therapeutically inappropriate ways, e.g., taking more than the prescribed dose; (2) the client reported the medications as lost or stolen; (3) the client's pharmacist reported client requests for additional benzodiazepines; (4) other prescribers reported the client seeking benzodiazepines from them; (5) a client's significant other reported benzodiazepine misuse; (6) a client self-reported misuse; and (7) evidence existed of benzodiazepine intoxication. Clients identified as misusers or abusers were compared to nonmisusers on twenty predetermined variables gathered from the index interview.

Findings

Seventy-one clients received benzodiazepines during the eighteen-month study period. Diagnostic categories of study participants were as following: major depression (75 percent); primary anxiety disorder (24 percent). One client received benzodiazepines for primary insomnia with no associated psychiatric disorder. The mean ±SD dose in diazepam (Valium) equivalents was 24±8 mg/day. The mean follow-up duration was approximately eight months, with mean duration of benzodiazepine use for the entire sample being about five months. Upon termination of the study, thirty-nine of the seventy-one participants were still using some form of benzodiazepine. No benzodiazepine abuse was detected in any subject, but 7 percent of the study group misused benzodiazepines.

Implications

The investigators of this study point out that, *with proper precautions*, benzodiazepines can be used for clients with primary anxiety disorder or major depressive disorder. It is essential to bear in mind that these study participants had no previous history of drug or alcohol abuse or dependence outside a major affective episode.

The implications for nursing are significant. For example, nurses working with clients on an in-patient unit must not only observe for the signs of potential benzodiazepine misuse/abuse but must also use knowledge of those signs within the context of client teaching. When family or significant others are available, discussion of benzodiazepine misuse or abuse will alert family or significant others to early signs of difficulty, allowing for early intervention.

This study also has direct implications for nurses who administer p.r.n. dosages of benzodiazepine to clients. It is essential to make a close and thorough assessment before administering p.r.n. dosages. Such assessment is likely to include severity and quality of presenting symptoms, precipitating factors, and effectiveness of alternative means of symptoms abatement. If alternative methods fail to reduce the severity of the symptom, the p.r.n. dosage may be a reasonable intervention. Once the medication is given, effectiveness in symptom relief needs to be assessed and documented, as does any emergent pattern of drug-seeking behavior. Such data are likely to provide nurses with valuable information for the interdisciplinary team, as well for the teaching efforts of nursing staff.

currently. Caffeine, however, interferes with the effectiveness of these drugs.

The effects are evident within the first days of treatment. These medications are absorbed much more rapidly and completely from the gastrointestinal tract than from intramuscular injection and are almost always administered orally. An exception is the use of intravenous diazepam to induce sleep before anesthesia or to manage status epilepticus. Peak levels of chlordiazepoxide are reached in the bloodstream two or four hours after oral ingestion and peak levels of diazepam are reached in one to two hours.

The major side effects of the benzodiazepines are related to their sedative qualities. Clients may complain of excessive drowsiness and must be cautioned against driving a car or operating other machinery.

Other drugs used to treat anxiety but generally less effective include the antihistamines diphenhydramine (Benadryl) and hydroxyzine (Vistaril, Atarax), the beta-blocker propranolol (Inderal), and methaqualone (Quāalude), a synthetic nonbarbiturate sedative. Methaqualone has been a much-abused drug, probably because of the intense euphoria associated with peak blood levels.

Another common use of benzodiazepines, especially librium, is in the detoxification of individuals addicted to alcohol. Given adequate doses of benzodiazepines to induce sedation (usually starting at 150 to 350 mg per day of chlordiazepoxide), alcoholic clients can be smoothly withdrawn by stepwise reductions in chlordiazepoxide dose over a one- to two-week period, without encountering alcohol withdrawal delirium or grand mal seizures.

Client Teaching and Nursing Considerations

Client teaching is an especially important element in the care of clients receiving antianxiety agents. As most people know, anxiety is a generally uncomfortable experience. Self-medication often becomes the relief-seeking behavior used by many people who suffer severe anxiety. Such a psychopharmacologic approach is *temporarily* helpful in the restoration of a person's capacities and internal comfort. When the client is able and ready to learn, however, other means of anxiety control *must* be taught. Many of the anxiolytic drugs (especially benzodiazepines) carry a potential for dependence and tolerance. Hence, nurses have a responsibility to help clients control anxiety in the most effective and safest way possible. The accompanying Client/Family Teaching box outlines a teaching plan for clients receiving benzodiazepines.

Psychobiology of Anxiolytic Drugs

Antianxiety drugs probably work through a process of synaptic activity involving a neurotransmitter called gamma aminobutyric acid (GABA), a common neurochemical in the brain and spinal cord. Benzodiazepines most likely potentiate GABA, producing muscle relaxation. This mechanism involves a complex process of presynaptic and postsynaptic receptor activity. Recent research has yielded information about the presence of a postsynaptic receptor commonly called the *benzodiazepine receptor*. As the term implies, benzodiazepines bind perfectly and with great specificity to this membrane, allowing for the sensation of relaxation.

Sedative-Hypnotic Drugs

The pharmacologic management of insomnia presents an interesting and challenging clinical problem. Many of the truly hypnotic drugs tend to have undesirable effects, including physiologic addiction, fatal overdose potential, and dangerous interactions with other medications because of liver enzyme induction. The first principle of treatment is to assess whether the insomnia is related to one of the major mental disorders, such as schizophrenia or major depression. If so, the insomnia can and should be treated as part of the larger problem, and sedative antipsychotics or antidepressants may be given at bedtime to accomplish this purpose.

Benzodiazepines

In the management of simple insomnia without an associated major mental disorder, the benzodiazepine compound flurazepam (Dalmane), 15 or 30 mg at bedtime, is the drug of choice. This drug is as free of toxicity as others in its class and therefore is both effective and safe. It is the one sleeping medication that does not seem to interfere with REM (rapid eye movement) sleep and therefore can be used on consecutive nights for approximately a month. Other benzodiazepine compounds that are used for their hypnotic qualities include triazolam (Halcion) and lorazepam (Ativan).

Barbiturates

Barbiturates are less commonly prescribed for their hypnotic effects. Their only advantage over the benzodiazepines is their low cost. Barbiturates, especially the short-acting types, such as secobarbital, are powerfully addicting substances. They are frequently used in

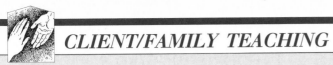

Medication Teaching Plan: Benzodiazepines

Brand Name: _____

Generic Name: _____

Administration: Your medication is taken by mouth.

Purpose: Your medication provides relief from symptoms of anxiety so you are able to participate in activities, use therapy more effectively, and take better care of yourself.

Target Symptoms: Your medication should decrease some symptoms you are having, such as: _____

_____

Other special instructions: Do not stop taking this drug without the assistance and advice of your physician. _____ is a medicine that must be slowly withdrawn. Drugs in this category are not intended for long-term use as physical and psychologic dependencies are possible.

Report the following symptoms to your therapist or primary care nurse: marked drowsiness, weakness, staggering gait, tremor, feeling of drunkenness.

The material, on both sides of this form, has been presented to me and discussed with me by: _____
Client's Signature _____ Date _____

Air, Food, Fluid

Food in your stomach will slow the absorption of this medicine.	Do not take medication with meals. If stomach upset is present, drink tea and broth and take soda crackers. Notify your nurse or physician if other stomach problems arise.
Effectiveness of this drug is lessened with excessive intake of caffeine or heavy tobacco smoking.	Drink decaffeinated beverages; avoid caffeinated colas, chocolate, or tea. Keep smoking to a minimum, if possible.
Alcohol increases the sedating effects of this drug.	Alcohol intake is not permitted during your hospitalization on this unit. Do not use alcohol after discharge, if you continue with this medication.

Personal Hygiene and Body Temperature

Possible rash/ itching skin	Notify your nurse or physician. Apply lotions to skin. Do not use soap that dries skin.

Rest/Activity

Dizziness	Lie down and rest. Get up slowly from lying position; dangle legs over edge of bed. Have your nurse check your blood pressure. Notify your physician or nurse.
Drowsiness	Drive your car or other vehicles with extra care. Plan for extra rest time. Do not take other medications unless approved by your physician.
Blurred vision	Notify your nurse or doctor. Use a magnifying glass for reading.

Solitude/Socialization

Unusual irritability or nervousness	Notify your physician or nurse. Ask your nurse for assistance in selecting an appropriate relaxation exercise.
Understanding your illness and medications	Talk with your nurse and physician to identify symptoms that are part of your illness or side effects from your medication.

SOURCE: Adapted from Langley Porter Psychiatric Institute Hospital and Clinics, 1984. University of California, San Francisco.

successful suicide attempts, since overdoses can cause severe central nervous system and respiratory depression. Barbiturates suppress REM sleep, leading to the phenomenon of REM deprivation and REM rebound—that is, after a week or two of treatment, they help induce the insomnia they were intended to control. Barbiturates also speed up the metabolism of anticoagulant and other drugs because they induce liver enzyme synthesis. This effect can be fatal. Long-acting barbiturates (phenobarbital) are very useful, however, in the detoxification of barbiturate addicts and the management of epilepsy.

The following groups of hypnotic preparations are commonly prescribed:

- Chloral derivatives (e.g., chloral hydrate)
- Piperidinediones (e.g., Doriden, Noludar)
- Alphatic alcohols (e.g., Placidyl)
- Antihistamines (e.g., Benadryl)

Client Teaching and Nursing Considerations

As with the benzodiazepines, sedative-hypnotic preparations are generally intended for either occasional or short-term use. These medications are appropriate for clients newly admitted to a psychiatric in-patient unit or for clients in outpatient therapy who develop sleep disorders. As other medications (e.g., antidepressants, lithium, neuroleptics) start to yield a therapeutic effect, however, the need for sedative-hypnotic medication should almost, if not completely, abate.

Nurses working with clients in these situations need to help them regulate their sleep patterns. Here are some strategies to reinstitute regular sleep patterns:

- Avoidance of caffeine and nicotine
- Exercise several hours before bedtime
- Relaxation techniques, including white noise
- Avoidance of alcoholic beverages before bed
- Warm baths
- Tryptophan-rich foods (see Chapter 13)
- A regular routine of retiring and rising
- Avoidance of light before sleep

It is essential that the nurse teaching relaxation techniques assess the client's sleep patterns and presleep routines to prescribe the correct technique to meet the client's needs. Ongoing evaluation of the effectiveness of the relaxation intervention allows for a change in approach if necessary.

Electroconvulsive Therapy

The topic of electroconvulsive therapy, more commonly known as ECT, almost always produces some discussion among health care providers. People rarely maintain a neutral stance in relation to ECT; to this day, the subject and procedure remain extremely controversial.

On the side of conservatism, many people refute the benefits of ECT, arguing that there is little scientific basis for the treatment and that producing deliberate seizure activity in the brain could *never* be therapeutic. Such arguments have an element of truth but often fail to consider the many people who have benefited from ECT. The liberal perspective often errs on the side of overenthusiasm for ECT, recommending its application in situations that are basically inappropriate.

A middle road does exist for the application of ECT in psychiatry today. Although it is reserved as a second-line therapy today because of the variety of psychopharmacologic interventions available, it remains a useful and therapeutic biologic alternative. The National Institute of Mental Health (NIMH) and the office of the medical applications of research of the National Institutes of Health (NIH) held a conference to explore issues of ECT's uses and to discuss areas of controversy related ECT. According to a report of the proceedings (Runck 1985), the conference explored the following issues: effectiveness, risks and adverse effects, appropriate uses of ECT, informed consent, proper administration of ECT, and research.

Electroconvulsive therapy was considered effective in the following clinical situations

- Severe delusional/endogenous depression
- Acute mania
- A subgroup of schizophrenics whose illness is of short duration and who demonstrate concurrent affective symptoms

ECT is unlikely to be effective for the following illnesses:

- Dysthymic disorder
- "Neurotic" depression
- Adjustment disorder with depressed mood
- Chronic schizophrenia

In discussing risks and adverse effects, Runck's report (1985) discussed a death rate of 2.9 deaths per 10,000 clients. Other risks are comparable to the risks of using brief anesthesia with muscle relaxants and the transient application of mechanical respiratory assistance. Possible adverse effects include the following:

- Transient confusion, memory loss, headache

- Transient hypotension, sinus tachycardia

- Negative perceptions, social stigma of clients receiving ECT

The procedure for the administration of ECT is relatively simple and routine today but nonetheless requires close assessment and observation of prepared staff. The procedure includes the following steps:

- Give no food/fluid before the treatment.

- Remove dentures, hairpins.

- Encourage the client to void before the procedure.

- Take vital signs.

- Give a methohexital (Brevital) injection to induce anesthesia.

- Give succinylcholine (muscle relaxant).

- Apply electrodes, using electrojelly.

- Give 1 to 130 volts for 0.1 to 0.5 seconds.

- Use mechanical means of respiration during the period following electrical impulse.

- Monitor seizure activity.

- Observe (postprocedure) for signs of respiratory difficulty.

- Reorient clients as they become alert and able to resume activities.

In the immediate postprocedure period, clients' memory will probably be affected by the procedure; most clients fail to remember the trip into the ECT procedure room. Other nursing concerns involve teaching the client and family or significant others what behavior to expect from the client after the procedure. Nurses may also work with clients, families, and significant others to discuss their concerns and provide accurate information about the procedure while attempting to allay anxiety.

Looking for Biologic Markers—Visual Imaging Techniques

Techniques and technology are available today that enable us to visualize the brain and its metabolic activities. The discussion that follows offers a synopsis of these techniques. While all of them are in use, some

have more clinical significance than others. In any event, the emergence of new technologies often directly affects nursing actions. If nothing else, nurses have a responsibility to teach clients about the examinations, much as medical-surgical nurses do with clients undergoing fluoroscopy or barium studies, for example.

Computed Tomography (CT Scanning)

Because the mind is not separate from the brain, assessment of behaviors must entail an examination of the biologic substrate for behavior. Usually, classic symptoms of neurologic dysfunction (e.g., headache, visual symptoms, seizures) do not prompt psychiatric assessment, and until recently, psychiatric symptoms did not routinely receive neurologic assessment. However, mood changes are often the earliest signs of neurologic dysfunction and merit close biologic assessment.

The CT scan is one means of visualizing gross pathology in the brain by taking very fine "photographs" of designated areas of the brain. The CT scan reveals "slices" or "cuts" of the brain, allowing for a very precise and thorough examination of the structures that make up the brain. More specifically, the CT scan examines the densities of given brain structures and compares these findings with those of normal controls.

In 1985 Brown and Kneeland reviewed a variety of studies involving the use of CT scans in psychiatry. They reported biologically observable changes via CT scanning in the following clinical entities:

- *Schizophrenia*—findings included ventricular enlargement, density changes in different parts of the brain, and cortical atrophy.

- *Affective disorders*—findings included ventricular changes and decreased cerebellar mass in some alcoholic bipolar clients.

- *Dementia*—findings demonstrated a lowered brain density.

Although these findings are of interest, they remain mainly academic at this time. Enlarged ventricles are not by themselves diagnostic of schizophrenia. However, the CT scan is an important examination in psychiatry because it allows for a clear assessment of the gross anatomy of the brain to determine potential causes for behavioral change.

In preparing clients for the procedure, nurses need to know whether the client's examination is to be done with or without injection of a contrast (dye) material.

The contrast injection, used in situations where a more defining and precise scan is desirable, adds the discomfort of an intravenous injection to the procedure.

The client needs to know the following facts about the CT scan:

• The scan lasts approximately 45 minutes.

• During the scan, the client lies on a movable stretcher.

• The CT scanner looks something like a huge doughnut, and the client's head is placed in the center or "hole of the doughnut."

• The machine moves to accommodate the electronic requests of the scanner's operator.

• It is essential that the client remain still throughout the procedure; medication sometimes helps the agitated client achieve that end.

• If an injection of contrast is used, the client may expect to feel transient "hot flashes" or experience an unusual taste; other, more severe symptoms may indicate an allergic reaction to the contrast.

• There are no restrictions on food or fluid intake prior to the examination.

Positron Emission Tomography (PET Scanning)

According to Brown and Kneeland (1985), PET scanning is a noninvasive way to measure physiologic and biochemical functions as they occur in live tissue. Scientists can watch brain metabolism through the use of a compound that is inhaled or injected and contains a radioactive "tag." Using a "tagged" glucose compound, for example, one can observe glucose use in the brain. Brown and Kneeland point out that glucose use is directly related to functional activity in regions of the brain. In some of the studies reviewed by Brown and Kneeland, PET scans have demonstrated the following:

• Decreased use of glucose in the frontal lobes of unmedicated schizophrenics

• Less use of glucose in the entire left cortex of select schizophrenics

• Less glucose use on the left side of the basal ganglia (see Chapter 6) than on the right

• Diminished glucose uptake in frontal and temporoparietal cortex (bilateral) in clients with Alzheimer's disease

PET scanning is used both for research and as a clinical diagnostic tool.

Magnetic Resonance Imaging (MRI)

MRI is a revolutionary technique introduced to clinical work in the recent past. What is new and innovative about this type of imaging is that it does *not* use ionizing radiation but yields pictures of superior quality to those of computed tomography.

According to Brown and Kneeland (1985), the principle is fairly straightforward. Atomic nuclei with an odd number of neutrons or protons act like magnets. Brown and Kneeland described the process as follows: "MRI images are formed by placing the appropriate part of the client's body within a stationary magnetic field, which causes the nuclei to align in the direction of the field. A radiofrequency pulse . . . is then applied." The result of the radio frequency pulse is an electric signal that yields an image (see Figure 32–3). The intensity of the image depends on the density of the nuclei being examined; pathologic lesions look different from normal tissue.

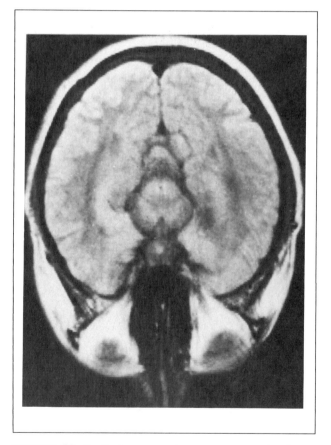

FIGURE 32–3 Nuclear magnetic resonance scan showing the central portion of the human brain. *SOURCE Courtesy Alan Jay Cohen, M.D., Clinical Instructor, Department of Psychiatry, University of California at San Francisco/San Francisco General Hospital.*

In preparing the client for an examination using MRI technology, the nurse may use the following guidelines:

- The MRI equipment is similar in appearance to that of the CT scanner.

- If the client is having MRI imaging of the head, explain that the head will be placed in the magnetic field, while the rest of the client's body remains on a stretcher outside the magnetic field.

- The client must remove all hairpins and jewelry, lest they be drawn into the magnetic field.

- Clients with metallic implants or metallic artificial joints may not be suitable for MRI as the magnetic field is likely to respond to the presence of metal in a way that could be detrimental to the client.

- The examination usually takes about 45 minutes, during which the client must remain still to prevent blurring of the images.

- Clients often become claustrophobic while in MRI; their whole body is in a tube. Teach clients to keep their eyes closed and to do deep breathing relaxation exercises.

The MRI has great potential for clinical work. Physicians have already been able to apply its refined technology to the presenting psychiatric difficulties of clients, and to translate its results into interventions aimed at relief of incapacity and suffering.

Other visual-imaging techniques continue to evolve, such as *brain electrical activity mapping* (BEAM) and *cerebral bloodflow techniques* (CBF).

While BEAM aims to enhance the clinical usefulness of the EEG, CBF explores the relationship between disturbed brain function, cerebral bloodflow, and metabolism of oxygen and glucose in the brain (Brown and Kneeland 1985). Current opinion is that while BEAM may be of use clinically in the near future, the likelihood of the same occurring with CBF is not as probable.

Psychosurgery

Like electroconvulsive therapy, *psychosurgery* conjures some very strong images in many people's minds. Since the inception of frontal lobotomies for the treatment of schizophrenia starting in 1936, psychosurgery has undergone major changes. Today, frontal lobotomies are mainly a thing of the past and essentially nonexistent in the United States. Modern psychosurgery continues in Western Europe, and consists of stereotaxic operations, performed at various locations in the limbic system (see Figure 32–4).

The desired effect of all psychosurgery is to diminish unpleasant affects. It has little impact on disintegrative symptoms such as hallucinations or delusions, but the client clearly is no longer threatened, frightened, or distressed by them. Postoperatively clients have little feeling for members of their families, their personal appearance, socially unacceptable behaviors, and their general future. These side effects are much diminished by the newer stereotaxic methods, however.

In the United States today, psychosurgery has been replaced with other biologic therapies, mainly psy-

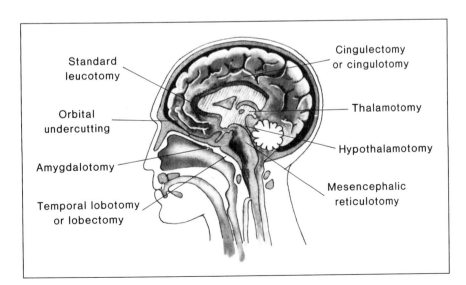

FIGURE 32–4   Psychosurgery sites.   SOURCE: Black, P., The rationale for psychosurgery.
The Humanist, July/August 1977, p. 7. Reprinted by permission.

chopharmacologic interventions. With the current upsurge in psychobiologic knowledge, the concept of psychosurgery seems outdated, but arguments continue over whether psychosurgery is an appropriate measure for those labeled criminal or sexual psychopaths.

Humanistic Interactionist Implications

"Humanistic psychiatric nursing practice is enhanced when scientific knowledge is delicately blended with an imagination that is sensitive, aware, and liberally educated" (Wilson and Kneisl 1983). Nothing could be closer to the truth of the nursing profession's relation to the psychobiologic therapies emerging today. Nurses need to be cautious to maintain the *art* of nursing, as the *science* of nursing's professional work in psychiatry thrusts us onto the threshold of the twenty-first century.

CHAPTER HIGHLIGHTS

• Biologic therapies have been in existence since ancient times, have taken various forms over the centuries, and are of extreme importance in psychiatric intervention today.

• Through a biologic perspective, any given individual's psychology is the result of neurochemical actions and reactions in the central nervous system.

• Biologic therapies work because of the changes they produce on cells of the central nervous system, permitting the emergence of new behaviors.

• Psychiatric nurses need to understand and remain abreast of current advances in psychobiology.

• *Psychotropic* drugs primarily affect the mind by exerting an effect on the cells of the central nervous system.

• In relation to psychotropic medication administration, nurses have responsibilities in the areas of assessment, intervention, and evaluation.

• Medication compliance is a complex phenomenon; nurses have used various teaching strategies in an attempt to improve client compliance.

• The major classes of psychotropic medications include antipsychotics (neuroleptics), antidepressants (TCA, MAOI), anxiolytics (benzodiazepines, etc.), antimania drugs (lithium, carbamazepine, valproic acid), and sedative-hypnotic medications (chloral derivatives, barbiturates, etc.).

• Electroconvulsive therapy is effective for several clinical entities; nursing care is essential for clients receiving this biologic therapy.

• Among the contemporary visual-imaging techniques, the ones that are most clinically useful are computed tomography and magnetic resonance imaging.

• While psychosurgery is still used in parts of Europe, it is rare in the United States; psychopharmacologic interventions are more commonly used in the United States.

REFERENCES

Brown RP, Kneeland B: Visual imaging in psychiatry. *Hosp Community Psychiatry* 1985;36(5):489–495.

Coccaro EJ, Siever LJ: Second generation antidepressants: A comparative review. *Clinical Pharmacol* 1985;25:241–260.

Derogatis LR: *Clinical Psychopharmacology*. Addison-Wesley, 1986.

Douyan R, Angrist B, Peselow E, Cooper T, Rotrosen J: Neuroleptic augmentation with alprazolam: Clinical effects and pharmacokinetic correlates. *Am J Psychiatry* 1989;142(2):231–234.

Garvey MJ, Tollefson GD: Prevalence of misuse of prescribed benzodiazepines in patients with primary anxiety disorder or major depression. *Am J Psychiatry* 1986;143(12):1601–1603.

Gorman JM, Liebowitz MR, Fyer AJ, Compeas R, Klein DJ: Treatment of social phobia with atenolol. *J Clin Psychopharmacol* 1985;5(5):298–301.

Green AI, Salzman C: Clozapine: Benefits and risks. *Hosp Community Psychiatry* 1990;41(4):379–380.

Kerr LE: Oral liquid neuroleptics: Administer with care. *Psychosocial Nurs Ment Health Serv* 1986;24(3):33–38.

Kneisl CR: *Wadsworth's Review of Nursing*. Wadsworth, 1985.

Massachusetts General Hospital: Buproprion: The second generation continues. *Biol Ther Psychiatry* 1985a;8(5):17–20.

Massachusetts General Hospital: Treating treatment-resistant depression: Antidepressants and stimulants? *Biol Ther Psychiatry* 1985b;8(6):13–18.

Osser DN: A systematic approach to pharmacotherapy in patients with neuroleptic-resistant psychoses. *Hosp Community Psychiatry* 1989;40(9):921–926.

Perry PJ, Garvey MJ, Kelly MW, Cook BL, Dunner FJ, Winokur G: A comparative trial of fluoxetine versus trazadone in outpatients with major depression. *J Clin Psychiatry* 1989;50:290–294.

Pope HG, McElroy SL, Nixon RA: Possible synergism between fluoxetine and lithium in refractory depression. *Am J Psychiatry* 1988;145(10):1292–1294.

Runck B: NIMH report: Consensus panel backs cautious use of ECT for severe disorders. *Hosp Community Psychiatry* 1985;36(9):943–946.

Selander JM, Miller WC: Prolixin group: Can nursing intervention groups lower recidivism rates? *J Psychosocial Nurs Ment Health Services* 1985;23(11):16–20.

Strahan A, Rosenthal J, Kaswan M, Winston A: Three case reports of acute paroxysmal excitement associated with alprazolam treatment. *Am J Psychiatry* 1985;142(7):859–861.

Tamminga CA, Gerlach J: New neuroleptics and experimental antipsychotics in schizophrenia, in Meltzer HY (ed): *Psychopharmacology: The Third Generation of Progress.* Raven Press, 1987.

Van der Kolk BA: Psychopharmacology: Uses of lithium in patients without major effective illness. *Hosp Community Psychiatry* 1986;37(7):675.

Wilson HS, Kneisl C: *Psychiatric Nursing,* ed 2. Addison-Wesley, 1983.

PART SIX

Applying the Nursing Process Across the Life Span

CONTENTS

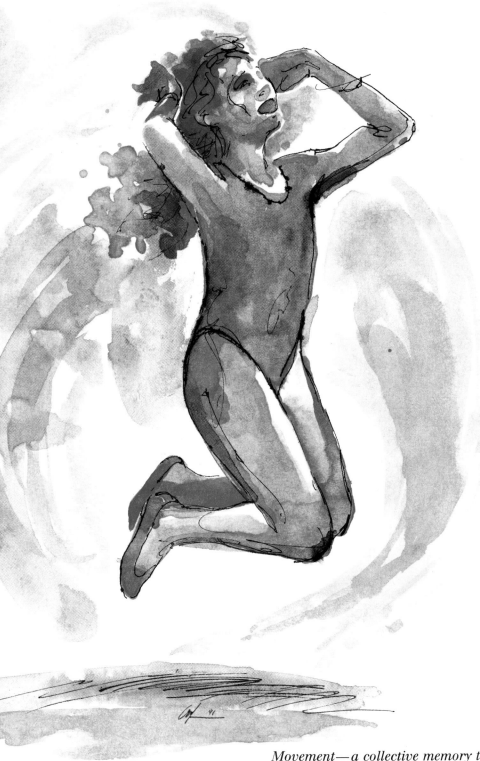

Movement—a collective memory that communicates emotions—
exists not always to soothe the spirit, but to express it.

Applying the Nursing Process with Children

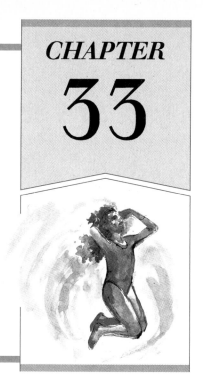

LEARNING OBJECTIVES

- Describe the generalist and specialist roles of the nurse in child psychiatry

- Discuss the common child psychiatric disorders

- Apply the nursing process to clinical situations with child psychiatric clients and their families

- Identify the role of the child psychiatric nurse in the various treatment modalities used with children

- Explain the responsibilities of the nurse in caring for children in a milieu

Beth Sipple

CROSS REFERENCES

Other topics related to this content are: Bulimia and anorexia nervosa, Chapter 20; Family assessment and family therapy, Chapter 30; Intrafamily physical and sexual abuse of children, Chapter 22; Milieu therapy, Chapter 31; Severity of psychosocial stressors for children and adolescents (Axis IV of DSM-III-R), Table 9–3 in Chapter 9; Suicide, Chapter 23.

Portions of the material in this chapter were contributed to the third edition by Janet Grossman and Kate Mayton.

THE PLIGHT OF THE estimated three million children believed to be suffering from serious emotional disorders can be summarized by stating that there are too many children (and families) in need of help, too few services available, and too few child psychiatric specialists to perform the services. This picture is made even bleaker by evidence suggesting that of the specialists available, at least one discipline, child psychiatric nursing, is being underused.

Child psychiatric nursing concerns itself with promotion of mental health in all children as well as treatment of emotionally disturbed children. There is a wide range of psychiatric disturbances in children. Some children are simply overwhelmed by everyday worries; others need constant supervision because they might hurt themselves or others or because their thought processes are disturbed.

Children with severe emotional disorders present a challenge that taxes the knowledge and resources of the psychiatric nurse. Children with these disorders typically experience problems in their families, schools, and communities. They tend to exhibit developmental delays that cause them to lag behind their peers. Their parents or significant others complain about their behavior or are frustrated by their lack of response. These children may also experience somatic problems typical of adults with psychiatric disturbances and may have communication difficulties or confused perceptions of reality.

Not all nurses understand psychiatric disorders, and some find it difficult to plan interventions with these children and their families. But since nurses often encounter these children, particularly those who are undiagnosed or untreated, knowledge of childhood disorders is important regardless of the nurse's area of clinical practice.

An understanding of childhood disorders also enhances practice in adult psychiatric nursing. Many disturbed adults have children with emotional problems or have difficulty with parenting skills. Psychiatric nurses are typically involved in family-centered care, which may include nursing activities such as conducting family therapy, supervising family visits, planning passes, providing family education, supporting family members in the milieu, and facilitating referrals for services for other family members.

Historical and Theoretic Perspectives

Child psychiatric nursing is a specialty area of psychiatric nursing. The specialty is relatively new, having its inception in the early 1950s, when graduate programs opened and training funds became available through the National Institute of Mental Health (NIMH). The early child guidance team did not include the nurse as a team member other than in the milieu. In some residential programs, the majority of milieu staff were from other disciplines, and only one nurse was included for each shift, primarily to attend to the physical needs of the children and administer medications. As the community mental health center movement developed, programs specifically for children began to offer appropriate roles for the child psychiatric nurse, including treatment, consultation, education, and medication supervision. However, these programs had great difficulty sustaining themselves. The small number of professional staff in these programs provided few opportunities and low visibility for the child psychiatric nurse. Because positions in child psychiatry were so limited, many of these nurses were also involved in the care of chronically institutionalized adults reentering the community.

The interdisciplinary team in the contemporary milieu consists of child psychiatrists, nurses, social workers, child psychologists, occupational therapists, recreational therapists, special educators, pediatricians, and child care workers. Other specialists are used for consultations as indicated, particularly child neurologists, speech and language specialists, child abuse teams, clergy, and physical therapists. It is not unusual for parents to need psychotherapy or psychoeducation themselves. In fact the child may have been referred to the child psychiatrist by the parents' own mental health worker or therapist. It is essential to coordinate efforts with the parents' therapists, particularly in the area of marital and family treatment.

Child Psychiatric Nursing Roles

New nursing roles emerging in child psychiatric specialization underscore the need for a medical-psychiatric approach because of the increased awareness and understanding of biochemical disorders and dual diagnosis. The term *dual diagnosis* is used to describe clients who have a primary medical and psychiatric diagnosis, such as a child who has both diabetes and a conduct disorder. Nurses who are experienced in working with medically ill people have a knowledge base that is useful in understanding the interaction of medical and psychiatric disorders. Medical conditions tend to be frightening and unfamiliar to members of other disciplines (e.g., social workers, teachers, and psychologists), who are more familiar with children who have a primary psychiatric diagnosis.

Nurses in child psychiatry explain laboratory tests to children, support children during these procedures, and administer antidepressants that require strict and systematic monitoring. These roles capitalize on the following characteristics of the child psychiatric nurse:

• Ability to address the interaction between physical and psychologic symptoms

• Experience in working with chronic populations (tertiary care)

• Knowledge and skills related to pharmacology (educating children and parents, monitoring side effects)

• Experience in nursing care of medical conditions such as seizure disorders, diabetes, and asthma

The Standards of Child and Adolescent Psychiatric and Mental Health Nursing Practice were developed to improve the quality of nursing care given by generalists and specialists in the field (see the accompanying Nursing Standards box). These standards—developed by the American Nurses' Association in cooperation with Advocates for Child Psychiatric Nursing, Inc.—pertain to all settings in which child and adolescent psychiatric nurses practice, apply to children and adolescents at all developmental levels, and are relevant in all social systems in which the child or adolescent is involved. A review of the standards reveals the following distinctive interlocking characteristics:

• A preventive approach to intervention

• Consideration of developmental variables

• Attending to interacting social systems

• Focus on nonverbal communication and activity

The standards also describe the specific roles of generalists and specialists in child psychiatric nursing as follows below (ANA 1985).

Generalists are nurses who are educated in basic professional nursing programs. These are some of the roles that child psychiatric nurse generalists assume:

• Milieu therapist who shares the responsibility for providing an atmosphere in which all activities and behaviors are focused on the therapeutic care of the child or adolescent

• Counselor or teacher of parents who have an emotionally disturbed or mentally retarded child or adolescent

• Collaborator with other mental health and psychiatric professionals in assessing the needs and planning for the care of a child or adolescent and family

• Responsible citizen and change agent who provides for the mental health needs of children and adolescents

• Promoter of mental health with individual children, families, and groups

• Participant in the research process and consumer of research findings relevant to child and adolescent psychiatric and mental health nursing

Clinical specialists are nurses who hold at least a master's degree in child and adolescent psychiatric nursing; have had supervised clinical practice at the graduate level; and demonstrate breadth and depth of knowledge, skills, and competence in the field. Certification is highly recommended for the specialist. Specialists may assume any of the generalist roles and may also assume, but are not limited to, these additional roles:

• Psychotherapist for individual children, groups of children, and families

• Clinical supervisor of client care staff and graduate nursing students

• Administrator of child and adolescent psychiatric and mental health nursing services

• Educator of nurses and other child care personnel in a variety of academic and clinical settings

• Consultant to professional and nonprofessional individuals or groups concerned with the general welfare, education, and care of children

• Researcher who contributes to the theory and practice of child and adolescent psychiatric and mental health nursing through research in this field or a related field

Biopsychosocial Factors

Problems that appear in children are not necessarily classified as psychiatric disorders. They may be conditions for which an appropriate diagnosis cannot be determined, for which no psychiatric disorder has been found, or for which a psychiatric diagnosis is not the current focus of treatment. For example, the child's problem might be rooted in parent-child difficulties and therefore is not a psychiatric disorder.

Etiology

Many factors contribute to the development of psychiatric disorders in children. The variables defined by researchers and clinicians depend on their theoretic framework, but nursing theorists view the etiology of psychiatric disorders as multidimensional. Etiologic factors generally fit the following four categories:

Genetic and Biophysical Factors   Genetic and biophysical influences of child psychiatric disorders

NURSING STANDARDS

ANA Standards of Child and Adolescent Psychiatric and Mental Health Nursing Practice

Professional Practice Standards

Standard I. Theory The nurse applies appropriate, scientifically sound theory as a basis for nursing practice decisions.

Standard II. Assessment The nurse systematically collects, records, and analyzes data that are comprehensive and accurate.

Standard III. Diagnosis The nurse, in expressing conclusions supported by recorded assessment and current scientific premises, uses nursing diagnoses and/or standard classifications of mental disorders for childhood and adolescence.

Standard IV. Planning The nurse develops a nursing care plan with specific goals and interventions delineating nursing actions unique to the needs of each child or adolescent, as well as those of the family and other relevant interactive social systems.

Standard V. Intervention The nurse intervenes as guided by the nursing care plan to implement nursing actions that promote, maintain, or restore physical and mental health, prevent illness, effect rehabilitation in childhood and adolescence, and restore developmental progression.

Standard V-A. Intervention: Therapeutic Environment The nurse provides, structures, and maintains a therapeutic environment in collaboration with the child or adolescent, the family, and other health care providers.

Standard V-B. Intervention: Activities of Daily Living The nurse uses the activities of daily living in a goal-directed way to foster the physical and mental well-being of the child or adolescent and family.

Standard V-C. Intervention: Psychotherapeutic Interventions The nurse uses psychotherapeutic interventions to assist children or adolescents and families to develop, improve, or regain their adaptive functioning, to promote health, prevent illness, and facilitate rehabilitation.

Standard V-D. Intervention: Psychotherapy* The child and adolescent psychiatric and mental health specialist uses advanced clinical expertise to function as a psychotherapist for the child or adolescent and family and accepts professional accountability for nursing practice.

Standard V-E. Intervention: Health Teaching and Anticipatory Guidance The nurse assists the child or adolescent and family to achieve more satisfying and productive patterns of living through health teaching and anticipatory guidance.

Standard V-F. Intervention: Somatic Therapies The nurse uses knowledge of somatic therapies with the child or adolescent and family to enhance therapeutic interventions.

Standard VI. Evaluation The nurse evaluates the response of the child or adolescent and family to nursing actions in order to revise the data base, nursing diagnoses, and nursing care plan.

Professional Performance Standards

Standard VII. Quality Assurance The nurse participates in peer review and other means of evaluation to assure quality of nursing care provided for children and adolescents and their families.

Standard VIII. Continuing Education The nurse assumes responsibility for continuing education and professional development and contributes to the professional growth of others studying children's and adolescents' mental health.

Standard IX. Interdisciplinary Collaboration The nurse collaborates with other health care providers in assessing, planning, implementing, and evaluating programs and other activities related to child and adolescent psychiatric and mental health nursing.

Standard X. Use of Community Health Systems* The nurse participates with other members of the community in assessing, planning, implementing, and evaluating mental health services and community systems that attend to primary, secondary, and tertiary prevention of mental disorders in children and adolescents.

Standard XI. Research The nurse contributes to nursing and the child and adolescent psychiatric and mental health field through innovations in theory and practice and participation in research, and communicates these contributions.

---

*Standards V-D and X apply only to the clinical specialist in child and adolescent psychiatric and mental health nursing.

SOURCE: *American Nurses' Association:* Standards of Child and Adolescent Psychiatric and Mental Health Nursing Practice. *1985. Reprinted with permission of the American Nurses' Association.*

include heredity, temperament, innate characteristics, congenital disorders, and constitution or health. The child is vulnerable to the strengths and weaknesses of each parent and to the separate effect of their combined genes. Hereditary influences are exemplified by the transmission of recessive genes for phenylketonuria, which causes mental retardation. Constitution or health variables are exemplified by the child's physical appearance and general state of health. The child born with fetal alcohol syndrome is an example of how innate factors resulting from mutation and regrouping of genes in the parents are then transferred to the child at conception. Premature birth is one type of congenital event that can affect behavior and social adaptation.

Social and Cultural Factors   The role of social and cultural factors in the etiology of psychiatric disorders has been acknowledged in the last thirty years. Gerald Caplan (1961), who has advocated primary prevention for adults and children, viewed psychiatric disorders as one of a set of social problems that must be handled at the community level.

The social and cultural variables affecting the child's mental health include the physical environment of the home and community, the family's socioeconomic resources, and cultural and social supports.

It is important to remember how dependent children are on their environment and especially on their families. As more is learned about family dynamics, it becomes increasingly clear that no one develops independently of family and social influences. Herzog (1970) has shown that in a family or life-style characterized by deprivation, high stress, or pervading social stigma, the children are more vulnerable to emotional, behavioral, and adjustment problems. The response of children to their environment is highly individualized. Rutter (1979) demonstrated that certain children are more negatively affected by adverse conditions than others. There is an interaction between vulnerability of the child and the degree of risk in the environment. Children may be vulnerable because of their constitutional or genetic makeup, temperament, sex, a physical or mental defect, or prenatal or perinatal insults. Sameroff and Chandler (1975) propose a continuum of caretaking causality; at one end are environments supportive enough to strengthen even the most vulnerable of children, while at the other end are environments too disordered to meet the needs of the most resilant child.

Family System Factors   Family system variables exert influence on the developing child through parenting styles, parent mental health or parent psychopathology, family relationships, and losses and separations. Parents shape their children's behavior by modeling and reinforcement through rewards and punishment. For example, modeling of antisocial behavior by a parent contributes to the child's refusal to follow rules in the school, home, and community.

Frequent moves and early loss of a parent through death or divorce impair the child's ability to form close relationships and make them prone to depression. Parent psychopathology such as depression or psychosis can result in failure to meet the child's basic needs or development of symptoms in the child similar to those of the parents. Physical or sexual abuse of the child by a parent typically results in chronic psychiatric disorders in the child such as self-destructive behavior, depression, or post-traumatic stress disorder. Dysfunctional family relationships, such as severe marital conflict or enmeshed relationships among child, parent, and grandparents, can create anxiety and confusion in the child.

Acquired Illness and Injury   Acquired illness and injury exert powerful influences on the emotional health of the child both through direct influence and through the secondary effect of interference with stages of personality and intellectual development. For example, accidental poisoning can lead to cognitive deterioration. Chronic diseases (e.g., asthma) developed in the perinatal period can severely restrict the child's physical activity and social experiences.

Mood Disorders

Mood disorders in children have become a popular topic in both professional and lay literature. Although there is widespread agreement in child psychiatry that depression exists as both a syndrome and an affect in children, there continues to be confusion about the clinical diagnosis, lack of knowledge about effective treatment, and uncertainty about incidence and etiology. Clinical work and research in the field of childhood depression are far behind the work in adult depression, which was spurred by findings in psychobiology and psychopharmacology. Despite these questions, mood disorders in children must be viewed as a major mental health problem. Depression is the most common psychiatric problem in children who attempt suicide, and youth suicide rates continue to rise.

The most common type of depression seen in children is secondary, or reactive, depression. This is the sadness that occurs in response to particular situations, including the trauma of hospitalization, surgery, or separation from a family member. Children might become depressed secondary to medical diseases, such as diabetes mellitus, asthma, and cardiac anomalies, or cognitive and behavioral problems. Children with learning disabilities frequently become depressed because of their frustration with school, particularly if the disorder is not recognized or special academic assistance is not provided. Depression that is not a response to the stress of an event is termed primary depression. Primary depression is a syndrome with identifiable symptoms; its etiology is not clearly understood, however.

It is important to distinguish between the child with feelings of depression and the child with a depressive syndrome. Many children feel sad at some point during a day, but the sadness does not last all day or for several days. For example, in an interview with a nurse, one 10-year-old girl said that she felt sad, but the sadness went away when she talked to her mother or when she woke up the next day. Unlike this child, depressed children have sad feelings that persist for significantly longer periods. One depressed child reported to the nurse that she could not remember the last time she felt happy or had a good time.

Causes of Mood Disorders in Children   Mood disorders may be caused by grief. Grief reactions in most children are not well understood. The timing of extended grief, which is considered pathologic in children, is not defined and may vary across developmental stages. Children also may rework grief reactions when they enter new developmental stages. Some children with major life changes, such as parental divorce or a move to a new community, fail to make transitions within a reasonable amount of time. In addition to having adjustment difficulties (such as failure to make friends or a decrease in school performance), the child may be sad. These situations, however, are not usually viewed as primary depression because the sadness is secondary to adjustment problems.

Mood disorders in children have been explained by genetic factors, biochemical factors, drugs, neurologic disorders, psychoanalytic theories, and learning theories. Twin and adoption studies provide genetic evidence for major depressive disorders. Family psychiatric history studies provide evidence for depression occurring throughout families. However, these occurrences in families could be related to genetic or environmental influences or both.

The biochemical studies revolve around depletion or elevation of noradrenaline and serotonin. These hypotheses have been tested more extensively in adults, and no theory predominates in children. Even the diagnostic usefulness of the dexamethasone suppression test in children is being questioned due to discrepant sensitivity and specificity across studies (Poznanski et al. 1987). Drugs such as stimulants can lead to depressive symptoms in children, as can cerebral hemisphere dysfunction and adrenal hyperplasia (Shaffer and Erhardt 1985).

Psychoanalytic theorists tended to reject the idea of depression in children. This was based on the belief that anger toward a lost object is repressed and results in guilt and loss of self-esteem leading to depression. Because the superego is not developed in the child, psychoanalysts believed guilt could not occur. Researchers first became interested in children's reactions to maternal separation and loss in the 1920s. Bowlby (1973) theorized that early loss can predispose a child to depression in later years. However, early loss is difficult to research, because there are many confounding variables.

Learning theorists discuss how depression in an individual is the result of inadequate reinforcement in the environment. Theorists are beginning to examine the reciprocity of depression in the marital couple, but efforts to develop a family systems model of depression that incorporates children are primitive at best.

Symptoms and Signs of Depression in Children   Children differ from adults in the biologic, developmental, and cognitive manifestations of depression, although depressive symptoms in adolescents are similar to depressive symptoms in adults. Little has been published on the developmental aspects of the clinical manifestations of depression in children. A few researchers are beginning to explore the possibility of a depressive syndrome even in infancy.

Children with mood disorders exhibit depressed affect or dysphoria, which generally lasts a minimum of one to four weeks. Poznanski (1982) described nonverbal signs of sadness such as fleeting smiles and a bland, frozen look. Even the most experienced nurses might not be able to identify sadness in the face of a child if they are looking for characteristic adult features. Poznanski also distinguished between verbal and nonverbal sadness, because children might appear sad but verbally deny these feelings. Children use a variety of terms such as *bad, gloomy, blue, empty,* and *not able to stand it* (Puig-Antich et al. 1980) to describe sad feelings. The nurse needs to listen carefully to the child's description.

Anhedonia, or the inability to enjoy oneself or have fun, is the most characteristic symptom of depression in children. Children who are questioned about their activities typically report several interests, whereas a depressed child might have difficulty thinking of one enjoyable thing. One depressed child, for example, spent many hours watching television but could not remember what he had watched. Children occasionally experience boredom, but a child who reports being bored 50 to 90 percent of the time is probably anhedonic.

By middle childhood, children with a positive self-concept can describe their appearance, schoolwork, and friendships positively. A child with a poor self-concept is more likely to describe personal characteristics negatively and report the use of derogatory nicknames by other children as if they were accurate.

Social withdrawal is also characteristic of depressed children but must be distinguished from the withdrawal of a child who has never developed good peer relationships. Many depressed children had good peer relationships at one time but now report that, "I have no friends," or "The kids don't like me." The withdrawn child might reject opportunities to play with other children or watch other children play.

Schoolwork is often impaired when a child is depressed, even though the child may previously have done well in school. The impaired schoolwork may be the result of the general apathy, an inability to concentrate, or distraction by internal stimuli.

Children who are depressed are often preoccupied with morbid thoughts, typically about themselves or others dying. For example, one child drew himself in a family drawing as if he was thinking of his grandmother who had died two years earlier. Suicidal thoughts, plans, or actions are also reported by depressed children. Children are influenced by their parent's suffering and mood. One 7-year-old girl tried to jump out of a car on a busy expressway. Her mother had also been depressed and suicidal following the imprisonment of the child's father, who had committed several violent crimes. Professionals and parents must acknowledge that children do think about suicide and may try to kill themselves.

Associated symptoms of depression include irritability, weeping, and somatic complaints. Irritable children are easily bothered by the smallest event. Some depressed children cry more than their peers, feel like crying frequently, or appear to be about to cry. Depressed children might complain of minor aches and pains that have no organic cause (Poznanski 1982).

Symptoms and Signs of Mania in Children
Depressed children occasionally have some symptoms of mania. Manic symptoms are difficult to diagnose in children, although in adolescents the symptoms resemble adult symptoms. One study identified the following manic symptoms in children (Puig-Antich et al. 1980):

• Elation, expansive mood: elevated mood and/or optimistic attitude about the future lasting four hours and being out of proportion to the circumstance

• Decreased need for sleep: less need for sleep than usual in order to feel rested

• Unusually energetic: more active than usual without expected fatigue

• Increase in goal-directed activity: more active in scholastic, social, or leisure activities (e.g., new projects, telephone calls, letter writing) compared with usual activity

• Grandiosity: increased self-esteem and approval of own worth, power, or knowledge compared with usual level

• Accelerated, pressured, or increased amount of speech: rapid or continual talking that can't be stopped

• Racing thoughts: thoughts racing through mind, having more ideas than usual or more ideas than can be handled

• Flight of ideas: accelerated speech with abrupt changes from topic to topic usually based on understandable associations, distracting stimuli, or play on words

• Poor judgment: excessive involvement in dangerous activities without recognition of potential for painful consequences

• Distractability: difficulty focusing attention on questions; jumping from one thing to another; failure to keep track of answers; and attentiveness to irrelevant stimuli

• Motor hyperactivity: constant movement, e.g., pacing up and down

Symptoms of depression and mania in children often characterize other psychiatric disorders in children. The diagnosis of a mood disorder is made on the basis of a composite of symptoms.

The topic of youth suicide is one of the most difficult issues for professionals. Suicide in children is discussed in Chapter 23.

Disruptive Behavior Disorders

The DSM-III-R lists three basic categories under the heading of disruptive behavior disorders. They are **attention deficit-hyperactivity disorder, oppositional defiant disorder,** and **conduct disorder.** The following criteria for these disorders help child psychiatric professionals not only to differentiate among the behavior disorders but also to sort out behavior that may be associated with other primary disorders. Children with affective disorders often act out with disruptive behavior. Also, because disruptive behavior is likely to come to the attention of school and police authorities, it is most often the immediate cause for referral for psychiatric services.

Knowledge of the sets of behaviors specific to each diagnostic category aids the nurse in the assessment phase. Few children exhibit all the behaviors in a category. More commonly, they exhibit behaviors across categories. In addition, normal healthy children may at times exhibit individual behaviors within diagnostic categories. The task of the multidisciplinary treatment team in child psychiatry is to take all aspects of the child's life into account in order to arrive at an understanding of the child's behavior difficulties. This understanding of the child and family guides the development of the individual treatment plan.

Attention Deficit-Hyperactivity Disorder

Attention deficit-hyperactivity disorder (ADHD) has these three characteristics: (1) Onset must occur before the age of 7 years, (2) it must not occur only during the course of autistic disorder, and (3) the episode must last six months or more and be characterized by at least eight of the following behaviors:

• Has difficulty remaining seated when required

• Fidgets with hands or feet or squirms in seat

• Has difficulty playing quietly and sustaining attention to tasks or play activities

• Talks excessively

• Shifts from one uncompleted activity to another and has difficulty following through on instructions from others (not due to oppositional behavior or failure of comprehension)—e.g., fails to finish chores

• Is easily distracted by extraneous stimuli

• Interrupts or intrudes on others (e.g., butts into other children's games)

• Blurts out answers to questions before they have been completed and has difficulty waiting turn in games or group situations

• Engages in physically dangerous activities without considering possible consequences (not for the purpose of thrill-seeking)—e.g., runs into the street without looking

• Is extremely messy or sloppy

• Loses things necessary for tasks or activities at school or at home (e.g., toys, pencils, books, assignments)

• Doesn't seem to listen when spoken to

Diagnostically, children with symptoms that meet the criteria for ADHD are a heterogeneous group. Within this population there is a high rate of co-occurrence of conduct disorder, oppositional defiant disorder, anxiety disorders, learning disabilities, intellectual impairments, and family psychopathology. ADHD may represent the symptomatic expression of a number of different disorders with different etiologies, courses, and treatment responses. The heterogeneity of client samples is a major limitation of most studies of ADHD.

Abnormalities of the noradrenergic, dopaminergic, and serotinergic systems have been proposed as neurobiologic predeterminants of ADHD. Research findings comparing unmedicated ADHD children with control groups have been inconclusive. It does appear that some dysfunction in noradrenergic metabolism or control must play a role in the disorder.

Drug therapy is effective in controlling the symptoms of ADHD. Psychostimulants are most commonly used. Drug therapy has been shown to improve attention, reduce activity level, reduce distractibility, improve interactions with others, and improve academic performance. The long-term effects of treatment on academic achievement and psychosocial adjustment remain unclear (Porter 1988).

Oppositional Defiant Disorder

Oppositional defiant disorder may occur between 3 and 18 years of age, must be of more than 6 months duration, and consist of a combination from a set of behaviors. The behaviors must be present other than during the course of another disorder like conduct disorder, or hypomanic or manic episode. These children frequently argue with adults; lose their temper; and are angry, resentful, spiteful, or vindictive. They often actively defy or refuse adult requests or rules (e.g., refuse to do chores at home), often deliberately do things that annoy other people (e.g., grab another child's hat), and are often touchy or easily annoyed. These children often swear or use obscene language, blame others for their own mistakes, and bully or are mean (other than physically cruel) to other children.

Conduct Disorder

Conduct disorder is the appropriate diagnosis if the individual is not 18 or older and the following behaviors have been present for a period of six months or more:

• Often is truant, "borrows" other children's possessions without permission in situations in which obtaining permission is expected, cheats in games with other children or in school work, and initiates physical fights

• May have run away from home overnight at least twice while living in parental or parental surrogate home, but not as a direct reaction to physical or sexual abuse, used a weapon in more than one fight, forced someone into sexual activity, or been physically cruel to animals or to other people (e.g., tied another child to a tree)

• May have deliberately destroyed others' property (other than fire-setting), deliberately engaged in fire-setting, and had voluntary sexual intercourse that began unusually early for general subculture

• May have regularly used tobacco, liquor, or other nonprescribed drugs and began regular use unusually early for general subculture

• Often lies (other than to avoid physical or sexual abuse); has broken into someone else's house, building, or car; has stolen outside the home without confrontation of a victim on more than one occasion (including forgery); or has confronted a victim (e.g., mugging, purse-snatching, extortion, armed robbery)

Tic Disorders

Tic disorders, which are often called habit spasms, are rapid, rhythmic, involuntary movements of individual muscle groups. Fifteen percent of all children develop transient tic disorders in the school years. These include such common symptoms as grimacing, eye blinking, nose puckering, and squinting. These disorders are more common in males, may run in families, and may occur in clusters. Stress, such as excitement and fatigue, may accentuate these habits.

Tourette's disorder is the most debilitating tic disorder. It is characterized by multiple motor and vocal tics. The motor tics almost always involve the head and may also involve the torso as well as the arms and legs. They are manifested by behaviors such as squatting, deep knee bends, twirling, hopping, skipping, jumping, eye blinking, and various touching behaviors. The vocal tics may include grunts, yelps, clicking sounds, barks, sniffs, coughs, stuttering, throat-clearing, snorts, or words. The most disturbing symptom to most observers, parents, and to older children with Tourette's disorder, is **coprolalia,** a complex vocal tic which consists of uttering obscenities and aggressive words and statements.

Assessment and treatment of these children are difficult and complicated. Cohen et al. (1985) have developed a detailed symptom checklist that nurses and parents can use to record specific motor and vocal symptoms. The most effective treatments for the motor and vocal symptoms are pharmacologic treatments such as neuroleptics. These medications have the potential to cause serious side effects, however, and the children need to be monitored carefully. The symptoms of Tourette syndrome are often exacerbated by stress or anxiety. Nurses can help by working with the family to understand how the child can better express feelings and learn more adaptive coping skills.

Elimination Disorders

The most common type of **elimination disorder is functional enuresis,** a chronic, involuntary passage of urine during sleep in children age 5 or older. Younger enuretic children may also have occasional or regular daytime incontinence or urinary frequency or urgency during the day. This condition, which is most common in males, should be differentiated from nocturnal incontinence caused by medical diseases such as diabetes or bladder infections. About one-fifth of enuretic children have psychiatric symptoms. Most enuretic children are distressed by the condition.

The most effective interventions with enuretic children include working with parents to discover the multiplicity of factors that may influence the child's inability to stay dry at night and during the day. Developmental issues or life situations that make the child anxious are important to explore. The child's age, the duration of the enuresis, and the child's motivation to overcome the problem are factors that affect the decision to implement behavioral interventions in isolation or in combination with pharmacologic treatment. For children over the age of 5 years tricyclic antidepressants are the drug of choice for enuresis.

Functional encopresis is defined as the repeated, involuntary passage of stool into clothing without the presence of any organic cause to explain the symptom. This fecal soiling occurs when bowel control is physiologically possible and after toilet training should have been accomplished. Encopresis is less common than enuresis and is more commonly associated with individual psychopathology. Treatment often involves vigorous bowel cleansing followed by a bowel retraining program combining medical and behavioral components plus specific treatment for any associated pathology.

Language and Speech Disorders

Most children achieve language by age 4 years. However, many neurophysical and psychologic disorders can interfere with speech and language. Childhood **language and speech disorders** can be separate, overlap, or coexist.

Speech abnormalities include voice, rhythm, and articulation disorders. These disorders are caused by a physical defect such as cleft palate, functional difficulties, processing difficulties, involuntary movements, and mental retardation. Language allows persons to communicate by putting perceptions and concepts of the world into words. Inadequate language skills can interfere with listening, speaking, reading, and writing in the learning situation. Language disorders include deviations in syntax (grammar), content (semantics), or pragmatics (use) from age-expected behavior. Language disorders can be primary or secondary to other conditions such as mental retardation, psychiatric disorders, hearing impairment, or deprivation.

Intervention for language disorders optimally begins within the first four years of life. Speech and language pathologists and audiologists diagnose and provide treatment, which can include a parent-child program, individual therapy, and group therapy. If children with language disorders are not treated, they are at risk for developing learning problems. The efforts of the specialists should be coordinated with those of schools, which typically offer a broad continuum of possible services. Children with these disorders usually need long-term services and monitoring but do very well with early intervention.

Autistic Disorder

Prior to the development of a classification system for psychiatric disorders in children, autism tended to be viewed as a psychotic disorder. This was related to the difficulty in reality testing and the grossly abnormal behavior displayed by autistic children. More recently, however, an appreciation of the pervasive effects on development of these children led to establishment of a new category, **pervasive developmental disorders. Autistic disorder** is the only subgroup of this category. Autism is a rare disorder and is more frequent in boys. However, a large number of children with other developmental disorders display autistic-like features. Less severe developmental disorders are quite common in children.

The diagnostic criteria include onset before 30 months of age, deviant social development, deviant language development, stereotyped behavior and routines, and the absence of delusions, hallucinations, and schizophrenic-type thought disorder. Deviant social development is most often demonstrated by a lack of emotional responsiveness and social reciprocity along with failure to bond. The parents may report that the child never differentiated the parents from other adults. The child does not come to the parents for comfort when ill, hurt, or tired. These children tend to treat people as inanimate objects.

Deviant language development is first seen in the child's inability to understand spoken language and lack of response to language. Babble, gesture, or mime may not be present or may be less than usual. Parents describe the child as not greeting them or as failing to mold or stiffening when they pick the child up. These children tend to produce little speech and are unable to carry on a conversation.

Stereotypic behaviors and routines are the third set of characteristics of autistic children. Rocking, hand flicking or twisting, and spinning are examples of stereotypic body movements. Autistic children may insist that the same routine be followed every time they participate in an activity such as shopping. They may become severely distressed over minor changes in the environment (e.g., a piece of furniture moved out of its usual place).

Mental retardation is present in about three-fourths of the children, and mentally retarded children may show some of the features of this disorder. Neurodevelopmental disorders such as poor coordination are often seen in autistic children.

Schizophrenic Disorder

Schizophrenic disorder can be found in children as young as age 5 years, but it is rare in children before age 6 or 8. Onset in adolescence is more common. Prepubertal onset of schizophrenia is in fact rarer than pervasive developmental disorders. Schizophrenic disorder in childhood is differentiated from pervasive developmental disorders by the presence of hallucinations, delusions, and disordered thought processes. Tanquay and Cantor (1986) describe children at least 6 years of age who have been diagnosed as schizophrenic (according to DSM-III-R criteria). These children have a thought disorder and symptoms including excessive anxiety, constricted affect, speech abnormalities, bizarre ideas and fantasies, morbid thoughts, lack of peer relationships, primitive defense mechanisms, and concrete thinking.

Incidence   The incidence of psychotic disorders in children is difficult to estimate because of the inconsistency of diagnostic measures. Studies agree that the disorder is rare, occurring in fewer than 1 of every 1000 children (Werry 1982). Psychosis in children is rare compared with the adult incidence. Males are more likely to develop schizophrenia prior to puberty. Schizophrenic disorder in children is so rare that the psychiatric nurse is unlikely to come in contact with such a child.

Symptoms and Signs   Schizophrenic disorder is a complex disorder with a variety of severe and bizarre symptoms, and it is difficult to diagnose. Researchers have not reached a general consensus regarding the associated characteristics and variations. Any child with a schizophrenic disorder exhibits only some of the characteristic symptoms.

Both hallucinations and delusions are rare before adolescence. In addition, research has shown little agreement about what constitutes a childhood hallucination. Hallucinations in children can be confused with other mental phenomena, such as fantasies, obsessions, imaginary play objects and companions, and dreams. Researchers have tried to distinguish between these processes and hallucinations by describing the characteristics of the hallucinations as bizarre and nonvolitional (Rothstein 1981). The following clinical example illustrates hallucinations and delusions as experienced by a child:

Doris, an 11-year-old, described hearing the voice of her mother calling her name and yelling at her, although her mother was not present. At times, she heard her own voice telling her to do things such as chores for her mother. She experienced her mother's voice as coming from outside her head and her own voice as coming from inside her head. She reported seeing a woman who looked like her mother and she thought was her mother.

She also believed that her mother was watching her. Doris described going to the bathroom in the morning and "daydreaming" that objects were weapons (e.g., Q-tips were sticks to stab people, and washcloths were used to smother people). All these experiences seemed real to Doris as they happened. Doris also believed that the world was coming to an end. She described hearing on the news that a hole was breaking apart pieces of the earth, and she thought this was going to happen. She also expressed concern that a heat wave might result in there not being enough air to breathe.

Schizophrenic disordered children exhibit developmental delays, particularly in speech. Speech may be monotonous, or the child may speak very little. The child may have eating and sleeping disturbances, with such behaviors as picky food preferences, taking prolonged periods to complete meals, and wandering around during the night. Mannerisms include activities such as pacing, rocking, and head banging. Repetitive behaviors are more frequently seen in children with schizophrenic disorder than in schizophrenic adults. Many questions about etiology (e.g., contribution of genetics and family social behaviors), manifestations (e.g., neurologic signs), and treatment remain unanswered. These questions continue to be pursued because of the severe disruption of the child's life (Tanquay and Cantor 1986).

The Nursing Process and Child Psychiatric Nursing

Child psychiatric nursing may be carried out in the outpatient psychiatric department, day program, or in-patient psychiatric unit of a medical center; a community mental health center or community agency; a therapeutic school; or a private practitioner's office. Children with a medical insurance card are most likely to be treated in a public agency. However, increasing numbers of children are being treated in medical centers because of the limited amount of outpatient reimbursement available from insurance carriers. Families in health maintenance organizations have limited access to psychiatric services, particularly in-patient services.

Schools are required by law to provide special education services for handicapped students, including those with psychiatric disorders. However, it is becoming increasingly difficult for school districts to provide tuition reimbursement for children to attend therapeutic schools (other than the services of that district) or to be placed in residential care.

Assessing

Nursing assessment in child psychiatry is a multistep process.

Basic Assessment of the Child   The basic assessment of a child has both psychosocial and physical components and is a necessary first step in initiating the plan of care. During this phase, the nurse gathers information from the parents as well as from the child client. The nurse needs to obtain not only such information as allergies and hygiene habits (about which children are usually poor historians) but also information on the child's and parents' views of the difficulties. Nursing assessment guidelines are provided in the accompanying Assessment box.

A physical condition may precipitate a behavioral problem, and so a complete physical examination is necessary to rule out any medical problems. For example, children with chronic physical conditions such as diabetes or asthma often adopt disruptive behaviors to cope with and regain control of their environment and their symptoms. A physical examination also establishes a baseline in the event psychopharmacologic treatment is indicated. The physical examination may also be used to determine if there are any physical findings possibly indicating sexual or physical abuse. Children with psychiatric disorders are frequently referred for neurologic evaluations to rule out disorders such as seizures.

From this initial assessment the nurse not only sets a care plan in motion but also determines what behaviors need to be assessed in greater depth in the second phase of assessment.

ASSESSMENT

Guidelines for Assessing Children

Demographic data: Name, age, date

Past history: Birth history, allergies, illnesses, medication

History of the presenting problem

Child's definition of the problem

Activities of daily living: Nutrition—weight, schedules, preferences; sleep—habits, sleep quality; elimination—habits, problems; handicaps, limitations

Physical assessment: Skin, head, hair, eyes, ears, nose, mouth, respiratory, cardiovascular, musculoskeletal, neurologic

Social assessment: Living arrangement, play activities, family health history, legal status, family visiting plan

Mental status: Mood, thought process, and content; hallucinations, perceptions; speech, orientation; suicidal ideation, homicidal ideation

Regular assessments of all children in all settings include evaluation of growth and development, physical health, academic skills, and risk factors. Assessment of these areas are the basis for primary prevention of psychiatric problems in children. Nurses are well prepared to participate in assessment of these areas and to educate others, such as parents, about the growth and development of the child. Nurses frequently are in a position to observe risk factors such as environmental factors, family characteristics, and characteristics that make the child vulnerable to risk (e.g., developmental disabilities, accidents, illnesses).

More comprehensive diagnostic assessments are indicated when children are demonstrating symptoms such as acting out, school failure, withdrawal, or inability to cope with tasks. The most comprehensive diagnostics are typically done in multidisciplinary diagnostic programs. A diagnostic evaluation may be conducted during a one-session interview with the child and parents or during several sessions. In addition, in-patient units provide a twenty-four-hour milieu in which to evaluate the child in the entire life space.

Life Space Interview The second phase of assessment—Redl (1966) calls it the **life space interview**—occurs in the milieu. Redl and many others maintain that it may take several interviews to obtain a complete assessment. The child is best assessed during normal daily routines and activities over a period of time. The initial time frame for in-patient care is a week to ten days with revisions based on ongoing assessment over the length of stay. Because the routines of most child units mimic the usual daily routines of children, the nurse is able to assess the child's social skills with peers and adults, self-care abilities, and mental status. The nurse then places this information in the context of the child's developmental stage to assess for age appropriateness. It is through these daily interactions that the nurse begins to understand how the child experiences the world. This ongoing nursing assessment gives the treatment team and family a better understanding of the child's integration of past experiences, current coping skills, and sense of self.

Family Assessment A family assessment is an essential part of a complete diagnostic workup of the child. The family assessment shifts the focus from the individual child to the family system. Each person is asked to identify what he or she sees as the problem in the family and what the family has done about it. An attempt is made to understand what the child's symptoms and current episode mean in terms of the family dynamics. Symptoms in other members or marital, sibling, or parent dyads are noted. An assessment is made of the potential for change within the system and the need for marital or family therapy. (See Chapter 30 for specifics.)

RESEARCH NOTE

Citation
Scahill L, Sipple B: Developmental history collection on a child psychiatric inpatient service. J Child Adolesc Psychiatr Ment Health Nurs 1990;3(2):52–56.

Study Problem/Purpose
The purpose of this study was to determine whether developmental and medical history data are being collected in a complete and consistent manner by child psychiatric nurses; whether nurses are clear about the data elements that make up a developmental history; and whether the data were being collected by clinicians other than nurses.

Methods
A sample of forty-one medical records was reviewed using explicit criteria to determine the quality of data being gathered. Prior to record review, nurses were asked to complete a questionnaire about views concerning relevance of developmental history to treatment planning.

Findings
Child psychiatric nurses felt that developmental history data are essential for developing individual treatment plans and that nurses should collect the data. Fifty percent of the nurses expressed uncertainty about how to conduct a developmental history interview. Forty-six percent of the medical records reviewed were missing global information concerning the child's developmental history. Nurses documented developmental information more frequently than did members of other disciplines. Nursing documentation following the introduction of a nursing admission form was more complete.

Implications
The findings illustrate the need for nursing staff education related to conducting a developmental history interview and developing a data-collection tool specifically for the child psychiatric in-patient population. One discipline needs to be responsible for collecting and recording the data. It makes most sense for nurses to assume the responsibility because nurses need the information to devise the plan of care. The systematic collection of developmental information upon admission can only enhance the quality of care on a children's psychiatric in-patient service.

Diagnosing

Ideally, the diagnostic assessment of the child culminates in the formation of both nursing and medical diagnoses, which are summarized in a multidisciplinary staff conference. Examples of psychiatric nursing diagnoses and DSM-III-R diagnoses related to children are discussed in the accompanying Case Study. The DSM-III-R Axis IV rating is made more specific to children by using the Severity of Psychosocial Stressors Scale: Children and Adolescents in Table 9–3 in Chapter 9. The child's general social, psychologic, and academic functioning is described using the Global Assessment of Functioning Scale (GAF Scale) in the box on page 172 in Chapter 9.

Planning and Implementing Interventions

Although the medical and nursing diagnoses may suggest certain standard interventions, each child must be considered individually. Intervention with the emotionally disturbed child and family involves an interdisciplinary approach determined by the child's age, developmental level, symptoms, parents' commitment, economic resources, and accessibility of services. Nurses are involved in either primary or collaborative roles in the various treatment modalities, including the following:

- Psychotherapy, play therapy
- Social skills training
- Psychopharmacology
- Milieu (routines, rules, peer pressure)
- Group modalities (including milieu meeting, group therapy, psychodrama)
- Occupational therapy (including art therapy, recreation therapy, sensory-motor integration)
- Parent approaches (including counseling, psychoeducation, family therapy, parent education, support groups)
- Placement (in a regular classroom with teacher consultation, therapeutic classroom, therapeutic day school, partial hospitalization, in-patient care, or residential care)

If the child is in a therapeutic milieu, the Joint Commission on Accreditation of Hospitals (JACH) mandates weekly multidisciplinary staff conferences on every client. The plan is developed at the initial conference and revised as indicated. The components of the multidisciplinary treatment plan include the following:

- Problems
- Goals (measurable, specific)
- Interventions (frequency)
- Responsible staff
- Target dates

Longitudinal follow-up of children with a severe emotional disorder is essential. Further episodes may be prevented by early detection of symptoms. In addition, children often regress following the return home from an in-patient hospitalization.

Nursing Goals   The following are some common nursing goals in working with children with severe psychiatric disorders:

- Develop a relationship with the parents and help them gain an accurate understanding of their child's strengths and weaknesses.
- Help the parents learn effective behavioral interventions and understand the principles that inform the interventions.
- Encourage the parents to be active members of the treatment team.
- Help the child develop more adaptive coping skills.
- Help the child express feelings in a helpful, productive manner.
- Provide opportunities for the child and parents to experience positive, successful interactions.
- Help the child develop relationships with others.
- Prevent the child from hurting self or others.
- Help the child maintain physical health.
- Promote appropriate reality testing by the child.
- Help the child communicate effectively.

Play Therapy   The treatment modality most widely used with children is **play therapy**. Play therapy lets children use their natural medium of expression to resolve conflicts. The play therapist adds the further resource of an accepting, understanding adult.

Functions of Play   Play has many functions. Children use play to:

- Master and assimilate past experiences over which they had no control
- Communicate with their unconscious constructs or needs

Text continues on p. 830

CASE STUDY

A Child with a Disruptive Disorder and a Mood Disorder

Identifying Information

Rob is a 9-year-old white, Protestant boy who is in the fourth grade. He is referred to the in-patient unit for diagnosis and treatment following an outpatient evaluation during which it was determined that his problems were too severe for outpatient management.

Client's Definition of Present Problem, Precipitating Stressors, Coping Strategies, Goals for Care

Rob and his parents defined the problem as his behavior, primarily his self-destructiveness and aggression toward others. The precipitants for the current crisis include several losses and illnesses in the nuclear and extended family and the potential loss of the father's work. Rob is coping poorly with the losses, and long-term marital problems are accentuated. Rob's understanding of the hospitalization is poor, as he feels he's here because others "pick on me." The goals include:
1. Preventing injury to self or others
2. Providing an intensive twenty-four-hour evaluation
3. Determining appropriateness of psychopharmacologic treatment
4. Providing family support and intervention
5. Encouraging effective peer socialization

History of Present Problem

For the past two months, Rob has shown evidence of suicidal ideation (e.g., writing a note saying "I want to kill myself.") He draws morbid pictures and worries about family members dying. He also writes "I hate myself." Rob recently threatened to take his father's pills so he wouldn't have to go to school. Rob withdraws to his room and cries. Rob has been aggressive toward his peers (e.g., trying to choke a child) and had been destructive of school property. Rob's peers tease him and call him names. Rob refuses to go to school on some days.

Rob was taking methylphenidate (Ritalin) for concentration problems but the medication was discontinued for the diagnostic evaluation. Rob appeared depressed and withdrawn while taking the Ritalin but became more volatile and aggressive once off the Ritalin. Rob's behavior problems have rapidly escalated following the illnesses and hospitalization of both parents and two grandparents and the death of one grandparent in the past seven months. Rob was placed on Ritalin seven months ago, and it was increased the month before the escalation of his symptoms. Rob previously did well academically, but this academic year his grades dropped. He enjoys bike riding, reading, and games. Peer relationships have been poor.

Psychiatric History

This is the first psychiatric hospitalization for this child. The only previous treatment was counseling in the school by a social worker in response to Rob's aggressiveness toward other children. Following the onset of the morbid and suicidal symptoms the school personnel referred the mother for outpatient treatment. There has been no previous psychiatric involvement with other family members. The Ritalin was prescribed by a neurologist.

Family History

The family has a routine for meal- and bedtimes. Rob's father is gone for long hours of working and often sleeps in the evening. Although Rob expressed no food dislikes, his mother states he is a "picky eater." He is small in stature but has not lost weight. He has difficulty falling asleep and at times complains of nightmares. Rob's impulsivity sometimes keeps him from doing tasks well, but his self-care is appropriate for his age.

▶

CASE STUDY (continued)

Social History

Rob lives in a suburban area with his parents who are in their twenties, and two siblings, 6 and 3 years old. Mrs V is a housewife who has a history of depression, anxiety, and medical problems. Mr V supports the family in a blue-collar job. The marital relationship is strained. The family lives in small quarters, and the siblings share a room. They live in the neighborhood where the father grew up, and the grandparents live close by. None of the family members has activities outside the home, and the family has few leisure activities in general. The family is isolated and extremely enmeshed with the extended family on both sides. Both parents were overprotected by their parents. Rob primarily plays with his siblings because no other children live in the area.

Family health has been poor recently. Four months prior to Rob's admission, his mother had a medical admission to the hospital. One month later, Rob's father suffered an industrial injury, resulting in a job change and financial uncertainty. Rob's paternal grandmother had an extreme weight gain following a move two years prior to his admission. Nine months prior to his admission, his maternal grandfather suffered a stroke. The maternal grandmother died two months prior to his admission after seven years with cancer.

A brother, age 6, is doing well in school and has friends, although he is impulsive and hyperactive and has mild developmental problems. A sister, age 3, is assertive and extroverted and is adjusting well in preschool and with her peers. The siblings are aggressive toward each other.

Significant Health History

Rob's physical health is good other than some difficulty in fine-motor coordination and mild anorexia reported by his mother. This well-groomed child showed no physical problems except for some minor bruises on his arm, which were reportedly self-induced. Because of staring periods, Rob was referred to a neurologist in preschool to rule out epilepsy. Findings were negative. Immunizations were up to date.

Rob was the product of an unplanned pregnancy, which ran a difficult course including hospitalizations toward term for toxemia. He was delivered by forceps, a 9 pound, 2 ounce baby. Developmental milestones were within normal limits. Walking and talking were early, and though toilet training was difficult, he was trained by age 3.

Rob's long history of behavioral problems began with temper tantrums at 6 months. At 3 he cut up the family sofa. The parents removed Rob from preschool because they felt the school could not handle his behavior. He continued to be a behavioral problem with poor socialization resulting in aggressiveness toward himself and others. Rob's concentration was poor, and he appeared depressed.

Current Mental Status

Appearance: well-groomed, neat and clean
Mood: energetic, excited, enthusiastic
Thought process: changes topics quickly
Thought content: appropriate to age and circumstance
Speech: has lisp, talks a lot
Orientation: good to three spheres
Eye contact: fair
Attention: fair
Memory: good

▶

CASE STUDY *(continued)*

Current Mental Status *(continued)*	Suicidal orientation: makes statements of intent to "punch myself because I'm no good"
	Homicidal ideation: he would like "to get really strong and let them (school bullies) have it."
Other Subjective or Objective Clinical Data	A dexamethasone suppression test was done at admission and was in the borderline range. After four weeks of intensive observation, Rob was given a trial dose of lithium. This was ineffective in controlling his mood swings. He was then switched to desipramine and maintained at a dose of 50 mg.

Diagnostic Impression

Nursing Diagnoses

Altered nutrition: Less than body requirements
Sleep pattern disturbance
Anxiety
Impaired social interaction
Altered role performance
High risk for violence: Self-directed
High risk for violence: Directed at others
Self-esteem disturbance
Hopelessness
Knowledge deficit
Ineffective individual coping
Altered parenting

DSM-III-R Multiaxial Diagnosis

Axis I: Cyclothymic disorder
           Attention deficit disorder
Axis II: Speech disorder (articulation)
Axis III: Fine motor deficits
Axis IV: 4-Severe
Axis V: Current GAF: 50
           Highest GAF past year: 60

NURSING CARE PLAN

A Child with a Disruptive Disorder and a Mood Disorder

Client Care Goals	Nursing Planning/ Intervention	Evaluation
Nursing Diagnosis: *Altered nutrition: Less than body requirements*		
Client will maintain or increase weight.	Structure meals and snacks. Help client make appropriate choices.	Maintains normal weight and enjoys meals.
Nursing Diagnosis: *Sleep pattern disturbance*		
Client will experience less anxiety at bedtime.	Use relaxation exercise at bedtime. Do not allow client to nap during the day.	Is able to sleep at regular intervals; feels safe in his bedroom.

NURSING CARE PLAN (*continued*)

A Client with a Disruptive Disorder and a Mood Disorder

Client Care Goals	Nursing Planning/ Intervention	Evaluation
	Provide extra support at bedtime.	
	Use extra time prior to bedtime to decrease physical activity.	
	Encourage client to talk about his fears.	
Nursing Diagnosis: *Anxiety*		
Client's anxiety level will decrease.	Provide ways for client to express feelings and worries.	Verbalizes feelings toward situations without feeling responsible for others.
Client will feel more secure.	Offer empathic comments about worries (e.g., "It must be hard to concentrate when you're worried about your Dad.")	
Nursing Diagnosis: *Impaired social interaction*		
Client will develop positive relationship with adult authority figures.	Assist client in developing new responses if necessary.	Shows evidence of decreased incidence of oppositional behavior.
	Broaden vocabulary relative to feelings. (Are you angry or hurt?)	
	Teach client to identify what upsets him.	
	Help client learn to remove himself from difficult situations and to tell adults he is having a difficult time.	
	Encourage client to talk about feelings rather than act out.	
Client will show improved social skills with peers, demonstrated by sharing, cooperation, healthy competition, and conflict resolution, as seen in a variety of milieu routines (meals, school, and play times).	Discuss basic expectations about social interactions with peers, stressing the basics of mutual respect and cooperation.	Maintains nonconflictual interactions with peers; appears to enjoy peer activities.
	Plan a program of gradually increased expectations of social interactions for the client.	
	Begin with interactions with staff, doing tasks and games so staff can instruct and provide role models for the client.	

▶

NURSING CARE PLAN *(continued)*

Client Care Goals	Nursing Planning/ Intervention	Evaluation
Nursing Diagnosis: *Altered role performance*		
Client will attend school and develop positive attitude toward school.	Provide constant and consistent feedback to client about how he is doing.	Consistently attends school; makes positive statements regarding school.
Client will attend to an activity long or well enough to complete tasks and progress in classwork.	Medicate as prescribed.	Maintains concentration and progresses in classroom.
	Provide a low-stimulus place to work in.	
	Provide tasks that can be accomplished in pieces or in a short time to help client feel successful.	
	Record success relative to intervention.	
	Provide feedback about success.	
Client will achieve in school consistent with his ability.	Refer for comprehensive educational psychologic testing of client's abilities related to school activities.	Functions at appropriate academic level.
	Implement recommendations.	
Client will compensate for his learning problem through awareness and development of new skills.	Provide learning materials that accent client's strengths in order to achieve academically. (The nurse acts in a supportive role and may work with client on individual academic tasks.)	Shows ability to learn new skills.
Nursing Diagnosis: *High risk for violence: Self-directed*		
Client will remain safe.	Inquire about suicidal thoughts, wishes, or plans.	Maintains decreased incidence of self-destructive and violent behaviors.
Suicidal thought content will decrease.	Provide verbal reassurance that you will not allow client to hurt himself or others.	
Client will develop new outlets for aggression.	Note and record observations of self-destructive behavior.	
Self-destructive behaviors will decrease.	Provide constant client supervision.	
	Place client on highest level of suicide precautions.	
	Review suicide level daily.	
	Do suicidal assessment during one-to-one with primary nurse (including physical assessment).	

▶

A Client with a Disruptive Disorder and a Mood Disorder

Client Care Goals	Nursing Planning/ Intervention	Evaluation
Nursing Diagnosis: *High risk for violence: Directed at others*		
Client will express feelings without harming another or losing control.	Develop a behavioral program to manage the aggressive impulses, using limit setting, time-outs, holding, and seclusion.	Maintains decreased incidence of problem behaviors; maintains self-control.
	State clearly and repeatedly that aggression is not tolerated and that staff are present to provide a safe place for all the children.	
Nursing Diagnosis: *Self-esteem disturbance*		
Client will begin to feel more positive about himself.	Help client label feelings. Reflect client's feelings.	Shows evidence of insight.
Nursing Diagnosis: *Hopelessness*		
Client will feel more hopeful about life.	Acknowledge client's feelings. Make connections with client's feelings and events. Record verbal statements about self.	Expresses positive thoughts about the future.
Nursing Diagnosis: *Knowledge deficit related to condition and treatment*		
Client will understand the medication at his developmental level. Client will understand his condition at his developmental level. Client will express negative and positive feelings associated with medication.	Inquire about client's understanding of medication and any changes associated with medication. Develop a teaching plan to teach client about his condition (e.g., depression). Provide opportunities for questions and discussion concerning condition, hospitalization and treatment. Reinforce client's attempts to learn about his condition. Encourage client to express feelings related to medication. Provide support and education when client receives venipunctures to measure blood levels of antidepressant medication by preparing and	Is able to describe the reason for his hospitalization and treatment. Complies to medication regimen and makes positive statements toward medications.

Client Care Goals	Nursing Planning/Intervention	Evaluation
	educating client and his parents, comforting and reassuring client during the procedure.	

Nursing Diagnosis: *Ineffective individual coping*

Client Care Goals	Nursing Planning/Intervention	Evaluation
Client will follow directions, including rules of conduct, without incident. Client will use alternate means of managing stress and/or anxiety precipitating acting out behavior.	Medicate as prescribed, since some behavior may recede spontaneously with medication (especially if secondary to a depression or other condition responsive to pharmacology; e.g., school phobia has been treated successfully with imipramine). Monitor behavior prior to and following medication.	Maintains decreased incidence of problem behaviors. Uses stress-management techniques to allay anxiety.

Nursing Diagnosis: *Altered parenting/Ineffective family coping: Compromised*

Client Care Goals	Nursing Planning/Intervention	Evaluation
Parents will understand client's normal and special needs. Parents will understand the action and monitoring of the medication. Parents will be prepared for handling the medication after discharge. Parents will begin to develop plan for suicide precautions at home. Client will feel nurtured and supported by parents. Parents will deal with their losses so that they do not provide additional stress for client. Parents will feel acknowledged and respected by the staff.	Meet with parents to understand treatment plan. Model support and nurturing of client. Attend the session between the physician and parents when medication is explained. Provide ongoing medication teaching for client and his parents, including the name of the medication, reason for taking it, description of what the child can expect, frequency and dosage, list of side effects (including serious and annoying effects), and potential for overdose. Plan for discharge, for example, safety, storage, and administration of medication; danger of sudden withdrawal from medication; when and how to report problems and take vital signs. Explain that plastic boxes with compartments for daily doses are available in pharmacies Reinforce seriousness of client's suicidal threats to parents.	Parents increase participation in treatment plan. Parents are supportive and nurturing. Parents describe use of medications, dosage, precautions, and side effects. Parents show evidence of planning for suicide precautions including a safe home environment and signed no-suicide contract.

NURSING CARE PLAN (continued)

Client Care Goals	Nursing Planning/ Intervention	Evaluation
	Reinforce parents' concern for client's safety.	
	Teach client and his parents about the unit philosophy and structure related to preventing suicide.	
	Establish no-suicide contract with client and his parents.	
	Develop a plan with parents for supervision during passes.	
	Encourage frequent and regular visits and phone calls.	
	Involve parents in client's care.	
	Provide support to parents (e.g., difficulty dealing with separation).	
	Educate parents about depression in children (e.g., symptoms and approaches).	

• Communicate with others

• Explore and experiment while learning how to relate to self, the world, and others

• Compromise between the demands of drives and the dictates of reality

Play therapy offers the child a safe place to explore all the uses of play, thus dealing with conflictual material, developing a healthy self-image, and learning about self in relation to the therapist (Figure 33–1). In short, play therapy offers the opportunity for growth under stable conditions.

Play is used in many different ways in child psychiatry:

• Recreation and socialization in day programs and in-patient milieus

• Rewards in therapeutic classrooms for children accomplishing their work (e.g., when you finish your math, you can play a board game with the staff)

• An activity during the child's one-to-one time with the primary nurse

• A method of evaluation or treatment of sensori-motor deficits

Role of the Play Therapist   The role of play therapist is not a passive one, but it is essentially nondirective. The child sets the pace and does the work. The therapist contributes personally as an accepting and understanding adult whose goal is to foster the child's development of self. The relationship between the child and therapist is a new experience for the child, one that does not translate effectively outside the play therapy situation. The therapist accepts these children fully as they are, yet maintains the belief that they can change and grow. As they begin to trust the relationship, children can use it as a context for trying out new ways of behaving and relating to themselves and others.

Dynamics of Play Therapy   The acceptance the therapist shows these children can help them evolve a new self-image. Fearful and passive children may be able to try out some assertive or aggressive behavior. Consistently aggressive children may explore new ways to meet their needs. Children who perceive themselves as worthless may eventually accept the therapist's message that they are valuable, worthwhile people. In some cases, it may be a matter of educating the child to the possibility of different interactive patterns. It is difficult for young children to think of

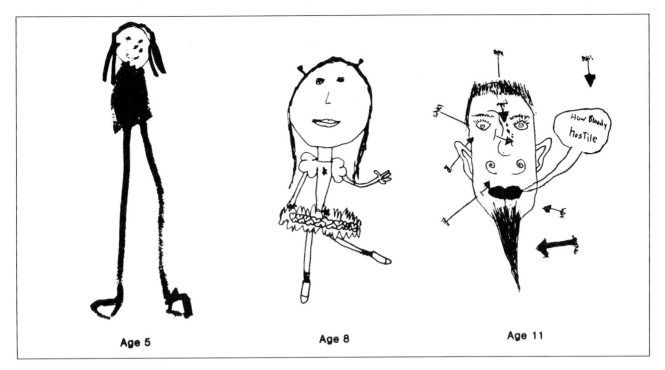

Age 5   Age 8   Age 11

FIGURE 33-1   Art therapy as a form of play therapy helps children communicate about their subjective reality in these self-portraits.

alternatives. They may believe that a dysfunctional family interactional pattern is the only possible one. Given a new pattern, they can explore new behavior. As they begin to resolve their conflicts and develop confidence and trust from the therapeutic relationship, their tension decreases, and they can expand their new awareness outside the therapeutic relationship.

Setting for Play Therapy   Ideally, play therapy is done in a well-equipped playroom. Toys might include dollhouse and furniture, puppets, dolls, blocks, art materials (Play-Doh, clay, paper, crayons, paints, marking pens), toy animals, telephone, cars and trucks, play kitchen, musical instruments, toy soldiers and guns, checkers and other games, and clothes for make-believe. (This kind of equipment is not strictly necessary. The nurse who is helping the fearful child overcome a terror of injections by letting the child handle the injection paraphernalia is also doing play therapy.) The toys stay in the playroom, and children use them there.

In the initial session, the therapist tells the children the playroom is for them to use as they please during the time they are there and sets the limits (usually the minimal ones of not hurting self or therapist or breaking equipment). Usually, therapists try to find out children's perceptions of what's going on by asking them why they are there. Therapists offer a brief description of their own understanding of the reason for the referral (e.g., "you're having trouble in school"). How things proceed from there is largely up to the child. Most children are eager to use the playroom situation and welcome the presence of an accepting, consistent, and understanding adult to resolve conflicts and try out different ways of relating to self and others.

The following example illustrates a child's use of play.

Twelve-year-old Laura had been sexually molested by her father. Her father was sent to prison for the sexual molestation of another preschooler. During Laura's therapy session, she asked the nurse therapist to go to the playroom. She built a fortress of large multicolored blocks. She put a chair inside the structure and sat down stating, "This is a dungeon. A rainbow dungeon." Her play demonstrated her ambivalent feelings toward her father (i.e., loss and resentment).

Group Therapy   Verbal group therapy with children tends to be most effective with adolescents or older prepubertal children. Verbal, insightful children are particularly good candidates. Children with a severe disruptive disorder may not be appropriate group candidates because they may disrupt the process and require the sole attention of the therapist. Activity therapy may be more effective with the prepubertal age group. For example, a psychiatric nurse-psychodramatist in an in-patient unit developed a sociodrama play group where children are encouraged to improve fairy tales, stories, or fantasies in a theater format followed by a discussion. (Psychodrama and sociodrama are discussed in Chapter 29.)

Psychopharmacology   Although the findings in psychopharmacology research with adults have been impressive (see Chapters 6 and 32), child psychopharmacology is less well developed. This can be explained by the typical lag between adult and child psychiatry, the unavailability of drug studies on children, and the concern for unknown developmental risks (e.g., some drugs can cause growth delay). Drugs have been used with children to decrease behavioral symptoms rather than to treat syndromes as with adults.

Medications Used with Children   Stimulants are the most commonly used medications with children and have been studied more often than other medications. Stimulants have been shown to increase ability to use cognitive skills, but not cognitive capacity, in hyperactive and normal children. These medications include methylphenidate (Ritalin) and pemoline (Cylert).

Antidepressants are used to treat depression, school phobia, attention deficit disorder, and enuresis. Even though several studies have demonstrated the effectiveness of tricyclics in a limited number of cases of enuresis, the exact mechanism is not known. Children may become tolerant, have symptom breakthrough, or have only temporary responses (Greenhill 1985). The Food and Drug Administration (FDA) limits the use of these medications with children because of cardiotoxicity. Imipramine (Tofranil) is the tricyclic antidepressant most commonly used with children as it is less cardiotoxic than other tricyclic medications. Nurses should administer these medications only under the orders of a physician with FDA exemption who uses strict procedure for monitoring cardiac effects and blood serum levels. Monoamine oxidase (MAO) inhibitors are not used with children because of the severe side effects and the difficulty in controlling children's diet.

Lithium has been found to be the·most effective drug for the treatment of mania. Since manic symptoms occur infrequently in children, this drug is not often used. Lithium is sometimes used to treat autistic, aggressive, and undersocialized conduct disordered children (Campbell 1985). This work is preliminary and there are few controlled studies.

Although frequently used in child psychiatry, neuroleptics do not have a specific target disorder in school-aged children. One study described the use of haloperidol (Haldol) in managing behavior such as fidgetiness, stereotypy, and hyperactivity in children with pervasive disorders (Campbell 1985). The most common use of neuroleptics in children is to sedate retarded children who are institutionalized, although this use is often inappropriate. Neuroleptics should be used sparingly with children because of side effects and unknown effects.

Nurses play an important role in monitoring the child on medication and educating the child and parents about the medication. Side effects should be monitored daily in in-patient settings and weekly in outpatient settings. Monitoring of side effects is discussed in Chapter 32.

Educating the Child and Parents   Drug holidays are used to assess the difference between drugged and drug-free states and to prevent growth delays. The child and the parents should be prepared for an increase in symptoms when the medication is removed. Record behavior of the child systematically and accurately to provide data by which the physician can make the decision about future medication. If the child is being treated in an outpatient setting, teach the parents and teachers to record the behavior. It is also necessary to assess the concerns the child has about side effects and stigmatization by peers related to the medication, or the child may fail to go to the school nurse to get the medication.

Assess parent's individual beliefs and fears about the medications. Parents are often concerned about the potential for the child to become dependent on medication, the side effects, and stigma. Give parents an opportunity to discuss their worries and questions and become informed about the medication. This time can be used to guide the parents toward a realistic view of the uncertainty of the medication so they will not anticipate a magical cure. Client information sheets on particular medications are helpful.

Milieu Nursing in Child Psychiatry   The majority of generalists in child psychiatric nursing work in in-patient settings. These settings provide the most intense methods of diagnosis and treatment. In-patient admission is indicated for children in the following situations:

• The child has threatened self (suicide, eating disorder) or others.

• Extreme family pathology interferes with the child's achievement of developmental tasks.

• Both physical and emotional disorders are present, and the contribution and interaction of each is unclear in terms of the child's difficulty.

• Extended and round-the-clock assessment is indicated.

• Outpatient treatment has not been effective.

• The child's behavior is progressively deteriorating (regression, psychosis).

Common to milieu treatment of children is the notion that the milieu is a safe environment for the child in which to accomplish the various therapeutic tasks of the treatment plan. Equally important is the child's need for a predictable environment. These needs are addressed in the structure and routines of a program, reinforced by behavioral management.

Child units have schedules that are very structured. Some components of the schedule, such as school, group therapy, and recreational therapy, are formally structured. Others are routines, such as early morning wakeup, meals, and bedtime, which tend to be more informal. Bedtime, for example, may be at 9:30 after 9:00 P.M. relaxation, with lights out at 10:00 P.M. Routines include washing up, brushing teeth, putting dirty clothes in the laundry. The children get some personal time to prepare for sleep by putting the day behind them and looking ahead to the next day.

The behavioral focus of the program allows the nursing staff to give continuous feedback to the children about the appropriateness of their behavior within each time frame. The children receive cues such as verbal praise, a sticker, or points, depending on developmental level, for appropriate behavior. Often these cues go together. For example, children who have a problem hitting others all the time may receive a sticker and verbal praise for no hits on an hourly basis until they connect their behavior to the reward. At that time the need for feedback may decrease to a less frequent schedule and to the need for only verbal reminders of the desired behavior.

At the same time staff are trying to reward children for positive behavior, they also need to know that negative behavior will not be tolerated. Typically when children cannot tolerate an activity they are asked to take a "time-out" from the activity by sitting on a chair until they are able to pull themselves together. If that does not work, the time-out may be taken in a "quiet room" free of objects and stimulation. If isolation is also too difficult, staff may use a restraining hold to help children calm down. As children are able to calm down, staff help them to see why they needed a time out and what they could do differently next time. The goal is to have children learn what precedes episodes during which they get out of control and learn ways to avoid the negative consequences of out-of-control behavior such as fights with other children. It is through effective limit setting that the nurse helps children separate their feelings from their behavior and learn more adaptive ways of expressing themselves.

Intensive Nursing Care   Child psychiatric units have a low staff-client ratio because of the intensive care these children require and the challenge of meeting the needs of children at different development levels. Children with psychotic disorders present some of the most difficult management problems. The Intervention box on page 834 gives an example of intensive nursing care in child psychiatry. Another example is the care of the suicidal child. See pages 567–568 in Chapter 23 for more information about suicidal children.

Countertransference in Child Psychiatric Nursing   Working with children, particularly children with emotional problems, may reactivate nurses' feelings about their family of origin or current family. Nurses may then react as if the client were part of that situation rather than responding to the current reality. Staff may also react to children or parents from their own stereotypes or beliefs rather than getting to know each child and parent as an individual. A third possibility is that the nurse can involve clients on the unit in conflicts or competition within the staff group itself. This phenomenon is known as countertransference. See also Chapter 26. The following vignette illustrates a common example of countertransference.

Eleven-year-old Cynthia had a history of living with extended family and several hospitalizations. Cynthia's mother was ambivalent toward her, often openly rejecting her (i.e., limited visitations and missed family sessions). Cynthia stimulated a lot of feeling among the staff about bad mothers and good mothers, and the staff was protective of the child and angry at the mother. The staff was encouraged to examine the mother's own deprivation by an abusive mother and the difficulties in raising this very troubled child.

Clinical supervisors and nursing managers can help staff reframe their view of the child and the family, identify personal experiences that limit their perception of the child, and identify unresolved staff issues. Through these explorations, staff can work more therapeutically with children and parents and increase their self-awareness.

Child disorders cannot be fully understood or managed without exploring the family context. Research studies have demonstrated that treating the family system produces more rapid and enduring changes.

Working with Families   Earlier milieu treatment tended to provide more of a custodial approach, while the current emphasis is on keeping the child involved with the family and helping the child return as quickly as possible to home and community. In-patient care is generally becoming more family oriented. Involving parents as active members of their child's treatment team has a profound impact on the degree to which the in-patient treatment has meaning to the child and the family. Each child participates in the routines and group activities of the unit, and individual treatment and family activities are planned according to the special needs of the child, involving the family as much as possible.

Professionals often fail to recognize the overwhelming and confusing feelings parents may feel when confronted with the decision to provide psychiatric services for their child. Parents often describe feelings of guilt, depression, anxiety, denial, and embarrassment. In addition, one parent must often

INTERVENTION

Guidelines for Working with the Psychotic Child

1. Assess degree of thought disorder (content and behavior):
   a. Record observations.
   b. Inform physician of escalations.
   c. Note response to psychopharmacology.
2. Encourage reality testing:
   a. Do not reinforce experiences that are not real.
   b. Make simple statements about experiences the child describes that do not exist.
   c. Direct attention to real experiences.
   d. Limit number of thoughts nurse will listen to and number of people available to listen to pressured thoughts.
   e. Help child avoid experiences that increase delusions.
   f. Avoid the use of jokes and puns commonly used with children.
   g. Avoid the unnecessary use of stimuli (such as intercoms or whispering between staff in child's room).
3. Encourage socialization:
   a. Interrupt isolation.
   b. Maintain eye contact with child.
   c. Provide instructions and rewards for appropriate behaviors in social situations.
4. Orient child to routines:
   a. Provide child with frequent data for orientation (such as calendar, clock, references to time and place, the reason for hospitalization, and introducing the staff to the child).
   b. Set up a structured routine for child's day. A chart of the routine could be drawn with clocks and pictures representing the activities.
   c. Discuss child's typical daily routine with the parents.
   d. Explain each procedure clearly and simply.
   e. Keep communication direct, concrete, and simple.
   f. Perform procedures in a consistent manner.
   g. Provide a minimum of changes in nursing staff (provide a primary nurse for each shift).
5. Provide a safe environment for the child:
   a. Supervise child frequently.
   b. Remove dangerous materials from child's room.

make this decision when the spouse is angry and nonsupportive of the plan. Grandparents frequently blame parents for the problem or push the parents not to follow through with treatment. The following example illustrates the anxiety and denial of the grandparents of a child with serious emotional problems:

The maternal grandmother of a suicidal child who was scheduled for admission to an in-patient unit tried to block the admission. She told her daughter just to send the child to stay with her for a while. The child psychiatrist and the child psychiatric nurse spent time with the parents discussing the pressure they experienced from the child's grandmother. They reminded the parents that psychiatric services are unfamiliar to the grandmother's generation. They also reviewed the basis for the recommendation of hospitalization. The parents were encouraged to make their own decision based on their experience with their child and their concerns for her safety. Possible explanations for the grandparents were suggested, and the professionals offered to be available to discuss the grandparents' questions and concerns.

Nursing staff often need to help parents plan their visits with the child to avoid perpetuating dysfunctional parent-child interaction. The following example illustrates the type of family problems encountered:

The staff in an in-patient milieu found they needed to help the parents of a 12-year-old boy plan the weekend day passes. The child reported he barely saw his parents while home on pass, and he generally returned early. His mother went to work, and his father had an outside activity. The child hung out at the local mall with his friends. This chain of events interfered with the goal of a transition of the child back into the family. The family therapist and primary nurse worked with the family unit to structure the passes to meet the goals of reentry and increase availability of the parents to the child.

Discharge Planning   Prior to discharge from in-patient hospitalization, the parents should meet with the interdisciplinary team to discuss the treatment plan. Components of the in-patient milieu program that have been helpful to the child are identified and then translated into appropriate interventions in the home environment. For example, the nurse works very closely with the parents to adapt time-outs, family meetings, and the bedtime routine to be realistic and meaningful at home. Parents need to be given this information verbally and in writing. A model for discharge planning is provided in the accompanying Client/Family Teaching box. In addition, conferences are typically held between the interdisciplinary team, the parents, and representatives from the child's community school to develop an individualized educational plan.

Aftercare   Aftercare refers to the plan and implementation for care and treatment after hospitalization of the child. Given the current limitations of third-party payment reimbursement for hospitalization, the priority in health care is abbreviated assessment and establishment of a plan of treatment within the context of limited or no outpatient benefits. Parents need to be involved in the decision-making process, and their wishes are the major determinant. All children who are hospitalized need some type of follow-up. The possible dispositions include:

- Discharge to home and return to the same school

- Foster care

- Day treatment program or special class

- Residential treatment

During the hospitalization, parents are encouraged to learn about their part in the child's difficulties. The parents' availability to the child and participation in the treatment usually predict the degree of cooperation that can be anticipated in the outpatient treatment.

CLIENT/FAMILY TEACHING

Discharge Planning with Parents

Discipline	Areas	Discipline	Areas
Child psychiatrist	Condition (simple explanation, course of condition)	Teacher	Summary of work accomplished
	Treatment needs (child, family)		Classroom behavior management
	Whom to tell and what (about hospitalization)		Homework management
	Medication		How to deal with child's reentry into community school
	Early warning signs to seek immediate help	Family therapist	Family contracts
	Medical care		Communication techniques
Primary nurse	Daily routine		Chores, responsibilities
	Limit-setting techniques		Family activities
	Positive reinforcement techniques		Structure
	Self-help skills		Problem-solving skills
	Socialization		Rules, consequences
Pharmacist/nurse	Dosage, administration of medication		Rewards, reinforcers
	Side effects of medication		
	Client medication information sheet		
	Methods to alleviate side effects of medication		

Parents and children tend to get anxious and fearful at the time of discharge. The child may be concerned about failing and being sent away again. Parents are worried the child may become symptomatic again and they will not be able to manage. The child and parents may experience a honeymoon period following discharge. During this period, the child shows little evidence of previous difficulties and seems to be making the transition well, and the parents may resist aftercare treatment. However, children often regress after a few months, and parents have difficulty maintaining the aftercare program developed in the hospital. The following is an example of the response of parents to the reemergence of their child's problems:

Following the discharge of an 11-year-old boy with attention deficit disorder and mood disorder, the parents reported everything was going well. School had begun, and the child started doing poorly on tests as he had prior to his admission. The parents were convinced he was going to be rehospitalized. They were frustrated by their own sense of incompetence and angry at the child for defeating himself. They generalized their worries to a longitudinal concern that the child would never accomplish anything worthwhile.

School Personnel The child reentering school needs help with explaining the absence to peers, since peers tend to be very curious about absences. Often parents put pressure on the child to keep the hospitalization a secret. However, school personnel who do not know the nature of the child's hospitalization are handicapped in facilitating the child's reentry. School personnel may need to maintain an important monitoring role for recurrence of symptoms, particularly if limited outpatient service is feasible. Reentry may be facilitated by participation in a reentry group, encouragement to participate in at least one peer extracurricular activity, and identification of a particular support person for the child in school.

Evaluating

The nurse looks to such routine data as vital signs, weights, sleep record, bowel and bladder charts, and other physical findings not only to confirm initial data base findings but also to note changes. Psychopharma-cologic treatments are followed especially closely because children reach toxic levels quickly and have many responses to medication not typical of the adult populations on which many drugs are initially tested. The more experienced nurse also develops an awareness of the physical findings that may be associated with emotional disturbance (e.g., encopresis and abdominal pains) as well as the physical problems that are accompanied by behavioral or psychiatric symptoms (e.g., Tourette disorder and seizure disorders).

The behavioral record provides another constant source of information for the child psychiatric nurse. Most treatment units make some provision for the periodic assessment of identified behaviors. To provide effective behavior management, the nurse must frequently evaluate the client's progress toward identified goals and the effectiveness of the reward system. Responsiveness to the individual needs of the client in a behavioral program enhances its effectiveness.

Because the therapeutic milieu treatment of children is characterized by an intense relationship between staff and clients and a consistent approach among staff interacting with the client, the exchange of information with colleagues is essential. The twenty-four hour assessment of the child going through various daily routines and interacting with others contributes invaluable information to the formulation of the plan of care for the family as well as the child. The nurse brings this information together to present a coherent plan, not one based on just a set of limited discrete observations by one person.

Finally, evaluations of child treatment must be compared to appropriate developmental markers. Frustration tolerance, for example, is far different in the 4-year-old than the 14-year-old. For this reason, evaluation of such behaviors must be made according to norms for age appropriateness. Individual and family norms also contribute to this problem. Often a child who exhibits what appears to be bad manners or poor boundaries with adults has been taught this behavior at home. Although children need to learn socially useful behavior, they also need to fit in with their families.

CHAPTER HIGHLIGHTS

• Child psychiatric nursing concerns itself with the promotion of mental health in all children as well as the treatment of the emotionally disturbed child.

• The role of the nurse in child psychiatry is changing as a result of the increase in focus on biochemical disorders and dual diagnoses.

• Standards of practice for generalists and specialists in child and adolescent psychiatric nursing have been published by the American Nurses' Association.

• The etiology of psychiatric disorders in children is multicausal and may include genetic and biophysical factors, social and cultural factors, family system factors, and acquired illness and injury.

• The manifestation of psychiatric disorders in children is influenced by the child's developmental level.

• Nursing assessment in child psychiatry is a multi-step process that includes basic assessment of the child (psychosocial and physical), life space interview, and family assessment.

• Nursing diagnoses specific to child psychiatric clients have been developed and are being refined.

• The treatment of psychiatric disorders in children must be family oriented and multidisciplinary in nature.

• Child psychiatric nurses are involved in primary or collaborative roles in various treatment modalities including play therapy, psychopharmacology, milieu, group therapy, parent counseling, and psychoeducation.

• The use of psychopharmacologic agents in children has not been well tested. These agents must be used cautiously and closely monitored.

• Discharge planning and aftercare facilitate the child's reentry into the community and may help prevent problems with adjustment and rehospitalization.

REFERENCES

Adkins AS: Helping your patient cope with Tourette syndrome. *Pediatr Nurs* 1989;15(2):135–137.

American Nurses' Association: *Standards of Child and Adolescent Psychiatric and Mental Health Nursing Practice*, ANA, 1985.

American Psychiatric Association: *Diagnostic and Statistical Manual of Mental Disorders* ed 3, revised. APA, 1987.

Asarnow JR et al.: Childhood-onset depressive disorders: A follow-up study of rates of rehospitalization and out-of-home placement among child psychiatric inpatients. *J Affective Disord* 1988;15(3):245–253.

Beitchman JH: Childhood schizophrenia: A review and comparison with adult onset schizophrenia. *Psychiatr Clin North Am* 1985;8(4):793–814.

Bowlby J: *Attachment and Loss*. Vol. 2, Separation: Anxiety and Anger. New York, Basic Books, 1973.

Burgess AW, Hartman CR, Kelly S: Assessing child abuse: The TRIADS checklist. *J Psychosoc Nurs* 1990;28:4–9.

Burgess AW, et al.: Child molestation: Assessing impact in multiple victims. *Arch Psychiatr Nurs* 1987;1(1):33–39.

Campbell M, Pali M: Measurement of tardive dyskinesia. *Psychopharmacol Bull* 1985;21:106–107.

Campbell M, Spencer EK: Psychopharmacology in child and adolescent psychiatry: A review of the past five years. *J Am Acad Child Adolesc Psychiatry* 1988;27(3):269–279.

Caplan G: *Prevention of Mental Disorders in Children*. Basic Books, 1961.

Clunn P: *Child Psychiatric Nursing*. Mosby, 1990.

Cohen D, Leckman J, Shaywitz B: The Tourette syndrome and other tics, in Shaffer D, Ehrhardt A, Greenhill L (eds): *The Clinical Guide to Child Psychiatry*. Free Press, 1985.

Eth S, Pynoos RS: *Post-Traumatic Stress Disorder in Children*. American Psychiatric Press, 1985.

Greenhill L: Pediatric pharmacology, Chapter 26 in Shaffer D, Ehrhardt A, Greenhill L (eds): *The Clinical Guide to Child Psychiatry*. Free Press, 1985.

Grossman J, et al.: *Alcoholism in Family Histories of Depressed Prepubertal Children*, unpublished manuscript. University of Illinois Medical Center, 1984.

Harnett NE: Conduct disorder in childhood and adolescence: An update. *J Child Adolesc Psychiatr Mental Health Nurs* 1989;2(2):74–77.

Herman JL, Perry JC, Van der Kolk B: Childhood trauma in borderline personality disorder. *Am J Psychiatr* 1989;146(4):490–495.

Herzog E, Lewis H: Children in poor families. *Am J Orthopsychiatry* 1970;40:375–387.

Hewitt K: Prevention of behavior problems in pre-school children: Preliminary considerations. *Health Visit* 1988;61(6):181–183.

Joshi PT, Capozzoli JA, Coyle JT: Low-dose neuroleptic therapy for children with childhood onset pervasive development disorder. *Am J Psychiatry* 1988;145(3):335–338.

Looney JG: *Chronic Mental Illness in Children and Adolescents*. American Psychiatric Press, 1987.

Oades RD: Attention deficit disorder with hyperactivity: The contribution of catecholaminergic activity. *Prog Neurobiol* 1987;29:229–236.

Peck M, Farberow N, Litman R: *Youth Suicide*. Springer Publishing, 1985.

Porter LS: The what, why, and how of hyperkinesis: Implications for nursing. *J Adv Nurs* 1988;13(2):229–236.

Pothier P, Norbeck J, Laliberte M: Child psychiatric nursing: The gap between need and utilization. *J Psych Soc Nurs* 1985;23:18–23.

Poznanski E: The clinical phenomenology of childhood depression *Am J Orthopsychiatry* 1982;52:308–313.

Poznanski E, et al.: *Cortisol Nonsuppression and Suicidal Ideation in Prepubertal Children*, unpublished manuscript. Rush-Presbyterian-St. Luke's Medical Center, 1987.

Puig-Antich J, Chambers W, Ryan W: *The Schedule for Affective Disorders and Schizophrenia for School-Age Children (K-SADS-P)*. Western State Psychiatric Institute and Clinic, 1980.

Redl F: *When We Deal with Children*. Free Press, 1966.

Rothstein A: Hallucinatory phenomena in children: A critique of the literature. *J Am Acad Child Psychiatry* 1981;20:623–635.

Rutter M: Invulnerability, or why some children are not damaged by stress. In *New Directions in Children's Mental Health*, ed. S. J. Shamsie. New York: SP Medical and Scientific Books, 1979.

Sameroff A, Chandler M: Reproductive risk and the continuum of caretaking causality, in Horowitz F (ed): *Review of Child Development Research*, vol. 4. University of Chicago Press, 1975.

Scahill L, Jekel JF, Schilling LS: Screening child psychiatry inpatients for communication disorders: A pilot study. *Arch Psychiatr Nurs* 1991;5(1):31–37.

Scahill L, Sipple B: Developmental history collection on a child psychiatric inpatient service. *J Child Adolesc Psychiatr Ment Health Nurs* 1990;3(2):52–56.

Seifer R, Nurcombe B, Scioli A, Grapentine WL: Is major depressive disorder in childhood a distinct diagnostic entity? *J Am Acad Child Adolesc Psychiatry* 1989; 28:935–941.

Shaffer D, Erhardt A, Greenhill L (eds): *The Clinical Guide to Child Psychiatry*. Free Press, 1985.

Tanquay P, Cantor S: Schizophrenia in children: Introduction. *J Am Acad Child Psychiatry* 1986;25:591–594.

Valente SM: Clinical hypnosis with school-age children. *Arch Psychiatr Nurs* 1990;4(2):131–136.

Webster-Stratton C: Interactions of mothers and fathers with conduct problem children: Comparison with a nonclinic group. *Public Health Nurs* 1989;6(4):218–223.

Weiner J, Hendren R: Childhood depression. *J Dev Behav Pediatr* 1983;4:43–49.

Weiss SJ: Personality adjustment and social support of parents who care for children with pervasive developmental disorders. *Arch Psychiatr Nurs* 1991;5(1):25–30.

Weissman M, et al.: Psychopathology in the children (ages 6–18) of depressed and normal parents. *J Am Acad Child Psychiatry* 1984;23:78–84.

Woolston J: Transactional risk model for short and intermediate term psychiatric inpatient treatment of children. *J Am Acad Child Adolesc Psychiatry* 1989;28(1):38–41.

Zimmerman ML: Art and group work: Interventions for multiple victims of child molestation. *Arch Psychiatr Nurs* 1987;1(1):40–46.

Applying the Nursing Process with Adolescents

Carol Bradley-Corpuel

LEARNING OBJECTIVES

- Relate the importance of using a humanistic interactionist framework to a comprehensive assessment of adolescent problems

- Describe the roles and functions of the nurse in outpatient and in-patient treatment settings for adolescents

- Describe the roles and functions of the nurse working with families of adolescent clients

- List at least four functions of the staff nurse working to maintain a therapeutic milieu

- Define the term *acting out*, giving an example of the adolescent's acting out a "life script"

- Construct a client contract for use with the adolescent in treatment

CROSS REFERENCES

Other topics relevant to this content are: ANA Standards of Child and Adolescent Psychiatric Mental Health Nursing, Chapter 33; Depression, Chapter 13; Drug abuse, Chapter 11; Eating disorders, Chapter 20; Family therapy, Chapter 30; Suicide, Chapter 23.

WHAT IS ADOLESCENCE? SOME sources define it simply as the time of physical and psychosocial development between the ages of 12 and 20. Others have described it as a period of "normal psychosis." Still others see it as an attempt by a tyrannical subculture to overtake adult America. It is not necessary to accept these last two definitions verbatim to understand their implications. Most people recognize the immense stress that occurs during adolescence and the importance it holds for that person's future.

Trying to understand the adolescent is a challenge to anyone. For the nurse who chooses to work with adolescents, the challenge offers considerable rewards. Nurses who can recollect their own experiences and reactions during this tumultuous time will better appreciate the adolescent's dilemma.

Theoretic Foundations

A sound theoretic knowledge base helps the nurse differentiate "normal" and "abnormal," usual and unusual, behaviors of the adolescent. In particular, the nurse can do a comprehensive assessment by focusing on the psychologic development of the individual and the evolution of the adolescent as a biopsychosocial being. The nurse can accomplish the first task with an understanding of developmental theory and the second with an appreciation of humanistic interactionist theory.

Developmental Theory

An understanding of developmental theory helps the nurse to identify deviations in the adolescent's growth and development processes and to intervene appropriately. The theories of Sigmund Freud, Erik Erikson, and Harry Stack Sullivan provide considerable insight into the adolescent's struggle to attain adulthood.

The development of the adolescent's sense of identity entails a preoccupation with self-image. It also entails a connection between future role and past experiences. In the search for a new sense of sameness and continuity, many adolescents must repeat the crisis resolutions of earlier years to integrate these past elements and establish the lasting ideals of a final identity. According to Erikson, these crisis periods or stages are reviews of the adolescent's sense of trust, autonomy, initiative, and industry, in that order. (See Chapter 4 for a discussion of the theories of Freud, Erikson, and Sullivan as they relate to adolescent growth and development.)

Humanistic Interactionist Theory

The nurse not only needs knowledge about developmental theories and psychobiology, but also needs to integrate humanistic interactionist principles into assessment and interventions to develop a trusting, caring interpersonal relationship with the adolescent client. The adolescent developmental period is a time in the individual's life when identity, values, and goals are in a state of flux. The nurse should take into account not only the immediate situation but also the impact of the developmental stage, social and cultural factors, family influences, and psychodynamic conflicts on the adolescent's behavior.

To do this the nurse should explore the meaning of the identified problem or behavior. The following questions can guide this exploration:

• What meaning does this behavior or problem hold for the adolescent?

• What message is the adolescent conveying through this behavior?

• What impact does this problem have on the client in this developmental stage? Is this a usual or unusual problem or behavior for the adolescent's peer group?

• How have resulting changes, if any, affected the adolescent and the adolescent's relationships with others?

• What goals does the adolescent have for the immediate and distant future?

• What personal strengths does the adolescent have to help deal with this problem?

• What considerations have the client and the nurse given to other developmental, familial, biologic, or sociocultural factors involved?

It is insufficient to base the nursing response to the adolescent's needs and dilemmas solely on behaviors without a more comprehensive evaluation of these other factors. This approach can lead to ineffective treatment, a temporary surcease of the initial behaviors with an upheaval of symptoms in another area, and possibly a sterile treatment environment without any meaningful therapeutic alliance. Only by considering all aspects of the adolescent client as a biopsychosocial being can the nurse truly understand the meanings of such behaviors to the adolescent and intervene effectively in the situation.

Historical Foundations

The role of the nurse in the care and treatment of adolescents has dramatically changed. Once regarded simply as a technician who monitored somatic therapies, the nurse is now acknowledged as a professional with numerous capabilities and skills that have a direct bearing on the favorable treatment outcome of adolescents.

The American Nurses' Association (ANA) now recognizes child and adolescent psychiatric and mental health nursing as a specialty area of psychiatric and mental health nursing practice. The ANA *Standards of Child and Adolescent Psychiatric and Mental Health Nursing Practice* (1985) are reproduced on page 813 in Chapter 33.

Whether a generalist or clinical specialist, the nurse in today's health setting integrates these characteristics and role responsibilities to intervene with the adolescent within the significant social system toward optimal social, emotional, cognitive, and physical development. Using expertise in identifying relevant deviations in the developmental process, the nurse works closely with the systems (family, school, community, and institution) on which the adolescent is emotionally and economically dependent.

The Role of the Nurse

The nurse can assume numerous roles within a variety of treatment modalities to help maintain the adolescent client's health and well-being and identify abnormal or problem-causing behavior during this difficult period of development.

In the Outpatient Setting

As a Community Health Nurse In the school, clinic, or community health agency, the nurse has excellent opportunities to observe the adolescent engage in the normal activities of daily living. The nurse has frequent occasion to counsel adolescents in the problems that confront them daily and to advise school or clinic staff members in their encounters with adolescents. The nurse who knows how to deal with normal adolescent problems will also be adept in identifying obstacles to effective resolution of emotional problems and suggesting further treatment.

School is the most influential experience in the adolescent's life outside of the home. The adolescent spends more waking time in school activities than in any other activity, and most of the adolescent's successes, problems, and conflicts are demonstrated in the school setting. Even adolescents who are supposedly "truant" from school are often on the school grounds, perhaps meeting their friends at lunchtime, playing cards in the library, or "hanging out" on the school steps. Such an "absent" student may suddenly appear at the school nurse's door because of "boredom" or a somatic complaint.

Unfortunately, the school nurse's role in the early recognition and treatment of predelinquent individuals has been minimized or has gone unrecognized. There are several reasons for this. First, school administrators and teachers tend to view the school nurse as a person who deals only with physical sickness and medical emergencies. They may not be aware that because of the intimate quality of a nurse-client relationship or the comprehensive and holistic nature of nursing assessments, the nurse may be helpful in exploring an area of conflict in the adolescent's life or intervening with a disruptive student. Such early intervention could prevent more serious problems in later years. Many studies have indicated a direct correlation between problems of early school life and the incidence of subsequent juvenile delinquency, depression, and suicidal behavior (Child et al. 1980, Harnett 1989, Pfeffer 1984, White et al. 1989). Here is a list of problems demonstrated by the adolescent in the school setting that call for early intervention:

- Antisocial behavior (e.g., stealing, setting fires, bullying others)

- Avoidant social behavior

- Chronic illness

- Depression

- Disruptive classroom behavior

- Drug abuse

- Excessive daydreaming

- Hypochondriasis

- Learning difficulties

- Poor school performance or dramatic shift in school performance

- Temper tantrums

- Truancy

Second, administrators tend to limit the nurse's activities to the school itself. They may see no need for the nurse to make home visits to meet with the sick student's family or view problems firsthand. Many school districts lack time and money to provide for counseling families or individuals in a formal setting. As the role of the independent nursing practitioner expands, and as legislation for third-party reimbursement for independent practice becomes a reality, nurses will be better able to assume more autonomy and responsibility and to meet the needs of the student more comprehensively and effectively.

Meanwhile, the nurse who is already employed in the school setting or community agency can seize every opportunity to provide an active school health program and to educate school administrators and faculty about the importance of preventive care. For example, the nurse in a viable school health program can provide preventive counseling not only to troubled adolescents in school but also to their preschool siblings during routine home visits. Nurses can establish productive relationships with teachers, help other faculty members encourage parent-teacher conferences, take an active part in developing the curriculum, and help adolescents on probation or parole return to school.

As a Nurse Counselor/Therapist
Whether in the clinic, home, school, or community health setting, the psychiatric nurse has many opportunities to organize individual, group, or family counseling sessions. Nurses can function within a variety of treatment roles, according to their experience and capabilities.

As an Individual Therapist   The nurse's qualifications and role in the clinic, school, or community setting may allow for counseling the adolescent on an individual basis. Sometimes the nurse can establish a trusting alliance and facilitate communication with the client. Sometimes, however, the adolescent is too threatened to talk openly with the nurse in this intimate setting. Some adolescents view the nurse as an authority figure and resist all efforts to communicate. The nurse may make more headway with this mode of treatment when it is used in conjunction with group therapy. Unless certified to provide this service, the nurse should counsel the adolescent only for the purposes of identifying the problem area and referring the client to a qualified professional for individual psychotherapy.

As a Group Therapist   It is usually most effective to work with adolescents in a group. Because the values, acceptance, and recognition of peers are so important during adolescence, the group can provide the support the student needs to deal with problems and effect change. In addition, involving the adolescent's peers helps dilute the conflict with adults that may exist in one-to-one work. In the school setting, health education groups can provide an acceptable forum for peer interaction and discussion of difficult topics. Otherwise, the nurse should practice as a group therapist only as a certified individual or with adequate supervision by a certified individual. Knowledge of group dynamics is crucial for the nurse to be an effective group leader.

As a Family Therapist   Being a parent of a "normal" adolescent is difficult at best. As the child grows into adulthood with all its perplexing questions and problems, parents normally worry about their child's safety and well-being. They may feel rejected because they are no longer needed in the same way. Because many parents of relatively normal adolescents share this plight, they can usually find receptive listeners who will give them comfort and support.

The problems of the parents of emotionally disturbed adolescents are more complicated. Many such parents have a strong sense of failure because their children did not turn out "right." Their feelings of guilt, frustration, and helplessness are likely to increase if their child is institutionalized. They have probably felt confused and resentful when experts offered them smug and guilt-provoking advice. Unlike the parents of other adolescents, they may have no one in whom to confide, either because they lack the support and understanding of others, or because their own self-reproach prevents them from seeking out confidants.

Meetings with family members may be indicated if the adolescent's role in the family seems to compound the problems presented in the school or agency setting. An important part of the problem-solving process is organizing initial interviews with parents and family members. The nurse can use the information gathered during these meetings to determine whether the problems stem from difficulties posed by the larger system (the family), and, if so, whether family therapy is indicated.

The nurse should show compassion and understanding for the parents' dilemma without blaming them or their offspring. Parents will be more receptive to family therapy and to exploring their part in the adolescent's problems if they sense that the nurse will support them, too. Stress and psychologic symptoms evidenced by parents can serve as markers for emotional or behavioral problems in adolescents (Compas et al. 1989). Any tendency to feel self-righteous or superior to the disturbed adolescent's parents is an obstacle to effective treatment. Such feelings are readily communicated to parents and can only validate their fear of blame and increase their reluctance to participate in therapy with their child. By the same token, the nurse should resist any temptation to overidentify with the parents, perpetuating the family system's problems. The adolescent and the family need a "neutral" party who can play an objective, knowledgeable, and supportive role in helping them change. The adolescent's chances for resolving the underlying conflicts and maintaining a healthy life are virtually nil if the family system remains unchanged.

Parents, school, and agency staff must understand the objectives and goals of treatment to appreciate the progress the client has made and avoid reinforcing the client's previously maladaptive behavior. The following incident illustrates the problems that arise when parents and school authorities, particularly those who must deal directly with behavior problems in the classroom, lack psychologic sophistication.

Jeremy, a 13-year-old boy, was referred to the school nurse because he was introverted and isolated. He made no contact with either his peers or teachers and rarely spoke unless addressed directly. After he had spent three months in group and individual therapy sessions with the nurse, Jeremy began to come to the grade counselor's office of his own accord to talk about his depression and the problems he had been having in his family. Both the grade counselor and the boy's family believed this to be an indication that his difficulties had worsened, and they began to complain to the nurse about his illness! Not only were Jeremy's parents and counselor ignorant of the goals of treatment and the behaviors expected to come with change, but apparently they were also uncomfortable with the changes in Jeremy's behavior and with the implications of these changes for their relationships with him.

The client's siblings may experience many different feelings. Sometimes they share in the parents' guilt and shame. Sometimes, however, they are pleased and relieved when the "troublemaker" is out of the family and hospitalized. The nurse should extend the same understanding to the siblings as to the parents and should help them see how each member of the family contributes to the problem. If the troubled adolescent is hospitalized, another member of the family, usually a sibling, may assume the role of the "bad" or "sick" person in the family, since the identified "bad" person is no longer at home. The nurse should be aware of this tendency. If the nurse is not skilled in assessing the need for family therapy or in providing this service, the family should be referred to a competent family therapist.

The nurse may identify a need for all of the above therapies in dealing with an individual's problem. In some cases, an informal discussion with the nurse is all that is warranted. In other cases, the nurse may identify problems that require considerable attention. Sometimes a period of unsuccessful treatment is necessary to determine that outpatient therapy is ineffective and that hospitalization is indicated. Before making such a recommendation, the nurse needs to establish a trusting relationship with the client and the parents.

In the In-Patient Setting

Admission into a hospital or other residential treatment facility may be indicated under the following circumstances:

• If the adolescent lacks sufficient ego strength to control impulsivity

• If the degree of destructive or antisocial behavior escalates beyond normal limits

• If the adolescent cannot form meaningful, stable relationships within the everyday environment (e.g., due to family dysfunction)

The existence of any one of the preceding conditions warrants counseling or professional treatment. A combination of two or more is likely to make treatment on an outpatient basis virtually ineffective and indicates the need for hospital or residential treatment.

Hospitalization of the disturbed adolescent has these advantages:

• It provides additional structure within which to handle the physically and psychologically destructive elements of the adolescent's behavior.

• It removes the individual from the stresses of a disturbed family environment.

• It offers opportunities for supporting existing ego strengths and for promoting whatever ability the client has for forming relationships.

Adolescents are sometimes institutionalized because their ideas are strange or threatening to their families, or because the responsible authorities seek to punish the adolescent's unacceptable behavior. The results can be disastrous. Therefore, it is important to make accurate assessments and to implement early treatment when indicated. The nurse plays a crucial role in making such assessments, undertaking appropriate interventions, and educating parents, teachers, and school officials to recognize such needs.

As a Staff Nurse in a General Hospital Setting
Adolescents with an emotional problem may have symptoms of physical illness and as a result may be admitted to a general hospital setting for evaluation and treatment. Clients with anorexia nervosa, in particular, may be referred for in-patient treatment on general adolescent medical units. Several hospitals have established innovative educational and work study programs for high school juniors and seniors (Johnsson 1990). Staff nurses in such a general hospital setting can take the opportunity to reach out to adolescents in these programs.

As a Consultant in a General Hospital Setting
Staff nurses from a psychiatric in-patient unit of a general hospital may be consulted by other nursing staff about emotionally disturbed adolescents who have been admitted to their general medical or surgical units. Some general hospital settings have clinical nurse specialists in psychiatric liaison positions to consult with nursing staff.

As a Staff Nurse or Clinical Specialist in the Psychiatric Setting   In the in-patient psychiatric setting, the staff nurse or clinical nurse specialist may assume any of the previously mentioned roles. Nurses in the in-patient setting also have numerous opportunities to observe and assess the family dynamics among the adolescent's family members and possibly to intervene. Nurses involved in family therapy sessions can perceive maladaptive ways of relating and take direct steps to work toward change. However, the nurse need not work within the structured format of a therapy hour to have an impact on the family system. The accompanying Intervention box delineates specific parent behaviors and corresponding interventions by the nurse in the therapeutic milieu.

Because in-patient nursing entails around-the-clock care, the nurse has the responsibility to maintain the therapeutic milieu. The role of the in-patient staff nurse includes the following:

• Maintaining the physical and psychologic safety of the unit

• Setting verbal and physical limits on the client's behavior

• Establishing meaningful one-to-one relationships with clients

• Identifying clients' strengths and promoting more adaptive coping skills

• Role modeling more socially acceptable behaviors

• Participating in group therapies and other structured activities

The Value of the Therapeutic Milieu

Many authors have described the importance of the therapeutic milieu, indicating the strong influence of the treatment environment on the treatment outcome. Chapter 31 discusses the development of the milieu concept.

Because of adolescents' needs for peer acceptance, their overwhelming uncertainties and fears, and their everchanging behaviors and attitudes about identity, the adolescents' chances for success in in-patient treatment are increased by a peer group setting. Much has been written about the value of the therapeutic milieu in dealing with adolescent problems, including the problems of drug abuse and similar destructive activities (Amini and Salasnek 1975, Amini et al. 1976, Lewis 1989). Without the social interaction and living-learning situations provided by the peer group, psychotherapy may be sterile and ineffectual.

The therapeutic community is a valuable experience for adolescents in treatment because of the following reasons:

• Adolescents more readily hear and accept limits from peers than from adults.

• Adolescents more readily respond to negative and positive feedback from peers.

• Shared goals and objectives facilitate group process and development of cohesion among adolescent group members.

• Group interaction allows for expression of appropriate feelings and identification with peers with similar feelings.

• Group interaction provides opportunities for learning how to develop relationships with others.

• Group structure allows for the testing of new, more adaptive behaviors.

• Adolescents receive feedback from the peer group and have the opportunity to give feedback in a supportive environment.

• The group format provides an opportunity to work out specific issues of conflict with adult group leaders while receiving the support and understanding of peers.

The Nursing Process and Adolescents

Adolescents present behaviors and problems unique to their developmental stage. Without knowledge and understanding about potentially difficult areas, the nurse may respond with confusion, anger, and even hostility, which will cause feelings of frustration and failure for both the nurse and the adolescent. The following pages contain numerous examples of either typical behaviors expected of the "normal" adolescent or problem behaviors that may provide the impetus for referral to a treatment setting, or both. In many situations the nurse may simply need attention drawn to the difficult issues encountered in working with adolescents. That information is given in the Assessment section. Situations that represent an identified problem necessitating treatment are categorized under Planning and Implementing Interventions.

Assessment

Accurate and comprehensive assessments can be obtained only by viewing the adolescent as a biopsychosocial being. Only by integrating knowledge from the biologic and psychologic sciences and humanistic

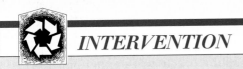

Guidelines for Intervening with Specific Parent Behaviors

Parent Behavior	Nursing Interventions	Parent Behavior	Nursing Interventions

Initiates loud verbal arguments during visits with adolescent	Stop the immediate behavior, pointing out the disruptiveness to the unit.
	
	Refer adolescent and family to family therapists to resolve differences and learn more adaptive ways of relating in supportive atmosphere of family therapy.
	
	Suggest that family therapist contract with family for one or more of the following:
	    Staff will monitor visits.
	    Family will bring up potentially volatile topics only within the structure of family meetings and not on the unit during visits.
	    Staff will intervene if arguments ensue on unit.
	    Staff may limit visiting time on unit.
		Is unable to set limits with adolescent during unit visits (is adversely influenced by manipulative attempts, tolerates verbal abuse, etc.)	Intervene if demands or behavior could yield physical harm, unit rule breaking, or other negative results.
			
			Point out problem and refer adolescent and parents to family therapy.
			
			Role model appropriate and effective limit setting with adolescent if necessary.
			
			Offer to discuss situation with parents and adolescent if desirable in immediate situation.
			
			Offer emotional support to parent who needs to talk.

Has history of physical violence against adolescent	Upon admission, contract with adolescent and family for no acts of violence against people or property. Monitor visits with adolescent on unit. Limit or deny passes with parents until progress is demonstrated. Depending on abilities with impulse control, refuse visiting privileges with adolescent until progress is seen in family therapy.	Has limited interaction with adolescent during unit visits	Initiate discussion among adolescent and family members related to visit and treatment goals. Refer problem and give observations to family therapists. Initiate discussion with parents to allow exploration of difficulty, if desired. Suggest that family members and adolescent discuss the problem in family therapy. Plan outings/special occasion celebrations to include families, if appropriate.

interactionist theory, can the nurse understand what a particular behavior means to the adolescent. Nurses who can recollect their own adolescent experiences—the conflicts and uncertainty as well as the elation and the triumphs—can better appreciate the adolescent's turmoil. It is equally important that the nurse discover who the individual adolescent is. Meanings of behavior, values, and actions can vary from client to client and may not reflect meanings or values held by the nurse. For example, the client who has trouble with competitive feelings may be reluctant to accept an invitation to play a game of Trivial Pursuit. In addition, since adolescents are between childhood and adulthood, they frequently have the feelings and choices of adulthood without an adult's abilities in verbal discourse and impulse control. As a result, adolescents may "act out" feelings and decisions nonverbally, in a childlike way. This is particularly true of the emotionally disturbed adolescent.

Acting Out

The concept of **acting out** is complex. The term has been used to describe a variety of behaviors, ranging from antisocial, destructive acts to unconscious impulses expressed in action rather than in symbolic words or symptoms. Acting out may, and often does, include destructive actions and seemingly undefinable behaviors. The term describes a re-creation of the client's life experiences, relationships with significant others, and resulting unresolved conflicts.

These are all components of what is commonly called the client's **life script,** which unfolds as the client relates, reacts, and behaves in accustomed ways. Through observation of and interaction with the client, the nurse can uncover the meanings that various behaviors and actions hold for the individual. For example, the child who has assumed the "black sheep" role in the family seeks to re-create that familiar role with others outside the home, particularly in the in-patient setting. The following clinical example illustrates one girl's relationship with her parents as replayed with the nursing staff on an in-patient unit.

Liza is 14 years old. She has been on the unit for six days. She is an attractive, engaging young person who has been friendly with both staff and clients. Liza has been on the periphery of several rule-breaking incidents but has not been directly involved. She has begun to establish close ties with Jim, a nurse, and engages in frequent lengthy discussions with him about her innermost feelings and fears. One evening she candidly talks to him about the callous way in which she was treated by one of the other nurses, a woman, in regard to a gynecologic problem. Liza says with undisguised fear and embarrassment that she is afraid the situation will repeat itself. She expresses great respect for Jim's knowledge and style and asks him to attend to any subsequent problems himself rather than report her dissatisfaction with Jane, the other nurse.

The implications for treatment are many. The most important factors for Jim to consider are what meaning Liza's behavior has for her and what would be the most therapeutically effective way to deal with the situation. The client's presenting problems and the expectation that the client will act out previous conflicts and life scripts have provided Jim adequate information on which to base an appropriate intervention. The client's attempt to seduce the nurse, and the need for nurses to examine their own behavior and motivations, are discussed in detail later in this chapter.

Jim recognizes the "pull" from Liza to feel that only he can adequately handle the situation. He remembers that Liza's home situation is chaotic. Liza's mother and father frequently fight over who is the better parent. Jim surmises that Liza also plays a part in these fights. The present situation seems to indicate that he is about to be played off against Jane, just as Liza perhaps plays one parent against the other. Jim responds by reiterating his concern for her dilemma and suggesting that Liza speak with Jane about the situation.

In this situation it is clear that the client is attempting to re-create her home situation, using two of the nurses to reenact the roles of her parents. Had Jim been seduced into playing the father's role in the script, he would have re-created the family's conflict on the ward. The ideal solution is for staff to interrupt this pathologic process by substituting a healthier way of resolving the problem. Thus, Jim does not react with compliance or with anger to Liza's attempts. Instead he recognizes the significance of her behavior and deals with the situation in a concerned yet healthy way, suggesting a resolution to the immediate problem that demonstrates respect for both Liza's and Jane's abilities to resolve the conflict.

Such situations are commonplace on an adolescent service. They require nursing staff to evaluate the client's psychodynamics and psychopathology as well as their own inner feelings and behavior. But these situations are not limited to the in-patient setting. This fact alone obliges nurses to be alert in observing and assessing verbal and nonverbal communication and to understand their own feelings and behavior in order to make accurate assessments and appropriate interventions.

Communication

Communication with adolescents is an art in itself. To become proficient in this area, the nurse must accept and understand the following:

• Adolescents tend to act out feelings and conflicts rather than verbalize them.

• Adolescents have an unconventional language of their own.

- Adolescents, especially disturbed ones, may use profanity frequently.

- Many clues can be obtained simply by observing the adolescent's behavior, dress, or environment.

The nurse who learns the skills of interviewing and the use of nonverbal cues and messages can use them comfortably and naturally in communicating with the adolescent.

Adolescents give many nonverbal cues to their specific emotional struggles, underlying confusion, or simply transitory moods. A glance around their rooms or a brief study of their dress can tell the nurse more than several direct questions would elicit. Sometimes adolescents give obvious cues. A client who wears a coat around the unit may be planning to run away. Other less obvious behaviors, which are often outside the client's conscious awareness or control, can also yield vital information. A sudden escalation of horseplay among the boys around bedtime is an example. The nurse would probably be correct in identifying this behavior as an expression of anxiety related to sexual identity and fears of homosexual feelings. Interactionist theory holds that the adolescent boy's newfound sexual feelings and changing body image provide unfamiliar ways of relating to members of his own sex. As a result, he regresses to preadolescent behavior, which served him well in handling close feelings then but now proves inappropriate. In this instance, firm limit setting is in order. The nurse should avoid interpreting the behavior or paying undue attention to the specifics. Testing and limit setting are discussed later in this chapter.

Adolescents seek to create a language all their own. This takes some understanding and acceptance. In seeking their identity, adolescents establish a form of communication unique to the group. To gain acceptance into the adolescent world, the adult must accept this need to employ ambiguous (to the adult) yet specific (to the adolescent) terms to express themselves. In many cases, the nurse must communicate with adolescents by using their own jargon.

This jargon often includes obscene and profane words. This is particularly true of disturbed adolescents, who have an especially difficult time expressing anger and fear appropriately. The words employed often reveal the nature of the emotional conflict. For example, a young male adolescent grappling with his sexual identity and aggressive feelings may resort to sexually graphic words when he feels anxious or afraid. The nurse may sometimes find it productive to use similar words to give explanations or to clarify communication. Understandably, some nurses have difficulty tolerating profane or sexually graphic language. However, nurses need to evaluate their clients' underlying reasons for using such language to help clients understand their feelings. Only then can they encourage clients to use more appropriate means of expression. If clients sense that the reason the nurse wants them to speak more appropriately is only to make the nurse more comfortable, the end result will not be satisfactory.

Adolescents in one study consistently identified the providing of information as a prime nursing behavior that was helpful to them (Paulson 1987). The adolescent psychiatric client often presents with symptoms of disturbed communication, which can affect all realms of daily living, particularly in relationships with peers, family members, and nonparental authority figures. Giving information is one way nurses can help decrease communication deficits and facilitate relationships with others. Other nursing behaviors are outlined in the section Planning and Implementing Interventions.

Anger and Hostility Expressions of anger and hostility are common on an adolescent ward. Anger expressed verbally usually takes the form of profanity. How effectively we deal with expressions of anger and hostility depends on how effectively we handle our own angry or hostile feelings. Nurses compromise their own effectiveness if they are uncomfortable with expressions of anger or hostility or view them as negative or to be avoided at all costs.

Nurse's Self-Assessment This brings up a subject that is rarely considered—anger felt and expressed by the nurse toward the client. The general focus on the client's need for understanding and good care seem to make it unacceptable for the nurse to display negative feelings toward the client. In the nursing care of adolescents, however, a constant all-giving and all-accepting attitude by the nurse, particularly during times of testing, would be not only nontherapeutic but also illogical and dishonest. Testing behavior is at an all-time high, and adolescents need honest feedback. The adolescent sometimes escalates the provocative behavior to evoke an angry reaction from the nurse. For nurses to pretend that they are not angry in such a situation is as undesirable for treatment as it would be for them to pretend that they were fond of the client. Honesty with one's feelings is a prime prerequisite in establishing and maintaining meaningful and productive relationships with adolescent clients. This does not mean that nurses should give vent to all their thoughts or impulses. They should be aware of their own reactions and use good judgment in handling them. The questions in the Nursing Self-Awareness box on page 848 could be of help in assessing the nurse's own ways of dealing with anger.

Anxiety and Resistance Normal adolescents frequently feel anxious as they experience change and inner turmoil in adapting to a new identity. The

NURSING SELF-AWARENESS

A Self-Awareness Inventory for Nurses Who Work with Adolescents

To increase self-awareness about the nurse's own way of dealing with anger:

- What kinds of things make me angry?

- How do I deal with my anger? Do I tend to ignore or hide it, or do I show that I am angry?

- Do I sometimes use profanity or act out my feelings in a physical way? How do I feel about others who do this?

- What do I think about how I handle anger?

- How do I feel about how I handle anger?

- How do I react to others when they are angry?

To increase self-awareness about the nurse's tendency to be seduced or manipulated:

- Is this client's friendliness compromising the professional role boundaries between us to "personalize" our relationship?

- Do I feel compelled to respond in a personal rather than a therapeutic way, possibly revealing information about my own life and lifestyle?

- Do I feel uncomfortable with the client's flattering comments or probing questions?

- Do I tend to forget that this person is a client?

- Is the client encouraging me to keep secrets from other staff or to "side" with client against other staff?

To increase self-awareness about the nurse's own sexual attitudes and feelings:

- How would I describe my adolescence as it related to my developing sexuality?

- What do I remember about the development and changes in my body?

- How did I feel about these changes?

- How would I describe my adolescent relationships with members of my sex?

- How would I describe my adolescent relationships with members of the opposite sex?

- What event stands out in my mind when I recall my sexual experiences during adolescence?

- How have these past relationships, events, and feelings influenced me today?

---

anxiety evidenced by the disturbed adolescent in treatment can indicate many other things. The changes required of the disturbed adolescent are much more threatening than those required of the normal adolescent. If treatment is to be successful, clients must look at the meaning of their behavior and must change many of their earlier interactional patterns. This can be frightening. For example, it is more comfortable to play the role of the "bad seed" or "bad kid," with its known pitfalls and expectations, than to attempt a change that entails many uncertainties and unknowns.

Clients feel threatened and anxious when the nurse does not act according to their expectations, because they must then find other ways of handling the situation. They must also deal with the anxiety. Frequently this anxiety is channeled into a game of "cops and robbers" as the client once again assumes a familiar role and maintains the negative or unhealthy image. The anxiety caused by unfamiliar roles is dissipated by further testing and acting out. The nurse should not take this as an indication that therapy is not working. It may simply indicate that the client needs to move ahead more slowly with insightful discoveries and needs the nurse's support in doing so.

The nurse should keep in mind that to such adolescents, "opening up" in a trusting way does not hold the same positive promise as it does for the nurse. The adolescent who has been rejected or experienced loss following close relationships in the past will feel wary of the nurse's expressions of interest or concern and will be cautious about repeating such experiences. These adolescents may respond to the nurse with testing behaviors, anger and mistrust, or outright rejection. Adolescents who expect rejection assume some control over the relationship if they reject others before being rejected themselves.

Sometimes nurses find it difficult to allow adolescents to grapple with their anxieties and fears. At other times, the nurse may not recognize the client's behavior as a symptom of anxiety or depression. The following clinical example demonstrates the value of a comprehensive assessment, of exploring all possible reasons for a client's resistance to the nurse's efforts before implementing action.

Kathy was the quietest and most aloof client on the ward. She had isolated herself from the other clients during the week that followed admission and avoided conversing with staff members outside meetings. One evening she seemed especially receptive to the new nurse, Ellie, who was able to interest her in a sewing project. Ellie, who was a new graduate, felt pleased that Kathy had responded warmly to her during their time together. The next day Kathy did not speak to Ellie and seemed to avoid her at all costs. Later Ellie noticed that the dress Kathy had been sewing was torn into shreds and stuffed into the wastepaper basket. Ellie interpreted this quite personally. She felt deeply hurt and rejected. In her discussion with her supervisor, Ellie showed her disappointment and anger. Her supervisor observed that, although the good time and feelings that Ellie and Kathy had shared the evening before were genuine, Kathy had not experienced many such times before with her parents or other adults. She suggested that Kathy was probably angry with Ellie for pointing up what she, Kathy, had missed. The supervisor suggested that Ellie be patient with Kathy. Perhaps later Ellie could reestablish the bond, and they would be able to talk about what had happened.

Fortunately, Ellie did not act on her angry feelings. Had she done so, she might have impulsively assessed Kathy's behavior as "hopeless," interpreting Kathy's anxiety and resistance as an inability to trust, or she may have begun to relate to the client in a vindictive way, withdrawing from Kathy in turn. Instead, she sought advice. Ellie's supervisor recognized that Ellie wanted badly to do well and needed positive feedback. She also realized that Ellie did not understand the nature of giving to emotionally disturbed adolescents. Had Ellie not sought advice, she might have acted on her angry feelings, further alienating Kathy and causing herself more anger and frustration. Without an understanding of Kathy's actions, Ellie would have continued to expect kindness in return for kindness and would have been keenly disappointed.

Seduction and Manipulation of the Nurse   In working with adolescents there is always a risk of seduction of the nurse, or being manipulated into relating in a nontherapeutic way. These factors contribute to the problem:

- The intimate nature of the nurse's involvement with the adolescent

- The narcissism inherent in this age group

- The nurse's all-accepting attitude in working with the adolescent

Narcissism in this age group is caused by the child's withdrawal from the parents and their value system. This withdrawal leads to a general self-centeredness, overevaluation of the self, heightened self-perception, decreased ability for reality testing, and extreme self-absorption. The result is that the people to whom adolescents turn become all-important and perfect in their eyes. Nurses may be strongly tempted to respond accordingly.

The dangers inherent in this situation are not simply the two possible extremes—total submission to temptation and participation in a sexual relationship with the client, or strong denial of temptation by maintaining a rigid, unapproachable stance that makes it impossible to establish a meaningful, trusting relationship. Neither of these extremes is unknown, but the greatest danger is actually intrinsic to the role of the helping professional. It is tempting to respond to the adolescent's idealized view, to be the "savior" who succeeded with this difficult person where everyone else has failed, to feel superior to the imperfect parents, the harassed school teacher, the skeptical juvenile judge, or the other staff on the unit. However, the nurse should not give in to such temptations. Complications will most certainly develop that at best will temporarily compromise the nurse's effectiveness and at worst will render the treatment program completely ineffective. Liza's example of acting out demonstrates this. Jim, the evening nurse, could have been seduced by Liza to collude with her against the day nurse, Jane, had he not been keenly aware of the possibility.

Nurses who work intensively with adolescents often face situations in which their own unresolved feelings are aroused. They must choose whether to act on these impulses or to explore their origin. Of course, one is not always conscious of these unresolved feelings. It would be absurd to expect nurses to be totally aware of the meaning of their behavior at any given moment. Nonetheless, the skilled clinician is usually acquainted with the issues or conflicts that have caused problems in the past. In doubtful cases, the knowledgeable nurse will seek consultation from such a clinician. The clinician can help the nurse assess the situation and understand what part the nurse may have played in initiating it. Nurses who wish to explore their personal conflicts further may then seek counseling or therapy. The nurse can use the questions in the earlier Nursing Self-Awareness box to assess the nature of such interactions with the client.

In addition, nursing staff would benefit from establishing one or more of the following to provide a consistent format for assessing and evaluating ongoing situations with adolescent clients:

- Each nurse's own ongoing supervision with preceptor or nurse supervisor

- A regularly scheduled meeting (perhaps monthly) for all nursing staff to discuss difficult situations and conflicting feelings

- A staff meeting (perhaps weekly) in which all disciplines identify interpersonal obstacles and plan interventions toward more optimal treatment

Given the nature of their work, the staff—particularly the nursing staff—undergo considerable stress as adolescents challenge accepted ideas and values. However, in a research study evaluating the levels of stress in an in-patient psychiatric adolescent unit, the nursing staff reported only low to moderate stress in what seemed to be high-stress situations (Campbell 1977). This raises the question of the extent to which staff members use denial in dealing with stressful issues and suggests that denial may indeed be necessary for those working with disturbed adolescents on a daily basis.

Sexual Behavior of the Adolescent   According to Jersild (1978, p 109), "Sexual development is a meeting ground of the biological, psychological, and moral influences that shape an adolescent's life." The nurse should not underestimate the importance of the adolescent's experimentation and attitude in sexual matters. Likewise, nurses should evaluate their own attitudes and feelings about sexual issues as they relate to their own past experiences and current activities. Conflicts in such matters or resentments left over from the past will certainly affect their decisions or interaction with the client regarding sexual matters. Again, while it is not necessary that the nurse resolve all these issues, it is highly desirable to be aware of areas of conflict that might make it difficult to view a situation objectively or set rational limits. Nurses may find the questions in the earlier Nursing Self-Awareness box helpful in increasing their self-awareness about sexual attitudes and feelings.

Until adolescents master their anxieties and fears about their sexual identity and gain control over sexual urges, they will exhibit a variety of behaviors and attitudes that may confuse or trouble the nurse. The following sections focus specifically on three related issues: heterosexual behavior, homosexual behavior, and pregnancy.

Heterosexual Behavior Heterosexual activity is normal and desirable during adolescence. However, the nurse who works with either normal or disturbed adolescents will sometimes see them engage in sexual activities that do not seem healthy or growth producing. For example, the adolescent girl who seeks punishment rather than true pleasure in her sexual exploits will display them in an overt, exhibitionistic way in a place where a particularly moralistic person will discover her and give her the reprimands she desires. She may be testing a parent's values in an attempt to resolve her own inner conflicts about this. Adolescents in an in-patient treatment setting where sexual intercourse is forbidden may engage in sexual intercourse where a staff member will be sure to discover them. The experience may reinforce their image of sexual behavior as "bad" behavior. Or it may simply provide a means of acting out their defiance of the rules, thereby earning the familiar "bad kid" label. The incident involving the nurse Barbara and the clients Laurie and Bill in the Planning and Implement-

ing Interventions section is an excellent example of this.

Homosexual Behavior   During preadolescence, people choose a member of the same sex with whom to experience intimate or loving feelings. This does not necessarily mean that a sexual relationship will ensue, although it often does. Homosexual activity may continue into the adolescent years.

Generally, however, adolescents begin to view homosexual feelings as a threat to the development of their identity. As result, they may ward off such feelings by engaging in frantic sexual activity with a member of the opposite sex. This is particularly true for boys. It is normal for the adolescent boy to be afraid of his own passive wishes and to label them homosexual. He has probably been brought up to identify with physical displays of strength or aggressive displays of power. Thus, an incident in which he feels threatened or powerless would produce feelings of sexual impotence, a fear of castration, a feeling of dependency or weakness, and a greater fear of homosexuality. The adolescent boy in treatment may act out these feelings, or he may attempt to reaffirm his masculinity with inappropriate displays of aggression or destructive behavior.

At the other extreme are adolescents who engage in predominantly homosexual activities. Many of these individuals find relationships with the opposite sex threatening or unrewarding and continue to seek intimacy with people of the same sex. Some feel more comfortable with companions of the same sex and are satisfied with these relationships. Others use their homosexual affiliation to express and act out hostility directed against their parents and their parents' values.

Since nurses who work with adolescents may encounter any of these situations, they must attempt to understand the meaning that homosexual behavior has for the client. The clients may need to explore their feelings and anxieties openly. Open discussion with an understanding yet knowledgeable professional may help to resolve many of the concerns and conflicts inherent in adolescent sexual behavior.

Clients who use homosexuality to express hostility toward their parents will undoubtedly act out with the staff as well. The nurse would be wise to remain objective and relatively nonjudgmental with these clients, allowing them to deal with the feelings of anger or depression that may result from addressing the conflict.

Although homosexual behavior during adolescence does not predict adult sexual preference, some adolescents make a lasting identification as homosexuals during these years. Such adolescents will not experience conflicts about homosexual relationships or need to flaunt them or act out with the staff in an angry or hostile way. In such cases, however, nurses may have to deal with their own negative feelings about homosexuality. It is important for the nurse to consider what their relationships mean to clients and to respect their right to make life-style choices for themselves.

Pregnancy   Adolescent pregnancy may reflect social and family expectations and unconscious motivations. Some teenage girls are quite pleased to be pregnant and suffer no emotional consequences from motherhood. In general, however, a conscious, deliberate decision to become pregnant at this age is manipulative. The goal may be to escape a difficult family situation, to express hostility toward parents, or to act out a life script in which the daughter is seen as "bad." The adolescent girl who did not receive adequate nurturing as a child could be acting out dependency needs by giving her baby the love and caring she herself did not receive. In so doing, she feels loved and cared for in turn.

The nurse should be sensitive to motivational factors in dealing with emotionally deprived adolescents. It is important to use existing educational tools and interpersonal relationships to help adolescent girls understand their needs and motivations in becoming pregnant. It is also important to educate teenagers of both sexes about sex and birth control. Many high schools are now recognizing this need and providing such information in birth control clinics or through health education classes. Too often parents and professionals alike deny the adolescent's sexual activity until an unwanted pregnancy occurs and it is too late to discuss the meaning of possible consequences of sexual behavior.

Dietary Problems and Eating Disorders   The eating habits and food preferences of disturbed adolescents can reveal a lot about the nature of their inner turmoil. A comparison between the client's diet and that of a nondisturbed adolescent may show little difference in variety but probably a great difference in quantity. Adolescents who have been deprived of early nurturing tend to eat more than other adolescents and probably place a higher value on mealtimes and on receiving their "share" of the food. The nurse may notice that adolescents consume more milk than usual during periods of stress or anxiety. In general, girls want to follow food fads or unreasonable dietary regimens to become slim and attractive. This usually gives the nurse an opportunity to engage in health teaching about food and exercise and to express a cooperative interest in their developing feminine identity. The eating disorders—anorexia nervosa, bulimia nervosa, and compulsive overeating—are discussed in Chapter 20.

Depression and Suicide   Both depression and suicide are thought to be underreported among adolescents. For every successful suicide, some researchers say, there are 200 attempts (Valente 1989). Moreover, there is real concern about a contagion of suicides, known as suicide clusters in which one suicide appears to set off another. Such clusters were reported in several communities in the last decade: In Fairfax, Virginia, eleven youths killed themselves during one school year; in Plano, Texas, seven adolescents died within a year; in Westchester County, New York, five teens killed themselves within one month. (See Chapter 23 for a complete discussion of adolescent suicide, including assessment and nursing intervention.)

Drug Use and Abuse   Experimentation with drugs among the adolescent population is widespread. Surveys have reported that 50 to 95 percent of the adolescent subjects have used drugs, including alcohol, at least once.

Adolescents give many reasons for using drugs: to experiment, to get high, to "get inside my head," to have fun, to understand more about life. Although the general public may disagree about whether drugs are harmful, the fact remains that using drugs—or at least experimenting with them—is acceptable to most adolescents.

How can the nurse determine when drug *use* becomes drug *abuse*? Generally, the adolescent who abuses drugs, including alcohol, exhibits at least one of the following characteristics:

• The adolescent's performance at school or work increasingly deteriorates.

• The adolescent is frequently caught high or in the act of getting high by parents or other authority figures.

• The adolescent increasingly resorts to drugs in times of stress or boredom.

• The adolescent has seriously deficient interpersonal relationships and can relate only when under the influence of drugs.

• The adolescent may lose interest in interpersonal relationships altogether, preferring to be high alone rather than to be with others.

Nurses are most effective when they can discern what the particular drug or high does for the client. A boy with a poor self-image and low-esteem may say that it makes him "feel like a man." A particularly shy or introverted girl may say that it makes her "outgoing and friendly." The nurse may discover that being high helps rid disturbed adolescents of angry or depressed feelings. Indeed, in the treatment setting, the client frequently resorts to smoking marijuana or "popping" uppers or downers to escape uncomfortable feelings.

RESEARCH NOTE

Citation

Schwartz RH, Wirtz PH: Potential substance abuse: Detection among adolescent patients. Clin Pediatr 1990;29(1):38–43.

Study Problem/Purpose

The purpose of the study was to pilot-test a revised self-administered brief screening tool to detect serious emotional or behavioral problems, particularly drug or alcohol abuse, in an adolescent population.

Methods

A revised thirty-item questionnaire, the Drug and Alcohol Problem (DAP) Quick Screen, designed to be accepted by adolescent clients in the clinic or physician's office, was pilot-tested on 355 adolescents, ages 14–18 years (median age of 16). These subjects all receive health care from a five-pediatrician group practice in Fairfax County, Virginia. Each youth was asked by the office receptionist to complete the questionnaire, answering "yes," "no," or "uncertain" to each item. They were also provided with a "yes or no" written choice for keeping all information confidential. Regardless of their answer, they were promised confidentiality even if they did not choose it. Parents who accompanied their offspring under age 18 were asked to first read a brief printed statement outlining the purpose of the project, requesting their consent for the child's participation, and agreeing to provide strict privacy to the teenager while completing the DAP Quick Screen. Scoring was based on a previous study, which used a forty-two-item prototype questionnaire comparing answers from 200 adolescents from the same pediatric practice with answers from 100 identified adolescent drug abusers at a drug abuse treatment facility. These groups had been matched for age and socioeconomic status. In this study those clients with a score of 6 or more were considered "high risk" for "red flag" behaviors, particularly

drug and alcohol abuse. Follow-up interviews were conducted with the adolescents who identified themselves by name and who scored 6 or higher. Telephone interviews were conducted with these subjects.

Findings

Ninety-six percent (341) of the subjects completed the screening questionnaire. Eighty-nine percent of these identified themselves by name. Fifteen percent (52) of the 341 responded "yes" to six or more items in the current study. Seventy-seven percent (40) of those clients who scored 6 or more identified themselves by name. A combination of only four key items on the questionnaire was able to select 70 percent of the high scores. These four questions identified the following: (1) use of tobacco products; (2) accusation by others of having an alcohol or drug problem; (3) school suspension; (4) riding in a motor vehicle with a driver who drank too much.

Implications

The DAP Quick Screen test appears to be a reasonably sensitive means of detecting adolescent problem behaviors in a primary care clinic or office setting. Whether a substantial number of physicians will accept or routinely use such a test is unknown. It would be important to couple such a test with a comprehensive follow-up and sensitive interviewing as well. Nurses in such settings can be instrumental in facilitating the tool's acceptance and use and in conducting the follow-up interviews. This method of a brief written questionnaire may meet with high acceptance by an adolescent population because accurate answers to direct queries regarding the extent of alcohol and drug consumption seem to be the exception rather than the rule. Such reports can be either greatly underreported or exaggerated, depending on the adolescent's needs at the time of the interview.

Diagnosing

The use of nursing diagnoses with adolescent clients can lend meaning and substance to the clients' behavior that might be overlooked with a DSM-III-R diagnosis alone. For example, a DSM-III-R diagnosis of "Disruptive behavior disorder, conduct disorder,

solitary aggressive type" identifies the nature of the adolescent's difficulty. By using the various subsystems provided by nursing diagnoses, the nurse can establish a more comprehensive picture of the client's difficulty and immediately become more goal-oriented in assessing and planning care. Moreover, in many treatment settings, mental health professionals are reluctant to give adolescents a DSM-III-R diagnosis during these formative years lest the adolescent be psychiatrically labeled (possibly erroneously). Such labeling may result in inadequate treatment, self-fulfilling prophecy, or both, in subsequent mental health contacts. Nursing diagnoses are identified with specific adolescent behaviors in the next section.

Planning and Implementing Interventions

Establishing a Contract with the Adolescent Contracts can be particularly useful with adolescents because they can feel powerless in a treatment setting, especially when "referred" by parents or the legal system. Moreover, with this increased sense of control over their own behavior adolescents become allies with the nurse in their treatment rather than the object of the nurse's treatment.

With most adolescents, a written contract is best, for these reasons:

• The goals and expectations are less easily forgotten.

• The process seems more formal and "serious" to the adolescent.

• There is less room for misinterpretation and manipulation.

Contracts seem especially helpful in situations of substance abuse, eating disorders, suicidal behavior, and impulsive or manipulative behaviors (as with some personality disorders). The case study on page 854 includes a contract for a depressed and withdrawn adolescent.

Whether verbal or written, the contract can be simply stated to promote clarity, consistency, and cooperation. Here is an example:

I will not take drugs or bring drugs into the unit.

I will not call or accept calls from my drug friends while in the treatment program.

I will go directly to my outpatient therapy appointment and return immediately to the unit.

I will not harm myself or others. If I feel like hurting myself, others, or property, I will tell the staff.

If written, the contract is signed by the client, dated, and cosigned by the nurse. The contract is renegotiated at regular intervals, hourly, daily, or weekly, depending on the goals, the severity of the symptoms, and the degree of compliance with the agreement. The form of the contract is less important than the way the nurse and the adolescent jointly set the goals and expectations, carry out the contract, set limits and renegotiate

changes, and evaluate the final outcome. See the nursing care plan on page 856. Chapter 26 discusses contracting with clients in general, and Chapter 23 discusses no-suicide contracts.

Anger and Hostility   Depending on the degree to which the client is experiencing and expressing anger and hostility, the nurse may choose any of a variety of interventions. These range from doing nothing other than observing the client's behavior, to physically restraining someone who is attempting destructive action. (See Chapter 21 for restraining strategies.) In some situations, a disturbed adolescent's ability to express anger directly to another person can be a sign of success in treatment. The choice of interventions also depends on the nurse's own experiences with such feelings, the nurse's knowledge and understanding of this client's life experiences with anger, and the external limits imposed by the agency.

In choosing an appropriate nursing intervention, the nurse can attempt to discover what meaning anger and hostility have for the client by asking the following questions:

• How has the adolescent handled anger in the past?

• Does the client have a history of aggression toward objects or persons?

• If so, what have been the consequences of this behavior?

• How does the adolescent feel following such a reaction?

• What kinds of things make the adolescent angry? Which of these would be most likely to occur on the unit or in our setting?

Steve had expressed great interest in building a model airplane. He had saved up his money and had taken a long time to choose "just the right one" at the hobby shop. After spending most of the afternoon constructing and painting it, he was interrupted by a phone call from his mother. She told him that she would not be able to attend the family meeting that week, giving a number of specious-sounding reasons. This was the third consecutive week that she had missed. Each time she gave questionable reasons for being unable to attend. Steve was disappointed and angry. He slammed down the receiver, yelling obscenities in response to the nurse's questions, and ran into his room. There he began to destroy the plane by throwing it repeatedly on the floor.

In the preceding example, Steve was not hurting himself or another. Although he did destroy property, the plane belonged to him, and he was free to do with it as he chose. The nurse resisted any impulse to stop Steve from damaging his plane. Since it was of

Text continues on p. 859

CASE STUDY

A Depressed Adolescent Client

Identifying Information

Cindy is a 15-year-old, single, white, female, nonpracticing Protestant, who is referred to the in-patient psychiatric unit by a social worker who is a friend of Cindy's mother. Cindy is a sophomore in high school. Third-party insurance will cover full cost of hospitalization.

Client's Definition of Present Problem, Precipitating Stressors, Coping Strategies, Goals for Care

Cindy is voluntarily admitted to the unit because "my mother says I'm impossible." She describes a three-year history of drug abuse, including marijuana, Valium, Seconal, and LSD. The precipitating stressor for this hospitalization was Cindy's slashing her wrist with a razor blade following an argument with her mother. Cindy says this is the first time she has "attempted suicide." Cindy reports that she frequently resorts to smoking marijuana or "sneaking" her mother's Valium when under stress, particularly following arguments with her mother. Her goals for treatment are "to gain control of my impulses and to learn more about myself." She says that she would like to get along better with her mother but says that is "unrealistic."

History of Present Problem

It is difficult to determine the exact date on which Cindy's problem first appeared (see Psychiatric History and Social History). It seems evident that her depression and related difficulties worsened around puberty at the age of 12, compounded by the abuse of drugs and the increased competitiveness among Cindy's siblings. Her parents state that she is now beyond control and they are at their "wit's end," having endured three years of "fighting, manipulation, and unhappiness."

Cindy describes herself as a "loner," who has few friends and keeps to herself at home and at school. She lives with her parents and two sisters. Cindy leaves the house each morning for school before the others are awake "to avoid the hassles with my mother and sisters." She has average to poor school grades. She reports frequent physical complaints, admitting that she frequently feigns illness to the school nurse to avoid certain classes. Cindy describes one female classmate to whom she feels close but states that their time together is brief and usually involves smoking marijuana in the morning just before school.

Psychiatric History

Cindy's parents have complained of difficulties with her "hyperactive, impulsive" behavior since she was 2 years old. According to her mother, Cindy was diagnosed at an early age as hyperkinetic following numerous visits to clinics and doctors' offices in quests for help for her uncontrollable behavior. Cindy's mother reports that Cindy could never be satisfied, cried all the time, and was never "still" once she was able to crawl.

During the past three years Cindy's difficulties have increased as she began to abuse drugs. Two months prior to this admission she underwent a four-week residential drug treatment program. The precipitant for this treatment was Cindy's suspension from school as a result of the school principal's discovery of Cindy and her friend smoking marijuana outside the cafeteria. The treatment modality was primarily a behavioral one, using a strict behavioral protocol of "time-outs" in a room alone or lost pass privileges for failure to attend or being late for meetings. The purpose of the program was educational. Meetings structured around films and discussions detailing the physical and legal risks of drug abuse consumed most of their waking hours. No attempts were made to explore the meaning of Cindy's drug-taking behaviors, her relationship to her parents, or the life events leading up to this

▶

CASE STUDY (continued)

difficult time. Cindy considers the program "helpful since I didn't take any drugs while I was there," but she acknowledges that she feels like a failure because she continues to use drugs.

Family History

Cindy lives with her parents, John and Kate, and two sisters (Katherine, 16 years old, and Janice, 14 years old). John is a chemist for a local pharmaceutical firm. Kate is a housewife. All three children are students at the same high school. On admission Cindy's parents explained that competition among the girls has been the primary problem at home, adding that Cindy's behavior makes it impossible to handle the problems. Since an early age Cindy has been identified as the "black sheep" of the family, according to Cindy. She has consistently been told she is "impossible" because she behaves badly and does poor to average schoolwork, whereas her sisters have both been honor students and model children, according to her parents. Cindy's mother, Kate, frequently made favorable comparisons between herself and Katherine, her oldest daughter. She made disparaging comparisons between Cindy and Kate's younger sister, who Kate felt had "stolen the show and my father away from me when I was 4 years old."

Social History

Although Cindy's pediatrician reports normal achievement of developmental milestones, Cindy's mother states she has always been "slow at everything." Her school record validates the report of poor to average grades, except for the third grade when Cindy achieved As and Bs. Cindy's teacher wrote in her report that Cindy's performance can improve with encouragement and personal attention. All accounts of Cindy's social development consistently support the idea of an isolated individual with few friends. Her leisure time has characteristically involved watching TV and occasionally spending time with her younger sister. According to Cindy, her three-year history of drug abuse has involved regular marijuana use one to two times a week, occasional use of Valium (5 mg tablet prescription for Cindy's mother), Seconal ("street reds") on two occasions, and LSD on two occasions. Cindy's mother insisted that Cindy was a heavy drug abuser "who takes anything and everything," but she acknowledged that the only times she was aware of Cindy's taking drugs had been those identified by Cindy on admission.

Significant Health History

Cindy's health history is unremarkable. She reports no allergies or hospitalizations. Her wrist slashing consisted of a superficial laceration of the left wrist, requiring no sutures in the emergency room.

Current Mental Status

Cindy is an alert, articulate bright female who is slightly overweight and appears older than her stated age. During the psychiatric examination she was cooperative and spontaneous, answering questions readily, although often giving vague responses necessitating more detailed inquiry. She was oriented to time, place, and person and denied having any hallucinations or delusions. Cindy performed adequately during most of the examination. She did rather poorly on serial sevens, however, making four mistakes in the four-minute period it took her to complete this exercise. Her explanations of proverbs were quite concrete. Cindy tended to minimize her depression, wanting to project a happy and healthy image to the interviewer. She revealed that her happiness is a front so that others would not know what is going on in her head. Cindy seems to have little insight into her current situation. Her primary defenses include denial, rationalization, and introjection.

CASE STUDY (continued)

Other Subjective or Objective Clinical Data

Cindy is on no prescription medications at this time. She denies any suicidal feelings but agrees to the terms of the client contract that she will tell staff if she feels like hurting herself.

Diagnostic Impression

A long-standing depression and extreme feelings of worthlessness stem from the treatment Cindy received from her parents as an abnormal, hyperative child. The onset of puberty combined with increasing competitiveness among the females in the family provided additional stress, leading to drug abuse and a suicidal gesture.

Nursing Diagnoses

Altered role performance
Chronic low self-esteem
High risk for violence: Self-directed
Hopelessness
Social isolation

DSM-III-R Multiaxial Diagnosis

Axis I: 300.40 Dysthymia, primary type, early onset
           305.20 Cannabis abuse
Axis II: 799.90 Deferred. (There is insufficient information to make any diagnostic judgment about an Axis II diagnosis or condition.)
Axis III: None
Axis IV: Psychosocial stressors:
           1. Onset of puberty with resulting physical and psychologic changes
           2. Increased competitiveness among siblings and mother with resulting arguments
           3. Suspension from school
           4. Suicidal gesture
           5. Four weeks out-of-home drug treatment with unsuccessful results
Axis V: Severity: 3-Moderate (predominantly acute events)
           Current GAF: 43
           Highest GAF past year: 55

NURSING CARE PLAN

A Depressed Adolescent Client

Client Care Goals	Nursing Planning/ Intervention	Evaluation
Nursing Diagnosis: Altered role performance		
Client will attend unit school program. Client will complete assignments. Client will ask for help when needed rather than passively fail to do work.	Implement behavioral contract, including school attendance and completion of assignments as criteria for rewards (e.g., "earned" time in room). Document daily difficulties and successes with school attendance and assignments in progress notes. Help identify her strengths and areas of interest.	On discharge, client attends school on a regular basis. Client asks for help with schoolwork rather than passively failing to do it.

NURSING CARE PLAN (continued)

Client Care Goals	Nursing Planning/ Intervention	Evaluation
	Encourage school participation and completion of work.	
	Give praise for assignments well done.	

Nursing Diagnosis: *Chronic low self-esteem*

Client will identify at least three strengths and discuss them in one-to-one and group therapy contacts.	Promote activities that use her strengths. Give praise for successes.	On discharge, client identifies at least three personal strengths.

Nursing Diagnosis: *High risk for violence: Self-directed*

Client will abstain from use of drugs or harmful substances. Client will talk with staff if she feels like hurting herself. Client will ask for one-to-one time with nurse on day and evening shifts. Client will ask for time to talk in groups (at least once daily) about her thoughts, feelings, and treatment plans.	Provide for physical safety of unit, ensuring that all sharp objects are confiscated. Search clients' and visitors' packages to ensure no drugs or harmful substances are brought onto unit. Implement behavioral contract regarding one-to-one contacts, group therapy participation, and increased freedoms. Spend time with her when she is not acting out. Do not wait for negative behaviors to give her attention. Reinforce positive behaviors. If client demonstrates a worsening of suicidal thoughts and diminished impulse control, assess need for limitations on privileges and freedoms (e.g., reverse status level; consider one-to-one observation, suicide precautions, visitor limitations). Document on day and evening shifts compliance and progress with plan.	On discharge, client talks with staff when she feels like using drugs or hurting herself. Client initiates such contacts without acting out her impulses or waiting for staff to approach her.

Nursing Diagnosis: *Hopelessness*

Client will recognize and accept sad, lonely feelings as long-standing problem. Client will talk about negative feelings rather than acting out.	Explore helpless, hopeless, sad, or lonely feelings. Attempt to correlate feelings with precipitating event (e.g., fight with sister).	On discharge, client states at least two feelings that are difficult to discuss with parents/ family members and identified ways in which she will approach them.

▶

NURSING CARE PLAN *(continued)*

Client Care Goals	Nursing Planning/ Intervention	Evaluation
	Document content and progress of one-to-one and group discussions.	
	Evaluate ability to correlate feelings with behavior.	
	If the client demonstrates worsening of feelings and social interaction, set limits and provide structure of one-to-ones. Document interventions and results.	

Nursing Diagnosis: *Social isolation*

Client Care Goals	Nursing Planning/ Intervention	Evaluation
Client will initiate social contact with peers at least once daily.	Establish mutually acceptable goals and objectives for socialization: e.g., "Who would you like to get to know here? How do you think you could approach her/him?"	On discharge, client initiates social contacts with peers.
Client will not isolate self in room except for "earned" time.		Client identifies uncomfortable feelings with others when they arise.
Client will ask for one-to-one time with nurse on day and evening shifts to discuss feelings.	Implement behavioral contract including reinforcement for positive behaviors (e.g., "earned" time in room alone for 15- to 30-minute periods).	
Client will participate in all planned social activities of unit.	Encourage to participate in social activities.	
Client will attend family meetings.	Evaluate progress with client regarding social interaction attempts, successes, and difficulties.	
	Encourage to explore feelings regarding interpersonal relationships with peers, parents, and other authority figures.	
	Encourage and support participation in group therapies.	
	Document nursing interventions and client results each shift in progress notes. With each attempt to initiate contact with peers, offer encouragement and constructive criticism, evaluating results with client.	

significant value to him, he later regretted having taken out his aggressions on it. However, the situation provided Steve with an opportunity to explore his actions, and he later asked the nurse why he would destroy something that he valued so much after his mother had disappointed and angered him. The parallel between this situation and hurting himself with drugs right after he had argued with his mother was only too apparent.

Incidents in which the nurse bears the brunt of a client's anger or hostility do not offer such obvious solutions. Disturbed adolescents may not think twice about addressing a female nurse as "bitch" and coupling such a greeting with a request for a favor. Adolescents direct insults and hostile remarks at nurses for many reasons, most of which have little to do with the nurses as people but a lot to do with them as adults or authority figures.

There are as many suggestions for intervention as there are people who will be involved in such exchanges. In choosing interventions, nurses should consider the meaning behind the client's behavior, their own relationship with this client, their own immediate feelings, and the result desired. For example, if the client calls the nurse "bitch" the first time they meet, the nurse may interpret this as a form of testing. She may choose to respond immediately with a bewildered look at this unwarranted display of hostility. Later, the nurse may approach the client, expressing a naive curiosity as to the origin of the hostile feelings: "Hey, I don't understand what happened between us a few minutes ago. We just met, and you're calling me a bitch. What's that all about?" This simple question conveys two messages. First, it indicates to the client that the nurse is not accustomed to this kind of salutation. Second, it indicates that the nurse is more interested in the motivation for the remark than she is in curtailing its use.

If the client resorts to name calling only when angry or under stress, the nurse may decide to ignore the words and deal only with the feelings involved. For example, if a client has angrily left an ongoing family meeting, and then calls the nurse a bitch, the nurse can probably assume that the anger is displaced. It is probably a result of overwhelming feelings experienced during the meeting. The nurse may elect simply to say, "I know you're not angry at me right now. It seems like the meeting is pretty heavy, though. Do you want to talk about why you don't want to be in there now?" In neither situation is the name calling intended as a personal affront. However, the way the nurse handles it determines both the outcome of the immediate situation and the nurse's chances of furthering the relationship with the client.

The adolescent's reaction to the nurse's intervention largely determines its effectiveness. For example,

with Steve, the boy who destroyed his plane, the nurse's goal was to help Steve understand the impulsive reaction that destroyed something he loved and to encourage a more appropriate and direct expression of anger at his mother. He was able to do this as well as draw a parallel between anger at his mother and his drug abuse, which hurt himself. If the nurse's goal had been simply to stop the destruction of his property, Steve could have felt even greater anger and frustration, and he might have turned his aggression toward himself, the nurse, or the environment. Certainly if Steve had escalated his destructive behavior, turning his aggression toward himself or others, then direct limit setting, including physical restraints, would have been indicated.

In first-time encounters with any client new to the setting, the nurse should not be surprised or dismayed about less-than-optimal success with intervention. It may take some time and trial and error to assess the client's behaviors and choose the most effective interventions. See the beginning of this section for a discussion of client contracts. The nursing care plan on page 860 is for clients who act out aggression against themselves, others, and/or property.

Testing and Limit Setting As young adolescents attempt to adjust to the upheaval in their emotional lives and begin to emancipate themselves from parental figures, a good deal of testing is to be expected. This is normal. However, the meaning that testing holds for the disturbed adolescent is a more complicated matter.

Adolescents who lack early nurturing have difficulty with interpersonal relations. In many cases, parents were emotionally unable to provide parenting. In other cases, they chose not to impose their values on their children. In either case, the children never developed the internalized values that reduce conflict and avert crisis in adolescence. This causes identity diffusions, which in turn result in emptiness, a lack of basic trust, and difficulties with intimacy on any level.

In the treatment setting, testing for these clients seems to consist of making limitless and absolute demands. Although these clients often react to imposed limits with cries of injustice, they often really seem to be asking for limits as an indication of caring.

Julie had been on the unit only two days. During that time she had seen several of the older clients run away from the unit, commonly known as going AWOL, and had witnessed the staff members' attempts to encourage those remaining on the ward to deal with whatever feelings they were experiencing. Toward the end of her second evening, Julie abruptly jumped up from a conversation with a nurse and ran toward the open door. The surprised nurse immediately followed, running down the stairs after her. A smiling Julie was waiting at the bottom step when the nurse arrived, quite breathless and thor-

Text continues on page 862

NURSING CARE PLAN

An Adolescent Client with Aggressive/Violent Behaviors

Client Care Goals	Nursing Planning/ Intervention	Evaluation
Nursing Diagnosis: High risk for violence: Directed at others		
Client will show increased impulse control.	Provide for physical safety of unit, ensuring that all sharp objects are confiscated.	Client is able to gain attention in positive, more adaptive ways.
Client will verbally express difficult feelings prior to acting out feelings and impulses.	Anticipate angry or potentially explosive situations, allowing time to talk about it, or at least acknowledge existence of present situation, e.g., "I think you're trying to get me angry now by throwing those things around the room. I would rather talk about what's happening between us."	Client asks directly for one-to-one time with assigned nurse and will set a later time if nurse not readily available.
Client will manifest more appropriate use of physical activities to cope with anxieties about potentially explosive situations.		Client asks for time to talk in groups (at least one per day) about thoughts, feelings, and treatment plans.
	Set firm limits on behavior while client can still hear them, before behavior escalates out of control. Expect that client will control actions.	Client talks with staff if feels like hurting self, others, or property rather than acting out impulses.
	Ask client to come to talk to nurse in quiet area away from peers. If client does not stop behavior, direct to room for "time-out" until calm.	
	If client continues to be violent against objects or threatens violence against others, tell client you are going to help with controls. Implement procedure for use of physical restraints or seclusion room.	
	Reinforce good behavior and give feedback at times when out of control, e.g., "I liked the way you handled John's provocative behavior today. You were cool when you told him that you were angry without storming around."	
	Spend time with client when not acting out. Do not wait for negative behavior to give attention.	

▶

NURSING CARE PLAN (continued)

Client Care Goals	Nursing Planning/ Intervention	Evaluation
	Document interventions, client response, and client's progress with impulse control and in potentially volatile situations.	
	With increasing anxieties and inability to deal with feelings, assess need for increasing levels of limits and structure, evaluating and documenting client's response with each level.	
	Evaluate and revise behavioral contract in collaboration with client.	

Nursing Diagnosis: *High Risk for violence: Self-directed*

Client will show increased impulse control to curb self-directed violence.	Directly address the underlying feelings of sadness, loneliness, confusion, ect., when appropriate.	Client responds to staff interventions designed to increase impulse control and curb violent acts.
	Ask other clients to give feedback in group meetings, particularly community meetings and small group therapy.	Client adheres to a no self-harm contract.
	Encourage more appropriate coping skills, e.g., use of physical activities.	
	Promote involvement with peers in activities and comment on socially acceptable behaviors.	
	Update and renegotiate no self-harm contract as necessary—at least daily as an initial plan.	
	Encourage client to accept responsibility for behavior rather than blaming other people or circumstances for problems or using anger to avoid dealing with painful feelings.	

SOURCE: Carrie McRae, RN, BSN, Langley Porter Psychiatric Institute, Unit B, San Francisco, California.

oughly confused, and began her barrage of questions. Julie quickly answered, "I just wanted to see if you cared enough to come after me."

In this situation no further action was necessary.

Sometimes the client may use annoying or destructive behavior to test the nurse. At these times, firm limit setting without further interpretation or exploration may be indicated. In other instances, the client may not be testing the nurse but may be reacting to some real threat or uncomfortable situation.

Joanne was quietly playing pool by herself when she noticed her therapist talking to a new female client. Her volatile nature gave way to jealousy and rage, and she immediately began to hit the billiard balls off the table, making a lot of noise and startling everyone around her. The nurse who had been observing her witnessed the change in her behavior and understood the reaction. Without questioning Joanne's apparent anger, she stepped up to the table and challenged her to a game, which Joanne immediately accepted. Since Joanne prided herself on her pool-playing ability, she quickly channeled her energy and competitive feelings into the game and won. She then sought out her therapist and happily announced her victory.

Had the nurse not understood what had triggered Joanne's outburst, she might have become angry with her for making noise. She might have seen this as a form of testing and might even have begun to set limits on Joanne's privilege of playing pool. This would certainly have produced a helpless and even angrier Joanne, who would probably have escalated her behavior. Since the nurse was perceptive and adept in handling such situations, the results were more satisfying to both parties. Because of the nurse's action, Joanne was able to save face by winning at pool and was not forced to feel more helpless.

Scapegoating

Scapegoating is common in many groups, but particularly in adolescent groups. It occurs in three stages.

1. Frustration generates aggression.

2. Aggression is displaced on relatively defenseless others.

3. Through a process of blaming, projecting, and stereotyping, this displaced aggression is rationalized and finally justified, since the identified scapegoat is "different" in some real way.

The members of a group tend to attack the scapegoat because they are afraid to attack the person on whom their feelings are actually focused.

Adolescents readily identify peers who are "different" and project on them their own fears and insecu-

rities about their changing images. The client identified as the scapegoat is the object of much teasing and many hostile remarks. The nurse should refrain from attempting merely to rescue the scapegoat, since this may augment the other clients' anger and frustration and encourage an escalation of the hostility. The nurse would be better to set limits on the behavior and then ask the group to focus on what is going on, to acknowledge the anxiety or other uncomfortable feeling that preceded the scapegoating incident. If possible, the nurse should anticipate the occurrence of scapegoating in times of stress and attempt to circumvent the process before it gets out of control.

The nurse should also be aware that identified scapegoats share some responsibility for their predicament by presenting themselves to the other clients in a different or provocative stance. In some instances the scapegoat of choice has an inner need to be punished and meets the group's urgent need to punish as well. The nurse can be valuable to these clients by helping them to explore whatever function this role serves for them. Examples of effective results in dealing with the scapegoating phenomenon are outlined in the nursing care plan on page 864.

Sexual Behaviors With a self-awareness and understanding of feelings and attitudes about sexual issues, the nurse can more readily plan interventions with sexual behaviors of the adolescent client.

Masturbation Masturbation is a normal sexual activity for people of all ages, from the beginning of sexual awareness to senescence. If the nurse has a relatively healthy attitude toward masturbation, it is not likely to cause problems unless the client masturbates in inappropriate places or uses masturbation to express hostility. The nurse is sometimes confronted with an adolescent boy who fondles his genitals when he is anxious or feels threatened. Understanding his behavior as an indication of anxiety, the nurse may elect to ignore the gesture and explore the nature of his anxiety with him. At other times, the boy may make a masturbatory gesture to convey contempt or hostility. In this case it would be ludicrous to feign indifference in response.

The nurse's reaction depends on all the previously mentioned factors, such as the client-nurse relationship and the behavior that preceded the gesture. Generally, however, it is wise to comment on the client's gesture, for example, by mentioning it as an attempt to "make me uncomfortable," and then to allow the client the opportunity to express his feelings verbally. It is unlikely that this intervention will produce a tumultuous outpouring of feeling resulting in immediate resolution. However, it does allow the nurse to acknowledge both the client's and the nurse's own feelings, perhaps paving the way for a more appropriate exchange in the future.

Heterosexual Behavior   The adolescent often uses sexual behavior as a means of acting out other conflicts and as a testing ground for the nursing staff's feelings and attitudes.

This is the third time Barbara, a nurse, had gone into Laurie's room to check on two clients, Laurie and Bill, who were an identified couple on the ward. Although there was a rule against clients having sexual intercourse with each other, Laurie and Bill had been discovered in the act each evening Barbara was on duty. Barbara found these discoveries disconcerting. She began to wonder whether she was the only staff member who checked on clients, since no one else had reported any sexual activity. She decided to bring the subject up in the next nursing care plan meeting to find a more effective way of dealing with the situation.

Imagine Barbara's surprise when the group agreed that Barbara was actually partly responsible for Laurie and Bill's acting out! While they supported Barbara, they evaluated the problem and gave Barbara feedback regarding her nonverbal messages. It seemed that her frequent checking on clients conveyed her expectation that they were up to something. Barbara acknowledged that she expected that sort of behavior from them and was quite afraid of discovering them in the act of intercourse. The group helped Barbara see that her own expectations were being met. Laurie and Bill were doing exactly what she expected them to do—maybe even wanted them to do. Laurie and Bill were following their scripts of being "bad" and expressing their hostility to Barbara. When Barbara heard how other staff members spent time with the couple to encourage them in indirect ways to join the larger group activities and compared her own behavior to that of her peers, it became apparent to her how obvious her anxiety and unconscious messages actually were! She then began to question her own attitudes about sexual matters and to explore why she feared discovering the couple engaged in sexual intercourse.

In the previous clinical example, the client couple used sexual behaviors to act out their own underlying feelings. Had Barbara's assessment been limited to the immediate situation, she would have focused only on their unacceptable behavior and would not have been open to the implications for her. By seeking out information and feedback from her peers she made a discovery about herself and realized more effective ways of anticipating and possibly circumventing such client behaviors rather than having to intervene after the fact. Had Barbara not asked for feedback, the problem would have continued with an increase in the sexual behaviors and in Barbara's frustration. The situation would have then demanded intervention by an astute supervisor or an empathetic colleague.

Homosexual Behavior   In situations where homosexual behavior is an expected developmental step or a life-style without expressions of anger or hostility toward parents or staff, little or no intervention from the nurse may be indicated. However, when homosexual behavior is used to act out feelings of impotence, or aggressive behavior is used to counteract feelings of intimacy, limits must be imposed.

The nurse would do well to anticipate such behavior and provide other ways for the adolescent to demonstrate his masculinity, perhaps by organizing a game of football or tennis, if he is fairly proficient at these skills, or engaging him in some other activity in which he excels. The point is to reestablish the adolescent's feeling of competency and control. Without such intervention his feelings of impotence will escalate to the point where he will most certainly act them out in a negative way. The client who uses homosexuality to express defiance against authority figures will most assuredly flaunt homosexual activities and consistently incur the anger, embarrassment, or both, of staff and clients alike.

Drug Abuse   The nurse will benefit from self-awareness and appreciation for the feelings that working with drug abusers can evoke. For example, the nurse who feels angry and punitive with the client who abuses drugs or overidentifies with the client and finds adventure in the client's drug stories cannot establish a therapeutic relationship with the client. Feelings of disdain or envy can compromise nursing care and, indeed, may make the client's treatment ineffective. Only by viewing drug abuse as a symptom of a broader illness can the nurse be effective in dealing with adolescents. Nurses who have contact with adolescents, especially in school or community settings, should familiarize themselves with the general effects of various drugs and the first aid treatment for each. These are thoroughly detailed in Chapter 11.

Evaluating

Evaluating nursing interventions with the adolescent client can be tricky for numerous reasons:

• The adolescent client may need to test the limit one more time following a nursing intervention to avoid appearing "too complaint" or to "save face" with the group.

• Although it is important to set limits with the adolescent, it is equally important to be flexible. To set a limit and immediately "draw the line" with the next infraction is to invite the adolescent to step over that line to test its seriousness.

• Quick judgments should not be made if immediate results are not obtained. Persistence and consistency are the keys to success.

• The behaviors that brought the adolescent to psychiatric treatment will continue long after treatment and nursing interventions are begun. Despite a well-designed nursing care plan and client contract, the

NURSING CARE PLAN

A Client Who Is a Scapegoat

Client Care Goals	Nursing Planning/ Intervention	Evaluation

Nursing Diagnosis: *Social isolation*

Client Care Goals	Nursing Planning/ Intervention	Evaluation
Client will increase peer group participation.	Encourage participation in group activities and offer opportunities for one-to-one exchanges with other clients.	Client participates in group activities and lessens need to be scapegoat for group.
Client will show decreased evidence of being "different" from peers.	Discourage monopolizing of staff members' time, pointing out how this isolates client from peers.	Client accepts offers to engage in activities with peers and will initiate offers.
Client will have more appropriate verbal expression of fears related to rejection or hostility from others.	Give feedback on how client's behavior affects others. Encourage peers to say how they feel when client rejects them, e.g., when client refuses to play pool with them.	Client recognizes pattern of being "different" and feeling outcast, e.g., "I want them to like me, but I never want to do the things they want to do."
	Intervene when peers are being sadistic toward client, pointing out the process rather than simply rescuing client.	Client spends less time with staff and feels more comfortable with peers.
	Encourage role modeling of healthy figures of client's sex on ward.	Client expresses anger and negative feelings in more direct ways.
	Encourage direct expression of feelings when client begins to act out anger or rejection passively.	Client checks out beliefs about others, identifying their motives for seeking contact with client and dealing more directly with own suspicious ideas.
	Help client check out motivations for staff members' or peers' behavior when client suspects rejection or hostile intentions.	
	Evaluate client's progress with peer relationships each day and evening shift.	
	Document course of assessments, interventions, and evaluations in progress notes.	

adolescent will resort to previous maladaptive ways, immature and impulsive acts, or destructive behaviors in the face of change, particularly if this change represents improvement or growth (e.g., an increase in privileges or an impending discharge). The nurse who thinks the nursing interventions are not effective may feel hopeless about progress and convey that hopelessness to the client and the rest of the treatment team.

• Use of a behavioral contract without understanding the underlying reasons or factors contributing to the adolescent's problems will result in a superficial approach with an equally superficial evaluation.

If the adolescent had the desire or the impulse control simply to "act right" after being given the rules and consequences, then the client would be doing so already, and psychiatric treatment would not have been necessary. The adolescent needs the structure and consistency of a nursing care plan and client contract without the rigidity that can be imposed by a "now or never" behavioral plan with absolute consequences.

The nurse can make a more adequate evaluation if aware of the social context and meaning of the behavior to the adolescent. For example, the nurse may be wrong in determining that an indicator of increased self-esteem for a female client would be to stop dyeing her hair purple. Perhaps dyeing one's hair an unusual color may have been an indication of low self-esteem during the nurse's adolescent years, but for the client in question, that may or may not be the case. For that adolescent client and her peer group, purple hair may be a well-defined status symbol.

Evaluation is determined to be effective or ineffective by the use of various subjective and objective behavioral criteria reflecting the client care goals. See the nursing care plans in this chapter for specific problems and their criteria for evaluation.

CHAPTER HIGHLIGHTS

• Adolescence is a stormy time of conflicting ideas and feelings when identity, values, and goals are in a state of flux. The individual is no longer a child with investment in play or parental approval but is not yet an adult with abilities in verbal discourse or impulse control.

• A comprehensive assessment of this developmental period and the adolescent's problems is possible with the use of principles related to the developmental stage, social and cultural factors, biologic factors, familial influences, and psychodynamic conflicts.

• In the home, school, or clinic environment, the general hospital setting, or the in-patient psychiatric setting, the nurse can perform a central role in counseling parents and families of adolescent clients.

• The nurse can maintain a therapeutic milieu by providing a physically and psychologically safe environment, setting verbal and physical limits on the client's behavior, establishing meaningful relationships with the adolescent, identifying clients' strengths, promoting more adaptive coping skills, role modeling more socially acceptable behaviors, and participating in therapy groups and structured activities.

• Adolescents can present "normal" behaviors and problems unique to this developmental stage that could give the nurse difficulty. To be effective with nursing interventions, the nurse needs to understand typical adolescent behaviors as well as extremes in behavior.

• Specific issues and problems frequently related to psychiatric nursing care of adolescents include attempts to manipulate the nurse into relating in a nontherapeutic way, use of unconventional language and profanity, testing and limit setting, anxiety and resistance, anger and hostility, scapegoating, adolescent sexual behavior, dietary problems, eating disorders such as anorexia nervosa, bulimia nervosa, and obesity, drug use and abuse, and suicidal behavior.

• *Acting out* is often misused to describe antisocial destructive acts. It may include destructive actions, but it is much more than that. The term describes a recreation of the client's life experiences, the relationships with significant others, and the resulting unresolved conflicts.

• Nurse interventions with adolescents may be most effective if designed within the format of a client contract.

• Scapegoating is common to adolescent groups. The key to effective intervention is identifying the need that the scapegoat has to be "different" and setting limits on the scapegoating behaviors.

• To evaluate behavior adequately, nurses should be aware of its social contexts and its meaning to the adolescent.

REFERENCES

American Nurses Association: *Standards of Child and Adolescent Psychiatric and Mental Health Nursing Practice.* American Nurses' Association, 1985.

Amini F, Salasnek S: Adolescent drug abuse: Search for a treatment model. *Compr Psych* 1975;16:379–389.

Amini F, Salasnek S, Burke EL: Adolescent drug abuse: Etiological and treatment considerations. *Adolescence* 1976;11:281–299.

Campbell C: Perception of stress by staff members in an adolescent milieu. Unpublished research, 1977.

Casey RJ, Berman JS: The outcome of psychotherapy with children. *Psychol Bull* 1985;98:388–400.

Compas BE, Howell DC, Phares V, Williams RA, Giunta CT: Risk factors for emotional/behavioral problems in young adolescents: A prospective analysis of adolescent and parental stress and symptoms. *J Consult Clin Psychol* 1989;57(6):732–740.

Erikson E: *Identity, Youth and Crisis.* W. W. Norton, 1968.

Goldsmith MF: Heart disease researchers tailor new theories—Now maybe it's genes that make people fat. *JAMA* 1990;263(January 5):17–18.

Harnett NE: Conduct disorder in childhood and adolescence: An update. *J Child Adoles Psych Ment Health Nurs* 1989;2(2):74–77.

Hogarth CR: *Adolescent Psychiatric Nursing.* Mosby, 1990.

Jersild AT: *The Psychology of Adolescence,* ed 3. Macmillan, 1978.

Johnsson J: Chicago's Mt. Sinai: Community rehab. *Hospital* 1990;January 5:39.

Jones M: *Beyond the Therapeutic Community: Social Learning and Social Psychiatry.* Yale University Press, 1968.

Lewis JE: Are adolescents being hospitalized unnecessarily? *J Child Adoles Psychiatr Ment Health Nurs* 1989;2(4):134–138.

Mahon NE: Developmental changes and loneliness during adolescence. *Top Clin Nurs* 1983;5:(April):66–76.

O'Toole AW, Loomis ME: Revision of the phenomena of concern for psychiatric mental health nursing. *Arch Psychiatr Nurs* 1989;3(October):288–299.

Pallikkathayil L, McBride AB: Suicide attempts: The search for meaning. *J Psychosoc Nurs* 1986;24(August):13–18.

Paulson N: Nursing behaviors perceived as helpful by adolescent patients treated on an inpatient psychiatric unit. Yale University School of Nursing, Master's Thesis, 1987.

Pfeffer CR: Clinical aspects of childhood suicidal behavior. *Pediatr Ann* 1984;13(January):56–61.

The school nurse's dilemma, interview. *J Psychosoc Nurs* 1984;22(August):31–34.

Schwartz RH, Wirtz PW: Potential substance abuse: Detection among adolescent patients. *Clin Pediatr* 1990; 29(1):38–43.

Trudeau DL: Special strategies for sexually abused adolescents in chemical dependency treatment. *Prof Counselor* 1989;3(6):30–33.

Trygstad LN: Stress and coping in psychiatric nursing. *J Psychosoc Nurs* 1986;24(August):23–27.

Valente SM: Adolescent suicide: Assessment and intervention. *J Child Adoles Psychiatr Ment Health Nurs* 1989;2(1):34–39.

Weisz JR, Weiss B: Assessing the effects of clinic-based psychotherapy with children and adolescents. *J Consult Clin Psychol* 1989;57(6):741–746.

Weisz JR, Weiss B, Alicke MD, Klotz ML: Effectiveness of psychotherapy with children and adolescents: A meta-analysis for clinicians. *J Consult Clin Psychol* 1987;55:542–549.

White JL, Moffitt TE, Silva PA: A prospective replication of the protective effects of IQ in subjects at high risk for juvenile delinquency. *J Consult Clin Psychol* 1989; 57(6):719–724.

Applying the Nursing Process with the Elderly

Colleen Carney Love

LEARNING OBJECTIVES

• Discuss three significant age-related demographic projections and their implications for future health services for the elderly

• Describe the normal physical and psychosocial changes accompanying the aging process

• List the major theories of aging and three main points of each

• Apply the nursing process to care of elderly clients

• List the important components of a multifactorial assessment of an elderly client

• Complete a psychosocial assessment of an elderly client

• Explain the importance of distinguishing between depression, dementia, and delirium

• Contrast the mood and affect of older persons experiencing ego integrity with those of elders experiencing despair

• Identify the most common DSM-III-R mental disorders and associated nursing diagnoses among elderly psychiatric clients

• Identify interventions that will foster ego integrity late in life

CROSS REFERENCES

Other topics relevant to this content are: Chronically mentally ill, Chapter 17; Elder abuse, Chapter 22; Organic mental disorders, Chapter 10; Psychotropic medications, Chapter 32; Substance abuse, Chapter 11, Suicide, Chapter 23.

NURSES HAVE ENORMOUS POTENTIAL to influence the health of the elderly. Of all the health professions, nurses have the most contact with elderly persons (Institute of Medicine 1983). Nursing's emphasis on interaction, humanism, and promotion of health, self-care, and autonomy are particularly important for meeting the unique biopsychosocial needs of the elderly. A report from the American Nurses' Association Council on Psychiatric and Mental Health Nursing addressed the need for the Division of Gerontological Nursing Practice and the Division of Psychiatric Mental Health Nursing Practice to work together to: (1) formally establish nursing's clinical authority in care of the aged; (2) lobby for public policy that enables the provider professional to control the practice environment, rather than be controlled by it; (3) improve the educational preparation of nurses to care for the aged; and (4) expand the profession's scientific and research base in this area (Joel, Baldwin, and Stevens 1989, p. 17).

The aim of this chapter is to provide a comprehensive discussion of health promotion, advocacy, and application of the nursing process to mental health care for the elderly. It provides a broad overview of important age-related, biopsychosocial nursing considerations for advocacy and health promotion in later life; discusses the DSM-III-R (1987) mental disorders commonly seen in later life; and presents guidelines for applying the nursing process to the mental health care of the aged.

Historical and Theoretic Perspectives

Roadblocks to Mental Health Services for the Elderly

The elderly are the most underserved population in need of supportive and tertiary mental health services. This discussion highlights four roadblocks (agism, myths, stigma, and access) to mental health services and examines the demographic realities that compel us to break down these disabling roadblocks through health promotion and client advocacy.

Ageism A primary roadblock to mental health services for older persons is **ageism,** which refers to negative, hostile attitudes toward the elderly (Butler 1980). In contemporary social environments, aging is often viewed with disdain and contempt. The elderly are criticized for being unattractive, incompetent, socially irrelevant, and unhealthy. For many years, the elderly were considered inappropriate candidates for mental health interventions. Freud's contention that the elderly lacked the needed mental elasticity for analysis was a major factor in forming an ageist bias among mental health professionals. This bias has until recently delayed advances in the study of mental health in late life. Ageism also stems from the belief that the elderly present a financial and emotional drain to the family and society. **Gerontophobia,** a phenomenon related to ageism, refers to fear in interacting with the elderly (Chaisson-Stewart 1985). Ageist attitudes can be internalized by elderly persons, causing decreased self-worth and self-esteem.

Researchers have identified six attitudes or countertransference responses elicited in therapeutic work with the elderly (Poggi and Berland 1985). These countertransference responses (see the accompanying Nursing Self-Awareness box) reflect ageist and gerontophobic influences that may deter a professional from engaging in mental health work with the elderly. These responses may also affect the quality of work of nurses who do interact with the elderly.

Nurses caring for the elderly must be aware of their feelings and make a conscious effort not to let countertransference responses influence clinical assessment and interventions with the elderly. Nurses can provide invaluable support, insight, and feedback to colleagues who are working with the elderly. We now know the elderly are as responsive to mental health services as any other age group. By modeling positive attitudes toward aging and by advocating quality of life and health care for the aged in all settings and at all levels of function, nurses can help dispel ageist and gerontophobic influences on health care of the elderly.

Myths Health professionals, and elders themselves, often equate growing old with growing sad, disengaged, and depressed. The myths that depression, disengagement, and senility are part of growing old all too often inhibit the elderly from seeking treatment for feelings and behaviors they think are a "normal" part of aging. Misled by these myths, professionals are less inclined to refer elderly clients for mental health services. We now know that advancing age does not condemn an individual to senility, isolation, loneliness, and depression. The majority of elderly persons live independently and contentedly well into late life.

Nurses can serve as advocates to the elderly by educating the public, health professionals, and the elderly themselves to differentiate between normal and pathologic states in later life. Dispelling the myths surrounding the aging process will help promote the notion that aging itself is not a "problem," so that

NURSING SELF-AWARENESS

Countertransference Responses from Working with the Elderly

- The work stirs feelings in the nurse about age and issues surrounding death.
- Working with the elderly touches on the nurse's conflicts about relationships with parents and parental figures.
- The nurse believes the elderly are too rigid and set in their ways and cannot change.

- The nurse feels skills are wasted because clients are old and want to die anyway.
- The nurse feels interventions are in vain because elderly clients may die during treatment rather than improve.
- The nurse's colleagues do not support work with the elderly for any of all of the above reasons.

when problems do arise, they will be identified and treated.

Stigma   Despite recent advances in mental health care, the stigma associated with mental illness remains very real to elderly people who were socialized when psychiatric treatment was less sophisticated than it is today. The elderly rarely seek psychiatric or mental health services and often deny or hide their psychic pain for fear of being labeled "crazy" or of losing control and being institutionalized.

Nurses have tremendous access to persons at all levels of the health care and social systems. By educating the public about mental disorders and state-of-the-art mental health care, nurses can decrease the stigma associated with mental illness and psychiatric treatment and thus help allay the fears of the elderly who require mental health services.

Access   Financial barriers, physical disability, and transportation problems limit older adults' access to health care services. Financing of health care for mentally ill elderly is a very real problem. Medicare, the major form of health care financing for the elderly, covers only a portion of the health care costs of its beneficiaries, and there is a notable lack of long-term care coverage and coverage for chronic problems. Outpatient and home care coverage for mental health services is limited at best. Many mental health services are not covered under Medicare at all. Even when services are reimbursed through Medicare, there is often a large copayment, which is a burden to those individuals without supplementary coverage. Financial problems often add to an elder's psychosocial stressors. Nurses must be active in lobbying for policy changes to improve access to health care through financing to cover acute and chronic illnesses as well.

Demographic Realities

The elderly population is growing faster than that of the nation as a whole. In 1980 the U.S. Bureau of Census reported that by the year 2000 there will be almost thirty-five million people aged 65 and over. Forty-two million persons will be 60 and over. The over-75 population, which includes the "middle-aged old" (71–80), the "old-old" (81–90), and the "very old-old" (91–100), is estimated to reach 17.4 million by the year 2000.

It is important to examine the age distribution of the over-65 population carefully. Grouping the elderly arbitrarily into an aggregate of all persons over the age of 65 tends to blur important distinctions between elderly age groups. The "old-old" group of elders tends to have the greatest incidences of depression, organic mental disorders, and chronic disabling illnesses. This group averages four to five times as many days in acute care hospitals as the national average, and 70 percent more than individuals aged 65 to 75 (Blazer 1980). Thus, the stereotypic **frail elderly,** who need many health care and maintenance services, constitute only 5 percent of the over-65 population. This differentiation by age group indicates that there is a large proportion of well elderly, particularly older women living alone (who outnumber single elderly men by 2.5 to 1), who will benefit from supportive psychosocial services.

The implications of a growing population of aging individuals are important for projecting needs and planning for social programs and fund allocation. The figures point to the need for greater numbers of health care professionals versed in the multiple needs of the elderly. Nursing's role in geriatrics and **psychogerontology** is expanding as the needs and real numbers of elderly increase (Ebersole 1985).

Theories of Aging

Defining mental health in late life is a difficult task. Many variables affect mental health as persons age, including:

- Health status and psychobiology
- Cultural factors
- Heredity
- The environment
- The family network
- Meaningful relationships
- Life losses
- Personality composition
- Economic and social support
- Spirituality
- Coping skills

Late-life research efforts and theory development have focused on biologic aging, development, psychology, and social and interactional factors to explain "normal aging." Yet the many variables to consider and the complex interface of physical and emotional factors necessarily impose limitations on any single theory of aging. The most frequently cited theories of aging, and the major points of each, are presented in the accompanying Theory box.

All the theories on aging must be viewed tentatively at this time because the research remains inconclusive. For example, the disengagement theory, which views withdrawal from social activities as a normal aspect of later life, is particularly controversial and potentially damaging to the elderly. When working with elderly individuals, the nurse must consider the individual needs and unique characteristics of each aging person rather than attempting to fit an individual into a theoretic mold.

Philosophic Perspectives

The Value of Interaction Each elder is unique. The philosophic tenets of humanistic interactionism provide us with a dynamic view of mental health in later life. This view focuses on the personal meaning each individual assigns to situations, behavior, life events, and relationships in his or her life. Essentially, interactionist theory tells us there is no one "right" way to age. Each person processes and interprets aging in an individual way. The following case studies illustrate the individuality of elders as they find personal meaning in their unique life situations:

The nurses respected 92-year-old Mrs Fee's need to refer to her diapers as "envelopes," and her desire to be "dressed for work," wear makeup, and carry a purse every day. Her many years as an executive secretary brought her much satisfaction and a sense of identity and self-esteem, which she maintains in her present situation by integrating aspects of her past.

Mr Floyd had never been socially active or considered a "joiner." He looked forward to the day when he would be able to retire and spend long idle hours relaxing, just "doing nothing."

Mrs Baptista became depressed for a time after her enforced retirement at age 65. She found herself bored and down in the dumps with the excess free time and decreased social contact. She came across a senior's organization and soon replaced her busy work schedule with active participation in elderly social activities and volunteer programs for handicapped children.

Mr Smith became despondent when he required nursing home care, interpreting it as a prelude to his death. His roommate, Mr Cliff viewed nursing home residency as a welcome haven, providing him with needed care, companionship, and three square meals a day.

Mental health for each elder is defined differently and expressed in unique ways. Through client interactions nurses can help elderly persons reflect on and integrate the past and find new meaning and purpose in the present.

Individuality versus Obsolescence A rich history of life experiences adds to the complexity and individuality of each elder. In the past, elderly people were revered for their knowledge and wisdom. In our present culture, information and technology are advancing so rapidly that the elderly are often viewed as obsolete and out of touch. Interactions influenced by ageist attitudes convey a sense of worthlessness and obsolescence, which is internalized by elderly persons and predisposes them to mental illness.

A long life is evidence of strength and wisdom. Certainly living to a ripe old age is indicative of adaptive strength and coping ability. The elderly have much to share with younger people. Contemporary elders have lived through more dramatic changes in culture and technology than any former generation. The elderly must be respected for their individual strengths and the life wisdom they have accumulated.

Ego Integrity versus Self-Despair Erikson (1963) noted that the developmental task of late life is to achieve a sense of ego integrity versus self-despair. People who look back on their lives with satisfaction and a sense of wholeness, accomplishment, and a life well lived have achieved ego integrity. They convey a sense of serenity and wisdom and a desire to change

THEORY

Theories of Aging

Theory	Key Ideas	Theory	Key Ideas
Biologic Theories		*Interactional Theories*	
Deliberate biologic programming	Cellular level theory of aging	Disengagement	Characterized by mutually satisfying withdrawal between older adults and society
	Diminished capacity for spontaneous change		Disengagement is seen as a gradual, intrinsic, inevitable process
	Each cell holds a finite capacity for reproduction and a preprogrammed termination		Cohorts prefer company of same age groups
	Aging is the result of intrinsic destiny		Little recognition of the heterogeneity of the elderly
	Decline of biologic, cognitive, and motor function is inevitable		Controversial theory widely debated
Wear-and-tear theory	Over time the human organism wears out	Activity theory	Contrasts with disengagement theory
	Structural and functional changes may be accelerated by abuse and stress accumulation		Activity is desired by the elderly
			Older adults remain active and involved
	The rate of organ system degradation varies from individual to individual		Lost roles and pastimes are replaced with meaningful substitutes
	Decremental model of aging		Assumes heterogeneity or individual uniqueness
Stress-adaptation	Emphasizes the effects of positive and negative stress on aging	Symbolic interactionist theory	The individual's experience is constructed socially through an ongoing process of interpretation
	Perception influences stress response		
	Stress may deplete reserves, predisposing to illness		The social context is crucial to understanding aging, since all values and meanings are dynamic and evolving
	Stress may lead to more effective adaptation and growth		
	Stress generally presumed to accelerate aging		

THEORY (continued)

Theory	Key Ideas	Theory	Key Ideas
	Satisfaction in life is influenced by the symbolic significance of things and social interactions encountered		Reintegration of unresolved conflicts desirable
	Expansive theory, useful for studying many aspects of the aging process		Successful integration of the past provides ego integrity and existential meaning
	Social values and views of aging influence each individual's experience		May result in anxiety, fear, and depression related to unresolved issues
Life review/reminiscence	Reminiscence is normal and universal		Acknowledges individual differences and uniqueness
	Past experiences return to the conscious level		Aging patterns differ from individual to individual
Personality Theories Erikson's eight stages of man	Developmental sequence of eight psychosocial stages of ego development	**Developmental Theories**	Elders desire control over living situation
	Each stage characterized by specific developmental tasks		Continuity of intimacy (including sexual activity)
	Predetermined structural order to maturation		Strive to maintain optimum level of health
	Assumes inborn coordination to average expectable environment		Desired contact with family and extended family
	Eighth stage: ego integrity versus despair		Pursue former and new activities
	Ego integrity requires integration of the past		Find meaning after retirement
Continuity theory	Personality is stable over time		Refinement of personal philosophy
	Habits, preferences, associations, commitments are relatively unchanged with age		Adjustment occurs to losses of significant others
	"You are like you always were, only more so"		

little of their past. Despair results when an elder experiences a sense of loss and meaninglessness, a feeling that life's goals have not been achieved. To foster trust and ego integrity, caregivers must convey respect and worth to the elderly. Nurses caring for elderly people in all settings can promote ego integrity in each unique elderly individual through interactions focusing on personal strengths and positive reminiscing. Teaching family members and caregivers to emphasize these personal strengths and to assist in the life review process will enhance the ego-strengthening social support available to the elderly.

Biologic Perspectives

The rate of physical aging, which begins at birth, varies tremendously among individuals. Different tissues and body systems vary widely in the rate at which they age. Some persons appear old at age 50, whereas others appear vibrant and energetic into their eighties and nineties (Busse and Blazer 1980). Factors believed to influence the aging process include heredity, cultural influence, the amount and regularity of exercise, past illnesses, the presence of chronic illness, and the stresses experienced throughout life.

Changes in physical functioning can dramatically affect a person's ability to cope with daily stress and perform the activities of daily living. Age-related metabolic, circulatory, nutritional, and neurochemical disturbances have been identified as physiologic antecedents in certain mental disorders.

While normal age-related changes cannot be prevented, nurses can assess the extent of these changes and help elderly clients adapt by encouraging ventilation of feelings about the aging process, suggesting environmental alterations, and increasing social support.

Psychologic Perspectives

Just as age-related physical changes vary from person to person, so do the psychologic changes that occur as one ages. The goal of research into the psychologic aspects of aging is to describe, understand, and predict the changes that come with age and differentiate normal age-related changes from abnormal, illness-related changes. While studying intelligence, memory, problem solving, learning ability, motor performance, personality, coping, and adaptation in later life, researchers have identified methodologic difficulties that are relevant to clinical practice. For example, tests valid for use in other age groups have been shown to lack validity in older subjects. The time of day and length of testing also influence performance of elders because of fatigue and boredom. The elderly are often intolerant of gadgetry such as stopclocks and computerized test formats. Nurses must consider the variety of backgrounds and life experiences when designing and interpreting tests results, thus making comparison across different age groups difficult.

Intelligence The idea that intelligence declines with age is widely debated among researchers. Disagreement centers around the timing and extent of age decrements, the causes of the decrements that do appear in the elderly, and the validity and reliability of IQ tests in measuring intelligence in older subjects (Belsky 1984). It now appears that the most important factors affecting intelligence have to do with the individual's lifelong patterns and abilities. Older persons who have been intellectually active in their lifetime and continue to be challenged intellectually and socially active and to relate well to others have been found to show a minimum decrease, and in some cases an increase, in IQ scores with advancing age (Braudis 1986).

Learning and Memory Learning and memory are closely related. It is commonly believed that as people age their memory starts "slipping," and they are not as quick to learn as they used to be. Elders often cite these changes themselves. According to the information-processing model, memory is an active process that passes through three stages: (1) encoding or receipt of the information, (2) storage of the information, and (3) retrieval of the information. One factor that has been noted to affect the storage and retrieval of information in older persons has to do with the use of **mental mediators.** Mediators are cues used to enhance memory and learning (Belsky 1984, p 132). Nursing students often use the phrase, "On old Olympus' towering top a Finn and German viewed all hops," to remember the twelve cranial nerves. This is an example of a mediator. Elderly subjects were found not to use mediators spontaneously to help them remember. When mediators were suggested to these subjects, however, their performance on tests improved. This information is useful for clinicians when helping the elderly to remember things.

Mr O'Brien began to forget his apartment keys when he left the house to go to the senior center for lunch every day. He never forgot his pipe and tobacco, however. The nurse at the center suggested Mr O'Brien mentally connect his tobacco pouch with his keys. She suggested that he get into the habit of putting his keys in his pocket at the same time he places his tobacco pouch there. This solved Mr O'Brien's problem of forgetting his keys.

As persons age, they tend to think and move more slowly than younger people. Part of this slower pacing is related to adaptation to sensory deficits and part to a more cautious approach to life. Older people perform better if information is meaningful to them.

When the elderly are permitted to pace themselves, rather than being rushed, their performance improves significantly. Nurses teaching elderly clients a new skill, such as progressive relaxation or assertion, may find the following guidelines useful:

• Present the information so that its utility to the client is clear.

• Allow clients to pace themselves.

• Provide time for repetition of material.

• Suggest mediators when appropriate.

• Be sincere and focus on small positive steps.

Overall memory, learning, intelligence, coping and adaptation, and personality remain relatively stable as individuals age. The elderly *can* be taught new ways of coping and handling the stressors of aging. Subtle, minimal changes are normal as people adapt to age-related changes in functioning and life experiences. Any marked variation in cognitive functioning or affective status of older people, whether sudden or progressive, should not be regarded as a normal part of aging. Gross alteration in mental status, personality, and cognition suggests the presence of a mental or physical disorder or both. The following section provides an overview of the most common mental disorders in later life.

Biopsychosocial Factors

Epidemiology

The ageist attitudes in our culture are responsible for many misperceptions about mental disorders in the elderly. Older people are believed to be more prone to mental disorders than the young. It is difficult to obtain exact incidence and prevalence rates of mental disorders in later life for several reasons. Often the elderly are difficult to reach with community-wide surveys. Researchers have noted that the elderly are reluctant to respond to research questions dealing with emotions. As mentioned earlier, the elderly often do not seek treatment, so elderly subjects are underrepresented in clinical samples. Different researchers diagnose mental problems differently, making comparisons between community-wide surveys difficult. Symptoms of mental illness in the elderly often differ from those of other age groups. While the DSM-III-R (APA 1987) has greatly enhanced our ability to make reliable and valid diagnoses of mental disorders, there are few age-specific categories for mental disorders in later life. Thus, in spite of the DSM-III-R's extensive detailed description of each problem category, clinicians and researchers continue to have difficulty applying the

written descriptions to symptoms in later life (Belsky 1984, Zung 1980).

The epidemiologic studies to date tell us that the elderly suffer no more than other groups from disorders, such as adjustment disorders, personality disorders, and grief reactions. The elderly do have a disproportionately high incidence of depression and are somewhat more likely to become paranoid. Organic brain syndromes, particularly the chronic organic dementias, are much more prevalent in the elderly. The elderly also frequently complain of sleep disturbances. Two recent areas of exploration, for which there is very little epidemiologic data at present, are substance abuse in later life and the chronically mentally ill elderly.

Mood Disorders

Mood disorders are primarily characterized by a disturbed affect or emotional experience. Mood disturbances in the elderly, as in other age groups, may present as:

• Sustained elation and hyperactivity, as seen in a manic episode

• Changes from elation to depression, as seen in a bipolar disorder

• Pervasive depressed mood not accompanied by mania, as seen in a major depression

Depression is the most prevalent and most treatable mental disorder in later life.

Depression in the Elderly Depression robs the elderly of late life satisfaction, inhibits ego integrity, and may substantially decrease an elder's life expectancy, since symptoms may precipitate or aggravate physical deterioration. Suicide rates among the elderly are more than three times the rates in the general population (Osgood 1985).

Although the signs and symptoms of depression are relatively consistent throughout the life span (see Chapter 13), certain characteristics of depression are particular to the elderly. It is crucial for clinicians to note that depression in the elderly, which responds well to treatment, may present with cognitive changes similar to those that accompany other organically based, irreversible disorders. Tyler and Tyler (1984) suggest that nearly half the elderly clients thought to be demented actually have a depressive disorder with misleading cognitive symptoms such as disorientation, agitation, and memory loss.

In addition to cognitive changes, another flag for depression in elderly persons is excessive preoccupation with physical symptoms, which is known as **somatization.** Expressing discomfort through the body may be more familiar to older persons than bringing forth symptoms of psychic pain. Chronic complaints of constipation, headaches, musculoskeletal pain, chest tightness and dyspnea with no physical basis, and chronic gastrointestinal upset may be the result of a depressed elder's unconscious shifting of attention away from distressing emotions to more "acceptable," familiar, and less stigmatized physical complaints. Clinicians have noted that because of the stigma associated with mental illness, depressed elderly clients sometimes "cover up" a dysphoric mood by maintaining meticulous grooming and feigning a cheerful affect (Love and Buckwalter, 1991). Nurses must be persistent and perceptive in looking for signs of depression. Depressed apathetic elders may believe they are supposed to feel blue and "down in the dumps" as they age. Nurses need to inform depressed elders and their families that depression is a pathologic condition often caused by biochemical imbalances. Interventions should be instituted to correct depressive states in the elderly as aggressively and comprehensively as in any other age group.

Suicide The depressed elderly are more prone to commit suicide than any other age group in the United States (Stenback 1980). The **lethality index** (ratio of suicide attempts to successful suicides) is also higher in the elderly, and these data do not even begin to tap the passive, indirect suicides accomplished by starvation and "accidental" overmedication. The dramatically high rates clearly indicate that suicide is a significant problem in later life.

Elders who present a greater suicide risk include:

- Elderly males

- The unmarried

- Caucasians

- Lower socioeconomic classes

- Elders with chronic pain and terminal illness

- The lonely and isolated in urban settings

- The elderly who use alcohol and medication to cope (Osgood 1985)

The suicidal elderly have been known to seek help (often for a vague or nonspecific physical problem) from physicians, clergy, and nurses prior to their self-destructive act. Thus, accurate assessment of suicide potential in the elderly is crucial and requires perception, active listening, and direct questioning. The suicidal elderly individual may present with:

- Verbal cues (e.g., "I'm going to end it all; life is not worth living; I won't be around much longer")

- Behavioral cues (e.g., completing a will, making funeral plans, "acting out," withdrawing, somatic complaints)

- Situational cues (e.g., recent move, loss of a loved one, diagnosis of a terminal illness) (Osgood 1985)

For more information on suicide and assessment of suicide potential including a lethality index, see Chapter 23. Osgood (1985) has written a comprehensive volume covering the topic of suicide in the elderly.

Adjustment Disorders The elderly often experience dramatic life changes because of losses through death, relocation, loss of independence, retirement, illness, and financial stress. One or a combination of life changes and losses may contribute to the development of an **adjustment disorder** in the elderly. The essential feature of an adjustment disorder is a maladaptive reaction to an identifiable psychosocial stressor (or stressors) that occurs within three months after the onset of the stressor and has persisted for no longer than six months (DSM-III-R). Adjustment disorders in the elderly may present with a variety of psychiatric symptoms including:

- Adjustment disorder with anxious mood

- Adjustment disorder with depressed mood

- Adjustment disorder with mixed emotional features

- Adjustment disorder with physical complaints

- Adjustment disorder with withdrawal

Organic Mental Syndromes and Disorders

The diagnostic group termed **organic mental syndromes** (OMS) refers to a temporary or permanent brain dysfunction that is either caused by an illness unrelated to a mental illness listed on the DSM-III-R Axis I or that has no known etiology. Organic mental disorder (OMD) are progressive pathophysiologic brain processes of known etiology. Both OMS and OMD cause a variety of psychologic, cognitive, and behavioral abnormalities. The elderly present with both OMS and OMD more than any other age group. The challenge for clinicians is to identify and treat reversible organic mental syndromes, whether they exist alone or with an irreversible condition.

Delirium Delirium refers to an acute confusional state that usually appears within hours or days. Delirium is characterized primarily by confusion and an obvious decrease in attention span and level of consciousness that may fluctuate over the course of the day. Other symptoms may include perceptual disturbances, psychomotor retardation or agitation, incoherent speech, and disorders of the sleep-wake cycle. When an elderly client becomes acutely confused, thorough and prompt assessment will often uncover a

Text continues on p. 881

RESEARCH NOTE

Citation

Gass KA, Chang AS: Appraisals of bereavement, coping, resources, and psychosocial health dysfunction in widows and widowers. Nurs Res 1989;38(1):31–36.

Study Problem/Purpose

This exploratory design used Lazarus and Folkman's (1984) model of stress and coping as a framework to examine aspects of bereavement in older widows ($n=100$) and widowers ($n=59$). The variables examined included resource strength (psychologic, social, and financial) and subject's appraisal of loss as either (a) a harmful loss without other losses, (b) a harmful loss with other anticipated threats (such as loss of independence or ability to manage without the person), or (c) a challenge and opportunity for growth.

In terms of bereavement or grieving period, the model posits that the bereaved individual's perceptions determine how the loss is appraised and influences what coping strategies and resources are available to the bereaved. Coping was defined as constantly changing cognitive and behavioral efforts to manage specific external and/or internal demands that are taxing or exceed a person's recourses. Coping was operationalized as either "problem-focused coping" (directed at practically managing or altering a problem causing distress) or "emotion-focused coping" (regulating the emotional response to the problem).

Six hypotheses were tested.

Findings

The study indicated that the way the bereaved individuals appraised their situation had a significant, direct influence on the coping style the subjects employed and the development of psychosocial health dysfunction during the bereavement period. Widowed persons who perceived bereavement as being accompanied by other anticipated threats (such as loss of independence) tended to use more problem-focused and emotion-focused coping and were at greater risk of developing psychosocial health dysfunction than those who perceived the loss as either a challenge or a significant loss not accompanied by other anticipated threats. The study also found that persons who employed more problem-focused coping demonstrated less psychosocial health problems than did persons who relied on emotion-focused coping. Resource strength directly influenced appraisal and indirectly influenced coping through appraisal. Widowed subjects with greater resource strength reported less psychosocial health problems than those with less resource strength. Men had greater resource strength than women in this study, which contributed to their lower perception of threat and fewer health problems. Sudden death of a spouse was directly related to fewer resources, which increased threat appraisal and psychosocial health problems. In contrast, persons who lost a spouse to a chronic illness had greater resource strength, which led to lower threat appraisal and better psychosocial functioning.

Nursing Implications

The Lazarus and Folkman model may be useful to professionals attempting to identify those individuals at risk of developing psychosocial health dysfunction following the loss of a spouse. As the population ages nurses will encounter bereaved individuals (particularly widows) more frequently. Nurses can help bereaved individuals to identify and augment resources available to them, and to use cognitive principles to appraise their situation realistically. Augmenting resources may include psychoeducation regarding the grieving process, encouragement of open expression of grief, spiritual support, opportunities for anticipatory grieving, and working through guilt associated with the loss. Fostering the use of problem-focused, reality-based coping strategies along with emotion-focused strategies to encourage clarification and control may help reduce psychosocial health dysfunction during the bereavement period.

CASE STUDY

A Client with Adjustment Disorder with Depressed Mood

Identifying Information

Mr Rozello is an 85-year-old Italian immigrant who is currently residing on the health-related floor in a long-term care facility. He is married to Mrs Rozello, age 80, who resides in the same facility on the skilled nursing floor. They are both devout Catholics.

The long-term care facility contacted a geropsychiatric nurse clinician to come to the facility to assess Mr Rozello, who had become increasingly unmanageable.

Client's Definition of Present Problem, Precipitating Stressors, Coping Strategies, Goals for Care

The Rozellos lived independently up until about a year ago, when Mrs Rozello suffered a massive stroke, leaving her comatose. She is described as having been a doting wife and a meticulous housekeeper. Despite living in this country since they were both 18, she spoke little English, relying on her husband for all interactions outside the immediate household. Since his admission Mr Rozello has refused to visit his wife and has demonstrated a variety of behavior changes, becoming progressively agitated and unmanageable. He has lost 15 pounds since admission. Mr Rozello's attending physician ordered diazepam 5 mg p.o. t.i.d. to control his anxious and combative tendency and temazepam p.r.n. for sleep. The medication seemed to decrease his agitation, although he became more withdrawn and confused during the day, refusing to participate in any activities. His disturbed sleep pattern remains unchanged; he wakes between 2:00 and 4:00 A.M. every morning and anxiously paces the hall, talking to himself.

Psychiatric History

Negative

Family History

Mr Rozello's parents were both laborers in Italy. He has lost contact with his only sibling, an older brother who resided in Italy. No other family information was available.

Social History

Mr Rozello immigrated to America with his wife when he was 18. Mr Rozello completed the equivalent of eighth grade in Italy before immigrating to the United States. He was employed as a mason for forty-seven years. He was affiliated with a fraternal organization for twenty-five years. Mr Rozello was active in several church-related activities up until several years before his admission to the facility. Mr Rozello is visited weekly by the parish priest, and several parishioners visit him occasionally. He has no surviving relatives and no close friends. Mr Rozello smoked cigars occasionally and drank one or two glasses of wine daily with dinner prior to admission. He has had no tobacco and no alcohol since admission.

Mr Rozello enjoyed gardening, tending his own grapevines and making wine annually, until his admission. He also mentioned that he enjoyed caring for the family dog, who died shortly before his wife became ill.

Significant Health History

Medical records revealed Mr Rozello had been essentially healthy during his adult years. Family health history was not available. He was on no medication at home. He has no allergies. His appetite has been poor since admission, and he had lost

Adapted from Love CC, Buckwalter KC: *Reactive depression*, in Mass MM, Buckwalter KC: Nursing Diagnosis and Interventions for the institutionalized Elderly. *Addison-Wesley, 1991.*

▶

CASE STUDY (continued)

15 pounds in the past eight months. He was treated for frequent fecal impactions for which he received Colace b.i.d. He had no physical limitations and had been physically active, gardening and taking daily walks with the family dog, prior to admission.

Current Affective and Mental Status

Mr Rozello appeared gaunt, disheveled, and tired, with uncombed hair and several days worth of stubble on his face. He emitted a pervasive feeling of despair with an undercurrent of anger and despondency. His mood was severely depressed. Mr Rozello was oriented in all spheres, with judgment and remote and recent memory intact. He scored 1 on the SPMSQ, which indicates intact intellectual functioning. His thoughts flowed logically, although he was easily distracted with some loosening of associations. Reality testing was intact, with no delusional thought content, nor signs of psychosis. He did not demonstrate any perceptual difficulty. His gait was obviously steady though slow. He spoke hesitantly of the many losses he had encountered in his life both long past and recently.

He noted that he and his wife had been sexually active occasionally until her illness. Currently he admits to decreased energy and libido.

When asked what things he did to get through difficult times in the past he looked puzzled and then explained he never considered his needs, since his wife's were more important. He indicated that his wife grieved quite openly and demonstratively, and he often felt the need to console her rather then himself. He noted their marriage was a good one and he loved his wife. When the subject of his wife's condition was mentioned, it became apparent that he felt irrationally guilty, blaming himself for not having insisted she see a physician when she had complained of dizziness. He abruptly blocked any further conversation about his wife's condition. Well into the assessment interview the following conversation between the nurse and Mr Rozello took place:

Nurse: Mr Rozello, do you ever think about killing yourself? — Assessment of suicidal ideation

Client: (Withdrawing, angrily) You think I'm crazy don't you? — Fear of stigmatization

Nurse: (Touching his arm, emphasizing her response with direct eye contact) Mr Rozello, You are *not* crazy. Everything you have said makes perfect sense to me. You are thinking very clearly and logically. — Validation, support, emphasis on strengths

(Pause) The staff and I are concerned about you because you seem blue and down in the dumps most of the time. You aren't eating or sleeping well. — Provides concrete evidence of disorder

You've lost weight, and these things suggest to me that you are feeling depressed. I can understand fully — Validation

why you are feeling blue. It seems very *normal* to me that you feel sad. (Pause) I would like to help you to — Expression of caring

feel better and maybe even be happy again. (Pause, nurse takes his hand) Sometimes when people have — Touch, contact, instillation of hope

suffered great losses in their life, they are able to feel — Validation

better if they can share their feelings with another — Education

person. You have been holding your sadness inside for a long time, and now it's affecting your health. — Empathy

(Pause) I would like to help you. You don't have to

CASE STUDY (continued)

suffer alone. I think together we can work this out. Would you be willing to share your feelings with me? (Long silence) Only you can tell us how you feel.

Reassurance

Seeking client input, reinforcing client's control

Client: (Withdraws his hand and wipes away a tear) If I could sleep better I'd feel better.

Shifting focus from feelings to somatic symptoms

Nurse: That's probably very true. Maybe a goal we could work on would be to help you sleep longer at night. (Pause) Do you think if you shared your upsetting feelings with me during the day you might feel more restful at night? (Long silence, no answer)

Validation, mutual goal setting
Redirecting

Reluctance, use of silence

Nurse: I imagine it feels uncomfortable for you to think about sharing your sadness with me. You don't know me very well. (Pause) Maybe we could start by talking about some of the good times you've had in your life? Would that feel more comfortable to you?

Validation, empathy, establishing trust by refocusing temporarily on less painful issues, being direct, using feeling words

Client: (Pause) Will you come every day?

Client's seeking clarification suggests acceptance

After much encouragement Mr Rozello agreed to see the nurse regularly. She continued the interaction and determined he was not suicidal.

Client Strengths/Signs of Growth

In excellent physical condition, chronic illness absent, completely mobile, agile, and fully ambulatory; nonsuicidal; resides on the Health-Related Unit, among many other highly functional peers; financially secure (SSI, private health insurance, and pension); has been assisting his roommate to the dining room recently; bilingual, had enjoyed translating magazines and newspapers to his wife; knowledgeable about gardening; possesses adaptive strengths, has endured significant losses in his life; had a solid marriage, good relationships with his neighbors in the community, and belonged to a fraternal organization much of his life, indicating the ability to maintain meaningful relationships; has strong religious beliefs; is physically attractive; has a rich life history, having immigrated from Italy; used to make his own wine; agreed to meet with the geropsychiatric clinician.

Diagnostic Impressions

Nursing Diagnoses

Dysfunctional grieving
Altered nutrition: Less than body requirements
Anxiety
Social isolation

DSM-III-R Multiaxial Diagnosis

Axis I: 309.00 Adjustment Disorder with Depressed Mood
Axis II: V71.09 No diagnosis on Axis II
Axis III: None
Axis IV: Psychosocial stressors: 5, Extreme (illness of wife, loss of independence)
Axis V: Current GAF:35
Highest GAF in the past year: 60

NURSING CARE PLAN

A Client with Adjustment Disorder with Depressed Mood

Client Care Goals	Nursing Planning/ Intervention	Evaluation
Nursing Diagnosis: *Dysfunctional grieving*		
Client will be begin expressing feelings, using feeling words.	Offer "feelings list" daily to help in feeling expression and identification.	Client engages in normal grief work: works through grief process, discusses reality of loss.
Client will explore guilt associated with wife's illness with staff.	Arrange for client to meet with geropsychiatric nurse twice a week.	Client visits wife, assists in her basic care, reads to her regularly.
Client will visit his wife.	Assist in recognition of grieving behavior during one-to-one interactions.	Client expresses feelings in preparation for wife's impending death.
Client will attend "griever's group."	Encourage "griever's group" membership.	
	Staff will meet with the client's parish priest to establish consistent approach and spiritual component.	
Nursing Diagnosis: *Altered nutrition: Less than body requirements*		
Client will begin eating small amounts 6× day.	Offer small frequent feedings.	Client regains 15 lbs.
Client will gain 2 lb/week.	Meet with dietitian twice a week for menu planning.	Client is free from impactions.
Client will have regular BM.	Provide liquid supplement as tolerated.	
	Offer small frequent feedings.	
	Give a glass of wine before dinner.	
	Encourage fiber and physical activity, give stool softener p.r.n.	
Nursing diagnosis: *Anxiety*		
Client will reduce pacing and combative behavior.	All staff will provide active listening.	Client accurately appraises stress level.
		Client expresses anger verbally.
Client will sleep past 5:00 A.M.	Encourage diversional activities through mutually developed plan with occupational therapist.	Client establishes adequate coping resources, such as renewed spiritual expression; increased IPR.
	Provide calm milieu; firm, calm staff.	Client seeks out one-to-one interactions once every day.

▶

NURSING CARE PLAN (continued)

Client Care Goals	Nursing Planning/ Intervention	Evaluation
	Reduce guilt through cognitive restructuring in 1 to 1 sessions.	
Nursing Diagnosis: *Social isolation*		
Client will explore ways needs can be met through interpersonal contact.	Respect client's need for time alone.	Client demonstrates precrisis communication skills per self evaluation.
	Recognize efforts to participate with positive feedback.	Client expresses one positive statement about self per day.
	Use touch appropriately.	Client expresses satisfaction with social interactions and name three sources of social support.
	Encourage budding interaction with roommate.	

specific organic factor or combination of factors such as infection; congestive heart failure; trauma; hepatic, pulmonary, and renal insufficiency; and drug toxicity.

The treatment of delirium, which is usually reversible, must be directed toward correcting the underlying disorder. Symptomatic treatment may be necessary, particularly if agitation, anxiety, perceptual disturbances, delusions, or other behavioral features are endangering the client's safety or interfering with the evaluation and treatment of the underlying disorder. Nursing interventions for a client with delirium include:

• Calm, consistent low level of stimuli (avoid sensory deprivation and overstimulation)

• Reassurance from trusted caregivers and significant others

• Physically secure, carefully monitored environment

• Night lights to aid orientation

• Judicial use of low-dose psychotropic medication

Dementia   **Dementia,** or loss of cognitive function, once thought to be an inevitable part of growing old, is now known to be a pathologic condition afflicting only 5 to 7 percent of the over-65 population (Mortimer et al. 1981). Certain reversible conditions that mimic dementia, known as **pseudodementia,** improve markedly with treatment. Causes of dementia-like symptoms (pseudodementia) include but are not limited to the following:

• Depression

• Metabolic and endocrine disturbances

• Infection

• Brain disorders such as parkinsonism, normal pressure hydrocephalus, focal lesions of the nondominant lobe, and subarachnoid hemorrhage

• Vitamin deficiencies

• Metal intoxication

• Systemic lupus erythematosus

• Any disabling disease

Although the dementias are irreversible, some have a progressively downward course ending in death. The causes of dementia vary and, as in the case of Alzheimer's disease, are not well understood. Multiinfarct dementia, caused by a series of small strokes, results in a variety of stepwise, focal, neurologic signs and symptoms.

Alzheimer's disease and multiinfarct dementia are the most prevalent dementias. **Senile dementia—Alzheimer's type (SDAT),** the fourth leading cause of death in the elderly, has received a great deal of publicity recently, heightening the public's awareness of the tragedy of dementia and its impact on family and caregivers. Zarit et al. (1985) note that since the time of increased publicity, increasing numbers of people have been incorrectly diagnosed with SDAT when in fact they have had a reversible dementia-like condition. The definitive diagnosis of SDAT can be made only on autopsy.

Family Burden Perhaps no other illness is as devastating to family members or caregivers as an irreversible dementia. The anguish of family members seeing loved ones becoming progressively more dependent is profound. The stress of looking after demented individuals, who often become delusional, suspicious, angry, and sometimes unmanageable, is being studied in a growing area of research called **family burden.** Coping abilities vary markedly according to the family's emotional, financial, and environmental resources. To prevent burnout and elder abuse, family members caring for a demented elder need emotional support and information about specific interventions aimed at problem solving and stress reduction. Nurses are in key positions to provide psychoeducative programs for the caregivers of demented individuals. Community support programs and publications are now available to provide emotional support, strategies, and practical information for persons choosing to care for a demented individual at home. Two useful publications are *The 36 Hour Day* (Mace and Rabins 1981) and *Alzheimer's Disease: A Guide for Families* (Powell and Courtice 1983). For further discussion of dementia and delirium, see Chapter 10.

It is crucial to perform a comprehensive physical and neurologic assessment whenever an elderly client presents with cognitive impairment. Nurses must become skilled at differentiating treatable disorders such as delirium and depression from irreversible dementia. It is also important to note that depression can exist with dementia or delirium, and the cognitive impairment may be worsened by the depressive overlay. Depression superimposed on dementia may cause increased cognitive problems, a situation described as **excess disability.** In these cases treatment with antidepressant medication may improve the cognitive status worsened by the depression. The accompanying Assessment box provides guidelines for distinguishing depression from dementia.

Anxiety Disorders

Anxiety is a universal sensation experienced subjectively as worry, fear, restlessness, and terror stemming from fear of a real danger or the anticipation of danger or a threat. Anxiety, particularly anxiety associated with panic disorder, is often accompanied by spontaneous somatic "fight-or-flight" phenomena including shortness of breath, palpitations, sweating, GI upset, and chest tightness. Anxiety that interferes with an individual's ability to function is considered an **anxiety disorder.** Anxiety is exceedingly common across age groups and increases in frequency with advancing age. For the elderly, the prevalence of panic disorder, obsessive compulsive disorder, and phobias combined ranged between 5.7 and 33 percent (Turnbull and Turnbull 1985).

Unfortunately, anxiety disorders are often missed in the elderly because, as with depression, the elderly often present with a predominance of physical complaints that mask the underlying disorder. Additionally, anxiety in the elderly is often the main feature of a depressive disorder, and too often the anxiety is treated but the depression persists, leading to a cycle of anxiety-depression and physical illness. Table 35–1 lists the different types of anxiety disorders and their central features. Anxiety disorders in the elderly must be differentiated from agitation secondary to adverse drug reactions (e.g., akathisia from neuroleptics) delirium, dementia, parkinsonism, paranoid disorders, hypoxia, and pain. Anxiety may also have predominant psychologic features, as seen in anxiety stemming from perceived powerlessness, fear, perceived loss of control and mastery, anticipated loss, despair, and grief reactions. The etiology of the anxiety state determines the appropriate treatment, which most often involves a combination of psychotherapy, relaxation training, behavior modification, systematic desensitization, social support, and judicious use of the appropriate class of psychoactive medication. Low-dose medication should be initiated when symptoms interfere with the elder's ability to benefit from the other psychoeducative and psychosocial "talk therapies."

Delusional Disorders

Delusions are defined as an important personal belief that is almost certainly not true and resists modification (Wilson and Kneisl 1984; p 75). The elderly are more prone than any other age group to persecutory and somatic delusions. Persecutory delusions involve the belief that the elder is under investigation, being harassed, or at the mercy of some powerful force. With somatic delusions the predominant theme is an imagined physical disorder or abnormality of appearance. Somatic delusions in older persons are frequently characterized by extremely morbid content.

Delusion processes in the elderly are often associated with delirium, depression, dementia, or anxiety disorders. In the elderly, persecutory delusions may be a response to a diminishing sense of self-mastery. Among the various symptoms exhibited by elderly people with psychiatric problems, delusions involving suspiciousness and persecutory ideation are among the most disturbing and unsettling for their families and caregivers. As older adults gradually give up important areas of function, such as financial management, cooking, and shopping, they may begin to develop delusions that people are robbing them or poisoning their food. They respond to these delusional processes by "dismissing" or rejecting their caregivers in an effort to regain control over these areas of life. Delusions may also result from internalized ageist

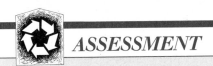

ASSESSMENT

Guidelines Differentiating Dementia from Depression

Affect

Observe the client's overall mood and self-presentation throughout the interview. Enlist interpretations from family and caregivers. "How has your mood been lately?"

Dementia Labile, fluctuating from tears to laughter, not consistent or sustained: may show apathy, depression, irritability, euphoria or inappropriate affect. Normal control impaired, suggestible to content of interview.

Depression Depressed, feelings of despair that are pervasive, persistent. May be anxious or hypomanic. Not influenced by suggestions. May be flat, withdrawn, sad, tearful.

Memory

Ask specific questions geared toward assessing recent and remote memory. Ask client to recall recent events, details from a classic, personal, or well-known story. Ask client to repeat a series of three or four words at five-, ten-, and fifteen-minute intervals.

Dementia Decreased attention. Decreased for recent events. Confabulation, covers up memory loss. Shows irritability when memory tested. Perseveration, dwells on certain topics inappropriately.

Depression Difficulty in concentration. Impaired learning of new knowledge. Decreased attention with secondary decrease in recent memory. May not respond when tested or will admit can't remember.

Intellect

Assess the client's cognitive functioning, taking into account cultural and educational factors, which will influence results. Ask the client to perform simple math equations and solve simple problems.

Dementia Impaired, decreased as tested by serial 7s, similarities, recent events. Decreased capacity for abstract thinking.

Depression Impaired but can perform serial 7s and usually remember recent events.

Orientation

Elicit level of orientation regarding person, time, place, date, etc. May vary with different times of the day.

Dementia Fluctuating with varying levels of awareness. Disoriented for time, place.

Depression May have some confusion, not as profound as in dementia.

Judgment

Ask the client to solve hypothetical problems (e.g., What would you do if you saw a fire across the street?)

Dementia Poor judgment with inappropriate behavior, dress. Deterioration of grooming, personal habits, and hygiene. Loss of bowel and bladder control.

Depression May be poor, especially if suicidal. May be careless with medication, and may risk personal safety.

Somatic Complaints

Ask the client specific questions regarding physical status. (How is your health?)

Dementia Fatigue, failing health complaints with vague complaints of pain in head, neck, back.

Depression Typical complaints as: decreases in sleep, appetite, weight, libido, energy, and constipation.

Psychotic Symptoms

Enlist interpretations from family and caregivers. Often (but not always) psychotic material will become evident during interview. (Are you being plotted against? Do you ever see/hear/smell things others do not?)

Dementia Mainly visual, hallucinations, delusions.

Depression May occur in psychotic depressions, mainly auditory hallucinations and delusions of a morbid quality.

SOURCE: Adapted from Zung WWK: *Affective Disorders, in Busse EW, Blazer DG (eds): Handbook of Geriatric Psychiatry. Van Nostrand Reinhold, 1980, p 357.*

TABLE 35–1   **Anxiety Disorders and Their Central Features**

Disorder	Central Features
Phobic disorders	Persistent, irrational fear/anxiety provoked by stimulus object, activity, or situation Avoidance of stimulus Fear recognized by client as irrational or excessive
Agoraphobia	Occurs with/without panic attacks Fear stimulus: being alone or in a public place where escape would be difficult or help hard to find
Social phobia	Fear stimulus: social situation involving possible embarrassment or humiliation
Simple phobia	Fear stimulus: situations similar to previous terrifying experience
Anxiety states	Persistent or recurrent anxiety not provoked by identifiable stimulus, generally nonsituational
Obsessive-compulsive disorder	Intrusive thoughts and/or repetitive behaviors performed under a sense of pressure Attempts to resist increased anxiety
Post-traumatic stress disorder	Acute and delayed reactions to a traumatic event Involves "reliving" the experience, emotional numbing, and development of somatic symptoms
Panic disorder	Sudden, unpredictable panic attacks involving intense apprehension and physical symptoms
Generalized anxiety disorder	Generalized, persistent anxiety for more than one month Includes three of the following: motor tension, autonomic hyperactivity, apprehension, and hypervigilance
Adjustment disorder with anxious mood	Nervousness/anxiety in reaction to identifiable psychosocial stressor

attitudes, sensory losses—particularly hearing impairment—and social isolation.

Caregivers must work to establish trust and consistency with delusional elders. It is important to assess the situation to validate that the persecutory and somatic content is not reality based. Clients need consistent social interaction, with caring, consistent reality orientation. Relieving social isolation and correcting sensory losses may solve the problem. Delusional processes associated with delirium often abate when the cause of the delirium is treated. Medication in small doses, geared toward relieving an underlying anxiety or depressive disorder, may be helpful, although compliance is often a problem due to the client's suspicion.

Substance Use Disorders

The extent of alcoholism and drug- and alcohol-related problems in the elderly is unknown. Typical signs of alcoholism, such as absence from work, difficulties in the family, and driving while intoxicated are often not apparent in older people, because they often are retired, live alone, and do not drive. It is

known that the elderly use a disproportionately high amount of prescribed hypnotics and over-the-counter sleep medications. Elderly persons also often take a variety of medications for one or more chronic medical conditions. **Polypharmacy,** or mixing medications, with or without alcohol use, is potentially dangerous and adds to the chance of untoward drug interactions in the elderly (Colling 1983).

There seem to be two categories of older drinkers. The first category includes those who have a long history of alcohol abuse. The second category, the late-onset, **reactive drinker,** includes those who drink in response to one or more age-related stressors, such as social isolation, loss of a loved one, and loss of social status (Blazer and Pennybacker 1984).

When older drinkers seek medical help for alcohol-related problems (e.g., malnutrition, injuries from falling, sleep problems), the alcoholism is rarely the presenting problem. Often a drinking problem is not diagnosed in an elderly client; the presenting symptoms are treated, and other symptoms are attributed to "normal" age-related changes. Glassock (1982) has suggested that a "conspiracy of silence" exists between the client, the client's family, and the health care provider to keep the client's drinking problem hidden and avoid the stigma associated with alcoholism.

Assessment for drug and alcohol abuse in elderly clients, especially socially isolated elders who have suffered recent life losses, should be approached with a high index of suspicion. Elderly alcoholics usually drink daily but in lower quantities than other age groups. Special problems may arise in older drinkers because of the:

- Decreased metabolic efficiency in older people
- Interaction of alcohol with medication
- Presence of chronic illness
- Sensory losses that occur with aging

 All elderly clients must be educated about the danger of mixing and altering medications. Nurses must approach elderly clients nonjudgmentally to educate them and their families about the risks of mixing medications and alcohol. Preventing reactive drinking may be accomplished by providing social support and preventive mental health services for elderly people who, by suffering one or more life losses, are at risk for social isolation and depression. For more information on substance use disorders see Chapter 11.

Disorders of Arousal and Sleep

The quantity and quality of sleep change with aging. In a comprehensive review of research on sleep and aging, the elderly demonstrated more frequent awakening during the night than younger adults, increased total time awake, and longer time spent in bed before finally falling asleep (Miles and Dement 1980). Changes in sleep patterns are believed to be related to changes in internal body rhythm (circadian asynchrony), emotional stress, physical illness, and drugs (Colling 1983). Over one-third of people over 60 complain of sleep disturbances (Woodruff 1985). The elderly have been found to nap more during the day and to use a disproportionately high amount of over-the-counter and prescription sleeping aids.

Problems with Use of Sleep Medication The chronic use of sedatives and hypnotics by elderly people has *not* been shown to improve the quality of sleep and can lead to many undesirable and dangerous side effects. The elderly excrete these drugs more slowly than the young and thus are prone to develop toxic effects, including delirium, daytime drowsiness, and loss of equilibrium. Respiration can be significantly disturbed with the use of sleeping medication, which may lead to a physiologically adaptive response of frequent arousal to stimulate respiration (Wynne et al. 1978).

Guides to Improve Sleep The following guidelines can be used to improve sleep in the elderly (Busse and Blazer 1980):

- Increased physical activity, particularly in the late afternoon and early evening hours, has beneficial effects.
- A cool room is usually more conducive to sleep than an overly warm room.
- A light bedtime snack containing calcium combined with sugar may help induce sleep.
- Stress reduction and progressive relaxation can be taught to older persons to help them relax.
- Elderly people should be encouraged to arise at the same time every day rather than try to catch up on lost sleep by "sleeping in" late in the morning.
- Elderly people should avoid napping during the day.
- The sleep "milieu" is very important in promoting sleep. Bed linen should be clean and made up each day.
- The elderly should spend as little time as possible in the bedroom during the day, thus associating the bedroom with sleep.

The Chronically Mentally Ill Elderly

A population of growing concern to clinicians, policy makers, and researchers is the **chronically mentally ill elderly** (CMIE). This subgroup, composed of elders with chronic schizophrenia and other chronic mental disorders such as bipolar disorder, has received little attention in the literature until only recently (Buckwalter and Light 1989, Strome 1989). Nursing homes have become the main institutional setting for these individuals, with an estimated 500,000 elderly persons with a chronic mental illness in nursing homes as of 1977 (Goldman, Feder, and Scanlon 1986). This number is predicted to increase as the population ages, posing unique challenges to nurses caring for these clients.

The CMIE have special needs and problems, including physical problems, personal and social limitations, compromised levels of neuropsychologic functioning, and underidentified concomitant physical illnesses. Strome (1989) notes that elderly persons with schizophrenia are a heterogeneous group ranging from individuals who present with symptoms either absent or well controlled to the floridly psychotic individuals who are refractory to treatment. The CMIE are the first aggregate of mentally ill to present with a long history of treatment with neuroleptics and consequently they are at risk for tardive dyskinesia and related involuntary movements of the face, mouth, and extremities; chronic constipation secondary to high anticholinergic side effects of the early low-potency neuroleptics; and the possibility of other heretofore unidentified problems related to long-term use of neuroleptics. The CMIE schizophrenic client may not cooperate in treatment; may present with self-harm impulses; and may not communicate heath care needs and symptoms to caregivers, thereby posing special management needs and concerns to nursing home staff. The CMIE client is at risk for all the chronic and acute illnesses of later life with the added disadvantages posed by mental illnesses and long-term effects of drug use. Additionally, most nursing homes are ill equipped to provide for the special needs of psychiatric clients. They may not have access to psychiatric and mental health nursing consultation. For more information on the chronically mentally ill elderly, see Chapter 17.

The Nursing Process and the Elderly

Assessing

The Nursing Assessment Interview The variety of theories on aging and the complex interface between physical, emotional, and environmental factors point to the importance of an individualized, multifactorial approach to assessment. The assessment information must be comprehensive and multidimensional. If available, a multidisciplinary team approach is usually most effective in securing comprehensiveness and providing validation of assessment impressions, leading to accurate diagnoses and effective intervention strategies.

The interview is the initial step in the assessment process and the most important procedure in differentiating between psychiatric disorders in the elderly. Interviewing requires skill and heightened sensitivity and typically takes more time with the elderly than with other age groups. The interviewer should attempt to make the interview pleasant for the elderly client, conveying a sense of respect and caring. The interviewer should be close to the client, use touch when appropriate to relieve anxiety, and be clear in stating the purpose of the interview and length of time it will take. A skilled diagnostician attends to verbal, nonverbal, and environmental cues, as well as the cognitive and behavioral aspects of the client. It may become necessary to repeat the purpose and time frame of the interview, since the elderly may forget during the interview.

Sensory loss, confusion, communication disorders, cultural influences, shame, and fear of stigmatization may inhibit expression of feelings by elderly persons. Older people may be unaware of changes in their behavior or expect negative changes as a "normal" part of aging. It is important to solicit interpretations

from family and staff members to help fill in aspects of the clinical picture and validate the information the client has provided.

The assessment information should include objective and subjective data regarding the client's physiologic status, psychologic status, cognitive status, and social and financial status. There are a variety of self-report screening tools designed for use specifically with the elderly. These require minimal special training to administer and help the nurse obtain subjective assessment information. These tools may also be used as objective evaluation instruments to measure the effectiveness of interventions. The **Iowa Self-Assessment Inventory** (Morris and Buckwalter 1988) is useful for obtaining a subjective functional assessment from elderly clients in a variety of settings. The **Geriatric Depression Scale** (Yesavage et al. 1982–1983) and the **Short Portable Mental Status Exam** (Pfeiffer 1975) are other examples of useful tools helpful in gaining information about depressive symptoms and mental status, respectively.

The following section provides guidelines for gaining subjective and objective assessment information about the client's physiologic, cognitive, emotional and psychosocial status.

Biologic Assessment Before a definitive psychiatric diagnosis can be made, all medically based illnesses that may present with psychiatric symptoms (e.g., depression, confusion, restlessness, and anxiety) must be ruled out. Additionally, a complete medical and neurologic workup is necessary to differentiate irreversible, untreatable dementing illnesses from reversible, treatable conditions (pseudodementia). It should be noted that nearly 50 percent of elderly emergency room admissions for "psychiatric" problems prove to have an underlying medical (organic) etiology, such as infection. In outpatient elderly populations, about 20 to 40 percent of clients with psychiatric symptoms have medical problems that cause or contribute to their disturbed mental state (Pies 1987). Therefore, all medical and nursing personnel must maintain a high index of suspicion whenever an elderly client presents with apparent psychiatric symptoms. A complete medical workup with subsequent ongoing medical supervision is essential for the elderly individual presenting with psychiatric symptomology.

Objective assessment information includes lab results, a complete history and physical including weight, vital signs, and a description of the physical appearance of the client. Standard diagnostic laboratory analysis should include complete blood chemistry, electrolytes, glucose, CBC, urinalysis, thyroid studies, BUN, creatinine, and liver function tests. The dexamethasone suppression test (DST) may be useful in identifying major depression in clients with early and/or mild-to-moderate dementia (Haggerty et al.

1988). Other procedures important for ruling out infectious processes, space-occupying lesions, drug toxicities, and cancers include chest radiography, drug toxicology screening, CT scanning, PET scanning, EKG, EEG, and lumbar puncture. In cases where normal-pressure hydrocephalus is suspected, a cysternogram is diagnostic. Dementia workup should include serologic tests for syphilis, folate, B_{12} levels, and trace minerals.

Subjective information includes clients' perceptions of their physical health and a description of their chronic illnesses, symptoms, and self-care activities.

Cognitive Status   A thorough mental status examination is essential. The *objective information* includes the *presence* and *extent* of cognitive impairment. The interviewer should include the family and caregivers to gain a description of the course of the mental changes. Did the changes happen gradually (e.g., SDAT, drug toxicity, metabolic imbalances), suddenly (e.g., depression, CVA, drug toxicity), or in a graduated, stepwise fashion (e.g., multiinfarct dementia)? Pfeiffer's (1975) Short Portable Mental Status Questionnaire (SPMSQ) is a simple, reliable, and valid ten-item cognitive performance evaluation tool (see Figure 35–1 on page 888). It was designed for use with the elderly and can be used by most nurses to assess and monitor cognitive changes in an elderly client. It is important to remember that the elderly are sensitive to fatigue, boredom, medication, and environmental influences, which can affect their mental status. The SPMSQ cannot distinguish delirium from dementia, however. Keep in mind that assessment tools designed for use with other age groups may not be accurate or complete for use with older persons.

Subjective information regarding cognitive status includes clients' own perceptions of their mental status. Questions to ask include: "How has your thinking been lately?" "Is your memory as good as it used to be?" "Have you been able to keep track of your medicines (days of the week, meals, time)?"

Psychologic/Emotional Status   *Objective data* regarding the client's psychologic and emotional status include the interviewer's impressions taken from both content and process aspects of the interview. This information overlaps significantly with the mental status exam information. Several aspects of this assessment require synthesis and inferences made from the history and subjective information provided by the client. Therefore, this assessment cannot be made with the same objectivity as an examination of the client's skin for example. The assessment summary should include descriptions, not labels. Overutilization of psychiatric terminology does not give an adequate picture of the client or the illness. Give examples of the client's behavior and, when appropriate, direct quota-

tions to substantiate inferences and to present a vivid picture.

The interviewer should describe the following:

• The client's overall mood, affect, and response to the interviewer

• Impressions from observing the client's interactions with family and others

• Coping skills and defenses used by the client

• Educational level, insight into illness, and pertinent cultural factors

• Components such as psychomotor activity, somatization, anxiety, judgment, substance abuse (past and present), obsessive-compulsive symptoms, irrational guilt, aggressive behavior, and impairment in concentration

• Speech, production and continuity of thought, emotional regulation, impulse control, suicidal ideation, and frustration tolerance

Be sure to include significant negative findings, such as absence of delusional thought processes, absence of suicidal ideation, and absence of hallucinations. The assessment should include not only pathology and problems but also health, adaptive strengths, and personal assets (ego strengths).

Strengths and Coping Strategies   Aging is a continuous process, punctuated by positive and negative stress-producing life events. The elderly are individuals who have learned to cope with stress. Information regarding an elder's coping strategies and strengths is as important as their psychologic symptoms. Bringing up the subject of adaptive strengths, you might begin by asking, "You have certainly lived a long, full life. Would you be willing to share some of your survival secrets with me?" Sample questions to gather information regarding the psychologic strengths of the elderly client are listed in the Assessment box on page 889.

Having gained an understanding of an elderly client's strengths and coping strategies (e.g., spiritual expression, listening to music, reading, reaching out to others), the nurse can foster these strengths and adaptive strategies by including them in the care plan and encouraging significant others and the client to mobilize them to deal with the situation at hand.

Sexuality   Sexuality is an important assessment area often overlooked by health care professionals. Sexual activity can and does continue into later life. Remember that sexuality does not refer only to sexual activity, it includes a broad multidimensional component of personhood and identity. Sexual expression includes body image, affection and love, flirtation, and social roles and interaction. Older people may abstain from sexual activity because they are denied the

Instructions: Ask questions 1–10 in this list and record all answers. Ask question 4A only if patient does not have a telephone. Record total number of errors based on ten questions.

+   -

____   1.   What is the date today?_____ (month/day/year)

____   2.   What day of the week is it?_____

____   3.   What is the name of this place?_____

____   4.   What is your telephone number?_____

____ 4A.   What is your street address?_____

____   5.   How old are you?_____

____   6.   When were you born?_____

____   7.   Who is the president of the U.S. now?_____

____   8.   Who was the president before him?_____

____   9.   What was your mother's maiden name?_____

____ 10.   Subtract 3 from 20 and keep subtracting 3 from each new number, all the way down.

_____

____   Total Errors
                        To be completed by interviewer

Patient Name:_____

        Sex: 1. Male   2. Female   Race: 1. White   2. Black   3. Other

Years of Education:_____

        1. Grade School   2. High School   3. Beyond High School

Interviewer's Name:_____

The total number of errors constitutes the score in the SPMSQ. The test is sensitive to educational attainment. For persons with 9–12 years of education, the following scoring applies:

        0-2 Errors: Intact intellectual functioning

        3-4 Errors: Mild intellectual impairment

        5-7 Errors: Moderate intellectual impairment

        8-10 Errors: Severe intellectual impairment

For persons with 8 or fewer years of education, one additional error is allowed for each scoring category. Persons with more than 12 years of education, one less error is allowed for each category.

FIGURE 35–1   Short Portable Mental Status Questionnaire (SPMSQ).   SOURCE: From Pfeiffer E: *The psychosocial evaluation of the elderly client, in Busse EW, Blazer DG (eds):* Handbook of Geriatric Psychiatry. *Van Nostrand Reinhold, 1980. Copyright © E. Pfeiffer, 1974.*

ASSESSMENT

Guidelines for Assessing Psychologic Strengths

What are some things you like about yourself?

What are some of the upsetting (stressful, difficult) times you can remember?

What did you do to comfort yourself when your (husband/wife) died?

How did you make it through the death of your son?

What kinds of things do you do to cheer yourself up?

What things make you happy? Content?

What do you do to nurture yourself?

What do you do to relax? To have fun?

What things do you think you can do to get you through these rough times?

How have the passing years affected your sexuality?

Do you enjoy sex as much as you used to?

Are you happily married?

What are you most concerned about right now?

How can I (we) help you through this difficult time?

not guarantee quality. Social support has important implications for recovery from psychologic disturbances. The more social support available, the better equipped an elderly person will be to overcome a stressful life event (Chaisson-Stewart 1985). Maintenance of an abundant, meaningful social network suggests strong interpersonal skills that can be mobilized to help negotiate late life stresses and losses. Formation of a new social network, when others have dissolved, is easier for an elderly person with the social skills and personal resources (e.g., assertiveness, friendliness, and warmth) to form new social bonds and friendships. Elderly people who have been unsuccessful or disinclined to develop strong ties and friendships may benefit from exploring the interpersonal factors that prevented them from reaching out to others in the past.

The elderly, who often survive on a low, fixed income, may be plagued by financial problems that affect their mental and physical health. Some communities have services that help the elderly manage finances and learn about financial aid and assistance programs. Removal of financial strain may dramatically improve the health of an elder pressured by inadequate funds and inexperience with financial management. Sample questions to gain information about the social and financial status of the client are listed in the accompanying Assessment box.

opportunity or they perceive negative social pressure and social norms regarding sexuality among persons their age. They may abstain out of fear of AIDS or other sexually communicable diseases. Broaching the subject of sexuality with an older person may be just the thing they need to allay fears and give them permission to explore an untapped source of pleasure they may have long since forgotten. Approach the topic in a tactful, caring, nonjudgmental manner. An elderly client who does not wish to discuss sexual issues most likely will make that clear, by stating it directly, not answering the question, or changing the subject. An older person who was socialized in a different, more conservative time may not feel comfortable discussing sex. However, bringing up the subject may give an elderly client the opportunity to explore his or her sexuality privately or with a significant other.

Social and Financial Status   The quality and quantity of social support (past and present) available to the elderly person must be assessed. Quantity does

ASSESSMENT

Guidelines for Assessing Social and Financial Status

How many phone calls do you get in a week?

How frequently do you receive visitors?

How frequently do you go visiting?

Are you happily married?

How would you describe your relationship with your (family, daughter, husband, wife, etc.)?

Who do you know well enough to go visiting at their home (room, if in nursing home)?

Do you have someone you can trust and confide in?

Do you find yourself feeling lonely?

Do you have someone who can drive you to the doctor or the hospital if you need it?

How is your financial situation? Do you worry about money?

Elder Abuse   It has been suggested that **elder abuse** is at least as serious, in terms of incidence, as child abuse (Hirst and Miller 1986). Elder abuse can take many forms, including active physical, emotional, or sexual maltreatment, as well as passive emotional neglect and omission on the part of the responsible person to provide for the normal physical and financial needs of the elder in their care. Hirst and Miller (1986) note that the elder at highest risk for abuse is often:

• Female

• Caucasian

• Physically and/or cognitively impaired

• Dependent

• Presenting behavior problems

The person at risk for abusing an elderly person is often:

• A family member (usually a daughter or son)

• Ill-equipped or reluctant to provide care

• Disorganized with marital problems

• An alcohol and/or drug abuser

• Lacking communications skills

• Lacking effective coping patterns

• Unrealistic in expectations of the older adult

The abused elderly may exhibit wariness of contact with adults, extreme withdrawal or aggressiveness in certain situations, infantile behavior, poor social interaction with peers, and ambivalent feelings toward family (Hirst and Miller 1986, p 30). Assessment of the elderly, particularly those seeking treatment in emergency rooms, must include observation for signs of abuse, including:

• Overmedication or deprivation of life-sustaining medications

• Falls and injuries, particularly bruises on face, arms, legs, and buttocks

• Malnutrition

• Extended periods of neglect or restraint evidenced by contracture pressure sores and long, curved fingernails and toenails

• Agitation when certain persons appear (family, friends, or caretakers)

The elderly rarely report abuse themselves out of fear of disbelief, reprisal, or institutionalization. The elderly often feel loyal to their abusers and may believe they deserve the maltreatment. Several tools have been developed to help with this essential portion of the assessment of the older adult (Ferguson and Beck

1983, Ross et al. 1985). Most states have mandatory reporting laws to protect the elderly from abuse. Nurses must be alert for signs of elder abuse and report any suspected cases in accordance with the legislation in their states. Through detection, education, clinical intervention, and research, nurses can reduce this serious threat to the health and quality of life of the elderly. See Chapter 22 for more information about Elder Abuse.

Informed Consent   The elderly are more often faced with health care decisions than are younger age groups. Sometimes **functional competency,** a term referring to clinical judgment regarding an individual's decision-making capacity (Stanley et al. 1988) is called into question. This poses special problems for caregivers faced with treatment decisions requiring informed consent. Whenever possible, elderly individuals and their significant others should be encouraged to plan ahead and formally assign a proxy decision maker (e.g., assignment of durable power of attorney and/or conservatorships). The laws vary from state to state. In cases where there is no legally assigned proxy decision maker for a cognitively impaired elder deemed unable to consent to medical procedures and treatment, the health care team together with the family must institute treatment according to the laws of the state.

Diagnosing

The following nursing diagnoses are integral to any nursing care plan for elderly clients with the following DSM-III-R Diagnoses. A brief discussion accompanies each of the diagnostic categories.

Major Depression
Low Self-esteem   Low self-esteem is a hallmark feature of depression. Not only do the elderly internalize social ageist biases, but they often are plagued with irrational guilt in the form of intrusive obsessional self-deprecating thoughts.

High Risk for Violence: Self-Directed   Feelings of hopelessness, low self-esteem, obsessive-compulsive symptoms, apathy, and powerlessness often contribute to suicidal ideation and gestures in the depressed elderly.

Activity Intolerance   Psychomotor agitation and/or psychomotor retardation are both symptoms of depression. Psychomotor agitation as seen in individuals with an agitated depression affects social interaction, self-care abilities, and the sleep-wake cycle. Psychomotor retardation is a commonly seen vegetative sign of depression in the elderly. These individuals also experience compromised self-care abilities, lack physical exercise, and are at risk of developing complications of decreased mobility.

Self-Care Deficit: Feeding   Many depressed elderly demonstrate dramatic weight losses, which in some cases indicate a passive suicide gesture. Less frequently, elderly individuals may experience a weight gain secondary to overeating and the decreased activity accompanying vegetative signs.

Altered Health Maintenance   The depressed elderly are at risk of developing physical health complications secondary to poor self-care and health maintenance habits.

Sleep Pattern Disturbance   More often than not, the elderly with depression experience sleep pattern disturbance, particularly early morning awakening. Occasionally, depressed elders report excessive sleeping.

Altered Thought Processes   Often the elderly present with cognitive changes, such as short-term memory loss, accompanying the depression. These changes are not often seen in younger age groups with depression. Concentration is often impaired, and lack of motivation hinders learning of new information.

Delirium

Sensory Perceptual Alterations   The hallmark feature of delirium is an acute change in level of consciousness. Often individuals with delirium present with hallucinations and delusions.

Impaired Social Interaction   Often, delirious elderly become combative or demonstrate bizarre behavior and gesturing.

Dementia

Impaired Verbal Communication   In later stages of SDAT, the elderly lose the ability to communicate verbally. In the case of multi-infarct dementia, the individual may become aphasic because of focal lesions.

Altered Role Performance   Social roles such as employee, professional, friend, spouse, and parent are lost to an individual whose cognitive functioning is impaired. These role losses create much grief in the individual as well as the significant others. As a result of these role alterations, financial and social support resources are often affected.

Self-Care Deficit   The progressive nature of SDAT causes the individual to lose the ability to perform activities of daily living. Eventually, the individual becomes totally dependent on others.

Impaired Social Interaction   Bizarre, compulsive, or disorganized social behaviors often characterize the middle and later stages of SDAT. Additionally, unpredictable behaviors of an explosive and potentially harmful nature known as "catastrophic reaction" often accompany SDAT.

Self-Care Deficit: Toileting   In the later stages of dementia, the client becomes incontinent of urine and stool.

Adjustment Disorder with Depressed Mood
See the Nursing Care Plan accompanying the Case Study, earlier.

Dysfunctional Grieving   The client becomes immobilized with the stress of the loss. Often depression ensues to the point that the only factor differentiating an adjustment disorder from major depression is the identified stressor that precipitated the loss.

Self-Care Deficits   Because of depression, individuals lose interest in and motivation to perform self-care activities. Grooming, hygiene, and activities of daily living are neglected. In extreme cases, the elder is at risk for developing other physical illnesses as a result of not taking medication and refusing to eat or engage in health care practices.

Altered Role Performance   The loss often leads to changes in social interaction and role performance, with potential for social withdrawal and loneliness and mental status changes due to lack of stimulation and validation.

Hopelessness   Hopelessness is a symptom of depression. The loss, coupled with the pervasive dysphoria, places the individual at risk of developing dependency and loss of function, as self-concept and motivation wane.

Anxiety Disorders

Ineffective Individual Coping   Often the anxiety symptoms impair an individual's ability to concentrate and think clearly, thus affecting judgment and often causing the client to decrease activities and avoid potentially stressful situations.

Activity Intolerance   Often the anxiety is accompanied by psychomotor agitation and restlessness.

Anxiety   Individuals with anxiety disorders experience fear, anxiety, and irritability to the point that they inhibit their usual pastimes and activities.

Delusional Disorders

Altered Thought Processes   Elderly individuals with delusional disorders often become paranoid and suspect others of trying to rob them, cheat them, or harm them in some way. They also often have delusional processes about their body or bodily functions. The delusional process often is accompanied by feelings of fear, paranoia, anger, and anxiety. Behavioral manifestations of these feelings may include suspiciousness, aggression, lashing out, social isolation, and unusual eating behaviors and "health" practices. Caregivers must sometimes go to great lengths to validate that the elder's claims are not reality based.

Impaired Social Interaction   Often the delusions are centered around family members and caregivers, making relationships strained if not impossible to maintain.

Planning and Implementing Interventions

There is a notable lack of studies comparing different nursing interventions used to treat mental disorders in later life. The few studies available concur that the elderly are more amenable to therapy than was previously believed. Several studies have demonstrated that a combination of psychotherapy and medication has been more efficacious in relieving depression in the elderly than either intervention alone. The studies available also support the use of reminiscence and life review, cognitive-behavioral approaches, group work, and somatic therapies. The choice of treatment is determined by the specific needs of the client and the nature of mental and physical disorders presented (Dye 1986). Financing and availability also influence treatment decisions.

Reminiscence and Life Review   Reminiscence and life review are useful interventions for clients experiencing self-esteem disturbance, grief, hopelessness, powerlessness, altered role performance, and social isolation. Reminiscing normally occurs to some degree throughout the life span, but the activity acquires special significance for elderly individuals (Ebersole 1976, 1978). Robert Butler used the term *reminiscence* and has noted that it is a universal activity in the elderly, reinforced by personal and environmental factors (e.g., personality, isolation, retirement, and relocation) and precipitated by the imminence of death (Butler 1963). Reminiscence provides a chance for working through issues from the past. Reminiscing is necessary for ego integrity, providing a means by which the elderly maintain a sense of identity and self-esteem. Life review, which is a part of the reminiscing process, may involve a more structured goal-oriented examination of the past.

Unfulfilled expectations, lifelong maladaptive patterns of interacting and coping, the unresolved death of a significant other, lack of accomplishment, "sins," ineffectiveness, rigidity, and failures are examples of issues that may need to be reckoned with as death approaches (Butler 1963).

When an elder expresses despair over the past, comments like, "Oh, just don't think about it," or "Why don't you focus on the happy times," while said with good intentions, may abruptly halt the resolution process necessary for reintegration of a distressing past. Nurses are socialized to supply answers, provide comfort, and relieve suffering. Encouraging an elderly person to work through painful and distressing memories may seem antithetical to the nurse's ethics of care and nurturance. However, it may be necessary for an elderly client to experience psychic pain during the integration process. Skilled, sensitive nursing interac-tions can facilitate the reintegration process for an elder by establishing a trusting, caring relationship in which active listening (even to repetitive material) and nonjudgmental validation prevail. The nurse's interactive role is to help the client find answers while moving through the life review process (Love and Buckwalter 1991).

Reminiscing can and should be stimulated for elders, individually and in groups. Creative uses of food, music, pets, and special events can facilitate the process and make it fun. Materials such as photo albums, journals, and tape and video recorders provide a means for elders so inclined to establish a permanent record of their life review, creating a legacy for those who follow.

Social Support and Group Interventions   Social support and group interventions are useful when working with clients who experience **Altered family processes, Knowledge deficit, Ineffective individual coping, Anticipatory and dysfunctional grieving, Powerlessness, Social isolation,** and **Spiritual distress.**

Loss of affiliation with significant groups (e.g., family, professional and work group, bridge club) and social support can lead to identity dissolution, isolation, loneliness, and despair in the elderly. Yalom (1975) identified "curative factors" in group psychotherapy, five of which are particularly beneficial to elderly persons. See the accompanying Intervention box.

Group therapy is considered by many to be the treatment of choice for the elderly. It is efficient, because eight to ten persons can benefit at one time. Long-term care facilities are ideally suited for group work because the members are easily accessible and transportation is not a problem.

Special Focuses of Group Work with Elders   A geriatric group may be designed for a variety of purposes. Severely depressed and cognitively impaired elders benefit from remotivation, resocialization, and reality orientation. Table 35–2 on page 894 provides a summary of the differences between groups with these different focuses. "Mixing affects" may be beneficial in stimulating withdrawn clients and calming anxious members. A cohort or specific age group focusing on reminiscing and life review may facilitate these processes for members reluctant to engage in reminiscing on a one-on-one basis. Movement, music, art, and role playing may bring forth creativity and expression of feelings (catharsis). The curative factors of "universality" and "instillation of hope" are beneficial for members of a "grievers" or widows group, in which the members can share their loss experiences.

Group work, when applied with sensitivity, caring, planning, organization, skill, and self-investment, can be fun and rewarding. Anecdotal evidence and an

INTERVENTION

Curative Factors in Group Interventions with the Elderly

Socialization	Provides replacement of meaningful relationships and stimulation of social skills. Allows for celebration of holidays and social events, reality orientation and reminiscing among cohorts. Provides opportunities to resume former roles (e.g., chairman, secretary, president).
Group cohesiveness	Refers to the "stick togetherness" characterized by group membership. Provides a sense of belonging (e.g., an old-old cohort group may begin to view themselves as the "biological elite" within a facility). Reaffirms ability to be liked and make friends. Provides for expression of affection and physical contact, esteem, and validation.
Universality	Provides a sense of, "We're all in this together." Enables members to see themselves in others and to share experiences, successes, and losses.
Instillation of hope	Compliments universality. Enables members to see others have suffered and survived similar situations. Members can share adaptive strengths and coping skills.
Altruism	Very important. Members are provided opportunities to feel needed and help others. Reinforces self-esteem. Often the support and advice received from peers is integrated more readily than "professional advice."

SOURCE: *Love CC, Buckwalter KC: Reactive depression, in* Nursing Diagnosis and Interventions for the Institutionalized Elderly. *Addison-Wesley, 1991.*

increasing body of research supports the effectiveness of this intervention with the elderly. Nurses are in key positions to explore this cost-effective, therapeutic intervention through ongoing research efforts.

Milieu Therapy   Milieu therapy, a broad, all-encompassing intervention, may be adapted to meet the needs of most of the nursing diagnostic categories. In particular, milieu therapy is appropriate for clients experiencing **Diversional activity deficit, Self-care deficit, Sleep pattern disturbance, Self-concept disturbance, High risk for violence, Altered thought processes, Powerlessness, and Impaired physical mobility.**

Behavioral principles and group process theory form the major theoretic foundation for constructing a therapeutic milieu. No other psychotherapeutic intervention has such strong implications for nursing in acute and long-term care facilities as the scientific structuring of the environment to promote health, foster individual strengths, and effect personal growth in clients and staff. Milieu therapy has preventive as well as therapeutic value and must be a major consideration in all settings providing services to elderly populations.

A geriatric milieu must be dynamic and evolving to meet the needs of each unique elder within a diverse and changeable client-staff community. Staff-related factors (e.g., nurse-client ratio, interpersonal variables, attitudes and interactions, staffing patterns and composition, and level of skill) have a profound influence on the prevailing atmosphere and therefore must be included in the milieu assessment and structuring. The Intervention box on page 895 provides a useful framework for organizing the complex concept of milieu into a workable format with some examples illustrating how to categorize interventions in the environment. Once categorized, the "milieu committee" (composed of staff and residents if at all possible) can determine which interventions should be manipulated or altered to promote health, foster growth, and prevent deterioration. The concepts of structure, containment, support, and validation may also be applied to home-based elders to ensure that their environment contains essential health promotion and preventive features.

Cognitive-Behavioral Therapy Cognitive-behavioral approaches to treatment are useful for the elderly experiencing **Ineffective individual coping, Fear, Powerlessness,** and **Self-concept disturbance.**

Vague, abstract, and "mysterious" approaches to therapy are not tolerated well by elderly persons. The elderly seek a therapeutic relationship that provides some reciprocity. Nurses caring for the elderly must

TABLE 35–2   **Differences between Remotivation, Resocialization, and Reality Orientation**

Reality Orientation	Resocialization	Remotivation
1. Correct position or relation with the existing situation in a community. Maximum use of assets	1. Continuation of reality living situation in a community	1. Orientation to reality for community living; present oriented
2. Called reality orientation and classroom reality orientation program	2. Called discussion group or resocialization to differentiate between a social function and a therapeutic need	2. Called remotivation
3. Structured	3. Unstructured	3. Definite structure
4. Refreshments and/or food may be served for identification	4. Refreshments served	4. Refreshments not served
5. Appreciation of the work of the world. Constant reminders of who and where clients are, why they are present, and what is expected of them	5. Appreciation of the work of the world. Reliving happy experiences. Encourages participation in home activities relating to subject	5. Appreciation of the work of the group stimulates the desire to return to function in society
6. Class range from 3 to 5, depending on degree/level of confusion or disorientation from any cause	6. Group range from 5 to 17, depending on mental and physical capabilities	6. Group size: 5 to 12
7. Meeting ½ hour daily at same time in same place	7. Meetings three times weekly for ½ to 1 hour	7. Meeting once or twice weekly for 1 hour
8. Planned procedure: reality-centered objects	8. No planned topic; group-centered feelings	8. Preselected and reality-centered objects
9. Response of resident is responsibility of teacher	9. Clarification and interpretation is responsibility of leader	9. No exploration of feelings
10. Periodic reality orientation test pertaining to residents' level of confusion or disorientation	10. Periodic progress notes pertaining to residents' enjoyment and improvements	10. Progress ratings
11. Emphasis on time, place, person orientation	11. Any topic freely discussed	11. Topic: no discussion of religion, politics, or death
12. Use of portion of mind function still intact	12. Vast stockpile of memories and experiences	12. Untouched area of the mind
13. Resident greeted by name, thanked for coming, and extended handshake and/or physical contact according to attitude in group	13. Resident greeted on arrival, thanked, and extended a handshake on leaving	13. No physical contact permitted. Acceptance and acknowledgment of everyone's contribution
14. Conducted by trained aides and activity assistants	14. Conducted by RN, LPN/LVN, aides and program assistants	14. Conducted by trained psychiatric aids

SOURCE: Adapted by permission of The Gerontologist/The Journal of Gerontology, from Barns E, Sack A, Shore H: The Gerontologist 1973;13:513.

invest themselves through active involvement and judicious self-disclosure to foster trust and a warm, caring relationship.

A combination of cognitive and behavioral approaches has been found to work best with the elderly. These approaches are "practical" and very specific, providing concrete goals (e.g., behavior change or correction of negative thought patterns) and ongoing evaluation of progress through self-monitoring of goal accomplishment.

Cognitive-behavioral therapy is based on the notion that the way we think about something influences the way we behave and feel. Negative patterns of thinking tend to be automatic and pervasive, coloring individuals' perceptions of the world around them and affecting their mood and self-esteem. Cognitive-behavioral therapy, used often and successfully with depressed older people, suggests that the depressed elder's unrealistic negative thought processes are central to becoming and staying depressed (Belsky 1984).

The box on page 896 lists common cognitive distortions and provides examples of alternatives the nurse might present to challenge the distorted thought processes of elderly clients.

Because cognitive-behavioral therapy focuses on symptoms and thought processes (rather than a hypothetical unconscious cause) and fosters a sense of self-responsibility and self-control, the elderly are often receptive and willing to try it. Furthermore, in cognitive-behavioral therapy, the elderly are not required to reveal their private thoughts to the clinician. Instead they focus on their problems and symptoms and receive advice from the clinician on how to make improvements. The advice gives the elderly a sense that they are getting something for their personal and financial investment. The self-monitoring of progress (often with a journal and/or homework assignments) provides inspiration for the elderly to proceed. For further information on cognitive-behavioral therapy see Yost et al. (1986).

(Guy, 1976) to assess for involuntary movements associated with tardive dyskinesia helps clinicians assess the presence of these psychotropic medication side effects. With proper staff development nursing staff may be trained to use this tool in a variety of settings.

It is generally recommended that the elderly client be started on dosages 30 to 50 percent of the recommended starting dosage for younger clients of similar size. The medication should be titrated until the desired therapeutic effect is established.

Ideally psychotropic drug therapy should be supervised by a geropsychiatrist. General medical practitioners unfamiliar with psychopharmacokinetics in the elderly often unknowingly overmedicate older clients. Among the elderly, psychotropic drugs are often prescribed inappropriately and the best drug within each class is often not selected (*Psychiatry Drug Alerts* 1989). A random sample of 1201 rest home residents found that 55 percent were taking at least one psychoactive medication and 11 percent were taking medications from two or more drug classes (Avorn 1989). Another study of 837 elderly in a rest home for deinstitutionalized psychiatric clients found that 82 percent were taking at least one antypsychotic drug and 15 percent were taking two neuroleptics. Half of the records of these residents included no notes by physicians on any mental health issue. Although 23 percent of the subjects taking neuroleptics showed signs of tardive movements, tardive dyskinesia was rarely mentioned. Nearly half of the staff in this rest home were unaware of the typical signs of tardive dyskinesia; they were unfamiliar with the parkinsonian effects and EPS seen with use of haloperidol; and they were unfamiliar with the categories (e.g., antidepressant, neuroleptic, sedative) into which six commonly prescribed psychoactive drugs (e.g., amitriptyline, chlorpromazine, diazepam) should be placed (*Psychiatry Drug Alerts* 1989).

Medication should never take the place of psychotherapeutic modalities. Psychotherapy should always be continued along with medications. For more information on psychopharmacologic interventions, see Dye (1986), Carnevali and Patrick (1986), and Chapter 32 of this text.

Electroconvulsant Therapy   The two- to three-week lag time between onset of antidepressant drug therapy and symptom relief is significant for severely depressed elders whose health is in danger. When suicide or starvation is a real threat, or when antidepressants are ineffective or contraindicated, electroconvulsant therapy (ECT) should be considered. The main criteria for selecting ECT as the treatment of choice in the elderly are severity of depression and need for immediate results (Zung 1980).

ECT is rapidly effective and safe with judicious screening and advances in the use of muscle relaxants and anesthesia. The unilateral method has been shown to decrease the confusion and recent memory loss associated with ECT. Essentially, ECT may serve as a lifesaving measure in the elderly. Ignorance and negative emotions associated with early, less sophisticated use of ECT should not enter into decisions regarding the appropriateness of this intervention with the severely depressed elderly.

Evaluating

As with assessment and diagnosis, evaluation in psychosocial nursing is based primarily on the client's appearance, behavior, and self-report. Realistic expectations and stated objectives should guide the evaluation process. Key parameters of evaluation include mood, affect and mental status. Whenever possible, involve the elderly in the evaluation process.

Mood and Affect   Subjective evidence of improvement in mood include clients stating they feel better, with increased sources of pleasure in daily activities and relationships. Objective signs of improved mood include expressive affect with more smiling and laughing appropriately. The range of affect is fuller and accompanied by less self-deprecating reference. Scores on depression and anxiety inventories show marked improvement over initial assessment scores and a decrease in somatization and obsessive signs.

Altered Thought Processes   Subjective indications of improvement include client reports that they are thinking more clearly and are better able to concentrate and remember recent and remote events. Individuals who presented with delusional processes and other signs of psychosis will note they feel more like themselves and will be able to make more accurate, reality-based interpretations. In clients with symptoms of mania, the euphoria, grandiosity, and expansiveness of mood will resolve into a more contained reality-based affect.

Objective indications of improved mental status and cognition include orientation to person, place, and time; improved mental status exam scores; and appropriate dress, behavior, and interpersonal interactions. Tests of judgment, abstract thinking, and recent and remote memory improve over initial presentation. Communication will improve and thought processes and content of speech will return to premorbid abilities. Clients will demonstrate tighter associations, improved ability to concentrate and to take in, process, and retain new information. It should be noted that improvement in thought process alteration is not a realistic goal for clients with an irreversible dementing illness.

Hopelessness   Expression of hope and self-acceptance, renewed involvement and motivation in activities, and planning for the future indicate improvement and replace dependency, apathy, and negative self-talk.

Self-Care Deficit   Clients will resume their premorbid level of self-care and health maintenance behaviors.

Activity/Rest Disturbances: Altered Psychomotor Activity   Vegetative signs will be replaced with more appropriately paced activities, movement, gait, speech, appetite, and sleep-wake cycle. Anxiety and fear will be replaced with subjective feeling of calmness, restfulness, and well-being.

Altered Nutrition: Less Than Body Requirements   Clients will report their appetites are returning to premorbid level, with increased pleasure associated with eating. Weight will return to normal range.

Risk for Violence: Self-Directed   Clients will report that suicidal ideation has markedly decreased if not resolved, and there will be less morbid preoccupation with death and dying.

CHAPTER HIGHLIGHTS

• The aging population is increasing at a faster rate than the general population.

• Most elderly people remain relatively healthy, active, and vital well into later life.

• The elderly are the most underserved population in need of mental health services due to ageist biases, stigmatization, myths regarding normal aging, and inaccessibility of care.

• Mental health in later life is linked closely to intrapersonal, environmental, and interpersonal interactive processes.

• Depression is the most prevalent, most treatable mental disorder in later life.

• Somatization, or excessive preoccupation with bodily functions, may be a sign of depression in an older adult.

• The chronically mentally ill elderly are the first clients to present with a history of long-term neuroleptic medication use.

• The suicide rate for elderly persons is nearly three times the rate of the general population.

• Electroconvulsant therapy may be a lifesaving intervention for severely depressed, suicidal older adults.

• Comprehensive, accurate, ongoing assessment is essential for differentiating treatable mental disorders from irreversible states.

• The elderly metabolize and excrete medication less efficiently, and are at risk for drug toxicity, which can mimic different mental disorders.

• Medication is not a substitute for psychotherapy. Medication should be prescribed primarily to enhance the effectiveness of psychotherapeutic interventions by reducing disabling symptoms.

• When the elderly are given psychotropic medication, they require only one-half to one-third the amount prescribed for younger adults of comparable weight, in doses divided over the course of the day.

• Family members caring for a dependent older adult need much emotional support and psychoeducative interventions.

• The elderly respond best to therapy that is goal oriented and practical and has built-in short-term goals that enable them to monitor their accomplishments and progress over time.

• For the older adult, social support and group affiliation is an important means for maintaining orientation, self-esteem, and a sense of identity and belonging.

• Reminiscing can be a significant therapeutic tool for enhancing self-esteem and maintaining a sense of identity in the older adult.

REFERENCES

American Psychiatric Association: *Diagnostic and Statistical Manual of Mental Disorders*, ed 3, revised. APA, 1987.

Avorn J: Use of psychoactive medication and the quality of care in rest homes: Findings and policy implications of a statewide study. *New Engl J Med* 1989;320:227–232.

Belsky JK: *The Psychology of Aging: Theory, Research and Practice*. Brooks/Cole, 1984.

Blazer DG: The epidemiology of mental illness in late life, in Busse EW, Blazer DG (eds): *Handbook of Geriatric Psychiatry*. Van Nostrand Reinhold, 1980.

Blazer DG, Pennybacker MR: Epidemiology of alcoholism in the elderly, in Hartford JT, Samorajski T (eds): *Alcoholism in the Elderly*. Raven Press, 1984.

Braudis EM: Later adulthood, in Edelman C, Mandle CL (eds): *Health Promotion Throughout the Life Span*. Mosby, 1986.

Buckwalter KC, Light E: New directions for psychiatric mental health nurses: The chronically mentally ill elderly. *Arch Psychiatr Nurs* 1989;3(1):53–54.

Busse EW, Blazer DG: Disorders related to biological functioning, in Busse EW, Blazer DG (eds): *Handbook of Geriatric Psychiatry*. Van Nostrand Reinhold, 1980.

Butler RN: The life review: An interpretation of reminiscence in the aged. *Psychiatry* 1963;26:65–76.

Butler RN: Meeting the challenges of health care for the elderly. *J Gerontol Nurs* 1980;8(February):87–96.

Carnevali D, Patrick M: *Nursing Management for the Elderly*, ed 2. Lippincott, 1986.

Chaisson-Stewart MG: *Depression in the Elderly: An Interdisciplinary Approach*. Wiley, 1985.

Cole M, Dastoor D: A new hierarchic approach to the measurement of dementia. *PSO* 1987;28(6):298–304.

Colling J: Sleep disturbances in aging: A theoretic and empiric analysis. *Adv Nurs Science*, October 1983, vol 6 1, pp 36–44.

Dye CA: *Assessment and Intervention in Geropsychiatric Nursing*. Grune and Stratton, 1986.

Ebersole PE: The therapeutic value of reminiscing with the aged. *Am J Nurs* 1976;76(August):601–602.

Ebersole PE: Establishing reminiscing groups, in Burnside IM (ed): *Working with the Elderly: Group Process and Techniques*. Duxbury, 1978.

Ebersole PE: Gerontological nurse practitioners; Past, present and future. *Geriatr Nurs* 1985;6:219–221.

Ebersole PE, Hess PA: *Toward Healthy Aging: Human Needs and Nursing Response*, ed 2. Mosby, 1985.

Erikson E: *Childhood and Society*, ed 2. W. W. Norton, 1963.

Ferguson D, Beck D: H.A.L.F.: A tool to assess elder abuse within the family. *Gerontol Nurs* 1983;4(5):301–304.

Goldman HH, Feder J, Scanlon W: Chronic mental patients in nursing homes: Reexamining data from the national nursing home survey. *Hosp Community Psychiatry* 1986;32(1):21–27.

Guy W. ECDEY Assessment Manual for Psychopharmacology, U.S. Government Printing Office, Washington, D.C., 1976.

Glassock JA: Older alcoholics: An underserved population. *Generations* 1982;192(Spring):23–24,64.

Gunderson JG: *Principles and Practice of Milieu Therapy 1983*. Aronson, 1983.

Haggerty JJ, Golden RN, Evens DL, Janowsky DS: Differential diagnosis of pseudodementia in the elderly. *Geriatrics* 1988;43(3):61–74.

Hirst SP, Miller J: The abused elderly. *J Psychosoc Nurs* 1986;24(October):28–34.

Illowsky BP, Kirch, DG: Polydipsia and hyponatremia in psychiatric patients. *Am J Psychiatry* 1989;145:6.

Institute of Medicine: *Nursing and Nursing Education: Public Policies and Private Actions:* National Academy Press, 1983.

Joel LA, Baldwin B, Stevens G: Report from the American Nurses' Association Council on Psychiatric Mental Health Nursing. *Gerontol Geriatr Ed* 1989:9 (3):17–25.

Love CC, Buckwalter KC: Reactive depression, in Mass M, Buckwalter KC (eds): *Nursing Diagnosis and Interventions for the Institutionalized Elderly*. Addison-Wesley, 1991.

Mace NL, Rabins PV: *The 36 Hour Day*. Johns Hopkins University Press, 1981.

McKay M, Davis M, Fanning P: Are you listening to yourself? Increase your self awareness for more control over your life. *Nurs Life*, Jan/Feb 1983, pp 57–63.

Miller F et al.: Formed visual hallucinations in an elderly patient. *Hosp Community Psychiatry* 1987;38(5): 527–529.

Miles LE, Dement WC: Sleep and aging. *Sleep* 1980;3: 119–220.

Morris WW, Buckwalter KC: Functional assessment of the elderly: The Iowa Self-Assessment Inventory, in Waltz CF, Strictland OL (eds): *Measurement of Nursing Outcomes*, vol. 1. *Measuring Client Outcomes*. Springer, 1988.

Mortimer JA, Schuman LM, French LR: Epidemiology of dementing illness, in Mortimer JA, Schuman LM (eds): *The Epidemiology of Dementia*. Oxford University Press, 1981.

Osgood NJ: *Suicide in the elderly*. Aspen Publications, 1985.

Pavkov J: Suicide in the elderly. *Ohio's Health* 1982; 34(1):21–28.

Pfeiffer E: A Short Portable Mental Status Questionnaire for the assessment of organic brain deficit in elderly patients. *J Am Geriatr Soc* 1975;23:443–441.

Pfeiffer E: The psychosocial evaluation of the elderly patient, in Busse EW, Blazer D (eds): *Handbook of Geriatric Psychiatry*. Van Nostrand Reinhold, 1980.

Pies, R: Psychiatric presentations of medical illnesses in the elderly. *Geriatr Med Today* 1987;(6)8:39–59.

Poggi RG, Berland DI: The therapist's reactions to the elderly. *Gerontologist* 1985;25(5):508–513.

Powell LS, Courtice K: *Alzheimer's Disease: A Guide for Families*. Addison-Wesley, 1983.

Psychiatry Drug Alerts January 1989;3(1):entire issue.

Psychiatry Drug Alerts March 1989;3(3):entire issue.

Roca R: Bedside cognitive examination: Usefulness in detecting delirium and dementia. *PSO* 1987;28(2):71–76.

Ross M, Ross P, Ross-Carson M: Abuse of the elderly. *Can Nurs* 1985;81(2):36–39.

Stanley B, Stanley M, Guido J, Garvin L: The functional competency of elderly at risk. *Gerontologist* 1988; 28:53–58.

Stenback A: Depression and suicidal behavior in old age, in Birren JE, Sloane RB (eds): *Handbook of Mental Health and Aging*. Prentice-Hall, 1980.

Strome T: Schizophrenia in the elderly: What nurses need to know. *Arch Psychiatr Nurs* 1989;3(1):47–52.

Thomas DR: Assessment and management of agitation in the elderly. *Geriatrics* 1988;43(6):45–50, 53.

Turnbull JM, Turnbull SK: Management of specific anxiety disorders in the elderly. *Geriatrics* 1958;40(8):75–82.

Tyler KT, Tyler HR: Differentiating organic dementia. *Geriatrics* 1984;39(3):38–50.

Verwoerdt A: Anxiety, dissociative and personality disorders in the elderly, in Busse EW, Blazer DG (eds): *Handbook of Geriatric Psychiatry*. Van Nostrand Reinhold, 1980.

Wilson HS, Kneisl CR: *Handbook of Psychosocial Nursing Care*. Addison-Wesley, 1984.

Woodruff DS: Arousal, sleep and aging, in Birren JE, Schaie KW (eds): *Handbook of the Psychology of Aging*. Van Nostrand Reinhold, 1985.

Wynne J, Block AJ, Hunt LA: Disordered breathing and oxygen desaturation during day time naps. *Johns Hopkins Med J* 1978;143:3–7.

Yalom ID: *The Theory and Practice of Group Psychotherapy*, ed 2. Basic Books, 1975.

Yanchick VA: Drug therapy, in Dye CA (ed): *Assessment and Intervention in Geropsychiatric Nursing*. Grune and Stratton, 1986.

Yesavage JA, Brink TL, Lum O, Huang V, Adley MB, Leirer VO: Development and validation of a geriatric depression rating scale: A preliminary report. *J Psychiatr Res* 1982–1983;17:37.

Yost EB, Beutler LE, Corbishley MA, Allender JR: *Group Cognitive Therapy: A Treatment Approach for Depressed Older Adults*. Pergamon Press, 1986.

Zarit SH, Orr NK, Zarit JM: *The Hidden Victims of Alzheimer's Disease*. New York University Press, 1985.

Zung WWK: Affective disorders, in Busse EW, Blazer DG (eds): *Handbook of Geriatric Psychiatry*. Van Nostrand Reinhold, 1980.

PART SEVEN

The Social, Political, Cultural, and Economic Environments for Care

CONTENTS

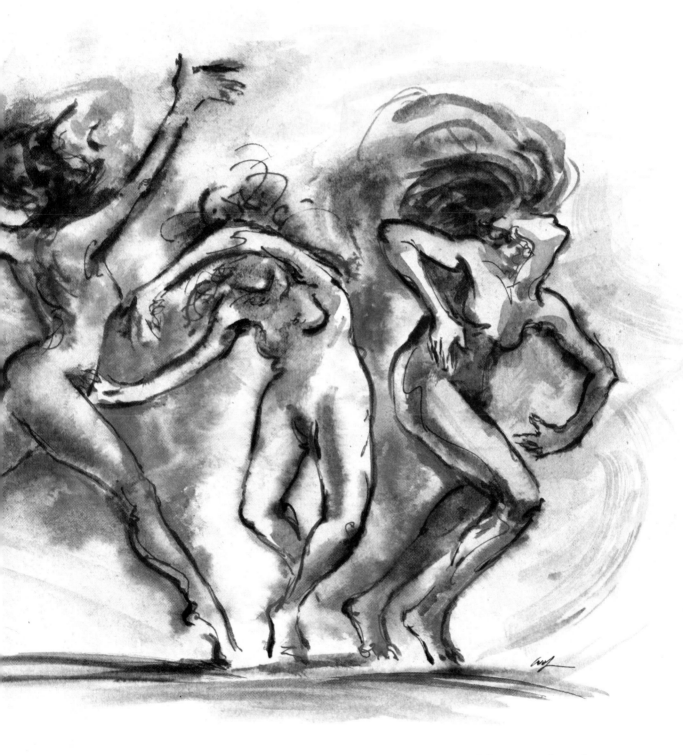

The harmonious movement of the group flows from the individual's sense of being and the group's spirit of common purpose.

Cultural Considerations

Sally A. Hutchinson

LEARNING OBJECTIVES

- State the relevance of cultural factors in psychiatric nursing practice

- Discuss cultural forces that influence mental health

- Explain the concepts of culture, holism, world view, ethnocentrism, and cultural relativism and their value for nursing practice

- Describe the process of obtaining a cultural profile

- Compare the three domains of heath care

- Identify the inherent dangers in cultural stereotyping

- Analyze the student's own cultural heritage and its effect on the nurse-client relationship

- Discuss some of the folk beliefs and healing practices of four minority groups

- Develop culturally aware strategies for implementing the nursing process

CROSS REFERENCES

Other topics relevant to this content are: Assessment, Chapter 9; Communication skills, Chapter 8; Ethics, Chapter 7; Nurse's values, Chapter 2; Psychiatric theories, Chapter 4.

Portions of the material in this chapter were contributed to the third edition by Carol Kneisl.

CULTURE PLAYS A MAJOR role in shaping how people think, behave, and feel. Culture determines how and by whom children are raised; how they are cuddled and fed; how they acquire rules of behavior; how they are punished; and how they learn about sex, gender roles, and marriage. Culture may affect personal psychology and shape character. Culture provides standards and values according to which we evaluate ourselves, our groups, and outsiders. Culture provides guidelines and rules for recognizing or diagnosing mental disorder and for its management and, sometimes, treatment (Foulkes 1980).

In a remote Eskimo village, a 34-year-old woman sits quietly, seemingly preoccupied with her own thoughts, in a trancelike state. Suddenly she leaps to her feet, throwing objects at the wall and heaping verbal abuse on her husband. His attempts to calm her do not work, and when he attempts to restrain her physically, she wrests herself from his grasp, tears off her clothing, and runs screaming out into the snow. Hearing her shrieks most of the adults of the village run after her across the snowfields. Although she initially outdistances them, she begins to tire, and the villagers finally catch up with her as she drops exhausted into the snow. They carry her back to her home where she falls into a deep sleep. When she awakens she recalls nothing of the episode. The people of the village are not surprised by her behavior. *Pibloqtok* can happen to anyone. No treatment is necessary; on awakening the next day the person behaves as usual.

On a busy downtown street walks a shy, introverted young Southeast Asian refugee, who has just been fired from his job as a restaurant dishwasher. The job was hard to come by in the first place, and now he and his family are faced with the discouraging prospect of trying to feed six people on the few dollars that remain from his last paycheck. At a crowded intersection the young man suddenly pulls a knife and begins to slash wildly at the startled people around him. He appears to be in a murderous rage and struggles with great strength, despite his small frame, against several people who are attempting to restrain and disarm him. A passing police cruiser picks him up and takes him to the police station. However, by this time he seems to be in a deep depression and fails to respond to their questions. The police take him to the community mental health center, where he is admitted to the in-patient unit and treated for depression. In Southeast Asia he would have been known as a victim of *amok,* the condition which gives us the phrase "run amok."

The behavior of the Eskimo woman and the Southeast Asian refugee has deep meaning for them and for others interacting with them. Both behaviors are examples of "culture-bound illnesses." Such illnesses vary from culture to culture and present as psychiatric problems to Western caregivers (Campinha-Bacote 1988).

In the Eskimo village, the hysterics of *pibloqtok* are a culturally sanctioned release in a society that stresses conformity and repression. In Western society, we might label the Eskimo woman as hysterical, sexually repressed, or acting out. In American psychiatric terminology, she might be said to be suffering from a dissociative disorder.

In the sixteenth century in Southeast Asia, *amok* referred to the behavior of brave fighters who chose to die in battle rather than lose. Those who ran amok fighting colonial oppression were honored and treated with respect. Although no longer socially acceptable, the cultural tradition remains, and maladjusted persons who have been humiliated still occasionally run amok, although episodes of amok are becoming less frequent. Outdated diagnostic practices in psychiatry might have led to a diagnosis of paranoid schizophrenia, or manic-depressive psychosis in the pre-DSM-III-R days.

In both of the examples above, the culture has an idea of what insanity *should* be and of the meaning of the behavior of its members. Culture shapes the very way we conceive of illness. Culture determines not only who is labeled mentally ill and under what circumstances, but also what treatment is given and who gives it. Therefore, a humanistic position in psychiatric nursing care must take account of culture and its influence on both client and nurse.

Relevance of Culture to Psychiatric Nursing Practice

This chapter pinpoints the relevance of culture to psychiatric nursing practice, discusses cultural complexity and diversity, biosocial factors and sociopolitical forces influencing mental health, folk beliefs and healing practices, the importance of cultural self-analysis for caregivers, and culturally aware strategies for nursing intervention blending insights from nursing, anthropology, sociology, and social psychology. It also explores the ways in which culture influences the perception, classification, process of labeling, explanation, symptoms, and treatment of what is called mental illness.

Historical Foundations

Psychiatric nursing has not traditionally focused on culture and its influence on psychiatric nursing practice. Various psychologic and psychoanalytic interpretations of client experience and behavior have predominated. The biochemical and physiologic aspects of mental illness have received increasing attention since the 1950s. But only within the last few years has culture been recognized as a relevant variable in nursing care. Note the following significant historical landmarks.

• 1940–1949: Experiences during and after World War II brought the reality of cultural differences home to military nurses. These nurses, hired by schools of nursing, brought cultural content to the curriculum.

• 1950–1959: Anthropologic and sociologic studies about nurses and nursing proliferated. Cornell University School of Nursing invited anthropologists and sociologists to lecture. Margaret Mead wrote an article for *Nursing Outlook* entitled "Understanding Cultural Patterns."

• 1960–1969: Nursing theorists focused on understanding how culture influences mental illness. Interest in indigenous (native) mental health workers (spurred on by the community mental health movement; see Chapter 38) and health care beliefs increased. This interest continues today, along with the desire to work toward giving culturally relevant care to different ethnic groups within our pluralistic society. Madeleine Leininger, a nurse anthropologist, developed and popularized the field of **transcultural nursing,** the study of different cultures, their health care belief systems, and their caring and curative practices. These understandings are used to provide culturally specific nursing care. During the sixties, several nurses obtained doctoral degrees in anthropology. In 1969, the Council of Nursing and Anthropology was established within the American Anthropological Association in an effort to bring together people with interests in both fields to study cultural practices relevant to nursing.

• 1970–1979: The Transcultural Nursing Society was established in 1974 and began presenting national transcultural nursing conferences in 1976. In 1977 the National League for Nursing (NLN) required cultural content in all nursing curricula. In 1978 the President's Commission on Mental Health expressed its belief in the value of traditional cultural health belief systems and indigenous healing practices. During that same year, the American Psychiatric Association created a Task Force on Cultural and Ethnic Issues in Psychiatry. The chief aims of the task force were to suggest culturally differentiated diagnostic and treatment techniques for various ethnic groups and to include cultural psychiatry in residency training programs for psychiatrists. In 1979 the NLN published a Position Statement on Nursing's Responsibilities to Minorities and Disadvantaged Groups. In this document the NLN advocated that nursing curricula include information on culture, that disadvantaged or minority group nursing students receive tutoring and assistance if needed, that hospitals hire nurses from different ethnic groups, and that research on nursing care of different ethnic groups be initiated.

• 1980: The American Nurses' Association established the Council on Intercultural Nursing to focus on minority issues in health care.

• 1989: The charter issue of the *Journal of Transcultural Nursing* was published.

Theoretic Foundations

To appreciate the relevance of culture to psychiatric nursing, we must understand several key concepts derived from anthropologic theory. These concepts offer a theoretic framework to guide nursing practice. Although they may appear simplistic and almost self-evident, in practice they are complex. They are much more clearly "felt" and understood when one works with or cares for a person from a different cultural group.

Holism

A distinguishing feature of anthropology and nursing, **holism** is the idea that every part of culture/behavior must be seen within the larger context. Only then can it make sense. From an anthropologic perspective a holistic view encompasses environment, material culture, world view, social structure, and symbolic systems and the interchanges among them. To isolate one component or subsystem is to ignore cultural complexity. We must transcend the individual parts in an effort to see the whole. In practice, nurses are considered to have a holistic approach if they view the client as participating in a specific environment, with its own material culture, ways of communicating, and beliefs about the world. Such nurses recognize that biopsychosociocultural variables influence health and therefore need to be assessed both separately and as part of the entire system.

Culture

Culture consists of the abstract values, beliefs, and perceptions of the world that lie behind people's behavior and are reflected by that behavior. Culture is shared by the members of a society, and when acted on it produces behavior considered acceptable in that society. Cultures are learned, through the medium of language, rather than inherited biologically, and the parts of a culture function as an integrated whole (Haviland 1983). The following incident illustrates the abstract concept of culture. The headline reads "A Tragedy in Santa Monica" (Reese 1985, p 10):

On a cold, windy afternoon last January, Fumiko Kimura walked slowly across the beach in Santa Monica, clutched her two young children to her and then, facing her native Japan, waded into the sea. Rescuers spotted the submerged bodies too late to save Kazutaka, four, and Yuri, six months, who gave a tiny gasp for breath and then died. But Kimura survived, consumed with anguish and resentment at herself and those who saved her. "They must have been Caucasians," she thought. "Otherwise they would have let me die."

This scenario, tragic from an American perspective, dramatically reveals how culture influences human beings. In America we view suicide as a negative, nihilistic act, a coward's way out. To take one's children is clearly murder and is against the law. In Japan, parent-child suicide is illegal, yet suicide is traditionally viewed as an honorable act. A mother who commits suicide with her children is more honorable than a mother who commits suicide alone, leaving her children to survive without her. The latter woman is viewed as "demonlike." Interestingly, Kimura's grief- and guilt-stricken husband also expressed envy of the bond his wife felt with their children. This story illustrates Margaret Mead's famous statement: "The worlds in which different societies (and individuals) live are distinct worlds, not merely the same worlds with different labels attached." Caring for culturally different clients requires nurses to be aware of this fact.

Culture refers more to the values and beliefs that underlie behavior than to the behavior itself. Culture is always in process, never static. According to Haviland (1983, p 33), subcultural variation is "a distinctive set of standards and behavior patterns by which a group within a larger society operates."

Value Orientations   Anthropologist Florence Kluckhohn developed the construct "value orientation" to describe systematic ways of thinking about human relationships, a sense of time, the relationships of people to nature. Value orientations are acquired during socialization in the family. People from subcultures are socialized to a different set of value orientations than those in the main culture. Value orientations affect adjustment. If they are radically different from those of mainstream North American culture, the result can be coping conflicts within the family, between spouses, and at work.

Subculture   There is some controversy about what constitutes a culture and a **subculture,** or culture within a culture. Recently researches have referred to the "culture" of the hospital, the operating room, or

the nursing school and the "subculture" of the mentally ill, the physically handicapped, or the elderly. Tripp-Reimer (1984) points out that simply sharing some common characteristics does not make people members of a culture or subculture. There must be considerably more homogeneity in the group for it to be considered a culture or a subculture. For example, the Choctaw Indians living on a reservation in Philadelphia, Mississippi, are a subculture because they share a language, values and beliefs, and behavioral patterns. They are part of the larger American Indian culture. In contrast, the physically handicapped are not a subculture because they have various disabilities, come from different socioeconomic levels, and may only rarely come into contact with other physically handicapped people.

A case can be made for viewing a hospital or part of it as a culture or subculture. The transient inhabitants of the hospital share a language, standards of acceptable behavior, and a similar world view. This can be seen even more clearly in speciality units, such as intensive care or psychiatric units. People can be viewed as working within a hospital culture while living within the American culture. Applying the term *culture* or *subculture* to these environments may help us understand a hospital, an emergency room, a school, or a church. Leininger (1970) and Spector (1979) view nursing as a subculture (the health care providers subculture) and document its definite set of beliefs, practices, habits, rituals, and values, often stemming from dominant American cultural values.

World View

A **world view** is the way a group of people (culture or subculture) see their social world, symbolic system, and physical environment and their own place in each. World view is revealed in people's religion, art, language, values, and health care beliefs and practices. A people's world view provides a sense of identity as an American Indian, a Puerto Rican, or a Masai tribesman. It promotes a group's survival and gives members a generally useful picture of the universe.

In a naturalist world view, which is held by hunters and gatherers, nature is respected. Animals are killed only for food, and even then they are valued and respected. Farmers, pastoralists, and modern humankind share an exploitative world view, in which the land and its products exist to be used or exploited. These two different belief systems, to live with nature or to control and improve it, clearly influence a group's approach to the world.

Snow (1974) proposes that Southern rural blacks essentially view the world as a hostile place with inaccessible resources. Consequently, they rely on supernatural solutions to health problems. Roberson (1985) disagrees with Snow, believing that the spiritual beliefs of Southern rural blacks indicate a positive world view—that God is beneficent and loving and, in spite of the difficulties in day-to-day life, God is always there. Roberson points out the interrelationship of religion and health and the ways religion helps people with the process of living.

Ethnocentrism

Ethnocentrism is the belief that one's own culture is more important and better than any other culture. It frequently takes the form of negative value judgments or selective reporting that criticizes or emphasizes negative aspects of other cultures (Beals 1979).

Health care providers need to confront their own ethnocentric, medicocentric, psychocentric views (see Kleinman et al. 1978). The following are examples of medicocentric beliefs:

• The doctor or nurse knows best.

• Clients must be compliant if they want to get better.

• If clients aren't compliant they don't want to get better and therefore are not worthy of our time.

• Psychiatric clients can be classified according to the DSM-III-R.

• Because of the nature of their illness, psychiatric clients are often noncompliant.

• The description of feelings and thoughts is very important in mental health.

These views are responsible for such professional beliefs as, "Why bother explaining her medication to her; she is ignorant," or "Hispanics have those crazy beliefs in their own witchdoctors. They never do what we say." Such ethnocentric beliefs, spoken or unspoken, inevitably create antagonism among clients and health care personnel. In the present litigious environment, antagonism can easily escalate to legal problems. To avoid this, nurses need to be aware of their own beliefs and values and recognize how these may be different from, not better than, those of the clients they care for. Taking a holistic view reduces the likelihood of ethnocentrism. In addition, a nurse who is aware of the potential for ethnocentrism can use this knowledge to educate and be a role model for others.

Cultural Relativism

Cultural relativism is the fundamental anthropologic concept that all cultures are equally valued. It argues against passing judgments about practices that are unfamiliar, strange, or even shocking to us, suggesting instead that all cultures can be evaluated only on their own values in context.

Combating ethnocentrism is not easy. It takes energy and work and constant assessment of oneself and society. Client problems need to be seen from a cultural relativist's perspective; that is, what does the problem seem like to the client? Only by understanding the client's view can nurses provide effective care. The next section addresses this problem.

Culturally Aware Strategies for Implementing the Nursing Process

Quality nursing care is culturally sensitive; that is, the nurse is aware of cultural issues that are important to the client and may affect the client's response to treatment. In planning nursing interventions the nurse does not follow a predetermined plan but plans care that is culturally congruent for each person. For example, if a Hispanic teenage girl is obese and wants to lose weight, the nurse would not hand her a printed 500-calorie diet plan but would work with her and a nutritionist to plan a diet based on the foods she prefers. The nurse would also discuss the care plan with the girl's father and would expect many family members at visiting time. If an Asian client who is a Buddhist wants time each day to meditate, the nurse would allow for that time in the care plan rather than imposing our frenetic Western pace in which every hour is filled with "constructive," "growth-producing" activity.

Taking a client's culture into consideration when planning care is not an easy task. It is time-consuming and requires patience, insight, and creativity on the part of the nurse.

Transcultural Nursing Premises

Cultural and social class differences between client and nurse may impede a nurse's best intentions. Henderson and Primeaux (1981) propose these fundamental transcultural nursing premises to help nurses avoid ethnocentric problems:

• Nurses cannot solve clients' problems, but they may be able to help clients solve their own problems.

• The easiest, least-creative response to transcultural conflict is to pretend that it does not exist.

• Every client behaves according to unwritten ethnic customs and traditions.

• Every successful effort by nurses to teach clients the elements of scientific medicine alienates clients

NURSING SELF-AWARENESS

Questions That Acknowledge Sociocultural Heritage

- What ethnic group, socioeconomic class, religions, age groups, and community do you belong to?
- What experiences have you had with people from ethnic groups, socioeconomic classes, religions, age groups, or communities different from your own?
- What were those experiences like? How did you feel about them?
- When you were growing up, what did your parents and significant others say about people who were different from your family?

- What about your ethnic group, socioeconomic class, religion, age, or community do you find embarrassing or wish you could change? Why?
- What sociocultural factors in your background might contribute to being rejected by members of other cultures?
- What personal qualities do you have that will help you establish interpersonal relationships with persons from other cultural groups? What personal qualities may be detrimental?
- What assumptions do you hold about the people who populate our world?

from relatives and friends who do not have this knowledge.

- Previous transcultural experience is a valuable asset when used as a general guide. However, such experience can be a liability if the nurse believes it provides the answer to every transcultural problem.

- Nurses will make mistakes in transcultural interactions, but they should learn from those mistakes and not repeat them.

Understanding One's Own Sociocultural Heritage

Gaining awareness of sociocultural differences requires that nurses first come to understand their own backgrounds and the influence of that background on their practice. Chapter 2 explored some dimensions of self-knowledge through an examination of the concept of professional and personal integration. This chapter urges nurses to acknowledge and explore their own sociocultural heritage. Nurses are better able to meet the sociocultural needs of a client when they acknowledge that a culture and a society influence their beliefs, values, attitudes, and behavior. The questions in the Nursing Self-Awareness box above are designed to facilitate acknowledgment of the nurse's own sociocultural heritage. Answering these questions honestly and completely is the important first step in self-awareness. The second step involves exploring beliefs and attitudes that may be different from or the same as those held by the client. Nurses might ponder the statements in the Nursing Self-Awareness box on page 908 (Henderson and Primeaux 1981, p 55).

Avoiding Misdiagnosis

Clients from different cultures may be misdiagnosed by Western health care providers. Culturally sensitive nurses can play a role in assessing clients' social, psychologic, and behavioral symptoms in the light of clients' own cultural norms. For example, a psychiatrist may diagnose a man who talks to the dead as schizophrenic, but for a Puerto Rican who believes in espiritismo, talking to the dead is a common practice. A client who is a charismatic Christian may lapse into an altered state of consciousness and speak in tongues. To interpret these behaviors as evidence of schizophrenia is inappropriate. Likewise, categorizing a refugee child who has experienced trauma and violence as mentally ill is revictimization. Obtaining a cultural profile helps to prevent misdiagnosis.

Assessing

Obtaining a Cultural Profile   Fong's (1985) CONFHER model is excellent for obtaining the client's *cultural profile*. Each variable in Fong's model is elaborated below, primarily in questions designed to elicit the relevant information. Some of this information can be gleaned from observation or from information on the chart. Some is more relevant to nurses caring for clients with biologic illnesses. Depending on the situation, some questions may be more useful than others. They should function as a comprehensive guide for gathering and assessing information and for planning care.

Fong suggests that before completing clients' cultural profiles, nurses should complete their own

NURSING SELF-AWARENESS

Exploring Specific Sociocultural Attitudes

- I accept opinions different from my own.
- I respond with compassion to poverty-stricken people.
- I think interracial marriage is a good thing.
- I feel uncomfortable in a group in which I am the ethnic minority.
- I consider failure a bad thing.
- I invite people I don't like to my home.
- I believe that the Ku Klux Klan has its good points.
- I set realistic life goals.
- I would enjoy serving as a juror in a rape case.
- I am concerned about the treatment of minorities in employment and health care.
- I feel uncomfortable in low-income neighborhoods.

- I prefer to conform rather than disagree in public.
- I value friendship more than money.
- I maintain high ethical standards as a professional.
- I would not object to premarital sex for my children.
- I spend a lot of time worrying about social injustices without doing much about them.
- I believe that almost anyone who really wants to can get a good job.
- I have a close friend of another race.
- I would rather attend a concert than an athletic contest.

---

cultural profiles to shed light on differences and similarities between client and nurse. The nurse can emphasize similarities to form a close therapeutic relationship. Differences may serve as topics for discussion. An open, ongoing dialog is beneficial for both parties because it promotes understanding of the other culture.

Communication Style

Does the client speak English fluently? If not, how limited is the client's ability to communicate in English?

Does the client understand common health terms such as *pain*, *fever*, and *nausea*?

Would the client like an interpreter or to have the question rephrased in simple English?

Can the client read and write in English?

Are there ethnic behaviors or styles of nonverbal communication to which the client adheres (e.g., the bowing of the head to show respect in the traditional Japanese culture, or frequent smiling and speaking softly in the Southeast Asian culture)?

Does the client mean what he or she says or, does the client give a pleasant, agreeable answer when a literal, factual answer might be unpleasant and embarrassing?

How much physical touching is appropriate in the client's culture?

Orientation

Does the client identify with a particular racial (e.g., Asian, African, or American Indian) or ethnic group (e.g., Chinese, Japanese, or Korean)?

Where was the client born?

Where has the client lived and for how long?

How long has the client or the client's ancestors been in America?

How closely does the client adhere to traditional habits and values of his or her cultural system?

The nurse should identify the client's beliefs about:

- Human nature (basically evil, both good and evil, or basically good)
- The relationship between humans and nature (people in subjugation to nature, in harmony with nature, or having mastery over nature)
- Time orientation (past, present, or future)
- The main purpose of life (being, being in becoming, or doing)

• People's relationships to one another (lineal, collateral, or individualistic)

Nutrition

Are there ethnic foods that the client prefers?

Are there foods the client is encouraged to eat when sick?

Are there foods to be avoided because of ethnic origin, health status, or illness?

Family Relationships

Who is in the family?

Is the client's definition of family nuclear, extended, or tribal?

Who is the head of the household?

Is the family matriarchal or patriarchal?

What is the role and position of women, the aged, male children, and female children within the household?

Who controls the rearing and socialization of children?

How are decisions made in the family?

Who manages financial matters?

How important is it to have the family nearby when the client is sick?

What are important social customs or taboos (e.g., table manners, forms of greetings, and customs between men and women or adults and children)?

What are family priorities and goals (e.g., family solidarity, more children, more money, more material possessions, better housing, higher social status, and optimal health)?

Where does the family live: inner city or suburbs; ethnic enclave; or white or black middle-class neighborhood?

Are art, music, and recreational amenities available?

Health Beliefs

Does the client rely on any self-care or traditional folk medicine practices?

Is the client currently being treated by a cultural healer (e.g., medicine man, Voodoo doctor, Chinese herbalist, or curandero)?

How does the client explain illness (e.g., germ theory, imbalance of yin and yang, or evil spirits)?

How does the client generally respond to pain (e.g., with stoic endurance, with loud cries, or with quiet withdrawal)?

How does the client respond to hospitalization?

Are there any illnesses that are more prevalent in the client's ethnic group (e.g., sickle cell anemia and hypertension among blacks, lactose intolerance among Asians and blacks, myopia among Chinese, or Tay-Sachs among Jews)?

Are there any diseases that the client would have increased resistance to because of ethnic background (e.g., cervical cancer among Jews or skin cancer among blacks)?

Education

Does the client prefer printed literature or audiovisual learning tools?

Does the client learn by trial and error or didactic methods?

What is the client's informal and formal education level?

What is the client's life experience?

Who in the family works?

What is the annual income of the family?

Does the family have health and dental insurance?

Religion

Does the client believe in God or gods?

Does the client have a religious preference?

What religious beliefs, sacred rites, and religious sanctions or restrictions does the client adhere to (e.g., beliefs of Christian Scientist, Seventh-Day Adventist, Buddhist, Native American Church, or West African Voodoo)?

What religious persons will be involved in the client's health care (e.g., Catholic priest, Buddhist monk, Islamic imam, or black minister)?

Understanding the Client's Beliefs and Practices Often health professionals are unaware of or insensitive to the reality that all clients have their own explanatory models of illness.

Illness Beliefs and Practices The following questions will help the nurse reveal the client's illness beliefs and practices (Randall-David 1985):

What do you think caused your problem?

Why do you think it started when it did?

What do you think your sickness does to your body?

How does it work?

How severe is your sickness? How long do you think it will last?

What are the main problems your sickness has caused for you?

Do you know anyone else who had this problem? What did they do to treat it?

Did you discuss your problem with any of your relatives or friends? What did they say?

What kinds of home remedies, medicines, or other treatments have you tried for your sickness? (Quantity, dosage, frequency, how prepared) Did it help? Are you still using it/them?

What type of treatment do you think you should receive?

What are the most important results you hope to receive from this treatment?

Do you think there is any way to prevent this problem in the future? How?

Is there any other information that would be helpful for designing a workable treatment plan?

It is far more useful to spend time getting answers to these questions and planning culturally relevant interventions than to waste time planning care that will be irrelevant to the client and thus ignored. Beside resulting in ineffective treatment plans, blocked communications will make both clients and professionals resort to their original stereotypes of each other.

 Medications and Compliance   One of the biggest problems identified by mental health professionals concerns psychiatric clients' noncompliance with medication orders. The frustrated professional cannot make the client understand that taking medicine "is necessary for the rest of your life" and "is what is keeping you out of the hospital." Amarasingham (1980) recognizes that clients have explanatory models not only about their illness but also about medications. She identifies common beliefs about medication in our culture:

- Medicine is necessary only as long as you feel sick.

- Diseases can be cured by diet manipulation or exercise.

- Medicine is a contaminating substance.

- Drugs are a "crutch"; it is virtuous not to take drugs.

- You may become immune to drugs if you take them often.

These beliefs directly influence whether a client complies with medication orders. The terms *complies* and *orders* reveal the medicocentric view that the client should do what doctors and nurses think is necessary. Because this method is ineffective, new strategies are required. The concepts of explanatory models, cultural

assessment, and negotiation are as useful with the problem of medications as with the more general problem of mental disorder. When medications are prescribed for psychiatric clients, the nurse should attempt to understand the client's beliefs and assumptions about the medication. Then the negotiation process described later in this chapter can begin.

Two problems in the nurse–psychiatric client interaction make the negotiation more difficult:

1. Psychiatric clients generally appear confused about the fact that taking medications helps keep them out of the hospital. Being out of the hospital generally implies wellness, and taking medication implies sickness. This apparent contradiction needs to be clarified over time.

2. Clients with psychiatric illnesses that require medication (depression, bipolar mood disorder, and schizophrenia) often are confused and disorganized and have memory impairment. Consequently, repeated negotiation and explanations are necessary.

The timing and environment for such interactions need to be taken into consideration. The environment should be peaceful and private and the client fairly lucid and relaxed, or the interaction will be unrewarding and ineffective.

Planning and Implementing Interventions

Negotiating Health Care Practices The goal of negotiating among professionals and the client and family about health care practices is to increase the effectiveness of treatment. A cultural assessment reveals the client's explanatory model of illness. The professional answers similar questions to clarify his or her own explanatory model for the client's "disease." Through discussions and negotiations the client and professional should come to an agreement about treatment. Ideally the treatment will be congruent with both models, and if not actually congruent it will not be counterproductive or harmful. For example, if a Hispanic client wants to eat certain foods to restore the balance and harmony that has gone out of his or her body due to illness and is also willing to take antidepressant medications, no harm is done and both client and professional are doing what they believe is correct. In contrast, if a hospitalized Buddhist refugee wants to meditate and remain isolated all day and night, additional negotiations will be needed. Perhaps a closely monitored outpatient treatment plan could be devised in which the client agrees to spend a certain number of hours a day with family or friends doing certain activities. The negotiation phase of the process requires excellent interviewing skills, creative listening, and ingenuity in adapting health care practices. However, the labor-intensive work of negotiating shared care plans will pay off in "compliance," and a close therapeutic relationship that is egalitarian rather than hierarchical.

Circumventing the Language Barrier An interpreter may be necessary if language is a barrier. If the client attempts to speak English, his or her thoughts may appear distorted when language is the real problem. There have been a number of documented instances in which persons have been diagnosed as mentally disordered and confined to a mental hospital because mental health professionals erroneously diagnosed a language problem or value difference as disordered thinking or psychosis. Nonverbal behavior may also be misinterpreted. The Intervention boxes on this page and page 912 provide specific guidelines for circumventing the language barrier.

Avoiding Cultural Stereotyping One person cannot be aware of all the cultural factors that should be taken into consideration in planning and implementing a particular psychiatric nursing intervention. A frequent solution to this dilemma is to go to the literature or the resource person likely to know the most about the culture in which we are interested. In doing so, however, we must put the data in the proper perspective. There is a danger of **cultural stereotyping**, that is, assuming that all members of one ethnic heritage are alike without taking steps to verify the assumption.

Acting as a Culture Broker   When nurses work with clients from different cultural groups, they can work toward assuming the role of culture broker or helping another person in that role. A **culture broker** essentially functions as a mediator between the people or groups from two cultures. Culture brokers are effective if they have knowledge of the two systems. There are two types of mediators: a hierarchical mediator, who works within the health care system, and a representative mediator, who is from the same ethnic community as the client (LaFargue 1985). The culture broker understands both the health care belief systems and the perspectives of client, family, and professional in the particular situation. Given this understanding, the culture broker essentially moves back and forth between groups to ensure client care that is effective, efficient, and viewed as helpful by the client. The culture broker can prevent problems merely by explaining to the professional a client's wish to have numerous visitors or worship in his or her own way with special candles and chanting. Or the culture broker may explain to the client and family that the chanting is fine but that there are hospital rules against candles because of the fire hazard. The aim is to have both sides understand and accept each other

INTERVENTION

Guidelines for Monolingual Providers in a Cross-Cultural Environment

- Unless you are thoroughly effective and fluent in the target language, always use an interpreter.
- Avoid using family members as interpreters.
- Learn basic words and sentences in the target language. Asking interpreters about words or comments that have not been translated prompts attention to detail.
- Use dictionaries of languages used by your client population. Beware of brief "definitions" that serve only as labels.
- Become familiar with special terminology. Specific beliefs, practices, and traditions are often referenced by indirect language or special terms. Local beliefs and moral tenets may lead to overemphasis on or underreporting of certain symptoms, issues, and events.
- Check the quality of translated health-related materials by having them back-translated.
- Meet with your interpreters on a regular basis. They will provide both a window and a mirror when you deal with another language and another culture.
- Personal information is often closely guarded and difficult to obtain. Clients often request a specific interpreter or even bring their own.
- Evaluate the interpreter's style and approach to clients. For special situations and problem cases, try to match the interpreter to the task.
- Be patient. Careful interpretation often requires the interpreter to use long explanatory phrases.

SOURCE: Adapted from Putsch R: Crosscultural communication. JAMA 1985;254:3347–3348.

and to negotiate the issues either group believes to be important.

Mobilizing Support Systems   Nurses need to assess a client's social support systems and mobilize them when necessary. Support systems are vital to a client's well-being and can be most useful in keeping them out of the hospital. Their functions can be incorporated into the nursing care plan.

INTERVENTION

Guidelines For Nurse-Interpreter– Client Interactions

- Address clients directly. Avoid directing all of your commentary to and through the interpreter.
- Be certain the interpreter is thoroughly involved with the client during an interview.
- Develop alternatives to gathering information by direct questions. People who are strangers to direct, Western-style inquiry may respond better to conversational modes.
- Invite correction and induce the discussion of alternatives: "Correct me if I'm wrong, I understand it this way . . . Do you see it some other way?"
- Pursue seemingly unconnected issues raised by the client. These issues may lead to crucial information or uncover difficulties with the interpretation.
- Come back to an issue if you suspect a problem and get a negative response. Be certain the interpreter knows what you want. Use related questions, change the wording, and come at the issue indirectly.
- Provide instructions in list format. Ask clients to outline their understanding of the plans.
- If alternatives exist, spell each one out.
- Emphasize by repetition.
- Clarify your limitations. The willingness to talk about an issue may be viewed as evidence of "understanding" it or the ability to "fix" it.
- Rumors, jealousy, privacy, and reputation are crucial issues in closely knit communities. Acknowledge the problem and assure the client of confidentiality.
- Unless the correct circumstances are devised, it may be impossible to address certain male/ female problems by way of discussion or physical examination.

SOURCE: *Adapted from Putsch R: Crosscultural communication.* JAMA 1985;254:3347–3348.

INTERVENTION

Guidelines for Language Use in Interpreter-Dependent Interviews

- Use short questions and comments. Technical terminology and professional jargon, such as "psychotropic medication," should be reduced to plain English.
- When lengthy explanations are necessary, break them up and have them interpreted piece by piece in straightforward, concrete terms.
- Use language and explanations the interpreter can handle.
- Make allowances for terms that do not exist in the target language.
- Try to avoid ambiguous statements and questions.
- Avoid abstraction, idiomatic expressions, similes, and metaphors. It is useful to learn about these usages in the target language.
- Plan what you want to say ahead of time. Avoid confusing the interpreter by backing up, inserting a proviso, rephrasing, or hesitating.
- Avoid indefinite phrases using *would, could, if,* and *maybe.* These can be mistaken for actual agreements or firm approval of a course of action.
- Ask the interpreter to comment on the client's word content and emotions.

SOURCE: *Adapted from Putsch R: Crosscultural communication.* JAMA 1985;254:3347–3348.

Using the knowledge she derived from her anthropologic research with mentally ill Hispanics, Garrison (1978) offers some practical suggestions:

- Mental health services should be localized in small neighborhood units, staffed by persons who are or can become thoroughly acquainted with the concrete social systems of that specific neighborhood.

- Acquaintance with the concrete social systems of the neighborhood can be brought about through interviews with clients in all degrees of disturbance. Influential, potentially helpful members of the community can be identified through reports from clients of their daily lives.

- Severely disturbed persons might be located alone or in pairs in community apartments as long as there are supportive others outside the household.

- Mapping the distribution of clients' residences within the area would show clusters of clients who might be organized into neighborhood-based groups or supportive networks.

• Supportive psychotherapy groups might be based in homes rather than the clinic, particularly in the homes of severely disturbed persons who require assistance to maintain the household.

• Neighbors, "good friends," Pentecostal people, spiritualist mediums, and bodega (a general store or apothecary in a Hispanic community) proprietors are particularly likely candidates to participate in recreated support systems, to provide or recommend foster home placement, or to alert mental health professionals to problems.

• "Living network therapy," or the maintenance of a network of natural associates in the neighborhood context, could probably be accomplished with no greater expenditure of money or professional time than is now spent on the same group of clients in medication maintenance.

• Quasi-groups and action sets can be mobilized in the support of clients, or can be cued to mobilize themselves in times of crisis for a client discharged into the community.

• Mental health services would probably be used more readily, and dropouts would be fewer, if time and attendance were structured less rigorously than is conventional in most mental health clinics. Walk-in services without fixed appointments and group activities without fixed membership are two examples of patterns congenial with those found in the natural community. Of course very chronic patients, no matter what ethnic group they represent, do not always keep appointments and therefore need assistance in getting regular care.

• Mental health services integrated with general medical clinics would be more acceptable to this population and probably better used than freestanding facilities.

Recognizing Characteristics of Culturally Relevant Services Flaskerud (1987, p 154) identifies these characteristics of culturally relevant services:

• Clients and therapists share the same cultural view of illness and the same language.

• Services are located in the client community.

• Services are available during weekend and evening hours.

• Brief, situation-oriented and crises-oriented therapy is offered.

• Family therapy is offered.

• Services or referrals for social, economic, or legal problems are offered.

• Referrals are made to culturally appropriate therapy.

• Referrals are made to traditional (folk) practitioners.

Therapy for psychologic problems that ignores the client's contextual situation—e.g., social, economic, and possibly legal difficulties—is inappropriate. A holistic approach that involves client advocacy with human services agencies is necessary.

Applying Research Findings Lawson (1986) reviewed research that concerns itself with racial and ethnic factors in pharmacotherapy and biologic psychiatry. The findings of these many research projects are as follows (socioeconomic status is controlled for in the first three studies):

• Black and Hispanic clients with bipolar mood disorder may hallucinate more than white clients. This may contribute to misdiagnoses of schizophrenia.

• Black schizophrenics may show more paranoia, hallucinations, and delusions than whites.

• Black clients with mood disorders may have more hallucinations, delusions, hostility, and somatization. Whites may have a greater degree of mania, depression, or guilt.

• Because depression is often unrecognized in racial and ethnic minorities, biologic assessment tools may be useful for diagnosis.

• Asians require lower dosages than whites for numerous psychotropic medications, such as lithium, antidepressants, and neuroleptics.

• Asians experience side effects at lower doses of psychotropic medications than blacks or whites.

• Asians show higher plasma levels of diazepam at a given oral dose than whites.

• Asians tolerate better the sedating effects of diphenhydramine.

• Hispanics require less antidepressant medication and report more side effects at dosages half the Anglo therapeutic dose.

• Black schizophrenics and depressed clients improve more than whites with phenothiazines and tricyclic antidepressants.

• Blacks have greater anxiety reduction with antianxiety and antidepressant agents.

• Blacks show more improvement with a tricyclic antidepressant in one week.

• Blacks who overdosed on amitriptyline had higher levels of antidepressants than whites who overdosed.

• Blacks show a significantly longer plasma lithium half-life and a higher ratio of red blood cell lithium to plasma lithium than whites or Asians.

Racial and ethnic differences have been found in serum creatinine phosphokinase (CPK), platelet serotonin, and HLA-A2. Consequently, when researchers aim to evaluate these biologic markers they must control for race. Lawson advocates more research on safe and effective doses of medications for different racial and ethnic groups. Not to do so and not to have different dose ranges for different ethnic groups can have dangerous consequences for clients.

Racial and ethnic factors also play a role in perceptual and diagnostic research. For example:

• An in-patient staff in one study perceived blacks as more violent than whites, although objective findings revealed blacks to be less violent.

• Other studies show blacks receive more p.r.n. medication and may spend more time in seclusion than whites.

• Blacks are more often diagnosed as schizophrenic when they really suffer from mood disorders (Jones and Gray 1986).

Jones and Gray believe such misdiagnoses result from cultural differences in language and mannerisms, difficulties in relating between black clients and white therapists, and the myth that blacks rarely suffer from mood disorders. They point out that in physical illness, physicians search for the causative agent and examine it in the context of symptoms. In psychiatry, by contrast, professionals can determine no causative agent, so they base diagnoses on signs, symptoms, and behaviors. Different illnesses may involve the same symptoms, and particular symptoms and behaviors are culturally determined in part, making diagnosis difficult. Misdiagnosis may occur because white therapists don't understand black clients' use of language and therefore may believe it is indicative of a thought disorder; they may view a black client's style of relating as a disturbance of affect and his or her mannerisms as bizarre.

Blacks are not the only group who may suffer from Western medicine's ethnocentrism. Three case studies of clients (Latin American, Asian, and Moslem) with minor depression revealed a different style of symptom expression from Western clients. They exhibited vegetative (anergia, sleep disturbance, weight loss) rather than cognitive and affective symptoms (Nikelly 1988). Thus, they are at risk for being misdiagnosed or overdiagnosed, e.g., of having depression when they really are experiencing culturally induced stress. Non-Western clients often focus on somatic problems that they expect to be treated with somatotherapy, an accepted mode of treatment in their culture. The DSM-III-R category of depression reflects a Western conception, based on our beliefs in egocentrism. In Western societies, it is permissible to reveal personal hurt, dependency, and despair. This is not true of cultures that are more group oriented. The central point in these case studies is that culture regulates how different illnesses manifest themselves.

Lefley (1990) reviewed research relevant to the relationship of culture to chronic mental illness. Some researchers and theorists have suggested that certain cultural beliefs and practices can influence positively the progress of clients with chronic mental illness. Some of these "cultural strengths" include world view, religion, alternative healing resources, values of interdependence, extended kinship structure, family support, and professionals' willingness to work *with* families. Lefley reports the following specific research findings:

• In developing countries, schizophrenia is briefer, less likely to recur, and less severe over time.

• Chronicity in North American culture may be due to our belief system that expects serious mental illness to be chronic.

• The facts that our culture is characterized by little social support and high stress may influence chronicity.

• In non-Western societies there is less social isolation, a more supportive and less intensely involved family milieu, and extended kinship networks that may affect chronicity positively.

• The church and supernatural belief systems provide natural support systems for the chronically mentally ill. The supernatural belief systems help explain mental illness.

• Relative to population distribution, African-Americans and American Indians have much higher admission rates than other racial and ethnic groups to state and county mental hospitals.

• Blacks are more likely to be diagnosed as schizophrenic and to connect with aftercare services, but they also receive fewer services than whites.

• Hispanics underuse ambulatory services but aggressive outreach increases their use of aftercare services.

• Women use in-patient facilities less than men.

• The race and sex of the client and the psychiatrist influence diagnosis even when clearcut DSM-III-R criteria are used.

• Psychosis is manifested differently in different cultures. Also, clients with the same illness (e.g., schizophrenia) report different symptoms. Black clients show more disorientation, hallucinations, and anger; white clients show more unsystematized delusions.

• Black and Hispanic clients with mood disorders have delusions and hallucinations more frequently than white clients.

• Even when age, sex, and education are controlled variables, the typical black depressed client "looks different" from the typical white depressed client.

• The black client with schizophrenia or dementia is less systematically impaired and shows fewer negative symptoms than whites; this may account for the perceived misdiagnosis.

• Black people do not like to take pills.

• Haitians prefer injections, viewing them as more powerful in counteracting the externally caused difficulties with their minds and/or bodies.

• Cubans and Puerto Ricans use many medications and often share medication among the family.

• The educational problem-solving approach mobilizes Hispanic families.

• Group therapy for American Indians and other group-centered cultures is useful especially if it clarifies feelings of "outsideness."

• Family network therapy is useful with American Indians and probably with other groups with extended families.

• Explaining mental illness as a physiologic imbalance that can be corrected by medication fits the belief system of Hispanic families.

• Purification rites can be therapeutic for American Indians or other groups who believe their illness occurred because they failed to propitiate malevolent spirits or to perform obligatory rituals.

• Rigid time schedules may be difficult for clients whose culture has different meanings and values about time.

Cultural variations exist in the experience, expression, diagnosis, and treatment of mental disorder. The previously mentioned research reveals that racial and ethnic factors are clearly linked to people's biologic makeup. In addition, racial and cultural bias can have serious consequences in terms of diagnosis and treatment. We need much more research in these areas to give safe and effective care—care that is culturally sensitive and emphasizes clients' and families'

strengths. Perhaps in the near future Good and Kleinman's (1985) suggestions that a cultural axis be added to the DSM psychiatric categories will be heeded. Thus, clients' cultural interpretations—their explanatory models—would be considered relevant in diagnosis and treatment.

Psychiatric researchers are attempting to make interview schedules and other mental health assessment scales that are culturally relevant (see Ebigbo 1982, Manson et al. 1985). The DSM-III-R and other psychologic inventories (e.g., MMPI) reflect Anglo-American medical belief systems and are often inappropriate for clients from other cultures. The specific problems of the instruments involve (a) lack of recognition of culturally important symptoms (b) lack of recognition of culturally organized clusters, and (c) the "category fallacy." "The 'category fallacy' . . . involves taking Western biomedical categories of disorder and applying their diagnostic criteria to other cultural groups without establishing the validity of those categories for that culture" (Guarnaccia, Rubio-Stipek, and Canino 1989). The aim is to generate the same kind of instruments that include culturally meaningful illness categories. To do this, we need knowledge of cultural specific disorders, knowledge as detailed as psychiatrists' knowledge of DSM-III-R diagnoses (Guarnaccia, Rubio-Stipek, and Canino 1989). Once valid instruments are developed, we can gain more information about psychiatric epidemiology, i.e., what illnesses are most prevalent in which groups.

Specific Folk Beliefs and Healing Practices of Selected Cultural Groups

Folk beliefs and healing practices are culture-specific ways of handling physical problems and emotional conflicts. For example, members of some cultural groups, such as Chicanos and Appalachian whites, believe that illnesses caused by witches' spells may not respond to drugs. This may account for a client's seeming noncompliance with a treatment plan. In some other ethnic groups—such as the Indians of North, Central, and South America; Chinese Americans; and Japanese Americans—herbal products are used to treat both physical and mental disorders. The culturally unaware mental health team member may not know that such herbs are being used or that they may produce both positive or negative interactions with medications.

Folk beliefs and healing practices reflect the world view of the particular culture. In most Western societies disease is viewed as the result of such natural phenomena as microbes, viruses, chromosomal abnormality, or chemicals. Many Third World people, however, believe that supernatural forces cause illness, and that cures can be effected by appealing to the supernatural force through witches or sorcerers or by controlling the force with magic.

Despite the fact that many people from different cultures become "westernized" in appearance and overt behavior when they move to the United States, they often retain their folk beliefs. One study of 450 college students in the United States and Ireland revealed that about 70 percent of the students relied on such magic as carrying good luck charms to an exam, crossing their fingers, having a lucky number, or knocking on wood. Reliance on magic can be seen even in technologically advanced groups. People often use magic to control things they feel they cannot control.

Being aware of **folk health care systems** helps the nurse provide better health care to particular groups of people. Culturally aware nurses are able to devise more meaningful nursing care plans and perhaps discover ways in which the middle-class Western system of health care can be humanized by incorporating folk beliefs and practices. The clinical example below demonstrates how an understanding of folk health care systems can be used to facilitate mental health treatment.

Henri, a 21-year-old Haitian refugee, was brought by his family to the emergency room of a large general hospital in Miami. Family members believed Henri was possessed by an evil spirit. They told the emergency room staff that they had been unable to control him for two days. He had been breaking dishes and glasses in the family's small apartment, shouting obscene curses in Creole at his mother, and attacking his brother on a number of occasions, screaming, "I am God the Son." Psychiatrists summoned by the ER staff prescribed massive doses of tranquilizers and arranged for his transfer to the in-patient psychiatric unit, where Henri remained for three more days with no decrease in his violent behavior. A surgical staff nurse who had been raised in Cuba and was familiar with santería (Cuba's folk blend of Catholicism and mysticism) heard of Henri's strange behavior. She suggested to one of her colleagues on the psychiatric unit that a voodoo practitioner might be helpful. After the psychiatric nurse confirmed that the family did believe in voodoo, she brought the suggestion to a team conference. After much heated discussion the team decided to try an exorcism by a voodoo priest if the family agreed. The exorcism was carried out at the offices of a community mental health outreach center in Miami's Little Haiti. The in-patient psychiatric staff who observed the exorcism ceremony found that their client became very quiet after it. Henri returned to their unit where professional treatment was continued, and he improved rapidly.

The unique aspect of this situation is that the psychiatric team was able to allow for a folk health care system that stood in opposition to the system of health care they espoused. There is a strong contradiction between professional and folk health systems in terms of the relationship between practitioners and clients. In folk systems, both practitioner and client define the nature of illness and health, while in professional systems practitioners are likely to have a monopoly on defining the nature of illness and health. The process of treatment is another basis for comparison. In folk systems, the process of treatment is a social act, whereas in professional systems it is a technologic act. The folk systems of some specific groups—black Americans, Hispanic Americans, Asian Americans, and American Indians—are discussed more thoroughly in the following sections.

Professional, Folk, and Popular Domains of Health Care

The *professional domain of health care* refers to psychiatrists, social workers, and nurses—institutionally sanctioned health care workers. These people generally focus on the disease process through a process of scientific assessment and diagnosis. As the professionals become enlightened to the possibly conflicting explanatory models of disease and illness, it is hoped they will learn to treat illness along with disease. Interestingly, 90 percent of clients who come to health care providers have already attempted to treat their illness with folk or popular methods.

Folk healers, the *folk domain of health care*, are healers such as root doctors, high priests from the cult of santería, or faith healers. Although these healers are considered nonprofessional, they are experts within their system. Some of the practices of these healers may sound bizarre, primitive, and unscientific, but the people who believe in them can document their healing abilities.

A young Hispanic girl had been admitted to the adolescent psychiatric unit for agitated behavior and apparent hallucinations and delusions. An interview revealed that she was being treated by a santería priestess (described later in the chapter). She chanted periodically, fondled a cluster of charms around her neck, and later told the nurse that she had been cured before by the priestess and she felt that with time the priestess would cure her again.

The effectiveness and power of folk healers should not be underestimated. A more useful approach is to find out everything possible about the healing practice to determine how it fits in with professional treatment. It is generally recognized that folk practitioners work on treating the illness and not the disease. Often if they view a problem as being out of their realm of expertise they will refer the client to a medical professional.

The *popular domain of health care* refers to family and friends who function in the role of healer by offering health information, emotional support, prayers, and advice.

P eg was a real "health nut" and believed that one's mental outlook was directly related to food intake and exercise. When her friends or family became depressed, she lectured them on exercising to increase endorphins and told them what kinds of foods promoted or prohibited sleep. According to Peg, almost any type of mental or physical problem could be treated by disciplined eating and exercise habits.

A client's explanatory model of illness does not simply derive from one or two domains of health care. It represents a blend of information from past and present experiences and education. Aiming for clarity in understanding the client's model encourages a therapeutic relationship based on mutual respect.

Racism

Racial prejudice has existed since the beginning of time and is present in all heterogeneous societies. Prejudice involves a stereotyping of groups and denigration of one group by another. "Racism is systematized oppression by one race of another . . . within every sphere of social relations—economic exploitation, military subjugation, political and cultural subordination . . . [These] interesting and developing processes operate so normally and naturally and are so much a part of the existing institutions of the society that the individuals involved are barely conscious of their operation" (Boggs 1989, p 138).

Racism and prejudice are emotional, not logical, and are learned very early in life. In our society, examples of racism and prejudice exist against women, gays, and ethnic and religious groups different from ourselves. Different theoretic explanations of racism exist, the most logical being that racism is the result of historical, cultural and economic forces. For in-depth information about racism, see Gordon Allport's classic study *The Nature of Prejudice* (1954). The following discussion of different racial and ethnic groups gives only a few examples of people who are frequently stereotyped and victimized by racial prejudice.

Discrimination and the Family in a Changing Society

As society changes, so do family structures. Today, the traditional, patriarchal, and intact family is no longer the predominant family structure. We have to redefine our concept of family to include gay families, single-parent families, blended families, communal families, and family structures of different ethnic groups. The family must be viewed in the context of culture. Once we understand this we are less likely to stereotype and discriminate against certain groups because of their differences. For example, rather than viewing the black family as a disorganized, single-parent, subnuclear, female-dominated social system (White 1989, p 380), we can assume another view—that it represents an extended family model. This model "consists of a related and quasi-related group of adults, including aunts, uncles, parents, cousins, grandparents, boyfriends, and girlfriends linked together in a kinship or kinlike network. This model of family life . . . captures the strength, vitality, resistance and continuity of the black family [and] the essence of black values, folkways, and lifestyles" (White 1989, p 382).

African Americans

Black Americans (also called African Americans), the largest racial minority group in America, are a large and diverse group of people who have one thing in common: African ancestors. Black Americans are young, old, poor, rich, rural, urban, tall, short, light, dark, religious, atheist, educated, and uneducated (Capers 1985). Ever since the slaves arrived in 1619, blacks have lived parallel to white American society. Capers (1985) points out that although they move in and out of white society, blacks are generally socialized among blacks and still suffer from racial prejudice and discrimination.

It is not easy to categorize the folk systems and healing practices of black Americans for a number of reasons. The system is a unique blend of African folklore, fundamentalist Christianity, the voodoo religion of the West Indies, and some tenets of both classic and modern medicine. Folk medicine is more likely to be important to black Americans who live in the southern United States or rural areas or who are recent immigrants, because they are less likely to have been thoroughly assimilated into the larger culture. However, folk practices may also be important to black Americans living in the urban Northeast and the West.

Health Care Beliefs and Practices   Blacks have historically been responsible for their own health care because the white North American health care system did not accept them. Thus, indigenous healing beliefs and practices are a core part of black culture. These health beliefs and practices did not originate in isolation but are integrally linked to the people's world view. Some of these beliefs are (Roberson 1985):

• Physical and mental illness and spiritual problems are all interrelated.

• Some illnesses are natural and can be treated by natural agents (herbs), whereas others are supernatural, that is, caused by witchcraft and evil people.

- Conflict in one's life can cause illness.

- Magic and witchcraft can counteract evil spells.

- People determine the cause of their illness and then go to the practitioner of their choice.

- People can be treated simultaneously by representatives of three domains of health care: a professional health care provider (professional domain); a faith leader or a root doctor (folk domain); and a grandmother or head of the family (popular domain).

- God is the ultimate healer.

- The bible has much useful information about health care.

- Prayer and belief in God are helpful healing strategies.

- Sin, stress, the devil, and a negative attitude may cause sickness.

Rootwork or Voodoo   For people who believe they have been hexed by another person, a **root doctor** (voodoo man or woman) is necessary to remove the hex or put a hex on someone else. The hex can cause illness, which frequently mimics mental disorder, by infusing the person with evil spirits. People believe they are hexed by ingesting food with something in it or by walking over the offending object. Plants, herbs, ground glass, and other substances can be used in putting on or neutralizing the hex ("fix," "mojo").

Voodoo is a Western African word that means god or spirit. According to voodoo, a religion, the spirits of the dead can visit the world of the living to bless or curse people. In Haiti, a blend of voodoo and Catholicism called *vodun* is of prime importance in the religious life of Haitian peasants. Voodoo priests (*houngan*) or priestesses (*mambo*) may exorcise evil spirits or may cause injury to an enemy by sticking pins into a wax image of the enemy. Voodoo and other forms of spiritualism are integral to the folk medicine of black Americans.

Faith Healing   Spiritual or faith healers deal with illness ascribed to spiritual or supernatural causes. The client may have somatic symptoms but will seek out a faith healer in one of two places.

1. In the community, faith healers function autonomously and are not part of organized religion.

2. Within a church, usually the Church of God, faith healers have revivals, during which people make testimonials or present themselves to be healed.

Family and Child-Rearing Practices   According to Hale (1980, pp 79–87), the child-rearing practices of the black family derive from the African culture and from adaptation to the racism and oppression black people face in America. These practices include:

- The teaching of children to live among white people without becoming white people (Nobles 1975)

- Strong bond between mother and child

- Children as valuable because they represent the continuity of life

- Dual socialization for black children, who must imitate the behavior of the culture in which they live and take on behaviors of the dominant culture to be upwardly mobile

- The black home as a sanctuary from society's wounds

- Strong motivation for children to achieve

- Strong religious orientation; the role of church as a socializing institution

- Black communication is emotionally charged and feeling-oriented

- Black children who are more feeling-oriented, people-oriented, and skilled at nonverbal communication than white children

- A low object orientation in black families

- A direct, often physical form of discipline (Peters 1981)

- High value on "mothering," whether the person is male or female (Peters 1981)

- Greater participation by the father in the child-rearing function as economic security increases (McAdoo 1981)

- Black fathers who socialize their children differently than white fathers, probably leading to the development of independence and high competence in daughters (McAdoo 1981)

- Black fathers who take an equal part in the child-reading decisions in the family (McAdoo 1981)

Nursing Practice Issues   To give good nursing care to black clients, nurses must understand the historical background and values and beliefs of black culture. Racism is an additional issue. The long history of racism has resulted in an often unarticulated and even unrealized lack of trust, with prejudice and often discrimination on both sides. Racism is rooted in our culture and cannot be denied. Griffith, a black psychiatrist, believes that the central problem throughout American life is that "black and white perceptions of reality, of what is important, are discordant" (1986, p 5). Therefore, white nurses must be sensitive to racial issues when working with black clients. Racism in psychiatric mental health care will increase clients' feelings of inadequacy, powerlessness, and frustration and can deprive them of a sense of control and hope (Brantley 1983). Such issues directly affect transference and countertransference and therefore should be confronted openly—for example, "How do you feel about having a white nurse?" Some black clients may desire a black nurse and, if possible, their request should be granted. If not, part of the therapeutic process can focus on dealing with the black-white problems. Black professionals working with black clients need to be careful not to overidentify with the client's aggression. Instead, they need to help the client view racism as a reality and to learn useful coping strategies (Brantley 1983). Psychiatric nurses in inpatient units have often discussed how black nurses and attendants are often much more effective than white staff with black male patients. Such realities should be considered when client assignments and interventions are initiated as the example below demonstrates.

John G, a 35-year-old black male, was brought into the locked unit screaming, kicking, and hallucinating. He was extremely paranoid and cowered in the corner for five days, withdrawing from the staff. He appeared frightened and became hostile and violent when approached. Bill, a black male attendant, was the only staff member who could talk with him. Bill began to check on John hourly and slowly began to increase the time he spent talking quietly and calmly to John. The bond between John and Bill was considered central to John's progress.

Nurses also need to recognize that cultural variables are directly related to client behavior. For example,

Georgia, a 50-year-old black woman, was admitted to the psychiatric unit for the third time for depression. An examination of her progress notes indicated she had been treated with a variety of antidepressants. An interview revealed she had severe financial problems that influenced her housing situation, she was in the middle of a crisis with one of her children, and her husband had recently died.

In this situation, which is common with poor blacks and poor people generally, antidepressants were not enough. Nurses need to assess the realities of a client's life and their relationship to the presenting illness. Instead of viewing Georgia as the disease category *depressed,* the nurse needs to plan intervention strategies that take into account the sociocultural variables. Helping her decide how to manage her finances and find an acceptable place to live are good beginning goals. When these basic needs are taken care of, the nurse can focus on Georgia's concerns about her child's crisis and her grief about her husband's death.

RESEARCH NOTE

Citation
Peltzer K: Causative and intervening factors of harmful alcohol consumption and cannabis use in Malawi. Int J Addictions 1989;24(2):79–85.

Study Problems/Purpose
The aim of this study was to identify culturally relevant factors in the causation of and intervention in harmful alcohol and cannabis use in Malawi.

Methods
Research assistants commuted to two communities almost every day for one month and several times a week for another month. As participant observers, they identified thirty individuals in each community with harmful alcohol consumption and cannabis use. Psychosocial assessment was done through informal interviews and participant observation. Sixty subjects were followed through monthly informal interviews and observations for six months with the aim of assessing intervention strategies.

Findings
Alcohol consumption and cannabis use were problems in both the Moslem and Christian communities. Of the ninety subjects 25 were female; 65 were male. The mean age was 34 years. Alcohol consumption increases after the monthly salary is received. As the month goes on, cheaper alcoholic beverages are consumed. An African socialization model that looks at three dimensions—the authority, the group, and the body-mind-environment dimension—was used to explain the causes of excessive alcohol consumption. In the follow-up of the sixty subjects, thirty-two did not improve, seven died, twelve improved, and nine could not be found.

Conclusion
Intervention strategies on a social and community level are no longer effective in the transitional Malawian. Only if the personality and life-style in a wider context are changed does the transitional drinker have a chance to become dry. Studies of the African healing churches that aid in basic life-style changes are needed.

Asian Americans

People whose ethnic heritage is identified with China, Japan, Korea, Southeast Asia, and such Pacific islands as Samoa, Guam, and the Philippines are identified as Asian American. According to Chang (1981), American nurses are more likely than ever before to have contact with clients from Asian backgrounds because of the recent influx of new immigrants from these countries. No one set of characteristics describes or categorizes Asian Americans, since there are similarities as well as differences among these various groups of people. Most of the specific examples in this section relate to Chinese Americans and Japanese Americans because together they constitute the largest Asian American population in the United States.

A strong Chinese influence pervades the folk systems of all Asian people. Traditional Chinese medicine is a well-organized system of medical theory with a strong philosophic character. It uses herbs, other flora, acupuncture, acupressure, massage, and nutrition principles, which also figure prominently in the holistic health movement. A resurgence of interest in traditional Chinese medicine in the People's Republic of China is resulting in the integration of these traditional forms of healing with Western biomedical science. "Barefoot doctors" in China are agricultural workers in rural communes who receive special training as part-time medical workers to provide integrated health care (Weisberg and Graham 1977). Unlike much of Western medicine, this form of health care focuses on preventing illness.

Health Care Beliefs and Practices Some of the health beliefs and practices of Asian Americans are:

• Health is present when natural forces are balanced; illness prevails if these factors are out of balance.

• There is no difference between physical and emotional illnesses.

• Mental disorder is stigmatized.

• The popular culture (family and friends) is used for mental health problems, which are reported as somatic complaints; hospitalization is suggested only for psychotic clients.

• As authorities, physicians and nurses are to be respected and obeyed. They tell the client what to do.

• Emotional control of feelings (fear, pain, anger) is good; self-assertion and expressions of individuality are not good.

• Treatments include herbs prescribed for specific ailments, nutritional therapy, moxibustion, cupping, acupuncture, and skin scraping.

Chinese folk medicine evolved from a systems view of the universe. Each organism in the universe interacts with and is affected by all others in the universe. The system derives its energy from the **yin** and **yang,** two opposing forces that must be perfectly balanced to maintain physical and mental health and social harmony (Campbell and Chang 1981). The yang is a positive force that produces light, warmth, and fullness, while the yin is a negative force that produces darkness, cold, and emptiness. In Asian American folk systems, some parts of the body are yang and others are yin. Yin and yang are also symbols for hot and cold, with yin being a cold energy force and yang a hot energy source. Hot foods are used to treat yin illnesses, and cold to treat yang illnesses. Many Hispanic Americans also share these beliefs.

Certain foods can restore balance, and herbs are also used to correct an energy imbalance. Louie (1985a) also describes other treatments.

• *Skin scraping:* Corn is dropped in water and rubbed over the skin—for heat stroke, headaches, indigestion, and colic.

• *Cupping:* A cup filled with heat is put on the skin and adheres due to the heat—for arthritis, stomach aches, bruises, and paralysis.

• *Moxibustion:* A plant is burned in a small wooden box and then the box is placed on the skin—for mumps, convulsions, nosebleeds, and backaches.

• *Acupuncture:* Needles are inserted into certain areas of the body—for many illnesses and for surgery.

• *Tai-chi exercises:* These are graceful, appear to be almost a slow motion ballet, and are performed regularly by many Chinese people.

Cao gio (coining), a treatment that is similar to skin scraping, is practiced by Cambodians and Vietnamese for fever or headache. The caregiver uses great pressure and rubs a coin up and down the person's body until red marks appear. In numerous instances children with such marks have been considered child abuse victims when they entered our Western health care system.

The Japanese code of behavior, Wabi-Sabi, has some similarities to the Chinese belief system. However, the professional should never assume that all Asians are alike. Differences among these varied cultural groups will be revealed in a cultural assessment and in the negotiation for treatment.

Family and Child-Rearing Practices Lu Jen Huang (1981) presents the Chinese Americans' history of adversity and oppression and their remarkably adaptive responses due, in part, to their strong nuclear and extended families. She notes the following characteristics of the Chinese American family:

- Usually, a close knit nuclear family

- Patriarchal authority

- Family loyalty patterns that contribute to discouragement of intermarriage

- Divorce a great shame and tragedy, especially for the woman

- Extended family with great respect for grandparents and ancestors

- Children who grow up with parents and extended family—e.g., babysitters unusual; children accompany adults on social and business occasions

- Strong control of aggression—sibling rivalry discouraged; older children to set examples for younger children and to give up pleasure in favor of someone else

- Lack of external expression of affection among family members except with infants or small children

- Filial piety and strict obedience to parents

Nursing Practice Issues Social harmony is of vital importance to Asian Americans. In an effort to maintain this harmony many avoid conflict and confrontation. This means they may smile and agree when they really disagree, and their conversation may appear vague and unfocused.

In assessing all Asian clients it is important to attempt to understand how they adjust to American society. Sue (1981) describes three possibilities:

1. The *traditionalists* retain their traditional values and reject Western beliefs and practices. Generally the older generation, traditionalists feel much conflict with the later generation, i.e., their children and grandchildren, who often give up some traditions.

2. The *marginal people* essentially "go native" and completely embrace Western values. Marginal people may have an identity crisis that is discovered during psychiatric treatment. Young refugees are often in this category. In an effort to cope, they put down traditional values and those who represent them because they appear so out of place in Western society.

3. *Asian Americans* are able over time to develop a new integrated identity while both retaining traditional beliefs and acquiring Western beliefs and practices.

The type of adjustment has implications for client care. For example, a marginal person may prefer individual therapy, whereas a traditionalist may accept only medication.

Asian medicine does not separate physical and mental illnesses the way Western medicine does. Rather, Asians express psychologic disharmony through somatic complaints such as headaches, dizziness, weakness, palpitations, and stomach aches. Because mental illness is stigmatized, clients prefer to see nurses, general practitioners, folk practitioners, and their family rather than psychiatrists or mental health workers (Flaskerud 1987).

Since the extended family unit is so important to Asians, and because the individual is subjugated to the group, individual psychotherapy may not be a useful treatment modality. Family therapy may be more useful if it emphasizes family dependence and role structures. Approaches that emphasize "communication, interpersonal feelings, feeling-touching maneuvers, introspection and egalitarian role relationships" should be avoided (Flaskerud 1987). Because Asians are private and do not generally discuss personal or family issues with strangers, an extended time period may be necessary for therapy. The nurse should be cautious in raising issues that appear conflictual or that evoke strong feelings (Louie 1985a). Because Asians will express their symptoms physically, many will want medication for relief.

Traditional Asians are suspicious of negotiation with a professional. They expect the professional to know best and prefer to be told what to do. Consequently, structure and education are useful.

Hospitalization poses a severe threat to Asians. Because they deplete all the family resources before they come to the hospital, the fear of separation from the family and the fear of death are present in the entire family system. Permitting the family to bring food and be involved in therapy is useful. Food is very symbolic to Asians. Certain foods even have medicinal purposes. In hospitals in China, families cook the food for their family members as often as possible. In China people don't say "How are you?" but "Have you eaten?" Drinking tea, an omnipresent ritual in the East, may help the client feel more welcome. Drinking tea together is an act of sharing, friendship, and social goodwill.

Asians feel that touching between strangers, boys and girls, or parents and children (after the age of 8) is inappropriate. Touching the head of a person may be construed as an attempt to rob the spirit. While Americans communicate with a wide range of facial expressions, Asians communicate primarily with their eyes.

Hiring Asian nurses and psychiatrists is a logical answer for Asian clients. However, Asian psychiatrists suggest that traditionalist clients may "lose face" by expressing their private thoughts and familial difficulties to an Asian therapist; a Western therapist would be more nonthreatening. As with blacks, the issue of countertransference (overidentification with or rejection of the client) is also significant (The Asian Pacific American 1978).

Two additional points are useful for nurses to know:

• Asians give gifts as appreciation rituals. They are offended if the gift is rejected.

• Our focus on time—the therapy "hour"—is offensive to Asians. They spend hours getting to know people and see predetermined abrupt endings as rude. More flexible time schedules are useful in enhancing a trusting relationship.

Native Americans

The category *Native Americans* refers to numerous groups of people in the United States who have different cultures but share the fact that they are our country's "native Americans" and have been oppressed by the American majority. In 1987 there were over 250 federally recognized tribes, 65 communities that have tribal status assigned by the states in which they are located, several dozen other communities that have not been formally recognized, and 209 Alaska Native villages (Manson et al. 1987). Some were sheepherders, others farmed or fished, and still others raised livestock. Most lost their land and consequently suffered from social and cultural disintegration. Today the various groups are in different stages of economic development. Generally, however, Indians are poor, or discriminated against, and have a high incidence of alcoholism and unemployment (ranging from 20–70 percent. Also, the median age of Native Americans (20.4 years) and Alaskan natives (17.9 years) is much lower than the median age of the U.S. population (30.3 years) (Manson et al. 1987). Violence, suicide and family breakdown are additional problems. Probably because of rapid culture change, some Indian tribes have been described as "self-destructing."

Health Care Beliefs and Practices Some general characteristics of Native American health care beliefs and practices are:

• Medicine and religion are inextricably linked.

• Illness occurs because a person is out of balance with nature and the universe.

• The native American church (the peyote religion) is essentially a healing ritual.

• The **shaman** (medicine man) heals with herbs and plants.

• Chanting, incantations, charms (to ward off evil), and fetishes are used in healing rituals, along with dance and the shaking of a rattle.

• Native American languages do not have clear-cut terms for mental disorders, which are seen as a lack of harmony.

• Private thoughts are kept to oneself.

In Native American culture, the world *medicine* can be equated with *mysterious*. It is linked to the supernatural religious experience central to the existence of the American Indian. According to Henderson and Primeaux (1981, p 244), it is impossible to separate Indian medicine and religion or to make distinctions between physical and mental illness.

The shaman is the central healing figure. Because the Native American theory of disease includes physical, social, psychologic, and environmental aspects, closely intertwined with spiritual and religious aspects, the germ theory is rejected. The shaman conducts a tribal healing ceremony, a highly ritualized and religious way of coping with illness and death. The shaman may also involve family members in the healing ritual, because family members (including a large extended family of cousins, aunts, uncles, etc.) are important sources of support during periods of crisis. It may be important to the family and to the client to have the healing ceremony carried out at the bedside of a hospitalized person. A medicine bundle containing charms or fetishes to ward off evil; a bag of herbs, plants, or roots to provide the curative aspect; a drum or rattle; and a special costume for the shaman may all be integral parts of the healing ceremony. The rattle may be shaken, or the drum beaten, while the healer chants the remedies revealed by the spirits.

Foods have symbolic meaning as well as nutritional value to Native Americans. For example, before visitors enter a home, the occupants sprinkle cornmeal on their shoulders to prevent them from bringing illness inside. Cornmeal may also be sprinkled around the bed of a hospitalized person or directly on the client (Henderson and Primeaux 1981, p 245).

A few authors have written about the concepts of disorder indigenous to certain Indian tribes. These authors point out the bias that exists because the descriptions of these disorders, also called culture-bound syndromes, are not analyzed within the cultural context. Studies that attempt to understand how these illnesses fit in with the life-style and world view of the people would be a useful contribution. Briefly, these disorders and their symptoms are (Trimble et al. 1984):

• *Windigo psychosis.* People with this disorder, have symptoms of melancholia and a craving for human flesh and believe that they have been transformed into a windigo, who has a heart of ice. There is disagreement over whether cannibalism really occurs.

• *Pibloqtok,* or active hysteria. In this convulsive hysterical seizure, the person at first is withdrawn and then becomes wildly excited, experiences convulsive seizures, and collapses. After sleep the individual appears perfectly normal and does not remember the experience. (See the first clinical example at the beginning of this chapter.)

• *Soul loss.* This disorder is characterized by sudden and repeated fainting, withdrawal, self-deprecation, and preoccupation with death and dead relatives.

• *Spirit intrusion.* A variety of symptoms are associated with spirit intrusion, including anorexia, insomnia, and apathy alternating with restlessness, crying spells, nostalgic dependency, dyspnea, pericardial sensations, and vague spastic pains. This disorder appears similar to what is known as agitated depression and is believed to be caused by evil spirits or ghosts.

• *Taboo breaking.* The disorder is brought on by broken taboos, usually involving sexual behavior. Symptoms can include mild weight loss, sleeplessness, fatigue, edema, headaches, heavy or irregular menstruation among women, mood swings, paranoia, and epilepticlike seizures.

• *Ghost sickness.* Believed due to evil power, ghost sickness can cause weakness; nightmares; feelings of danger, futility, and suffocation; confusion; loss of appetite; fainting; dizziness; and fear.

Dietary deficiencies are also suggested as possible causes for windigo psychosis and pibloqtok.

Family and Child-Rearing Practices   Price (1981) notes the cultural diversity of Native Americans but also presents their similarities—their precedence in North American, their rural residence on reservations, and their problems with the paternalism of the U.S. government. He discusses the following family and child-rearing practices of the native-oriented Menomini ("wild rice people" of Wisconsin).

• Social institutions helped bind the society together—e.g. clans, chiefs, councils, religious associations

• Personal characteristics of equanimity, emotional control (even under duress), autonomy, humor, and hospitality are valued.

• Children are received as reincarnated elders.

• Children and old people are close to the supernatural power that pervades all things.

• Naming is ceremonious and very important.

• Children are treated with tolerance and permissiveness—e.g., gradual weaning, casual toilet training, mild discipline.

• Children participate in social events.

• Elders tell the children stories about proper behavior.

• The group is child oriented because their purpose is to transmit traditional culture.

Nursing Practice Issues   In caring for Native Americans, the nurse needs always to be aware of the meaning given to nature and the environment. Keeping this in mind, the nurse can thoughtfully develop a nursing care plan that takes these needs into consideration. Perhaps a home health nurse can care for clients in their own environment. Nurses can also permit many family members to visit in the hospital since the family is so important. Permitting the shaman or an Indian healer to come into the hospital for curing rituals may also aid the client's recovery.

Hispanic Americans

By the year 2000 Hispanics will make up 40 percent of the United States population. The Hispanic population is generally young and has difficulties with education, housing, and employment, all of which affect their mental health needs (Hispanic Americans 1978). The Hispanic American population includes a number of diverse ethnic groups from Spanish-speaking countries in Central and South America and some Caribbean islands. It would be an error to assume that all Spanish-speaking groups share the same beliefs. Some of the subcultural differences between Mexican Americans, Puerto Ricans, and Cubans, for example, are discussed below.

It is important to recognize that many Chicanos (Mexican Americans) are not immigrants but were born in the United States. Many live in the Southwest. Puerto Ricans are United States citizens and enter and leave the country as they desire. They tend to live in New York and other areas of the Northeast. Many Cubans left their homes for political reasons and now reside in southern Florida. The group differences are directly related to their varied histories. Even the most apparent communality, language, is not always shared, since several Spanish dialects are spoken in the United States.

Health Care Beliefs and Practices   The list below summarizes many of the health care beliefs and practices of Hispanic Americans:

• The family is central to Hispanic culture. If a problem exists, the family is the first source of support.

• Older family members (especially males) must be consulted before treatment or hospitalization is accepted.

• Families keep very sick family members at home for a long time. (This can be a problem with certain physical illnesses, schizophrenia, or bipolar mood disorder.)

• If a person is hospitalized, the family wants to care for and eat and spend the night with the person. They want to share in the suffering.

• Males are responsible for elders, women, and children, so they require authority over the system and family members.

• Three concepts are basic to a Hispanic's way of life: *respeto* (intrinsic worth of the individual and subsequent pride in oneself), *cariño* (giving and receiving love at the same time), and *dignidad* (strong belief in the dignity of individuals and their value as human beings (Hispanic Americans 1978).

• Independence and interdependence are positively valued.

• There is no differentiation between physical and emotional illnesses because the mind and the body are inseparable.

• Mental illness (hospitalization or a medical diagnosis) implies stigma and loss of respect.

The fundamental belief of espiritismo is that all who have ever lived reside in the spiritual world and continue to influence the living. Facilitating communication between the two worlds can help minimize conflict and solve problems. Animal sacrifices may be used to give thanks or to appease the supernatural beings. In Miami, Florida, police are being educated about the cult of santería, including the belief of animal sacrifice, so they can be more effective when they are called to a "disturbance" (which often is a group of people practicing santería).

According to Sandoval (1983), santería offers a type of magic to people who can use it to control the supernatural forces that threaten their lives. Santería is a source of power and strength, a form of support for the believers.

Curanderismo **Curanderismo** is a folk healing system derived from Aztec Indian and Spanish cultures. The **curandero,** or folk healer, functions in the role of adviser to the Mexican-American family (especially the father) and the client. The curandero is chosen by God to help people with folk illnesses such as *susto, mal de ojo,* or *empacho* (indigestion, a ball in the stomach). Unlike espiritismo, curanderismo has no relationship to evil spirits; the curandero functions more like a health care provider in that good will and the aim of holistic care are there.

The major philosophic premises of curanderismo are (Maduro 1983, p 868):

• Disease or illness may follow strong emotional states (such as rage, fear, envy, or mourning of painful loss).

• Disease or illness may result from being out of balance or harmony with one's environment.

• A person is often the innocent victim of malevolent forces.

• The soul may become separated from the body (loss of soul).

• Cure requires the participation of the entire family.

• The natural world is not always distinguishable from the supernatural.

• Sickness often serves the social function, through increased attention, and rallying of the family around a person, of reestablishing a sense of belonging (resocialization).

• Latinos respond better to an open interaction with their healer.

• The popular system (family and friends) is the first system people turn to for help, the second is a folk healer, and the third is a medical professional.

• People are innocent victims of malevolent external or internal forces.

• **Susto** (fright sickness) has a natural cause.

• Many folk beliefs have a religious basis; accidents and illnesses are caused by the wrath of God or a saint, by the evil eye (*mal de ojo*), or *susto*.

• A hot-cold (*caliente-frio*) imbalance of body humors is responsible for disease.

Mal de Ojo **Mal de ojo** is thought to be the result of a witch purposefully casting a spell or a person involuntarily injuring a child by looking admiringly at the child. Magical amulets of coral and jet, scapulars of the saints, and tiny bags of salt or garlic around the neck or wrist are used to help protect one from the evil eye. The fear of severe injury or death from the evil eye is so great that it may contribute to what Engle (1971) calls a *lethal life situation,* an otherwise sudden and unexplained rapid death under conditions of psychologic stress.

Espiritismo and Santería Among Mexican Americans, Cubans, and Puerto Ricans, the **espiritisto,** spiritualist, or medium, is believed to be capable of putting a person in touch with the dead. **Espiritismo,** a religious cult of European origin, is a way to counteract or prevent *mal de ojo* and is also concerned with moral behavior. In contrast to the *espiritisto,* the Cuban *santero,* who is a practitioner of **santería** (the unique blend of Catholicism and mysticism referred to in the earlier clinical example of Henri), is not concerned with the client's moral behavior. Both espiritistos and santeros prescribe folk remedies, such as teas, herbs, salves, and lotions, which may be purchased in a *botánica,* a store that sells these items along with religious articles such as statues and scapulars.

Santería is a healing practice that essentially is a combination of African (Yoruba) religion, Catholicism, and espiritismo. The many cults of santería are different, but all worship the Oricha-Santo, a divinity that evolved from the blending of the Yoruba god (Oucha) and a Catholic saint. People who "make saints" are initiated into the cult of santería for a cost of up to several thousand dollars. These people may or may not become practicing priests. Initiation is a lengthy ritualistic process. Noninitiated believers may pay for an espiritisto to heal them. Meetings occur in the espiritisto's home in a room that may have an altar, pictures of saints, and candles. Many complex rituals are performed, depending on the nature of the presenting symptoms. Occasionally several mediums are present, and all help in the communication between the material and the spirit world.

Hot-Cold Theory of Disease   The hot-cold theory of disease espoused by many Hispanic Americans stems from the classic theory spelled out by Hippocrates, the father of medicine. According to the theory, it is necessary to balance blood, phlegm, black bile, and yellow bile (the four body humors) to achieve or maintain health. In her discussion of the health care needs of Spanish-speaking clients, Murillo-Rohde (1981) identifies the characteristics of each of these body humors in relation to both temperature and moisture: Blood is hot and wet, phlegm is cold and wet, black bile is cold and dry, and yellow bile is hot and dry. When the four humors are balanced and the body is warm and somewhat wet, the body is healthy. When the humors are not balanced and the body is very hot, cold, dry, wet, or any combination of these, the body may become diseased.

Treatment by using the proper "hot" (*caliente*) or "cold" (*frio*) foods, herbs, or medicines is thought to restore the body to its normal balance. Hot diseases are treated by cold foods, herbs, or medicines, and vice versa.

"Bad air" is another explanation for illness that seems to be related to the hot-cold theory of disease. "Bad air" is often night air, particularly cold air or a cold draft, thought to cause illnesses such as earache, rheumatism, facial paralysis, and tuberculosis. There is no simple explanation of "bad air," however, since it also seems to be connected to some extent with the belief that *aire* is an evil spirit, the result of witchcraft, or a dangerous emanation from a corpse or from the moon (moonlight).

Family and Child-Rearing Practices   Alvarez, Bean, and Williams (1981) point out that the size of the Mexican-American family is its most noticeable feature. They describe the following family and child-rearing practices:

• The culture is more person-oriented than goal-oriented; people are warm and emotional.

• Hispanics are less materialistic and competitive than Anglos and are oriented to the present. Material goods are only a means to an end.

• People are mannerly, polite, courteous and show deference, in contrast to Anglo practices of openness, harshness, and directness.

• The family is important to all members; an extended family is common.

• The needs of the family may take precedence over individual needs.

• The family is a place of refuge. A person who needs help will go first to a family member.

• Male dominance is valued. The father has absolute dominance over the mother and children. All major decisions are his responsibility.

• Machismo—in part sexual virility or maleness—is emphasized. Boys have more freedom than girls. Machismo also involves courage, honor, respect for others, and the belief that one should care fully for one's family and remain involved with the extended family.

• Younger people are subordinate to older people and hold them in great respect.

• Women are subservient to men and have the primary roles of homemaker and mother.

• As adolescents, girls are chaperoned to be protected from sexual advances of young men.

• Older children help with work in the family, caring for young siblings, and so on.

• Children are to be models of respect. Discipline is strict.

Nursing Practice Issues   Hispanic Americans, unlike Asian Americans or Native Americans, are an effusive people who want health care professionals both to show respect (*respeto*) and to be friendly (*personalismo*). Shaking hands and smiling are expected. The nurse who admires a child should also touch that child; not to do so may inspire fear of the evil eye.

In assessing a client who believes in spirits, witches, or santería, the nurse needs to determine if the client's beliefs are acceptable to santería or the subculture. If the belief system is out of the ordinary for the client's family or friends, the possibility of a mental disorder is greater. Symptoms attached to witchcraft or the supernatural often mimic mental disorder.

Initial interviews should include the entire family, and the nurse needs to assume an authoritative role at first. Hispanics want advice and suggestions and rely on the authority of the professional. Although North Americans openly discuss sex with caregivers, Hispanics view sex as a private topic. The nurse needs to ascertain what topics the individual or family is comfortable discussing. More sensitive areas may be saved until later. Remember also that Hispanics frequently have somatic symptoms that may indicate anxiety or depression.

After assessing whether the client is experiencing a culture conflict, the nurse determines how the conflict affects the client's mental state. Hispanics (and others from other cultural groups) often feel pressures to remain Hispanic but must become Americanized to survive. They feel familial demands not to leave the culture yet may date Anglos. All this causes discomfort and possible identity problems.

Hispanics who are still tied to their culture and believe in santería or go to a curandero may feel too embarrassed or guilty to tell the nurse. The nurse should convey acceptance of this and ask directly if they are seeking help from other sources. Then perhaps all the healers can work together for the benefit of the client, or at least the nurse can make sure that one treatment or medication is not counteracting another.

Some researchers have suggested having health clinics in the **barrio** (Hispanic neighborhood) because Hispanics prefer not to go to a mental health clinic that is distant. Research has shown that they, more than whites or blacks, take advantage of neighborhood mental health services.

Recognition that the Hispanic culture is heterogeneous should help prevent cultural stereotyping. Efforts to understand and accept the client's world view and values will help ensure a positive therapeutic encounter.

Immigrants and Refugees

In the last decade the United States has become home for increasing numbers of immigrants and refugees. *Immigrants* often leave their country by choice with varying degrees of distress; *refugees* are actually fleeing their homes, usually because of social or political upheaval. Recent immigrants generally are from China, the Middle East, and South America; refugees have flooded the United States from Cambodia and Haiti.

Both immigrants and refugees arrive in the United States in an extremely vulnerable condition. However, refugees who have witnessed a devastating war in which friends and loved ones have been killed or injured are by far the most vulnerable. In addition, women may be more conflicted by immigration because they may have had to leave their parents or young children behind; they may be victims of violence or sexual abuse, and after settlement they may have

more trouble assimilating compared to younger people and even their own children (Ogur 1990). Increased rates of mental illness are the result of such physical and psychic trauma and of sociocultural disintegration. Refugees and immigrants who appear disturbed are often taken to a psychiatric hospital. To plan culturally relevant care, nurses need an appreciation for the stresses they have undergone and are experiencing.

According to Lipson and Meleis (1985), immigrants and refugees initially experience a personal and social disorganization that may culminate in a cultural exhaustion syndrome. Being in a new and totally different world where people speak and act strangely and where they (immigrants and refugees) are usually not understood is extremely stressful. **Culture shock** is another term used to describe the feelings of depression and frustration that result from immersion in a totally different environment. The nurse may also experience culture shock when working in a different country or caring for many clients from another culture, as in a refugee center. The more different the host culture, the more potential there is for problems (Lipson and Meleis 1985).

Refugees must first meet their basic needs for survival—food, work, a home; this requires considerable energy but keeps them occupied. After these needs are met, more generalized anxiety and depression may occur. Physical illness and somatic problems are common. Ideally, a nurse coming in contact with an immigrant would obtain a cultural profile. However, if there is not enough time (for example, if a client is admitted for a psychiatric evaluation in the emergency room), a few key questions are useful (Lipson and Meleis 1985, p 50):

How long has the client been in the country? Where did the client grow up?

What language does the client speak? How well does the client know English?

What is the client's nonverbal communication style?

What are the client's religious practices?

What is the client's ethnic affilation and ethnic identity?

Who makes decisions in the family?

What systems of social support exist for the client?

On the basis of this interview and a brief mental health assessment, the nurse can begin to assess if and how cultural exhaustion or the stress of immigration contributes to the total picture. Interviews often have to be conducted with the help of an interpreter (see the Intervention boxes earlier in this chapter). Care that is relevant and focuses on the problem as perceived by the client will have a greater possibility of being effective. As nurses increase their understanding of what refugees and immigrants experience, they can better plan for their clients' needs.

CHAPTER HIGHLIGHTS

• Culture (learned behavior) shapes the way we conceive of illness. Culture determines not only who is labeled mentally ill and under what circumstances but also the nature of the treatment and the identity of the helper.

• Recently culture has been recognized as a relevant variable in nursing care.

• Understanding the following key concepts from anthropology is vital in appreciating the relevance of culture to psychiatric nursing: holism, culture, world view, ethnocentrism, cultural relativism.

• Culturally relevant and sensitive nursing care requires that the nurse take a client's culture into consideration when planning care.

• Obtaining a cultural profile and eliciting the client's explanatory model of illness are vital steps in the nursing process.

• Nurses need to be careful not to stereotype clients from different cultural groups.

• Nurses are in a good position to function as culture brokers and to mediate between people or groups from two cultures.

• Being aware of clients' folk health care systems will help the nurse provide better health care to particular groups of people.

• Understanding the three domains of health care—professional, folk, popular—and the client's use of them is helpful to the nursing process.

• Natural support systems are vital to a client's well-being.

• Racial and ethnic factors are linked to people's biologic makeup, which directly affects their responses to medication.

• Cultural heritage also affects what health care professionals believe about clients and how they care for clients.

REFERENCES

Ailinger R: Beliefs about treatment of hypertension among Hispanic older persons. *Topics Clin Nurs* 1985;7:26–31.

Allport G: *The Nature of Prejudice.* Addison-Wesley, 1954.

Alvarez D, Bean F, Williams D: The Mexican-American family, in Mindel C, Habenstein R: *Ethnic Families in America.* Elsevier, 1981.

Amarasingham L: Social and cultural perspectives on medication refusal. *Am J Psychiatry* 1980;137:353–58.

The Asian Pacific American. *Cultural Issues in Contemporary Psychiatry* (tape). Smith, Kline and French, 1978.

Aylesworth L, Ossorio P, Osaki L: Stress and mental health among Vietnamese in the United States, in Endo R, Sue S, Wagner N (eds): *Asian-Americans: Social and psychological Perspectives.* Basic Books, 1978.

Beals A: *Culture in Process.* Holt, Rinehart and Winston, 1979.

Boggs J: Uprooting racism and racists in the United States, in Colombo G, Cullen R, Lisle B (eds): *Rereading America.* St Martin's Press, 1989.

Brantley T: Racism and its impact on psychotherapy. *Am J Psychiatry* 1983;140:1605–1608.

Brink P: Value orientations as an assessment tool in cultural diversity. *Nurs Res* 1984;33:198–203.

Campbell T, Chang B: Health care of the Chinese in America, in Henderson G, Primeaux M (eds): *Transcultural Health Care.* Addison-Wesley, 1981.

Campinha-Bacote J: Culturological assessment: An important factor in psychiatric consultation-liaison nursing. *Arch Psychiatr Nursing* 1988;2(4):244–250.

Capers C: Nursing and the Afro-American client. *Topics Clin Nurs* 1985;7:11–17.

Chang B: Asian-American patient care, in Henderson G, Primeaux M (eds): *Transcultural Health Care.* Addison-Wesley, 1981.

Chapman J, Chapman H: *Psychology of Health Care: A Humanistic Perspective.* Wadsworth Health Sciences, 1983.

Chaves D, LaRochelle D: The universality of nursing: A comprehensive framework for practice. *Int Nurs Rev* 1985;32:10–13.

Colombo G, Cullen R, Lisle B: *Rereading America.* St Martin's Press, 1989.

Dougherty MC, Tripp-Reimer T: The interface of nursing and anthropology. *Am Rev Anthropol* 1985;14:219–241.

Ebigbo P: Development of a cultural specific (Nigeria) screening scale of somatic complaints indicating psychiatric disturbance. *Culture Med Psychiatry* 1982:6:29–34.

Egan M: A family assessment challenge: Refugee youth and foster family adaptation. *Topics Clin Nurs* 1985;7:64–69.

Eisenthal S et al.: Adherence and the negotiated approach to patienthood. *Arch Gen Psychiatry* 1979;36:393–398.

Engle G: Sudden and rapid death during psychological stress: Folklore or folk wisdom? *Ann Intern Med* 1971;74:771–782.

Flaskerud J: Perceptions of problematic behavior by Appalachians, mental health professionals, and lay non-Appalachians. *Nurs Res* 1980;29:140–149.

Flaskerud J: A proposed protocol for culturally relevant nursing psychotherapy. *Clin Nurs Specialist* 1987;1(4):150–157.

Fong C: Ethnicity and nursing practice. *Topics Clin Nurs* 1985;7:1–10.

Foreman J: Susto and the health needs of the Cuban refugee population. *Topics Clin Nurs* 1985;7:40–47.

Foulkes E: The concept of culture in psychiatric residency education. *Am J Psychiatry* 1980;137:811–816.

Frank J: Foreword, in Kiev A (ed): *Magic, Faith, and Healing.* Free Press, 1964.

Garrison V: Support systems of schizophrenic and non-schizophrenic Puerto Rican migrant women in New York City. *Schizophr Bull* 1978;4:561–596.

Good B, Kleinman A: Epilogue: Culture and depression, in Kleinman A, Good B: *Culture and Depression.* University of California Press, 1985.

Griffith E: Blacks and American psychiatry. *Hosp Community Psychiatry* 1986;35:5.

Guarnaccia P, Rubio-Stipek M, Canino G: Ataques de nervios in the Puerto Rican diagnostic interview schedule: The impact of cultural categories on psychiatric epidemiology. *Culture Med Psychiatry* 1989;13:275–295.

Hale J: The Black woman and childrearing, in Rodgers-Rose L: *The Black Woman.* Sage, 1980.

Harwood A: *Ethnicity and Medical Care.* Harvard University Press, 1981.

Haviland W: *Cultural Anthropology.* Holt, Rinehart and Winston, 1983.

Henderson G, Primeaux M (eds): *Transcultural Health Care.* Addison-Wesley, 1981.

Hispanic Americans. *Cultural Issues in Contemporary Psychiatry* (tape). Smith, Kline and French, 1978.

Huang L: The Chinese-American family, in Mindel C, Habenstein R: *Ethnic Families in America.* Elsevier, 1981.

Hutchinson SA, Wilson HS: American nurses on safari: An illustration of coping with cultural complexity. *Pub Health Nurs* 1985;2(3):153–158.

Jones B, Gray B: Problems in diagnosing schizophrenia and affective disorders among blacks. *Hosp Community Psychiatry* 1986;37:61–65.

Kleinman A, Eisenberg L, Good B: Culture, illness and care: Clinical lessons from anthropologic and cross-cultural research. *Ann Intern Med* 1978;88:251–258.

LaFargue J: Mediating between two views of illness. *Topics Clin Nurs* 1985;7:70–77.

Lawson W: Racial and ethnic factors in psychiatric research. *Hosp Community Psychiatry* 1986;37:50–53.

Lefley H: Culture and chronic mental illness. *Hosp Community Psychiatry* 1990;41(3):277–286.

Leighton A: Culture and Psychiatry. *Can J Psychiatry* 1981;26:522–529.

Leininger M: *Nursing and Anthropology: Two Worlds to Blend.* John Wiley and Sons, 1970.

Lin T: Psychiatry and Chinese culture. *West J Med* 1983;139:862–874.

Lipson J, Meleis A: Culturally appropriate care: The case of immigrants. *Topics Clin Nurs* 1985;7:48–56.

Louie K: Providing heath care to Chinese clients. *Topics Clin Nurs* 1985a;7:18–25.

Louie K: Transcending cultural bias: The literature speaks. *Topics Clin Nurs* 1985b;7:78–84.

MacDonald A: Folk health practices among north coastal Peruvians: Implications for nursing. *Image* 1981;13:51–55.

Maduro R: Curanderismo and Latino views of disease and curing. *West J Med* 1983;139:868–884.

Manson S et al.: Psychiatric assessment and treatment of American Indians and Alaska natives. *Hosp Community Psychiatry* 1987;38(2):165–1783.

Manson S et al.: The depressive experience in American Indian communities: A challenge for psychiatric theory and diagnosis, in Kleinman A, Good B (eds): *Culture and Depression.* University of California Press, 1985.

McAdoo J: Involvement of fathers in the socialization of Black children, in McAdoo H: *Black Families.* Sage, 1981.

McGoldrick M, Rohrbaugh M: Researching ethnic family stereotypes. *Family Process* 1987;26(1):89–99.

Mead M (ed): *Cultural Patterns and Technical Change,* UNESCO. New American Library, 1955.

Murillo-Rohde I: Hispanic American patient care, in Henderson G, Primeaux M (eds): *Transcultural Health Care.* Addison-Wesley, 1981.

Nichter M: Idioms of distress: Alternatives in the expression of psychosocial distress: A case study from south India. *Culture Med Psychiatry* 1981;5:379–408.

Nikelly A: Does DSM-III-R diagnose depression in non-Western patients? *Int J Social Psychiatry* 1988;34(4):316–320.

Nobles W: Africanity in Black families. *The Black Scholar.* June, 1975.

Ogur B: Mental health problems of translocated women. *Health Care Women Int* 1990:11(1):43–47.

Orque M, Bloch B, Monrroy L: *Ethnic Nursing Care.* Mosby, 1983.

Papajohn J, Spiegel J: *Transactions in Families.* Jossey Bass, 1975.

Peltzer K: Causative and intervening factors of harmful alcohol consumption and cannabis use in Malawi. *Int J Addictions* 1989;24(2):79–85.

Peters M: Parenting in Black families with young children, in McAdoo H: *Black Families.* Sage, 1981.

Price J: North American Indian families, in Mindel C. Habenstein R: *Ethnic Families in America.* Elsevier, 1981.

Putsch R: Cross-cultural communications. *JAMA* 1985; 254:3344–3348.

Randall-David E: *Mama Always Said: The Transmission of Health Care Beliefs among Three Generations of Rural Black Women,* dissertation. University of Florida, Gainesville, Florida, 1985.

Reese M: A tragedy in Santa Monica. *Newsweek* May 6, 1985, p 10.

Reeves K: Hispanic utilization of an ethnic mental health clinic. *J Psychosoc Nurs* 1986;24(2):23–26.

Roberson M: The influence of religious beliefs on health choices of Afro-Americans. *Topics Clin Nurs* 1985; 7:57–63.

Rozendal N: Understanding Italian American cultural norms. *J Psychosoc Nurs* 1987;25(2):29–33.

Ruiz M: Open-closed mindedness, intolerance of ambiguity and nursing faculty attitudes toward culturally different patients. *Nurs Res* 1981;30:177–181.

Sandoval M: Santeria. *J Fla Med Assoc* 1983;70:620–628.

Schor J: Wabi-sabi. *JAMA* 1984;252:3173.

Schwartz D: Caribbean folk beliefs and Western psychiatry. *J Psychosoc Nurs* 1985;23(11):26–30.

Snow L: Folk medical beliefs and their implications for care of patients. *Ann Intern Med* 1974;81:82–96.

Sobralske M: Perceptions of health: Navajo Indians. *Topics Clin Nurs* 1985;7:32–39.

Spector R: *Cultural Diversity in Health and Illness.* Appleton-Century-Crofts, 1979.

Stern P: Solving problems of cross-cultural health teaching: The Filipino childbearing family. *Image* 1981;13:47–50.

Sue D (ed): *Counseling the Culturally Different: Theory and Practice.* Wiley, 1981.

Trimble J et al.: American Indian concepts of mental health, in Pederson P, Santorious N, Marsella A (eds): *Mental Health Services and the Cross-Cultural Context.* Sage, 1984.

Tripp-Reimer T: Barriers to health care: Variations in interpretation of Appalachian client behavior by Appalachian and non-Appalachian health care professionals. *West J Nurs Res* 1984;4:179–191.

Tripp-Reimer T: Reconceptualizing the construct of health: Integrating emic and etic perspectives. *Res Nurs* 1984;7:101–10-9.

Tripp-Reimer T, Brink P, Saunders J: Cultural assessment: Content and process. *Nurs Outlook* 1984;32:78–82.

Tripp-Reimer T, Dougherty M: Cross-cultural nursing research. *Am Rev Nurs Res* 1985;3:77–104.

Weisberg M, Graham J: *A Barefoot Doctor's Manual.* Cloudburst Press of America, 1977.

Westermeyer J: Clinical considerations in cross-cultural diagnosis. *Hosp Community Psychiatry* 1987;38(2):160–165.

White J: Black family life, in Colombo G, Cullen R, Lisle B (eds): *Rereading America.* St Martin's Press, 1989.

Wilson HS, Hutchinson SA: Contemporary mental health care in the People's Republic of China. *Am J Nurs* 1983;83(3):393–395.

Zhi-Zhang L: Traditional Chinese concepts of mental health *JAMA* 1984;252:3169.

Legal Issues and Clients' Rights

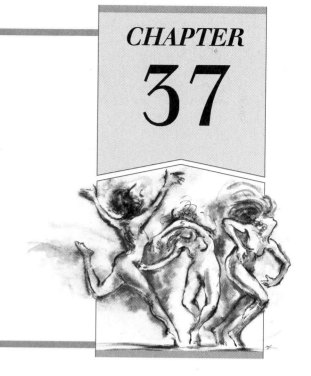

LEARNING OBJECTIVES

- Describe the historical roots of current mental health law
- Relate mental health legislation to humanistic psychiatric nursing practice
- Describe the relationship between the legal and civil rights of mental health clients and humanistic psychiatric nursing practice
- Identify and discuss advocacy interventions in psychiatric nursing
- Identify the major components of mental health legislation
- Analyze key court decisions about mental health laws
- Identify liability issues and safeguards
- Compare the four major rules or tests that are used in an insanity defense

Joanne Keglovits

CROSS REFERENCES

Other topics relevant to this content are: Clients' rights regarding electroconvulsive therapy, medication, and other biologic therapies, Chapter 32; Deinstitutionalization, Chapter 38; Ethical dilemmas, Chapter 7; History of moral treatment, Chapter 1; Milieu aspects, Chapter 31; Monitoring treatment compliance among the chronically mentally ill, Chapter 17.

JUDICIAL, LEGISLATIVE, POLITICAL, AND economic decisions profoundly influence mental health practice. Many factors bring about changes in the understanding and practice of mental health intervention. These changes challenge the psychiatric nurse to examine central issues, such as the definition of *mental health*, decision-making, clients' and society's rights, liability, and accountability. This examination requires a surrender of past ideas and generally improves care, but it often confuses the boundaries of mental health practice and the law. This confusion entraps mental health professionals, lawyers, families, clients, and the public in a muddle of conflicting policies and procedures.

The individual rights of minority groups, including the mentally disordered, have taken on new meaning over the past twenty years. Many of the values implied by a humanistic perspective are now mandated by law. These values, however, blur the boundaries between public and individual good, voluntary and involuntary treatment, and informed and uninformed consent, and this blurring of boundaries makes the development and implementation of policies difficult. In addition, a client's right to privacy, to receive and refuse treatment, and to define happiness and growth pivot on society's values.

This chapter attempts to bring some clarity to the ever-changing relationship between the law and mental health services so that nurses can not only practice with confidence but also exercise their power as citizens and professionals to influence the direction of mental health care.

Historical and Theoretic Foundations

Before reviewing contemporary legal practice, this chapter takes a brief historical look at the relationship between the law and the state of mind known by many names, including madness, lunacy, and mental illness.

Laws develop in a social context, ideally in response to the problems and needs of the governed. Traditionally, mental disability was considered a private matter, except where either public safety or legal issues (usually regarding property) were at stake. Only in the last few hundred years has society been seeking out its mentally disturbed members to do something for them.

Greek and Roman Law

Greek and Roman law took account of "mad" people chiefly in relation to protection of the community and protection of the mad person's property. From Plato's

Laws we learn that the insane were generally not held responsible for criminal actions. Slaves defective in mind or body could not be sold, and a fine was levied against both slaveholders and families who let their mad members loose in the city.

English Law

In early England the feudal lord assumed guardianship of a mentally disordered person and control of the person's property. After consolidation of the crown in the thirteenth century, this function was assumed by the king, who, as *parens patriae* (father of his country), was considered the protector of the personal and property interests of his subjects. The parens patriae doctrine is one rationale for present-day commitment statutes.

Law in Colonial America

The North American colonists brought to the New World not only their worldly possessions but also much of the culture and tradition of their mother countries. Mental disorder was generally not recognized as a major medical problem or a pressing social concern in the United States in the seventeenth and eighteenth centuries. North American society was still largely rural, and in most cases the insane could be dealt with in an informal manner.

Early Commitment Laws

In the second quarter of the nineteenth century, a number of factors combined to make traditional and informal mechanisms ineffectual. It was a time of immigration of ethnic minorities, of rapid population growth, and of periodic economic depressions and unemployment. The emphasis was on the establishment of institutions to take care of those who could not take care of themselves. This could take the form of the poorhouse, almshouse, jail, or asylum. Massachusetts and New York established state hospitals in which to segregate and treat the insane.

The movement for state mental hospitals was also accelerated throughout the country by the crusade of Dorothea Dix. Dix's determination about this single issue gained her a broad base of support, and she was eventually responsible for founding or enlarging over thirty mental hospitals. (See Chapter 1.)

Even though mental hospitals increased in size and number, **commitment** procedures continued to be easy and informal, without much concern for the individual's right to liberty. During the 1840s, two lawsuits in particular captured the legal profession's, and to a certain extent the public's, attention regarding the problem of personal liberty and wrongful civil commitment. In 1845, Josiah Oakes, using the common law right of *habeas corpus* (a writ requiring the agency holding a person in custody to show that it is doing so legally and properly), successfully petitioned the Massachusetts Supreme Court for his release from McLean Asylum in Massachusetts on the grounds that he had been illegally committed by his family. In its decision, *Matter of Oakes*, 8 Law Rptr 123 (Mass Sup Ct 1845), the court acknowledged that no person should be deprived of life or liberty without due process of law and that both dangerousness and need for treatment were commitment criteria.

This decision is said to have set a new precedent for the detention of the alleged insane. The old standard of "detention of the violent" was not applicable in this case. Oakes had been detained for "therapeutic reasons," because he was thought to suffer from hallucinations and was conducting his business affairs in an unsound manner. The charge grew out of the fact that Oakes, an elderly and generally judicious man, had become engaged to a woman of questionable character shortly after his wife's death.

The second case that drew attention, particularly from physicians and hospital employees who were regularly involved in commitment proceedings, was that of Hinchman (Brakel et al. 1985). Hinchman, an inmate at the Friends' Asylum in Philadelphia, instituted a civil suit for wrongful detention. The suit was filed against his family, the physician, and the hospital employees involved in his commitment. In addition to regaining his freedom, he succeeded in obtaining damages.

Commitment legislation was seen as necessary not only to safeguard the prospective client but also to protect hospital employees. With recovery rates declining and reports that a large number of insane persons were still in almshouses despite the increase in the number and cost of asylums, mental hospitals came under attack. The publication of exposés by former mental clients added fuel to the fires of public mistrust of these hospitals.

Much of the lunacy legislation enacted in the United States during the 1870s was a reaction to public distrust of mental hospitals. The emphasis in the legislation was on preventing the commitment of sane individuals. Once the question of sanity was settled, protective legislation usually ended. The model for lunacy legislation was the criminal law system, with its procedural safeguards of sworn complaints, open hearings, and jury trials. Unlike criminal sentences, however, commitments were for an indefinite period of time. Civil rights were automatically taken away during confinement.

In 1890 New York passed the State Care Act, making the state primarily responsible for the cost of hospitalizing its indigent clients. Other states followed suit, and the state system continued to predominate until the middle of the twentieth century.

Twentieth-Century Mental Hygiene Laws

Despite many advances in psychiatric theory and treatment, nineteenth-century legal practices remained on the statute books of most states well into the twentieth century. Over the years, however, commitment procedures lost many of their protective elements. After World War II, prominent psychiatrists and psychiatric organizations began attacking these commitment laws on the ground that they were hindering the delivery of good psychiatric care to the mentally ill. Words such as *escapee* and *parole* were believed to stigmatize the mentally disordered, and jury trials were said to be traumatizing rather than helpful. Leaders of this reform movement in the late 1940s and early 1950s reasoned that "railroading" or wrongful commitment was a myth.

One of the results of this movement was the model legislation published in 1952 by the National Institute of Mental Health, which advocated:

- Increased use of admission on a voluntary basis

- Admission on medical certification

- Nonjudicial proceedings for involuntary hospitalization

- Opportunities for clients to protest after admission

Many states followed the recommendations and updated their mental health statutes. New York State added a new statewide agency, the Mental Health Review or Information Service, to make sure the procedural rights of involuntary clients were followed.

In the last twenty years the courts have had an impact on the direction of mental health legislation and state statutes. As a review of history tells us, the courts have traditionally been concerned with the possibility of wrongful commitment. Little attention was paid to the restrictions placed on the legal and civil rights of an individual once hospitalized. In recent years, however, the courts have become more concerned with the substantive rights of a hospitalized individual, including the right to treatment, the right not to perform institutional labor, and retention of civil rights such as the rights to communication, visitation, religious activities, and medical self-determination. This is reflected in many state statutes, along with an emphasis on procedural safeguards centering on involuntary commitment.

The Client Advocacy Role of the Psychiatric Nurse

Gaps between Theory and Practice

The rights clients have in theory and those in actual practice are often quite different. Richard Price and Bruce Denner (1973, p 7) aptly comment on this phenomenon: "Although Pinel was able to remove the chains from the inmates of the Bicêtre by declaring that they were mentally ill, today may people lose a substantial portion of their human and civil rights when the same declaration is made about them." This discrepancy between rights in theory and practice is often cited but has received little systematic attention.

This discrepancy exists for two basic reasons: (1) the struggle between client and provider rights and authority and (2) the "medical model" approach. For example, Szasz and others contend that within the medical model an individual is labeled "mentally ill" because of certain behavior or "symptoms." The label implies that sickness will prevent the client from knowing what is good in the way of treatment.

The gap between the rights clients have in theory and in practice may be the result of a knowledge deficit on the part of treatment providers. The remedy is simple: educate the treatment providers so that they in turn can educate their clients. Another possibility that may not be so amenable to an easy solution is that direct care treatment providers are threatened by the expansion of clients' rights. When asked to comment on a California court's mandated review of psychoactive medication for involuntary clients, over 90 percent of nursing staff said the new regulation not only hampered treatment but made their job both more difficult and more dangerous (Hargreaves et al. 1987).

In 1985, legislation was enacted and funding became available to states for external protection (i.e., protection other than by treatment providers) and advocacy programs. This funding was extended in 1988 for another three-year period. These state advocacy programs have the authority to investigate reported incidents of neglect and abuse of the mentally ill in public or private hospitals, residential facilities, and nursing homes. See the Research Note for an example of an advocacy service for community residents.

Although laws can protect certain aspects of human rights, there is a far greater area that laws cannot protect. Laws rarely have a direct effect on a person's beliefs, values, and attitudes, which to a great extent determine whether the letter or the spirit of the law will be carried out. Psychiatric nurses practicing from a humanistic perspective are often in a position to advocate both the letter and the spirit of clients' rights.

Physical and Psychologic Abuse of Clients

Clients are particularly vulnerable to both physical and psychologic abuse and often do not have the ability or power to defend themselves. There is little actual data on how much client abuse exists in treatment settings. One advocate group ranked client abuse to be the most frequent rights violation complaint. Another ranked it third. These are the types of abuse reported to occur with some frequency:

• Supplying clients with drugs or alcohol in return for favors

• Making privileges contingent on favors from clients

• Slapping and kicking clients when staff felt frustrated

• Using restraints when other less intrusive alternatives were available

• Verbal harassment including threats, sarcasm, and other "put-downs"

• General threats of harm if clients do not behave "appropriately" or as they are told

• Inhumane physical facilities

Advocacy Strategies for Psychiatric Nurses

Psychiatric nursing intervention would be directed at some of the identifying causes that may lead to client abuse, including:

• Unsuitability of certain staff who do not have the patience or understanding to work with clients having trouble with control

• A buildup of stresses that have reduced both the staff's patience and ability to problem solve (burnout)

• An actual lack of knowledge of other means of interacting with clients in a high-stress situation

Other areas of advocacy include:

• Educating clients and their families about their legal rights

• Monitoring treatment planning and delivery of service for abuse of clients' rights

• Evaluating policies and procedures regarding clients' rights infringement

RESEARCH NOTE

Citation
Freddolino P, Moxley D, Fleishman J: An advocacy model for people with long-term psychiatric disabilities. Hosp Community Psychiatry 1989; 40(11):1169–1174.

Study Problem/Purpose
The purpose of this study was to examine the impact of one advocacy model, Client Support and Representation (CSR), on recipients of mental health services in a community setting. It was hypothesized that recipients of CSR services would be better able to cope with the stresses of daily living and thereby reduce their need for hospitalization.

Methods
Over a three and one-half year period, 359 men and women between the ages of 18 to 65 were recruited prior to discharge from psychiatric and residential programs and randomly assigned to an experimental (*n*=222) or a control group (*n*=137). The experimental CSR model included an initial and continuing identification of problems by the client along with at least one weekly telephone contact and one monthly meeting. Problem identification was targeted to those areas correlated with successful community living, such as housing, income and benefits, employment, legal issues, medication, physical and mental health needs, transportation, and personal social and family issues. From the problem list clients were asked to identify specific goals and were encouraged to be as active as they could in attaining those goals. CSR services were available for six months.

Information about mental health service utilization was collected for the period two months before and twelve months after recruitment. For clients in the experimental group, a detailed list of needs, identified problems, and resolved problems was maintained. The self-report Hopkins symptoms checklist, used to monitor psychiatric symptoms, was administered at the recruitment interview and then again after two, five, and twelve months.

Findings
Clients in the CSR program were hospitalized significantly fewer days than clients in the control group. However, once the advocacy services terminated, the differences in hospitalization rates between the two groups disappeared. Client problems clustered around the nuts and bolts of community living, such as income, benefits (Supplemental Social Security, delayed checks, and so on), housing, legal issues (bad debts to utilities, credit cards, traffic violations). Requests for help obtaining health services (physical, mental, and dental) and employment came next in terms of client priority.

Implications
Advocacy services have traditionally focused on rights protection, with an emphasis on abuse and neglect in an in-patient setting. This study identified an advocacy model that helped frequent users of mental health services to live more successfully in the community. The proposed model is similar to the advocacy function of case management, in that it responds to needs identified by clients. However, unlike case managers, advocates are not involved with clinical issues and do not act as service coordinators or identify with mental health services. CSR advocates are free to fulfill their primary roles of educator, mentor, and coach to help clients act for themselves as much as possible in problem solving and goal attainment.

• Making sure clients have the necessary information to make an informed decision or give an informed consent

• Questioning other health professionals when their care is based more on stereotypic ideas than an assessment of the client's needs

• Speaking out for safe practice conditions when threatened by budget cutbacks

Overview of Mental Health Laws and Judicial Decisions

The two functions of law are social control and conflict settlement. These are best understood as a political mechanism. The four primary sources of law in this country, at both the state and federal level are: (1) constitutional law, (2) statutory law, (3) administrative law, and (4) common law.

Constitutional law legitimizes statutory, administrative, and common law. *Statutes* are the written laws passed by the legislatures in response to the perceived need for social regulation. Each state has a mental health statute. Individuals or groups can influence the process not only by voting for specific candidates but also by testifying before committees and submitting written proposals or briefs for public hearings on proposed changes in mental health legislation. Nursing practice acts are another example of statutory law. Each state has statutes spelling out procedures for mental hospital admission and discharge. Some states also have statutes on the medical and legal rights of individuals once they are in the hospital.

Administrative law comes from the rules and regulations promulgated by administrative departments and offices as they operationalize the broadly worded statutes into standards. For example, each state mental health statute also has an accompanying book of regulations spelling out the implementation process.

The fourth source of law is *common,* or court-made, law. Common law develops as the courts decide specific cases. A ruling by a court establishes precedent for all lower courts within its jurisdiction. Interpreting the statutes and their compliance with basic constitutional rights is the primary function of the United States Supreme Court. A Supreme Court ruling sets precedent for all courts in the United States. The Supreme Court accepts only a small percentage of the cases referred to it and will accept only those cases involving a right guaranteed by the Constitution. The Supreme Court usually chooses and rules on narrow issues. However, the decision sets precedent for further litigation.

The review of mental health laws and judicial decisions underscores the fact that there is great variability from state to state.

Admission Categories

The two major categories of hospitalization are **voluntary admission** and **involuntary commitment**. Admission and release procedures differ accordingly. They are described below and compared in Table 37–1.

Voluntary Admission   All states now have some provision for voluntary admission. Voluntary admission comes about by written application for admission by prospective clients, or someone acting in their behalf, such as a parent or guardian. As the word *voluntary* implies, the client has a right to demand and obtain release. However, all states but California have what is called a "grace period" in which the client agrees to give notice, usually in writing, of intention to leave. Depending on the statute, this grace period can last from twenty-four hours (in Arizona) to fifteen days (in Oklahoma). It is justified on the ground that the hospital staff needs time to examine the client to determine whether a change to involuntary status is indicated. The extra time also gives family and staff the opportunity to persuade the client to remain voluntarily. This "conditional provision" is seen by some as a covert form of involuntary hospitalization.

There are now statutory assurances in over half the states, compared with just nine a decade ago, that voluntary clients must be adequately informed of their rights and status.

Informal voluntary admission, an alternative to the structure and personal concessions required in voluntary admission, is an option in at least ten states, including New York, Pennsylvania, Connecticut, and Illinois. This procedure is akin to that required in a medical admission. The prospective in-patient verbally requests admission and is free to leave the institution at any time. Informal voluntary admission procedures are more likely to be an option in general and pri-

TABLE 37–1   **Voluntary and Involuntary Hospitalization Compared**

	VOLUNTARY ADMISSION			INVOLUNTARY COMMITMENT	
	Informal	*Voluntary*	*Emergency*	*Temporary*	*Extended*
Released	Anytime	Usually conditional	Average after 3 to 5 days	48 hours to 6 months	After from 60 to 180 days or an indeterminate time
Use	Limited	Increasing	Increasing	Increasing	Decreasing
Criteria for admission	Client request	Client request	Usually client dangerousness	Client dangerousness or need of care and treatment	Client dangerousness or need of care and treatment

vate facilities than in state institutions, and they account for a small percentage (less than 1 percent to 9 percent) of all admissions in states that have this provision.

Involuntary Commitment The state's ability to hospitalize or commit an individual involuntarily is sanctioned by one of two state powers:

1. Police power enables the state to hospitalize people who are considered dangerous to others because of their illness.

2. Parens patriae power enables the state to take on the role of protector and assume responsibility for people considered dangerous to themselves or unable to care for themselves in a potentially dangerous situation because of a mental disability.

Most states provide for more than one involuntary hospitalization procedure. Involuntary hospitalization can come about if the designated body, such as a court, an administrative tribunal, or the required number of physicians find that the prospective client's mental state meets the statutory criteria for involuntary commitment. The criteria vary from state to state according to the type of involuntary hospitalization. However, all state involuntary commitment statutes can be expected to include one or more of the following criteria:

- Dangerous to self or others

- Unable to provide for basic needs

- Mentally ill

In an increasing number of states (now 25), involuntary commitment is justified only if the individual is dangerous to self or others because of a mental disorder. The remaining states augment this by stating that the client's need for care and treatment may also justify commitment. See Brakel et al. (1985) for specific state laws governing civil commitment.

Involuntary hospitalization can be divided into three categories: (1) emergency, (2) temporary or observational, and (3) extended or indeterminate. Civil commitment to outpatient psychiatric treatment is also possible in a number of states.

Emergency Emergency involuntary hospitalization is available in all but Alabama, Arkansas, and Mississippi. It is a temporary measure with limited, short-range goals, and it deals largely with the prevention of behavior likely to create a "clear and present" danger to the client or others. Under common law any official or private person has the right to detain a dangerous mentally disordered person.

Some formal application is required to initiate emergency detention. In some states any citizen may make the application. In others it is limited to police officers, health officers, and physicians. Because this type of involuntary admission is an emergency measure and is warranted only until the appropriate legal steps can be taken, the statutes limit the amount of time an individual can be detained. The limits range from twenty-four hours in states such as Arizona, Georgia, and Michigan to twenty days in New Jersey. The usual practice is to allow detention for three to five days.

Temporary or Observational Temporary or observational involuntary hospitalization can be described as the involuntary commitment of an allegedly mentally deranged individual for a specified period of time to allow for adequate observation so that a diagnosis can be made and treatment instituted. The actual time period varies. It can be as short as forty-eight hours (in Alaska) and as long as six months (in West Virginia).

In some states, any citizen can make an application for the temporary hospitalization of a person in need of aid. Others require a family member or guardian, a health or welfare officer, or a physician to apply. Temporary hospitalization may be brought about by the medical certification of one or two physicians or may require further approval by a judge, justice, or district attorney in some jurisdictions.

At the end of the observation period, several options are available. The treating physician may (1) discharge the client, (2) have the client stay voluntarily, or (3) file an application for extended hospitalization. In at least nine states, observational hospitalization is mandatory before a court ruling in favor of extended hospitalization.

Extended or Indeterminate Indeterminate or extended involuntary hospitalization can come about through either judicial or nonjudicial procedures. *Judicial* hospitalization procedures require that a judge or jury determine whether the person is mentally ill to a degree that requires extended hospitalization. If so, the court orders the client hospitalized for an extended period (60 to 180 days) or an indeterminate time.

Proceedings are usually initiated by an application for hospitalization of an allegedly mentally ill person. About half the states permit any responsible person or citizen to make or swear to the application. Others allow only one or more of the following groups: relatives, public officers, physicians, and hospital superintendents. Supporting medical evidence may or may not be required at the time of application.

Most states having judicial hospitalization procedures make some provision for a prehearing medical examination in addition to the medical certification required to support the application. In all forty-eight jurisdictions having judicial hospitalization procedures, it is mandatory to notify the person proposed to be hospitalized of the proposed hearing. The large majority of states also require notice to the client's attorney, family, or guardian.

A hearing is mandatory in most states, although a few states leave it to the client to request it. While the client's presence is required at the hearing in a few states, most states merely permit attendance if it is not thought to be harmful to the client's condition or if the client in fact demands it. Few states require the hearing to be held in a courtroom. Most say the place is entirely discretionary.

Jury trials are no longer mandatory in any state, but fifteen states still have provisions for the use of a jury to decide the question of hospitalization.

Nonjudicial procedures for extended or indeterminate involuntary hospitalization include both administrative and medical certification, but such procedures are much less prominent on the statute books than they were a decade ago. Three states (Nebraska, South Dakota, and West Virginia) have provisions for administrative hospitalization procedures. Extended hospitalization is brought about by an administrative board, which basically follows the same procedure used in judicial hospitalization.

Involuntary hospitalization by *medical certification*, an alternative to the more traditional judicial commitment, is possible in eight states and the District of Columbia. It is usually advocated for clients who are incapable of consenting to voluntary treatment, although they do not protest hospitalization. The need for hospitalization is usually determined by an examination by one or more physicians and documented by a medical certificate. All states having medical certification provide either for judicial proceedings if the client contests the hospitalization at any time after certification or for expanded habeas corpus proceedings.

Involuntary Outpatient Commitment A growing number of states have modified their statutes and regulations to allow for court-ordered outpatient treatment. Although this option is not widely used at present, Perlin (1989) predicts it will be one of the growth areas in involuntary law in the near future. In most states allowing for involuntary outpatient commitment, the criteria are similar to that necessary for in-patient commitment; i.e., proof of mental illness and dangerousness. A few states have passed statutes permitting preventive commitment, considered by legal scholars to be a variation of involuntary outpatient commitment. In these instances outpatient commitment is used to avert a further deterioration of the person's mental health that would require in-patient hospitalization. Jemelka et al. (1989), in a review article on the mentally ill in prison, suggest involuntary outpatient commitment as one way to ensure that mentally ill offenders follow through with outpatient treatment once they are released from prison. Conditional release, a concept related to outpatient commitment, is discussed later in this chapter.

Dilemmas Associated with Involuntary Commitment Involuntary hospitalization is an exercise of power and like all power can be abused. Because of this potential for abuse, commitment criteria are important. In this country, a person's loss of liberty can be justified only under certain circumstances. Loss of individual freedom through incarceration is generally accepted as justified if one is charged with a crime. In the past individuals were quarantined if they had a contagious disease such as tuberculosis. Today debates continue regarding the restriction of activities of HIV-infected individuals and the public's right to safety.

As the review of mental health statutes shows, a degree of "dangerousness" is the favored justification for loss of liberty by involuntary hospitalization. The "dangerousness" criterion is not without its inherent problems. Some of these are considered to be:

• Definitions of "dangerousness" vary from state to state.

• It is impossible to predict dangerous behavior reliably.

• In the absence of other criteria, "dangerousness" will be overused to justify admission.

• The stigma of *dangerous* will be added to that of *mentally ill*.

• The stereotype of *mentally disabled* will be reinforced and thus will work against the development of community programs.

• The media will be encouraged to continue selective reporting of instances in which mental illness and criminal behavior appear to be linked.

• Clinical practice shows "dangerous" individuals are often not treatable, while the most treatable individuals are not dangerous.

Discharge or Separation from a Mental Institution

A client can separate from a mental institution in one of three ways: discharge, transfer, and escape.

Discharge Like admission, discharge from a mental hospital can have various layers of complexity. Discharges occur in one of two ways—conditionally or absolutely.

Conditional As implied by the word *conditional*, complete discharge in this situation depends on whether the person fulfills certain conditions over a specified period of time, usually six months to a year. Compliance with outpatient care, demonstrated ability and willingness to take medications, and ability to meet the needs of daily living are a few of the many possible prerequisites.

An individual who is unable to meet the specified conditions can be reinstitutionalized without going through any legal admission procedure. An individual committed for an extended or indeterminate time is more likely to be a candidate for conditional than absolute discharge.

Absolute   The legal relationship between the institution and the client is terminated by an absolute discharge. If the client should require readmission to the hospital at any time, even a few hours after discharge, a new hospitalization proceeding would be required.

An absolute discharge can be brought about in three ways:

1. An administrative discharge is issued by the hospital officials.

2. A judicial discharge is ordered by the courts.

3. A writ of habeas corpus is ordered by the courts on the client's application.

As a rule, the authority for discharging involuntary clients rests in the hands of the hospital superintendent, and these clients are given administrative discharges. However, a few statutes extend this power to the central agency responsible for supervising mental institutions in the state, such as the Department of Mental Hygiene. The client has no formal method of initiating an administrative discharge.

Twenty-seven states have provisions for judicial discharge, which is initiated by an application to the court by the client, the client's family, or any citizen who is in disagreement with hospital authorities over the client's need to be hospitalized. A few states require the application to be accompanied by a medical certificate supporting the idea that the client is ready for discharge. In many states, judicial discharge does not depend on complete recovery. A degree of improvement may be sufficient. Twenty-one states guard against frequent applications for discharge by the same clients by imposing a three-month to one-year waiting period between requests.

All but a few states recognize the right of clients, or persons acting in their behalf, to question, by means of a writ of **habeas corpus,** the legality of their detention in a mental hospital. This writ, dating back to English common law, is available not only to mental clients but also to any person deprived of liberty through illegal detention. The question of the need for continued confinement of the client is not addressed by habeas corpus in most states. Some courts have expanded the writ to include an examination of the client's mental status at the time of the proceedings. In these cases the basic criterion for further detention or release is the client's present mental status. This expanded use of the writ is reflected in the statutes of at least sixteen states.

Transfer   Transfers account for approximately 3 percent of the separations from a mental facility. Most are transfers within the state and county mental health system. A smaller number are transfers from state to federal facilities or from one state to another.

Escape   A client may take the initiative and decide to terminate the relationship with the institution by informally leaving the hospital grounds. This is commonly referred to as escape, **elopement,** or being AWOL (absent without leave). Voluntary clients cannot generally be returned to the hospital against their will. However, involuntarily committed clients may be brought back to the hospital against their will with the assistance of the police, if necessary.

Rights of Clients

The current concern for clients' rights has not developed overnight. It actually has been evolving since the 1960s, when there was an increased interest in the underrepresented minority groups including blacks, the poor, women, and the mentally disabled.

In 1980 the United States Congress passed the Mental Health Systems Act, which included a model mental health client's bill of rights. This model bill of rights is summarized in the accompanying Advocacy box. The Omnibus Budget Reconciliation Act of 1981 brought about the repeal of parts of the Mental Health Systems Act but did retain the bill of rights.

Right to Treatment   The first argument for a right to treatment for involuntarily committed individuals came from Morton Birnbaum, a lawyer and a physician, in an article published in 1960. However, the ground-breaking cases did not come from the familiar circles of civil commitment but from individuals who had been sidetracked from the prison system into hospitals.

Rouse v Cameron   The first case to address the right to treatment issue directly and gain national attention was *Rouse v Cameron*, 373 F2d 451 (DC Cir 1966). In 1962, Charles Rouse had been brought to trial for carrying a dangerous weapon, which is a misdemeanor in the District of Columbia and carries a maximum sentence of one year. Instead of being convicted and sent to trial, Rouse pleaded "not guilty by reason of insanity," and was sent to the maximum security pavilion at Saint Elizabeth's Hospital for treatment. Under District of Columbia law, the plea of

ADVOCACY

Mental Health Systems Act Bill of Rights

1. Right to appropriate treatment in the least restrictive setting.

2. Right to individualized treatment plan, subject to review and reassessment. To include assessment of mental health services needed after discharge.

3. Right to active participation in treatment, with the risk, side effects, and benefits of all medication and treatment to be discussed, as well as treatment alternatives.

4. Right to give or withhold consent. May be treated without personal consent only in emergencies or with the consent of a guardian after incompetency has been determined by a court.

5. Right to be free of experimentation unless it follows the recommendations of the National Commission on Protection of Human Subjects.

6. Right to be free of restraints except in an emergency and unless restraints are specifically part of the treatment plan, always subject to the participation and consent requirements. Applies also to behavior-modification techniques involving restraints and seclusion.

7. Right to a humane environment.

8. Right to confidentiality of mental health information.

9. Right of access to personal treatment records unless two mental health professionals believe it to be detrimental.

10. Right to as much freedom as possible to exercise constitutional rights of association and expression. Restriction of specific visitors is allowed only if freely documented and part of the treatment plan.

11. Right to information about these rights in both written and oral form, presented in an understandable manner at the outset of treatment and periodically thereafter.

12. Right to assert grievances through a mechanism that includes the power to go to court.

13. Right to obtain advocacy assistance.

14. Right to criticize or complain about conditions or services without fear of retaliatory punishment or other reprisals.

15. Right to referral to complement the discharge plan.

insanity takes away criminal responsibility and subjects the defendant to an automatic involuntary commitment.

Four years later, Rouse questioned his detention by means of a writ of habeas corpus on the ground that he had not received any psychiatric treatment. His lawyer argued that he was entitled to treatment in exchange for loss of liberty. State laws vary tremendously on how the person committed by reason of insanity obtains release. Some state statutes require the person to remain committed until pardoned by the governor. Others require the person to meet the same criteria for discharge as any other civilly committed individual.

Judge David Bazelon, speaking for the United States Court of Appeals for the District of Columbia, stated that involuntary commitment is imposed because it is assumed that the criminal offender needs treatment for a mental condition. If treatment is not given, as in Rouse's case, the court held, the offender is deprived of basic rights. Although Judge Bazelon said Rouse was entitled to treatment on the basis of the present District of Columbia statute, he indicated that there might be a constitutional basis for the right as well. Whenever possible, however, courts will base their decisions in statutory rather than constitutional grounds.

Nason v Bridgewater Another important decision was the Supreme Judicial Court of Massachusetts ruling in *Nason v Bridgewater*, 233 NE2d 908 (Mass 1968). John Nason, a man indicted for murder, had been sent to Bridgewater State Hospital because he was found incompetent to stand trial. After spending five years at Bridgewater, the Massachusetts facility for the dangerously insane, he filed a writ of habeas corpus for his release on the ground that he was not receiving adequate treatment, and he requested transfer to another facility. Through expert testimony, Nason's attorneys were able to show that staffing at Bridgewater was so grossly inadequate that Nason was simply receiving custodial care. The court acknowledged the existence of a constitutional right to treatment, at least for incompetent people awaiting trial, and even went on to suggest what a proper treatment plan for Nason would be.

While *Rouse* and *Nason* may have had little impact on the actual delivery of care in most institutions around the country, they did articulate the right to treatment and provided a statutory and tentative constitutional rationale for that right.

Wyatt v Stickney The next step in the move to establish a right to treatment through the court system was taken in Alabama in 1970, with the filing of *Wyatt v Stickney*, 344 F Supp 373 (MD Ala 1972). It was the first class suit successfully brought against a state's entire mental health system. The issue was detention without treatment of individuals committed civilly and involuntarily. The court established that involuntary clients have a constitutional right to individualized treatment that will give each of them a realistic chance to be cured or at least improve. The court found that the treatment program in Alabama state institutions was deficient in three fundamental areas. It did not provide:

1. A humane psychologic and physical environment

2. Qualified staff to administer adequate treatment

3. Individualized treatment plans

To remedy these defects, the court promulgated a lengthy and detailed set of standards, including:

• Provisions against institutional peonage (against institutional use of clients for work)

• A number of protections to ensure a humane psychologic and safe physical environment

• Minimum staffing requirements

• Establishment of a human rights committee at each institution

• A requirement that every client have a right to the least restrictive setting necessary for treatment

If the standards could not be met and clients were denied adequate treatment, the court stated, they had to be released from custody. In the words of Judge Johnson, "to deprive any citizen of his or her liberty upon the altruistic theory that confinement is for human therapeutic reasons and then fail to provide adequate treatment violates the very fundamentals of due process" (*Wyatt v Stickney*, 325 F Supp 781, 785 [MD Ala 1971]).

Donaldson v O'Connor   Another important development in the constitutional right to treatment controversy was *Donaldson v O'Connor*, 493 F2d 507 (5th Cir 1974). Kenneth Donaldson, an involuntary patient in a Florida mental hospital for over fourteen years, brought suit against the hospital superintendent, alleging that the superintendent had maliciously deprived him of his constitutional right to liberty. At trial, the jury found that (1) Donaldson had received not merely inadequate treatment but no treatment at all, (2) he was not dangerous, (3) acceptable community alternatives were in fact available for Donaldson, and (4) the doctor, knowing all this, had "maliciously" refused to release him.

On appeal, the federal court of appeals held that there is a constitutional right to treatment, and it awarded $38,000 in compensatory and punitive damages to Donaldson. However, the United States Supreme Court declined to affirm the court of appeals finding of constitutional right to treatment. The court said that the case raised a single question concerning

every person's constitutional right to liberty—that is: Does one have the right to be discharged from custodial care if not dangerous to self or others, the right not to receive treatment if one can survive safely in freedom? The unanimous answer was yes (*O'Connor v Donaldson*, 43 USLW 4929 [1975]).

In February 1977, at the age of sixty-seven, Kenneth Donaldson was awarded $20,000 from two defendant psychiatrists. Donaldson's lawsuit had been undertaken in the public interest by the American Civil Liberties Union and the Mental Health Law Project, and a ruling in early May 1977 entitled Donaldson to recover reasonable attorneys' fees. Donaldson has written a book about his confinement, *Insanity Inside Out* (1976).

The concept of right to treatment is an outgrowth of the philosophic point of view that the deprivation of liberty, whether voluntarily or involuntarily, must have an overriding purpose. Review of court cases indicates the right to treatment came about because there was no overriding purpose: Because of overcrowded conditions, inadequate staffing, financial and programmatic deficiencies, there were not enough resources to deliver the bare minimum of treatment. "Right to treatment" ensures that clients are not in a treatment setting for custodial purposes only. The necessary elements in a treatment-oriented program are:

• Physical examination and social and psychologic assessment on admission and then as indicated

• Treatment plans with clear objectives and interventions

• Evidence of client participation in treatment planning and consent for all treatment methods

• Up-to-date medical records

• Treatment in as normal an environment as possible

• Staff in adequate numbers and with sufficient training to provide quality care

• Availability of treatment that meets the client needs identified in the treatment plan

• Necessary support services such as dental, speech, physical, and rehabilitation therapy

• Ongoing treatment plan evaluations

• Programs to help clients develop skills needed for independent versus institutional living

• Adequate discharge planning to a less restrictive setting, according to client's needs

Some of the unresolved problems or questions regarding the "right to treatment" issue are the cost in tax dollars and the difficulty in providing effective treatment for all conditions. If effective treatment does not exist, is custodial care enough?

Right to Refuse Treatment The courts articulated a committed client's right to treatment over a decade ago. More recently the courts have been asked to rule on whether the client in a mental institution has the right to refuse treatment.

One of the first cases is that of *Price v Sheppard*, 239 NW 2d 905 (Minn 1976), in which electroconvulsive therapy was felt to be an "intrusive" treatment and not allowed to be given against a competent client's wishes. The two best known cases are *Rennie v Klein* and *Rogers v Okin*.

Rennie v Klein *Rennie v Klein* was initiated in December 1977 by John Rennie, an involuntarily committed client at a New Jersey state hospital who claimed that the hospital and the New Jersey Department of Human Services were violating his constitutional rights by forcibly administering medication. Mr Rennie had objected to the side effects produced by chlorpromazine (Thorazine) and lithium carbonate.

Judge Stanley Brotman ruled that involuntarily committed clients have a qualified right to refuse psychotropic medication (New Jersey statutes already stated that voluntary clients have an absolute right to reject medication). His decision was based on the constitutional right to protect their mental processes from governmental interference. Judge Brotman, impressed by the side effects of psychotropic medication, stated, "Individual autonomy demands that the person subjected to the harsh side-effects of psychotropic drugs have control over their administration" (*Rennie v Klein* 462 F Supp at 1145).

Judge Brotman did qualify the right to refuse, listing four factors to be considered in overriding a client's objection:

• *Safety.* Is the client a physical treat to other clients or staff?

• *Competency.* Is the client competent to make treatment decisions?

• *Less restrictive means.* Do less restrictive means of treatment exist, and are they available?

• *Risk versus benefit.* What are the risks of permanent side effects from the proposed treatment?

In 1979 Mr Rennie's complaint was amended to include class-action allegations, and the court went on to add more specific steps to be followed in implementing an involuntarily committed client's qualified right to refuse treatment. These included:

• Notify clients that they have a right to refuse medication.

• Provide clients with information regarding potential side effects of the medication.

• Obtain written consent prior to initiation of medication.

If written consent is withheld by a client already declared "legally incompetent" by the court or certified "functionally incompetent" by a treating psychiatrist, the decision to medicate forcibly would be referred to a client advocate. It would be in the client advocate's discretion to request a hearing before an independent psychiatrist, who would base a decision on the four factors mentioned above. In the case of a competent though involuntarily hospitalized person, a hearing before an independent psychiatrist would be required at which the client would have the right to legal counsel.

Rogers v Okin Another important case in the establishment of a client's right to refuse medication is *Rogers v Okin*, 478 F Supp (D Mass 1979). In 1975 a class-action suit was initiated by clients at Boston State Hospital, who contended that their constitutional rights were being violated by the hospital's practice of using forced seclusion and medication in nonemergency situations. Judge Joseph Tauro issued a temporary restraining order against the use of seclusion and medication without the client's informed consent. In the case of a person declared incompetent by the court, informed consent would need to be elicited from the client's guardian. This restraining order applied to both voluntary and involuntary clients. In 1979, after a lengthy trial, the court made the temporary restraining order permanent.

Judge Tauro based his decision on the constitutional right to privacy (right to be left alone) and the first amendment right to freedom of thought. While Judge Tauro recognized that safety considerations might necessitate forcible administration of medication, he allowed much less discretion on the part of the hospital staff than did Judge Brotman in *Rennie*. Only in emergencies that create a substantial likelihood of physical harm to the client or others could medication be forcibly administered. Judge Tauro did not include a set of procedures to be followed in the case of client refusal, as had been done in *Rennie*. Instead, hospital staff were directed to apply to the court for a competency hearing and subsequent appointment of a guardian for clients they believed were incompetent to make treatment decisions. The decision in *Rogers* is considered to be more far-reaching than that in *Rennie*, since it grants competent clients and guardians of incompetent clients an absolute right to refuse medication in nonemergency situations.

Other recent court decisions support a qualified right to refuse psychotropic mediation, unless a legitimate emergency exists. It is vital to remember that overriding a client's right to refuse treatment is legally complicated and related to safeguards in place to manage such situations. These safeguards protect the rights of all people.

Dilemmas Associated with Right to Refuse Treatment There are a number of areas of judicial disagreement in the right to refuse treatment that will create dilemmas for the mental health professional. For example, there is no common definition of the term *psychiatric emergency*. The traditional definition of *emergency* refers to an overt and immediate threat to a person's life. The contemporary definition centers on the immediate, impending, and significant deterioration of the client's condition.

Another area of controversy is: At what point can the state override an involuntarily committed client's right to refuse psychotropic medication in a nonemergency? Is it only when a person has been judged incompetent, or does danger to self or others provide a legitimate reason under the state's police power to administer treatment?

In the case of an incompetent individual, there is disagreement over who should decide for the person and what standard should be used. Is it to be a guardian, the hospital staff, or the judiciary? Is the standard to be what the best interests of the client seem to be as judged by an informed outsider, or is it what the client would want if competent to make the choice?

Here are some criteria a court is likely to use in ruling on a case involving the right to refuse treatment:

- **Client competency.** If the client is competent, informed consent is possible.

- **Intrusiveness of treatment.** As the intrusiveness increases, so does the court's scrutiny.

- **Permanence of treatment effect.** If side effects are adverse and permanent, a court is less likely to override refusal.

- **Experimental nature of treatment.** The treatment must have scientific merit, and the client must give informed consent.

- **Risk-benefit ratio.** The benefits of treatment must outweigh the risk.

- **Motivation for treatment.** The treatment cannot be used to punish or "quiet" the client for the staff's benefit.

- **Motivation for refusal.** Religious objections are usually upheld.

Despite the difficulties and issues raised by the client's right to refuse treatment, some very real positive outcomes are:

- Clients must be involved in treatment choices, process, and outcome.

- Clients must be informed of choices and offered alternatives.

- Staff must acquire a second opinion on potentially harmful procedures.

Least Restrictive Alternative The idea of least restrictive alternative has become an important component of both the deinstitutionalization and clients' rights movements. The term **least restrictive alternative** (LRA) generally refers to the placement of clients in the therapeutic setting that will provide care while allowing maximum freedom.

The first of these was *Lake v Cameron*, 364 F2d 657 (DC Cir 1966). Mrs Lake, a 61-year-old woman, had difficulty caring for herself because of confusion secondary to arteriosclerotic brain disease. While not considered a danger to others, she did wander when confused and was subsequently admitted to St Elizabeth's Hospital. The court ruled that Mrs Lake did not need twenty-four-hour psychiatric supervision and a less restrictive form of treatment should be found. Ironically, even though Mrs Lake won her case, she ended up dying at St Elizabeth's because no other facility was available.

While in principle the right to LRA is relatively straightforward, its implementation is often not so clear-cut. Work is being done on defining the concept (see Killebrew et al. 1982, Ransohoff et al. 1984) so that the restrictiveness of a given setting can be measured more accurately.

The ANA's Standards for Psychiatric and Mental Health Nursing Practice expect that the nurse will "set limits in a humane and least restrictive manner to assure the safety of client and others." To help nurses begin to judge the restrictiveness of an intervention, Garritson (1983) suggests consideration of the following dimensions, which are discussed below:

- Treatment setting

- Institutional policy

- Enforcement

- Treatment

- Client characteristics

Treatment Setting Treatment setting is evaluated on such criteria as the limitations it places on physical freedom (locked or unlocked), choice of activities, and the presence of "adult status" as shown by locked bedrooms and unsupervised use of private bathroom facilities. In this scheme, total institutions would be considered the most restrictive, half-way houses less so, and family or independent living the least.

Institutional Policy Institutional policy is the degree of restriction imposed by the rules and regulations necessary to run the institution. Criteria to evaluate a setting would include such items as the amount of supervision in daily living tasks, the amount of client involvement in treatment planning, and the priority of activities that increase the client's autonomy.

Enforcement The enforcement dimension includes the methods sanctioned to enforce the institution's rules. Is coercion or threat of punishment used? Is the standard for socially acceptable behavior higher in the institution than it would be in the client's own environment? For example, a nurse says to a client, "We don't use that foul language here . . . I don't think you're ready for that pass." How readily and to what extent is the client's autonomy compromised to meet organizational needs?

Treatment The treatment dimension has to do with the intrusiveness of the treatment used. Pychosurgery and electronconvulsive therapy would be considered more intrusive than medication. Long-acting medication such as fluphenazine decanoate would be considered more intrusive than oral medication. The clarity of treatment goals is also a consideration. Nebulous or nonexistent goals increase restrictiveness.

Client Characteristics The client's characteristics or illness is seen by some as restricting behavior to a much greater degree than any locked door. Some believe it is simplistic to think that moving a client from an institutional setting to the community will automatically result in less restriction. Without effective community-based treatment, including safe housing, the chronically ill clients frequently end up in "psychiatric ghettos." (See Chapter 17.)

Communication and Visitation

All but three states (Alabama, Mississippi, West Virginia) have some statutory provisions on client correspondence. The basis for laws granting communication rights is that such communication can expose cases of wrongful hospitalization. Generally, communication is unrestricted or guaranteed to named public officials or the central hospital agency for the state. Twenty-seven states extend this guarantee to include correspondence with attorneys. Most states require that any correspondence limitation be part of the client's clinical record. Approximately half the states require the client to have reasonable access to writing materials and postage.

All but five states (Alabama, Mississippi, Pennsylvania, Virginia, and West Virginia) have some statutory provisions concerning visitation. However, hospital authorities are generally given broad discretionary powers to curtail this right. Before implementing any restriction in communication or visitation the nurse should ask: Is it fair and reasonable? Could I defend it to a noninvolved professional?

Restraints and Seclusion

Though improvements in treatment have decreased the use of mechanical or physical restraints, such restraints still play a role in some treatment programs. Most states have attempted to regulate their use by statute. Twenty-six states specify that restraints can be used when the client presents a risk of harm to self or others. Eight states also permit the use of restraints for therapeutic purposes. Some states specifically say restraints are not to be used for punishment or staff convenience. In those states not having statutory provisions regarding restraints the procedures to be followed usually are found in the administrative regulations.

Half the states have laws relating to seclusion. Prevention of harm to self or others is the most common criterion, followed by treatment or therapeutic reasons. Colorado specifically prohibits the use of seclusion but does allow a time-out period. The use of either restraints or seclusion must be documented in the client's medical record in most states.

Electronconvulsive Therapy and Psychosurgery

In almost all states, electronconvulsive therapy (ECT) is closely regulated by statute. Most state statutes specify that ECT can be administered only if informed consent is obtained from the client. In the case of an incompetent client, consent must be obtained from the guardian or next of kin. The client's right to refuse ECT is specifically mentioned in many state statutes.

Psychosurgery, referred to in various state statutes as "brain surgery," "lobotomy," or "experimental" or "hazardous" procedures, is also closely regulated by state statute. Most state statutes specify that psychosurgery can be performed only if informed consent is obtained from the client. In a number of states, psychosurgery can be done only upon a court order if the client is incompetent. The client's right to refuse psychosurgery is also specifically mentioned in many state statutes.

Periodic Review

Thirty-one states and the District of Columbia have some provision for periodic review of involuntary clients. Periodic review provides some protection for the individual against spending more time than necessary in the hospital. Review is required every thirty days in some states, every year in others. A few states require review "as frequently as necessary," or "from time to time." The actual scope of the review is usually not governed by statute. The trend in recent years has been away from hospitalization for indeterminate periods of time. In New York and California, short-term commitment is the rule, and court review is necessary to extend commitment for another short period.

Participation in Legal Matters

Contracts Clients committed to a mental hospital generally maintain their right to make a valid contract, unless they have also been judged incompetent. In most states, commitment proceedings are separate from those for competence. Therefore, an individual who is "legally incompetent" is not necessarily subject to commitment, and an individual committed to an institution is not automatically legally incompetent. Even though the issue of contracts may seem clear-cut, in reality, a client's right to contract may be restricted by the administrative regulations of hospitals and state mental health agencies. A contested contract would most likely be a matter for the court to decide.

Wills To make a valid will, an individual must:

• Be aware of making a will

• Be familiar with the property being disposed of

• Know the names, identities, and relationship of the people named in the will

An individual with a psychiatric diagnosis, whether in or out of the hospital, can make a valid will as long as these requirements are met. Psychosis with accompanying delusions does not by itself negate a valid will. The delusions have to produce a significant distortion of the person's perception of the property, family, or personal relationships to invalidate the will.

Marriage and Divorce According to statute and common law, a valid marriage contract hinges on the individual's possession of sufficient mental capacity to give consent. Sufficient mental capacity implies that the person:

• Understands the nature of the marriage relationship

• Knows the duties and obligations involved

The statutes of a small number of states prohibit marriage by mentally disordered persons because they are believed to be incapable of making a contract. More states, however, prohibit marriage by the mentally disordered on the grounds that they are "insane" or "of unsound mind," without specifically defining these terms. Despite these prohibiting statutes, few states even try to enforce the prohibition outside mental institutions.

Most states have provisions for annulment or divorce on the ground of prenuptial mental disability. Within the last twenty-five years, divorce on the grounds of postnuptial mental disability has been incorporated in the statutes of most states.

Voting The majority of states do not actually prohibit hospitalized persons from voting. In fact, some specifically preserve this right by legislation. The institutionalized are eligible to register to vote in twelve states. In eighteen others the ability to vote depends on a hospitalized client's legal competence. Only in Maryland and Missouri are individuals confined to an institution ineligible to vote. All states except Louisiana allow absentee voting by disabled persons. The hospitalized client's right to vote is probably more restricted by caretaker and community apathy than it is by statute.

Right to Drive Statutes on driving privileges are difficult to interpret. Most states will not issue a driver's license to mentally disturbed persons. In some states this restriction also applies to epileptics, drug addicts, and alcoholics. Several states suspend a driver's license as soon as the individual enters a mental institution. Other jurisdictions limit the restriction to individuals admitted involuntarily, while still others base suspension on legal competence.

Right to Practice a Profession The ability of a hospitalized client to practice a profession is usually impaired simply by the physical confinement. However, the majority of states have some statutes prohibiting the practice of a profession by a mentally disturbed person. The vagueness of the statutes often makes it difficult to know when they are applicable. As a rule, it is up to the professional licensing board to suspend or revoke the license of a member who is believed to be too mentally incapacitated to practice a profession safely, even though not hospitalized.

Rights of Children or Minors

The rights of children, along with those of other groups frequently considered politically powerless, have been the subject of judicial and legislative action over the last twenty years. Up until this time children or minors had few rights of their own. Under early common law, children were the parent's "property" and owed them strict obedience.

In most states an individual is considered a minor or juvenile if younger than 18 years of age. As a minor the person is considered legally incompetent. Legal consent for medical treatment must come from parents or guardian. There are, however, a number of exceptions to this general rule of presumed legal incompetence in some state statutes. These include the rights to:

• Seek treatment for drug abuse

• Consent to contraception

• Seek psychiatric treatment

Other factors, such as military service, marriage, emancipation, pregnancy, and parenthood, may also affect the age at which a minor may be considered competent.

The most controversial issue of a minor's role in the mental health system involves involuntary commitment. Like adults, minors can be committed to a mental hospital against their will. But, unlike adult admissions, the admission of a minor who objects is considered "voluntary" if the parents have authorized it. Because of the realization that parents may not always be acting in the best interests of the child, a number of lawsuits challenging this practice were filed in the 1970s. It was argued that "voluntary" admission of minors without procedural safeguards was unconstitutional, and that a court hearing should always be held to determine if commitment is warranted. The Supreme Court had already ruled in 1967 *In re Gault* (387 US 1) that juveniles in the criminal justice system were entitled to some of the same procedural safeguards accorded adult defendants. Many states did change their commitment statutes to include procedural safeguards. However, in the 1979 case of *Parham v J.R.* (442 US 584), the United States Supreme Court upheld the rights of parents to admit their children to psychiatric facilities as long as a "neutral factfinder" (physician) believes medical standards for admission have been met.

The trend for inclusion of procedural safeguards, though slowed by the ruling in *Parham v J.R.*, continues as an increasing number of states have modified their "voluntary" parental commitment statute by one or more of the following factors:

• Lowering the age of required consent: In four states (Alaska, Idaho, Vermont, and Pennsylvania) the age is 15 or older. The majority of states specify 16 to 18. In New Jersey alone is 21 years the age of consent.

• Requiring consent of the child.

• Providing for a court hearing if the child protests.

• Providing for self-initiated institutionalization for minors: In New Mexico a child 12 years or older qualifies for self-initiated hospitalization, six other states cite age 14 years, and the rest are divided between 16 and 18 years of age.

Therapist-Client-Public Relations

Confidentiality Almost all states have a specific statute regarding confidentiality of client information, and the specific steps to be taken for release of that information. The confidential nature of the client information is also cited in the American Nurses' Association Code of Ethics, as it is in most professional codes.

The goal of confidentiality is to ensure the client's privacy. There is a significant amount of stigma attached to being the recipient of psychiatric treatment. Though professionals may argue that this is unfair, it is a fact. Because of this, it is important that clients be the ones to give out this information about themselves. Instructors, students, supervisors, or team members who receive information about a client in the course of supervision or in providing treatment for the client are also obligated to treat this material as confidential.

For disclosure of information to occur, a client needs to sign a release form. To be a valid release, the client must be told as specifically as possible what information is to be released. The client should know the following prior to signing:

• What information is going to be released?

• Who needs it?

• Why do they need it?

• When will they need it?

• How will it be used?

Emergency situations may arise. For example, a client may be in a car accident or take an overdose while out on pass and end up being treated in another hospital's emergency room. In these situations, release of information can occur without the client's approval. It is important to document such a breach of confidentiality.

Confidentiality of information is not easy to maintain. Medical records are generally kept, not in locked files, but at an easy access point in the nurses' station. Medical files usually travel all over the hospital with the client and are often available for the perusal of others not directly involved in the client's treatment. The increased use of computers for communication and data storage, along with the information requested by the government, third-party payers, and employers, often poses a threat to a client's privacy. More mundane incidences of breaches of confidentiality occur when staff talk about clients in the halls, elevator, and cafeteria.

Privileged Communication **Privileged communication** is a narrower concept than confidentiality. It is established by state statute to protect possibly incriminating disclosures made by the client to specified professionals. Privileged communication has traditionally existed between husband and wife, attorney and client, clergy and church member, and physician and client. In some states, communications between psychologist and client are also accorded privileged status. Arkansas, New York, Oregon, Vermont, and Wisconsin recognize privileged communication between nurse and client. The privilege is the client's and can be claimed only if a therapeutic relationships exists. The professional can reveal the information at the client's request.

Each state that grants a privilege also specifies exceptions to that privilege. The most common exceptions include:

• When the therapist suspects child abuse

• When the therapist is seeking civil commitment

• When the court orders the exam

• When the client introduces a defense of mental illness into litigation proceedings (likely to happen in child custody disputes, malpractice suits against therapists, personal injury suits, workers' compensation cases, and will contests)

• When the client poses a danger to others (establishes the therapist's duty to warn)

Disclosure to Safeguard Others An exception to confidentiality and privilege that has developed from a recent California Supreme Court decision illustrates the competition between two responsibilities of the mental health professional:

1. Confidentiality to the client

2. Protection of the public from the "violent" client

The court's ruling underlines the mental health professional's responsibility to balance the two.

In *Tarasoff v Regents of the University of California*, 13 CAL3d 177, 529 P2d 553, 118 Cal Rptr 129 (1974), the parents of Tatiana Tarasoff successfully sued the University of California, claiming that a psychotherapist on the staff of the university's student counseling center had a responsibility to warn their daughter that his client, Prosenjit Poddar, had threatened to kill her when she returned from a trip abroad. At the time, the psychologist did notify campus security officers that he believed his client was dangerous and should be involuntarily committed for observation and treatment. However, Poddar appeared rational to the police and promised them he would stay away from Ms Tarasoff. Poddar terminated treatment, and two months later killed Tatiana Tarasoff.

The suit was brought on two accounts: (1) failure to warn Tarasoff, and (2) failure to detain Poddar for treatment. Although the suit was dismissed by the lower courts, on appeal the California Supreme Court reversed the dismissal, saying that, despite the unsuccessful attempt to confine Poddar, the therapist knew that Poddar was at large and dangerous and had a duty to warn Tarasoff of the danger. The court recognized the client's right to confidentiality but said this must be weighed against the public's need for safety against violent assault, especially when an individual in danger can be identified. The *Tarasoff* concept or at least some version of it has continued to be reaffirmed in a number of state and federal jurisdictions. In two cases, therapists were held liable for not taking some action to protect potential unidentified victims.

Appelbaum (1985) suggests a change from the idea of "a duty to warn" to that of a "duty to protect." The accompanying Intervention box shows a model to help mental health caregivers decide on a course of action in implementing the duty to protect.

Situations in which reporting by physicians to authorities is required by law include child and elder abuse, knife or gunshot wounds, certain contagious diseases, and the driving of a car by a person with unstable epilepsy. In court cases so far a client's voicing of suicidal ideation does *not* create a duty to warn. The duty to warn or protect applies only when there is danger to others.

The "duty to warn" has stirred up controversy in the mental health community. There is concern about the fact that clients with aggression problems will drop out of therapy, not use it effectively, or be less likely to seek treatment for fear of being betrayed. Remember also that no mental health professional can reliably predict the future violence of a mentally disordered person.

Liability and the Psychiatric Nurse

Criminal and civil are the two main classes of law. *Criminal law* pertains to behavior considered to be a threat to the order of society as a whole, such as murder, assault, and robbery. *Civil law* is concerned with the legal rights and duties of private parties.

An important division of civil law is known as *tort law*. The term **tort** comes from the Latin word meaning twisted. A tort is a wrongful act resulting in injury for which the injured party files a civil suit requesting legal redress, usually in form of monetary damages. Torts may be intentional, as in assault, battery, defamation of character, invasion of privacy, false imprisonment, fraud, and misrepresentation; or unintentional, as in negligence.

Medical **malpractice** refers to the negligent acts of health care professionals when they fail to act in a responsible and prudent manner in carrying out their professional duties.

As the practice of nursing moves toward greater independence and accountability, nurses are more likely to be named as defendants in lawsuits. Some reasons for increases in claims against mental health professionals are:

• The emphasis on clients' rights in recent court decisions

• The public's more open attitude and greater expectations of treatment

• The new legal duties identified in the therapist-client relationship, such as the "duty to warn"

• The publicity given the sizable sums awarded in some psychiatric malpractice cases

According to the American Psychiatric Association, the most frequent sources of claims (listed in order of decreasing frequency) for psychiatrists are:

• Client suicide

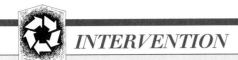

INTERVENTION

Model for Implementing the Duty to Warn or Protect

Do	How
Assess dangerousness.	Compare data to factors believed to correlate with dangerous behavior, such as increasing use of drugs and/or alcohol, current and past threats of violence and/or assaultive behavior, presence of command hallucinations.
	Ask: Is the threat serious? Are the threats repeated? Are the means to carry out the threat available? Can the victim be identified? Is the victim accessible?
Select a course of action to protect the victim.	Consider either voluntary hospitalization or, if necessary, initiate involuntary commitment.
	If the client is already hospitalized, is a more secure unit needed to prevent escape?
	If the client is an outpatient, is medication needed? Are more frequent visits needed? Is a more intensive outpatient care needed, such as a day program?
	Because threats often involve family members, is intensive, systems-oriented therapy indicated to include the intended victim?
	If containment or control is not possible, contact identified victim. Consider also alerting the police.
Implement decision.	Continue to monitor: If initial course of action fails, take other measures. Be sure to document this decision-making process in the client's record.

- Improper treatment
- Ineffective or improper medication
- Breach of confidentiality
- Wrongful commitment
- Injuries from electronconvulsive therapy
- Sexual misconduct
- Failure to obtain consent

The basic elements of every nursing malpractice suit are:

- The client claims that a special duty of care is owed; that is, a nurse-client relationship existed.

- Because of this the nurse is required to meet a specific standard of care.

- The nurse's failure to meet that standard resulted in injury or harm.

- The client claims compensatory damages.

The most important legal element in a nursing malpractice case is whether the nurse met the required standard of care. A court may determine the expected standard of care by the profession's standards of practice and testimony of expert witnesses.

The case of *Abille v U.S.* (482 F Supp 703 Calif) illustrates a breach of the American Nurses' Association's Standards of Psychiatric and Mental Health Nursing Practice and emphasizes the importance of written communication between nurse and physician.

Aramul Abille was admitted to a U.S. Air Force base hospital after becoming increasingly depressed and suicidal secondary to the reserpine used to treat his hypertension. As a new client, he was not allowed to leave the unit. Four days later the nursing staff assumed without a verifying written medical order (later a verbal order would be claimed) that Mr Abille was allowed to leave the unit with permission of the nurse on duty. Mr Abille left the unit unescorted to attend Mass and returned without incident. The following morning he was allowed to go to breakfast unescorted. This time he committed suicide by jumping from a seventh floor window. The court ruled that the nurse involved with Mr Abille's care breached the standard of care due under Alaska law. The nurse failed to exercise reasonable care to protect a suicidal client against foreseeable harm to himself.

Another case shows the importance of nursing observation and documentation, even though in this case it did not prevent a tragedy.

Distraught with problems and a pending divorce, Matthew Wassner was voluntarily admitted to a psychiatric hospital. During this admission he expressed thoughts of suicide and also thoughts of killing his wife and her mother. Three weeks after his discharge he was readmitted again voluntarily after a suicide attempt. Nurses' notes revealed close observation of Mr Wassner and his repeated homicidal threats. Three weeks after his second admission, he was given a pass. He subsequently secured a gun and shot and killed his wife and her friend. He was tried and convicted on two counts of murder. The children brought a wrongful death action against the hospital, seeking damages for the murder of their mother by their father. The court granted substantial damages to the children. No liability was attributed to the nurses involved, but the physician was judged negligent.

 In another case the court found that a nurse who forcibly administered medication to a competent adult client had committed an intentional tort.

The client was involuntarily committed to a mental hospital. She was a practicing Christian Scientist and refused medication. The court held that medication could be given over the client's religious objections only if she were harmful to herself or others. The court allowed her damages for assault and battery.

It is important to remember the nature and purpose of hospital records and to follow prudent, appropriate, and ethical procedures in record maintenance. Records that have been changed for whatever reason need to include the date, the reason for the change, and the signature of the person making the change. A dishonest change could result in the charge of fraud or misrepresentation as in *Pisel v Stamford Hospital et al.* 430 A2d (Conn 1980).

A 23-year-old woman was admitted with a diagnosis of schizophrenia. She spent three days in a furnitureless quiet room for safety reasons. On the fourth day the bed was returned to the room, but no rationale was noted in the chart. A few days later, an order on the client's chart for an antipsychotic medication was not noted, and the client was without medication for three days. The client was later found in a semicomatose condition with her head lodged between the side rails and mattress. Subsequently, the nursing director ordered the nursing staff to "rewrite" the nursing notes. The substituted record clearly conflicted with other records and staff testimony. A $3.6 million verdict against the hospital has been upheld.

Many factors contribute to the initiation of a malpractice suit by a client. As long as a nurse is involved in practice, lawsuits are a possibility. The nurse may be sued without necessarily being singled out. A number of ways to protect against a successful lawsuit are to:

• Be aware of provisions in the state nurse practice act.

• Follow standards of care.

• Know the relevant law.

• Review hospital procedures and policies with both the standards of care and relevant law in mind, clarify any conflict with legal counsel if necessary, and then follow procedures

• Document the nursing process, chart accurately and precisely, and chart any significant change as soon as possible. Remember that any omission is presumed not to have occurred.

• Chart objectively, avoiding phrases like "doing well" or "having a good day."

• Question the physician about any ambiguous orders before carrying them out.

• Be sure to adequately describe methods used in client education and evaluation of client's comprehension.

• Make sure your nursing documentation reflects the precautions taken during intensive nursing actions such as one-to-one or the use of seclusion or restraints.

• Never alter a client's record after the fact.

• Have malpractice insurance.

Intersection of Psychiatry and Criminal Law

Psychiatry also affects the resolution of such legal questions as the credibility of witnesses, competency to make a will or contract or to stand trial, compensation of injured persons, custody of children, and, most controversial, criminal responsibility.

Competency to Stand Trial

Competency to stand trial is based on our common law tradition that defendants must have the mental capacity to defend themselves in a court of law. The process of determining competency to stand trial is the issue most frequently leading to the hospitalization of individuals in the criminal justice system. Until 1972, pretrial commitment was widely used as the final disposition. The defendant failed to become "competent" and remained in the institution indefinitely. Such was the case in *Jackson v Indiana*. The defendant was a 27-year-old retarded, hearing-impaired, mute individual who was accused of stealing property valued at nine dollars and confined to a maximum security unit awaiting trial. Because of his disabilities, it was doubted that he would ever become competent to stand trial. In its ruling, the United States Supreme Court set out some general limitations on the length of pretrial commitments, saying a person cannot be held more than a "reasonable period of time." If the person is unlikely to become competent to stand trial, the civil commitment standards must be met, or the person must be released.

A psychiatric nurse clinician is qualified in some states to perform competency evaluations by interviewing the defendant to determine his or her understanding of the nature of the legal process, recognition of the consequences of the accusation, and ability to assist counsel in the defense.

A competency evaluation no longer requires an in-patient stay and may be done in a prison outpatient setting. While not many nurses may actually do competency evaluations, nurses employed in public mental hospitals may work with clients transferred from the prison system for treatment to regain their competency.

Insanity Defense

All civilized cultures have had some form of insanity defense. It has been recognized in English courts for over 700 years. Insanity tests or rules that are influential or currently in use include wild beast, M'Naghten, irresistible impulse, Durham or "product," and model penal code.

Wild Beast Test   The wild beast test, articulated in 1723, essentially said a man must be so totally deprived of his understanding and memory that he knows no more of what he is doing than an infant or wild beast. The wild beast test remained the standard for judging responsibility until a case involving the assassination attempt of a head of state in 1800. The defense successfully argued that if the person's mental condition either produced or caused the criminal act, the person should not be held legally responsible for it. This was considered a landmark decision because it broke with the idea that a person must be totally deprived of reason, and did not link insanity with the inability to tell right from wrong. Subsequent cases did not follow this precedent but reverted back to the wild beast test. However, this reasoning is found in the Durham test or "product rule" of 1954.

M'Naghten Rule   From the trial of *The Queen v Daniel M'Naghten* in 1843 came a set of rules that for many years has provided the basis for the majority of American federal and state courts' decisions on the insanity plea.

Daniel M'Naghten was a Scottish woodcutter who felt persecuted by the Tories, who were in power. He believed they were following him, preventing him from sleeping, accusing him of crimes, and planning to murder him. He decided to take action and shoot the prime minister, but he mistakenly shot the prime minister's secretary.

The jury found M'Naghten not guilty by reason of insanity. Even though M'Naghten was committed to an asylum and spent the rest of his life there, his acquittal was met with anger and outrage, much like the recent outcry in the Hinckley acquittal (discussed later in this chapter). M'Naghten's attack had been the fifth attempt on a political figure in forty years, and the government and press believed the court's action would not help to stem this tide. The fifteen judges of the common law court were called to task for their ruling and asked to clarify and tighten the concept of criminal responsibility. Their clarification has come to be known as the **M'Naghten rule,** which states that for an insanity plea to be valid, the defendant at the time of committing the offense must have been functioning under such a defect of the mind, or reasoning power, as not to know the nature and quality of the act or that it was wrong.

The M'Naghten rule was adopted in the federal and most state courts in the United States by 1851. Until recently, only New Hampshire had judged insanity pleas by a rule not in line with the M'Naghten formula.

Irresistible Impulse Test   The claim that the M'Naghten rule focused exclusively on cognition led to the development of the **irresistible impulse** doctrine as a supplement to the M'Naghten rules in some states. The irresistible impulse test refers to a person's inability, because of a mental disorder, to control behavior even though that person may know it is wrong. A popular question asked in making the determination is: "Would the person have yielded to that impulse had a policeman been at his (her) elbow?"

Durham Test or "Product Rule"   In 1954 the Supreme Court of Appeals for the District of Columbia handed down its decision in *Durham v US*, discarding the M'Naghten rule and introducing another basis for determining criminal responsibility. Known as the "product rule," this had actually been articulated by the New Hampshire Supreme Court in 1870. The rule stated that a person is not criminally responsible if the behavior at the time of the crime was a "product" of mental illness. The Durham rule did not gain wide acceptance and was generally discarded in 1972.

American Law Institute's Model Penal Code   In 1955 the **American Law Institute (ALI)** drafted the **Model Penal Code** test, which states that a person is

Myths and Realities of the Insanity Defense

Myth: Many criminal defendants plead insanity and most are acquitted.

Reality: The insanity plea is rarely used; acquittals are extremely rare.

Myth: The insanity defense causes major problems for the criminal justice system.

Reality: The insanity defense has a minor practical role in the criminal justice system but a very important moral role.

Myth: Mentally ill people are dangerous and are capable of violent behavior at any time.

Reality: The overwhelming majority of the 35 million mentally ill people in this country are neither dangerous nor unpredictable; they are victims of stigma.

Myth: Most insanity defendants are murderers who commit random acts of violence.

Reality: Most of the crimes committed by insanity defendants are nonviolent crimes. Only 14 percent of insanity defendants are charged with homicide or other violent crimes, most of which are directed not at strangers but at family members and authority figures.

Myth: The insanity defense allows defendants to fool juries and escape punishment.

Reality: The overwhelming majority of acquittees suffer from the most serious forms of mental illness.

Myth: The insanity defense is a rich man's defense.

Reality: Most insanity defendants are likely to be as poor as most other criminal defendants.

Myth: Insanity trials are a "circus" of conflicting expert testimony that confuses the jury.

Reality: Most insanity cases reflect agreement among the experts, the defense, and the prosecution; few go to trial, and even fewer go to a jury. The celebrated cases are the exception, not the rule.

Myth: Most insanity acquittees go free immediately or within a short time after trial.

Reality: The majority of acquittees are confined for significant periods of time.

Myth: Insanity acquittees repeat the same crime when they are released.

Reality: Crimes committed by insanity acquittees upon release tend to be less violent in nature. Recidivism rates are no higher than for convicted felons.

Myth: The "guilty but mentally ill" verdict means that the defendant will receive mental health treatment.

Reality: A "guilty but mentally ill" verdict does not guarantee treatment beyond what a convicted felon would receive.

---

not responsible if because of a mental disease he or she lacks the capacity either to appreciate the criminality (wrongfulness) of an act or to conform his or her conduct to the requirements of the law. The ALI formulation includes both cognitive (knowledge) and volitional (control) criteria. It is used in all federal circuit courts and was used in the Hinckley case. More than half the states also use these criteria. Approximately one-third of the states use some variation of the M'Naghten rule and irresistible impulse test. New Hampshire is the only state still using the product rule.

Proposals since the Hinckley Verdict

Despite its infrequent use, the insanity defense is the subject of much debate since the 1982 "not guilty by reason of insanity" verdict in the trial of John Hinckley, Jr., would-be assassin of President Ronald Reagan. The verdict drew a mixed reaction from the American public. Some believed Hinckley to be insane.

Others felt frustrated that punishment had not been administered. To some people the success of the insanity plea seemed linked to the ability to afford an expensive legal defense.

Prior to the Hinckley verdict, the insanity defense had been raised in a number of other sensational cases. The media focus on the "Twinkie defense"—so called because of the argument that junk food affected Dan White's mental functioning and diminished his responsibility in the murder of a San Francisco mayor and councilman—did not exactly portray psychiatry in a positive light. David Berkowitz, a bizarre multiple murderer known as "Son of Sam," was initially found incompetent to stand trial. Once competent, he surprisingly pleaded guilty to second-degree murder, and the insanity issue was never presented at trial.

Prior to more effective treatment of mental disorders, a verdict of not guilty by reason of insanity (NGRI) saved a person from the death penalty but not from lifelong incarceration. With modern treatment, however, individuals who are found NGRI are often released or discharged quite early. Movie and television portrayals of ex-mental clients as "mad killers" and "homicidal maniacs" have primed the public to fear the worst.

Since the Hinckley verdict there have been various proposals to limit drastically or abolish the insanity defense. Montana and Idaho have already done so. The National Commission on the Insanity Defense was an independent commission established by the National Mental Health Association to broaden the public debate on the insanity defense and make recommendations of its own. From its investigations, public hearings, and analysis, the commission concluded that much of the outcry for change in the insanity defense is based more on myths and displaced frustration over the multiple problems of the criminal justice system than on facts. The myths and realities of the insanity defense are summarized in the accompanying box.

No definitive answers are available on the fate of the insanity defense, which reflects society's ambivalence and discontent with this issue. However, it is a moral and ethical dilemma worthy of the attention of psychiatric nurses.

CHAPTER HIGHLIGHTS

• Law develops in a social context—ideally in response to the problems and needs of the governed.

• Factors influencing the development of laws about the rights of mentally disturbed persons include the state of medical knowledge, the community's acceptance of some responsibility, and the legal profession's sensitivity to the social and civil liabilities that befall the mentally disturbed.

• Knowledge of existing mental health legislation is essential for nurses to become politically active and protect the legal rights of individuals using mental health services.

• Mental health legislation varies considerably from state to state. In every state, mental hygiene laws identify procedures for admission to and discharge from mental hospitals, but only some states deal with the medical and legal rights of hospitalized persons.

• Members of the health professions are being held increasingly accountable for their behavior. They need to become familiar with the state laws that govern their responsibilities and actions.

• Contemporary issues concerning rights of hospitalized clients include access to communication, use of restraints and seclusion, use of psychosurgery and electroconvulsive therapy, and provision for periodic review of involuntary clients.

• Contemporary legal issues important in humanistic psychiatric nursing practice include involuntary admission criteria, the right to treatment, civil rights of hospitalized persons, client-therapist relations, the controversial right to refuse treatment, and treatment in the least restrictive alternative.

• Theory about rights of mental clients often is not reflected in practice.

• Effective implementation of client's rights frequently depends on awareness, support, and advocacy by the psychiatric nurse.

• Mental health statutes and court decisions impact on the practice of psychiatry. Psychiatry also affects the resolution of such legal questions as the credibility of witnesses; competency to make a will, contract, or to stand trial; custody of children; and, most controversial, criminal responsibility.

REFERENCES

Alexander R: The right to treatment in mental and correctional institutions. *Social Work* 1989;34(2):109–112.

Appelbaum P: The right to refuse treatment with antipsychotic medications: Retrospect and prospect. *Am J Psychiatry* 1988;145(4):413–419.

Appelbaum P: *Tarasoff* and the clinician: Problems in fulfilling the duty to protect. *Am J Psychiatry* 1985;142:425–429.

Bach JP: Requiring due care in the process of patient deinstitutionalization: Toward a common law approach to mental health care reform. *Yale Law Journal* 1989;98(6):1153–1172.

Bender BM, Murphy D, Mark B: Caring for clients with legal charges on a voluntary psychiatric unit. *J Psychosoc Nurs* 1989;27(3):16–20.

Bernstein MR, Miller RD, VanRydrock GJ: The impact of the right to refuse treatment on a forensic patient population: 6 month review. *Bull Am Acad Psychiatry Law* 1989;17(2):107–119.

Birnbaum M: The right to treatment. *American Bar Association Journal* 1960;46:499–505.

Bloom JD: The character of danger in psychiatric practice: Are the mentally ill dangerous? *Bull Am Acad Psychiatry Law* 1989;17(3):241–254.

Brakel SJ, Parry J, Weiner BA: *The Mentally Disabled and the Law*. American Bar Foundation, 1985.

Brooks AD: Law and ideology in the case of Billie Boggs. *J Psychosoc Nurs* 1988;20:22–25.

Brown P, Smith CJ: Mental patients' rights: An empirical study of variation across the United States: *Int J Law Psychiatry* 1988;11:157–165.

Code for Nurses with Interpretive Statements. American Nurses' Association, 1976.

Cournos F: Involuntary medication and the case of Joyce Brown. *Hosp Community Psychiatry* 1989;40(7):736–740.

Croxton TA, Churchill SR, Fellin P: Counseling minors without parental consent. *Child Welfare* 1988;67(1):3–14.

DeCoste B: The many faces of advocacy: Victory and peace. *Am J Nurs* 1990;90(1):80–81.

DeLeon Siantz ML: Children's rights and parental rights: A historical and legal ethical analysis. *J Child Adolesc Psychiatr Ment Health Nurs* 1988;1(1):14–17.

Donaldson K: *Insanity Inside Out.* Crown, 1976.

Freddolino P, Moxley D, Fleishman J: An advocacy model for people with long-term psychiatric disabilities. *Hosp Community Psychiatry* 1989;40(11):1169–1174.

Garritson SH: Degrees of restrictiveness in psychosocial nursing. *J Psychosoc Nurs* 1983;21:9–16.

Guidry J, Rinck W, Rinck C: Persons with developmental disabilities and tardive dyskinesia: A historical perspective and an examination of state policies responding to litigation questions. *J Psychiatry Law* 1988;Winter:625–659.

Haimowitz S: HIV and the mentally ill: An approach to the legal issues. *Hosp Community Psychiatry* 1989;40(7):732–736.

Hargreaves WA et al.: Effects of the Jamison-Farabee consent decree: Due process protection for involuntary psychiatric patients treated with psychoactive medication. *Am J Psychiatry* 1987;144(2):188–192.

Hiday V, Scheid-Cook TL: A follow-up of chronic patients committed to out-patient treatment. *Hosp Community Psychiatry* 1989;40(1):52–59.

Jemelka R, Trupin E, Chiles JA: The mentally ill in prison. *Hosp Community Psychiatry* 1989;40(5):481–491.

Killebrew JA, Harris C, Kruckeberg K: A conceptual model for determining the least restrictive treatment-training modality. *Hosp Community Psychiatry* 1982;33:367–370.

McFarland B, Faulkner LR, et al.: Chronic mental illness and the criminal justice system. *Hosp Community Psychiatry* 1989;40(7):718–723.

Mental Health Systems Act: Summary and analysis. *Mental Disability Law Reporter* 1980;4:383–390.

Miller RD, Doren DM, VanRybrolk G, Maier G: Emerging problems for staff associated with the release of potentially dangerous forensic patients. *Bull Am Acad Psychiatry Law* 1988;16(4):309–319.

Monahan J: Risk assessment of violence among the mentally disordered: Generating useful knowledge. *Int J Law Psychiatry* 1988;11:249–257.

Morrison EF: Victimization in prison: Implications for the mentally ill inmate and for health professionals. *Arch Psychiatr Nurs* 1990;28(8):25–30.

Myths and Realities: A Report of the National Commission on the Insanity Defense. National Mental Health Association, March 1983.

Nelson S, Berger V: Current issues in state mental health forensic programs. *Bull Am Acad Psychiatry Law* 1988;16(1):67–75.

Parry J et al.: *Mental Disability Law: A Primer,* ed 3. American Bar Foundation, 1988.

Perlin ML: *Mental Disability Law: Civil and Criminal.* 3 vol. Michie Company, 1989.

Price R, Denner B: *The Making of a Mental Patient.* Holt, Rinehart and Winston, 1973.

Rachlin S: Rethinking the Right to Refuse Treatment. *Pychiatr Ann* 1989;19(4):213–219.

Ransohoff P, et al.: Restrictivenss of care among the severely mentally disabled. *Hosp Community Psychiatry* 1984;35:706–709.

Rosenbaum A, Appelbaum P: *Tarasoff* and the researcher: Does the duty to protect apply in the research setting? *Am Psychol* 1989;44(6):885–894.

Rubenstien L, Gattozzi A, Goldman H: Protecting the entitlements of the mentally disabled: The SSDI/SSI legal battles of the 1980s. *Int J Law Psychiatry* 1988;(11):269–278.

Schmidt MJ, Geller J: Involuntary administration of medication in the community: The judicial opportunity. *Bull Am Acad Psychiatry Law* 1989;17(3):283–292.

Schmidt W, Otto R: A legal and behavioral sciences analysis of statutory guidelines for children's mental health and substance abuse services: The Florida case. *J Psychiatry Law* 1988;Spring:9–65.

Schwartz HI, Vingiano W, Perez CB: Autonomy and the right to refuse treatment: Patients' attitudes after involuntary medication. *Hosp Community Psychiatry* 1988;39(10):1049–1054.

Smith SR, Meyer RG: *Law, Behavior, and Mental Health: Policy and Practice.* New York University Press, 1987.

Standards of Psychiatric-Mental Health Nursing Practice. American Nurses' Association, 1982.

Szasz T: *Law, Liberty and Psychiatry.* Macmillan, 1963.

Weiss FS: The right to refuse: Informed consent and the psychosocial nurse. *J Psychosoc Nurs* 1990;28(8):25–30.

Zonona H, Applebaum PS, Bonnie R, Roth L: Statutory approaches to limiting psychiatrists' liability for their patients' violent acts. *Am J Psychiatry* 1989;146(7):821–828.

Community Mental Health

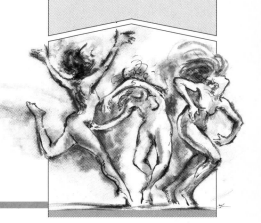

LEARNING OBJECTIVES

- Identify the social conditions that led to the development of the community mental health movement

- Discuss the impact of legislation on community mental health

- Explain six concepts basic to community mental health philosophy

- Relate the ANA Psychiatric-Mental Health Nursing Standards of practice and professional performance to community mental health nursing

- Identify community mental health nursing roles appropriate to the educational preparation, skills, and experience of the individual nurse

- Describe community mental health nursing roles and functions in terms of primary, secondary, and tertiary levels of prevention

- Evaluate the problems of the community mental health and deinstitutionalization movements

- Discuss examples of innovations in community care of the severely and chronically mentally disordered

Holly Skodol Wilson
Carol Ren Kneisl

CROSS REFERENCES

Other topics relevant to this content are: Chronically mentally ill, Chapter 17; Families, Chapter 30; Family burden in schizophrenia, Chapter 12; History, Chapter 1; Legal issues, Chapter 37.

THE TWO PEOPLE DESCRIBED below have something in common: their experiences with a system for delivery of mental health services called **community mental health**. This chapter explores the dimensions of their experience in which the locus of care has shifted in three decades from large, often isolated, state institutions to the community itself. This chapter also addresses continuing problems and current issues that have resulted from this shift.

In the cavernous interior of a large railroad terminal, a 39-year-old woman makes her home on an old wooden bench, surrounded by three large plastic bags that hold all her earthly possessions. She hears voices inside her head and see frightening things such as snakes and abandoned babies. She is one of an estimated tens of thousands of homeless men and women in New York City thought by various observers to be former residents of state psychiatric hospitals. In another metropolitan area, a 62-year-old man walks to a storefront clinic in his neighborhood where he tells the receptionist in his native Italian that his pill bottle is empty and he needs another prescription.

Turning Points in Psychiatric Care

The community mental health movement is often referred to as the third revolution in psychiatry (the first was the provision of treatment for, rather than incarceration of, the mentally ill; the second was the emphasis on intrapsychic causes, an outgrowth of psychoanalysis). However, a number of other turning points have been responsible for creating the social conditions that led to the development of the community mental health movement:

• In the late 1700s, Philippe Pinel of Paris cast off the chains and irons that bound the mentally disordered and ushered in the era of moral management and mental institutions (the first revolution).

• At the turn of this century, Sigmund Freud of Vienna developed a method of investigation, therapeutic technique, and body of scientific concepts and propositions called psychoanalysis (the second revolution).

• During World War II, almost 2,000,000 late adolescent and young adult men were found unfit for military service because of psychiatric and neurologic findings, and large numbers of military personnel and veterans required psychiatric treatment and hospitalization.

• The National Institute of Mental Health was created in 1946, heralding the beginning of a new federalism in the provision of mental health services.

• Drug treatment for mental illness began in the early 1950s.

• In 1955 the National Mental Health Study Act established the Joint Commission on Mental Illness.

• In his 1963 message to Congress, President John F. Kennedy called for a "bold, new approach" to the problems of mental illness and mental retardation.

This chapter is concerned with the events that began in 1955 and shaped the social movements that we know as deinstitutionalization and community mental health. It also suggests future directions.

Historical Perspectives on the Community Mental Health Movement

The emergence of the community mental health movement can be traced through these events:

• In the ten years following the end of World War II, the in-patient population of state psychiatric institutions grew from 450,000 to 550,000. New institutions were built and old ones became more crowded. This had a profound impact on the economic health of many states and drew the attention and concern of politicians at local, state, and national levels. They were the moving force responsible in 1955 for legislating the National Mental Health Study Act that established the Joint Commission on Mental Illness and Health. This group was charged with the responsibility of studying the mental health needs of the nation and making recommendations for a national mental health program.

• Psychotropic drugs, especially tranquilizers, were being increasingly used. They helped staff members manage large numbers of clients in crowded conditions. Research into chemotherapy and the etiology of mental illness seemed to promise that an answer or cure could be discovered any time.

• Group therapy and short-term (five to six sessions) individual psychotherapy instituted to treat large numbers of military personnel began to be used for other segments of the population. Mental health professionals began to consider options other than costly long-term individual psychotherapy or long-term hospitalization.

• Milieu therapy, sometimes called sociotherapy, began to develop based on the efforts of Maxwell Jones, who established therapeutic communities in English hospital settings (1953), and Alfred Stanton and Morris Schwartz (1949) and Milton Greenblatt, Richard H. York, and Esther Lucille Brown (1955), who studied milieus in the United States.

By 1961, the Joint Commission on Mental Illness and Health had presented its report, *Action for Mental Health,* to Congress. The report concluded that psychiatric services in this country were woefully inadequate. The landmark recommendations of the group called for:

• A shift from institutional to community-based care

• A more equitable distribution of mental health services

• Preventive services

• Consumer participation in both the planning and delivery of mental health services

• The hiring and training of citizens in the community as nonprofessional mental health workers

• The education of increased numbers of mental health professionals

• Public support for research

• Shared federal, state, and local funding for the construction and operation of a system of community mental health centers

The Community Health Center Act authorized 150 million dollars in federal funds to be matched by state funds over three years for the construction of comprehensive community mental health centers. A center could continue to receive federal support in decreasing proportions for an eight-year period. It was expected that after this time centers would be able to operate on state and local funds and fees received from services.

The Community Mental Health Centers Act did not work as planned. Some states and local municipalities did not have funds to match those available at the federal level. Some centers, especially those in poverty areas or predominantly rural areas, were unable to generate sufficient revenue through fees. Services that generated little or no income, such as public education and mental health consultation, began to suffer.

President Carter established a twenty-member President's Commission on Mental Health in 1977. The *Report to the President of the President's Commission on Mental Health* (1978) focused on the following major areas:

• Providing community-based services as the keystone of the mental health system

• Improving community support systems and networks among families, neighbors, community organizations, and existing service components

• Establishing national health insurance that would include coverage for mental health care

• Encouraging mental health coverage (including outpatient) in all health insurance plans

• Continuing the phaseout of large public mental hospitals and improving services in those remaining

• Providing funding to increase the number of mental health professionals, especially those working with minorities, children, and the aged

• Establishing a center with a strong emphasis on primary prevention within the National Institute of Mental Health

• Protecting the human rights of persons in need of mental health care

• Improving the delivery of services to underserved populations and high-risk populations, such as minorities and the chronically ill, through a new federal program

• Developing an advocacy program for the chronically mentally ill

• Increasing support for research related to mental health and illness

• Providing health education to the public and increasing the public understanding of mental health problems

• Centralizing the evaluation efforts of governmental agencies concerned with mental health

The Community Mental Health Systems Act of 1980 was a major achievement of the outgoing Carter administration. It was designed to implement the recommendations made by the president's commission authorizing the funding of **community mental health centers,** services to high-risk populations, ambulatory mental health care centers, a prevention unit and associate director for minority concerns at NIMH, rape research and services, and recommending a model mental health patient's bill of rights. The severely mentally disordered continued to inhabit state institutions, and those with less acute problems used the services of federally funded community mental health centers. There was little coordination between these two systems. Clients discharged from state institutions often failed to receive follow-up services, and certain populations—the chronically mentally ill, the elderly, and youth—fell between the two systems. This act was intended to coordinate federal and state efforts.

The 1980 Community Mental Health Systems Act was essentially repealed in 1981 when the 97th

Congress passed the new Reagan administration's Omnibus Budget Reconciliation Act (PL97–35). The new budget placed the mental health services programs formerly administered by NIMH into an alcohol, drug abuse, and mental health services **block grant,** shifting the decision-making about allocation of funds to the states and decreasing the federal role in coordination.

The decrease in the federal budget has had far-ranging effects on the community mental health movement. It cuts funding for community mental health centers and other mental health care delivery programs.

In 1977 the NIMH began its **Community Support Program (CSP)** designed to assist states and communities to develop long-term comprehensive **community support systems (CSS)** for people with long-term mental illness. Financial assistance in the form of grants was provided to state mental health agencies to improve their service system activities. What began as a pilot effort soon developed into a national program (Mosher and Burti 1989). By 1986 CSP extended its activities to provide funds for community services demonstration projects that bring a systems view to community mental health. A CSS is more than a network of services. It represents a philosophy about the way services should be delivered to the chronically and persistently mentally ill that has contributed to what are currently growing family and consumer movements. The elements of CSS are:

• Mental health treatment directed to helping clients manage symptoms, manage medications, recognize signs of relapse, and cope with daily living

  • Crisis response services

  • Health and dental care

  • Housing

  • Income support

  • Peer support

• Family and community support on an individual and group basis directed at helping clients cope with life problems and stresses

  • Rehabilitation services

  • Protection and advocacy

  • Client identification and outreach

Psychosocial rehabilitation, supported apartment programs, and case management (central notions of CSP) are gaining in popularity and availability in the 1990s (NIMH 1987).

On October 1, 1983, the single largest payer for health care services (Medicare) started paying hospitals according to a system called **prospective payment**

(PP). With that development, hospitals of this nation embarked on a new and uncharted course.

Cost-based, retrospective reimbursement is a complicated term for the way hospital care had been paid for prior to October 1983. It was a system that current policy makers argue rewarded hospitals for spending more. "Retrospective payment for services put most of the financial risk on the payer and provided hospitals with incentives to maximize use" (Davis 1984). The concept of prospective payment is presumably intended to provide incentives for efficient hospital management. If a hospital is paid a fixed amount for each client admitted for a hysterectomy, for example, it has an incentive not to exceed that specified payment for each type of client. The assumption is, of course, that **diagnostically related groups (DRGs)** (groups of diagnoses for which a set payment is made) correlate well with use of hospital resources. At the time of this text's publication, psychiatric care DRGs grow in their influence on decisions.

Original Concepts

The original basic philosophy of the community mental health movement was that health care is a right and, therefore, mental health services should be available to all people. The six concepts basic to community mental health are discussed below.

Systems Perspective

The systems perspective provides a holistic view of people and their environment and has already been described in other chapters. Basic to community mental health is the notion that people constantly interact with the environment. A systems perspective requires broadening the scope of mental health care beyond the individual to the system (community) as a whole with holistic awareness of the biologic, psychologic, and sociocultural forces that influence interacting systems.

Levels of Prevention

Since its origin, the community mental health movement has emphasized prevention. Gerald Caplan (1964) adapted the concepts of preventive medicine for application to psychiatry in general and to community mental health in particular. The levels of prevention in mental health care—primary, secondary, and tertiary—are the foundation for the nursing role in community mental health, and are described later in this chapter.

Interdisciplinary Collaboration

The essential services of community mental health cannot be totally provided by the members of any one discipline or paraprofessional group. Blurring of roles between and among mental health professionals is even more apparent in community mental health programs. It can be traced to the 1961 report of the Joint Commission on Mental Illness and Health that recommended that nurses provide brief, short-term psychotherapy to psychiatric clients. While some nurses in some sections of the country were already doing so, this report further legitimized their psychotherapy role. The 1963 legislation funded graduate level clinical specialist programs to prepare nurses at the psychotherapist level. The lines between psychiatric nursing and the other mental health professions became even more indistinct and even psychiatric nurses have experienced difficulty in defining what is unique to nursing. Fortunately, increased nursing research and the development of nursing theories have helped define this area for psychiatric nurses.

Consumer Participation and Control

Consumer participation and control was another ideal community mental health movement. Although the 1961 Joint Commission report recommended community involvement and was supported by the subsequent legislation, the practical aspects were not clear.

In many instances, citizen participation continued as it had in the past; socially prominent citizens, wealthy contributors, and health care providers continued to serve on the governing bodies of mental health agencies. The 1975 amendments provided clarifying guidelines for citizen participation by requiring governing bodies of new community mental health centers to be composed of people living in the area served by the community mental health center, at least half of whom should not be health care providers. In addition, it required that centers in operation before 1975 appoint community members in an advisory capacity to their governing boards. This legislation aimed to ensure that the services provided by community mental health centers would respond to the needs of the citizens. This demonstrated both the philosophic and policy commitment to a decision-making role for the citizens of a given community.

Members of the community also participate in other ways. Some indigenous nonprofessionals have been employed by community mental health programs as human service workers. Because they understand the problems of the community and the language and customs of ethnic groups specific to that community, they have been quite successful in delivering personalized mental health services. The most meaningful participation has been through consumer advocacy self-help groups such as the **National Alliance for the Mentally Ill (NAMI)**.

Comprehensive Services

The community mental health philosophy is committed to providing a full range of comprehensive services to all the members of a community.

The community as client was defined in terms of **catchment areas**, geographically circumscribed areas comprising a city, or several rural communities, with from 75,000 to 200,000 residents. This divided a population into segments whose mental health needs could be met by a specifically designed system of services. Optimally, the segments were supposed to be small enough to promote collaborative relationships within the system of services.

Continuity of Care

Continuity of care means that, while providing comprehensive services to clients, caregivers also assume the responsibility of monitoring or assisting clients in their move from one program to another. In traditional mental health care systems, separate programs rarely interface, and clients may feel that they have been shuttled from one mental health agency to another. In some instances, clients become discouraged or embarrassed about obtaining needed services. Others are unable to be persistent or seek help in the first place. The continuity of care concept in community mental health was intended to correct these problems. Unfortunately, the community mental heath movement has not fulfilled its promise in relation to the concept.

Nursing Roles in Community Mental Health

Community mental health nursing roles consist of a wide scope of activities from the maintenance of mental health and prevention of illness to treatment and rehabilitation. In the broadest sense of the words, the community is the client. Because people are constantly interacting with the environment, when community mental health nurses provide direct services to individual clients, they also direct attention toward the client's community.

Applying the ANA Standards

One of the ANA Psychiatric Nursing Professional Performance Standards provides an umbrella for community mental health nursing practice at the clinical specialist level:

Standard 10: Utilization of Community Health Systems
The nurse participates with other members of the community in assessing, planning, implementing, and evaluating mental health services and community systems that include the promotion of the broad continuum of primary, secondary, and tertiary prevention of mental illness.

While demonstrating competence in meeting Standard 10 has been determined by the ANA to be in the province of the specialist, the community mental health nurse generalist uses all the other standards as guidelines for practice.

Levels of Community Mental Health Nursing

There is no one set of skills, educational preparation, or nursing experience that determines who is and who is not a community mental health nurse. Both generalists and specialists practice in community settings. They are identified by their commitment to the philosophy and concepts presented earlier in this chapter. However, their roles vary according to the educational preparation, skills, and experience they possess.

Primary, Secondary, and Tertiary Prevention

Community mental health nurses hold the principles of primary, secondary, and tertiary prevention as central to their clinical work.

• **In primary prevention**, the nurse is concerned with preventing new cases of mental disorder by counteracting harmful stressors. Nursing activities are directed toward fostering mental well-being and identifying potential stressors and segments of the population that may be at high risk.

• **In secondary prevention**, the nurse attempts to shorten the duration of a mental disorder through early case-finding and treatment and to reduce its prevalence in a given segment of the population.

• **In tertiary prevention**, the nurse implements treatments and rehabilitative services for clients who have been diagnosed as mentally disordered.

Table 38–1 gives specific examples of community mental health nursing roles and functions in all three levels of prevention.

Community Mental Health and Deinstitutionalization: Continuing Problems and Current Issues

Deinstitutionalization and the community mental health movement, called "a bold new approach" by President John F. Kennedy in the 1960s, grew out of political, social, and economic circumstance. Although these concepts mean different things to different people, the consensus is that deinstitutionalization resulted in the discharge of large numbers of clients from mental hospitals and the avoidance of and decrease in hospitalization of mentally ill people, many of whom would have been hospitalized in mental institutions thirty years ago. The community mental health movement refers to changes in the delivery of mental health services.

The shifts in number and location of clients and the changes in mental health services have not resulted

---

TABLE 38–1   Community Mental Health Nursing Roles and Functions

Primary Prevention	Secondary Prevention	Tertiary Prevention
Identifying potentially stressful conditions in the community and high-risk populations	Providing brief psychotherapy to individuals, groups, and families	Helping plan for a client's discharge from the hosptial
Holding effective parenting classes for adolescent parents, at day-care centers, in schools	Suicide prevention hot line counseling and staffing crisis intervention programs	Coordinating and monitoring follow-up care in home, half-way house, foster care home, or other transitional service
Holding divorce therapy groups for couples, families, and individuals	Providing counseling to victims of violence and their significant others	Teaching clients self-care activities before discharge from the hospital using psychosocial rehabilitation
Providing mental health consultation to health care providers	Holding stress reduction groups for health care providers	Serving as a client advocate
Providing mental health education to members of the community	Case-finding and referring clients in need of treatment	Providing individual, group, and family psychotherapy
Consulting with self-help groups	Providing emergency mental health services	Referring clients to self-help groups or aftercare services
Being politically active in relation to mental health issues	Intake, screening, and assessment of clients	Staffing partial hospitalization programs

RESEARCH NOTE

Citation

Wilson HS: Deinstitutionalized Residential Care for the Mentally Disordered: The Soteria House Approach. *Grune & Stratton, 1982.*

Study Problem/Purpose

In the absence of conventional, elaborate, psychiatric control structures (such as formalized authority lines, hierarchical division of labor, formal organizational goals, schedules, therapies, and locked doors), how are problems of social control solved?

Methods

Data were collected using field research strategies. These strategies included 200 hours of field observation, eleven in-depth interviews with eight staff members, analysis of all available documents related to the facility (e.g., grant proposals, journal articles, correspondence, and records), attendance at four formal presentations about the setting, review of a documentary film, and self-examination of the investigator's own experiences.

Findings

Conventional, formal techniques for social control are negated and avoided at Soteria House. Instead of restrictive, controlling approaches to manage others' behaviors, an infracontrol process emerges. Infracontrol consists of three implementing processes: presencing, fairing, and limiting intrusion. *Presencing* refers to ways in which the physical presence of other people influence and shape resident behavior. *Presencing* consists of mere physical presence, purposeful monitoring, and active intervention. *Fairing* refers to the management and distribution of work according to an implicit understanding of fairness. *Limiting intrusion* refers to the process of restricting involvement and control by external agencies in the activities of Soteria House.

Implications

The deinstitutionalization movement aimed to provide vigorous early treatment to mentally disordered individuals close to their home and aimed to avoid the debilitating impact of prolonged hospitalization with its loss of social and interpersonal skills. Yet community mental health treatment has become governed by rigid standards, policies, procedures, and regulations. Clients are screened, labeled, medicated, and discharged with the same lack of attention to their self-control and self-determination as occurred in institutional treatment. Soteria House operationalized the deinstitutionalization philosophy and showed that successful experience provides direction to nurses wishing to intervene in a less rigid, controlling, and routinized fashion. The Soteria approach has the capacity to humanize care of the increasing numbers of chronically mentally disordered. Additionally, humane treatment philosophies and techniques are applicable in all health care settings.

---

in improved care. Kennedy's "bold new approach" is now characterized as:

- "A disaster by any measure used" by the Public Citizen Health Research Group and the National Alliance for the Mentally Ill

- A bureaucratized clearinghouse, where "dispatching and processing" clients has replaced "storing" them (Wilson 1982)

- "An abdication of responsibility due to shortcomings in legislation, lack of funding and the unanticipated impact of discharged clients on communities" (Bassuk and Gerson 1978)

- A misnomer by Talbott (1979), who substituted the term **transinstitutionalization** to refer to the circumstances in which chronically mentally ill people have been shifted from "a single lousy institution to multiple wretched ones."

Talbott (1979) characterizes the outcomes as follows:

- The dramatic appearance of large numbers of dirty, hallucinating strange faces on city streets, in low-cost ghettos, and deteriorating neighborhoods; in his words, "naked men dancing on Broadway and bag ladies on Park Avenue"

- Transfer of thousand of clients to nursing homes

- Mental health service patterns of use characterized by "falling between the cracks," a lack of follow-up, and "the revolving door" of continued readmissions

An analysis of data collected at NIMH yielded three conclusions about deinstitutionalization:

1. Outpatient care had not replaced in-patient care.

2. Public institutions have not been replaced by community-based facilities.

3. Private resources have not replaced public ones as the bearer of cost for the mentally ill.

Persistent Problems

Aviram (1990) defines the most stressing problems and current issues for community care of the chronically mental ill as follows:

* Homelessness and problems of residence.

* Issues related to relying on strictly medical interpretations of mental illness. These interpretations do not take into account that many of the problems are clearly related to the welfare system and therefore limit systemwide biopsychosocial perspectives.

* Financing of services through individual contacts. This structure creates a negative organizational incentive to provide services to those regarded as "difficult" clients. This system of financing, coupled with scarcity of resources, has led to the practice of "creaming" or "skimming" the best and most stable clients. Under such conditions, the severely and persistently mentally ill (SMI) who are most needy are the most seriously neglected.

* Insufficient research knowledge about psychiatric rehabilitation programs that limits financial independence and self-sufficiency of people with mental disorders, particularly with respect to work skills and employment.

* The burden on families. Even those mentally ill persons who do not live with their families create a family burden by their presence in the same community. Organizations of families of the mentally ill and such self-help groups as NAMI often act as watchdog and critic and sometimes create a conflict between family groups and mental health professionals. Yet all agree on the need for improvement in community services.

Alternatives to Deinstitutionalization

The psychiatric community has learned some important lessons from its experience with **deinstitutionalization** and the community mental health movement over the last decades. Caregivers have learned to think about the needs of the mentally ill, particularly the chronically mentally ill (CMI) or the **severely and persistently mentally ill (SMI)** in new ways. We have learned about:

* The importance of social support

* The necessity of involving natural or family caregivers

* The importance of planning creative, residential alternatives.

* The need to direct treatment approaches to both the disorder itself and the associated disability through social skills training

* The possibility that nursing could provide a cadre of specialists in psychoeducation and chronic care management to transform these lessons into renewed opportunities for mental health care.

Deinstitutionalization is one of the most important developments in the history of psychiatry, yet the well-intentioned reform movement has from its beginning been plagued by a variety of problems.

The Case Manager

The concept of the case manager advanced by the Community Support Program of NIMH was an important innovation in the care of the long-term mentally ill in the community. Case managers are expected to coordinate services and ensure their delivery to meet the needs of the mentally ill. Many of the basic features of this newly created position are grounded in the tradition of social work. Although some saw the case manager as a panacea for all the problems of community care for the seriously mentally ill, major difficulties have stemmed from the ambiguous role.

The case manager is expected to be the primary care agent, the human contact between the client and the bureaucracy, the advocate for the client, and simultaneously, the representative to the formal organization. Critics feel that if case managers are to fulfill their potential, they would need the resources, administrative authority, and salaries that would attract professionals to this role (Aviram 1990).

Psychoeducational Approaches for Family Caregivers

Theoretic and scientific interest in the relationships between support and outcomes for disabled and dependent disordered clients have resulted in another post-deinstitutionalization innovation known as the **psychoeducational approach** (Anderson et al. 1981; 1986). Reports from successful treatment programs for the chronically ill underscore the importance of mobilizing interpersonal and environmental supports to maintain biologic, psychologic, and social functions and community tenure (Test and Stein 1978). Erosion of social supports leaves the disabled vulnerable to extreme isolation and to the recidivism, treatment inadequacy or instability, and social disaffiliation that this isolation frequently implies.

Goals The psychoeducational approach to family treatment has two basic goals:

1. Decreased client vulnerability to environmental stimulation through a program of educated maintenance chemotherapy and other treatment regimens

2. Increased predictability and stability of the family environment achieved by decreasing the anxiety of family members about the client, increasing their knowledge about chronic mental disorders, and increasing their repertoire of strategies to deal with the problems that need confident management

When rehospitalization rates are used to reflect outcomes, the rate is significantly less in families who have undergone psychoeducation than in control groups whose family members were treated exclusively with drug or surgical therapy (Anderson et al. 1981).

Phases in the Psychoeducation Approach The two goals of psychoeducation can be achieved through interventions that fall into four somewhat overlapping categories:

1. Connecting

2. Survival skills training

3. Individualization

4. Continuation or disengagement

Connecting Psychoeducation with families of chronically disordered and dependent clients is based on the central premise that families can be a pivotal resource for the care and long-term management of their relatives if they are given emotional and practical support and information. The approach begins as early in contacts with the family system as possible with sessions devoted to connecting, or building an alliance, with the family. Such sessions typically include discussion of the pain, frustration, embarrassment, and anger associated with the burdens of caring for a chronically disordered, disabled, and dependent relative. The intent of these sessions is to obtain a good grasp of the type and degree of difficulties experienced by the family. The nurse in this role should realize that most families have met at least one health professional who has implied that they directly or indirectly caused their relative's illness. For this reason, the nurse should strive to be viewed as the family's ombudsman. Moreover, the nurse should realize that feelings of helplessness and hopelessness prevail even among caring and concerned families and should emphasize

the family's strengths and power to influence the course of things positively. The family's performance of care tasks can have a positive effect on the client and become important to keeping the client alive, out of the hospital, or at a higher level of self-care adaptive functioning. The final task of this initial phase in the psychoeducational approach is to establish a mutual agreement about the goals, content, length, rules, and methods of family counseling. The point here is to establish a treatment contract.

Survival Skills Training Often survival skills training takes the form of multiple family workshops that provide information about the symptoms, onset, course, and outcome of the client's disability and about different families' experiences living with it. It is important to distinguish between factual data and opinions about these topics. Information about medications should include the mechanisms of action, main effects, and possible side effects. The nurse should stress the evidence that medication compliance is associated with control and even survival but encourage each family to weigh the costs and benefits of all and any medications. Information about management should include how to set reasonable limits, decrease overstimulation, avoid blow-ups, create helpful structures such as labels for those with Alzheimer's disease, and reevaluate and modify expectations for the client. The nurse should support family members' needs to normalize their own lives as much as possible and to establish networks for social and psychologic support as well as practical help.

Individualization The individualization category of family meetings customarily includes both client and caregiving family. The overall goal of these meetings is to apply strategies to the individual situation. The sessions usually address family boundaries and client responsibilities.

The goals with respect to family boundaries are to increase structure in the family (i.e., the boundaries between the client and the family) and decrease the boundaries between the family and sources of social support. The goal with respect to client responsibilities is to increase the client's assumption of self-care tasks and enhance competencies in these areas. Problems often center on the client's lack of energy and motivation to decrease dependency and increase self-care levels and the family's guilt about providing for their own needs rather than concentrating on the client's needs. The psychiatric nurse can provide invaluable help by becoming a **broker for community resources,** directing and coordinating family members toward respite care, support groups, and the like.

Continuation or Disengagement Usually when maximally effective family functioning has been attained, the family either moves into more conventional family therapy or elects "maintenance sessions," which become less frequent and ultimately terminate.

The intent of these sessions is to maintain initial gains and to abort potential new problems by anticipating stress and reinforcing knowledge about the client's illness—be it schizophrenia, substance abuse, or Alzheimer's disease—its characteristics, and family burdens.

Model Community Support Programs

Several community support programs that incorporate both case management and psychoeducational approaches are currently regarded as relatively successful. These include New York City's Fountain House, which began forty-two years ago as a meeting place for former mental clients. Each day, about 400 people visit the landscaped grounds and tastefully furnished buildings. In addition, Fountain House provides shelter for more than 200 people citywide in group homes and apartments. According to many, however, the core of Fountain House is its work program. Members perform almost all the chores at the complex. Those who do well are placed in part-time entry-level jobs at some thirty-one companies, including law firms, ad agencies, and banks. Unfortunately, the impact of this model mental health program is all too limited. Fountain House can accept only one of every five people who apply for membership.

Another innovative community mental health program was developed in Madison, Wisconsin, by Stein, Test, and their colleagues (1978). Their program was called **PACT (Program for Assertive Community Treatment)**. The phases of this model program, which began in the early 1970s, were improving public hospital care, releasing clients early to the community, maintaining difficult clients in the community, and eventually reorganizing the system of care. At the heart of the Stein and Test approach were the following features:

• Willingness to deemphasize traditional office- and facility-based practice to provide care in the community

• Extensive and flexible use of multidisciplinary teams to cope with needs of severely ill clients by making use of community services

• Assertive adaptability, i.e., recognition that there is no "quick fix" for the problems of designing service systems for the severely mentally ill and that successful care models must address change on many levels.

Despite the relative successes of a few demonstration models, such as those described above, critics charge them with paternalism, coercion, and other practices that foster dependency and disability in the interest of social control. Yet, they have demonstrated the value of supportive functions such as assertive outreach, repeated crisis intervention, and dynamic

family involvement among people who are trying to "make it crazy." Estroff's (1981) ethnography, *Making It Crazy*, although not intended as a critique of the PACT model, clearly illustrates how disempowered, dependent, and impoverished some clients remain even in "innovative" model community programs.

Future Directions: Toward True Innovation

Case management, psychoeducation, and the model programs for training in community living described above are among the essentials for community mental health services in the 1990s. Additional strategies such as psychosocial rehabilitation, supervised housing, and the like must be developed according to what Mosher and Burti (1989) identify as the "three umbrella principles" for community mental health programs of the future:

1. *Contextualization,* or keeping clients in as close contact with their usual geographic and interpersonal surroundings as possible, thus enhancing support from the client's family network

2. *Preservation and enhancement of personal power and control* among clients by providing information, exercising advocacy, helping to identify options, and in general keeping client engaged in a self-care process

3. *Normalization,* or supporting clients as they apply problem-solving skills to activities of daily living, such as work and housing options, in order to foster a sense of personal efficacy through real accomplishments, no matter how small, in a normal world.

In a future characterized by cutbacks in resources, increased needs for self-determination, family caregiving, and power based on knowledge and information, psychiatric nurses have a unique opportunity to bring true innovation to the programs needed in community mental health.

CHAPTER HIGHLIGHTS

• The community mental health movement (known as "the third revolution" in psychiatry) is a social movement as well as a system for the delivery of community-based mental health services.

• Landmark recommendations made in 1961 by the Joint Commission on Mental Illness and Health drew the attention and concern of politicians and mental health professionals toward the woefully inadequate psychiatric services in the country.

• Millions of dollars of federal funding were provided for the construction of comprehensive community mental health centers, mental health research, and training programs for mental health care providers.

• Other major studies, such as the 1978 report of the President's Commission on Mental Health, gave visibility to the professional competence of nurses in mental health care and made significant recommendations toward coordinating the two-tiered system of mental health care that had evolved.

• In the two-tiered system of mental health care the severely mentally ill continued to inhabit state institutions, and those with less acute problems used the services of community mental health centers. Certain populations (recently discharged clients, the chronically mentally ill, the elderly, youth, and minority groups, for example) fell between the two categories and were not served.

• In 1980 Community Mental Health Systems Act (which was intended to coordinate the two-tiered system) could not be implemented without a change in the political and economic climate. In addition, decreases in the federal budget caused increasing concern over the possible demise of community mental health programs.

• Introduction of prospective payment systems in the form of DRGs may lead to changes in psychiatry's future.

• The basic philosophy of the community mental health movement is that health care is a right, and, therefore, mental health services should be available to all people.

• Six concepts central to community mental health are (1) a systems perspective; (2) an emphasis on prevention; (3) interdisciplinary collaboration, balancing flexible role boundaries with unique areas of expertise; (4) consumer participation and control; (5) the provision of comprehensive services to the community as client as defined by geographic catchment areas; and (6) continuity of care for clients in their movement from one program to another.

• Community mental health nursing roles include such diverse activities as effective parenting classes; divorce therapy groups; suicide prevention counseling; case finding; planning for a client's discharge; teaching self-care activities; staffing partial hospitalization programs; and providing individual, group, and family psychotherapy.

• The ANA Standards provide guidelines for both nursing generalists and specialists who practice in community settings.

• Conventional treatment under the community mental health system has become a highly prescriptive, elaborately formal structure of policy, regulations, and

standards in which the old state hospital warehouse has been replaced by a similarly bureaucratic clearinghouse.

• Part of the community mental health system's dilemma is that is must protect the community and, at the same time, guarantee the client's rights.

• Deinstitutionalization is simultaneously the *fact* that the resident population of state hospitals has decreased about 62 percent, and a *philosophy* of civil-libertarian emphasis on clients' rights and expanded-care services based in the client's communities.

• Shifting the location and funding arrangements for the chronically and severely mentally disordered has not solved their problems.

• Case management, psychoeducation, and a few model service programs have been recognized as achieving some degree of success.

• Genuine innovation is needed to devise alternative care approaches, particularly for the severely and chronically mentally disordered.

• Principles suggested as essential to community mental health in the future are contextualization, empowerment, and normalization.

REFERENCES

Anderson CM, Hogarty GE, Reiss DJ: The psychoeducational family treatment of schizophrenia, in Goldstein M: *New Directions for Mental Health Services.* Jossey Bass, 1981.

Anderson CM, Reiss DJ, Hogarty GE: *Schizophrenia and the Family.* Guilford Press, 1986.

Aviram U: Community care of the seriously mentally ill: Continuing problems and current issues. *Community Ment Health J* 1990;226(1):69–88.

Bachrach LL: A conceptual approach to deinstitutionalization. *Hosp Community Psychiatry* 1978;29:573–578.

Bachrach LL: Planning mental health services for the chronic patient. *Hosp Community Psychiatry* 1979;30:387–92.

Bassuk EL, Gerson S: Deinstitutionalization and mental health services. *Sci Am* 1978;238:46–53.

Beigel A: Planning psychiatry's future. *Hosp Community Psychiatry* 1986;37(6):551–554.

Berns JS, Hamilton MS: Nursing role in community mental health, in Jarvis LL (ed): *Community Health Nursing: Keeping the Public Healthy* FA Davis, 1981, pp 319–353.

Caplan G: *Principles of Preventive Psychiatry.* Basic Books, 1964.

Davis CK: The status of reimbursement policy and future projections, in Williams C (ed): *Nursing Research and Policy Formation: The Case of Prospective Payment.* American Academy of Nursing, 1984.

Estroff S: *Making It Crazy: An Ethnography of Psychiatric Clients in an American Community.* University of California Press, 1981.

Goldman HH: Defining and counting the chronically mentally ill. *Hosp Community Psychiatry* 1981;32:21–27.

Greenblatt M, York RH, Brown EL: *From Custodial to Therapeutic Patient Care in Mental Hospitals.* Russell Sage Foundation, 1955.

Mosher LR, Burti L: *Community Mental Health Principles and Practice.* Norton, 1989.

National Institute of Mental Health: Toward a model plan for a comprehensive community-based mental health system. DHHS, 1987.

Reinke B, Greenley JR: Organizational analysis of three community support program models. *Hosp Community Psychiatry* 1986;37(6):624–629.

Report to the President of the President's Commission on Mental Health. Vol. I. US Government Printing Office, 1978.

Stein LI, Test MA (eds): *Training in the Community Living Model: A Decade of Experience.* Jossey-Bass, 1985.

Talbott JA: Deinstitutionalization: Avoiding the disasters of the past. *Hosp Community Psychiatry* 1979;30:621–624.

Test MA, Stein LI: Community treatment of the chronic patient: Research overview. *Schizophr Bull* 1978;14:350–364.

Thompson KS, Griffith EEH, Leaf PJ: A historical review of the Madison model of community care. *Hosp Community Psychiatry* 1990;41(6):625–634.

Wilson HS: *Deinstitutionalized Residential Alternatives for the Severely Mentally Disordered: The Soteria House Approach.* Grune & Stratton, 1982.

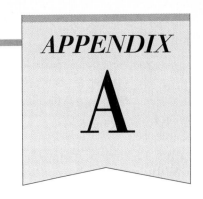

DSM-III-R Classification: Multiaxial Categories and Codes

All official DSM-III-R codes are included in ICD-9-CM. Codes followed by a * are used for more than one DSM-III-R diagnosis or subtype in order to maintain compatibility with ICD-9-CM. A long dash following a diagnostic term indicates the need for a fifth digit subtype or other qualifying term. The term *specify* following the name of some diagnostic categories indicates qualifying terms that clinicians may wish to add in parentheses after the name of the disorder. The abbreviation NOS = Not Otherwise Specified.

The current severity of a disorder may be specified after the diagnosis as:

Mild
Moderate } currently meets diagnostic criteria
Severe

In partial remission (or residual state)

In complete remission

Disorders Usually First Evident in Infancy, Childhood, or Adolescence

Developmental Disorders

Note: These are coded on Axis II.

Mental Retardation

317.00	Mild mental retardation
318.00	Moderate mental retardation
318.10	Severe mental retardation
318.20	Profound mental retardation
319.00	Unspecified mental retardation

Pervasive Developmental Disorders

299.00	Autistic disorder. *Specify* if childhood onset
299.80	Pervasive developmental disorder NOS

Specific Developmental Disorders

Academic skills disorders

315.10	Developmental arithmetic disorder
315.80	Developmental expressive writing disorder
315.00	Developmental reading disorder

Language and speech disorders

315.39	Developmental articulation disorder
315.31*	Developmental expressive language disorder
315.31*	Developmental receptive language disorder

Motor skills disorders

315.40	Developmental coordination disorder
315.90*	Specific developmental disorder NOS

Other Developmental Disorders

315.90*	Developmental disorder NOS

Disruptive Behavior Disorders

314.01	Attention-deficit hyperactivity disorder

Conduct disorder

312.20	Group type
312.00	Solitary aggressive type
312.90	Undifferentiated type
313.81	Oppositional defiant disorder

Anxiety Disorders of Childhood or Adolescence

309.21	Separation anxiety disorder
313.21	Avoidant disorder of childhood or adolescence
313.00	Overanxious disorder

Eating Disorders

307.10	Anorexia nervosa
307.51	Bulimia nervosa
307.52	Pica
307.53	Rumination disorder of infancy
307.50	Eating disorder NOS

Gender Identity Disorders

302.60	Gender identity disorder of childhood
302.50	Transsexualism. *Specify* sexual history: asexual, homosexual, heterosexual, unspecified
302.85*	Gender identity disorder of adolescence or adulthood, nontranssexual type. *Specify* sexual history: asexual, homosexual, heterosexual, unspecified
302.85*	Gender identity disorder NOS

Tic Disorders

307.23	Tourette's disorder
307.22	Chronic motor or vocal tic disorder
307.21	Transient tic disorder. *Specify:* single episode or recurrent
307.20	Tic disorder NOS

Elimination Disorders

307.70	Functional encopresis. *Specify:* primary or secondary type

Source: American Psychiatric Association: *Diagnostic and Statistical Manual of Mental Disorders*, ed 3, revised. APA, 1987.

307.60 Functional enuris. *Specify:* primary or secondary type. *Specify:* nocturnal only, diurnal only, nocturnal and diurnal

Speech Disorders Not Elsewhere Classified

307.00* Cluttering
307.00* Stuttering

Other Disorders of Infancy, Childhood, or Adolescence

313.23 Elective mutism
313.82 Identity disorder
313.89 Reactive attachment disorder of infancy or early childhood
307.30 Stereotypy/habit disorder
314.00 Undifferentiated attention-deficit disorder

Organic Mental Disorders

Dementias Arising in the Senium and Presenium

Primary degenerative dementia of the Alzheimer type, senile onset

290.30 With delirium
290.20 With delusions
290.21 With depression
290.00* Uncomplicated (Note: code 331.00 Alzheimer's disease on Axis III)

Code in fifth digit: 1 = with delirium, 2 = with delusions, 3 = with depression, 0* = uncomplicated

290.1x Primary degenerative dementia of the Alzheimer type, presenile onset, _____ (Note: code 331.00 Alzheimer's disease on Axis III)
290.4x Multi-infarct dementia, _____
290.00* Senile dementia NOS. *Specify:* etiology on Axis III if known
290.10* Presenile dementia NOS. *Specify:* etiology on Axis III if known (e.g., Pick's disease, Jakob-Creutzfeldt disease)

Psychoactive Substance-Induced Organic Mental Disorders

Alcohol

303.00 Intoxication
291.40 Idiosyncratic intoxication
291.80 Uncomplicated alcohol withdrawal
291.00 Withdrawal delirium
291.30 Hallucinosis
291.10 Amnestic disorder
291.20 Dementia associated with alcoholism

Amphetamine or similarly acting sympathomimetic

305.70* Intoxication
292.00* Withdrawal
292.81* Delirium
292.11* Delusional disorder

Caffeine

305.90* Intoxication

Cannabis

305.20* Intoxication
292.11* Delusional disorder

Cocaine

305.60* Intoxication
292.00* Withdrawal

292.81* Delirium
292.11* Delusional disorder

Hallucinogen

305.30* Hallucinosis
292.11* Delusional disorder
292.84* Mood disorder
292.89* Posthallucinogen perception disorder

Inhalant

305.90* Intoxication

Nicotine

292.00* Withdrawal

Opioid

305.50* Intoxication
292.00* Withdrawal

Phencyclidine (PCP) or similarly acting arylcyclohexylamine

305.90* Intoxication
292.81* Delirium
292.11* Delusional disorder
292.84* Mood disorder
292.90* Organic mental disorder NOS

Sedative, hypnotic, or anxiolytic

305.40* Intoxication
292.00* Uncomplicated sedative, hypnotic, or anxiolytic withdrawal
292.00* Withdrawal delirium
292.83* Amnestic disorder

Other or unspecified psychoactive substance

305.90* Intoxication
292.00* Withdrawal
292.81* Delirium
292.82* Dementia
292.83* Amnestic disorder
292.11 Delusional disorder
292.12 Hallucinosis
292.84* Mood disorder
292.89* Anxiety disorder
292.89* Personality disorder
292.90* Organic mental disorder NOS

Organic Mental Disorders Associated with Axis III Physical Disorders or Conditions, or Whose Etiology Is Unknown

293.00 Delirium
294.10 Dementia
294.00 Amnestic disorder
293.81 Organic delusional disorder
293.82 Organic hallucinosis
293.83 Organic mood disorder. *Specify:* manic, depressed, mixed
294.80* Organic anxiety disorder
310.10 Organic personality disorder. *Specify* if explosive type
294.80* Organic mental disorder NOS

Psychoactive Substance Use Disorders

Alcohol

303.90 Dependence
305.00 Abuse

Amphetamine or similarly acting sympathomimetic

304.40 Dependence
305.70* Abuse

Cannabis

   304.30   Dependence
   305.20* Abuse

Cocaine

   304.20   Dependence
   305.60* Abuse

Hallucinogen

   304.50* Dependence
   305.30* Abuse

Inhalant

   304.60   Dependence
   305.90* Abuse

Nicotine

   305.10   Dependence

Opioid

   304.00   Dependence
   305.50* Abuse

Phencyclidine (PCP) or similarly acting arylcyclohexylamine

   304.50* Dependence
   305.90* Abuse

Sedative, hypnotic, or anxiolytic

   304.10   Dependence
   305.40* Abuse
   304.90* Polysubstance dependence
   304.90* Psychoactive substance dependence NOS
   305.90* Psychoactive substance abuse NOS

Schizophrenia

Code in fifth digit: 1 = subchronic, 2 = chronic, 3 = subchronic with acute exacerbation, 4 = chronic with acute exacerbation, 5 = in remission, 0 = unspecified.

Schizophrenia

   295.2x   Catatonic, _____
   295.1x   Disorganized, _____
   295.3x   Paranoid, _____. *Specify* if stable type
   295.9x   Undifferentiated, _____
   295.6x   Residual, _____. *Specify* if late onset

Delusional (Paranoid) Disorder

   297.10   Delusional disorder. *Specify* type: erotomanic, grandiose, jealous, persecutory, somatic, unspecified

Psychotic Disorders Not Elsewhere Classified

   298.80   Brief reactive psychosis
   295.40   Schizophreniform disorder. *Specify:* without good prognostic features or with good prognostic features
   295.70   Schizoaffective disorder. *Specify:* bipolar type or depressive type
   297.30   Induced psychotic disorder
   298.90   Psychotic disorder NOS (atypical psychosis)

Mood Disorders

Code current state of Major Depression and Bipolar Disorder in fifth digit: 1 = mild, 2 = moderate, 3 = severe, without psychotic features, 4 = with psychotic features (*specify* mood-congruent or

mood incongruent), 5 = in partial remission, 6 = in full remission, 0 = unspecified.
   For major depressive episodes, *specify* if chronic and *specify* if melancholic type.
   For Bipolar Disorder, Bipolar Disorder NOS, Recurrent Major Depression, and Depressive Disorder NOS, *specify* if seasonal pattern.

Bipolar Disorders

Bipolar disorder

   296.6x   Mixed, _____
   296.4x   Manic, _____
   296.5x   Depressed, _____
   301.13   Cyclothymia
   296.70   Bipolar disorder NOS

Depressive Disorders

Major depression

   296.2x   Single episode, _____
   296.3x   Recurrent, _____
   300.40   Dysthymia (or depressive neurosis). *Specify:* primary or secondary type. *Specify:* early or late onset
   311.00   Depressive disorder NOS

Anxiety Disorders (or Anxiety and Phobic Neuroses)

Panic disorder

   300.21   With agoraphobia. *Specify* current severity of agoraphobic avoidance. *Specify* current severity of panic attacks
   300.01   Without agoraphobia. *Specify* current severity of panic attacks
   300.22   Agoraphobia without history of panic disorder. *Specify* with or without limited symptom attacks
   300.23   Social phobia. *Specify* if generalized type
   300.29   Simple phobia
   300.30   Obsessive compulsive disorder (or obsessive compulsive neurosis)
   309.89   Post-traumatic stress disorder. *Specify* if delayed onset
   300.02   Generalized anxiety disorder
   300.00   Anxiety disorder NOS

Somatoform Disorders

   300.70* Body dysmorphic disorder
   300.11   Conversion disorder (or hysterical neurosis, conversion type). *Specify:* single episode or recurrent
   300.70* Hypochondriasis (or hypochondriacal neurosis)
   300.81   Somatization disorder
   307.80   Somatoform pain disorder
   300.70* Undifferentiated somatoform disorder
   300.70* Somatoform disorder NOS

Dissociative Disorders (or Hysterical Neuroses, Dissociative Type)

   300.14   Multiple personality disorder
   300.13   Psychogenic fugue
   300.12   Psychogenic amnesia
   300.60   Depersonalization disorder (or depersonalization neurosis)
   300.15   Dissociative disorder NOS

Sexual Disorders

Paraphilias

302.40	Exhibitionism
302.81	Fetishism
302.89	Frotteurism
302.20	Pedophilia. *Specify:* same sex, opposite sex, same and opposite sex. *Specify* if limited to incest. *Specify:* exclusive type or nonexclusive type
302.83	Sexual masochism
302.84	Sexual sadism
302.30	Transvestic fetishism
302.82	Voyeurism
302.90*	Paraphilia NOS

Sexual Dysfunctions

Specify: psychogenic only, or psychogenic and biogenic. (Note: If biogenic only, code on Axis III.) *Specify:* lifelong or acquired. *Specify:* generalized or situational.

Sexual desire disorders

302.71	Hypoactive sexual desire disorder
302.79	Sexual aversion disorder

Sexual arousal disorders

302.72*	Female sexual arousal disorder
302.72*	Male erectile disorder

Orgasm disorders

302.73	Inhibited female orgasm
302.74	Inhibited male orgasm
302.75	Premature ejaculation

Sexual pain disorders

302.76	Dyspareunia
306.51	Vaginismus
302.70	Sexual dysfunction NOS

Other Sexual Disorders

302.90*	Sexual disorder NOS

Sleep Disorders

Dyssomnias

Insomnia disorder

307.42*	Related to another mental disorder (nonorganic)
780.50*	Related to known organic factor
307.42*	Primary insomnia

Hypersomnia disorder

307.44	Related to another mental disorder (nonorganic)
780.50*	Related to a known organic factor
780.54	Primary hypersomnia
307.45	Sleep-wake schedule disorder. *Specify:* advanced or delayed phase type, disorganized type, frequently changing type

Other dyssomnias

307.40*	Dyssomnia NOS

Parasomnias

307.47	Dream anxiety disorder (nightmare disorder)
307.46*	Sleep terror disorder
307.46*	Sleepwalking disorder
307.40*	Parasomnia NOS

Factitious Disorders

Factitious disorder

301.51	With physical symptoms
300.16	With psychological symptoms
300.19	Factitious disorder NOS

Impulse Control Disorders Not Elsewhere Classified

312.34	Intermittent explosive disorder
312.32	Kleptomania
312.31	Pathological gambling
312.33	Pyromania
312.39*	Trichotillomania
312.39*	Impulse control disorder NOS

Adjustment Disorder

Adjustment disorder

309.24	With anxious mood
309.00	With depressed mood
309.30	With disturbance of conduct
309.40	With mixed disturbance of emotions and conduct
309.28	With mixed emotional features
309.82	With physical complaints
309.83	With withdrawal
309.23	With work (or academic) inhibition
309.90	Adjustment disorder NOS

Psychological Factors Affecting Physical Condition

316.00	Psychological factors affecting physical condition. *Specify* physical condition on Axis III

Personality Disorders

Note: These are coded on Axis II.

Cluster A

301.00	Paranoid
301.20	Schizoid
301.22	Schizotypal

Cluster B

301.70	Antisocial
301.83	Borderline
301.50	Histrionic
301.81	Narcissistic

Cluster C

301.82	Avoidant
301.60	Dependent
301.40	Obsessive compulsive
301.84	Passive aggressive
301.90	Personality disorder NOS

V Codes For Conditions Not Attributable to a Mental Disorder That Are a Focus of Attention or Treatment

V62.30	Academic problem
V71.01	Adult antisocial behavior

V40.00   Borderline intellectual functioning. (Note: This is coded on Axis II)
V71.02   Childhood or adolescent antisocial behavior
V65.20   Malingering
V61.10   Marital problem
V15.81   Noncompliance with medical treatment
V62.20   Occupational problem
V61.20   Parent-child problem
V62.81   Other interpersonal problem
V61.80   Other specified family circumstances
V62.89   Phase of life problem or other life circumstance problem
V62.82   Uncomplicated bereavement

Additional Codes

300.90   Unspecified mental disorder (nonpsychotic)
V71.09*   No diagnosis or condition on Axis I
799.90*   Diagnosis or condition deferred on Axis I

Multiaxial System

Axis I   Clinical syndromes
            V codes
Axis II   Developmental disorders
            Personality disorders
Axis III   Physical disorders and conditions
Axis IV   Severity of psychosocial stressors
Axis V   Global assessment of functioning

Severity of Psychosocial Stressors Scale: Adults

Note: This is coded on Axis IV.

Code	Term	Examples of Stressors	
		Acute events	Enduring circumstances
1	None	No acute events that may be relevant to the disorder	No enduring circumstances that may be relevant to the disorder
2	Mild	Broke up with boyfriend or girlfriend; started or gaduated from school; child left home	Family arguments; job dissatisfaction; residence in high-crime neighborhood
3	Moderate	Marriage; marital separation; loss of job; retirement; miscarriage	Marital discord; serious financial problems; trouble with boss; being a single parent
4	Severe	Divorce; birth of first child	Unemployment; poverty
5	Extreme	Death of spouse; serious physical illness diagnosed; victim of rape	Serious chronic illness in self or child; ongoing physical or sexual abuse
6	Catastrophic	Death of child; suicide of spouse; devastating natural disaster	Captivity as hostage; concentration camp experience
0	Inadequate information, or no change in condition		

Severity of Psychosocial Scale: Children and Adolescents

Note: This is coded on Axis IV.

Code	Term	Examples of Stressors	
		Acute events	Enduring circumstances
1	None	No acute events that may be relevant to the disorder	No enduring circumstances that may be relevant to the disorder
2	Mild	Broke up with boyfriend or girlfriend; change of school	Overcrowded living quarters; family arguments
3	Moderate	Expelled from school; birth of sibling	Chronic disabling illness in parent; chronic parental discord
4	Severe	Divorce of parents; unwanted pregnancy; arrest	Harsh or rejecting parents; chronic life-threatening illness in parent; multiple foster home placements
5	Extreme	Sexual or physical abuse; death of a parent	Recurrent sexual or physical abuse
6	Catastrophic	Death of both parents	Chronic life-threatening illness
0	Inadequate information, or no change in condition		

Global Assessment of Functioning Scale (GAF Scale)

Note: This is coded on Axis V.

Consider psychological, social, and occupational functioning on a hypothetical continuum of mental health-illness. Do not include impairment in functioning due to physical (or environmental) limitations.

Note: Use intermediate codes when appropriate, e.g., 45, 68, 72.

Code

90
│
81
Absent or minimal symptoms (e.g., mild anxiety before an exam), good functioning in all areas, interested and involved in a wide range of activities, socially effective, generally satisfied with life, no more than everyday problems or concerns (e.g., an occasional argument with family members).

80
│
71
If symptoms are present, they are transient and expectable reactions to psychosocial stressors (e.g., difficulty concentrating after family argument); no more than slight impairment in social, occupational, or school functioning (e.g., temporarily falling behind in schoolwork).

70
│
61
Some mild symptoms (e.g., depressed mood and mild insomnia) *or* some difficulty in social, occupational, or school functioning (e.g., occasional truancy, or theft within the household), but generally functioning pretty well, has some meaningful interpersonal relationships.

60
│
51
Moderate symptoms (e.g., flat affect and circumstantial speech, occasional panic attacks) *or* moderate difficulty in social, occupational, or school functioning (e.g., few friends, conflicts with coworkers).

50
│
41
Serious symptoms (e.g., suicidal ideation, severe obsessional rituals, frequent shoplifting) *or* any serious impairment in social, occupational, or school functioning (e.g., no friends, unable to keep a job).

40
│
31
Some impairment in reality testing or communication (e.g., speech is at times illogical, obscure, or irrelevant) *or* major impairment in several areas, such as work or school, family relations, judgment, thinking, or mood (e.g., depressed man avoids friends, neglects family, and is unable to work; child frequently beats up younger children, is defiant at home, and is failing at school).

30
│
21
Behavior is considerably influenced by delusions or hallucinations *or* serious impairment in communication or judgment (e.g., sometimes incoherent, acts grossly inappropriately, suicidal preoccupation) *or* inability to function in almost all areas (e.g., stays in bed all day; no job, home, or friends).

20
│
11
Some danger of hurting self or others (e.g., suicide attempts without clear expectation of death, frequently violent, manic excitement) *or* occasionally fails to maintain minimal personal hygiene (e.g., smears feces) *or* gross impairment in communication (e.g., largely incoherent or mute).

10
│
1
Persistent danger of severely hurting self or others (e.g., recurrent violence) *or* persistent inability to maintain minimal personal hygiene *or* serious suicidal act with clear expectation of death.

Psychotropic Drugs in Common Usage

Eileen Trigoboff
Nan Rich

Index of Drugs

Product Information

Note: The information that follows has been selectively abstracted from the sources listed under "References" for use as an educational aid and does not cover all possible uses, actions, precautions, side effects, or interactions of this medicine. It is not intended as medical advice for individual problems.

Generic name: alprazolam
Brand name: Xanax
Classification: Antianxiety; benzodiazepine; skeletal muscle relaxant
Common uses: Anxiety disorders; relief of anxiety associated with depression; panic disorder
Should not be used if: Client is pregnant or nursing; client has narrow-angle glaucoma, hepatic, or renal disease.

Possible side effects: Drowsiness; fatigue; ataxia; dizziness; orthostatic hypotension; ECG changes; tachycardia; blurred vision; tolerance; physical and psychologic dependence; may aggrevate symptoms in some depressed patients.
Possible drug interactions: Increases central nervous system depression from other drugs, including alcohol, antipsychotics, antihistamines, antidepressants, anticonvulsants,

971

barbiturates, and narcotics. Nicotine, caffeine, valproic acid, and rifampin decrease alprazolam's effectiveness.

Nursing considerations: Assess anxiety level; potential for addiction; history of allergies and or medical problems; watch for symptoms of overdose, such as intoxication, disinhibition, impairment in judgment and memory, depressed vital signs; evaluate blood pressure reclining and standing, blood studies, hepatic studies, I&O. Educate client about potential for injury from operating cars or machinery, abrupt withdrawal, and combining with CNS depressants. Refer to Client/Family Teaching: Benzodiazepines, Chapter 32.

Usual dosage: 1.5–4 mg/day, should be gradually increased from 0.25–0.5 mg/day in 2–3 divided doses. Take with food to reduce GI symptoms.

Onset: 30–60 minutes, peaks in about 1 hour.

Generic name: amantadine HCl
Brand name: Symmetrel
Classification: Antiparkinsonian; cyclic primary amine
Common uses: Prophylaxis and/or treatment of extrapyramidal reactions; parkinsonism; symptomatic treatment of influenza caused by A influenza virus strains.
Possible side effects: Headache; dizziness; drowsiness; fatigue; orthostatic hypotension; CHF; blurred vision; leukopenia; nausea and vomiting; dry mouth; urinary frequency or retention; peripheral edema; skin mottling; photosensitivity; depression; psychosis; hallucinations.
Possible drug interactions: Additive with other anticholinergic drugs and CNS stimulants; thiazide-type diuretics may decrease excretion and lead to toxic buildup of amantadine.
Nursing considerations: Assess I&O; give after meals for better absorption; evaluate therapeutic response, skin problems, respiratory status or allergic reactions; advise gradual changes in body position to avoid orthostatic hypotension, avoidance of abrupt discontinuation of drug and caution in activities that require concentration.
Usual dosage: PO (adults 13–64)— 100 mg BID or 200 mg as a single daily dose; reduced dose for children, elders, and patients with renal impairment.
Onset: For therapeutic effect, two weeks is required, then it takes effect in 4–48 hours, peaks in 1–4 hours, and will last 12–24 hours.

Generic name: amitriptyline
Brand names: Amitril; Elavil; Emitrip; Endep; Enovil; Levate; Meravil; Novotriptyn: Rotavil
Classification: Tricyclic antidepressant; tertiary amine
Common uses: Major depression; depressive phase of bipolar disorder; chronic pain; and various types of headaches.
Should not be used if: Client is taking MAO inhibitors; pregnant or lactating; under 12 years of age; has a history of hypersensitivity to tricyclics; is in recovery phase of myocardial infarction; has untreated angle-closure glaucoma.
Possible side effects: Drowsiness; dizziness; orthostatic hypotension; tachycardia; hypertension; heart block; CHF; cardiovascular collapse; ECG changes; agranulocytosis; thrombocytopenia; leukopenia; dry mouth; constipation; weight gain; and urinary retention. Other less common effects are noted.

Possible drug interactions: Potentiates CNS depressants, including alcohol, barbiturates, and benzodiazepines; severe systemic reactions with MAO inhibitors; nicotine increases amitriptyline metabolism; thyroid medications may interact to produce arrhythmias and tachycardia.
Nursing considerations: Assess initial vital signs and weight, monitor throughout therapy; be aware of sudden changes in mood, which may indicate lethality. Evaluate for symptoms of blood dyscrasias, including sore throat, fever, malaise, unusual bleeding or bruising; and symptoms of overdose, such as confusion, agitation, irritability. Caution client to be careful when operating machinery, standing up, and in exposure to the sun. Refer to Client/Family Teaching: Tricyclic Antidepressants, Chapter 32.
Usual dosage: Initially 75–100 mg/day for adults, less for elders and adolescents; increasing to 150–200 mg/day. Maintenance doses may be as low as 25–40 mg/day.
Onset: May take 2–4 weeks to see therapeutic results, will peak 2–12 hours after administration, and lasts for weeks.

Generic name: amoxapine
Brand name: Asendin
Classification: Tricyclic antidepressant; dibenzoxazepine derivative-secondary amine
Common uses: Major depression with psychotic symptoms; depression associated with organic causes; depressive phase of bipolar disorder; and mixed symptoms of depression and anxiety.
Should not be used if: Client is hypersensitive to tricyclics; pregnant or lactating; under 14 years of age; taking MAO inhibitor; in an acute recovery period following a myocardial infarction. Use caution with patients having history of seizures, prostatic hypertrophy, cardiovascular, hepatic, renal, or respiratory difficulties, or who are elderly, debilitated, or psychotic.
Possible side effects: Drowsiness; dizziness; orthostatic hypotension; blurred vision; nasal congestion; tachycardia; myocardial infarction; ECG changes; dry mouth; constipation; urinary retention; and many other less common problems.
Possible drug interactions: Potentiates CNS depressants, including alcohol, barbiturates and benzodiazepines; severe systemic reactions with MAO inhibitors; nicotine increases amoxapine metabolism; thyroid medications may interact to produce arrhythmias and tachycardia.
Nursing considerations: Assess initial vital signs and weight, monitor throughout therapy; be aware of sudden changes in mood, which may indicate lethality. Evaluate for symptoms of blood dyscrasias, including sore throat, fever, malaise, unusual bleeding or bruising; and symptoms of overdose, such as confusion, agitation, irritability, and physical signs. Caution client to be careful when operating machinery, standing up, and in exposure to the sun. Refer to Client/Family Teaching: Tricyclic Antidepressants, Chapter 32.
Usual dosage: Initially, 50 mg two or three times daily. Increase to 300 mg/day. NTE 400–600 mg/day, depending on available supervision.
Onset: Therapeutic effect in 2–4 weeks, thereafter blood level peaks 90 minutes after ingestion.

Generic name: benztropine mesylate
Brand name: Cogentin
Classification: Antiparkinsonian; anticholinergic
Common uses: Parkinsonism; extrapyramidal symptoms associated with antipsychotic drugs (not including tardive dyskinesia); prevention of extrapyramidal side effects.
Possible side effects: Drowsiness; dizziness; blurred vision; dry mouth; constipation; paralytic ileus; and other physical problems.
Possible drug interactions: May increase CNS depression with alcohol, barbiturates, narcotics, and benzodiazepines. May decrease antipsychotic effects of the phenothiazines or haloperidol. May increase anticholinergic effects of any other drug with anticholinergic properties.
Should not be used if: Client is hypersensitive; pregnant or lactating; under 3 years of age; routinely exposed to elevated external temperatures; has cardiac or GI problems; has glaucoma or urinary obstructions; has hypertension or hyperthyroidism.
Nursing considerations: Assess for symptoms of Parkinson's disease, such as tremors, muscular weakness and rigidity, drooling, shuffling, flat affect, and disturbance in balance or posture; extrapyramidal symptoms are similar with the addition of akinesia (muscular weakness), akathisia (restlessness), dystonia (involuntary muscular movements), oculogyric crisis (rolling back of the eyes), and tardive dyskinesia (bizarre facial and tongue and/or body movements). Evaluate for constipation, GI disturbance, or paralytic ileus, which may be life threatening. Educate client to avoid OTC medications until physician agrees, to avoid driving or other activities that require intense concentration, and not to stop medication abruptly.
Usual dosage: May be given PO or IM. For Parkinsonism, begin at 0.5–1.0 mg and increase gradually to smallest effective dose. Maximum daily dose is 6 mg/day. For extrapyramidal symptoms, give 1–4 mg daily or BID.
Onset: PO—onset, 1–2 hours; duration 24 hours. IM—15 minutes; duration 6–10 hours.

Generic name: bupropion
Brand name: Wellbutrin
Classification: Monocyclic antidepressant; amino ketone type
Common uses: Clients with depression who fail to respond or who cannot tolerate alternative antidepressant treatments. Not recommended as a first choice.
Should not be used if: Client is hypersensitive; taking MAO inhibitors; pregnant or lactating; under 18 years of age; has a history of seizure disorder, cranial trauma, bulimia, or anorexia nervosa. Use caution if client has cardiovascular, hepatic, or renal problems or if client is suicidal, psychotic, elderly, or debilitated.
Possible side effects: Agitation; insomnia; headache; migraine; tremors; seizures; blurred vision; sedation; dizziness; tachycardia; dry mouth; constipation; nausea; vomiting; weight loss; anorexia; leukopenia; and other not so common physical problems. Slight increase in BP; orthostatic hypotension; slight weight loss.
Possible drug interactions: Drugs that alter hepatic enzyme activity may decrease metabolism of bupropion; levodopa may increase incidence of adverse effects; MAO inhibitors enhance toxicity of bupropion; drugs that lower seizure threshold may increase risk of seizures.
Nursing considerations: Assess for lethality and sudden mood elevation that may precede suicide attempt; vital signs and weight; malaise. Evaluate history of seizures, allergies, glaucoma, alcohol/drug consumption, contraceptive use. Educate client to understand precautions about illness, medications, and precautions that must be taken in regard to driving and operation of machinery.
Usual dosage: PO (adults)—initially 200 mg/day given as 100 mg BID, increased to a maximum of 450 mg over several weeks of treatment.
Onset: May take up to 4 weeks for clinical efficacy, peaks in 1–3 hours and stays in the system for 1–2 weeks.

Generic name: buspirone
Brand name: Buspar
Classification: Antianxiety agent
Common uses: Generalized anxiety states
Should not be used if: Client is hypersensitive; using MAO inhibitors; elderly or debilitated; pregnant or lactating; under 18 years of age. Use caution with clients who have hepatic or renal dysfunction. Clients should be withdrawn from benzodiazepines or sedative/hypnotics before therapy with buspirone.
Possible side effects: Drowsiness; dizziness; headache; nervousness; nausea; and several other less common problems.
Possible drug interactions: Use with MAO inhibitors may elevate blood pressure.
Nursing considerations: Assess extent of anxiety, lethality, presence of side effects. Evaluate history for allergies, contraceptive use, childbearing status, alcohol/drug abuse. Educate client to take care in activities that require concentration and to avoid potential hazards. This medication is less sedating than benzodiazepines.
Usual dosage: PO (adults)—5 mg TID, to be increased at intervals of 2–3 days, NTE 60 mg/day, usually effective dose: 20–30 mg/day.
Onset: Therapeutic levels may be reached in 7–10 days; it peaks in 40–90 minutes; its duration in the body is unknown.

Generic Name: carbamazepine
Brand Name: Tegretol
Classification: Anticonvulsant
Common uses: Seizure disorders; trigeminal neuralgia
Should not be used if: Sensitivity to tricyclic antidepressants; baseline hematologic abnormalities or receiving other myelotoxic drugs; history of bone marrow depression. Use caution if client has history of cardiac damage, liver disease, increased intraocular pressure.
Possible side effects: Sedation; anticholinergic effects; dizziness; drowsiness; blurred vision; speech disturbances; abnormal involuntary movements; GI distress; muscle relaxation; antiarrhythmic action; antidiuretic effects; nystagmus; minor hematologic changes; hypotension; aggravation of hypertension; pruritus; photosensitivity; diaphoresis; chills.
Possible drug interactions: Serum concentrations of anticonvulsants may be decreased; calcium-channel blocking agents (verapamil) may be increased to toxic level;

erythromycin decreases clearance of carbamazepine; doxycycline should not be given concomitantly; serum concentration of warfarin decreased; MAO inhibitors not recommended; reliability of oral contraceptives may be adversely affected.

Nursing considerations: Tasks requiring mental alertness or physical coordination may become difficult; assess for carbamazepine toxicity if erythromycin is also utilized; discuss contraception; assess elimination patterns; assure proper hydration.

Usual dosage: Oral suspensions produce higher peak concentrations. Children 6–12 years: 50 mg 4 times/day; Over 12 and adults: 400 mg/day to 1.2 grams/day.

Onset: Peak plasma concentration within 2–8 hours.

Generic name: chloral hydrate

Brand name: Notec; Aquachloral Supprettes; Cohidrate; Novochlorhydrate

Classification: Sedative-hypnotic; CNS depressant; chloral derivative

Common uses: Insomnia; moderate anxiety; preoperative sedation; anxiety associated with drug withdrawal.

Should not be used if: Client is hypersensitive; pregnant or lactating; elderly or debilitated; has severe hepatic, renal, or cardiac disease, gastritis, esophagitis, peptic or oral ulcers, history of porphyria or drug abuse.

Possible side effects: Drowsiness; dizziness; skin rashes; nausea and vomiting; diarrhea; leukopenia; physical and psychologic dependence.

Possible drug interactions: Potentiates action of other CNS depressants such as alcohol and opiates; increases effects of anticoagulants; in combination with furosemide, may produce blood pressure changes; flushing and diaphoresis.

Nursing considerations: Assess level of anxiety/agitation, sleep patterns, lethality, presence of side effects. Evaluate history of allergies, use of contraceptives, childbearing status, use of drugs/alcohol. Educate about need for medication, caution in operation of cars and machinery.

Usual dosage: PO (adults)—insomnia, 500–1000 mg at bedtime.

Onset: Effective in 30–60 minutes, lasts 4–8 hours.

Generic name: chlordiazepoxide

Brand name: Librium

Classification: Antianxiety; benzodiazepine

Common uses: Temporary relief of anxiety; acute alcohol withdrawal

Should not be used if: Client is hypersensitive to benzodiazepines; using other CNS depressants; pregnant or lactating; an infant; in shock or coma; elderly; or debilitated. Use caution with clients with narrow-angle glaucoma, hepatic or renal dysfunction, a history of drug abuse/addiction, or lethality.

Possible side effects: Drowsiness; fatigue; ataxia; dizziness; shock; cardiovascular collapse; and many other less common physical effects.

Possible drug interactions: Other CNS depressants produce additive CNS depression; effects of chlordiazepoxide are increased by cimetidine and decreased by valproic acid; oral contraceptives are contraindicated; phenytoin is increased in the system; the effects of levodopa are increased; digoxin's excretion is decreased; antitubercular

drugs have contradictory effects; disulfiram decreases clearance of chlordiazepoxide.

Nursing considerations: Assess vital signs, reclining and standing; lab values; level of anxiety; lethality; presence of side effects; childbearing status; contraceptive use. Evaluate for history of allergies, drug/alcohol abuse, glaucoma. Educate client to understand the problems of the disease and use of medication, take drug with food, use caution in operation of automobiles and other machinery. Refer to Client/Family Teaching: Benzodiazepines, Chapter 32.

Usual dosage: PO (adults)—5–25 mg TID or QID for anxiety; PO (adults)—50–100 mg for acute alcohol withdrawal; maximum daily dose 300 mg/day.

Onset: Is effective in 15–30 minutes and peaks in 2–4 hours.

Generic name: chlorpromazine

Brand name: Thorazine; Chlorazine; Klorazine; Ormazine; Promapar; Promaz; Thor-Prom

Classification: Antipsychotic/neuroleptic; antiemetic; phenothiazine

Common uses: Management of psychotic disorders such as schizophrenia; manic phase of bipolar disorder (until lithium takes effect); brief reactive psychosis; intractable hiccups; severe behavior problems in children; nausea and vomiting; pre- and postoperative sedation.

Should not use if: Client is hypersensitive to phenothiazines; comatose or CNS-depressed; taking CNS depressants; pregnant or lactating; under 2 years of age; has bone marrow depression, blood dyscrasias, subcortical brain damage, Parkinson's disease, liver, renal, or cardiac insufficiency, severe hypo- or hypertension. Use caution for clients with a history of seizures, prostatic hypertrophy, diabetes, hypocalcemia, severe reactions to insulin or ECT; who may be exposed to extreme temperatures or organophosphate insecticides; if client is withdrawing from alcohol or barbiturates.

Possible side effects: Sedation; headache; extrapyramidal symptoms; tardive dyskinesia; blurred vision; neuroleptic malignant syndrome, orthostatic hypotension; skin rashes; photosensitivity; dry mouth; nausea; vomiting; increased or decreased appetite; constipation agranulocytosis; leukopenia; anemia; thrombocytopenia; pancytopenia; laryngeal edema; laryngospasm; bronchospasm; suppression of cough reflex.

Possible drug interactions: Additive effects with CNS depressants and anticholinergic drugs; with epinephrine, may reverse action and lead to decreased blood pressure and tachycardia; aluminum or magnesium hydroxide may decrease absorption; the effects of lithium and levodopa may be decreased; may be neurotoxic in combination with lithium; may increase plasma levels of propranolol and metoprolol; cimetidine may decrease the effectiveness of phenothiazines; clonidine may produce severe hypotension; caffeine may counteract antipsychotic effects.

Nursing considerations: Assess therapeutic effects of medication; level of sedation; vital signs; childbearing status; ability to carry out activities of daily living. Evaluate lab values for symptoms of blood dyscrasias, extrapyramidal symptoms, tardive dyskinesia, symptoms of neuroleptic malignant syndrome, history of allergies and drug/alcohol consumption. Educate about nature of illness and use of medications; caution client to be careful when operating vehicles and machinery, and in processes that involve concentration. Refer to Client/Family Teaching: Antipsychotics, Chapter 32.

Usual dosage: PO (adults)—10 mg TID or QID, or 25 mg BID or TID; increased by 20–50 mg until symptoms are controlled; maximum daily dose of 200 mg.

Onset: 30–60 minutes, peaking in 2–4 hours and lasting 4–5 hours.

Generic name: clomipramine
Brand name: Anafranil
Classification: Tricyclic antidepressant
Common uses: Severe obsessive-compulsive disorder; depressive symptoms; panic disorder, or phobic disorder, but only if OCD is the primary diagnosis and strongly dominates the clinical picture.
Should not be used if: Client is hypersensitive to tricyclic antidepressants; using MAO inhibitors; in acute recovery from myocardial infarction; pregnant or lactating; under 18 years of age. Use with caution for clients with a history of seizures; urinary retention, glaucoma, cardiovascular disorders, hepatic or renal insufficiency, psychosis, acute intermittant porphria, or who are elderly or debilitated.
Possible side effects: Drowsiness; dizziness; mania; tremors; lowered seizure threshold; blurred vision; orthostatic hypotension; delayed ejaculation; anorgasmia; cardiac arrest; dry mouth; constipation; agranulocytosis; neutropenia; pancytopenia; and many other less common physical symptoms.
Possible drug interactions: Potentiates CNS depressants, including alcohol, barbiturates, and benzodiazepines; severe systemic reactions with MAO inhibitors; methylphenidate, phenothiazines, haloperidol, and cimetidine increase clomipramine serum levels; quinidine, procainamide, disopyramide potentiate adverse cardiovascular effects of clomipramine; smoking increases clomipramine metabolism; disulfiram decreases clomipramine metabolism; the absorption of levodopa and phenylbutazone is delayed; warfarin increases prothrombin time; dicumarol increases in the plasma; thyroid medications may interact to produce arrhythmias and tachycardia.
Nursing considerations: Assess initial vital signs (BP, lying down and standing) and weight, monitor throughout therapy; be aware of sudden changes in mood that may indicate lethality, note presence of obsessions and compulsions. Evaluate for symptoms of blood dyscrasias, including sore throat, fever, malaise, unusual bleeding or bruising, and symptoms of overdose, such as confusion, agitation, irritability, and physical signs. Educate client as to nature of disease, need for medication as withdrawal from medication may cause recurrence, properties of medication, including length of time drug takes to reach effective levels, to be careful when operating machinery and motor vehicles, standing up, and in exposure to the sun. Refer to Client/Family Teaching: Tricyclic Antidepressants, Chapter 32.
Usual dosage: OCD PO (adults)—75–150 mg/day in three divided doses.
Onset: Peak plasma in under 2 hours, takes effect in 5–10 weeks.

Generic name: clonazepam
Brand name: Klonopin; Rivotril
Classification: Anticonvulsant; benzodiazepine derivative
Common uses: Prophylactic treatment of seizures; panic attacks; mild sedation
Should not be used if: Client is hypersensitive to benzodiazepines; lactating, has acute angle-closure glaucoma, chronic respiratory or severe liver disease. Use caution if client is pregnant, elderly, or debilitated; depressed or suicidal; has a history of drug abuse/addiction.
Possible side effects: Drowsiness; ataxia; behavior problems; nausea/vomiting; constipation; blood dyscrasias; increased salivation; nystagmus; diplopia; respiratory depression; and several other less common physical effects.
Possible drug interactions: Additive with other CNS depressants; may increase absence seizures with valproic acid; phenobarbital, phenytoin, and carbamazepine decrease the effect of clonazepam; disulfiram increases its effect but may also lead to toxic reactions.
Nursing considerations: Assess vital signs; lab values; lethality; presence of side effects. Evaluate history of allergies, glaucoma, drug and alcohol consumption, childbearing status. Educate about usefulness of medication and disease process, caution needed in operation of vehicles and machinery. Refer to Client/Family Teaching: Benzodiazepines, Chapter 32.
Usual dosage: PO (adults)—initially 15 mg/day in three divided doses; may be increased to 20 mg/day.
Onset: Takes effect in 20–60 minutes; peaks in 1–2 hours; lasts from 6–12 hours.

Generic name: clorazepate
Brand name: Tranxene
Classification: Antianxiety; benzodiazepine
Common uses: Anxiety disorders and anxiety symptoms; partial seizures (adjunctive management); acute alcohol withdrawal
Should not be used if: Client is hypersensitive to benzodiazepines; taking other CNS depressants; pregnant or lactating; under 9 years of age. Use caution with elderly or debilitated patients; those with hepatic or renal dysfunction; a history of drug abuse/addiction; depression or lethality.
Possible side effects: Drowsiness; fatigue; ataxia; dizziness; and many other less common effects.
Possible drug interactions: Additive with other CNS depressants; effects increased by cimetidine; nicotine and caffeine decrease effects; neuromuscular blocking agents increase respiratory depression; reduces excretion of digoxin, increasing potential for toxicity; antacids reduce effectiveness.
Nursing considerations: Assess anxiety level; potential for addiction; history of allergies and/or medical problems; watch for symptoms of overdose, such as intoxication, disinhibition, impairment in judgment and memory, depressed vital signs. Evaluate blood pressure reclining and standing, blood studies, hepatic studies, I&O. Educate client about potential for injury from operating cars or machinery, abrupt withdrawal, and combining with CNS depressants. Refer to Client/Family Teaching: Benzodiazepines, Chapter 32.
Usual dosage: For anxiety, PO (adults)—15–60 mg/day in divided doses.

Onset: Takes effect in 30–60 minutes and peaks in 1–2 hours.

Generic name: clozapine
Brand name: Clozaril
Classification: Antipsychotic; tricyclic dibenzodiazepine derivative
Common uses: Management of psychotic symptoms in schizophrenic patients for whom other antipsychotics have failed.
Should not be used if: Client is hypersensitive to tricyclics; CNS-depressed or comatose; has myeloproliferative disorders, severe granulocytopenia.
Possible side effects: Agranulocytosis; sedation; salivation; dizziness; headache; tremors; sleep problems; akinesia; fever; seizures; sweating; akathisia; confusion; fatigue; insomnia; dry mouth; constipation; nausea; abdominal discomfort; vomiting; diarrhea; tachycardia; hypotension; hypertension; urinary abnormalities; leukopenia, neutropenia, eosinophilia.
Possible drug interactions: Anticholinergic effects increased with other anticholinergic drugs, in combination with antihypertensive drugs produces increased hypotension; potentiates CNS depressive drugs; bone marrow suppression is increased with antineoplastic medications; plasma concentration of warfarin, digoxin and other protein-bound drugs.
Nursing considerations: Evaluate for symptoms of blood dyscrasias, including sore throat, fever, malaise, unusual bleeding or bruising. Assess initial vital signs and weight, monitor throughout therapy; be aware of sudden changes in mood, which may indicate lethality; skin turgor, presence of side effects including pseudoparkinsonism, constipation and/or urinary retention. Educate about disease process, uses of medication and side effects. Caution client to be careful when operating machinery and motor vehicles, standing up and walking until stabilized, and in exposure to excessive external or environmental temperatures including hot tubs and showers; avoid use of OTC medications, alcohol or CNS depressant medications until cleared by doctor. Refer to Client/Family Teaching: Antipsychotics, Chapter 32.
Usual dosage: PO (adult)—initially 25 mg/day QD or BID; may increase to 300–450 mg/day gradually over 2 weeks, NTE 900 mg/day.
Onset: May take 2–4 weeks for therapeutic effect.

Generic name: diazepam
Brand name: Valium; Valrelease
Classification: Antianxiety; benzodiazepine
Common uses: Anxiety disorders; acute alcohol withdrawal; skeletal muscle spasms; convulsive disorders (adjunctive therapy); status epilepticus; preoperative sedation and relief of anxiety; anterograde amnesia.
Should not use if: Client is hypersensitive to benzodiazepines; using other CNS depressants; pregnant or lactating; an infant; in shock or coma; elderly or debilitated. Use with caution if client has narrow-angle glaucoma, hepatic or renal dysfunction, a history of drug abuse/addiction or lethality.
Possible side effects: Drowsiness; fatigue; ataxia; dizziness; shock; cardiovascular collapse; agranulocytosis; and many other less common physical effects.

Possible drug interactions: Other CNS depressants have additive depressant effects; cimetidine and valproic acid increase effects of diazepam; oral contraceptives and antitubercular drugs have contradictory effects; nicotine and caffeine decrease effects of diazepam; serum levels of phentoin may be increased; the effects of levodopa are decreased; excretion of digoxin may increase potential for toxicity.
Nursing considerations: Assess vital signs reclining and standing; lab values; level of anxiety; lethality; presence of side effects; childbearing status; contraceptive use. Evaluate for history of allergies, drug/alcohol abuse, glaucoma. Caution client that drug may become habit forming, to take drug with food, to use caution in operation of automobiles and other machinery; drug should not be used longer than four months unless directed by a physician; consult with physician before taking any OTC preparations in conjunction with diazepam. Refer to Client/Family Teaching: Benzodiazepines, Chapter 32.
Usual dosage: PO (adults)—2–10 mg BID or QID.
Onset: Takes effect in 30–60 minutes; peaks in 1–2 hours.

Generic name: diphenhydramine
Brand name: Benadryl; Bendylate; Benylin; Compoz; Fenylhist; Surfadil
Classification: Antihistamine with anticholinergic and sedative side effects
Common uses: Relief from allergies, cold symptoms, extrapyramidal side effects, Parkinson's disease, motion sickness, nausea and vomiting, dizziness; for mild sedation.
Should not be used if: MAO inhibitors have been used in previous 2 weeks. Use caution with clients with pregnancy, lactation, asthma, heart or lung disease, glaucoma, ulcers, difficulty urinating, high BP, seizures, hyperthyroidism; under 6 years of age.
Possible side effects: Sedation; dry mouth and mucous membranes; vision problems; difficulty urinating; muscle weakness; excitement (especially in children); nervousness.
Possible drug interactions: Potentiates alcohol and other CNS depressants; MAO inhibitors prolong and intensify anticholinergic effects.
Nursing considerations: If a dose is missed, do not double dose; caution advised in tasks requiring alertness, I&O.
Usual dosage: Usual daily dose range 75–200 mg, nighttime sleep aid dosage 50 mg.
Onset: Takes effect and peaks in 1 hour, lasts for 4–6 hours.

Generic name: disulfiram
Brand name: Antabuse
Classification: Alcohol deterrent; aldehyde dehydrogenase inhibitor
Common uses: Chronic alcoholism (aversion therapy)
Should not be used if: Client is hypersensitive to thiuram derivatives; has severe myocardial disease, coronary occlusion, psychoses; has recently received or is receiving metronidazole, paraldehyde, alcohol or alcohol-containing preparations; use caution with clients who have hepatic or renal insufficiency, diabetes mellitus, seizure disorders, cerebral damage, history of rubber-contact dermatitis, chronic or acute nephritis, hepatic cirrhosis,

abnormal EEG results, multiple drug dependence, hypothyroidism; or who are pregnant.

Possible side effects: Drowsiness; headache; metallic or garlic-like aftertaste; hepatotoxicity; blood dyscrasias; disulfiram-alcohol reaction, which includes tachycardia, hypotension, flushing, dyspnea, headache, nausea and vomiting.

Possible drug interactions: Mild to severe life-threatening reactions with alcohol-containing preparations (including topical), increased effects of diazepam and chlordiazepoxide; phenytoin intoxication, prolonged prothrombin time with oral anticoagulants; unsteady gait or marked changes in behavior with isoniazid; acute toxic psychosis with metronidazole; additive CNS stimulation with marijuana; with barbiturates and paraldehyde, increased serum concentration and possible toxicity; combination with tricyclic antidepressants may produce acute organic brain syndrome and enhance the disulfiram-alcohol reaction; decreased clearance of caffeine.

Nursing considerations: Assess baseline vital signs and weight; mood, appearance, orientation, and behavior; assess for symptoms of alcohol withdrawal, oral contraceptive use, childbearing status. Evaluate alcohol and drug use, history of allergies, diabetes, cardiac disease, epilepsy, hypothyroidism, liver disease, psychosis, adverse side effects (symptoms can occur within 5–10 minutes after ingestion of alcohol). Educate about condition and need for therapy, medication effects and contraindications. Refer to Chapter 11.

Usual dosage: PO (adults)—initial dosage 250–500 mg/day in a single dose for 1–2 weeks. Not to exceed 500 mg/day.

Onset: Takes effect in 3–12 hours, lasts up to 14 days.

Generic name: doxepin HCl
Brand name: Adaptin; Sinequan
Classification: Tricyclic antidepressant; debenzoxepin; tertiary amine
Common uses: Major depression with melancholia or psychotic symptoms; depression associated with organic disease and alcoholism; depressive phase of bipolar disorder; psychoneurotic anxiety; mixed symptoms of anxiety and depression.
Should not be used if: Client is hypersensitive to tricyclic antidepressants; taking a MAO inhibitor; in acute recovery phase after myocardial infarction; pregnant or lactating; under 12 years of age; has untreated angle-closure glaucoma, a history of urinary retention. Use caution if client has cardiovascular, hepatic, or renal problems or if client is suicidal, psychotic, elderly, or debilitated.
Possible side effects: Drowsiness; dizziness; orthostatic hypotension; tachycardia; myocardial infarction; heart block; CHF; ECG changes; cardiovascular collapse; dry mouth; constipation; urinary retention; agranulocytosis; thrombocytopenia; leukopenia; and several less common problems.
Possible drug interactions: Potentiates CNS depressants, including alcohol, barbiturates, and benzodiazepines; severe systemic reactions with MAO inhibitors; nicotine increases doxepin metabolism; thyroid medications may interact to produce arrhythmias and tachycardia; cimetidine, phenothiazines, and haloperidol increase doxepin serum levels; oral contraceptives decrease effects of doxepin; disulfiram decreases doxepin metabolism, absorption of levodopa, and phenylbutazone is decreased; plasma concentration of dicumarol is increased.
Nursing considerations: Assess for lethality and sudden mood elevation that may precede suicide attempt, vital signs, weight, malaise. Evaluate history of seizures, allergies, glaucoma, alcohol/drug consumption, contraceptive use. Educate client to understand precautions about illness, medications, and precautions that must be taken in regard to driving and operation of machinery. Refer to Client/Family Teaching: Tricyclic Antidepressants, Chapter 32.
Usual dosage: PO (adults)—initial dosage 10–25 mg TID; usual optimal dose 75–150 mg/day; entire dose may be taken at bedtime.
Onset: May take from 2–4 weeks, peaks in less than 2 hours and lasts for weeks in the system.

Generic name: fluoxetine
Brand name: Prozac
Classification: Bicyclic antidepressant
Common uses: Major depressive disorder
Should not be used if: Client is hypersensitive; pregnant or lactating. Use caution if client has a history of seizures, lethality, being underweight, hepatic or renal insufficiency, drug abuse, a recent MI; if client is elderly or debilitated.
Possible side effects: Headache; nervousness; insomnia; drowsiness; anxiety; tremors; dizziness; fatigue; rash; nausea; diarrhea; dry mouth; anorexia; weight loss; anemia; thrombocytopenia; leukopenia; thrombocythemia; excessive sweating.
Possible drug interactions: Prolongs half-life of diazepam; potential for hypertensive crisis with MAO inhibitors; with tryptophan, there may be increased central and peripheral toxicity, agitation, restlessness, GI distress; fluoxetine increases activity of warfarin.
Nursing considerations: Assess for suicidal ideation, sudden elevation in mood, mental status, symptoms of blood dyscrasias. Evaluate vital signs, weight, history for drug/alcohol abuse, glaucoma, childbearing status. Educate client about disease process and value of medication therapy, possible side effects, when to expect results, to be cautious with machinery or motor vehicles.
Usual dosage: PO (adults)—initial dose 20 mg/day given in the morning, may be increased after several weeks if no improvement is noted; doses above 20 mg/day should be administered BID (morning and noon); maximum daily dose of 80 mg/day.
Onset: Takes effect in 3–5 weeks, will peak in 6–8 hours and remains in the system for weeks.

Generic name: fluphenazine
Brand name: Prolixin HCl; prolixin decanoate
Classification: Antipsychotic/neuroleptic; phenothiazine; piperazine
Common uses: Acute and chronic psychotic disorders; schizophrenia
Should not be used if: Client is hypersensitive to phenothiazines, sulfites, or tartrazine; comatose or CNS depressed; taking large amounts of CNS depressants; hyper/hypotensive, under 12 years of age; pregnant or lactating; client has bone marrow depression, subcortical brain damage, Parkinson's disease, hepatic, renal or cardiac insufficiency.

Use caution with clients who have a history of seizures, respiratory, renal, hepatic, thyroid, or cardiovascular disorders, prostatic hypertrophy, glaucoma, diabetes, hypocalcemia, a history of severe reactions to insulin or ECT; clients who are exposed to extremes of temperatures or organophosphate insecticides or who are elderly or debilitated.

Possible side effects: Sedation; headache; extrapyramidal symptoms; tardive dyskinesia; blurred vision; neuroleptic malignant syndrome; orthostatic hypotension; skin rashes; photosensitivity; dry mouth; nausea; vomiting; increased or decreased appetite; constipation; agranulocytosis; leukopenia; anemia; thrombocytopenia; pancytopenia; laryngeal edema; laryngospasm; bronchospasm; suppression of cough reflex.

Possible drug interactions: Cumulative effects with other CNS depressants; decreases effects of levodopa; additive anticholinergic effects; decreased antipsychotic effects with anticholinergic agents; barbiturates may decrease effects of fluphenazine; may be toxic with epinephrine; clonidine may produce acute brain syndrome; magnesium/aluminum containing antacids reduce absorption/effectiveness; lithium decreases plasma levels and effectiveness, may be neurotoxic; decreased phenytoin metabolism; increased risk of toxicity; cimetidine decreases effectiveness of fluphenazine; possibility of severe hypotension with clonidine; increased seizure potential with piperazine.

Nursing considerations: Assess therapeutic effects of medication; level of sedation; vital signs; childbearing status; ability to carry out activities of daily living. Evaluate lab values for symptoms of blood dyscrasias; evaluate for extrapyramidal symptoms, tardive dyskensia, symptoms of neuroleptic malignant syndrome, history of allergies and drug/alcohol consumption. Educate about nature of illness and use of medications; caution in operation of vehicles and machinery, and in processes that involve concentration. Refer to Client/Family Teaching: Antipsychotics, Chapter 32.

Usual dosage: Fluphenazine HCl, PO (adults)—initial dose 0.5–10 mg/day in divided doses Q 6–8 hours. Optimal effect usually under 20 mg/day, occasionally 40 mg/day is required. Fluphenazine decanoate (adults), 12.5–25 mg IM every 1–3 weeks. Conversion approximately 12.5 mg of fluphenazine decanoate every 3 weeks for every 10 mg fluphenazine HCl daily.

Onset: PO (HCl)—takes effect in 60 minutes, peaks in 1.5–2 hours, lasts for 6–8 hours; IM (HCl)—takes effect in 60 minutes, peaks in 0.5 hour, lasts 6–8 hours; IM (decanoate)—takes effect in 1–3 days, peaks in 1–2 days, lasts for 1–3 weeks.

Generic name: flurazepam
Brand name: Dalmane
Classification: Sedative-hypnotic; benzodiazepine derivative
Common uses: Short-term use for insomnia, characterized by difficulty falling asleep, frequent nocturnal awakening, and/or early morning awakening.
Should not be used if: Client is hypersensitive to benzodiazepines; pregnant or lactating; under 15 years of age. Use caution with elderly or debilitated patients, those with anemia, hepatic or renal dysfunctions, a history of drug abuse/addiction, are depressed/suicidal, are using other CNS depressants, or have low serum albumin.
Possible side effects: Residual sedation; dizziness; confusion; headache; lethargy; weakness; paradoxical excitement; blurred vision; encephalopathy; rashes; nausea and vomiting; diarrhea; constipation; agranulocytosis; tolerance; physical and psychologic dependence.
Possible drug interactions: Other CNS depressants, antipsychotics, antidepressants, antihistamines, anticonvulsants, and cimetidine are all cumulative in effect with flurazepam; neuromuscular blocking agents may increase respiratory depression; disulfiram may increase the duration of action.
Nursing considerations: Assess lab values and baseline vital signs, sleep patterns, suicidal ideation, childbearing status, presence of side effects. Evaluate history of allergies or glaucoma, current and past history of alcohol/drug use, oral contraceptive use, mental status, blood dyscrasias. Educate about illness and need for medication, about other techniques for sleep induction, to avoid driving, operation of hazardous machinery or other functions that require concentration until drug is stabilized, other safety precautions such as raised side rails on the beds, active metabolites are retained in the body for several days.
Usual dosage: PO (adults)—15–30 mg at bedtime.
Onset: Takes effect in 15–45 minutes; peaks in 30–60 minutes and stays in the system for days.

Generic name: haloperidol
Brand name: Haldol; Haldol Enthante; Peridol/Haloperidol Decanoate
Classification: Antipsychotic/neuroleptic; butyrophenone
Common uses: Management of acute and chronic psychosis; control of Tourette syndrome; symptoms of dementia in the elderly; short-term treatment of hyperactive children; prolonged treatment of chronic schizophrenia.
Should not be used if: Client is hypersensitive to haloperidol or tartrazine, comatose or severely CNS depressed, taking other CNS depressants; pregnant or lactating; under 3 years of age; has bone marrow depression, blood dyscrasias, subcortical brain damage, Parkinson's disease, respiratory, hepatic, renal, thyroid or cardiovascular disorders, severe hypo/hypertension. Use caution with clients with history of seizures, prostatic hypertrophy, glaucoma, diabetes, hypocalcemia, acute illness or dehydration; clients who are elderly or debilitated, exposed to extreme environmental temperatures, or have severe reactions to insulin or ECT.
Possible side effects: Sedation; headache; extrapyramidal symptoms; tardive dyskinesia; blurred vision; neuroleptic malignant syndrome; orthostatic hypotension; photosensitivity; dry mouth; anorexia; constipation; paralytic ileus; impaired liver function; hypersalivation; agranulocytosis; leukopenia; anemia; laryngeal edema; laryngospasm; bronchospasm; suppression of cough reflex; diaphoresis; and many other less common physical symptoms.
Possible drug interactions: CNS depressants have an additive effect; anticholinergic agents have additive anticholinergic and decreased antipsychotic effects; barbiturate anesthetics have increased incidence of excitatory effects and hypotension; barbiturates may decrease antipsychotic ef-

fects; metyrosine potentiates extrapyramidal side effects; the efficacy of levodopa is decreased; additive cardiac depressive effects with quinidine; the antihypertensive action of guanethidine is decreased; the hypotensive action of propranolol and metoprolol is increased; lithium may produce neurologic toxicity or encephalopathy; with epinephrine may decrease blood pressure; phenytoin may decrease the effects of haloperidol; carbamazepine decreases the effects of haloperidol; methyldopa leads to increased sedation and abnormal mental symptoms; caffeine may counteract antipsychotic effect.

Nursing considerations: Assess mental status, ability to carry out activities of daily living, presence of spastic facial movements or unusual vocal utterances, symptoms of blood dyscrasias, extrapyramidal symptoms, symptoms of neuroleptic malignant syndrome, baseline vital signs and weight. Evaluate history for allergies, childbearing status, oral contraceptive use, drug/alcohol use, signs and symptoms of cholestatic jaundice. Educate about nature of illness and effective use of medication, to avoid hot tubs and showers and to get up slowly to avoid orthostatic hypotension, to use a sunscreen during exposure. Educate about nature of side effects and to report problems, to avoid driving or operation of machinery that requires concentration until more stable, that constipation may occur and should be reported, to avoid OTC preparations until physician is consulted. Refer to Client/Family Teaching: Antipsychotics, Chapter 32.

Usual dosage: PO (adults)—tablets or concentrate 3–5 mg BID or TID; daily dosages of up to 100 mg may be necessary for severely resistant patients. IM (adults)—2–5 mg Q 4–8 hours, may be administered as often as Q 60 minutes if client is severely agitated. Maintenance with IM decanoate is initially 10–15 times the daily oral dosage, to a maximum of 100 mg per dose every 4 weeks.

Onset: PO—erratic in length of time to effective therapy, peaks in 2–6 hours, full therapeutic effects may not be observed for 4–8 weeks; IM—takes effect in 30–60 minutes, peaks in 10–20 minutes, and stays in the system for 4–8 hours. IM decanoate—peaks in 6–7 days and will remain effective for 3–4 weeks.

Generic name: hydroxyzine
Brand name: Vistaril; Atarax; Atozine; Durrax; Vamate
Classification: Antihistamine; antianxiety; piperazine derivative
Common uses: Anxiety; relief from allergies; pruritus; nausea and vomiting; motion sickness
Should not be used if: Caution should be exercised in clients with pregnancy or lactation; asthma; heart disease; glaucoma; ulcers; difficulty urinating; high BP; seizures; hyperthyroidism.
Possible side effects: Sedation; decreases mental alertness and physical coordination; dry mouth; headache; increased anxiety; ischemia.
Possible drug interactions: Enhances alcohol and other CNS depressants; epinephrine should not be used to administer vasopressor effects; MAO inhibitors prolong and intensify anticholinergic effects.
Nursing considerations: Caution client to be careful when doing taks requiring alertness; falsely elevated urine

hydroxycorticosteroids. Evaluate for vital signs, assure proper hydration, I&O.
Usual dosage: 75–100 mg/day to 200–400 mg/day.
Onset: 15–30 minutes, effects for 4–6 hours.

Generic name: lithium carbonate
Brand name: Lithane; Eskalith; Lithonate; Lithotabs; Lithobid; Lithium Citrate; Lithonate-S
Classification: Antimanic; alkali metal ion salt
Common uses: Manic phase of bipolar disorder; maintenance therapy to prevent or diminish intensity of subsequent manic episodes; depression associated with bipolar disorder.
Should not be used if: Client has severe renal or cardiovascular disease, dehydration, sodium depletion, brain damage, or is pregnant or lactating. Use caution with elderly clients, those having thyroid disorders, diabetes mellitus, urinary retention, a history of seizure disorder.
Possible side effects: Fine hand tremors; fatigue; dizziness; confusion; restlessness; headache; lethargy; drowsiness; ECG changes; acne; rash; hypothyroidism; excessive weight gain; anorexia; nausea and vomiting; diarrhea; dry mouth; thirst; polyuria; glycosuria; diabetes insipidus; reversible leukocytosis (WBC 10,000–15,000).
Possible drug interactions: Aminophylline; mannitol; acetazolamide; sodium bicarbonate; drugs high in sodium content may increase renal elimination and decrease effectiveness of lithium; haloperidol may cause encephalopathic syndrome and result in brain damage; neuromuscular blocking agents prolong effects of skeletal muscle relaxation; paroxicam, indomethacin, and nonsteroidal anti-inflammatory drugs produce significant increases in plasma lithium levels thereby increasing potential for toxicity; thiazide diuretics decrease renal clearance of lithium, thus increasing risk of toxicity; phenothiazines produce decreased antipsychotic effect and/or increased lithium excretion; phenytoin and carbamazepine may have adverse neurological effects; iodides have additive hypothyroid effects; increased dietary sodium increases renal elimination of lithium while decreased dietary sodium decreases renal excretion of lithium, thus increasing risk of toxicity.
Nursing considerations: Assess mood and behavior, baseline vital signs and weight, lab values, lethality. Evaluate renal and thyroid function tests and baseline ECG in collaboration with physician, any physical symptoms that the client displays; wrists and ankles for edema; hydration; neurologic state. Educate client and family about the disease and the effective use of medication, including side effects and when to notify physician; about taking medication with meals to avoid GI upset; to use contraception; not to operate machinery until lithium levels are stable; to avoid increasing normal fluid intake. Refer to Client/Family Teaching and Nursing Care Plan: Lithium Carbonate, Chapter 32.
Usual dosage: Acute mania—PO (adults): 600 mg TID or QID. Maintenance therapy—PO (adults): 300–1200 mg/day in divided doses.
Onset: Normalization of symptoms is usually apparent after 1–3 weeks. Takes effect rapidly after stabilization, peaks in 0.5–3 hours, duration is variable.

Generic name: lorazepam
Brand name: Ativan
Classification: Antianxiety agent; benzodiazepine
Common uses: Anxiety; irritability in psychiatric or organic disorders; insomnia
Should not be used if: Client is hypersensitive to benzodiazepines; using other CNS depressants; pregnant or lactating; under 12 years of age; in shock or coma; elderly or debilitated. Use with caution if client has narrow-angle glaucoma, hepatic or renal dysfunction, a history of drug abuse/addiction, or lethality.
Possible side effects: Drowsiness; fatigue; ataxia; dizziness; constipation; dry mouth; ECG changes; tachycardia; orthostatic hypotension; blurred vision; and many other less common physical effects.
Possible drug interactions: Other CNS depressants produce additive CNS depression; effects of lorazepam are decreased by nicotine and caffeine; neuromuscular blocking agents increase respiratory depression; digoxin excretion is reduced, thus increasing potential for toxicity.
Nursing considerations: Assess vital signs, lying and standing; lab values; level of anxiety; lethality; presence of side effects; childbearing status; contraceptive use. Evaluate for history of allergies, drug/alcohol abuse, glaucoma. Educate client to understand the problems of the disease and use of medication, not to take drug for everyday stressors, to take drug with food, to use caution in operation of automobiles and other machinery, to avoid use of alcohol and OTC medications until physician is consulted, not to discontinue medication abruptly. Refer to Client/Family Teaching: Benzodiazepines, Chapter 32.
Usual dosage: PO (adults)—2–3 mg BID or TID. IM form available.
Onset: Takes effect in 15–45 minutes, peaks in 2 hours, duration is variable.

Generic Name: molindone HCl
Brand Name: Moban
Classification: Tranquilizer; antipsychotic; dihydroindolone
Common uses: Management of psychosis
Should not be used if: Severe CNS depression; known sensitivity to drug; pregnant or lactating; under 12 years of age.
Possible side effects: Blurred vision; glaucoma; constipation; akathisia; akinesia; dry mouth; decreased sweating; headache; drowsiness; orthostatic hypotension; tachycardia; difficulty talking; mask-like face; restlessness; stiff extremities; trembling; tardive dyskinesia; muscle spasms; neuroleptic malignant syndrome; agranulocytosis.
Possible drug interactions: Antacids and diarrhea medication decrease absorption; potentiates alcohol and other CNS depressants; may decrease absorption of phenytoin or tetracyclines.
Nursing considerations: Assess for neuroleptic malignant syndrome; allergic reaction to sulfite. Caution client to be careful when doing tasks requiring alertness. Educate about use of care to avoid becoming overheated. Assure good hydration, I&O. Refer to Client/Family Teaching: Antipsychotics, Chapter 32.
Usual dosage: Initially 50 mg/day to 225 mg/day; maintainence doses 15–150 mg/day.
Onset: Peak within 1 hour, duration of action 36 hours.

Generic name: oxazepam
Brand name: Serax
Classification: Sedative–hypnotic; benzodiazepine
Common uses: Anxiety; agitation during alcohol withdrawal
Should not be used if: Caution in prescribing for clients who are pregnant or lactating, have kidney or liver disease, allergy to aspirin or tartrazine (yellow dye).
Possible side effects: Drowsiness; muscle incoordination; fatigue; dizziness; confusion; restlessness; excitement; muscle spasms; nightmares; dose dependent CNS adverse effects.
Possible drug interactions: Nicotine decreases effectiveness; alcohol potentiates sedation and dizziness; levodopa-treated patients may experience decreased control of parkinsonian symptoms. Closely observe patients on anticonvulsants.
Nursing considerations: Caution client to be careful when doing tasks requiring alertness; this medication may become habit forming; if a dose is missed do not double dose; some evidence that ataxia and risk of falls is increased in geriatrics; gradual tapering off medication; the need for continued use should be reassessed regularly. Refer to Client/Family Teaching: Benzodiazepines; Chapter 32.
Usual dosage: 30–60 mg/day, for severe anxiety or agitation associated with ETOH withdrawal 45–120 mg/day in divided doses.
Onset: 15–45 minutes, duration 7–8 hours.

Generic name: perphenazine
Brand name: Trilafon
Classification: Antipsychotic; phenothiazine
Common uses: Symptomatic management of psychotic disorders; severe nausea and vomiting in adults.
Should not be used if: Sulfite sensitivity, under 12 years of age.
Possible side effects: Dizziness; orthostatic hypotension; dry mouth; muscle spasms; slow or difficult speech; tremors; shuffling gait; drooling; restlessness; weakness; blurred vision; constipation; difficulty urinating; tardive dyskinesia; photosensitivity; decreased body temperature regulation; drowsiness; tachycardia; agranulocytosis, pruritus; depositions of pigment in body tissues and fine particulate matter in lens and cornea; GI distress.
Possible drug interactions: Potentiating effects of alcohol and other CNS depressants; lowered seizure threshold therefore dosage adjustment on anticonvulsants; lithium used concurrently may cause unusual adverse neurologic effects; do not use with metrizamide.
Nursing considerations: Caution client to be careful when doing tasks requiring alertness; avoid overheating. Assess for extrapryamidal reactions; track elimination patterns; observe for unusual hematologic occurrences. Due to enhanced response, CNS depressants (alcohol, etc.) cannot be used; with hypocalcemia increased dystonia occurs; assure proper hydration; may be necessary to continue antiparkinsonian medication after discontinuance of drug; protect medication from light. Educate about tardive dyskinesia. Refer to Client/Family Teaching: Antipsychotics, Chapter 32.
Usual dosage: 12–24 mg/day to 16–64 mg/day.

Onset: For prompt control of severe symptoms, IM administration recommended; specific onset information not available.

Generic name: phenelzine sulfate
Brand name: Nardil
Classification: Antidepressant; monoamine oxidase inhibitor
Common uses: Atypical, nonendogenous, or neurotic depression; depression accompanied by anxiety; clients unresponsive to other antidepressants (usually not drug of choice).
Should not be used if: Client is hypersensitive to MAO inhibitors; a paranoid schizophrenic; pregnant or lactating; over 60/under 16 years of age; has pheochromocytoma, CHF, diseases of cardiovascular, renal, or hepatic systems, hypertension, a history of severe headaches. Use caution with clients with history of seizures, lethality, schizophrenia, diabetes mellitus, angina pectoris, hyperthyroidism or who are agitated/hypomanic, suicidal, sensitive to tartrazine (FD&C yellow No. 5).
Possible side effects: Hypertensive crisis; dizziness; headache; drowsiness; blurred vision; orthostatic hypotension; hypertension; cardiac dysrhythmias; dry mouth; constipation; weight gain; photosensitivity; flushing; increased perspiration; urinary frequency; anorexia.
Possible drug interactions: Specific food (containing tyramine, tryptophan); drink and other medications may cause severe reactions; alcohol is to be avoided; OTC or prescription cold, hay fever or weight-reducing medication, other MAO inhibitor or tricyclic antidepressant; fluoxetine may result in severe adverse effects; amphetamines; may be additive with CNS depressants; elevated BP with Buspirone; exaggerated effects of general anesthetics; caution with disulfiram.
Nursing considerations: Diet must be regulated to prevent dangerous reactions (e.g., sudden hypertension); know and teach symptoms of hypertensive crisis (severe headache, palpitation, neck stiffness, nausea, sweating, visual disturbances); closely monitor blood pressure; assess lethality; assure proper hydration; medication may take several weeks to begin effect; caution advised in tasks requiring alertness; evaluate for lethality; protect medication from excessive exposure to heat and light; medication must be discontinued 7–14 days prior to elective surgery. Refer to Client/Family Teaching: MAO Inhibitors, Chapter 32.
Usual dosage: 45 mg/day–90 mg/day, maintenance therapy as low as 15 mg/day.
Onset: Maximum benefit 2–6 weeks.

Generic name: phenobarbital
Brand name: Bar; Barbita; Eskabarb; Floramine; Luminal; Orpine; Solubarb; Stental; Luminal sodium
Classification: Sedative-hypnotic; anticonvulsant; barbiturate; CNS depressant
Common uses: Moderate anxiety states; insomnia; seizures (long term); status epilepticus; pre/post operative sedation.
Should not be used if: Client is hypersensitive to barbiturates; has hepatic, renal, cardiac, or respiratory disease; a history of previous drug addiction or of porphyria; use caution with clients who are anemic, elderly, or debilitated, depressed/suicidal, pregnant, lactating; or ammonia intoxication.

Possible side effects: Drowsiness; dizziness; lethargy; residual sedation; agranulocytosis; thrombocytopenia; respiratory depression; laryngospasm; bronchospasm; tolerance; nausea and vomiting; and other less common physical and psychologic problems.
Possible drug interactions: Additive with other CNS depressants, chloramphenicol, MAO inhibitors, valproic acid, cimetidine, disulfuram all increase effects of phenobarbital; with phenytoin the effects of either drug may be increased or decreased; the effectiveness of oral contraceptives, oral anticoagulants, corticosteroids, digitoxin, and doxycycline are decreased; with furosemide there is a risk of orthostatic hypotension; phenobarbital decreases levels of griseofulvin.
Nursing considerations: Assess sleep patterns, seizure activity, suicidal ideations, baseline vital signs, laboratory tests; evaluate effectiveness of therapy, history of alcohol and drug use, childbearing status/contraceptive use, presence of adverse reactions, client and family's response to diagnosis. Educate family and client concerning diagnosis, need for medication, possible effects of medication, dangers of operating vehicles or machinery, while medication is effective.
Usual dosage: PO (adults)—15–30 mg BID or TID. PO (children)—2 mg/kg TID.
Onset: PO—takes effect in 20–60 minutes; peaks in 8–12 hours and lasts from 6–10 hours.

Generic name: phenytoin, phenytoin sodium
Brand name: Dilantin; Di-Phen; Diphenylan
Classification: Anticonvulsant; hydantoin; antiarrhythmic
Common uses: Tonic-clonic (grand mal) and partial seizures with complex symptomatology; grand mal seizures associated with status epilepticus or occurring during or following neurosurgery; autonomic seizures; cardiac arrhythmias.
Should not be used if: Client is hypersensitive to phenytoin; lactating; has sinus bradycardia; heart block; absence (petit mal) seizures and seizures related to hypoglycemia. Use with caution for clients with hepatic or renal dysfunction, diabetes mellitus, hypotension, myocardial insufficiency, or who are elderly, pregnant or debilitated.
Possible side effects: Nystagmus; ataxia; drowsiness; decreased alertness; hypotension; arrhythmias; circulatory collapse; cardiac arrest; skin rashes; hypertrichosis; exfoliative dermatitis; nausea and vomiting; blood dyscrasias; gingival hyperplasia.
Possible drug interactions: Trimethoprim, amiodarone, benzodiazepines, disulfiram, isoniazid, phenylbutazone, chloramphenicol, cimetidine, sulfonamides, salicylates, acute alcohol intake, phenothiazines all increase the effects of phenytoin, thus increasing the risk of toxicity; barbiturates, diazoxide, rifampin, antineoplastic agents, chronic alcohol abuse, antacids, calcium gluconate, carbamazepine decrease the effects of phenytoin; effects may increase or decrease with phenobarbital, valproic acid, sodium valproate; phenytoin decreases effects of corticosteroids, oral contraceptives, digoxin, furosemide, doxycycline, dopamine, and levodopa; phenytoin increases effects of primidone.
Nursing considerations: Assess baseline vital signs, seizure activity, laboratory values, for presence of skin rashes,

adverse reactions and side effects. Evaluate history of past and present disease states, drug/alcohol use, allergies, contraceptive use and childbearing status. Educate family and client about the disease process, need for and properties of medication, dangers of operating motor vehicles and machinery while drug is active in the system.

Usual dosage: PO (adults)—100 mg TID or QID (MDD 600 mg).

Onset: PO—Takes effect in 0.5–2 hours; peaks in 1.5–3 hours and lasts from 6–12 hours.

Generic name: propranolol HCl
Brand name: Inderal
Classification: Antihypertensive; antianginal; anti-arrhythmic; beta-adrenergic blocker
Common uses: Hypertension; angina pectoris; cardiac arrhythmias; migraine headaches; essential tremor; acute exacerbation of schizophrenic disorder and anxiety states; action tremors (drug-induced), tardive dyskinesia; acute panic symptoms; intermittent explosive disorder.
Should not be used if: Client is hypersensitive to beta-adrenergic blocking agents; pregnant or lactating; has heart block greater than first degree, cardiogenic shock, CHF, overt cardiac failure, bronchial asthma, bronchospasm, severe COPD, allergic rhinitis during the pollen season, Raynaud's syndrome, malignant hypertension, sinus bradycardia. Use with caution if client has diabetes mellitus, myasthenia gravis, Wolff-Parkinson-White syndrome, thyrotoxicosis, impaired hepatic or renal function, inadequate cardiac function, sinus node dysfunction, or is undergoing surgery.
Possible side effects: Dizziness; fatigue; insomnia; weakness; bradycardia; peripheral arterial insufficiency; hypotension; first and third degree heart block; intensification of AV block; nausea; diarrhea; agranulocytosis; depression; bronchial obstruction; bronchospasm; laryngospasm; and many other less common problems.
Possible drug interactions: Catecholamine depleting drugs produce additive reduction in sympathetic tone, resulting in hypotension, bradycardia, vertigo, syncope; digitalis glycosides produce additive depression of AV conduction, potentiation of bradycardia; the effects of sympathomimetics are decreased; antimuscarinics and tricyclic antidepressants antagonize propranolol's cardiac effects; smoking increases clearance of propranolol; diuretics and other antihypertensives increase hypotensive effects; prolongs hypoglycemic effects of insulin; severe rebound hypertension when propranolol is discontinued abruptly; increased effects of chlorpromazine, cimetidine, oral contraceptives, furosemide, hydralazine, succinylcholine and tubocurarine; phenytoin, rifampin, phenobarbital, and other barbiturates decrease levels of propranolol; thyroid hormones decrease its effects; isoproterenol, norepinephrine, dopamine, dobutamine reverse its effects; aluminum hydroxide gel reduces its absorption; ethanol slows its absorption; phenothiazines are additive pharmacologically.
Nursing considerations: Assess baseline vital signs, including weight, orthostatic blood pressure, extremities for coldness and paresthesia. Evaluate blood pressure and pulse before administration of drug, history of allergies, drug/alcohol use, use of oral contraceptives/childbearing status,

presence of adverse reactions (including symptoms of CHF). Educate client and family about illness, need for medication, and side effects, caution in operation of motor vehicles and other machinery.

Usual dosage: PO (adults)—wide range of dosages from 10–30 mg/day TID/QID for cardiac arrhythmias to 80–120 mg/day TID for exacerbation of schizophrenia or anxiety states.

Onset: Takes effect in 30 minutes, peaks in 60–90 minutes and lasts for 4–6 hours.

Generic name temazepam
Brand name: Restoril
Classification: Sedative-hypnotic; benzodiazepine
Common uses: Relief of anxiety; short-term treatment of insomnia; acute alcohol withdrawal; adjunct with anticonvulsants for seizure control.
Should not be used if: Client is pregnant or lactating. Use caution with geriatric, liver disease patients.
Possible side effects: Drowsiness; ataxia; weakness; confusion; agitation; GI complaints; urinary retention; dry mouth; increased appetite; increased salivation; constipation; menstrual irregularities.
Possible drug interactions: Alcohol, psychotropic drugs, anticonvulsants, antihistaminics and other CNS depressants are enhanced; levodopa-treated patients may experience decreased control of parkinsonian symptoms; closely observe patients on anticonvulsants.
Nursing considerations: Relatively slow GI absorption, therefore may be more effective 1–2 hours before bed. Caution client to be careful when doing tasks requiring alertness, this medication may become habit forming, if a dose is missed do not double dose, some evidence that ataxia and risk of falls is increased in geriatrics. Assess for contraceptive use, gradual tapering off medication, sleep pattern; the need for continued use should be reassessed regularly. Refer to Client/Family Teaching: Benzodiazepines, Chapter 32.
Usual dosage: 15–30 mg/day
Onset: Onset 15–45 minutes, duration of action 7–8 hours.

Generic name: thioridazine HCl
Brand name: Mellaril; Millazine; SK Thioridazine
Classification: Antipsychotic/neuroleptic; phenothiazine; piperidine
Common uses: Psychotic disorders; moderate to marked depression with variable degrees of anxiety (short term); multiple symptoms such as agitation, anxiety, depression, sleep disturbances, tension, and fears in geriatric patients; hyperkinesis, combativeness, and severe behavioral problems in children.
Should not be used if: Client is hypersensitive to phenothiazines, sulfites, or tartrazine; comatose or severely CNS depressed; pregnant or lactating; under 2 years of age; has bone marrow depression, blood dyscrasias, subcortical brain damage, Parkinson's disease, liver, renal, and/or cardiac insufficiency, severe hypotension or hypertension. Use caution with clients who have a history of seizures, respiratory, renal, hepatic, thyroid and cardiac disorders, prostatic hypertrophy, glaucoma, diabetes, or if exposed to extreme environmental temperatures, have a history of severe reactions to insulin or ECT, or who are elderly or debilitated.

Possible side effects: Sedation; headache; extrapyramidal symptoms; blurred vision; neuroleptic malignant syndrome; orthostatic hypotension; cardiac arrest; ECG changes; arrhythmias; pulmonary edema; circulatory collapse; skin rashes; photosensitivity; exfoliative dermatitis; dry mouth; nausea and vomiting; constipation; paralytic ileus; agranulocytosis; leukopenia; anemia; thrombocytopenia; pancytopenia; laryngeal edema; laryngospasm; bronchospasm; suppression of cough reflex; and other less common symptoms.

Possible drug interactions: Cumulative effects with other CNS depressants; decreases effects of levodopa; additive anticholinergic effects, decreased antipsychotic effects with anticholinergic agents; barbiturates may decrease effects of thioridazine; may be toxic with epinephrine; clonidine may produce acute brain syndrome; magnesium/aluminum containing antacids reduce absorption/effectiveness; lithium decreases plasma levels and effectiveness, may be neurotoxic; decreased phenytoin metabolism, increased risk of toxicity, cimetidine decreases effectiveness of thioridazine; possibility of severe hypotension with clonidine; increased seizure potential with piperazine.

Nursing considerations: Assess therapeutic effects of medication; level of sedation; vital signs; childbearing status; ability to carry out activities of daily living. Evaluate lab values for symptoms of blood dyscrasias, extrapyramidal symptoms, tardive dyskensia, symptoms of neuroleptic malignant syndrome, history of allergies and drug/alcohol consumption. Educate about nature of illness and use of medications; caution in operation of vehicles and machinery, and in processes that involve concentration. Refer to Client/Family Teaching: Antipsychotics, Chapter 32.

Usual dosage: PO (adults)—50–100 mg TID initially; may be gradually increased to maximum daily dose of 800 mg, then reduced gradually to maintenance dose.

Onset: Takes effect in 30–60 minutes; peaks in 2–4 hours; lasts for 4–6 hours.

Generic name: thiothixene
Brand name: Navane
Classification: Antipsychotic/neuroleptic; thioxanthene
Common uses: Psychotic disorders; schizophrenia; acute agitation
Should not be used if: Client is hypersensitive to thioxanthenes or phenothiazines, comatose or severely CNS-depressed, taking large amounts of CNS depressants, hyper/hypotensive; under 12 years of age; pregnant or lactating; has bone marrow depression, subcortical brain damage, Parkinson's disease, hepatic, renal or cardiac insufficiency. Use caution with clients who have a history of seizures, respiratory, renal, hepatic, thyroid, or cardiovascular disorders, prostatic hypertrophy, glaucoma, diabetes, hypocalcemia, a history of severe reactions to insulin or ECT; clients who are exposed to extremes of temperatures or organophosphate insecticides or who are elderly or debilitated.
Possible side effects: Sedation; headache; extrapyramidal symptoms; tardive dyskinesia; blurred vision; neuroleptic malignant syndrome; glaucoma; orthostatic hypotension; skin rashes; photosensitivity; contact dermatitis; dry mouth; nausea and vomiting; anorexia; constipation; agranulocytosis; leukopenia; anemia; thrombocytopenia; pancytopenia; laryngeal edema; laryngospasm; bronchospasm; suppresion of cough reflex; and other less common symptoms.

Possible drug interactions: Cumulative effects with other CNS depressants; decreases effects of levodopa; additive anticholinergic effects, decreased antipsychotic effects with anticholinergic agents; barbiturates may decrease effects of thiothixene; may be toxic with epinephrine; clonidine may produce severe hypotension; magnesium/aluminum containing antacids reduce absorption/effectiveness; lithium decreases plasma levels and effectiveness, may be neurotoxic; decreased phenytoin metabolism, increased risk of toxicity; cimetidine decreases effectiveness of thiothixene; increased seizure potential with piperazine; caffeine counteracts antipsychotic effects.

Nursing considerations: Assess mental status, therapeutic effects of medication, level of sedation, vital signs and weight, childbearing status, ability to carry out activities of daily living. Evaluate lab values for symptoms of blood dyscrasias and cholestatic jaundice; extrapyramidal symptoms; tardive dyskinesia; symptoms of neuroleptic malignant syndrome; history of allergies and drug/alcohol consumption. Educate about nature of illness and use of medications, caution in operation of vehicles and machinery, and in processes that involve concentration. Refer to Client/Family Teaching: Antipsychotics, Chapter 32.

Usual dosage: PO (adults)—initial dose 2–5 mg/day; increased to maximum daily dose of 60 mg; usual optimal dose 20–30 mg/day.

Onset: Takes effect slowly, peaks in 2–8 hours, lasts for 12–24 hours.

Generic name: trazodone HCl
Brand name: Desyrel
Classification: Antidepressant
Common uses: Depression; anxiety; sleep disturbances; alcohol dependence
Should not be used if: Initial phase of MI recovery; pregnant or lactating; under 18 years of age.
Possible side effects: Drowsiness; dry mouth; dizziness; orthostatic hypotension; muscle aches; sinus bradycardia; akathisia; anemia; early menses; delayed urine flow; hypersalivation; impotence; impaired speech; increased appetite; increased libido; nausea and vomiting; rash; priapism.
Possible drug interactions: Alcohol, barbiturates and other CNS depressants may be enhanced; antihypertensive medication may require dose reduction; digoxin and phenytoin levels may increase.
Nursing considerations: Caution client to be careful when doing tasks requiring alertness; medication has been associated with incidence of priapism; should be taken shortly after food. Assess lethality, depression, side effects, alcohol/drug abuse. Evaluate history of allergies.
Usual dosage: Initially 150 mg/day, increased to 400 mg/day (to 600 mg/day for inpatients)
Onset: Therapeutic levels reached in 7–14 days, peak after 1 hour (if taken on empty stomach); 2 hours (if taken with food).

Generic name: triazolam
Brand name: Halcion
Classification: Hypnotic; benzodiazepine

Common uses: Relief of anxiety; short-term management of initial insomnia; muscle spasm; epilepsy.

Should not be used if: Client is pregnant or lactating; depressed. Use caution with clients with impaired renal or hepatic function or chronic pulmonary insufficiency; under 18 years of age.

Possible side effects: Sedation; dizziness; lightheadedness; headache; nervousness; ataxia; nausea and vomiting; confusion.

Possible drug interactions: Alcohol, psychotropic drugs, anticonvulsants, antihistaminics and other CNS depressants are enhanced; may interact with disulfiram; cimetidine reduces plasma clearance; levodopa-treated patients may experience decreased control of parkinsonian symptoms; closely observe patients on anticonvulsants.

Nursing considerations: This medication may become habit forming; if a dose is missed do not double dose. Caution client to be careful when doing tasks requiring alertness. Evaluate for signs of OD (slurred speech, confusion, shakiness, SOB or trouble breathing, severe drowsiness, severe weakness, staggering), which may occur at 4 times maximum therapeutic dose; sedative effect may decrease over time; contraceptive use. Assess lethality, rebound insomnia after discontinuance; abrupt discontinuance should be avoided. Refer to Client/Family Teaching: Benzodiazepines, Chapter 32.

Usual dosage: 0.125–0.25 mg for elderly, debilitated; 0.25–0.5 mg HS

Onset: Peak in 1.3 hours, duration in body under 5.5 hours.

Generic name: trifluoperazine

Brand name: Stelazine; Suprazine

Classification: Antipsychotic; phenothiazine

Common uses: Management of psychotic disorders; short term treatment of non-psychotic anxiety.

Should not be used if: Sulfite sensitivity; metrizamide being administered. Use caution with clients with severe cardiovascular disorders, seizure history, lactating mothers, children with acute illnesses or dehydration, geriatric, debilitated, renal or hepatic disease, glaucoma, prostatic hypertrophy, hypocalcemia; safety during pregnancy has not been established.

Possible side effects: Akathisia; blurred vision; decreased alertness; dizziness; dry mouth; muscle spasms; slow or difficult speech; tremors; shuffling gait; drooling; restlessness; weakness; blurred vision; constipation; difficulty urinating; tardive dyskinesia; photosensitivity; decreased body temperature regulation; orthostatic hypotension; tachycardia; agranulocytosis; pruritus; pigment depositions in various body tissues; deposits of fine particulate matter in lens and cornea; breast engorgement with lactation.

Possible drug interactions: Additive or potentiating with other CNS depressants; lowered seizure threshold therefore dosage adjustment on anticonvulsants; lithium used concurrently may cause unusual adverse neurologic effects; do not use with metrizamide.

Nursing considerations: Geriatric clients may be more susceptible to hypotension and neuromuscular reactions; monitor for phenytoin toxicity (this medication lowers the seizure threshold). Caution client to be careful when doing tasks requiring alertness. Assess elimination patterns, avoid overheating; protect liquid medication from light. Assess for extrapyramidal reactions. Educate about tardive dyskinesia and photosensitivity. Refer to Client/Family Teaching; Antipsychotics, Chapter 32.

Usual dosage: Psychotic disorders—Adults 2–4 mg/day up to 40/mg day, Children 6–12 years 1–2 mg/day. Non-psychotic anxiety: Adult—2–4 mg/day not to exceed 6 mg/day, 12 weeks.

Onset: Optimum therapeutic response usually within 2–3 weeks.

Generic name: trihexyphenidyl HCl

Brand name: Aphen; Artane; Hexaphen; Trihexane; Trihexidyl

Classification: Antiparkinsonian agent; anticholinergic; synthetic tertiary amine

Common uses: All forms of parkinsonism (adjunctive therapy); extrapyramidal symptoms (except tardive dyskinesia) associated with antipsychotic drugs.

Should not be used if: Client is hypersensitive to anticholinergics; under 3 years of age; has angle-closure glaucoma, pyloric or duodenal obstruction, stenosing peptic ulcers, prostatic hypertrophy or bladder neck obstructions, achalasia, myasthenia gravis, ulcerative colitis, toxic megacolon, tachycardia secondary to cardiac insufficiency or thyrotoxicosis. Use with caution if client is elderly or debilitated, pregnant or lactating, exposed to extreme environmental temperatures, has narrow angle glaucoma, hepatic, renal, or cardiac insufficiency, hyperthyroidism, hypertension, autonomic neuropathy, or a tendency toward urinary retention.

Possible side effects: Drowsiness; dizziness; blurred vision; nervousness; dry mouth; nausea; constipation; paralytic ileus; and numerous other less common problems.

Possible drug interactions: Other drugs with anticholinergic properties increase anticholinergic effects, which may produce anticholinergic toxicity manifested by confusion, overt psychosis, visual hallucinations, hot dry skin, dilated pupils; decreases absorption of levodopa and digoxin; increased CNS depressant effects; decreases therapeutic effect of chlorpromazine, phenothiazines, and haloperidol; MAO inhibitors increase effects of trihexyphenidyl; antacids decrease its absorption; decreased antipsychotic effect with phenothiazines and haloperidol.

Nursing considerations: Assess baseline vital signs and weight, oral contraceptive use and childbearing status, symptoms of Parkinson's disease, such as tremors, muscular weakness and rigidity, drooling, shuffling, flat affect, and disturbance in balance or posture; extrapyramidal symptoms are similar with the addition of akinesia (muscular weakness), akathisia (restlessness), dystonia (involuntary muscular movements), oculogyric crisis (rolling back of the eyes), and tardive dyskinesia (bizarre facial and tongue movements with stiff neck and difficulty in swallowing). Evaluate for constipation, GI disturbance, or paralytic ileus which may be life-threatening. Educate patient to avoid OTC medications until physician agrees, to avoid driving or other activities that require intense concentration and not to stop medication abruptly.

Usual dosage: For drug-induced side effects, usual daily dose range 5–15 mg.

Onset: Takes effect in 1 hour, peaks in 1.5 hours, lasts for 6–12 hours.

Generic name: valproic acid

Brand name: Depakote

Classification: Anticonvulsant

Common uses: Management of simple and complex absence seizures (petit mal); adjunct to other anticonvulsants

Should not be used if: Safe use during pregnancy has not been established; caution in lactating women.

Possible side effects: Nausea and vomiting; sedation; drowsiness; ataxia; headache; hepatic effects including hepatotoxicity, hyperammonemia, hyperglycinemia, prolonged bleeding time; transient alopecia, generalized pruritus.

Possible drug interactions: Additive with CNS depressants including other anticonvulsants; increased phenobarbital plasma concentrations with possible severe CNS depression; barbiturates require observation for neurologic toxicity; clonazepam produces petit mal; potentiates MAO inhibitors; aspirin and warfarin also decrease bleeding time.

Nursing considerations: May impair ability to perform hazardous activities requiring mental alertness or physical coordination; overdosage may cause somnolence or coma. Evaluate seizure activity.

Usual dosage: Initially 15 mg/kg daily, maximum 60 mg/kg daily

Onset: Therapeutic effects in several days to more than one week.

REFERENCES

American Hospital Formulary Service, American Society of Hospital Pharmacists, 1990.

Bailey, David, Cooper, S, Bailey, Deborah, *Therapeutic Approaches to the Care of the Mentally Ill,* F.A. Davis Company, 1984.

Gitlin, MJ, *The Psychotherapist's Guide to Psychopharmacology,* The Free Press, 1990.

Lader, M, Herington, R, *Biological Treatments in Psychiatry,* Oxford Medical Publications, 1990.

Physician's Desk Reference, ed 44. Medical Economics Company, Incorporated, 1990.

Skidmore-Rota, L, *Mosby's 1991 Nursing Drug Reference,* C.V. Mosby Company, 1991.

Townsend, MC, *Drug Guide For Psychiatric Nursing,* F.A. Davis Company, 1990.

GLOSSARY

Abnormal Involuntary Movement Scale (AIMS) An assessment instrument for quantifying iatrogenic movements resulting from psychotropic drugs.

Abreaction A process in which repressed material, particularly a painful experience or conflict, is brought back to a person's awareness. The person then not only recalls but also relives the repressed material, which is accompanied by affective response.

Abuse Misuse of a drug that can be discontinued at will.

Accommodation Adjustment of the organism to an object in the environment; incorporation of an experience as it is.

Acquaintance (or date) rape Rape by an acquaintance, friend, lover, boyfriend, or husband.

Acquired immune deficiency syndrome (AIDS) A contagious and fatal condition of immune system depression for which there is no known cure.

Acting out Term used to describe a recreation of the client's life experiences, relationships with significant others, and resultant unresolved conflicts. Acting out may include, but is not limited to, destructive actions.

Active progressive relaxation A strategy that helps people identify tense muscle groups by distinguishing between sensations from purposeful muscle tensing and conscious muscle relaxing.

Adaptation The result of interchange between the organism and environment involving modification of the organism that enhances its ability for further interchange; involves assimilation and accommodation.

Addiction A cluster of cognitive, behavioral and physiologic symptoms that indicate that a person has impaired control of psychoactive substance use. Called psychoactive substance dependence in DSM-III-R.

Adjustment disorder Maladaptive reaction to an identifiable psychosocial stressor.

Adrenocorticotropic hormone (ACTH) Brain hormone that is not suppressed in depressed clients, reflecting a limbic system dysfunction associated with disturbances in mood, affect, appetite, sleep, and autonomic nervous system activity.

Adult ego state In transactional analysis theory, the ego state responsible for the objective appraisal of reality and the capacity to process data.

Affect Emotion or feeling; the tone of one's reaction to persons and events.

Affection need The interpersonal need to establish and maintain a satisfactory relation between self and other people with regard to intimacy and liking.

Affective disorders A specific group of psychiatric diagnoses that are predominantly characterized by disturbances in mood accompanied by a full or partial manic or depressive syndrome. Called mood disorders in DSM-III-R.

Ageism Negative, hostile attitudes toward the elderly.

Aggressive behavior Behavior that offends and alienates others.

Agnosia Difficulty recognizing everyday objects.

Agoraphobia The fear of being in places or situations from which escape might be difficult or embarrassing or in which help might not be available in the event of a panic attack.

AIDS Dementia Complex (ADC) The most common neurologic disorder in persons with AIDS. Symptoms range from mild memory loss to severe global confusion, loss of motor skills, depression, mood swings, psychotic symptoms, and hysteric reactions.

AIDS-related complex (ARC) The condition of having some clinical symptoms diagnosed as AIDS-related, but without the formal indicators of AIDS as defined by the Centers for Disease Control.

AIDS Service Organization (ASO) A community-based organization whose primary mission is to provide education about HIV and/or to provide services to people affected by the HIV epidemic.

Akathisia One of the classes of side-effects caused by neuroleptic drugs. Signs of this condition include motor restlessness, an urge to pace, a need to shift weight, or an inability to stand or sit still.

Al-Anon A support group for spouses and parents of alcoholics.

Al-Ateen A support group for teenage children of alcoholics.

Alcoholic In popular usage, one whose continued or excessive drinking results in impairment of personal health, disruption of family and social relationships, and loss of economic security. Alcoholism is believed by many to be a disease with strong genetic links.

Alcoholic hallucinations Auditory hallucinations reported as occurring approximately 48 hours after heavy drinking by alcohol-dependent clients.

Alcoholics Anonymous (AA) A self-help organization that uses a twelve-step program to assist alcoholics in achieving and maintaining sobriety.

Alcohol withdrawal syndrome The constellation of physiologic and behavioral symptoms that occur when an addicted individual stops drinking.

Algorithms Behavioral steps, or step-by-step procedures, for the management of common problems to provide structured, standardized guidelines for decision making.

Alliance for the Mentally Ill A national support group for families of the mentally ill, with many local and state affiliates. Provides educational programs and political action.

Alternate nostril breathing A general relaxation exercise that helps a person reduce tension and sinus headaches by inhaling and exhaling through alternate nostrils one at a time.

Alzheimer's disease A chronic, progressive disorder that is the major cause of degenerative dementia in the U.S. With the progression of the condition there is often memory and judgment loss, loss of interest, and carelessness. The cause of the disease is unknown, and there is no known treatment. Diagnosis is based on changes in the brain, plaques, and neurofibrillary tangles. It is recorded as a physical disease on Axis III of DSM-III-R.

Ambivalence Simultaneous conflicting feelings or attitudes toward a person or object.

American Law Institute's Model Penal Code (ALI) States that a person is not held responsible for his or her behavior if he or she lacks the capacity to appreciate the wrongfulness of the act or to conform his or her behavior to the requirements of the law. Used in more than half the states and all federal circuits.

American Nurses' Association (ANA) Classification of the Phenomena of Concern for Psychiatric/Mental Health Nursing A refinement of psychiatric nursing diagnoses developed by an ANA appointed panel of specialists and termed "PND-I" by the authors of this text.

Amnestic syndrome A category of OMS in which relatively selective areas of cognition (short and long-term memory) are impaired.

Androgyny Human characteristics and behaviors that are not limited to a specific gender.

Anger rape Rape distinguished by physical violence and cruelty to the victim. The ability to injure, traumatize, and shame the victim provides the rapist with an outlet for his rage and temporary relief from his turmoil.

Anhedonia The inability to experience pleasure.

Animism In a child's cognition, attributing human attributes to objects.

Anorexia nervosa Refusal to maintain body weight over a minimal normal for age and height accompanied by disturbance in body image.

Antabuse (disulfiram) A drug given to alcoholics that produces nausea, vomiting, dizziness, flushing, and tachycardia if alcohol is consumed.

Anterograde amnesia Amnesia for short-term memories; remote memories remain intact. Present in blackouts, a symptom of alcoholism.

Anticholinergic side-effects Side-effects caused by the use of neuroleptic medications, including symptoms such as dry mouth, constipation, urinary retention, blurred vision, and dry mucous membranes.

Anticipatory guidance A process that aims to help persons cope with a crisis by discussing the details of the impending difficulty and problem solving before the event occurs.

Antidepressant medications Psychopharmacologic preparations used to treat symptoms of depression and depressive equivalents. Most common antidepressants come from the tricyclic or monoamine oxidase inhibitor classes.

Antipsychotic medications Psychopharmacologic preparations used to treat symptoms of disintegrated thought, perception, and affect; also called neuroleptics, they include the following classes: phenothiazine, thioxanthene, butyrophenone, dihydroindolone, dibenzoxazepine.

Antisocial Behavior that is counterproductive or hostile to the well-being of society in general.

Antisocial personality disorder A personality disorder with the essential feature of a pattern of irresponsible and antisocial behavior.

Anxiety Nonspecific, unpleasant feeling of apprehension and discomfort that can be communicated interpersonally and that prompts the person to take some action to seek relief.

Anxiety disorders Patterns in which anxiety is either the predominant disturbance or a secondary disturbance that is confronted if the primary symptom is taken away.

Anxiolytic medications Psychopharmacologic preparations used in the abatement of anxiety-related symptoms. Drug classes in this group include benzodiazepines, beta-blockers, antihistamine sedatives, sedatives with hypnotic effects, and propanedides.

Anxious–fearful A category of personality disorders that includes avoidant, dependent, compulsive, and passive-aggressive.

Apathy Lack of feeling, concern, interest, or emotion.

Aphasia Difficulty searching for words.

Apraxia Inability to perform previously known, purposeful, and skilled activities.

Assault A physical attack that results in physical injury.

Assertiveness Asking for what one wants or acting to get what one wants in a way that respects the other person.

Assertiveness training An approach to therapy that is usually accomplished in groups to help people who tend either to be passive and discount themselves or to be too aggressive. Assertiveness techniques and exercises are designed to teach individuals to ask for what they want and to refuse requests from others without feeling guilty.

Assimilation Adjustment of an object in the environment to the organism; taking in experience to the extent that one can integrate it.

Attention-deficit hyperactivity disorder Developmentally inappropriate inattention, impulsiveness, and hyperactivity.

Autistic Relating to private, individual affects and ideas that are derived from internal drives, hopes, and wishes. Most commonly refers to the private reality of persons labeled schizophrenic as opposed to the shared reality of the external world.

Autistic disorder A severe pervasive developmental disorder with onset in infancy or childhood characterized by impaired social interaction, impaired communication, and a markedly restricted repertoire of activities and interests.

Autoerotic asphyxia An often fatal paraphilia in which the person decreases the flow of blood to the brain during masturbation, releasing the stricture at the point of orgasm.

Autogenic training A systematic training program of structured exercises to reduce stress-related conditions, modify the reaction to pain, and reduce or eliminate stress disorders.

Avoidant personality disorder A personality disorder with the essential feature of a pervasive pattern of social discomfort, fear of negative evaluation, and timidity.

Axon The part of the neuron that conducts impulses away from the cell body.

Barrio Hispanic neighborhood.

Beck's Depression Inventory A 21-item multiple choice questionnaire on which clients rate themselves on variables related to depression, such as sadness, weight loss, fatigue, guilt, suicidal ideas, social withdrawal, insomnia, etc.

Behavior modification A method of reeducation or treatment mode based on the principles of Pavlovian conditioning and further developed by B. F. Skinner; an effort to change behavior patterns through techniques that manipulate stimuli.

Behavioral contract An agreement between client and staff that clearly identifies expected client behaviors and expected staff behaviors.

Behaviorist model of psychiatry A model, based on the research of Ivan Pavlov and J. B. Watson, that is sometimes called "stimulus-response learning" or "behavioral conditioning." It assumes that psychiatric symptoms are clusters of learned behaviors that persist because they are rewarding to the individual.

Bender-Gestalt Test A psychological test that asks clients to reproduce, as best they can, nine geometric designs that are printed on separate cards. Believed useful in identifying organic brain damage.

Bestiality See zoophilia.

Binge The rapid ingestion of a large amount of food in a short time period, usually two hours or less. Foods selected are generally high caloric and easy to ingest, such as snack foods and ice cream.

Bioenergetics Techniques for reducing muscular tension by releasing feelings, consisting of physical exercises and verbal techniques.

Biofeedback A technique for gaining conscious control over unconscious body functions such as blood pressure and heartbeat to achieve relaxation or the relief of stress-related physical symptoms; involves the use of self-monitoring equipment.

Bioperiodicities Biologic rhythms ranging from microseconds of biochemical reactions for nerve activity to the menstrual cycle or the entire life span.

Biparental failure A family situation in which the male parent fails to offset the child's troubled relationship with the mother by providing positive experiences for the child.

Bipolar disorders One or more manic episodes accompanied by one or more depressive episodes.

Bisexuality Sexual preference for same or opposite sex interactions; has sexual activity with either.

Bizarre delusion Belief involving a phenomenon that a person's culture would regard as totally implausible, e.g., thought broadcasting or being controlled by a dead person.

Blackouts A term for anterograde amnesia experienced by alcoholics; some believe blackouts are an acute brain syndrome due to dehydration of brain tissue.

Blended family A family in which one or both marital partners have previously been divorced or widowed and bring with them their children from the former relationship.

Blind spot (psychologic) An area of a person's personality of which the person is totally unaware. Unperceived areas are often hidden by repression so that one can avoid painful emotions.

Block grant A shift of decision-making about allocation of funds for mental health to the states under the Reagan administration's 1981 Omnibus Budget Reconciliation Act.

Blunted affect (emotions) An extreme restriction in emotional expression; only minor degrees of emotional intensity are evident.

Body dysmorphic disorder Preoccupation with an imagined defect in appearance, or grossly excessive concern over a slight physical anomaly.

Body image An individual's concept of the shape, size, and mass of his or her body and its parts; the internalized picture that a person has of the physical appearance of his or her body.

Body scanning Focusing separately on all parts of the body to note the location of any tension or tightness.

Borderline personality disorder A personality disorder with the essential feature of a pervasive pattern of unstable self-image, interpersonal relationships, and mood.

Boundary The personal limits one utilizes to differentiate between one event and another; for example, one's boundaries keep one from experiencing another person's pain.

Broker for community services One who directs and coordinates family members of the CMI toward respite care, support groups, and the like.

Bulimia nervosa Recurrent episodes of binge eating accompanied by purging and persistent overconcern with body shape and weight.

Burnout A condition in which health professionals lose their concern and feeling for the clients they work with and begin to treat them in detached or dehumanizing ways. It is an attempt to cope with the intense stress of interpersonal work by distancing.

Cao gio Also called "coining," this folk practice is used by people from the Far East for treatment of fever or headache. The caregiver rubs a coin up and down the person's body with great pressure until red marks appear.

Cardiac neurosis A combination of anxiety, tension, and the signs and symptoms of cardiac disease in the absence of underlying cardiovascular pathology; a type of hypochondriasis.

Care-partners A term coined by gay persons to describe those persons to whom they are emotionally committed in a long-term relationship.

Catalysts Unconflicted members of a group who are able to move the group on to the next phase of group work.

Catatonia A disturbance in psychomotor behavior that can either take the form of stupor, in which the client appears unaware of the environment, or rigidity, in which the client may maintain a rigid posture and resist efforts to be moved.

Catatonic A term used to describe an unusual behavioral state in which the disordered person assumes a fixed position and may remain in that state for hours; most commonly related to specific forms of schizophrenia.

Catatonic excitement An activity disturbance in schizophrenia in which the client moves excitedly but not in response to environmental influences.

Catatonic posturing A motor behavior change in which the client holds bizarre postures for periods of time.

Catchment area A geographically circumscribed area identified as the service area for a community mental health center.

Catharsis A basic process in psychotherapy, in which the client freely puts personal feelings, thoughts, daydreams, and interpersonal problems into words. The process usually produces a feeling of relief.

Cathexis In psychoanalysis, the attachment of emotion to an object, person, or idea. It may be positive or negative emotion (love or hate).

Cerebellum The second largest portion of the human brain, which is divided into two sections and is located posterior to the cerebrum.

Cerebrum The most superiorly located, largest section of the brain; divided into two connected hemispheres.

Certification A method of attesting to competence, usually by a professional organization.

Checking perceptions A communication skill in which the therapist shares how he or she perceives and hears the client and asks the client to verify these perceptions. Perception checks are used to make sure that one person understands the other.

Chief complaint The client's own words for his or her presenting problem as expressed in the course of an intake interview or psychiatric history.

Child ego state In transactional analysis theory, the ego state that represents the archaic relics of early childhood.

Child within A phrase that represents the thoughts, needs, and feelings of a child who exists within an adult.

Choria Quick, jerky, purposeless involuntary movements. The primary motor disorder seen in Huntington's disease.

Chronic disorders Diagnostic categories that carry a high potential for persistent and severe impairment; clients often called "the chronically mentally ill" (CMI).

Chronically mentally ill (CMI) The population whose continuing or episodic functional impairment may be attributed to serious psychiatric disorder, regardless of specific diagnosis or living situation.

Chronically mentally ill elderly (CMIE) A subgroup composed of elders with chronic schizophrenia and other chronic mental disorders; this group is expected to increase as the population ages.

Chronobiology The study of biorhythms or periodic processes. Disturbances in biorhythms are thought to influence some mental disorders.

Circadian rhythms Cycles of approximately 24-hour duration in humans that control diurnal fluctuations in sleep, body temperature, plasma concentration of cortisol, and other hormones.

Circularity A characteristic of family system behavior in which each person's behavior is viewed as cause and effect at the same time.

Circumstantial communication See circumstantiality.

Circumstantiality A disturbance in associative thought processes in which a person digresses into unnecessary details and inappropriate thoughts before communicating a central idea.

Clang associations Associations between thoughts based on the sounds of words rather than their meanings; a form of thought disturbance found among clients with schizophrenia.

Clarifying Asking the client to give an example to clarify a meaning in order to understand the basic nature of the client's statement.

Client government Strategy of milieu therapy in which hospitalized clients use the democratic process to govern themselves.

Clinical ecology An alternative to traditional environmental medicine; entails assessment/treatment of physical/psychologic disorders that have been triggered secondary to exposure to certain foods, chemicals, and inhalants in the environment.

Clinical specialist in psychiatric nursing A graduate of a master's program providing specialization in the clinical area of psychiatric/mental health nursing.

Co-alcoholic A term coined by Al-Anon referring to the spouses and families of alcoholics.

Codependence The dependence of one adult on a second adult who is usually an addict.
A group of learned behaviors that prevents individuals from taking care of themselves and has at its core a preoccupation with the thoughts and feelings of others.

Cognitive therapy Therapeutic approach based on the principle that one's thought process can affect feelings. The goal of this therapy is to help the client recognize thought patterns that lead to dysphoric feelings.

Cohesion A sense of belonging, the result of all the forces acting on members to remain in a group.

Co-ism A phrase implying that every member of an alcoholic's family is emotionally impaired.

Commitment The legal process by which a person is confined to a mental hospital, usually associated with involuntary hospitalization. Also a sense of dedication and responsibility.

Community mental health center The executive locus for applying community mental health concepts. Centers include in-patient facilities, partial hospital facilities (day, night, or weekend), out-patient department, emergency services, consultation, and education programs.

Community mental health movement System for delivery of mental health services often referred to as the third revolution in psychiatry.

Community Mental Health Systems Act 1963 legislation authorizing 150 million dollars in federal funds over three years to construct comprehensive community mental health centers.

Community Support Program (CSP) A program started in 1977 by the NIMH to assist states and communities to develop long-term comprehensive community support systems for people with long-term mental illness.

Community Support System A network of comprehensive services that includes mental health treatment, crisis response services, housing, dental care, and so on for the persistently mentally ill.

Competitive frame of reference A system in which no two people can be thinking, feeling, or doing the same thing at the same time.

Complementary relationships Relationships based on the enjoyment of differences and interdependence. They may deteriorate when one partner controls what the complementarity is and how it is maintained.

Complementary transactions Transactions in which the transactional stimulus and the transactional response occur on identical ego levels.

Complex partial seizure A seizure that usually originates in the temporal lobe and involves limbic system structures; these seizures consist mainly of automatisms that last up to five minutes.

Compulsion An uncontrollable, persistent urge to perform an act repetitively in an attempt to relieve anxiety; performed in response to an obsession, according to certain rules, or in a stereotyped fashion.

Concrete communication Overly symbolic communication or inability to think and communicate abstractly; thought to be a sign of preoccupation with unreal or delusional material.

Conditioned response Behavior that occurs as a consequence of rewarding conditions that act as a stimulus.

Condom Barrier protection placed on the penis to prevent transmission of body fluids during sexual activity.

Conduct disorder DSM-III-R disruptive behavioral disorder seen in children.
A persistent pattern of conduct in which the basic rights of others and major age-appropriate societal norms or rules are violated.

Confidentiality Treating as private the information clients provide about themselves so that no harm will befall the client for having disclosed the information; includes releasing information about clients only with their permission.

Conflict A clash between opposing forces. It may be conscious or unconscious, intrapersonal or interpersonal.

Conflicted member A member of a group whose posture toward authority or intimacy is inflexible, rigid, or compulsive.

Confrontation A communication that deliberately invites another to self-examine some aspect of behavior in which there is a discrepancy between what the person says and does.

Consultation-liaison The provision of psychiatric and mental health expertise regarding a client or problem area at the request of another health professional.

Contract A set of expectations agreed on by two or more people about what each will contribute to the relationship.

Control need The interpersonal need to establish and maintain a satisfactory relation between self and others with regard to power and influence.

Conversion disorder Alteration or loss of physical functioning that cannot be explained by any known pathophysiologic mechanism; apparently an expression of a psychologic conflict or need.

Coping behavior The behaviors persons under stress use in struggling to improve their situations.

Coprolalia Repeating socially unacceptable, usually obscene, words or phrases; a complex phonic tic.

Cotherapy The sharing of responsibility for therapeutic work, usually in groups or with families.

Counterdependency Behavior that stems from a need to deny dependence longings. May be displayed as aggressiveness, extreme independence, or other maneuvers that distance others.

Countertransference Sigmund Freud's term for irrational attitudes taken by an analyst toward a patient. It may create problems in psychotherapeutic work. The therapist needs to become aware of countertransference and seek consistent supervision to intervene when it occurs.

Couples therapy A contemporary term for what used to be known as marital therapy. Acknowledges the existence of interactional dyads not necessarily based on marriage.

Creutzfeldt-Jakob disease A presenile dementia affecting the cerebral cortex through cell destruction and overgrowth. The cause is believed to be a slow-acting viral agent.

Crisis A situation in which customary problem-solving or decision-making methods are no longer adequate; a state of psychologic disequilibrium. A crisis may be a turning point in a person's life.

Crisis counseling (intervention) A counseling strategy designed to be brief (five to six sessions) and issue oriented. It may be individual, group, or family therapy.

Crossed transaction A transaction in which a change in ego state occurs terminating a complementary relationship.

Cultural relativism The belief that all cultures are equally valued and that they can be evaluated based only on their own values.

Cultural stereotyping Assuming that all members of one ethnic group are alike.

Culture Abstract values, beliefs, and perceptions of the world that lie behind behavior and are reflected by behavior. Culture is *learned* behavior.

Culture-bound syndromes Concepts of mental disorders that exist only within a given culture, such as windigo psychosis.

Culture broker A person who functions as a mediator between two people or groups from different cultures.

Culture shock The feelings of depression and frustration that are the result of being immersed in a totally different environment.

Curanderismo A folk healing system in Hispanic cultures derived from Aztec Indian and Spanish cultures.

Curandero(a) A folk healer in Hispanic cultures who is able to treat susto (fright) and other folk illnesses.

Custodial care The process of maintaining people in an institution though not for treatment purposes.

Cyclothymia Chronic mood disturbance of at least two years' duration involving numerous hypomanic episodes and numerous periods of depressed mood or loss of interest and pleasure that is not sufficient to meet the criteria of major depression or a manic episode.

Cytomegalovirus encephalitis (CMV) A viral, opportunistic infection commonly manifest as retinitis, colitis, and respiratory syndromes.

Decanoate A form of injectable neuroleptic that is released into the body over a period of approximately two weeks.

Deep breathing Moving the diaphragm downward in order to fill the lungs completely with air.

Defense mechanisms Operations outside of a person's awareness that the ego calls into play to protect against anxiety; the psychoanalytic term for coping mechanisms; also called mental mechanism. A glossary of terms containing defense mechanisms and their definitions is included in DSM-III-R (1987).

Dehumanize To detract from or interfere with unique human qualities to think, plan, create, relate to others, and experience a sense of autonomy and separateness from others.

Deinstitutionalization A humanitarian philosophy committed to community-based care for the mentally ill, which has resulted in decreased census of the state mental hospitals and emergence of community-based treatment facilities.

Delirium A reversible, acute confusional state that usually appears within hours or days.

Delirium tremens (DTs) An acute psychotic state usually occurring after a prolonged and copious intake of alcohol.

Delusional disorder Termed paranoid disorder in DSM-III; mental disorder with essential feature of persistent, nonbizarre delusion that is not due to any other mental disorder; hallucinations are not prominent; delusions may be erotomanic, grandiose, jealous, persecutory, and somatic.

Delusions An important personal belief that is almost certainly not true and resists modification.

Dementia An organic mental syndrome that is often chronic. Onset is usually acute although it may be gradual. Recent memory becomes impaired first; personality change is apparent and brain damage is evident.

Dementia praecox Kraepelin's term for schizophrenia, meaning "early senility."

Dendrite The part of the neuron that conducts impulses toward the cell body.

Denial A defense mechanism, or coping mechanism, by which the mind refuses to acknowledge a thought, feeling, wish, need, or reality factor.

Dependent personality disorder A personality disorder with the essential feature of a pervasive pattern of dependent and submissive behavior.

Depersonalization An alteration in the perception or experience of the self in which the usual sense of one's reality is temporarily lost or changed; feeling as if one is in a dream, detached, or an outside observer of one's body or mental processes.

Depersonalization disorder The occurrence of persistent or recurrent episodes of depersonalization severe enough to cause marked distress.

Depressive disorder One or more major depressive episodes without the history of a manic or hypomanic episode.

Derealization A feeling of being disconnected from the environment; sometimes manifested by a feeling that the environment has changed.

Desensitization A counterconditioning technique used by behaviorists to overcome fears by gradually increasing exposure to the fearful stimuli.

Devaluation Sustained criticism used to defend against feelings of inadequacy.

Developmental/maturational crisis A turning point during which usual coping patterns are inadequate; a crisis that occurs in response to stress common to a particular period in human life cycle.

Developmental phases/stages Universally experienced series of biologic, social, and psychologic events that occur on a timetable and include specific tasks or challenges to be met.

Developmental task A challenge that arises during predictable life periods calling for the person to use skills, resources, and supports to achieve the goal inherent in the task.

Deviance Behavior outside the social norm of a specific group.

Dexamethasone suppression test (DST) Test used in diagnoses of endogenous depression (chronic depression not caused by external factors like grief or loss). Involves administering a single dose of dexamethasone followed by blood and/or urine monitoring of cortisol levels. In depressed people the dexamethasone does not suppress adrenocortical functioning.

Diencephalon Consists of the portions of the brain located between the cerebral hemisphere and the midbrain, its main structures include the thalamus and hypothalamus.

Disability Any restriction or lack (resulting from an impairment) of ability to perform an activity in the manner or within the range considered normal for a human being.

Disengagement A family pattern characterized by unresponsive and unconnected interactions between members. Structure, order, and authority may be absent or weak.

Disinhibition A condition seen in conjunction with benzodiazepine administration in which a person demonstrates irritability, often verbal hostility, and possibly violent outbursts.

Displacement A defense or coping mechanism in which a person discharges pent-up feelings on persons less threatening than those who initially aroused the emotion.

Disruptive behavior disorders Behavior disturbances that are distressing to others and interfere with the child's social functioning.

Dissociation A defense or coping mechanism that protects the self from a threatening awareness of uncomfortable feelings by denying their existence in awareness.

Dissociative disorders Characterized by a disturbance or alteration in the normally integrative functions of identity, memory, or consciousness.

Dopamine hypothesis The biochemical hypothesis that schizophrenia may be related to overactive neuronal activity that is dependent on dopamine; increased dopamine activity is associated with increased schizophrenic symptoms.

Double bind A complex series of paradoxical interactions in which one person demands a response to a message containing mutually contradictory signals while the other person is not able to comment on the incongruity or to escape from the situation.

Dramatic-erratic A category of personality disorders that includes histrionic, narcisstic, antisocial, and borderline.

DRGs (diagnostically related groups) The list of conditions on which prospective hospital cost payment is calculated; intended to predict resource use.

Drug holidays Planned and carefully executed withdrawals from psychotropic medications; especially common in cases where neuroleptic medications are used.

DSM-III-R Abbreviation for the revised third edition of the

Diagnostic and Statistical Manual of Mental Disorders published by the American Psychiatric Association in 1987.

Dual diagnosis   The simultaneous existence of a major psychiatric condition and a medical condition.

Dualism   A philosophic perspective that views an individual as two irreducible elements: mind and body.

Dumping   Moving the chronically mentally disordered from an institution into the community without providing for continuity of care.

Dysarthria   Difficulty in speaking.

Dyspareunia   Pain with sexual activity, commonly associated with sexual intercourse.

Dysphoria   A sense of disquiet or restlessness.

Dysthymia   Chronic disturbance of mood involving depressed mood for at least two years.

Eccentric   A category of personality disorders that includes paranoid, schizoid, and schizotypal.

Ego   A concept of the organized part of personality that screens stimuli from the outside world and controls internal demands. As intermediary between the unconscious and the world, it includes defensive, cognitive, and executive functions. Consciousness resides in the ego, but some of its operations are out of the person's awareness.

Egocentric thought   In a child's cognition, everything is considered from child's point of view.

Egodystonic homosexuality   Homosexual arousal that is distressing to the individual who explicitly states a desire for heterosexual arousal patterns.

Egosyntonic   A perspective on oneself that does not motivate seeking change.

Elder abuse   Maltreatment of an older individual ranging from passive neglect of physical and emotional needs to overt physical, mental, or sexual assault.

Electra complex   In psychoanalytic theory, incestuous attachment of girls to their fathers during the phallic stage (from 3 to 6 years of age). Parallels the Oedipus complex for boys.

Elimination disorders   Disorders that involve a child or adolescent's inability to achieve bowel or bladder training at the appropriate age level.

Elopement   The departure or flight of a client from a psychiatric hospital.

Empathy   The ability to feel the feelings of other people so that one can respond to and understand their experiences on their terms. It is distinguished from sympathy by lack of condolence, agreement, or pity.

Enabler   Family member in an alcoholic's or addict's life whose behavior contributes to the continuation of chemical use.

Enmeshment   A family pattern characterized by a fast tempo of interpersonal exchange, overcontrol, and intrusiveness, usually from parent to child.

Episodic memory   The processing and storage of information, such as recalling the events of the day.

Espiritismo   A religious cult of European origin that can counteract or prevent mal de ojo and is concerned with moral behavior.

Espiritista   A spiritualist in Hispanic cultures who is able to put people in touch with the dead.

Ethnocentrism   The belief that one's own culture is more important than, and preferable to, any other culture.

Euthanasia   The intentional termination of a life of such poor quality that it is considered not worth living; can be active or passive.

Evocative memory   The ability to understand that an unseen object or person still exists when out of sight.

Excess disability   The increased cognitive impairment seen when depression and/or delirium occurs in a demented individual.

Exhibitionism   Intentional exposure of one's genitals to a stranger or unsuspecting person accompanied by sexual arousal and masturbation either during or after the experience.

Expressed Emotion (EE)   A characteristic of families of schizophrenics who are highly critical, hostile, or overinvolved with their afflicted relative. High EE is associated with more frequent relapses.

Expressive aphasia   Difficulty in finding words and naming objects.

Extended family   All persons related by birth, marriage, or adoption to the nuclear family.

Extrapyramidal side-effects (EPS)   Side-effects caused by the use of neuroleptic medications, including three separate classes: parkinsonism, dystonias, and akathisia.

Extrapyramidal system   A system of descending motor tracts that originate from various regions of the cerebral cortex and subcortical areas. Because these tracts do not travel through the pyramids of the medulla, they are called extrapyramidal.

Factitious disorders   Physical or psychologic symptoms that are consciously and voluntarily produced by the client.

Faith healers   Religious people who deal with illness ascribed to spiritual or supernatural causes.

Family burden   The stress created in a family caring for a demented individual.

Family life-style   A family's biased perception of the outside world and its automatic means of coping with this world. It is the front or facade the family presents to others.

Family myths   Well-integrated unchallenged beliefs, shared by all family members, about each other and their positions in family life.

Family of origin   The family in which an individual grew up.

Family theme   A family's perception of its development and history.

Fantasized nurturing parent   An internal construct of a loving and benevolent person developed by the child as a means of dealing with the experience of inconsistent or abusive parenting.

Fantasy   A defense mechanism that is a sequence of mental images, like a daydream. It may be conscious or unconscious. It is considered by some to be an individual's attempt to resolve an emotional conflict.

Feedback   The process by which performance is checked and malfunctions corrected; a regulatory function in the communication process, requiring two persons—one to give and one to receive it.

Female sexual arousal disorder   Failure to attain or maintain adequate lubrication during sexual activity and/or lack of a subjective sense of sexual excitement during sexual activity.

Feminism A viewpoint that examines the impact of being female and exhorts the rights of females.

Fetal alcohol syndrome (FAS) Physical and mental defects found in babies of alcoholic women.

Fetish The sexualization of a specific body part such as feet or hair, or the desire for a specific inanimate object such as shoes, leather, or rubber for sexual arousal.

Fight-flight Aggression (fight)–withdrawal (flight) response to stress.

Flat affect (emotions) A lack of emotional expression.

Folk domain of health care Nonprofessional healers such as root doctors, faith healers.

Frail elder Dependent, chronically ill older person.

Frotteurism Intense sexual arousal associated with acts or fantasies of rubbing against a nonconsenting partner.

Frustration The thwarting or delaying of an important ongoing activity or the attainment of an important goal.

Functional assessment Assessing a client's level of self-care.

Functional competency A term referring to clinical judgment regarding an individual's decision-making capacity.

Functional encopresis Repeated involuntary or intentional passage of feces into places not appropriate for that purpose.

Functional enuresis Repeated involuntary or intentional voiding of urine into bed or clothes after an age at which continence is expected.

Games In transactional analysis, ulterior transactions with concealed motivations.

Gender identity The sex role assignment as masculine, feminine, or ambivalent; generally based on external genital identification at birth.

Gender role The socialization and demonstration of the sexual behaviors expected of a given sex.

General adaptation syndrome (GAS) The objectively measurable structural and chemical changes produced in the body when stress affects the whole body. The GAS occurs in three stages: (1) alarm, (2) resistance, and (3) exhaustion.

General systems theory A conceptual framework that can be applied to living systems or people and that integrates the biologic and social sciences logically with the physical sciences.

Generalized anxiety disorder A disorder characterized by "freefloating" unrealistic or excessive anxiety about two or more life circumstances; manifested by autonomic hyperactivity (sweating, dizziness), irritability, and musculoskeletal tension.

Geriatric Depression Scale A tool for assessing depressive symptoms in elderly clients.

Gerontophobia Fear of contact and dealing with the elderly.

Ghettoization Movement of the mentally ill to restricted areas such as central business areas offering single room rentals.

Global assessment of function (GAF) A ninety-point scale used as Axis V of DSM-III-R to assess a client's psychologic, social and occupational function. Ratings are made for the current level at the time of evaluation and for the highest level in the past year.

Group dynamics The interactions among members of a group; the forces that underlie group interaction.

Group therapy Psychotherapy of several clients at the same time in the same session. It may emphasize examination of the interpersonal relationships of members of the group to see how they usually interact with others.

Groupthink The mode of thinking engaged in by people who are members of a highly cohesive in-group in which uniformity and agreement are given such priority that critical thinking is impossible or unacceptable; term coined by Irving Janis.

Hallucination A false perception, the most common of which are auditory and involve hearing voices; other types of hallucinations are tactile, somatic, visual, gustatory, and olfactory. A sensory impression in the absence of external stimuli that occurs during the waking state.

Handicap A disadvantage resulting from an impairment or a disability that limits or prevents the fulfillment of an individual's normal role.

Hidden agenda A personal goal that is unknown to others and is at cross-purposes with dominant group goals.

Histrionic personality disorder A personality disorder with the essential feature of a pervasive pattern of excessive emotionality and attention seeking.

HIV-related condition The third category in the HIV trajectory, including individuals who have begun to experience the physical effects of immune system deterioration but do not meet the criteria for a formal diagnosis of AIDS.

HIV-seropositive The second category of individuals affected by HIV who have received validation of HIV status through test results but as yet exhibit no symptoms associated with immune system suppression.

HIV trajectory The spectrum of possible disease progression or stages associated with HIV infection.

Holism A philosophic perspective that views the person as an integrated whole whose parts share an organic and functional relationship.

Homelessness Absence of housing. In an extreme form, homelessness refers to street dwellers. A more moderate type of homelessness involves movement between temporary forms of housing such as emergency shelters.

Homeostasis The principle that all organisms react to changing conditions in an effort to maintain a relatively constant internal environment; in general systems theory, the characteristic of systems to strive to maintain a dynamic equilibrium, or balance, among various forces that operate within and on it.

Homophobia The unrealistic fear of homosexuality and homosexuals that stems from myths and stereotypes associated with homosexuality.

Hoodoo men/women See root doctors.

Hot line A telephone crisis counseling service often used in crisis intervention centers to provide immediate contact between a person in crisis and a counselor.

Human immunodeficiency virus (HIV) The extremely tiny but virulent retrovirus that causes AIDS. It consists of a double-layered shell or envelope full of proteins, surrounding a bit of ribonucleic acid (RNA).

Humanism A view of human beings that values the individual's freedom of choice. In psychiatric nursing practice, a philosophy of devotion to the interests of human beings wherever they live and whatever their status. It reaffirms the spirit of compassion and caring for others and constructively and wholeheartedly affirms the joys, beauties, and values of human living.

Huntington's disease A genetically transmitted disease involving both motor and cognitive changes; an example of a condition with subcortical dementia.

Hypertensive crisis Dangerously high blood pressure, precipitated by the combination of monoamine oxidase inhibitor antidepressants and foods rich in tyramine.

Hypervigilance Increased state of guardedness or watchfulness.

Hypochondriasis Preoccupation with the fear of having or the belief that one has a serious disease despite medical reassurance.

Hypomanic episode A distinct period in which the predominant mood is elevated, expansive, or irritable but less severe than manic episode and without delusions.

ICU psychosis Intensive care syndrome combining depression, withdrawal, anxiety, hallucinations, delusions, paranoia, and delirium.

Id In psychoanalytic theory, all inherited psychic properties of the person, most notably the instincts and drives.

Identification A defense mechanism; the wish to be like another person and to assume the characteristics of that person's personality.

Identity diffusion The failure to integrate various childhood identifications into a harmonious, adult, psychosocial identity; the "as if" personality.

Illusions Misperceptions and misinterpretations of externally real stimuli. Visual and auditory illusions are much more common than tactile, olfactory, and gustatory illusions.

Impairment Any loss or abnormality of psychological, physiological, or anatomical structure or function.

Imparting information A communication skill in which the nurse makes statements that give needed data to the client and therefore encourages further clarification based on additional input.

Inappropriate affect Affect that is discordant with the content of a client's speech or ideas.

Inclusion need The interpersonal need to establish and maintain relationships with others.

Individuals at risk The first category in the HIV trajectory.

Induced psychotic disorder A mental disorder with the essential feature of a delusional system that develops in a second person as a result of association with a first person who already has a psychotic disorder (historically known as *folie à deux*).

Informational confrontation Describing the visible behavior of another person.

Informed consent A client's right to have treatment explained in order to agree with it or to refuse it.

Infradian Biorhythms longer than twenty-four hours.

Inhibited female orgasm Persistent or recurrent failure to attain orgasm during sexual activity.

Inhibited male orgasm Delay or lack of ejaculation even with intense sexual stimulation over a lengthy period of time.

Inhibited sexual desire disorder Persistent low interest or lack of interest in any form of sexual activity.

Insanity An obsolete medical term for psychosis or mental illness. Continues to be used in legal terminology.

Institutionalization The process of decline in functioning characterized by dependency, apathy, resignation, and inability to manage daily living outside an institution and created by an environment that controls all individual decision making, negates independence and autonomy, and segregates inmates from the mainstream community.

Intellectualization A defense mechanism in which intellectual processes are overused to avoid closeness or affective experience and expression. It is closely related to rationalization.

Interaction process analysis A verbatim, progressive recording of the verbal and nonverbal interactions between client and nurse within a given time.

Interpersonal communication Communication that takes place between two persons and in small groups; person-to-person communication.

Interpretive confrontation Expressing thoughts and feelings about another's behavior and drawing inferences about the meaning of the behavior.

Intoxication Maladaptive behavior and substance-specific syndrome due to ingestion of a psychoactive substance.

Intrafamily physical abuse Violence within the family.

Intrafamily sexual abuse Inappropriate sexual behavior, instigated by an adult family member or surrogate family member, whose purpose is to arouse the adult or a child sexually. Behaviors can range from exhibitionism, peeping, and explicit sexual talk to touching, caressing, masturbation, and intercourse.

Intrapersonal communication The level of communication that occurs when people communicate with each other.

Introjection The process of accepting another's values and opinions as one's own if they contradict the values one had previously held.

Involuntary commitment The legal process by which a person is confined without consent to a mental hospital. There are three categories: (1) emergency, (2) temporary, and (3) extended. Criteria vary from state to state.

Iowa Self-Assessment Inventory A tool for obtaining a subjective functional assessment from elderly clients.

Irrational self-talk In rational-emotive therapy, the untrue thoughts with which one describes and interprets the world to oneself; usually catastrophic interpretations of an event or the need to live up to an absolute standard.

Irresistible impulse The inability of a person to control his or her behavior as a result of a mental disorder even though he or she may know it is wrong. Supplements M'Naghten rule in an insanity plea in a few states.

Isolation A primary defense mechanism in which affect and impulse are separated and pushed out of consciousness.

Kaposi's sarcoma An opportunistic malignancy that is the second most common opportunistic condition among persons with AIDS. May affect the skin and several internal organs including the brain.

Kinesics The study of body movement (for example, facial expressions, gestures, and eye movements) as a form of nonverbal communication.

Kluver-Bucy-like syndrome A syndrome occurring in the terminal phase of Alzheimer's disease including hyperorality, blunting of emotions, bulimia, and attempts to touch objects in sight.

La belle indifférence An inappropriate lack of concern about a disability. Seen in certain clients with conversion disorder. Literally means "beautiful indifference."

Labile affect A pattern of observable behaviors that express emotion characterized by repeated, rapid, abrupt shifts.

Learned helplessness (excessive dependence) A condition in which a person attempts to establish and maintain contact with another by adopting a helpless, powerless stance.

Least restrictive alternative Imposition of the least amount of limitation or interference on an individual's thought and decision-making, physical activity, and sense of self as necessary to provide both maintenance care and active treatment.

Lethality assessment A systematic method of assessing a client's suicide potential.

Lethality index The ratio of suicide attempts to successful suicides.

Libido In psychoanalytic theory, the sexual drive; see sexual desire.

Life script Expectations for the client's life that have evolved over time due to the client's life experiences and relationships with significant others. The life script can affect numerous areas of living, e.g., the client's choices for career, life mate (to have or not to have), and patterns of behavior.

Life space interview Assessment of the child during normal daily activities and routines over a period of time.

Limbic system Is considered to be the "emotional brain." The parts of the limbic system include the hippocampus, lingulate gyrus, isthmus, hippocampal gyrus, and uncus.

Limit-setting The reasonable and rational setting of parameters for client behavior that provide control and safety.

Linking A communication skill in which the nurse responds to the client in a way that ties together two events, experiences, feelings, or people. It may be useful in connecting the past with current behaviors.

Long-term survivors People who have outlived the average projections for survival after a diagnosis of HIV disease or AIDS.

Loose associations Thinking characterized by speech in which ideas shift from one subject to another that is unrelated.

Looseness of associations A phenomenon commonly observed in schizophrenia where an apparently unrelated idea or experience reminds a person of some other experience or idea.

Magical thinking The belief that one's thoughts, words, or actions will produce an outcome that defies normal laws of cause and effect.

Maintenance roles Group roles oriented toward building group-centered attitudes among the members and maintaining and perpetuating group-centered behavior.

Major depressive episode Depressed mood or loss of interest or pleasure in all or almost all activities for a period of at least two weeks.

Mal de ojo "The evil eye" thought to be the result of a witch purposefully casting a spell or a person involuntarily injuring a child by looking admiringly at it.

Male erectile disorder Persistent erection problems during 25 percent or more of sexual activity.

Malleus Maleficarum (The Witches' Hammer) A 1487 textbook of both pornography and psychopathology that labeled dissenters and the mentally ill as witches and recommended burning at the stake to destroy the devil's host or witch.

Malpractice Negligent act of professionals when they fail to act in a responsible and prudent manner in carrying out their professional duties.

Mania A mood characterized by hyperactivity, excitement, agitation, euphoria, excessive energy, decreased need for sleep, and impaired ability to concentrate or complete a single train of thought.

Manic episode A distinct period during which the predominant mood is elevated, expansive, or irritable.

Mantra A syllable, word, or name that is chanted over and over during meditation.

Masochism See sexual masochism.

Masturbation Manual stimulation of genital organs or other body parts. The act may be for the purpose of erotic stimulation commonly resulting in orgasm but is not limited to that (e.g., may be a conscious expression of hostility toward the nurse or may be an unconscious expression of the client's anxiety).

Mediators Cognitive cues to enhance memory and learning.

Medical-biologic model of psychiatry A model based on classification that emphasizes systematic observation, naming, and classification of symptoms, and views emotional-behavioral disturbances as diseases like any other disease. Abnormal behavior is assumed to be directly attributable to a disease introduced from outside the body or an internally developed biochemical change.

Meditation A method of achieving a state of deep rest and increasing alpha wave brain activity enabling one to focus on one thing at a time in order to achieve inner peace and harmony.

Medulla oblongata The specialized segment of neurologic tissue that attaches the brain to the spinal cord.

Mental disorder A clinically significant behavioral or psychologic syndrome or pattern that occurs in a person and is associated with distress or disability or with an increased risk of suffering death, pain, disability, or an important loss of freedom; is not an expectable response to a particular event or experience.

Mental hygiene movement The development of preventive psychiatry and the formation of child guidance clinics based on the social consciousness of the early 20th century.

Mental status examination Usually a standardized procedure with the primary purpose of gathering data to determine etiology, diagnosis, prognosis, and treatment.

Midbrain Lies between the cerebral hemispheres and the pons. Within the midbrain are specialized centers for vision, hearing, and the modulation of wakeful/sleepful periods.

Midlife crisis Period of disequilibrium between 35 and 45 years of age during which people discover visible signs of aging and experience feelings of boredom, dissatisfaction with the way life has developed, and uncertainty about the future.

Milieu therapy The purposeful use of people, resources, and events in the patient's immediate environment to promote optimal functioning in activities of daily living, development/improvement of interpersonal skills, and capacity to manage outside the institutional setting.

Minnesota Multiphasic Personality Inventory (MMPI) Complex, lengthy psychologic test consisting of 550 questions and yielding a clinical profile of the client's personality structure.

Mirroring Imitating the client's behavior.

Mixed message Communication in which the verbal and the nonverbal aspects contradict one another.

M'Naghten rule Legal rule to determine whether a psychiatrically ill person is responsible for a criminal act he or she committed. Based mainly on whether the person knew the "nature and quality" of the act and that doing it was "wrong." Used in about one-third of the states.

Mnemonic disturbances Inability to remember recent events; may extend to profound memory loss for both recent and past events.

Monistic view A philosophy that asserts that the mind and body are one.

Mood A prolonged emotion that colors the whole psychic life.

Mood disorders A group of disorders with the essential feature of disturbance of mood accompanied by a full or partial manic or depressive syndrome. Previously called affective disorders in DSM-III.

Moos Word Atmosphere Scale A tool used to describe treatment environments according to factors of the atmosphere such as involvement, support, spontaneity, autonomy, practical focus, personal focus, order, clarity, control, and expression of anger.

Moral treatment A movement for psychiatric reform that considered mental illness a disease and proposed its "moral management" in therapeutic surroundings; humane treatment rather than punishment for the mentally ill.

Multiaxial system The five axes of DSM-III and DSM-III-R.

Multi-infarct dementia Dementia due to significant cerebrovascular disease; patchy deterioration.

Multiple personality disorder The existence of two or more distinct personalities or personality states within a person that recurrently take control of the person's behavior.

Multiplex relationships Relationships that have two or more functions or activities, in contrast to uniplex relationships.

Mutual self-help groups A type of social support provided through group interaction by persons currently undergoing the same type of event or situation.

Narcissistic personality disorder A personality disorder, the essential feature of which is a pervasive pattern of grandiosity, hypersensitivity to the evaluation of others, and lack of empathy.

Narcoanalysis Psychotherapeutic treatment to uncover repressed memories and affects under partial anesthesia induced by intravenous barbiturates, for example.

Narcotic Anonymous (NA) A 12-step self-help program for addicts.

National Alliance for the Mentally Ill (NAMI) See Alliance for the Mentally Ill (AMI).

Negative reinforcement In behaviorist/learning theory, alteration of an adversive stimulus to increase the probability that a behavioral response will occur.

Negative symptoms Schizophrenic symptoms including flattening of affect, loss of motivation, and poverty of speech.

Negative transference Client reactions in therapeutic work based on negative feelings (hate, bitterness, contempt, annoyance, etc.) left over from unsatisfying past relationships.

Negotiated reality The creation of a mutually understood, common ground.

Neologism A private, unshared meaning of a word or term. Neologisms are frequently characteristic of the language of schizophrenic individuals.

Neurofibrillary tangles Characteristic in Alzheimer's disease, the tangle is composed of interneurons that have increased in thickness and twisted into tangled masses of fibrous strands or bundles in the temporal lobe.

Neuroleptic Medications also known as "antipsychotics."

Neuroleptic malignant syndrome (NMS) An infrequent yet extreme condition that occurs in clients who are severely ill and is believed to be the result of dopamine blockade in the hypothalamus. Symptoms of this syndrome include: diaphoresis, muscle rigidity, and hyperpyrexia.

Neuroleptic threshold The optimal dose of a medication at which a client responds, taking into consideration Parkinsonian side effects.

Neurolinguistic programming (NLP) A communication model derived from theory in linguistics, neurophysiology, psychology, cybernetics, and psychiatry.

Neuron The cell that transmits electrical impulses throughout the body, but specifically characteristic of the nervous system.

Neurosis A pre-DSM-III-R category of mental disorders characterized by anxiety and avoidance behavior.

Neurosyphilis A dementia that is the direct result of untreated syphilis.

Neurotic conflict In psychoanalytic theory, the consequence of a traumatic experience in which client experiences ideas or feelings that are incompatible with his or her ego; believed to generate anxiety and use of defense mechanisms.

Neurotransmitter A highly specialized neurochemical that allows transmission of an electrical impulse from one neuron to the next across the synapse.

New chronic patient Term applied to younger, community-based clients who appear difficult to treat in conventional services.

Non-assertive behavior Timid, ineffective behavior.

Nonoxynol-9 Ingredient in spermicidal foams, creams, and jellies.

Nonverbal communication Communication between two or more people without the use of words. Facial expressions, gestures, and body postures are examples.

Normal pressure hydrocephalus A presenile dementia affecting 5 percent of those diagnosed as demented; may be incorrectly diagnosed as Parkinson's disease.

Norms The set of unwritten rules of conduct or prescriptions of behavior established by members of a group.

North American Nursing Diagnosis Association (NANDA) Nursing organization responsible for reviewing, studying, and accepting specific nursing diagnoses that cover all clinical practice areas.

NSGAE (Nursing Adaptation Evaluation) A proposed alternative to Axis V or additional Axis VI for DSM-III-R or DSM-III.

Nuclear family The "traditional" family consisting of two parents in a time-limited, two-generational relationship consisting of a married couple and their children by birth or adoption. A relatively recent development in human history.

Nursing "The diagnosis and treatment of human responses to actual or potential health problems" (ANA 1980).

Nursing diagnosis The conceptualization of a client's need, problem, or situation from the unique perspective of the theoretical constructs in the discipline of nursing.

Nursing process The conscious, systematic set of cognitive behavioral steps that comprise the clinical act in nursing practice.

Obesity Bodily weight 20 percent more than ideal weight, as defined by charts established by life insurance companies.

Objective data Verifiable information collected from other sources than client and significant family, including psychologic test results and laboratory test findings.

Object loss The forced, often traumatic, separation of a person from a significant object of attachment.

Object permanence The capacity to understand that an absent person or object will return.

Object relation The emotional attachment one person has for another as opposed to feelings for oneself.

Obscene phone caller A person who calls non-consenting victims and breathes heavily, makes sexual noises, or uses explicit language to upset, disgust, or shock the victim.

Obsession A persistent idea, thought, or impulse that cannot be eliminated from consciousness by logical effort even though the person recognizes it as the product of his or her own mind.

Obsessive compulsive personality disorder A personality disorder with the essential feature of a pervasive pattern of perfectionism and inflexibility.

Occulogyric crisis One of the manifestations of an acute dystonic reaction in which the affected person demonstrates a fixed gaze, often upward.

Oedipal conflict/Oedipus complex In psychoanalytic theory, the major process of the phallic stage from 3 to 6 years of age in which incestuous feelings are attached to the opposite sex parent and aggressive feelings are directed to the same sex parent.

Omnipotence Fantasies of greatness or power.

One-to-one relationship A mutually defined, collaborative, goal-directed client-therapist relationship for the purpose of crisis intervention, counseling, or individual psychotherapy.

Opisthotonos A manifestation of an acute dystonic reaction in which the affected person demonstrates spasms of the neck and back, forcing the back to arch and the neck to bend backward.

Opportunistic infection Infection caused by an organism that may be common in the environment but causes disease only in a person with a poorly functioning immune system.

Oppositional defiant disorder A pattern of negative, hostile, and defiant behavior (without violation of the rights of others) to an extent more common than in others of the same mental age.

Oral character The individual with unresolved conflicts of the earliest life stage of development (a sense of trust as theoretically defined by Erik Erikson). These insatiable needs may be displayed through overeating, verbal pessimism, sarcasm, and mistrust of others.

Organic anxiety syndrome Prominent, recurrent panic attacks or generalized anxiety caused by a specific organic factor.

Organic brain disease (OBD) A term for brain disorders that was used in the mid-20th century. Included defects in cerebral vessels and the brain itself.

Organic brain syndrome (OBS) An older term, replaced by organic mental disorder and organic mental syndrome, that categorizes multiple disorders of the brain related to defects in the brain or its vessels.

Organic delusional syndrome Presence of delusions due to a specific organic factor.

Organic hallucinosis Presence of prominent persistent or recurrent hallucinations due to a specific organic factor.

Organic mental disorders Designate particular organic mental syndromes in which the etiology is known or presumed.

Organic mental syndrome (OMS) A temporary or permanent brain dysfunction without reference to etiology.

Organic mood syndrome Prominent and persistent depressed, elevated, or expansive mood due to a specific organic factor.

Organic personality syndrome Persistent personality disturbance due to a specific organic factor.

Orientation phase The beginning phase of a one-to-one relationship characterized by the establishment of contact with the client.

Other-aided Having as a focus another person's needs and wants, always concentrating on someone else in order to proceed with life.

Overload In communication theory, sensory input that exceeds a person's tolerance level or capacity.

Pace To go with or match the patient at whatever rate he or she is moving, talking, or feeling.

Panic An acute attack of anxiety associated with personality disorganization.

Panic disorder with agoraphobia Recurrent panic attacks accompanied by the fear of being in a situation from which escape might be difficult or embarrassing or help might not be available.

Panic disorder without agoraphobia Recurrent panic attacks without the avoidance behavior that results from agoraphobia.

Paradox A self-contradictory communication; for example, the demand "Stand up for yourself!"

Paranoid personality disorder A personality disorder with the essential feature of a pervasive and unwarranted tendency to interpret the actions of people as deliberately demeaning or threatening.

Paraphilia Persistent or necessary association of a specific nonhuman object or activity that involves giving or receiving pain, or activity with a nonconsenting partner, to experience full sexual arousal and satisfaction.

Paraphrasing An activity or communication skill in which the nurse restates what she or he has heard the client communicating. It offers an opportunity to test the nurse's understanding of what the client is attempting to communicate.

Parataxic mode Earliest experiences of the infant in which all the baby knows consists of momentary experiences, undifferentiated feeling states without connections, or sense of self as a separate being.

Parens patriae Enables the state to take the role of protector and involuntarily hospitalize individuals "for their own good."

Parent ego state In transactional analysis theory, the ego state that incorporates the feelings and behaviors learned from parents or authority figures.

Parkinsonian syndrome An adverse reaction that resembles Parkinson's disease resulting from the effects of antipsychotics on the extrapyramidal tracts of the CNS.

Parkinson's disease A condition involving tremors and rigidity without cognitive involvement, recently associated with ultimate dementia for one in three clients over time.

Passive-aggressive personality disorder A personality disorder with the essential feature of a pervasive pattern of resistance to demands for adequate social-occupational performance.

Passive progressive relaxation A relaxation strategy wherein the muscles are relaxed in sequence.

Pedophilia The sex object is a child. Manipulation or fondling of the child's genitals is usually involved.

Perception The experience of sensing, interpreting, and comprehending the world; a highly personal and internal act.

Perseveration Persistent repetition of words, ideas, or subjects.

Personal space The "invisible bubble" of territory around a person's body into which intruders may not come.

Personality Deeply ingrained patterns of behavior that include the way one relates to, perceives, and thinks about the environment and self.

Personality disorders Enduring patterns of perceiving, relating to, and thinking about the environment and oneself that become inflexible and maladaptive and cause either significant functional impairment or subjective distress; coded on Axis II of DSM-III-R.

Personality traits Lifelong personality patterns that do not significantly interfere with one's life but may charm, annoy, or frustrate others.

Pervasive developmental disorders See autistic disorder.

Phantom experience The sensation of feeling a part of the body that is no longer there.

Phantom pain Perception of pain in a body part that has been surgically or accidentally separated.

Phenothiazines One of the classes of neuroleptic or antipsychotic medications.

Phobia An excessive, persistent, irrational fear of an object or situation that causes the person to avoid the object or situation.

Pick's disease Presenile dementia with age onset in the mid fifties; possibly a genetic predisposition.

Pinpointing Calling attention to statements, inconsistencies among statements, or similarities or differences in points of view, feelings, or actions.

Play therapy Therapy used with children, usually of preschool and early latency ages. The child reveals problems on a fantasy level with dolls, toys, and clay. The therapist may intervene with explanations about the child's responses and behavior in language geared to the child's comprehension.

Pleasure principle In psychoanalytic theory, the tendency for the id to seek pleasure and avoid pain. The demands of the pleasure principle become modified by the reality principle, and the individual thereby develops the capacity to delay immediate release of tension or achievement of pleasure.

Pneumocystis carinii pneumonia A common opportunistic infection in persons with AIDS and the most frequent cause of death.

Polypharmacy The mixing and matching of medication seen in elderly persons who often have a variety of chronic medical problems.

Pons The neurologic structure that is located above the medulla; contains the centers for cranial nerves 5, 6, 7, and 8 and aids in the regulation of respirations.

Poppers Volatile amyl and butyl nitrates in breakable glass capsules inhaled to enhance sexual pleasure.

Popular domain of health care Family and friends who function in the role of healer by offering health information, emotional support, prayers, and advice.

Positive reinforcement In behaviorist theory and operant conditioning, an environmental event that rewards and thus increases the probability of a behavioral response.

Positive symptoms Schizophrenic symptoms, including hallucinations, delusions, and thought disorders.

Positive transference Client reactions in therapeutic work based on positive feelings (love, affection, respect, trust) from satisfying past relationships.

Post-traumatic stress disorder Reexperiencing with intense terror, fear, and helplessness a psychologically distressing event that is outside the range of usual human experience.

Postural hypotension A clinical phenomenon in which, after receiving certain psychotropic medications, the affected person's blood pressure decreases, especially when standing up from a lying or sitting position. Hypotension is most common with aliphatic and piperidine antipsychotic preparations.

Poverty of content of speech Speech that is adequate in amount but conveys little information because of vagueness, empty repetitions, or use of stereotyped or obscure phrases.

Power rape Rape distinguished by the rapist's intent to command and master another person sexually, not to injure the victim.

Primary Caregivers (PCGs) Persons who are generally responsible for providing or coordinating daily care for a person who cannot perform self-care activities.

Primary data source The client himself or herself as the provider of assessment information.

Primary degenerative dementia, Alzheimer's type See Alzheimer's disease.

Primary gain The mechanism in conversion disorder whereby the psychological need or conflict is kept out of awareness.

Primary prevention Elimination of factors that cause or contribute to development of disease or disorder.

Primitive idealization Assigning unrealistic powers to an individual on whom one is dependent.

Privileged communication Legal term, established by state statute to protect possibly incriminating disclosures made by the client. The privilege is the client's, the professional can reveal the information at the client's request.

Problem solving A specific form of intellectual activity used when an individual faces a situation he or she is unable to handle in terms of past learning. Problem-solving strategies are considered crucial in any psychotherapeutic endeavor. They consist of the following sequential steps: observation, definition, preparation, analysis, ideation, incubation, synthesis, evaluation, and development.

Processing A complex and sophisticated communication skill in which direct attention is given to the interpersonal dynamics of the nurse-client experience. Process comments focus on the content, feelings, and behavior experienced within the nurse-client relationship.

Professional domain of health care Traditional Western institutionally sanctioned health care workers such as a psychiatrist, nurse, and social worker.

Professional Service (Standards) Review Organization (PSRO) Required by Congress to implement quality control methods in health care delivery systems; a mode of evaluation.

Program for Assertive Community Treatment (PACT) An innovative community mental health program developed in Madison, WI by Stein, Test, and their colleagues in the early 1970s.

Progressive relaxation A method of deep muscle relaxation based on the premise that muscle tension is the body's physiologic response to anxiety-provoking thoughts and muscle relaxation blocks anxiety.

Progressive supranuclear palsy (PSP) A presenile subcortical dementia resulting from cell atrophy in the midbrain portions of the brain; no known cause or treatment.

Projection An unconscious defense mechanism in which what is emotionally unacceptable to the individual is rejected and attributed to others.

Projective identification The placement of one's aggressive feelings onto another, thereby justifying expressions of anger and self-protection.

Projective test A personality test that evokes projection in the response of the person tested.

Prospective payment A shift in American health care policy initiated by Medicare in 1983 away from cost-based retrospective reimbursement for hospital costs toward fixed payment based on diagnostically related groups (DRGs).

Prototaxic mode Process of perceiving experience that appears as the infant matures so that parts are recognized; however, there is still no ability to see logical connections (follows parataxic mode).

Proxemics The study of the space relationships maintained by people in social interaction, including the dimensions of territoriality and personal space.

Pseudodelirium Presence of symptoms of delirium when no organic cause can be found.

Pseudodementia Affective disorders, particularly depression, that mimic symptoms of dementia.

Pseudohostility Chronic conflict, alienation, tension, and inappropriate remoteness among members of a family. The problems of family life are denied in an attempt to negate the hostility among the members.

Pseudomutuality A method of family functioning in which the members act "as if" it is a close, happy family when in fact it is not.

Psychiatric audit A means of evaluation in which criteria for quality care are compared with actual practice as recorded on the client's chart.

Psychiatric history A set of interview questions oriented to the medical model, designed to elicit information about an individual's present and previous psychiatric experiences. Information may be provided by family, friends, and others about the client, resulting in a variety of perceptions.

Psychiatric nurse According to the American Nurses' Association, a registered nurse in a psychiatric setting who possesses a minimum of a bachelor's degree.

Psychiatric nursing A specialty within the nursing profession in which the nurse directs efforts toward the promotion of mental health, the prevention of mental disturbance, early identification of and intervention in emotional problems, and follow-up care to minimize long-term effects of mental disturbance.

Psychiatric Nursing Diagnoses, ed 1 (PND-I) Used in this text to refer to The American Nurses' Association classification system of specific nursing diagnoses that comprise the phenomena of concern for generalist and specialist psychiatric-mental health nursing (1987).

Psychic determinism In psychoanalytic theory, the tenet that none of human behavior is accidental, that emotional and behavioral events do not happen randomly or by chance. Each psychic event is believed to be determined by the ones that preceded it.

Psychoanalysis A theory of human development and behavior and a form of psychotherapy developed by Sigmund Freud and his followers. It is a form of insight therapy that relies on the technique of free association to explore the dynamic, psychogenic, and transference aspects of a client's personality.

Psychoanalytic model of psychiatry An approach founded by Sigmund Freud, holding that all psychologic and emotional events are understandable. The meanings behind behavior are sought from childhood experiences that are believed to cause adult neurosis. Therapy in this model consists of clarifying the psychologic meanings of events, feelings, and behavior and thereby gaining insight.

Psychobiology The study of the biochemical foundations of thought, mood, emotion, affect, and behavior.

Psychodrama A form of group psychotherapy, developed by Jacob Moreno, that uses dramatic techniques and the language and setting of theatrical productions to achieve psychotherapeutic goals.

Psychoeducation An approach used with family caregivers that emphasizes goals of (1) decreasing client vulnerability to environmental stimulation through educated maintenance chemotherapy; (2) increasing family stability by increasing both knowledge and coping strategies.

Psychoendocrinology The study of the relationships between behavior, endocrine function, and human biology.

Psychogenic amnesia A sudden inability to recall important personal information that is too extensive to be explained by ordinary forgetfulness.

Psychogenic fugue Sudden, unexpected travel away from home or customary work locale with assumption of a new identity and inability to recall one's previous identity.

Psychogerontology Study of mental health and illness in later life.

Psychoimmunology An exploration of relationships between the central nervous system, the immune system, behavior, and human biology.

Psychophysiologic disorders Disorders having both physiologic and psychologic components.

Psychosis A state in which a person's mental capacity to recognize reality, communicate, and relate to others is impaired, thus interfering with the person's capacity to deal with life demands.

Psychotic disorders not elsewhere classified A category of diagnoses for clients who present with psychotic features yet do not fully exhibit characteristics of the schizophrenic, delusional, or major mood disorders.

Psychotic transference   A situation in which the relationship with the therapeutic person supersedes all other relationships.

Purge   To evacuate the gastrointestinal tract through self-induced vomiting or use of emetics, laxatives, or enemas.

P.W.A.s   Persons with AIDS.

Questioning   A very direct communication activity that may be useful when the nurse needs specific information from the client. There are two types: (1) Open-ended questioning focuses on the topic but allows freedom of response; and (2) closed-ended questioning limits the client's responses to yes or no. When used to excess, questioning acts to control the nature and extent of the client's responses.

Rape   Any forced sex act with key factor being lack of adult consent.

Rape trauma syndrome   A syndrome of specific responses to the experience of being raped; also a nursing diagnosis.

Rapid ejaculation   The absence of voluntary control of ejaculation; the man or the couple define this as a problem with their satisfaction.

Rationalization   A defense or coping mechanism in which a person falsifies experience by constructing logical or socially approved explanations of behavior.

Reaction formation   A defense or coping mechanism in which unacceptable feelings are disguised by repression of the real feeling and reinforcement of the opposite feeling.

Reactive drinking   Late-onset alcohol abuse associated with developmental transitions and life losses in the elderly.

Reality principle   In psychoanalytic theory, largely a learned ego function whereby people develop the capacity to delay immediate release of tension or achievement of pleasure. This is Sigmund Freud's term for the practical demands of society, which are often in conflict with the individual's own wishes.

Receptive aphasia   Difficulty grasping complex concepts.

Recidivism   A tendency to relapse into a previous mode of behavior. For psychiatric clients, recidivistic concerns focus on relapse of psychiatric illness with a reemergence of symptoms.

Reciprocity   In social support, the extent to which each person gives and receives in the exchanges that occur between the two people.

Reflected appraisals   In Harry Stack Sullivan's interpersonal theory of psychiatry, the means by which one's self-view is learned through interaction with significant others.

Reflecting   A communication skill in which the nurse reiterates either the content or the feeling message of the client. In "content" reflection, the nurse repeats basically the same statement as the client. In "feeling" reflection, the nurse verbalizes what seems to be implied about feelings in the client's comment.

Reinforcement   Term from behaviorist or learning theory that refers to altering environmental stimuli to increase the probability that a behavioral response will occur; can be positive as a reward or negative as a removal of adversive stimuli.

Relapse   The term used to refer to recidivism among alcoholics and addicts after a period of abstinence.

Repression   A coping mechanism in which unacceptable feelings were kept out of awareness.

Residual deviance   Term from sociologist Thomas Schiff's theory of mental disorder referring to diverse forms of deviance that do not fit under any other explicit label.

Resistance   All the phenomena that interfere with and disrupt the smooth flow of feelings, memories, and thoughts. In the traditional psychoanalytic sense, anything that inhibits the client from producing material from the unconscious. Resistance is often cited by psychotherapists to "explain" unsuccessful treatment of a client.

Reticular activating system   Located within the reticular formation; receives information from the cord and relays it via the thalamus to all parts of the cerebral cortex. It plays a major role in states of consciousness.

Revolving door syndrome   Short hospital stays with rapid turnover and a pattern of readmission.

Rigidity   Lacking in flexibility; unyielding; a need to be precise and accurate.

Role taking   A process through which people empathize with one another.

Rolfing   Structural realignment of the body in proper relationship to the field of gravity; a body-mind therapy.

Root doctors (hoodoo men/women)   Folk health practitioners who use plants, ground fibers, and various herbs to put an evil spell on another or to neutralize an evil spell.

Rorschach test (inkblot test)   A personality test in which a person says whatever comes to mind as he or she looks at a series of ten standardized cards with inkblots on them. It is believed to reveal many aspects of the individual's personality structure and emotional functioning.

Sadism   See sexual sadism.

Sadistic rape   Rape distinguished by brutality as a necessary ingredient for the rapist to become sexually excited.

Safer sex practices   Practices that can be instituted during sexual activity to reduce the risk of transmission of HIV or other sexually transmitted diseases.

Santeria   In Hispanic cultures, a religion comprised of a unique blend of Catholicism and mysticism. A Santero(a) is a practitioner/priest of Santeria.

Scapegoating   A process by which an individual or group of individuals is identified as different from others and becomes the object of the group's fears, frustrations, or anger.

Schema *(plural, schemata)*   Internal representation of some specific action, according to Piaget's cognitive theory. Beginning in infancy, they evolve to operational schemata of higher order in adolescence when abstract thinking occurs.

Schismatic family   A family in which the children are forced to join one or the other camp of two warring spouses.

Schizoaffective disorder   A mental disorder that appears to be both schizophrenia and a mood disturbance but does not meet DSM-III-R criteria for either.

Schizoid personality disorder   A personality disorder with the essential feature a pattern of indifference to social relationships and a restricted range of emotional experience and expression.

Schizophrenia   A mental disorder with essential features of characteristic psychotic symptoms during the active phase of the illness, functioning below highest level previously achieved, failure in social development, and a duration of at least six months.

Schizophreniform disorder A mental disorder that shares all essential features with schizophrenia except that the duration, including all phases, is less than six months.

Schizotypal personality disorder A personality disorder with the essential feature of a pervasive pattern of peculiarities of ideas, appearance, and behavior and deficits in interpersonal relatedness.

Seasonal affective disorder (SAD) A major depressive episode with seasonal pattern.

Secondary data sources Charts, test results, and family members who provide assessment information about a client.

Secondary gain The mechanism in conversion disorders that allows the client to avoid distressing or uncomfortable activities while receiving support from others.

Secondary prevention The early detection and treatment of disease and disorder.

Seduction of the nurse An attempt by the client to manipulate the nurse to relate in a nontherapeutic way. This manipulation and the end result may be of a sexual nature, but it usually takes the form of nonsexual behaviors. For example, it may involve flattery to get the nurse to do special favors for the client or to ignore maladaptive behavior usually warranting limit setting.

Selective inattention A filtering out of stimuli under conditions of moderate and severe anxiety.

Self-actualizing people According to Maslow, people who make full use of their talents and potentialities; those doing the best they can understand themselves better than other people, and do not allow their own desires to distort their judgment.

Self-awareness A sense of knowing what one is experiencing. It is a major goal of all therapy.

Self-disclosure Being open to personal feelings and experiences; sharing information and feelings with others.

Self-fulfilling prophecy An idea or expectation that is acted out, largely unconsciously, thus "proving" itself.

Self-hypnosis Putting oneself into a hypnotic state, often used to achieve significant relaxation, to make positive suggestions for changes in one's life, or to uncover forgotten events that continue to influence the person.

Self-system (self-dynamism) One of Harry Stack Sullivan's central concepts—that the self is a construct built out of the child's experience. It is made up of "reflected appraisals" learned in contacts with other significant people.

Semantic memory Knowledge memory that allows people to synthesize and think about events. Used in language, abstraction, and logical operations.

Senile dementia The term used for all organic brain disorders before the 20th century.

Senile plaques Starch-like protein materials deposited in brain tissues in Alzheimer's clients. The extracellular plaques are composed of a cluster of degenerating nerve terminals.

Separation-individuation The process of identifying oneself as different from the primary caretaker while maintaining an emotional attachment to that person.

Severely and persistently mentally ill (SPMI) Clients with chronic functional impairment due to a mental disorder.

Sexual addiction A progressive disease with sex as the drug of choice to numb pain. The addict spends 50 percent or more of all waking hours dealing with sex.

Sexual aversion disorder Persistent or recurrent extreme aversion to and avoidance of all or almost all genital sexual contact with a sexual partner.

Sexual masochism The need to experience emotional or physical pain in reality or fantasy to have sexual arousal.

Sexual sadism The need to inflict emotional or physical pain or humiliation in activity or fantasy to have sexual arousal.

Shaman Medicine man.

Shaping An intervention procedure in behaviorist/learning theory in which reinforcement is manipulated to bring the client closer and closer to a desired behavior.

Ships of fools Boatloads of mad people set out to sea during the early Renaissance period.

Short Portable Mental Status Examination A tool for assessing the mental status of elderly clients.

Simple phobia Persistent fear of a specific stimulus object or situation accompanied by an immediate anxiety response.

Simpson Neurological Scale An assessment instrument for quantifying EPS.

Skewed family A family in which one spouse is severely dysfunctional and the other spouse, usually aware of the dysfunction of the partner, assumes a passive, peacemaking stance to preserve the marriage.

Social-interpersonal model of psychiatry A model of psychiatry whose advocates believe that crucial social processes are involved in the development and resolution of disturbed behavior. It focuses on the larger and more general context of deviant behavior and on the processes by which an individual comes to be labeled or identified as deviant.

Social margin A conceptual term describing clients who slip through the cracks of the mental health care system.

Social phobia Persistent fear of one or more social situations in which the person is exposed to scrutiny by others and fears acting in a way that will be humiliating or embarrassing.

Social selection The concept that the social disadvantages of the chronically mentally ill are the result of their illness.

Social skills training An intervention program for schizophrenics focusing on such skills as introducing oneself, starting and ending a conversation, asking for assistance, and other simple yet essential social interactions.

Social support Emotional and tangible support given and received through interpersonal interactions among people who know one another.

Somatization Excessive preoccupation with physical symptoms often associated with depression in the elderly.

Somatization disorder Recurrent and multiple somatic complaints for which medical attention has been sought; apparently not due to physical disorders.

Somatoform pain disorder A disorder in which physical symptoms suggest the presence of a physical disorder in the absence of organic findings; there may be positive evidence or a strong presumption of associated psychologic factors.

Splitting A defense mechanism that prevents one from uniting the good (love) and bad (hate) aspects of oneself or of one's image of another person. The person views himself or herself as all good or all bad, failing to integrate the positive and negative qualities of the self and others into a cohesive image.

Stanford-Binet Scale A commonly used intelligence test for children, consisting of a series of tasks of increasing difficulty.

Stimulus Term from behaviorist or learning theory that refers to an event, condition, or situation that precedes a response or behavior.

Stress A broad class of experiences in which a demanding situation taxes a person's resources or capabilities causing a negative effect.

Stressor The source of stress, the demanding situation.

Stress-vulnerability models Models that look at relapses among the chronically mentally ill in terms of an interaction between individual vulnerability and environmental stressors.

Structuring An attempt to create order or evolve guidelines.

Stupor A motor behavioral change in schizophrenia in which the client holds the body still and is unresponsive to the environment.

Subcortical dementia The personality cognitive changes seen in Huntington's disease. May include violent emotional outbursts, inability to solve problems and process information quickly, and poor concept formation.

Subculture Culture within a culture that shares a language, values, beliefs, and behavioral patterns.

Subjective data Information reported by the client and significant others in their own words.

Substance abuser A person who experiences problems with health, work, family, and social relations as a result of drug or alcohol use.

Subsystem In family systems theory, a triad, dyad, or other group of members who are linked together in some special association in the family.

Suicidal attempt A serious suicide try involving definite risk. The outcome frequently depends on the circumstances and is not under the person's control.

Suicidal cluster A contagion of suicides in which one suicide appears to set off another.

Suicidal gesture A more serious warning than a suicidal threat. May be followed by a carefully planned suicidal act that attracts attention without seriously injuring the subject.

Suicidal threat A statement of suicidal intent accompanied by behavior changes indicative of suicidal ideation.

Suicide The taking of one's own life. It is considered destructive aggression turned inward.

Summarizing A communication skill in which main ideas are highlighted. Summarizing reviews for client and nurse what the main themes of the conversation were. It is useful in helping the client to focus thinking.

Superego In psychoanalytic theory, a special agency of the ego that embodies rules (conscience) and values (ego ideal) resulting from influences of parental figures.

Suppression A defense or coping mechanism in which unacceptable feelings and thoughts are consciously kept out of awareness.

Suspiciousness An attitude of doubt about the trustworthiness of objects of people.

Susto Fright sickness present in some Hispanic groups, believed to be from a natural cause such as viewing something very unpleasant.

Symbolic interactionism A distinctive approach to the study of human conduct based on the premises that (1) human beings act toward things on the basis of the meaning that the things have for them, (2) the meaning of things in life is derived from the social interactions a person has with others, and (3) people handle and modify the meanings of the things they encounter through an interpretive process.

Symmetrical relationships Relationships based on maintaining equality between members. They allow for respect and trust but may deteriorate into competition.

Synapse The microscopic gap between neurons.

Synaptic vesicles Small liquid filled sacs located on the membranes of neurons at the synapse. The synaptic vesicles contain neurotransmitter substances.

Synergy The characteristic of a system such as a family that the whole is greater than the sum of its parts.

Syntaxic mode A process of perceiving experience in which a child learns to use language in a consensually validated way, i.e., with reference to meaning accepted by the listener (follows parataxic mode).

Systematic desensitization A process in which a person is exposed serially to a predetermined list of anxiety-provoking situations, graded in a hierarchy from the least to the most frightening, with the goal of reducing the anxiety these situations cause.

Tangential communication Expressions or responses that are irrelevant to the content of the topic at hand.

Tangential response An inappropriate response to a statement in which the content of the statement is disregarded. The reply is directed toward either an incidental aspect of the initial statement, the type of language used, the emotions of the sender, or another facet of the same topic.

Tardive dyskinesia Usually a nonreversible and late-onset complication of antipsychotic medications. Characteristically, this condition is evidenced by the presence of abnormal, involuntary movements of the face, jaw and tongue that produce bizarre grimaces, lip smacking, and protrusion of the tongue.

Task roles Group roles that facilitate group efforts in the selection, definition, and solution of a group problem.

Termination phase (of one-to-one) The end phase of the one-to-one relationship characterized by the termination of contact with the client.

Territoriality The assumption of a proprietary attitude toward a geographic area by a person or a group.

Tertiary prevention Reducing impairment and disability associated with disease and disorder.

Tetrahydroaminoacridine (THA) A potent anticholinesterase drug undergoing trials for restoration of some cognitive function in early Alzheimer's disease.

Thematic Apperception Test (TAT) A projective psychological test in which clients are shown pictures of people in various emotional situations and asked to describe what is happening in the picture.

Theory A set of interrelated constructs or propositions that present a systematic explanation of phenomena.

Theory for practice A set of interrelated propositions that specify actions and intended consequences in a situation.

Theory of nursing A comprehensive general theory that addresses the definition of the domain and scope of nursing.

Therapeutic alliance A conscious relationship between a helping person and a client in which each implicitly agrees that they need to work together to help the client with personal problems and concerns.

Therapeutic community Creation of an environmental milieu in which the hospitalized client can have a corrective interpersonal experience by recreating and resolving obstacles to constructive social relationships; traditional hierarchical roles and authority structures are minimized; originally attributed to Maxwell Jones.

Therapeutic contract The client's definition of personal goals for treatment, plus the nurse's professional responsibilities.

Therapeutic touch The specific transfer of energy in a therapeutic manner in which some of the excess energies of the healer are directed to the client, or energy is transferred from one place to another in the client's body.

Therapeutic use of self The ability of the psychiatric nurse to use theory and experiential knowledge along with self-awareness and the ability to explore one's personal impact on others.

Thought blocking Stopping the expression of a thought midway.

Thought broadcasting Belief that thoughts, as they occur, are broadcast from one's head to the external world.

Thought insertion The belief that thoughts that are not one's own are being inserted into one's mind.

Thought stopping A method of overcoming obsessive and phobic thoughts by first concentrating on the unwanted thoughts and, after a short time, stopping or interrupting the unwanted thoughts.

Thought withdrawal The belief that thoughts have been removed from one's head.

Thyrotropin-releasing hormone (TRH) infusion test A test used in the assessment of depression. Depressed clients show a blunted thyroid-stimulating hormone response to TRH despite otherwise normal thyroid.

Tic disorders Disorders characterized by involuntary, sudden, rapid, recurrent, nonrhythmic, stereotyped, motor movement or vocalization.

Token economy A behavioral approach that rewards clients for desired behavior using token reinforcers such as food, candy, and verbal approval.

Tort A wrongful act resulting in injury for which the injured party is requesting compensation through a civil suit.

Torticollis One of the manifestations of an acute dystonic reaction characterized by an uncontrollable twisted neck.

Tourette's disorder Multiple motor and one or more vocal tics; may involve touching, squatting, twirling, grunts, barks, sniffs, and coprolalia.

Toxoplasmosis A parasitic opportunistic infection.

Traits (personality traits) Enduring patterns of perceiving, relating to, and thinking about the environment and oneself.

Transactional analysis (TA) A system introduced by Eric Berne that has four components: (1) structural analysis of intrapsychic phenomena, (2) transactional analysis proper, (3) game analysis, and (4) script analysis—used in both individual and group psychotherapy.

Transcultural nursing The study of different cultures, their health care belief systems, and their caring and curative practices.

Transference In psychoanalytic theory, an unconscious phenomenon in which feelings, attitudes, and wishes originally linked with significant figures in one's early life are projected onto others who have come to represent these figures in one's current life.

Transinstitutionalization Movement of the mentally ill from one custodial setting to another.

Transsexualism Persistent discomfort and sense of inconsistency between psychologic gender identity and anatomic gender.

Transvestic fetishism Cross dressing required for sexual arousal prior to masturbation or coitus.

Triangulation In family systems theory, the process of forming a triad. Dysfunctional triangulation is a major concept in the Bowen approach to family therapy.

Trust Feeling confident that another person will behave in ways that will bring beneficial consequences.

Type A personality A highly competitive, driving personality often associated with coronary disease, angina pectoris, and myocardial infarction.

Type I schizophrenia A type of schizophrenia characterized by "positive symptoms" of schizophrenia, including hallucinations, delusions, and thought disorder; thought to be associated with biologic abnormality of dopamine receptors; responds well to psychotropic medications.

Type II schizophrenia A type of schizophrenia characterized by "negative symptoms" of flattening of affect, loss of motivation, and poverty of speech; shows little response to neuroleptic treatment.

Ulterior transaction A transaction that occurs on both overt (social) and covert (psychologic) levels.

Ultradian Biorhythms shorter than 24 hours.

Unconflicted member (independent member) A group member who is able to assess situations and alter roles or behavior appropriately.

Unconscious In psychoanalytic theory, the part of the mind that is out of awareness and helps to determine personality.

Underload A situation that occurs when delay or lack of information interferes with one person's ability to comprehend the message of another.

Undoing A secondary defense operation in which a compulsive act is performed in an attempt to prevent or undo the consequences anticipated from a frightening obsessional thought or impulse.

Uniplex relationship Relationships that have only one function or activity, in contrast to multiplex relationships.

Universality Ethical principle that one will make the same moral decision regardless of the persons or place involved.

Vaginismus Sexual disorder marked by involuntary spasm of the vaginal muscles making sexual intercourse difficult or impossible.

Validity A quality of an instrument important to evaluating its worth. It means that the instrument measures what it is supposed to measure.

Values clarification A systematic, widely applicable method of helping learners become aware of their beliefs and values, choose among alternatives, and match stated beliefs with actions.

Vegetative signs of depression Symptoms accompanying depression such as psychomotor retardation, anorexia, constipation, lethargy, diminished libido, poor concentration, and insomnia; thought to be associated with cortisol regulation.

Victimatology The study of victims of violent assault.

Violence Behavior by an individual that threatens or actually does harm or injury to people or property.

Visualization Using a person's own imagination and positive thinking to reduce stress or promote healing.

Vocational rehabilitation Provision of supported employment opportunities for people with psychiatric disabilities.

Voluntary admission A legal process by which a person chooses to be admitted to a mental hospital; requires written application by the person or someone acting in his or her behalf, such as a parent or guardian.

Volunteer linking A social support intervention that involves using a person who has experienced a similar event or situation to provide temporary support and assistance to someone currently undergoing the same type of event or situation.

Voyeurism Watching an unsuspecting person while that person is undressing, grooming, or having sexual activity; associated with masturbation during or after the activity.

Wechsler Intelligence Scale A commonly used intelligence test.

Wernicke-Korsakoff syndrome A syndrome usually associated with alcoholism and characterized by confusion, disorientation, and amnesia with confabulation.

Working phase The middle phase of the one-to-one relationship characterized by the maintenance and analysis of contact.

Working relationship The framework within which a client constructs behavioral change.

Works The intravenous drug user's needle and syringe.

World view Refers to how a group of people (culture or subculture) see their social world, symbolic system, and physical environment and their own place in each of them.

Writ of habeas corpus A means by which a person can challenge the legality of his or her detention.

Yin and yang In Oriental philosophy, two opposing forces that must be in perfect balance for physical and mental health and social harmony to be maintained.

Zoophilia (bestiality) Selection of animals as actual or fantasized sexual partners.

Zung's Self-Rating Depression Scale A scale of 20 descriptors of depression on which clients rate themselves. Useful in determining the depth or intensity of depression.

INDEX

Note: *t* following a page number indicates a table; *i* following a page number indicates an illustration

Numbers

5-Hydroxyindoleacetic acid (5–HIAA), 399
5-Hydroxytryptamine. *See* Serotonin
6-Hydroxydopamine (6HD), 60

A

AA. *See* Alcoholics Anonymous
AASECT (American Association of Sex
    Educators, Counselors, and
    Therapists), 364
Abandonment, 413, 640. *See also*
    Regression
  in disengaged families, 730
  of mentally ill, 8
Abdellah, Faye, 73
  nursing theory, 74, 75
Abille v U.S., 947
Abnormal Involuntary Movement Scale
    (AIMS), 774, 778*i*–779*i*
Abstract reasoning and thinking. *See*
    Reasoning; Thinking
Abuse. *See* type, for example, Client abuse;
    Intrafamily sexual abuse
Accidental disasters
  assessing, 683
  as crisis, 677, 683–685
  diagnosing, 683
  evaluating, 685
  intervening, 683–685
  planning for, 683–685
Accreditation, clinical experience for, 17
Acetylcholine, 60, 108
  in Alzheimer's disease, 186, 187
  in progressive supranuclear palsy (PSP),
    190
Ackerman, Nathan, 12, 728
ACoA perspective of codependency, 579–
    580

Acquired immune deficiency syndrome. *See*
    AIDS
ACTH. *See* Adrenocorticotropic hormone
Acting out
  by adolescents, 846
  in one-to-one relationships, 619–620
Action for Mental Health (1961), 12–13,
    18, 955
Active euthanasia, 126
Active listening, 32
Active values, 28
Activity intolerance (diagnosis)
  in the elderly, 890, 891
  in schizophrenic clients, 271–272, 283
Activity theory of aging, 871
Activity therapy groups, 718
Activity/rest disturbances: Altered
    psychomotor activity, in the elderly,
    898
Acute confusional states. *See* Delirium
Acute dystonic reactions, 772
  timing, symptoms, treatment, nursing
    implications, 775*t*
Adaptation, 81. *See also* General adaptation
    syndrome
Adaptation theory, 76
Adaptin. *See* Doxepin
ADC. *See* AIDS dementia complex
Addiction
  abuse versus, 216
  attitude toward, 125
  codependence and, 578
  sexual, 354–355
  susceptibility to, 238
Addison's disease, 448
Additive drug effects, 238
ADH (Antidiuretic hormone), 896
Adjustment disorders
  with anxious mood, central features, 884*t*
  with depressed mood, 113
    case study, 877–879
    diagnoses, 891
    nursing care plan, 880–881

DSM-III-R categories, 969
  in the elderly, 875
Adler, Alfred, 11, 64, 70, 689
Administrative discharge, 938
Administrative law, 934–935
Admission. *See* Voluntary admission and
    Involuntary commitment
Adolescents, 840–865
  anxiety disorders, 966
  assessing, 844–851
  behaviors, 571, 846–851
  depression in, 571, 815
  diagnosing, 852–853
  DSM-III-R disorders, 965–966
  in Erikson's eight stages, 66*t*
  evaluating outcomes, 863, 865
  gender identity, 352
  hallucinogens susceptibility, 238
  in-patient treatment, 843
  intervening, 853–863
  mandating services for, 13*t*
  marijuana use by, 231
  milieu therapy for, 844
  nurses' roles with, 841–844
  nursing care plan for aggressive/violent
    behaviors, 860–861
  nursing process, 844–865
  planning, 853–863
  rights of, 944–945
  schizophrenia onset in, 819
  stressors, 570
    severity scale, 170*t*
  substance abuse by, 218, 231, 238–239
  suicide, 568–570, 571
    assessing, 570
    risk factors, 571
  theoretic foundations, 840
Adrenal cortex, stress and, 81
Adrenal glands, stress and, 81
Adrenaline, 229
Adrenocorticotropic hormone (ACTH),
    stress and, 81
Adult children of alcoholics, 240, 579–580